Clinical Diagnosis in
Ophthalmology

Clinical Diagnosis in Ophthalmology

JACK J KANSKI
MD, MS, FRCS, FRCOphth

Honorary Consultant Ophthalmic Surgeon
Prince Charles Eye Unit
King Edward VII Hospital
Windsor, UK

ELSEVIER
MOSBY

MOSBY
ELSEVIER
An affiliate of Elsevier Inc

First published 2006

ISBN 0323037615

British Library Cataloguing in Publication Data
A catalogue record for this book is available from the British Library

Library of Congress Cataloging in Publication Data
A catalog record for this book is available from the Library of Congress

Notice
Medical knowledge is constantly changing. Standard safety precautions must be followed, but as new research and clinical experience broaden our knowledge, changes in treatment and drug therapy may become necessary or appropriate. Readers are advised to check the most current product information provided by the manufacturer of each drug to be administered to verify the recommended dose, the method and duration of administration, and contraindications. It is the responsibility of the practitioner, relying on experience and knowledge of the patient, to determine dosages and the best treatment for each individual patient. Neither the Publisher nor the author assume any liability for any injury and/or damage to persons or property arising from this publication.

The Publisher

Printed in China
Last digit is the print number: 9 8 7 6 5 4 3 2 1

The Publisher's policy is to use **paper manufactured from sustainable forests**

Commissioning Editor: Paul Fam
Project Development Manager: Belinda Kuhn
Project Manager: Susan Stuart
Design Manager: Andrew Chapman
Illustration Manager: Mick Ruddy
Illustrator: Antbits
Marketing Managers: Lisa Damico, Gaynor Jones

CONTENTS

PREFACE

It has been said that 'one picture is worth a thousand words'!

In ophthalmology, visual recognition is often a major factor in making a correct diagnosis and memorizing medical facts. Most textbooks are limited by the number of illustrations and therefore tend to show only typical cases. However, in many instances the same clinical condition may manifest a wide variety of appearances, and it is only with experience that a wealth of information for diagnosis and teaching can be acquired.

The main purpose of the atlas is to present a spectrum of clinical signs, both ocular and systemic, from trivial to severe. It is hoped that this will enable the clinician to acquire new knowledge, as well as to reinforce existing understanding of disease processes. It should be emphasised that *Clinical Diagnosis in Ophthalmology* is not a textbook and does not include descriptions of symptoms and treatment although, where appropriate, special investigations are included.

JJK

Windsor 2005

ACKNOWLEDGEMENTS

I am extremely grateful to medical colleagues for supplying me with the new images for this book. I am also particularly indebted to several medical photographers who frequently do not receive their deserved recognition for contributions to medical texts. Although the source of the images is indicated in the text, I would especially like to acknowledge the following for making a major contribution to *Clinical Diagnosis in Ophthalmology*.

Irina Gout MD, MScOphth, PhD
Prince Charles Eye Unit, Windsor, UK

Chris Barry CRA
Lions Eye Institute, Perth, Australia

Kulwant Sehmi FRPS, ABIPP, AIMI
Moorfields Eye Hospital, London, UK

Patrick Saine CRA
Dartmouth Hitchcock Medical Center, Lebanon, New Hampshire, USA

Rhonda Curtis CRA, COT, FOPS
Washington University Medical School, St Louis, Missouri, USA

Stanislaw Milewski MD, MA, FACS
University of Connecticut, USA

Lawrence Merin RBP, FIMI
Vanderbilt University Medical Center, Nashville,Tennessee, USA

Pablo Gili MD
Area de Cirugia Unidad de Oftalmologia, Madrid, Spain

Usha Kaul Raina MD, FRCS (Edin), FRCOphth
Maulanta Medical College, New Delhi, India

Anne Bolton BA, BIPP, DATEC
Oxford Eye Hospital, Oxford, UK

Leslie MacKeen BSc, OA, CRA
Hospital for Sick Children, and Massie Labs, Toronto, Canada

Andrew Pearson MRCP, FRCOphth
Prince Charles Eye Unit, Windsor, UK

Ronald Marsh MD, FRCS, FRCOphth
Western Eye Hospital, London, UK

Sue Ford ARPS, AIMI, RMIP
Western Eye Hospital, London, UK

Andre Curi MD
Federal University of Minas Gerais, Brazil

Illustrations from

Albert, DM; Jakobiec, FA. Principles and Practice of Ophthalmology, WB Saunders, © 1994.
1.5, 1.112, 1.278, 14.21, 16.35a, 16.35b, 16.35c

Ansell, BM; Rudge, S; Schaller, JG. A Colour Atlas of Paediatric Rheumatology, Wolfe, ©1991.
6.230

Bouloux, P-M. Clinical Medicine Assessment Questions in Colour, Wolfe, ©1993.
12.151, 16.58

Boruchoff, S. Anterior Segment Disease, Butterworth-Heinemann, ©2001.
6.192, 6.194

Byer, NE. The Peripheral Retina in Profile: a Stereoscopic Atlas, Criterion Press, Torrence, CA, ©1982.
11.4, 11.7, 11.10, 11.11, 11.18

Casey, TA; Sharif, KW. A Colour Atlas of Corneal Dystrophies and Degenerations, Wolfe, ©1991.
6.117, 6.122, 6.132, 6.133, 6.151, 6.153, 6.155, 6.156, 6.157, 6.158, 6.159, 6.162, 6.163, 6.164, 6.172

Emond, RT; Welsby, PD; Rowland, HA. Colour Atlas of Infectious Diseases 4e, Mosby, ©2003.
3.80, 10.43

Forbes, CD; Jackson, WF. Color Atlas and Text of Clinical Medicine, Mosby, ©2003.
1.139, 6.25, 10.214, 12.89, 12.143, 12.152, 16.41

Gass, JDM. Stereoscopic Atlas of Macular Diseases: Diagnosis and Treatment, Mosby, ©1997.
10.291, 14.79, 14.83

Goldman, L; Ausiello, D. Cecil Textbook of Medicine, Saunders, ©2004.
6.190, 10.235, 10.236, 12.87

Hayes, PC; Finlayson, NDC. Colour Guide Medicine, Churchill Livingstone, ©1994
10.73, 10.215

Kanski, JJ. Clinical Ophthalmology: a Systematic Approach 5e, Butterworth-Heinemann, ©2003.
1.3, 1.28, 1.29, 1.31, 1.40, 1.46, 1.105, 1.146, 1.13, 1.164, 1.165, 1.166, 1.171, 1.172, 1.175, 1.178, 1.184, 1.187, 1.192, 1.194, 1.195, 1.196, 1.197, 1.200a, 1.200b, 1.214a, 1.214b, 1.214c, 1.224, 1.227, 1.229, 1.228, 1.243, 1.249, 1.273a, 1.273b, 2.3, 2.5, 2.6, 2.8, 2.13, 2.16, 2.17, 2.21, 2.22, 2.23, 2.24a, 2.24b, 2.25, 2.26, 2.47, 2.48, 2.54a, 2.54b, 2.54c, 2.55, 2.56, 2.58, 2.59, 2.60a, 2.60b, 2.61a, 2.61b, 2.73, 2.87, 2.89, 2.99, 2.100, 2.109, 2.112, 2.113, 2.114, 2.118, 2.125, 2.127, 2.132, 2.133, 2.134a, 2.134b, 2.146, 2.147, 2.151, 2.158, 2.160, 2.173, 2.174, 2.182, 3.8, 3.11, 3.13, 3.14, 3.15, 3.19, 3.20, 3.21, 3.23, 3.25, 3.27, 3.28, 3.30, 3.37, 3.38, 3.45, 3.47, 3.57, 3.59, 3.62, 3.63, 3.67, 3.71, 3.75, 3.76, 3.79, 3.83, 3.85, 3.101, 3.109, 3.110, 3.114, 3.116, 3.118, 3.119, 3.125, 3.126, 3.149, 3.150, 3.158, 3.162, 3.165, 3.179, 3.180, 3.187, 3.190, 3.196, 3.200, 3.203, 3.207, 4.4, 4.8, 4.14, 4.19, 4.20, 4.25, 4.26, 4.28, 4.29, 4.38, 4.41, 4.42, 4.49, 5.1, 5.17, 5.18, 5.19, 6.1, 6.6, 6.7, 6.13, 6.16, 6.21, 6.27, 6.29, 6.33, 6.35, 6.38, 6.40, 6.41, 6.42, 6.43, 6.44, 6.51, 6.53, 6.59, 6.60, 6.61, 6.62, 6.64, 6.66, 6.67, 6.70, 6.71, 6.72, 6.84, 6.85, 6.88, 6.89, 6.92, 6.94, 6.95, 6.96, 6.97, 6.99, 6.104, 6.107, 6.108, 6.112, 6.114, 6.120, 6.121, 6.122, 6.125, 6.128, 6.132, 6.136, 6.139, 6.141, 6.143, 6.144, 6.147, 6.149, 6.152, 6.167, 6.168, 6.169, 6.170, 6.195, 6.196, 6.205, 6.208, 6.213, 6.220, 6.231, 6.241, 6.242, 6.250, 6.257, 6.259, 7.1, 7.4, 7.11, 7.14, 7.16, 7.22, 7.23, 7.27, 7.32, 7.33, 7.36, 7.44, 7.46, 7.49, 7.55, 7.56, 7.69, 7.73, 7.74, 7.102, 7.103, 7.105, 7.107, 7.111, 7.113, 7.116, 7.119, 7.120, 8.15, 8.16, 8.17, 8.18, 8.27, 8.40, 8.43, 8.53, 8.56, 8.57, 8.68, 8.70, 8.72, 8.74, 8.85, 8.87, 8.88, 8.94, 8.110, 8.120, 8.121, 8.123, 8.129, 8.131, 8.132, 8.133, 8.136, 8.147, 8.148, 8.149, 8.150, 8.154, 8.155, 8.157, 8.160, 8.162, 8.164, 8.166, 9.17, 9.19, 9.22, 9.23, 9.33, 9.37, 9.41, 9.43, 9.50, 9.58a, 9.58b, 9.60, 9.80, 9.83, 9.93, 9.100, 9.107, 9.108, 9.109, 9.112, 9.114, 9.117, 9.131, 9.132, 9.138, 9.145, 9.147, 9.148, 9.150, 9.155, 9.168, 9.179, 10.21, 10.28, 10.29, 10.34, 10.36, 10.38, 10.40, 10.41, 10.44, 10.56, 10.70, 10.72, 10.89, 10.107, 10.110, 10.122, 10.125, 10.127, 10.151, 10.154, 10.164, 10.177, 10.186, 10.191, 10.196, 10.203, 10.205, 10.210, 10.216, 10.219, 10.221, 10.223, 10.226, 10.229, 10.230a, 10.230b, 10.239, 10.240, 10.241, 10.245a, 10.245b, 10.245c, 10.245d, 10.247,

10.248, 10.257, 10.266, 10.275, 10.286a, 10.286b, 10.287, 10.289, 10.293, 11.4, 11.7, 11.9, 11.10, 11.11, 11.13, 11.14, 11.15, 11.18, 11.20a, 11.20b, 11.27, 11.28, 11.29, 11.38, 11.39, 11.52, 11.55, 12.9, 12.18, 12.28, 12.29, 12.61a, 12.61b, 12.61c, 12.61d, 12.66, 12.79, 12.80, 12.82, 12.83, 12.84, 12.85, 12.86, 12.90, 12.98, 12.99, 12.100, 12.101, 12.110, 12.112, 12.114, 12.118, 12.140, 12.145, 12.156, 12.165, 12.166, 12.171, 12.191, 12.193, 13.11a, 13.11b, 13.11c, 13.38, 13.45a, 13.45b, 13.45c, 13.45d, 13.46a, 13.46b, 13.46c, 13.46d, 13.57a, 13.58, 13.83, 13.91, 13.92, 13.93, 14.73a, 14.73b, 14.73c, 14.73d, 14.99, 14.100, 14.101, 14.102, 14.103, 14.108, 15.53, 16.33a, 16.33b, 16.40, 16.42, 16.43, 16.44a, 16.44b, 16.44c, 16.44d, 16.44e, 16.45a, 16.45b, 16.45c, 16.49a, 16.49b, 16.49c, 16.52, 16.53, 16.55, 16.57, 17.13a, 17.13b, 17.15a, 17.15b, 17.16, 17.18, 17.19, 17.24a, 17.24b, 17.24c, 17.26, 17.29a, 17.29b, 17.29c, 18.36, 18.50, 18.51, 18.67, 18.68, 18.72, 18.78, 18.80, 18.83, 18.86, 18.90, 18.91

Kanski, JJ; Milewski, SA; Damato, BE; Tanner, V. Diseases of the Ocular Fundus, Elsevier Mosby, ©2005.
9.101a, 9.101b, 9.101c, 9.102a, 9.102b, 9.102c, 9.151, 10.150, 10.172, 10.189a, 10.189b, 10.260a, 10.260b, 10.260c, 10.265a, 10.265b, 10.281a, 10.281b, 10.281c, 10.283a, 10.283b, 10.283c, 10.291, 10.292a, 10.292b, 10.292c, 10.292d, 11.16, 12.115a, 12.115b, 12.115c, 12.158, 12.174a, 12.174b, 12.174c, 12.152, 13.40, 13.49, 13.63, 13.87a, 13.87b, 13.87c, 13.88a, 13.88b, 13.88c, 13.100a, 13.100b, 13.100c, 13.102, 13.103, 13.106, 13.107, 13.109, 13.113a, 13.113b, 13.120, 14.1, 14.6, 14.7, 14.12, 14.14, 14.15, 14.19, 14.27, 14.30, 14.31, 14.32, 14.33, 14.40, 14.41, 14.44, 14.47a, 14.47b, 14.54, 14.55, 14.57, 14.61, 14.62, 14.63, 14.64, 14.66, 14.67, 14.69, 14.70a, 14.70b, 14.70c, 14.72a, 14.72b, 14.72c, 14.76, 14.79, 14.80, 14.82a, 14.82b, 14.82c, 14.83a, 14.83b, 14.89, 14.92, 14.105, 14.107, 14.110a, 14.110b, 14.111, 14.113, 14.114a, 14.114b, 14.115, 14.117, 14.118, 14.119, 14.120, 15.2, 15.8, 15.17, 15.19, 15.20, 15.28, 15.32a, 15.32b, 15.32c, 15.40, 15.41, 15.59, 15.60, 15.61, 15.62, 15.63, 15.69, 15.70, 15.71, 16.1, 16.5, 16.7, 16.15, 16.16, 16.18

Mir, MA. Atlas of Clinical Diagnosis, Saunders, ©2003.
3.97, 4.11, 4.13, 6.26, 6.187, 6.188, 6.189, 7.71, 7.72, 8.100, 9.133, 10.75, 10.76, 10.104, 10.212, 10.213, 10.48, 16.36, 16.37, 16.59, 9.128, 10.42

Moll, JH. Colour Guide Ophthalmology, Churchill Livingstone, ©1992.
4.45, 4.47, 4.48, 5.2, 12.106, 13.95, 13.96

Podos, SM; Yanoff, M. Textbook of Ophthalmology, vol 9, Mosby, ©1991.
10.171

Silbert, JA. Anterior Segment Complications of Contact Lens Wear 2e, Butterworth-Heinemann, ©2000.
1.33, 1.39, 1.45

Trend, P; Swash, M; Kennard C. Colour Guide Neurology, Churchill Livingstone, ©1992.
9.156, 9.172

Watson, P; Hazleman, BL; Pavésio, C; Green, WR. Sclera & Systemic Disorders 2e, Butterworth-Heinemann, ©2004.
3.144, 4.3, 4.29, 4.30, 4.31, 4.32, 4.39:

Zitelli, BJ; Davis, HW. Atlas of Pediatric Physical Diagnosis, Mosby, ©2002.
2.157, 2.161, 2.162, 2.163, 3.180, 4.51a, 4.51b, 4.51c, 4.51d, 4.53a, 4.53b, 6.23a, 6.23b, 6.30a, 6.30b, 6.31a, 6.31b, 6.31c, 6.32, 6.186, 6.235, 8.146, 9.134, 9.24a, 9.24b, 9.136, 10.176, 10.185, 10.232a, 10.232b, 10.232c, 12.104, 12.105, 14.22, 15.9a, 15.9b, 15.9c, 15.9d, 15.9e, 15.10a, 15.10b, 15.10c, 15.11a, 15.11b, 15.44, 17.10, 17.6a, 17.6b, 17.6c, 17.6d

CHAPTER 1

EYELIDS

DISORDERS OF LASHES

Trichiasis

Trichiasis is a very common acquired condition characterised by inturning of lashes arising from normal sites of origin. It may be idiopathic or secondary to chronic lid margin disease. It should not be confused with pseudotrichiasis associated with entropion.

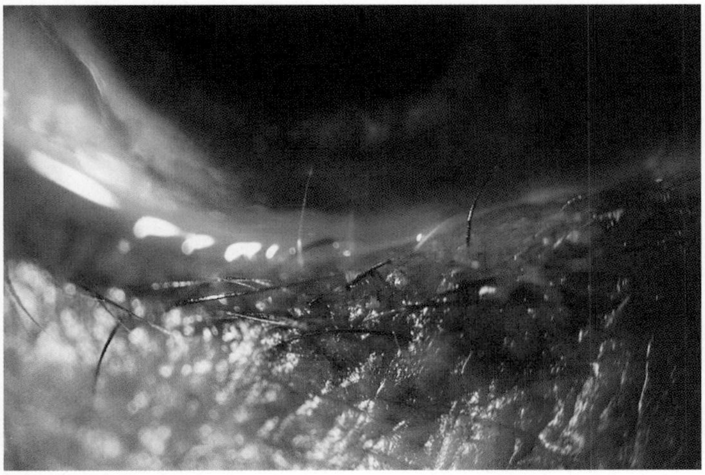

Fig. 1.1 Idiopathic trichiasis.

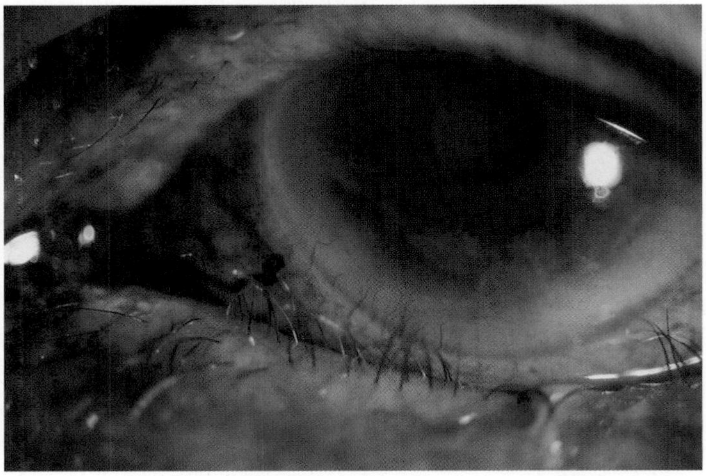

Fig. 1.2 Severe long-standing trichiasis causing inferior corneal scarring.

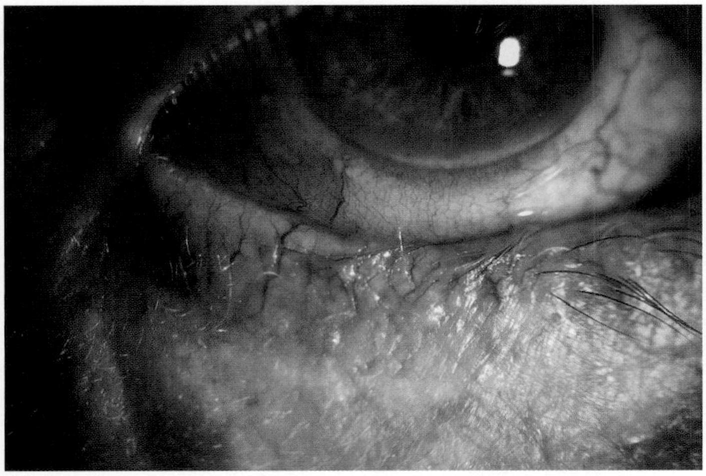

Fig. 1.3 Trichiasis and misdirection of lashes due to severe chronic anterior blepharitis.

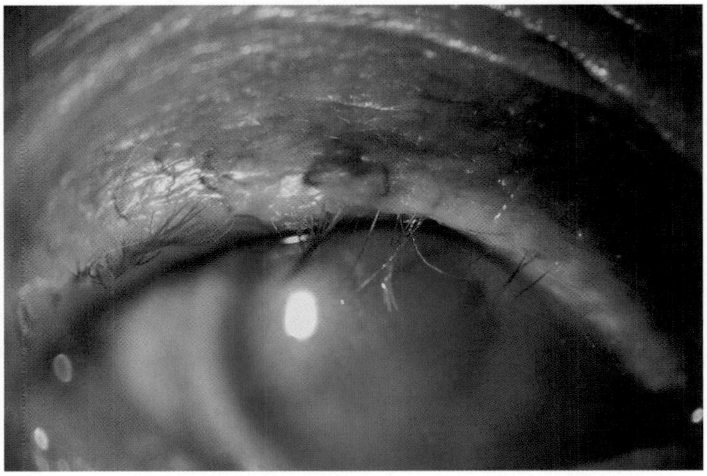

Fig. 1.4 Trichiasis of the upper lid and corneal scarring due to herpes zoster ophthalmicus.

Congenital distichiasis

Congenital distichiasis is a rare condition that may be sporadic or dominantly inherited. A minority of patients also manifest chronic lymphoedema, spinal arachnoid cysts and congenital heart defects (lymphoedema–trichiasis syndrome).

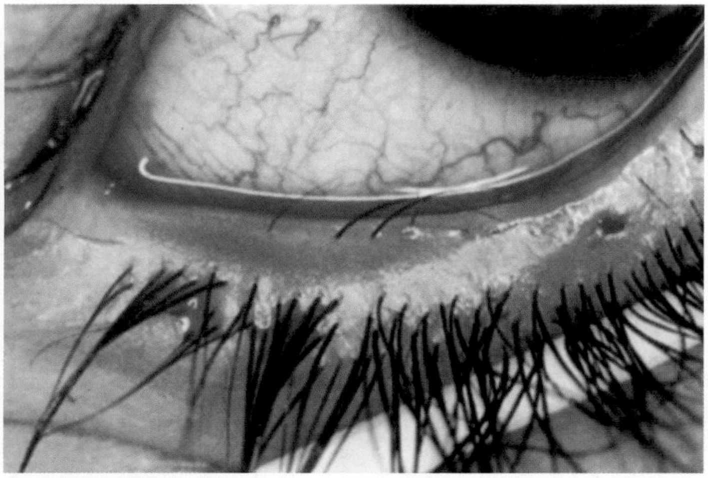

Fig. 1.5 A partial or complete second row of lashes emerging at or slightly behind the meibomian gland orifices. The aberrant lashes tend to be thinner, shorter and less pigmented than normal cilia and are often directed posteriorly. (Courtesy of D. M. Albert and F. A. Jakobiec.)

Acquired distichiasis (metaplastic lashes)

Acquired distichiasis is caused by metaplasia and dedifferentiation of the meibomian glands to become hair follicles in patients with cicatrising conjunctivitis.

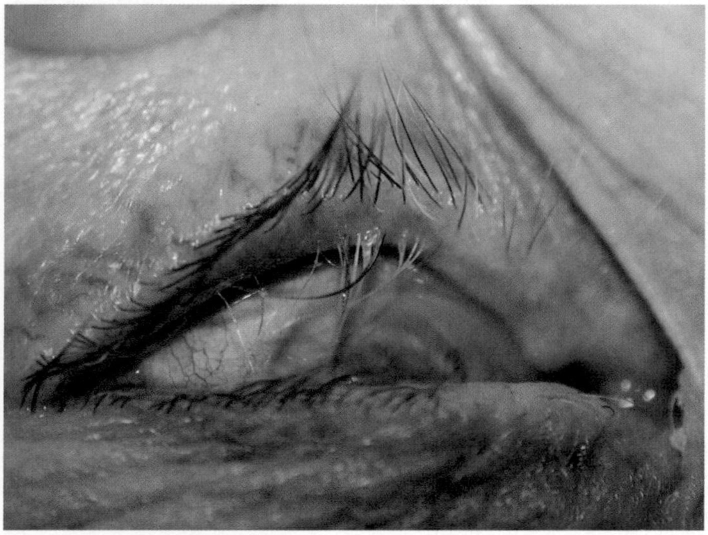

Fig. 1.6 A variable number of lashes that originate from meibomian gland orifices.

Lash ptosis

Lash ptosis may be idiopathic or associated with the floppy eyelid syndrome, dermatochalasis or long-standing facial palsy.

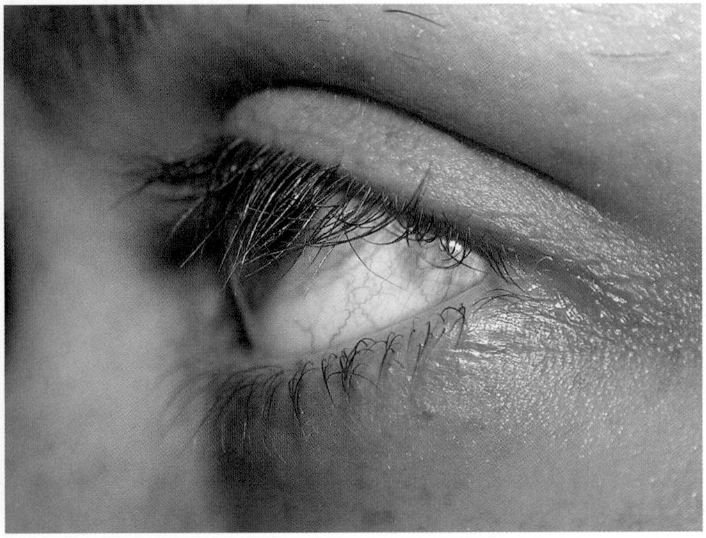

Fig. 1.7 Downward displacement of normal lashes.

Ectopic lash

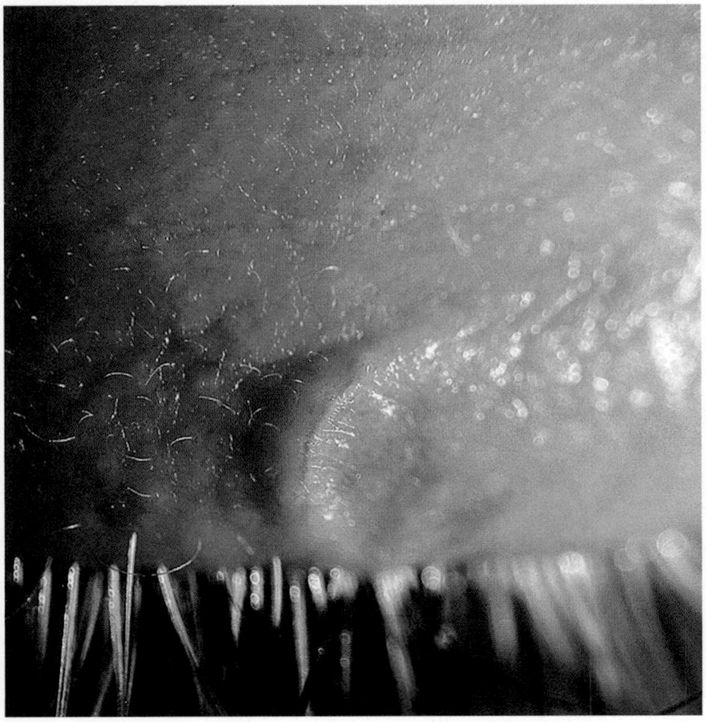

Fig. 1.8 Subcutaneous lash.

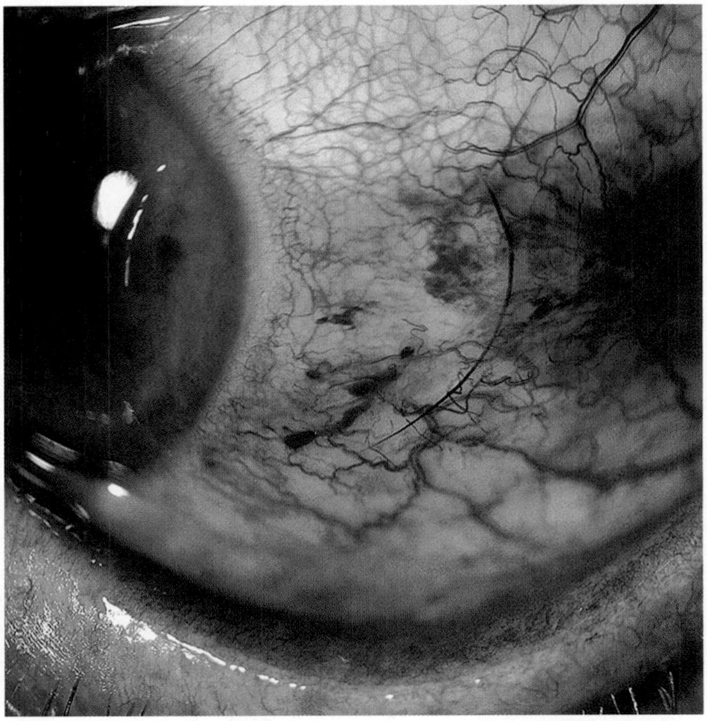

Fig. 1.9 Subconjunctival lash.

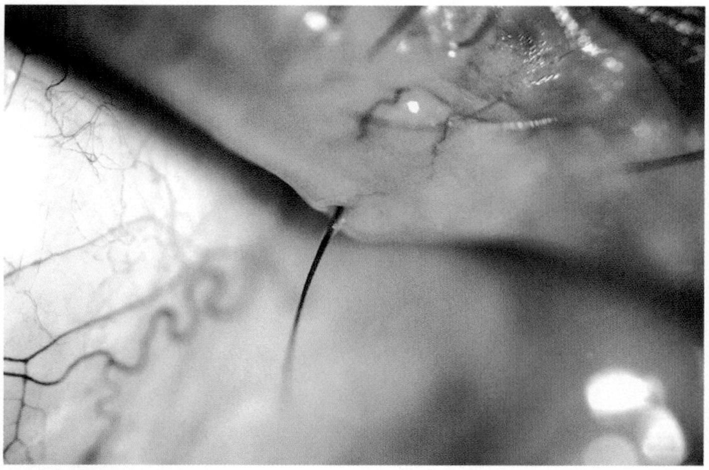

Fig. 1.10 Lash in a punctum may cause irritation on blinking.

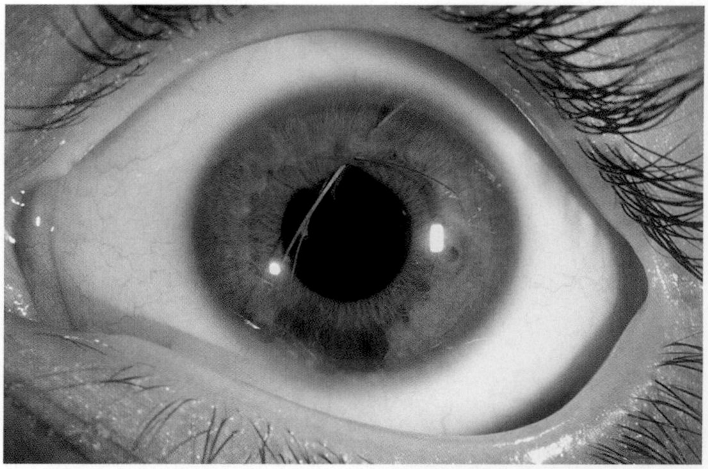

Fig. 1.11 Lash introduced into the anterior chamber during surgery. (Courtesy of L. Merin.)

Madarosis

Madarosis is a decrease in number or complete loss of lashes.

Local causes

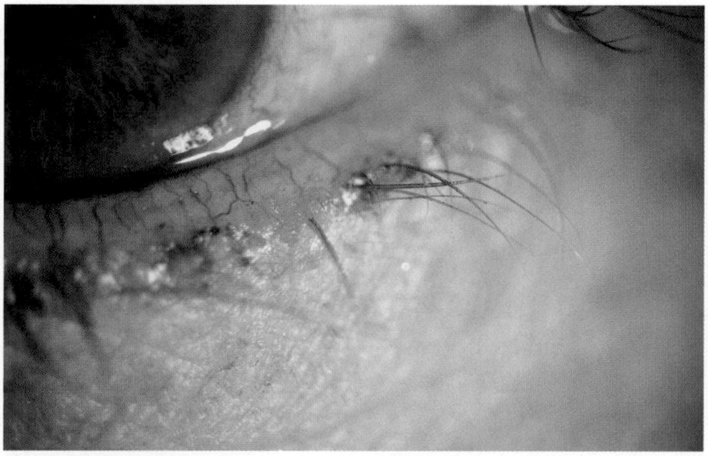

Fig. 1.12 Severe long-standing anterior blepharitis.

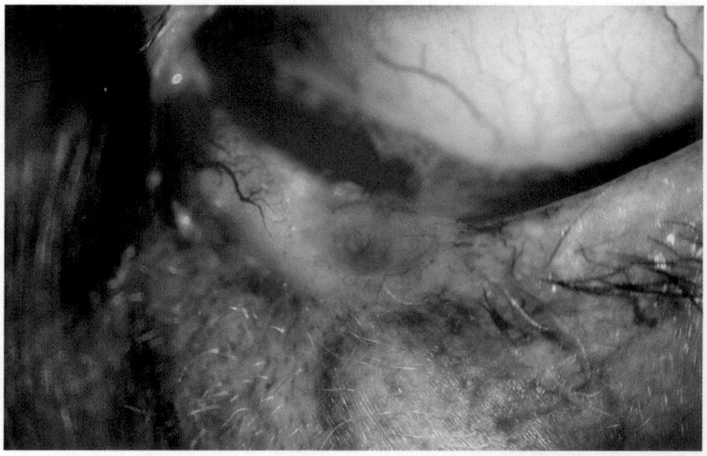

Fig. 1.13 Destruction of lashes by infiltrating lid tumours.

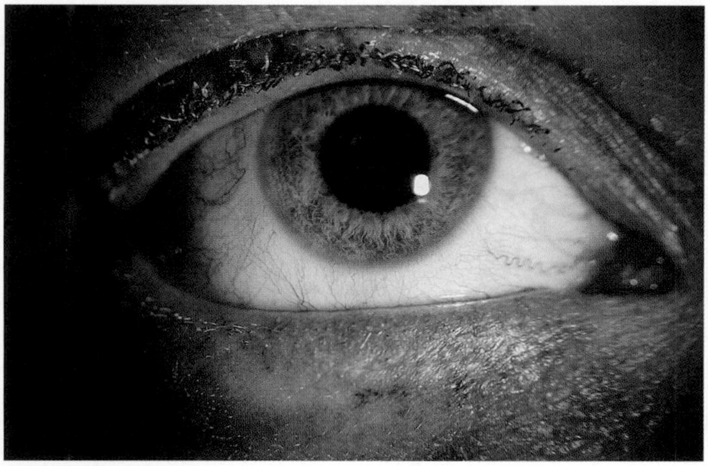

Fig. 1.14 Thermal burns.

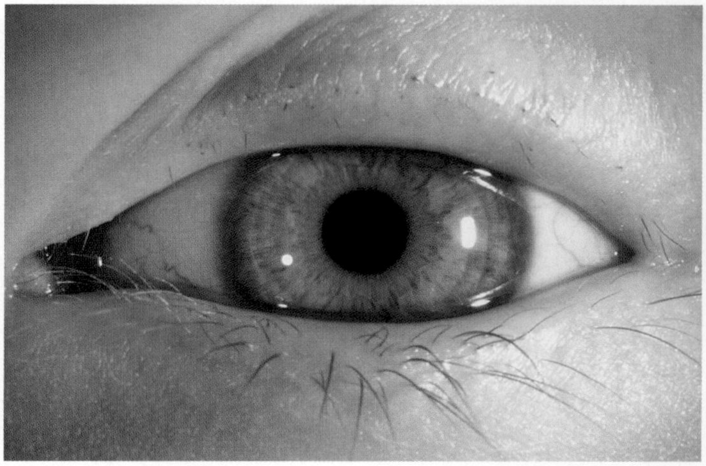

Fig. 1.15 Trichotillomania – habitual hair removal. (Courtesy of L. Merin.)

Associated systemic conditions

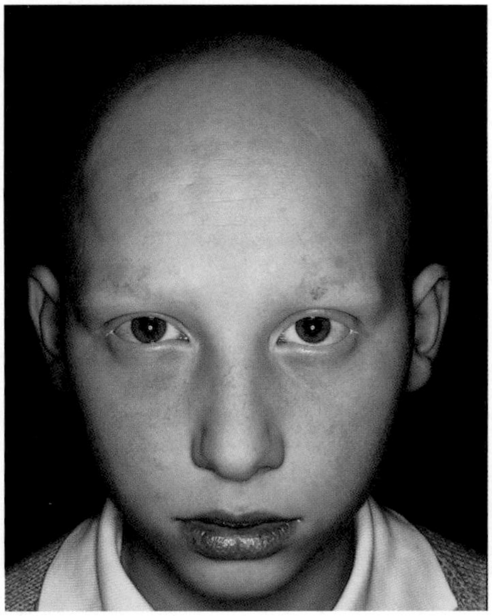

Fig. 1.16 Generalised alopecia.

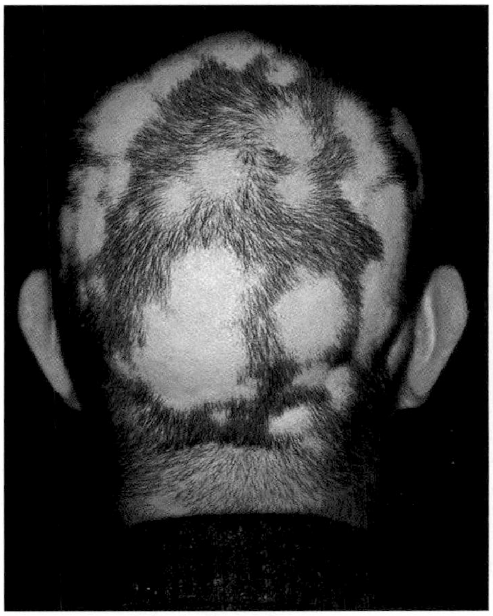

Fig. 1.17 Alopecia areata.

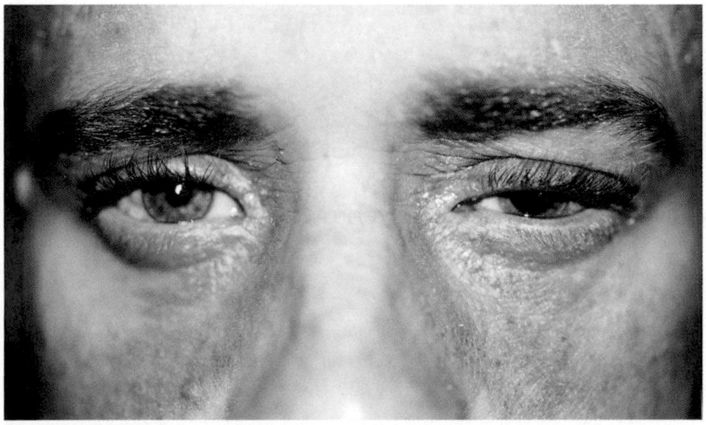

Fig. 1.18 Atopic dermatitis, characterised by itchy erythema, scaling and lichenification.

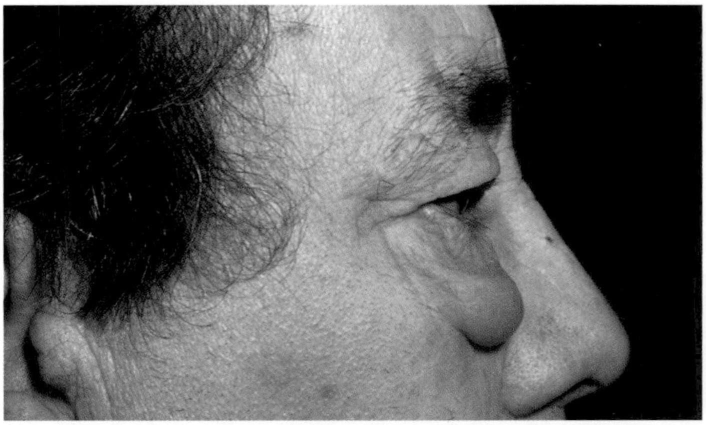

Fig. 1.19 Myxoedema, which may also cause loss of eyebrows and puffiness of periorbital skin.

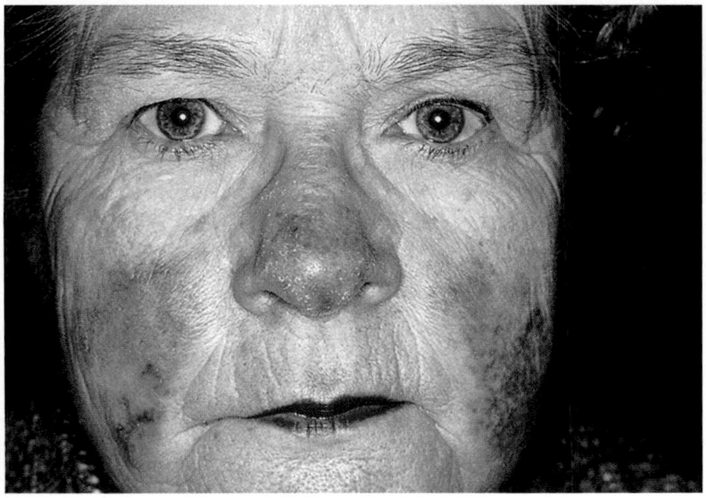

Fig. 1.20 Systemic lupus erythematosus, which may be associated with a characteristic 'butterfly' facial skin rash.

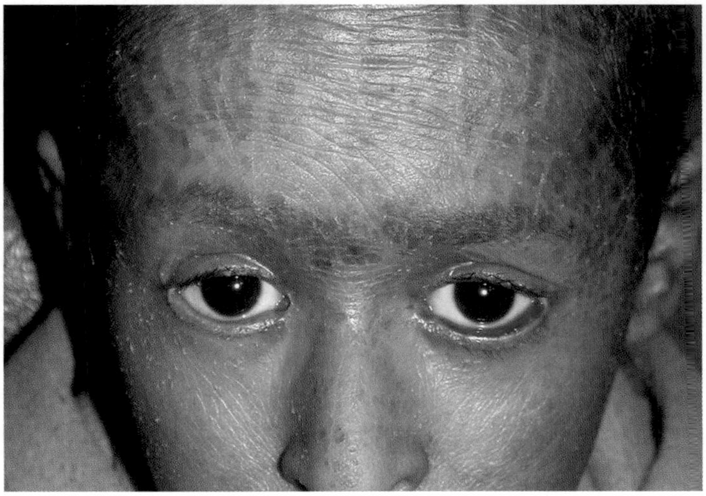

Fig. 1.21 Ichthyosis, characterised by itchy, dry and scaly skin. (Courtesy of A. Pearson.)

Seborrhoeic blepharitis

Seborrhoeic blepharitis may occur in isolation or in association with staphylococcal blepharitis (mixed anterior blepharitis).

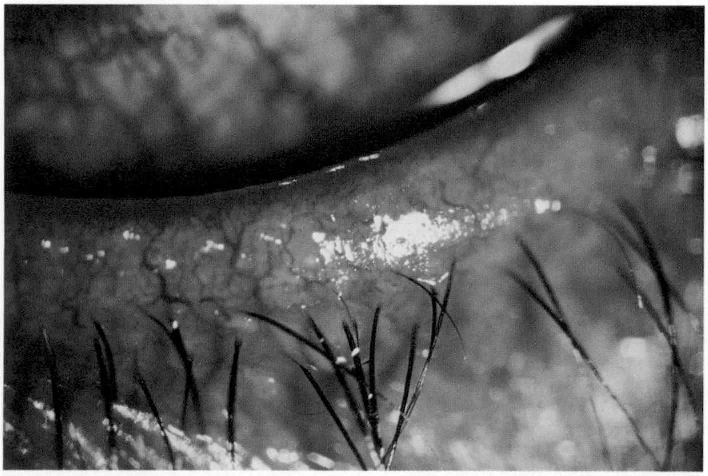

Fig. 1.30 Hyperaemic and greasy anterior lid margins.

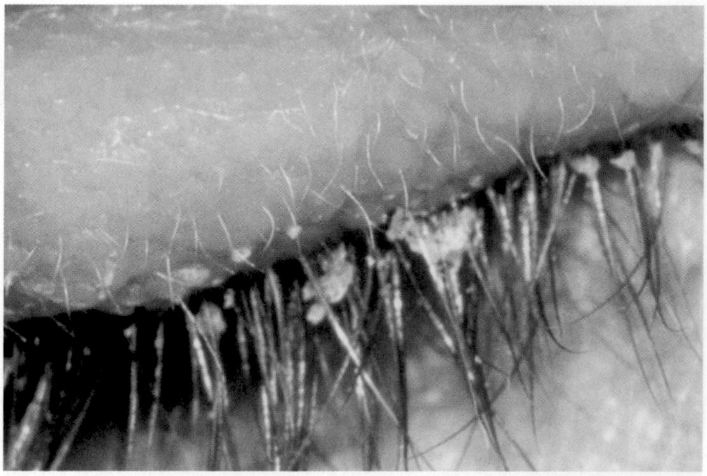

Fig. 1.31 Soft scales located anywhere on the lid margin and lashes. (Courtesy of J. A. Silbert.)

Association

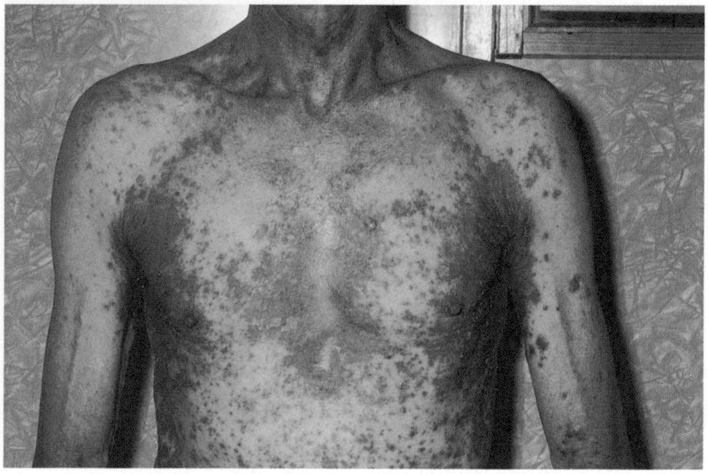

Fig. 1.32 Seborrhoeic dermatitis, characterised by a red scaly rash that classically affects the scalp (dandruff), central face, nasolabial folds, eyebrows and central chest.

Posterior blepharitis

Posterior blepharitis is a manifestation of meibomian gland dysfunction. It may occur in isolation or in association with anterior blepharitis (mixed anterior and posterior blepharitis).

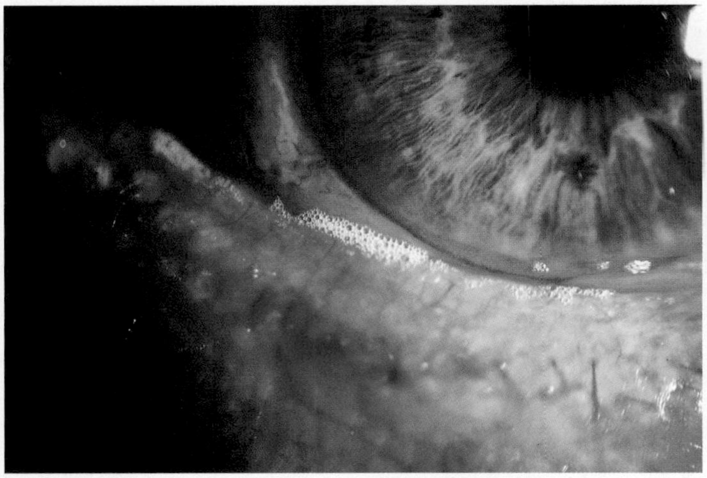

Fig. 1.33 The tear film is oily and in severe cases froth accumulates on the lid margins or inner canthi.

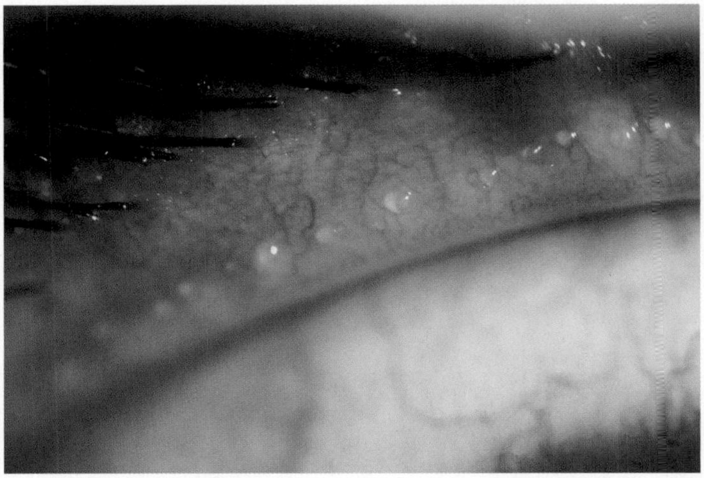

Fig. 1.34 The meibomian gland orifices are capped by small oil globules.

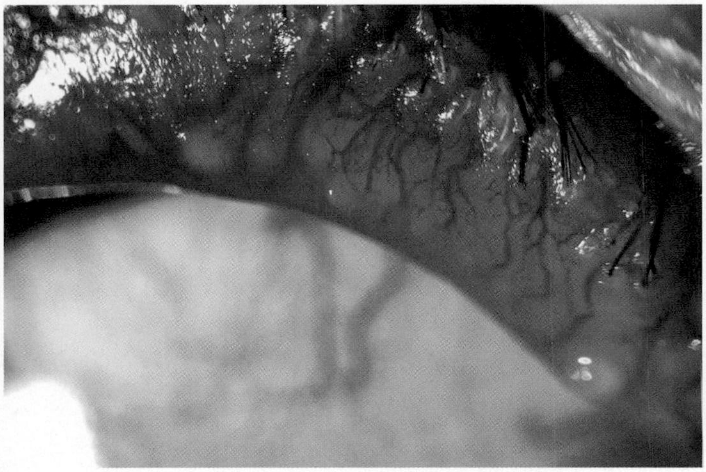

Fig. 1.35 The posterior lid margin shows hyperaemia, telangiectasia and patchy obstruction of meibomian gland orifices.

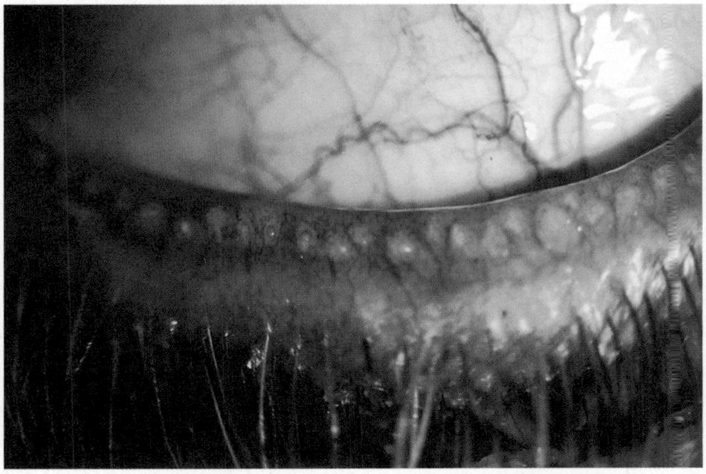

Fig. 1.36 Extensive obstruction of meibomian gland orifices and lid margin telangiectasia.

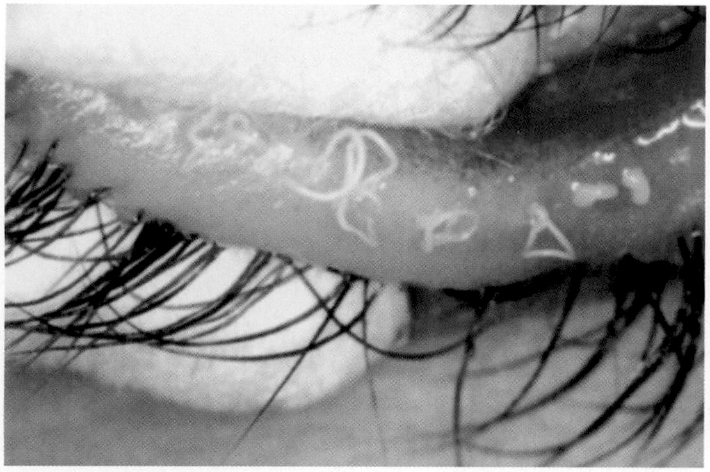

Fig. 1.37 Inspissated, toothpaste-like plaques expressed from meibomian glands. (Courtesy of J. A. Silbert.)

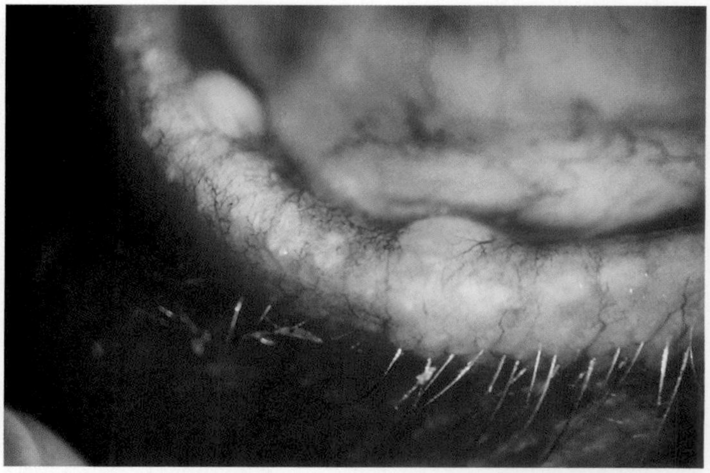

Fig. 1.38 Multiple small chalazia and thickening of the posterior lid margin.

Association

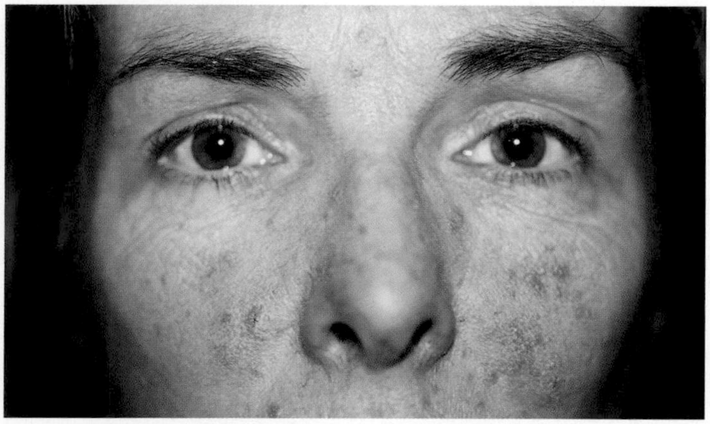

Fig. 1.39 Acne rosacea, characterised by itching, flushing and telangiectasia of facial skin.

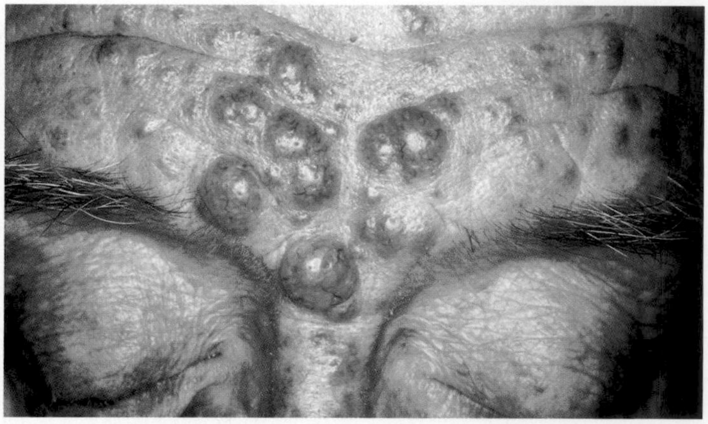

Fig. 1.40 More severe rosacea with hypertrophy of sebaceous glands.

Angular blepharitis

Angular blepharitis is an uncommon condition caused by *Moraxella lacunata* or *Staphylococcus aureus*.

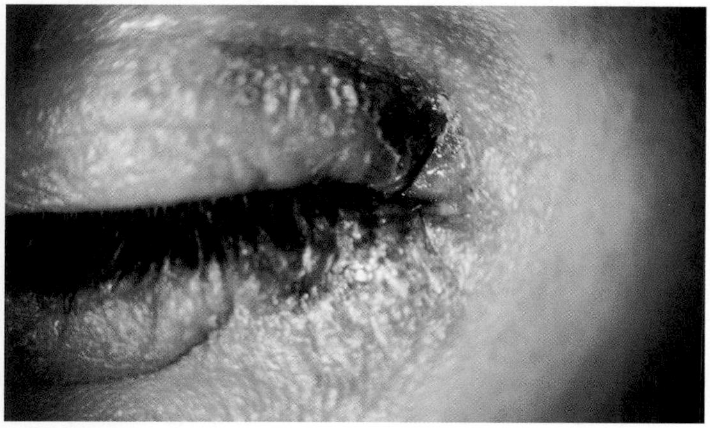

Fig. 1.41 Red, scaly, macerated and fissured skin at one or both canthal regions.

Blepharitis due to infestations

Phthiriasis palpebrarum

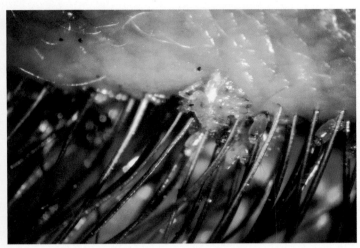

■ **Fig. 1.42** The lice (*Phthirus pubis*) are anchored to the lashes by their thick claws. The ova and their empty shells appear as brownish, opalescent pearls adherent to the base of the cilia.

Demodex folliculorum

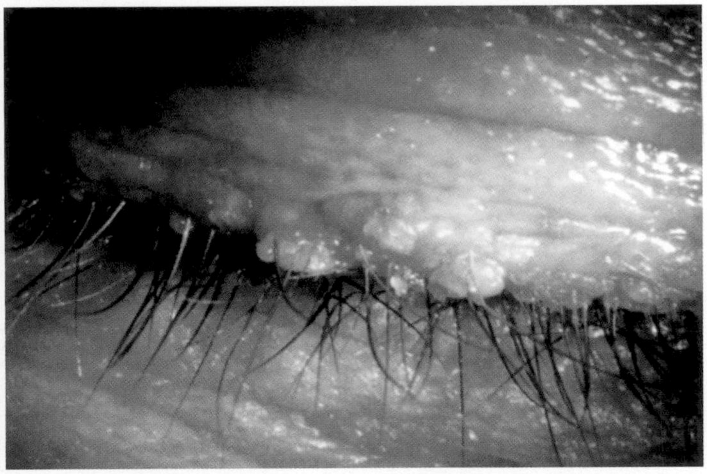

■ **Fig. 1.43** Semi-transparent, thin, tube-like crusting of the lashes and lid margin. (Courtesy of J. A. Silbert.)

ALLERGIC DISORDERS

Acute allergic oedema

Acute allergic oedema may be caused by insect bites, angioedema and urticaria.

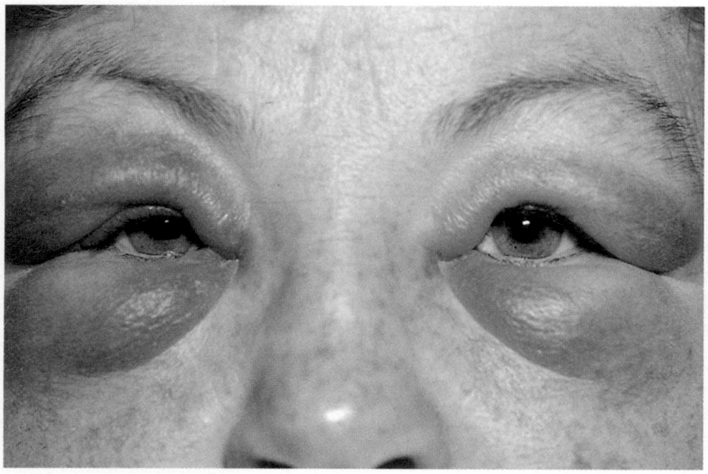

Fig. 1.44 Bilateral, painless, erythema and pitting lid oedema.

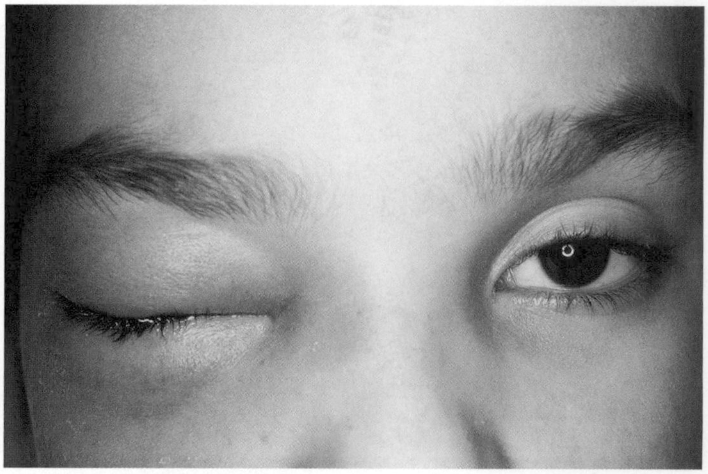

Fig. 1.45 Unilateral allergic oedema due to an insect bite.

Contact dermatitis

Contact dermatitis is caused by sensitivity to topical medication.

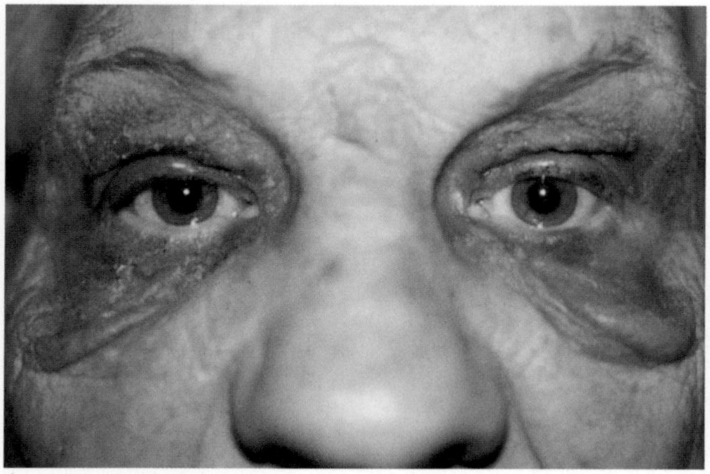

Fig. 1.46 Erythema and mild oedema associated with tearing and itching.

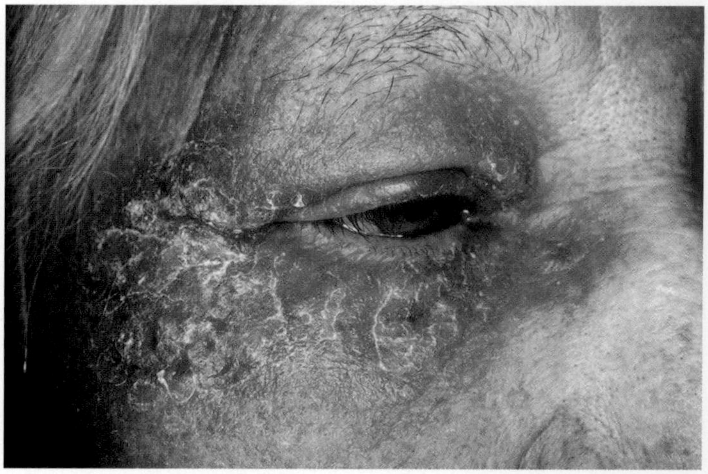

Fig. 1.47 If the cause is not withdrawn the oedema subsides but the erythema persists and the skin becomes thickened and crusty.

Atopic eczema (dermatitis)

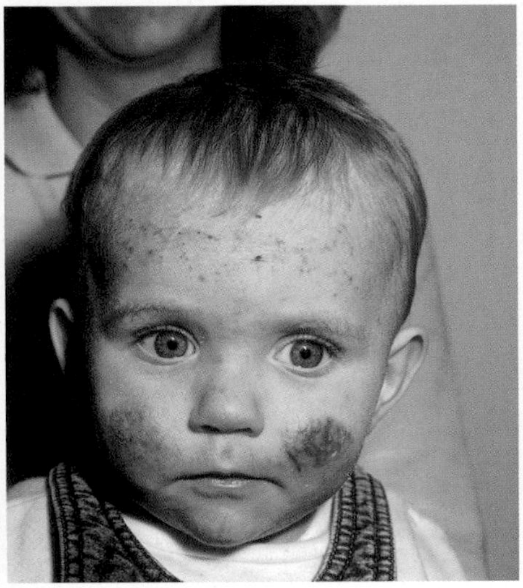

Fig. 1.48 Facial eczema is usually seen in infants.

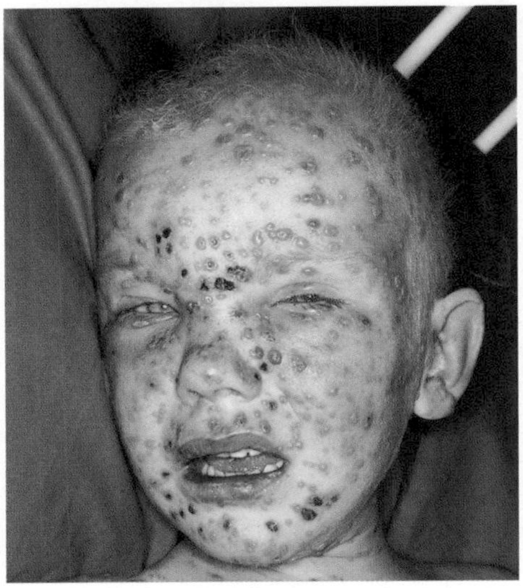

Fig. 1.49 Extensive herpes simplex infection in a child with eczema (eczema herpeticum).

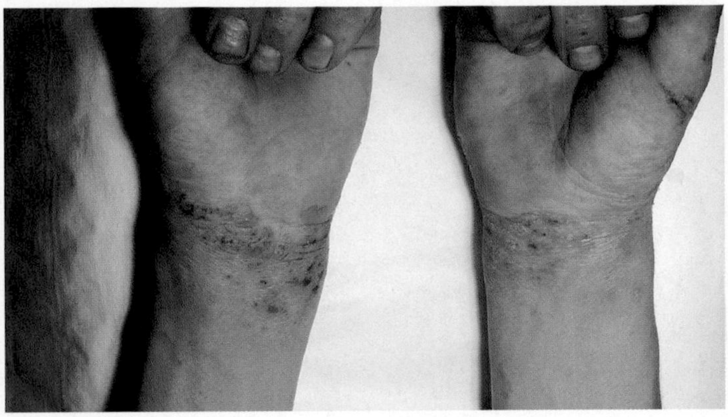

Fig. 1.50 Flexural eczema usually develops later in childhood.

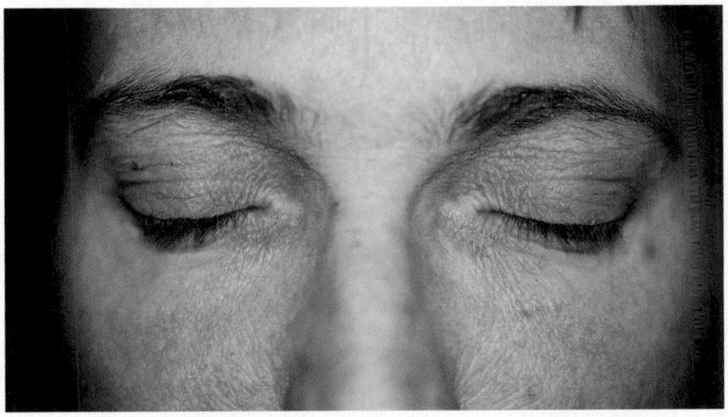

Fig. 1.51 Eyelid involvement is characterised by thickening and vertical fissuring of the lids.

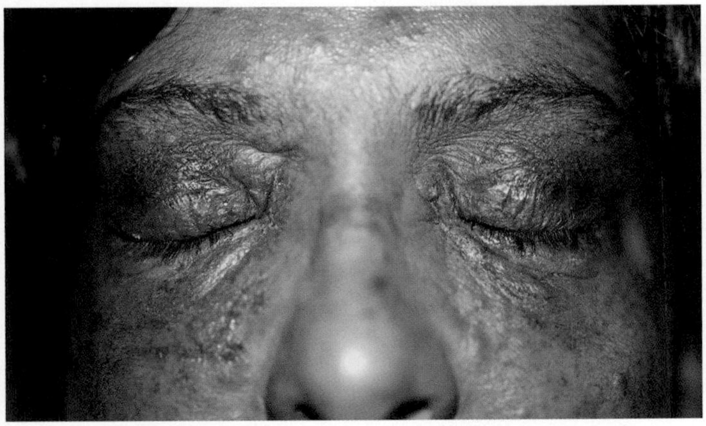

Fig. 1.52 Very severe lid involvement which may be associated with staphylococcal blepharitis, angular blepharitis and madarosis.

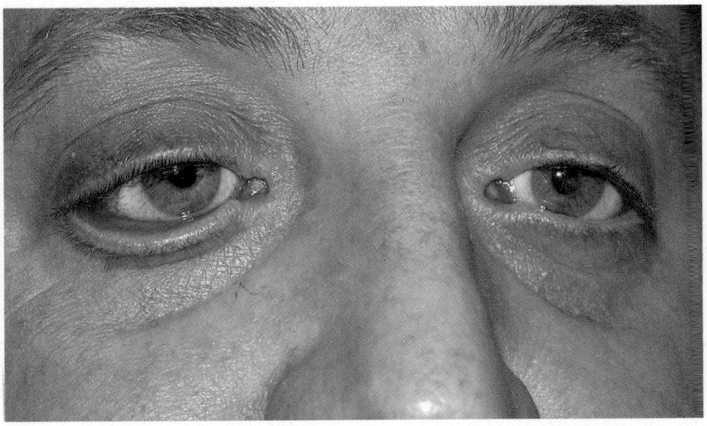

Fig. 1.53 Atopic eczema causing cicatricial ectropion. (Courtesy of A. Pearson.)

Ocular associations

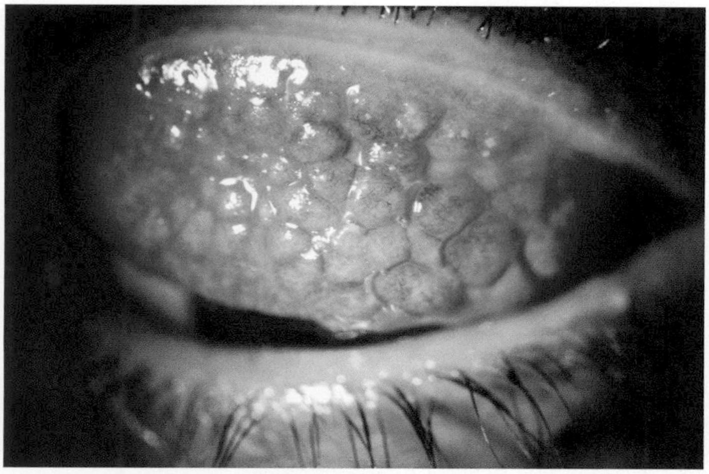

Fig. 1.54 Vernal disease in children, characterised by superior tarsal 'cobblestone' papillae.

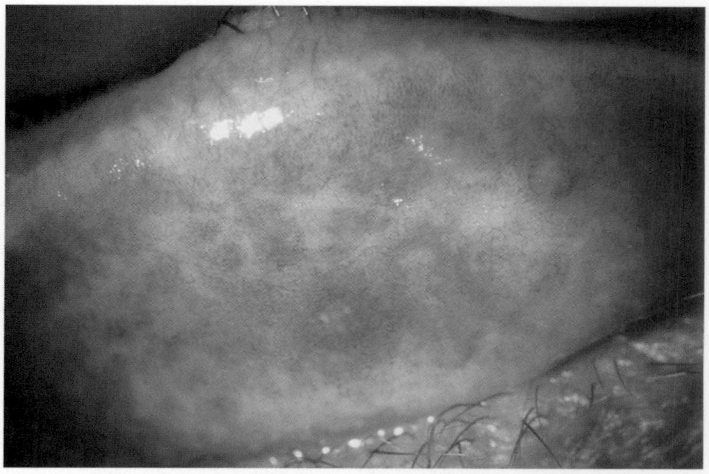

Fig. 1.55 Chronic keratoconjunctivitis in adults, characterised by a featureless tarsal conjunctiva. (Courtesy of S. Tuft.)

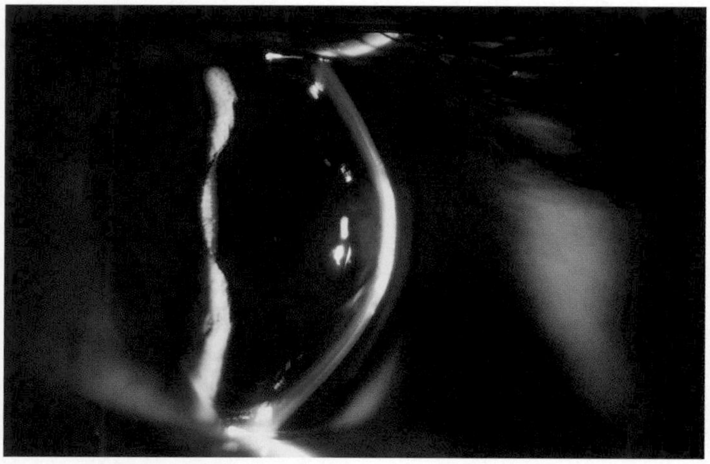

Fig. 1.56 Keratoconus.

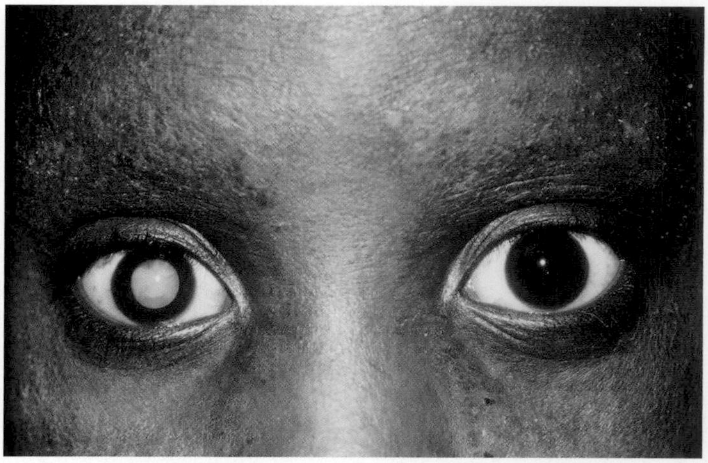

Fig. 1.57 Presenile cataract. (Courtesy of S. Ford and R. Marsh.)

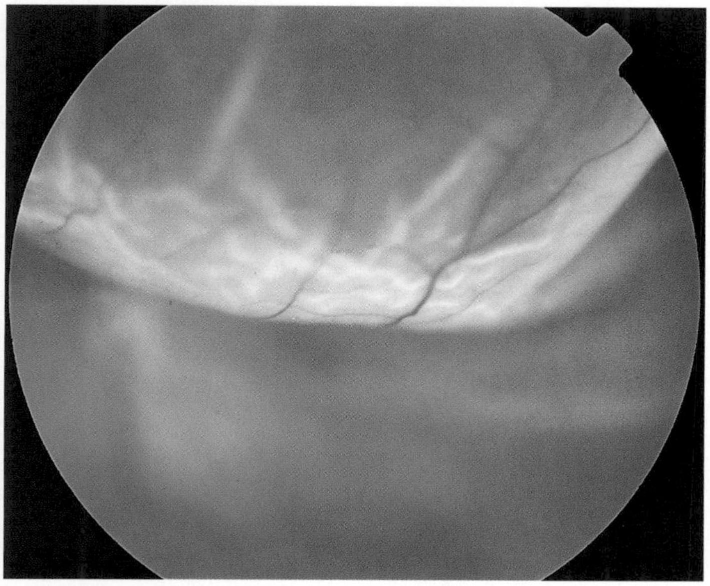

Fig. 1.58 Retinal detachment is uncommon.

VIRAL INFECTIONS

Herpes zoster ophthalmicus

Involvement of ophthalmic division of the trigeminal nerve by shingles is referred to as herpes zoster ophthalmicus.

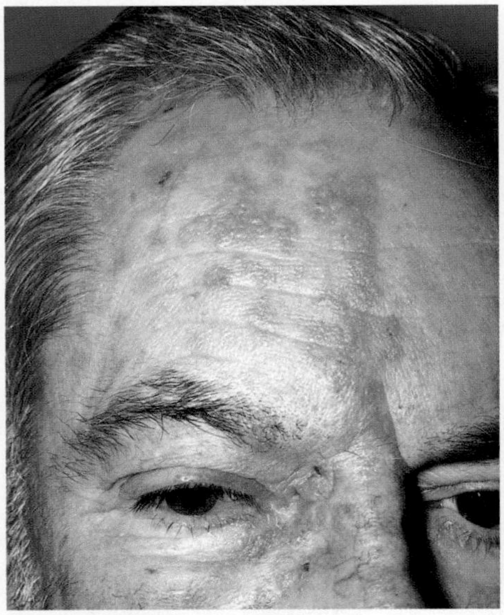

Fig. 1.59 Presentation is with a unilateral painful maculopapular rash.

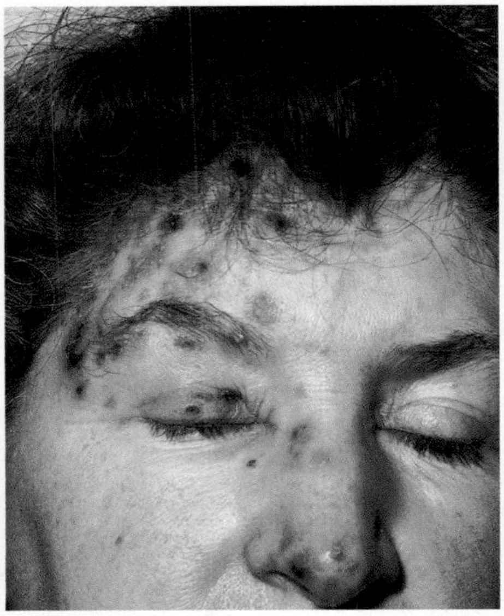

Fig. 1.60 Vesicles and pustules develop within a few days. Involvement of the external nasal nerve, which supplies the tip of the nose, is associated with an increased risk of ocular complications.

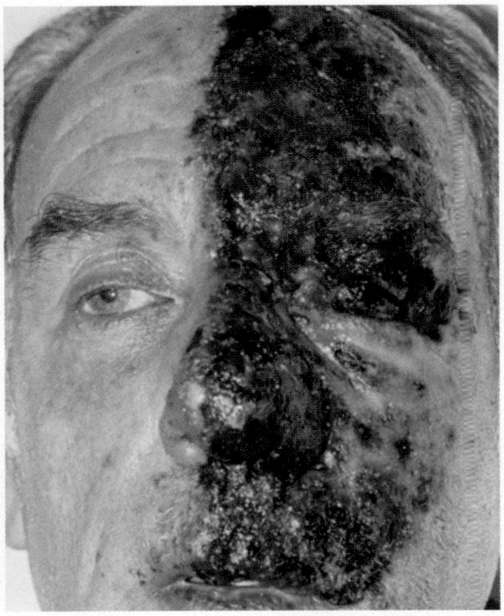

Fig. 1.61 Involvement of both ophthalmic and maxillary divisions is uncommon.

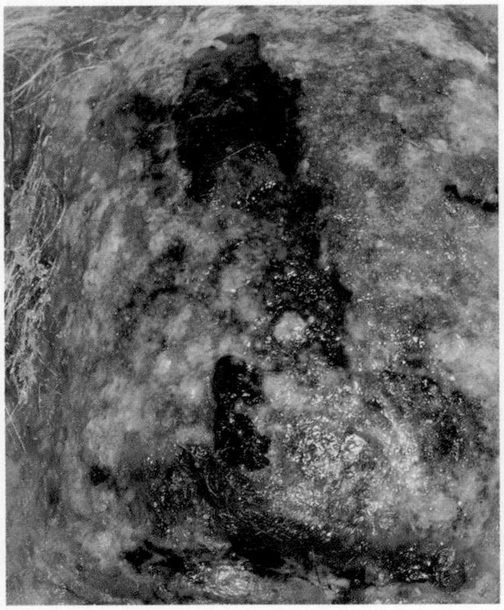

Fig. 1.62 Confluent haemorrhagic lesions in severe disease.

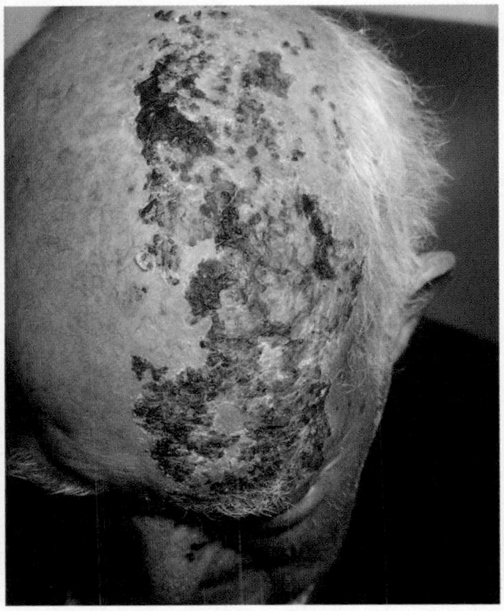

Fig. 1.63 Severe crusting.

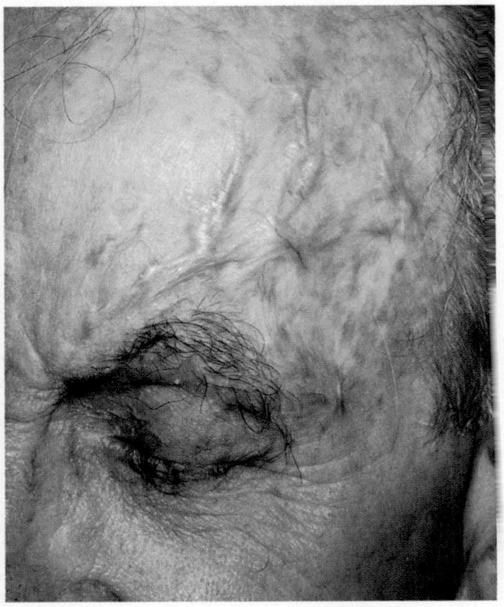

Fig. 1.64 Residual scarring of the forehead may be associated with postherpetic neuralgia (Courtesy of S. Ford and R. Marsh.)

Ophthalmic complications

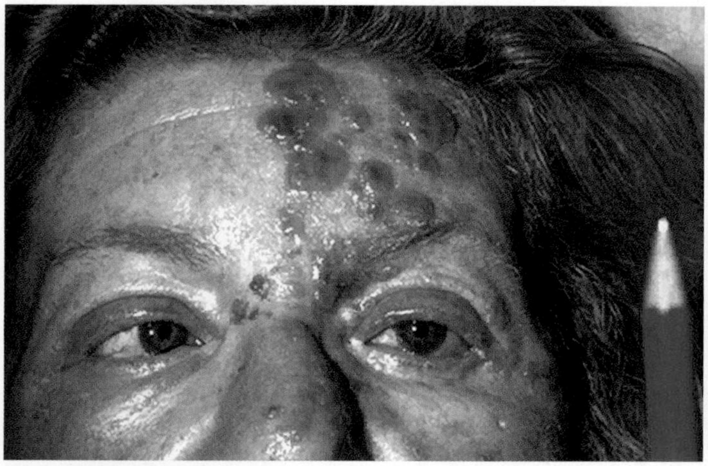

■ **Fig. 1.65** Ocular motor palsies, such as a left sixth shown here, are uncommon. (Courtesy of S. Ford and R. Marsh.)

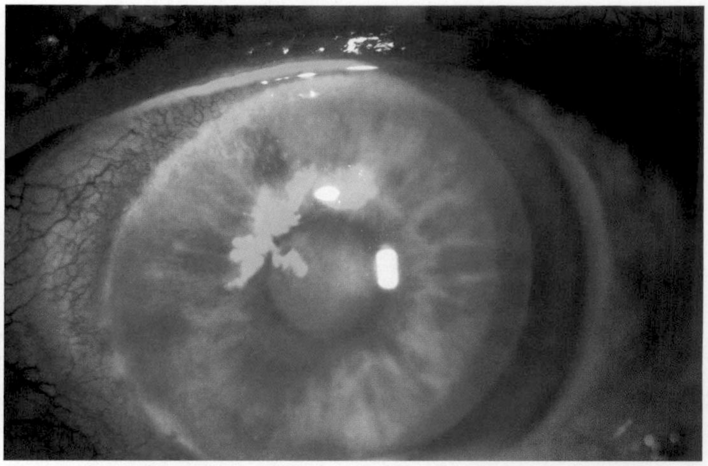

■ **Fig. 1.66** Acute epithelial keratitis characterised by dendritic or stellate lesions. (Courtesy of S. Ford and R. Marsh.)

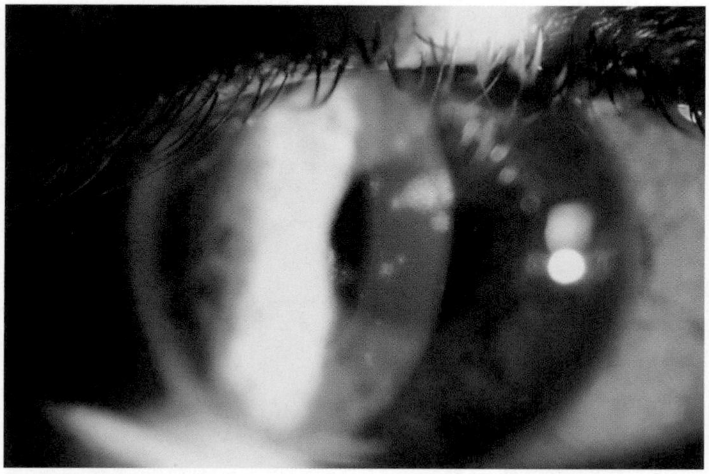

■ **Fig. 1.67** Nummular keratitis. (Courtesy of S. Ford and R. Marsh.)

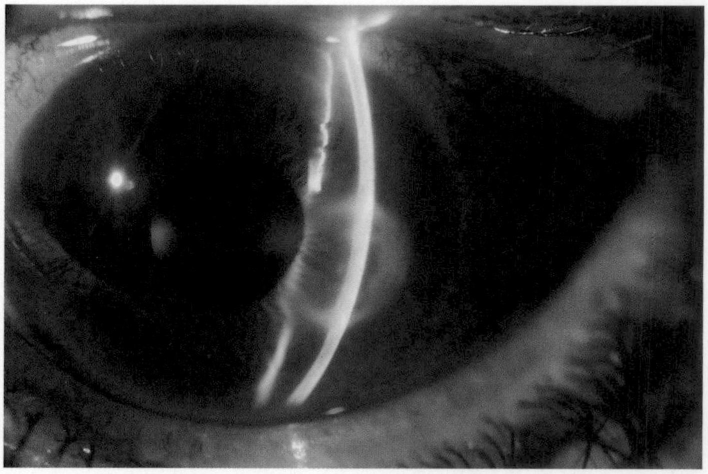

■ **Fig. 1.68** Disciform keratitis, which may be eccentric. (Courtesy of S. Ford and R. Marsh.)

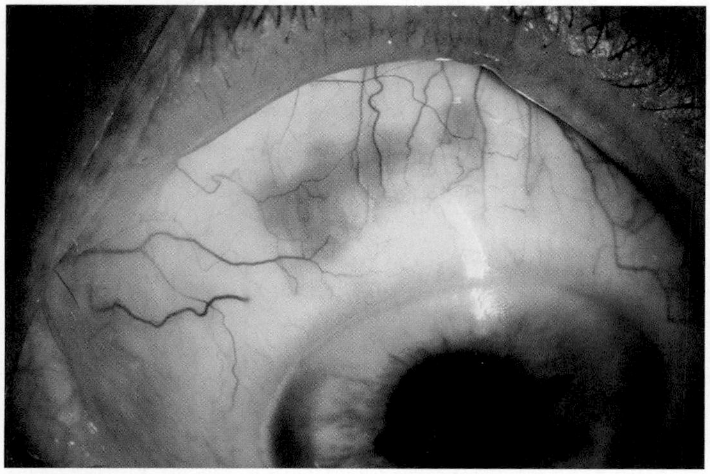

■ **Fig. 1.69** Scleritis may result in patchy scleral thinning. (Courtesy of S. Ford and R. Marsh.)

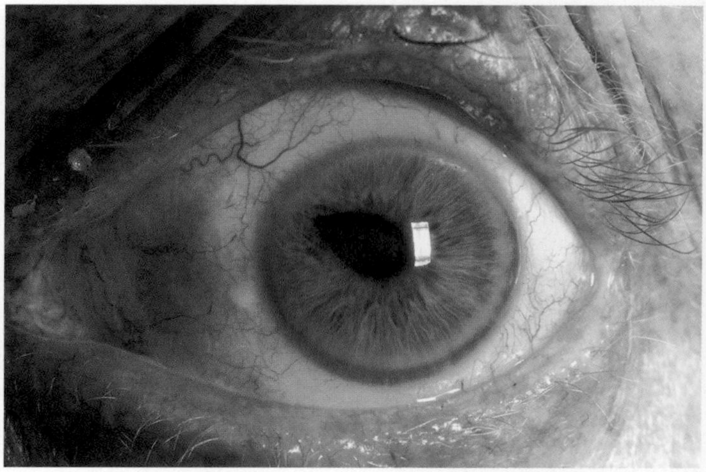

■ **Fig. 1.70** Anterior uveitis may give rise to iris distortion and atrophy. (Courtesy of S. Ford and R. Marsh.)

Herpes simplex

The eyelids may be involved in primary herpes simplex infection which typically occurs in childhood.

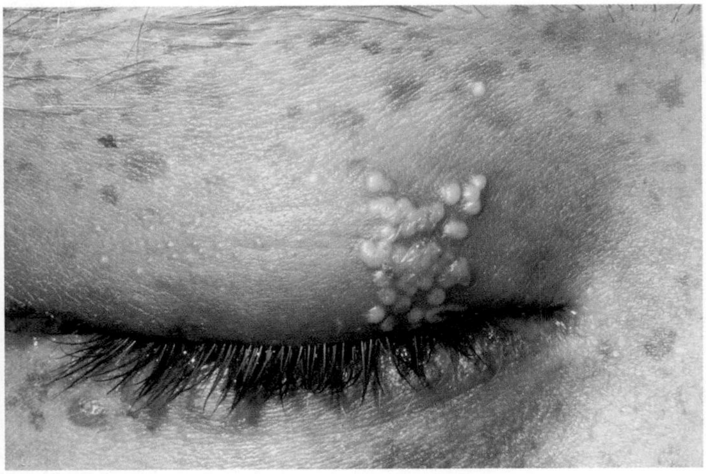

Fig. 1.71 Presentation is with crops of small vesicles.

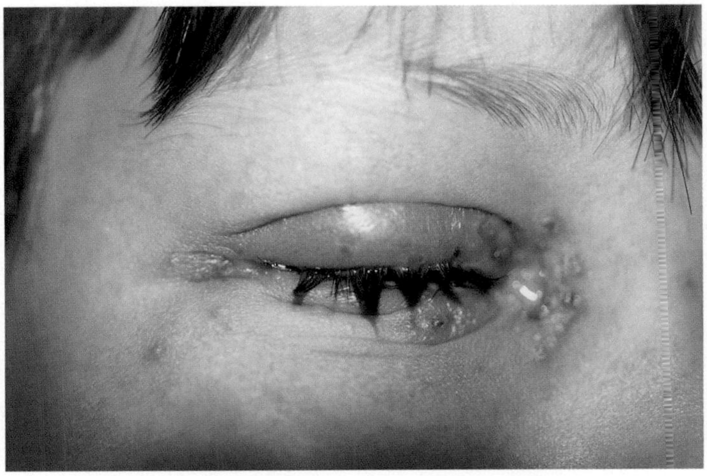

Fig. 1.72 Herpetic vesicles and lid oedema.

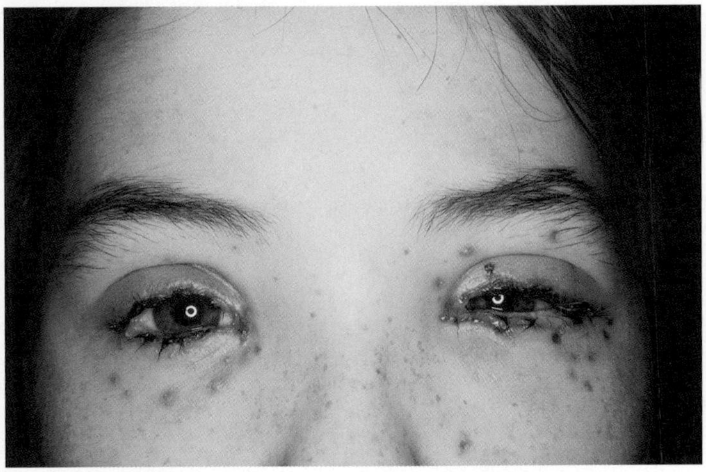

Fig. 1.73 Blepharoconjunctivitis, which may be associated with epithelial keratitis. (Courtesy of S. Ford and R. Marsh.)

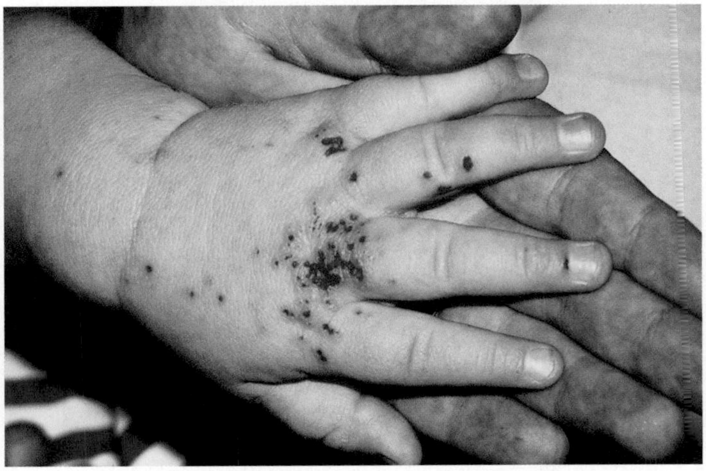

Fig. 1.74 Herpetic vesicles on the hand.

Molluscum contagiosum

Molluscum contagiosum is caused by an oncogenic poxvirus.

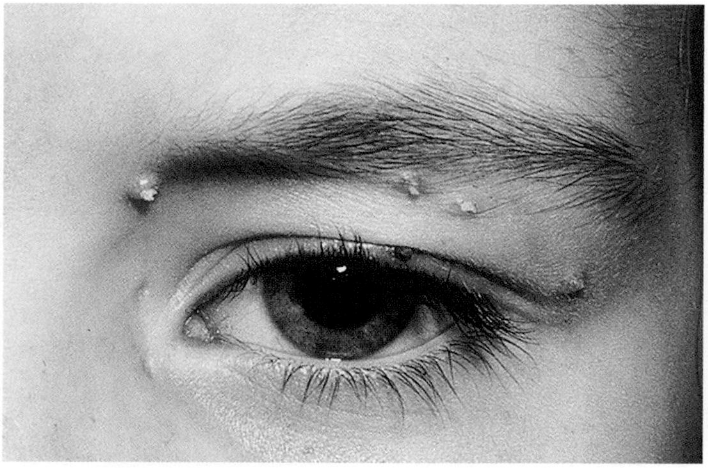

Fig. 1.75 Multiple, small molluscum nodules.

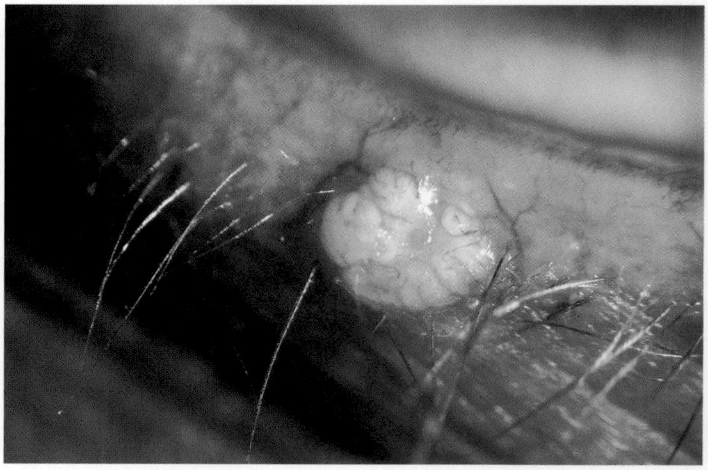

Fig. 1.76 Solitary, small, pale, waxy, umbilicated nodule on the eyelid.

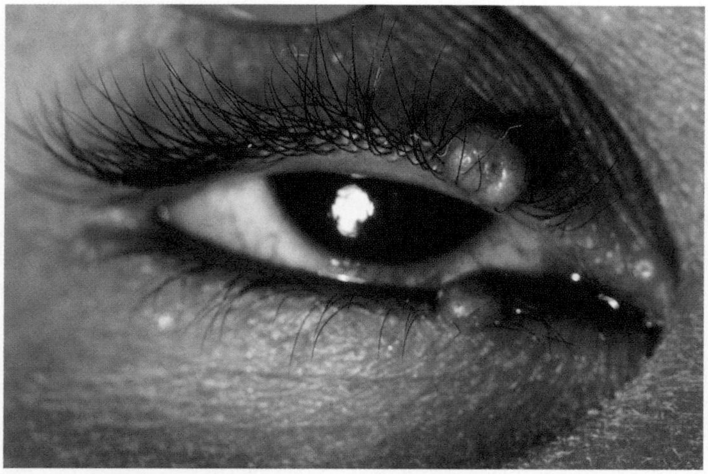

Fig. 1.77 Patients with immune deficiency may manifest multiple large lesions.

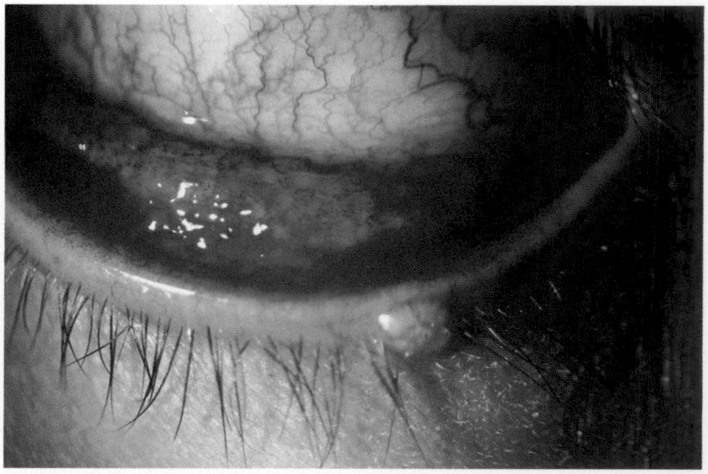

Fig. 1.78 Secondary ipsilateral chronic follicular conjunctivitis may develop if the lesion affects the lid margin.

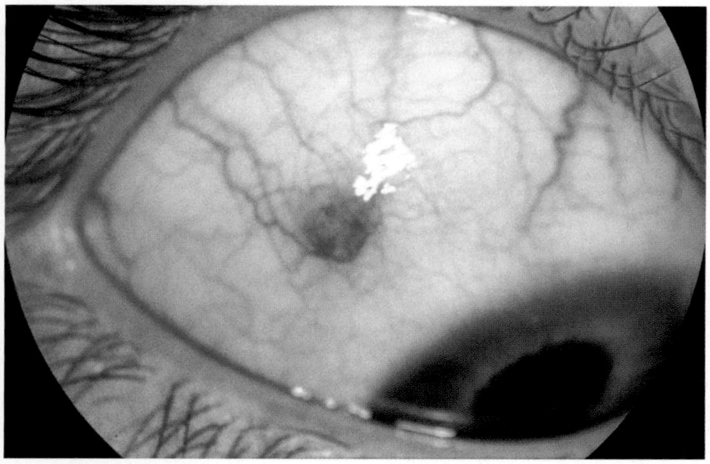

Fig. 1.79 A conjunctival molluscum nodule, which is very rare. (Courtesy of R. Murray.)

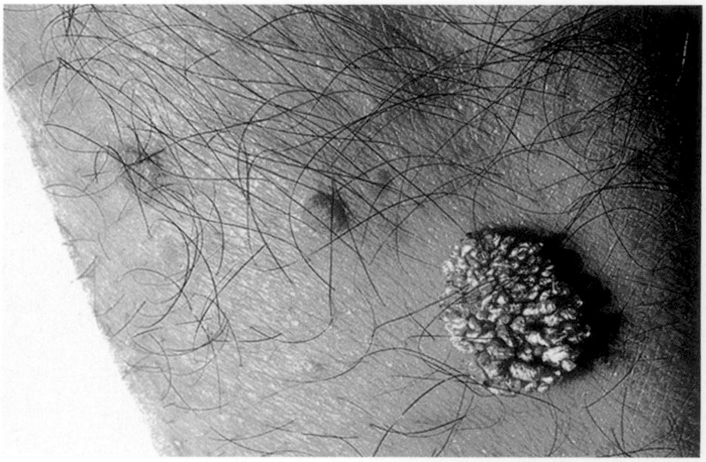

Fig. 1.80 Several small and one very large molluscum lesion.

BACTERIAL INFECTIONS

Internal hordeolum (acute chalazion)

An internal hordeolum is a small staphylococcal abscess involving meibomian glands.

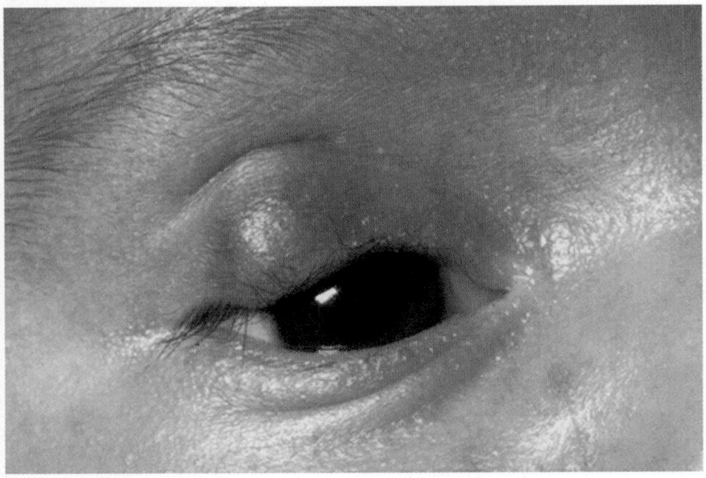

Fig. 1.81 A tender swelling within the tarsal plate with overlying cutaneous erythema.

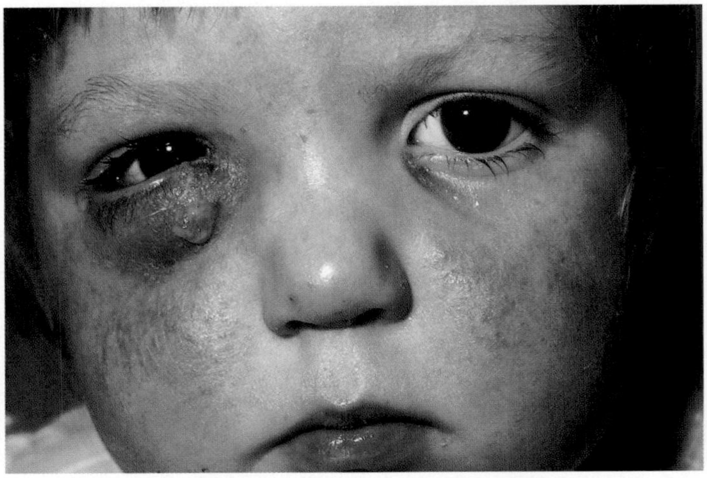

Fig. 1.82 The lesion may enlarge and then discharge either posteriorly through the conjunctiva or anteriorly through the skin.

External hordeolum (stye)

An external hordeolum is an acute staphylococcal abscess of a lash follicle and its associated gland of Zeis or Moll.

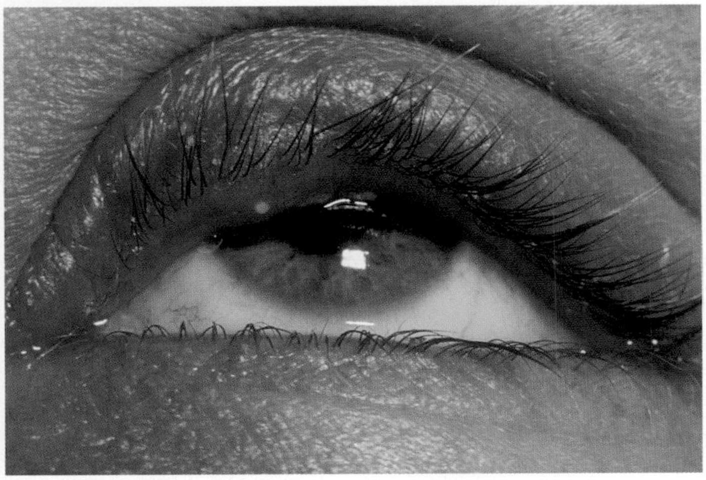

Fig. 1.83 Tender swelling in the lid margin that points through the skin. (Courtesy of S. Tuft.)

Preseptal cellulitis

Preseptal cellulitis is an infection of subcutaneous tissues anterior to the orbital septum that typically affects children.

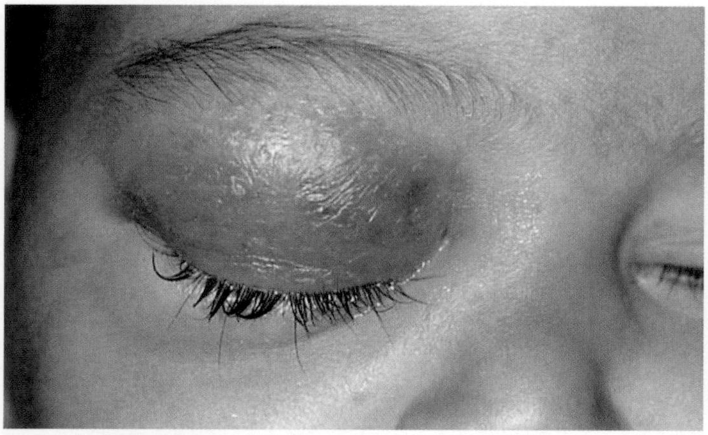

■ **Fig. 1.84** Unilateral, tenderness, oedema and erythema. (Courtesy of U. Raina.)

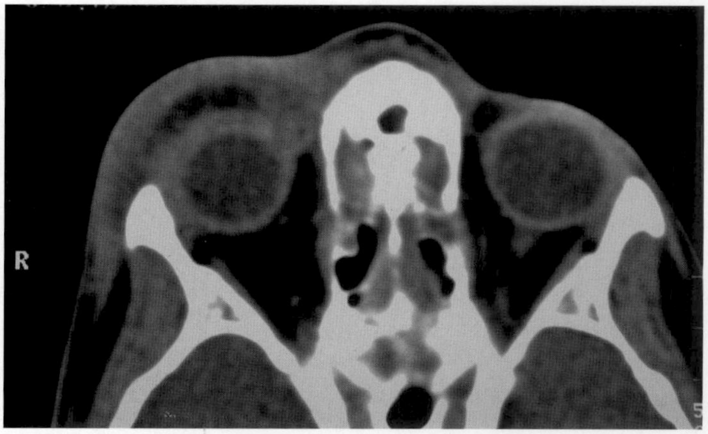

■ **Fig. 1.85** Axial CT shows opacification anterior to the orbital septum and lack of involvement of orbital tissues. (Courtesy of A. Pearson.)

Impetigo

Impetigo is a superficial skin infection caused by *Staphylococcus aureus* or *Streptococcus pyogenes*.

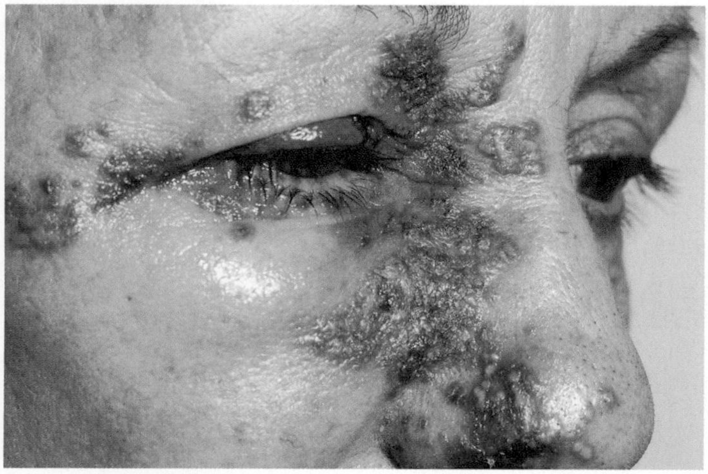

■ **Fig. 1.86** Erythematous macules, which rapidly develop into vesicles.

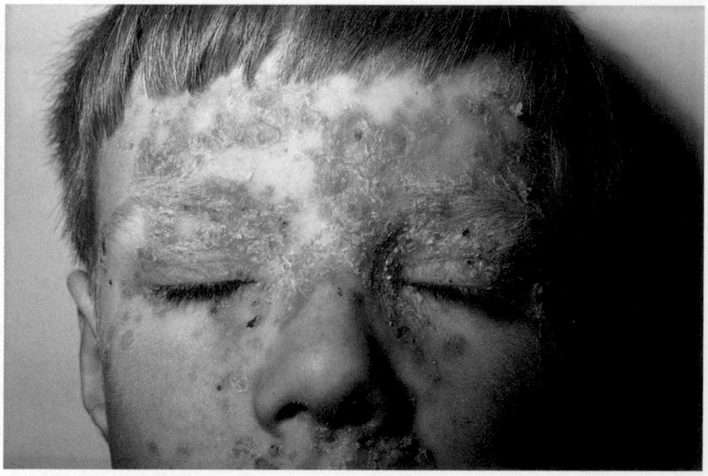

■ **Fig. 1.87** Golden-yellow crusting following rupture of vesicles.

Erysipelas (St Anthony fire)

Erysipelas is an acute subcutaneous spreading cellulitis caused by *Streptococcus pyogenes* through a site of minor skin trauma.

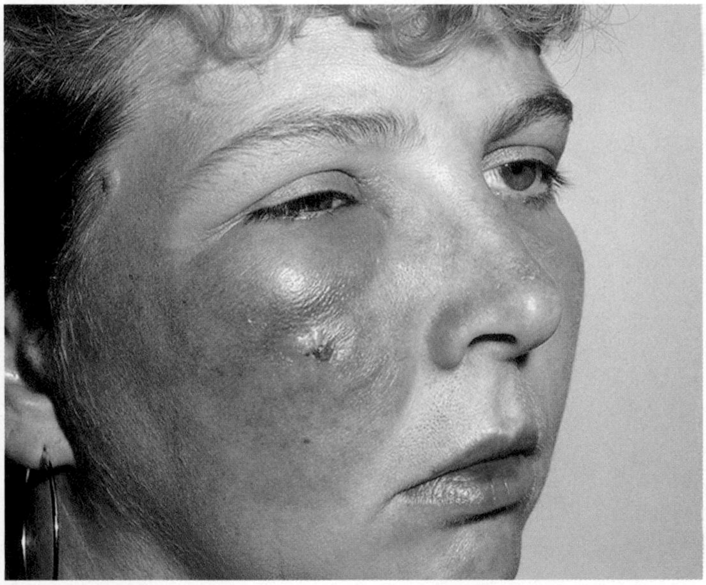

Fig. 1.88 An expanding, well-defined, indurated, erythematous subcutaneous plaque.

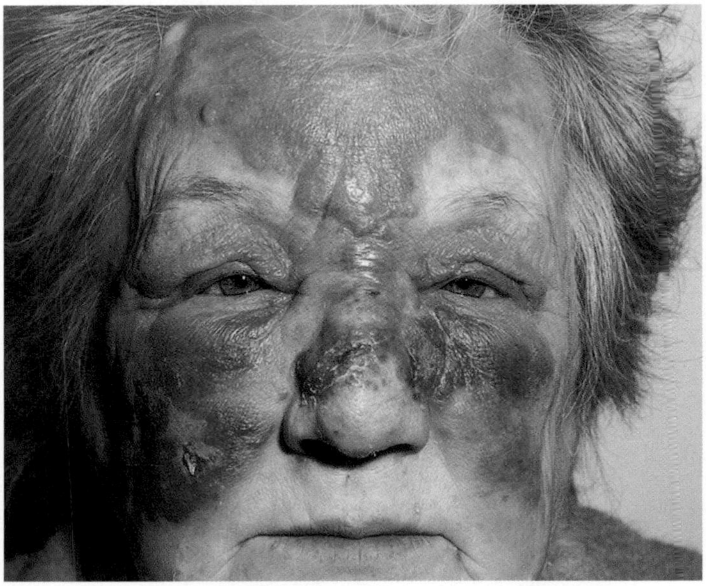

Fig 1.89 A butterfly configuration is characteristic.

Necrotising fasciitis

Necrotising fasciitis a rapidly progressive necrosis, initially involving subcutaneous soft tissues and later the skin, which is usually caused by *Streptococcus pyogenes* and occasionally *Staphylococcus aureus.*

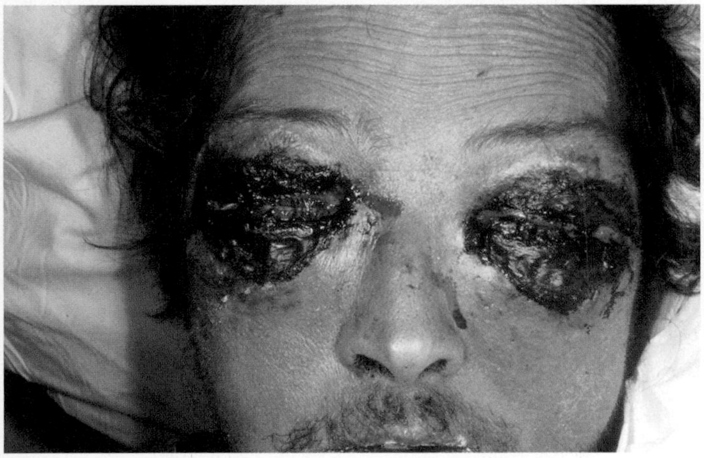

Fig. 1.90 Black discoloration of skin due to gangrene secondary to underlying thrombosis.

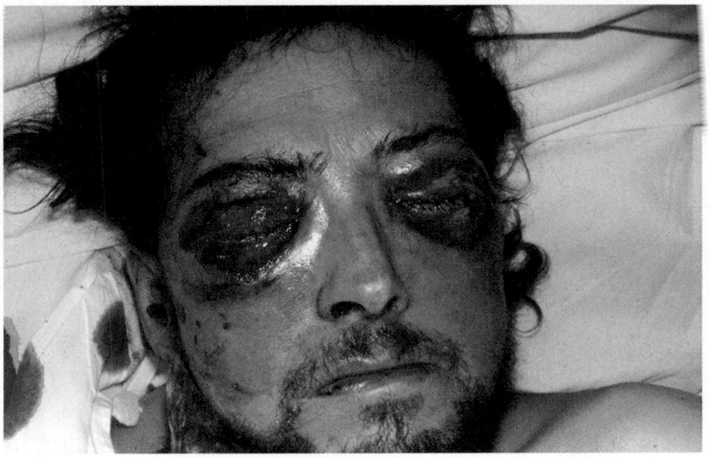

Fig. 1.91 Appearance following debridement.

CYSTS

Meibomian cyst (chalazion)

A chalazion is a chronic, sterile, lipogranulomatous inflammatory lesion caused by blockage of meibomian gland orifices and stagnation of sebaceous secretions.

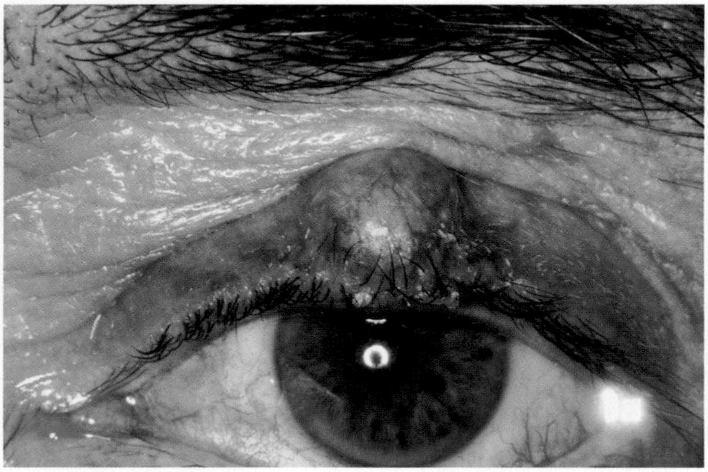

Fig. 1.92 A non-tender, roundish, firm lesion within the tarsal plate.

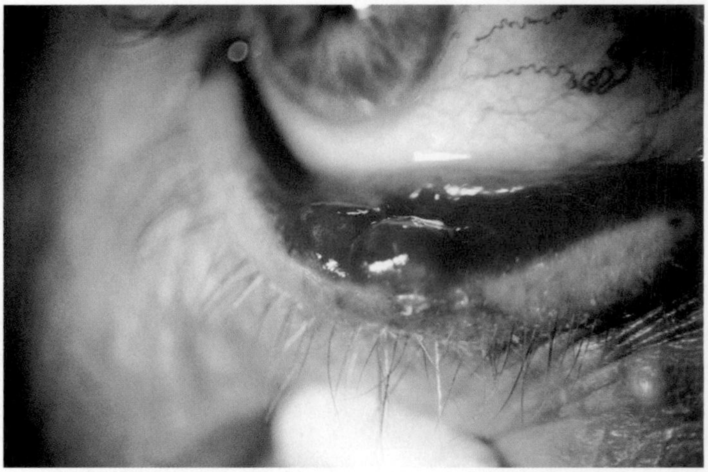

Fig. 1.93 Eversion of the eyelid may show a polypoidal granuloma if the lesion has ruptured through the tarsal plate.

Cyst of Moll (apocrine hidrocystoma)

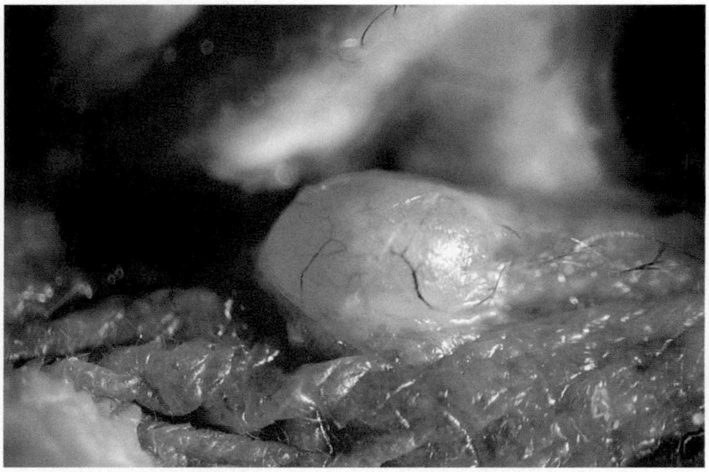

Fig. 1.94 A small, round, non-tender, fluid-filled lesion on the anterior lid margin.

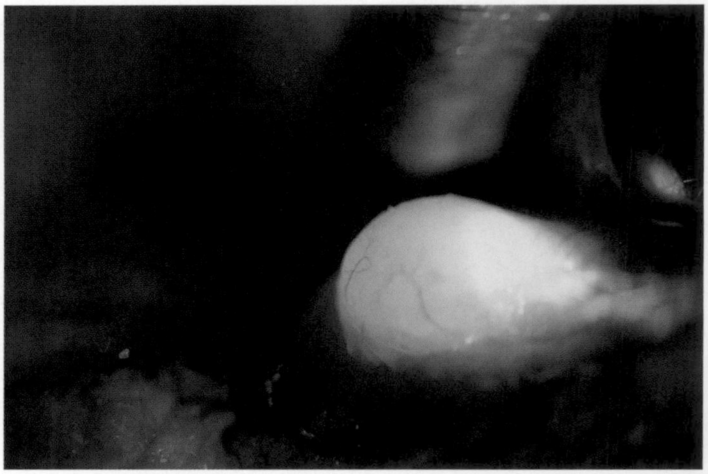

Fig. 1.95 The cyst is translucent.

Eccrine sweat gland hidrocystoma

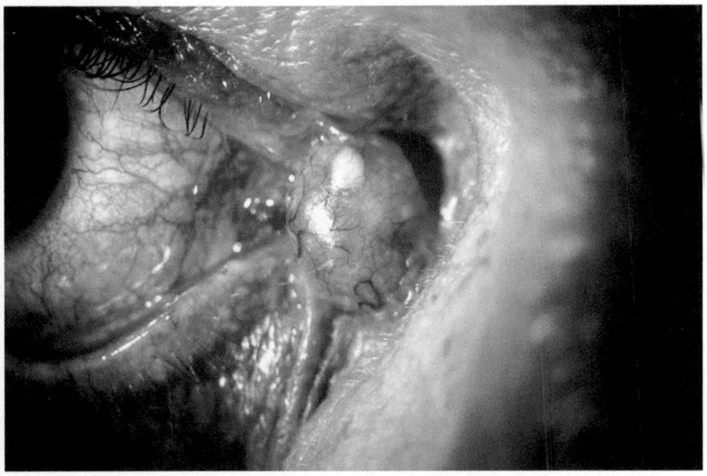

Fig. 1.96 This is similar in appearance to a cyst of Moll except that it is not confined to the lid margin.

Cyst of Zeis

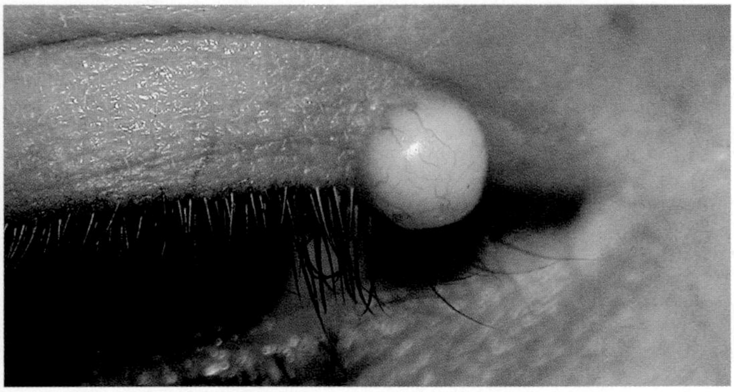

Fig. 1.97 A small round, non-tender lesion on the lid margin that contains sebaceous secretions and is therefore not translucent. (Courtesy of A. Pearson.)

Sebaceous cyst

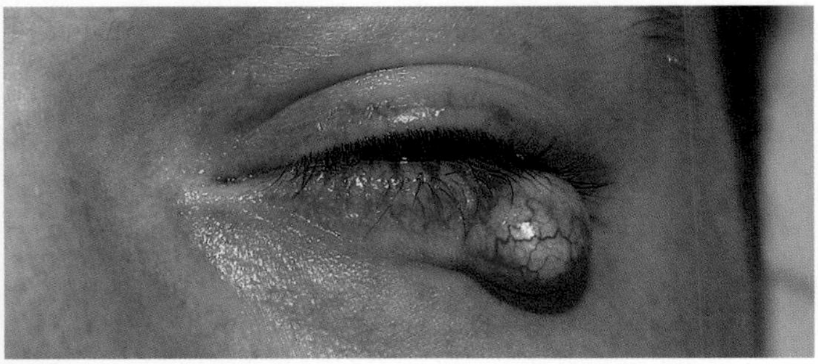

Fig.1.98 A central punctum with retained cheesy secretions. (Courtesy of A. Pearson.)

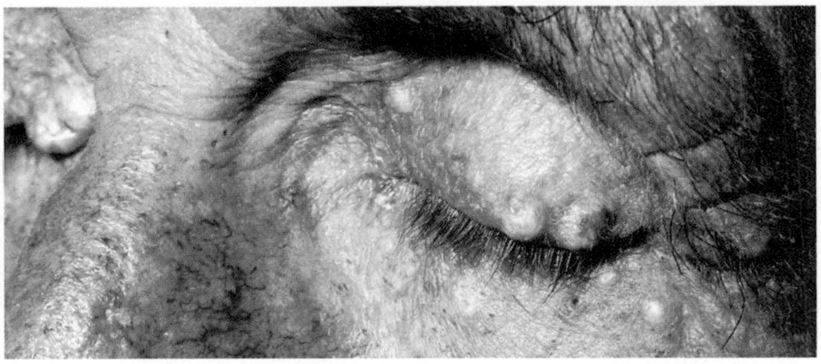

Fig. 1.99 Multiple small sebaceous cysts.

Epidermal inclusion cyst

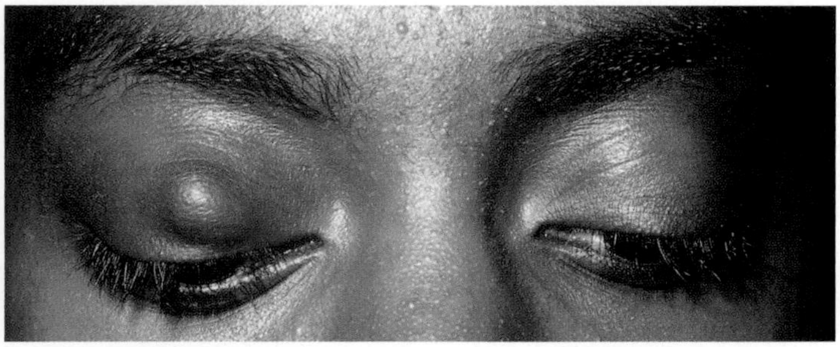

Fig. 1.100 A slowly growing, firm subepithelial nodule, which is frequently solitary and often antedated by trauma or surgery. (Courtesy of S. Ford and R. Marsh.)

Comedo (blackhead)

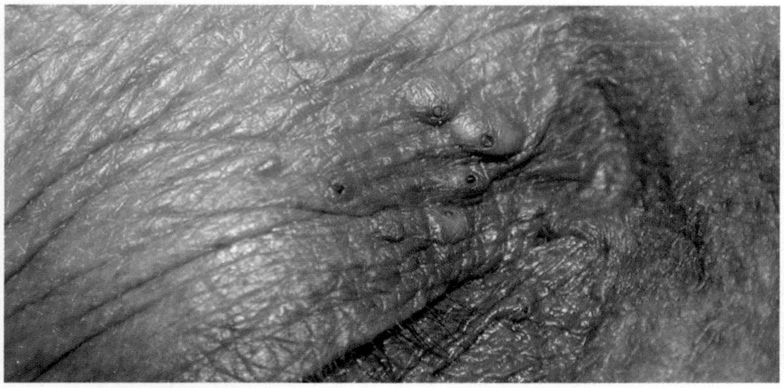

Fig. 1.101 These typically occur in patients with acne vulgaris and are caused by occlusion of sebaceous glands. (Courtesy of A. Pearson.)

Milia

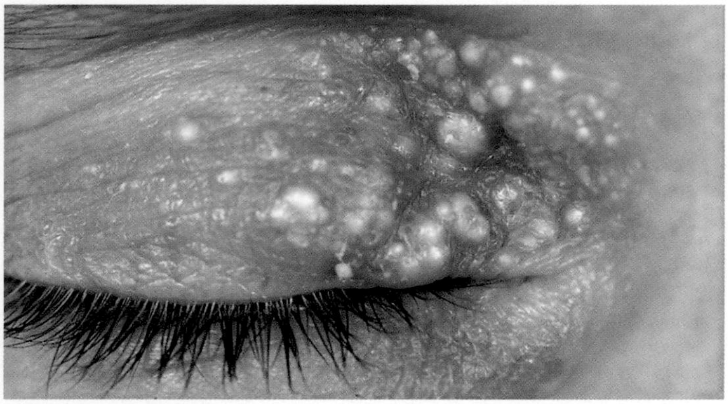

Fig. 1.102 Crops of tiny, white, round, superficial cysts derived from hair follicles or sebaceous glands.

BENIGN TUMOURS

Viral wart (squamous cell papilloma)

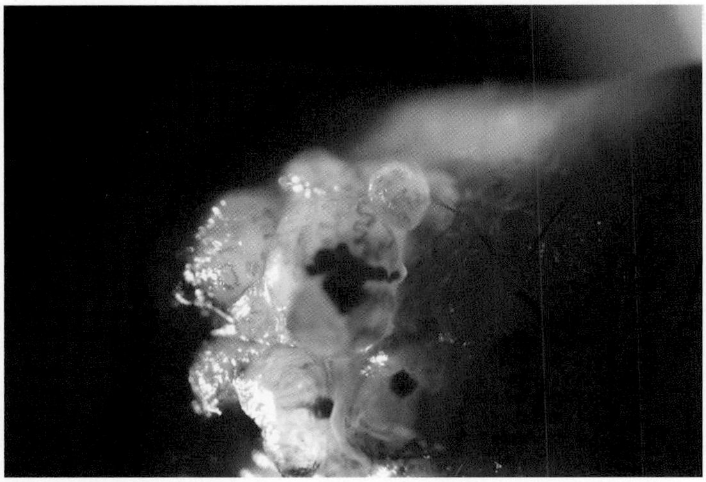

■ **Fig. 1.103** A pedunculated papilloma with a characteristic raspberry-like surface.

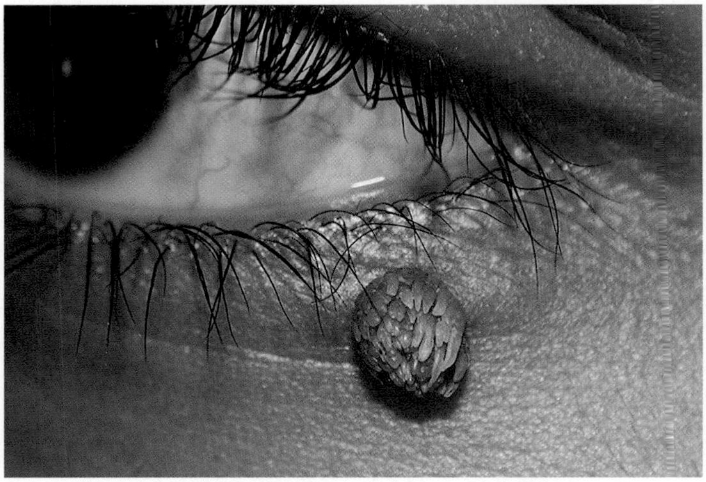

■ **Fig. 1.104** A small, pigmented pedunculated papilloma. (Courtesy of A. Pearson.)

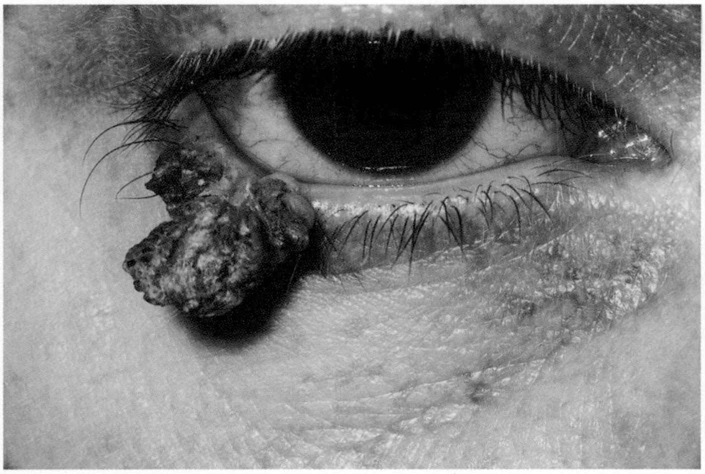

■ **Fig. 1.105** A very large pigmented papilloma.

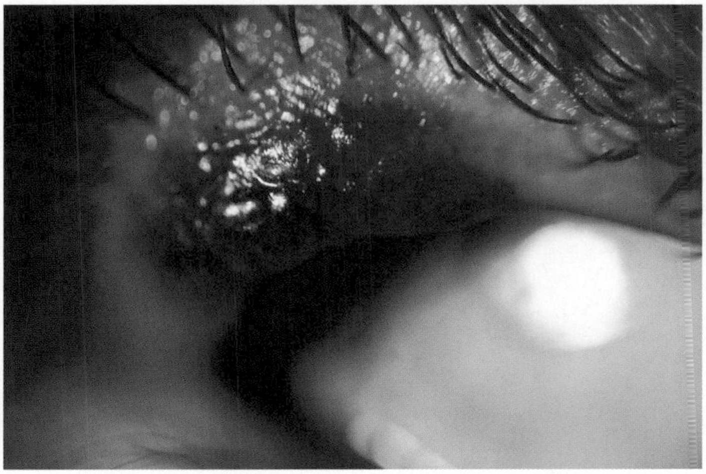

■ **Fig. 1.106** A broad-based (sessile) papilloma.

Seborrhoeic keratosis (basal cell papilloma)

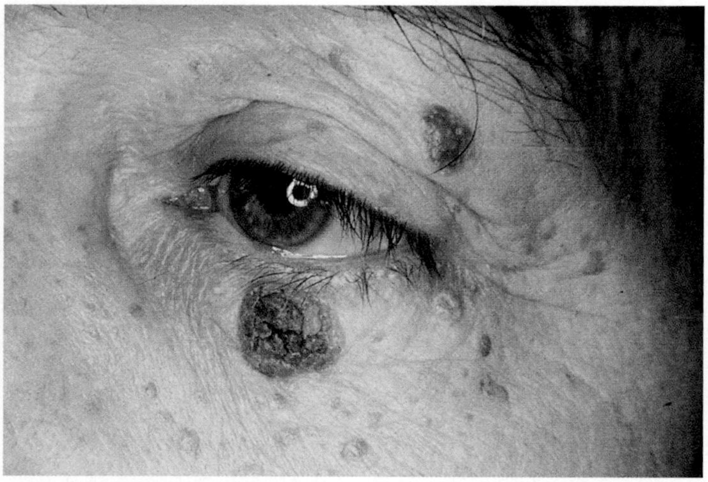

■ **Fig. 1.107** A discrete, greasy, brown, flat, round or oval lesion with a friable verrucous surface and a 'stuck-on' appearance.

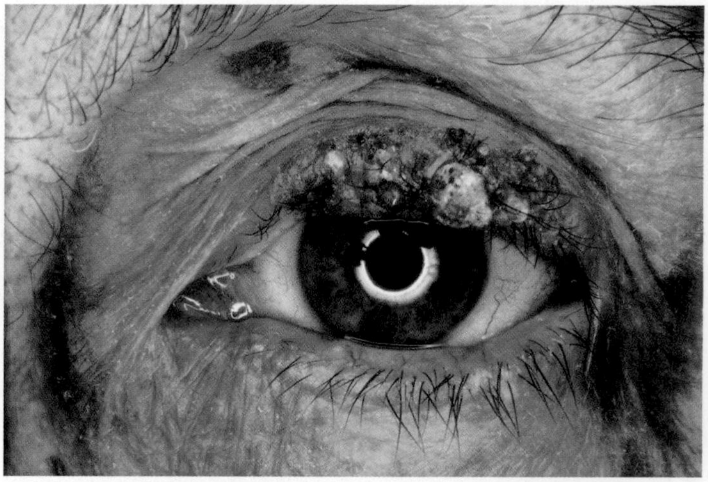

■ **Fig. 1.108** Peduncular seborrhoeic keratosis is less common.

Dermatosis papulosa nigra

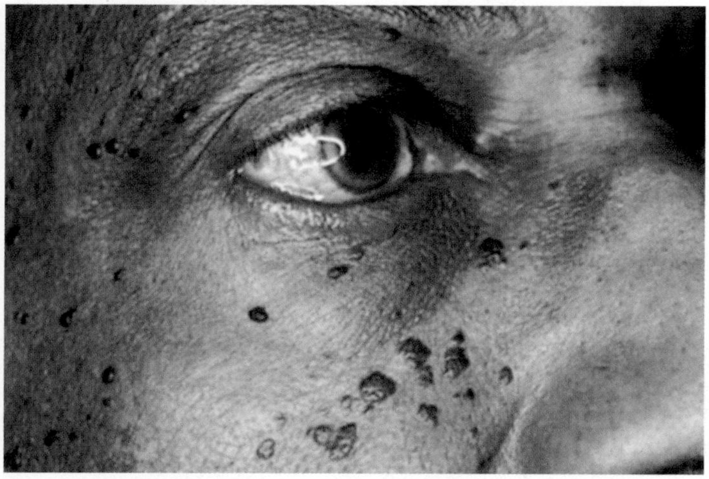

■ **Fig. 1.109** A variant of seborrhoeic keratosis characterised by pigmented lesions in a black person. (Courtesy of D. M. Albert and F. A. Jakobiec.)

Inverted follicular keratosis

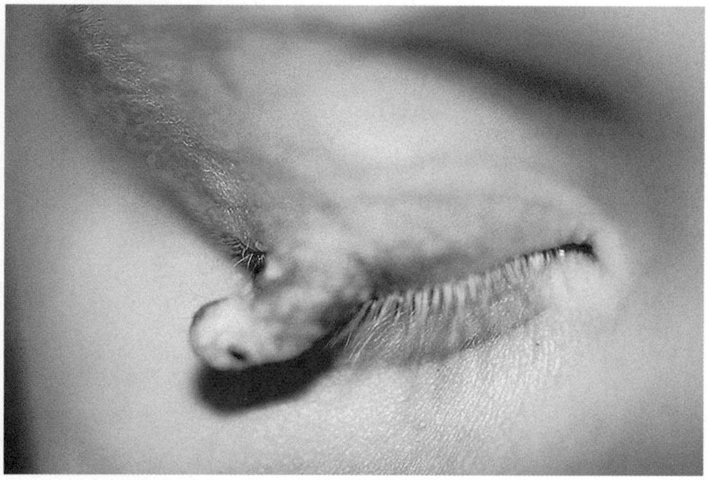

■ **Fig. 1.110** A small, fast-growing wart-like or nodular lesion which shows the same histological characteristics as basal cell papilloma.

Syringoma

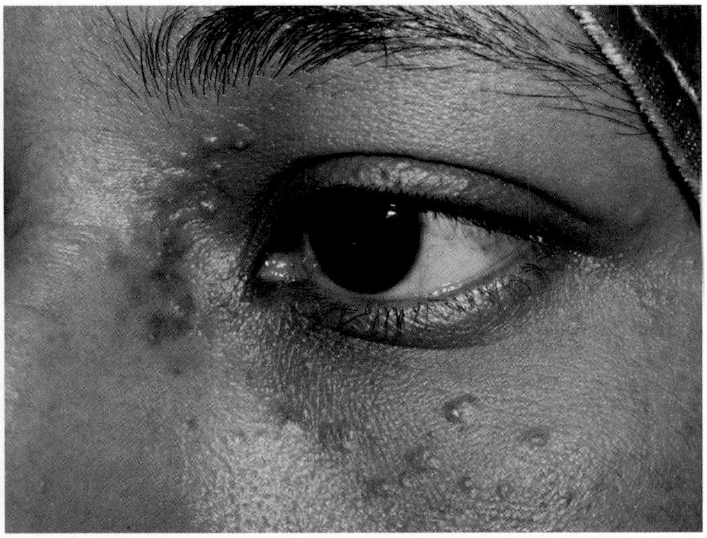

■ **Fig. 1.111** A common eccrine sweat gland tumour consisting of small papules.

Pyogenic granuloma

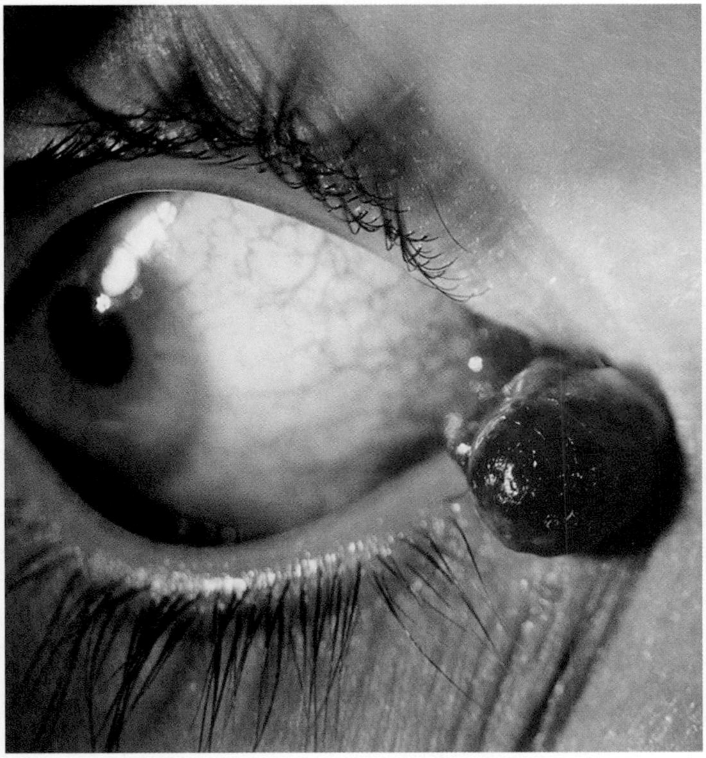

■ **Fig. 1.112** A fast-growing, vascularised, pinkish mass of granulomatous tissue usually antedated by surgery, trauma or infection.

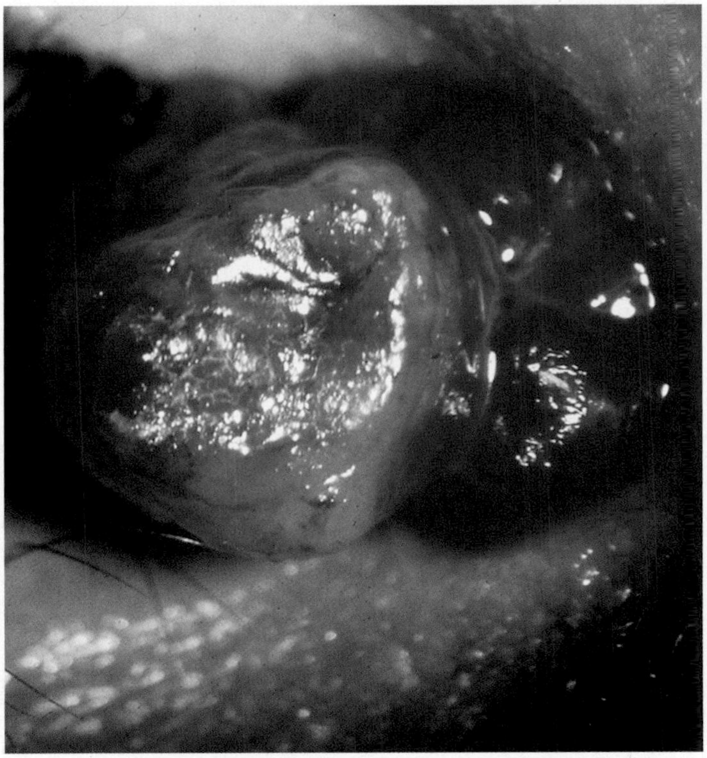

■ **Fig. 1.113** A large pyogenic granuloma. (Courtesy of S. Ford and R. Marsh.)

Acquired melanocytic naevus

Dermal

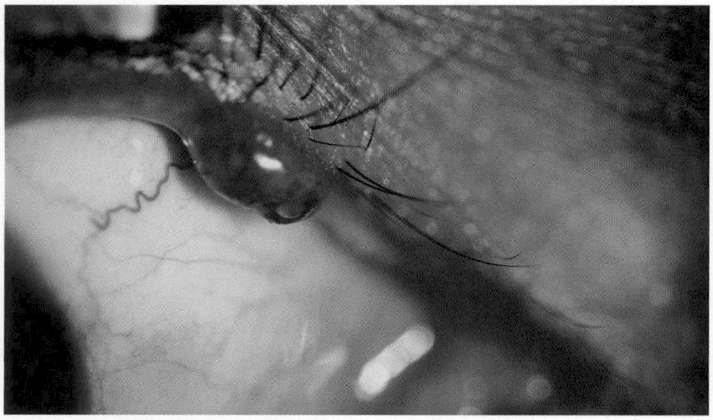

Fig. 1.114 A brown-black, elevated lesion often with a papillomatous configuration.

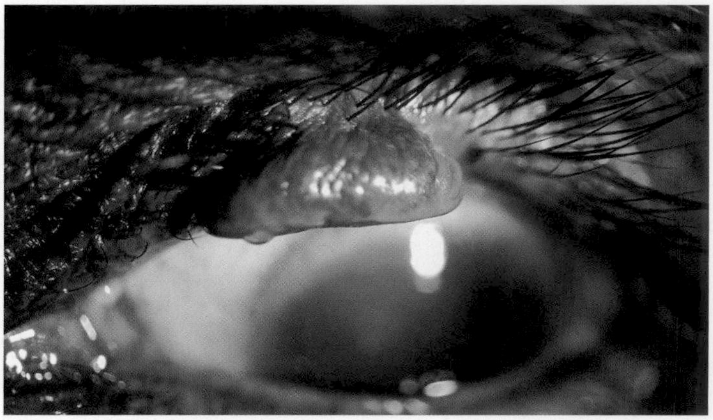

Fig. 1.115 A large, pigmented dermal naevus.

Junctional

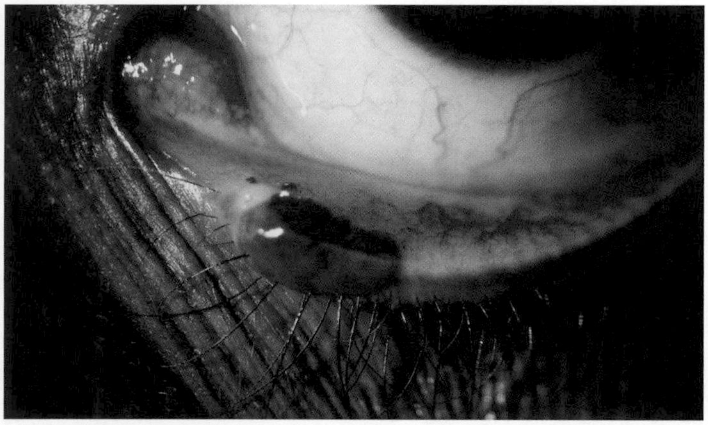

Fig. 1.116 Usually flat, well-circumscribed lesion which is uniformly brown in colour.

Compound

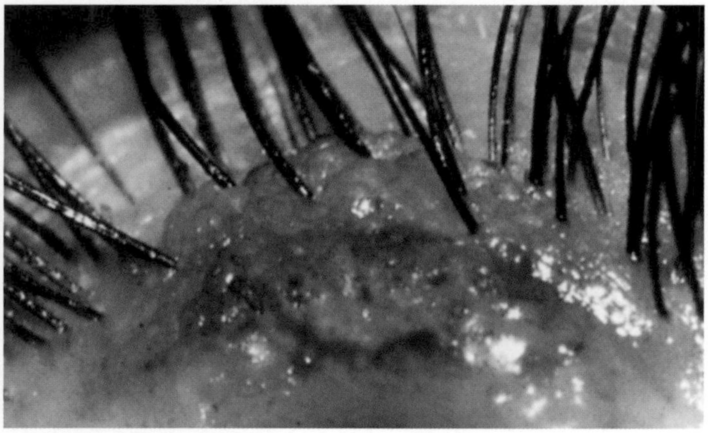

Fig. 1.117 This has both dermal and junctional components and is usually brown.

Unusual naevi

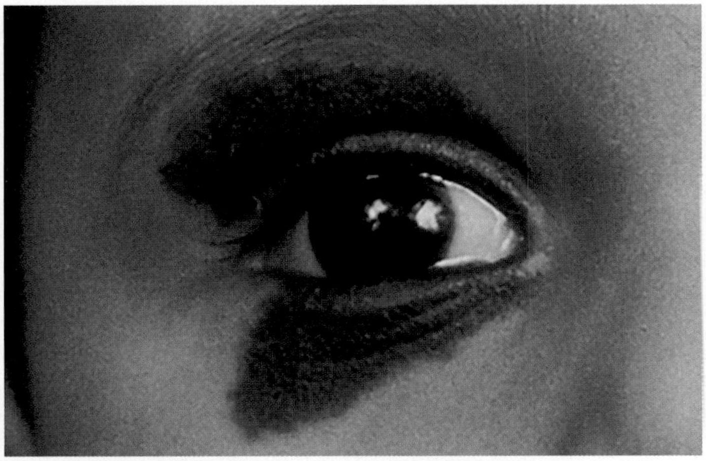

■ **Fig. 1.118** Congenital 'kissing' naevus. (Courtesy of N. Raik.)

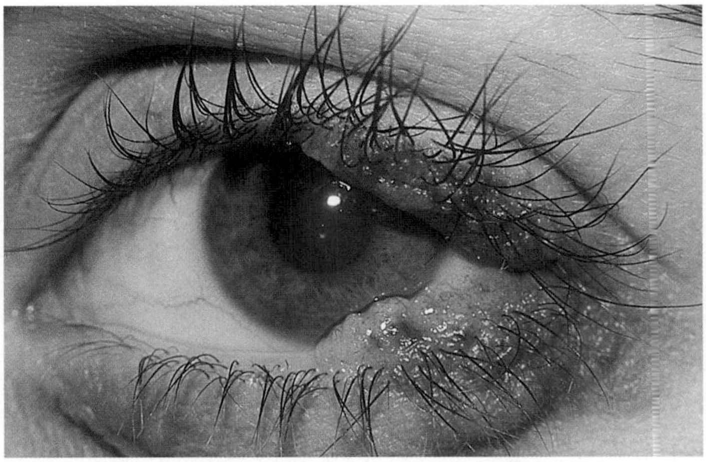

■ **Fig. 1.119** Acquired papillomatous 'kissing' hairy naevus. (Courtesy of S. Webber.)

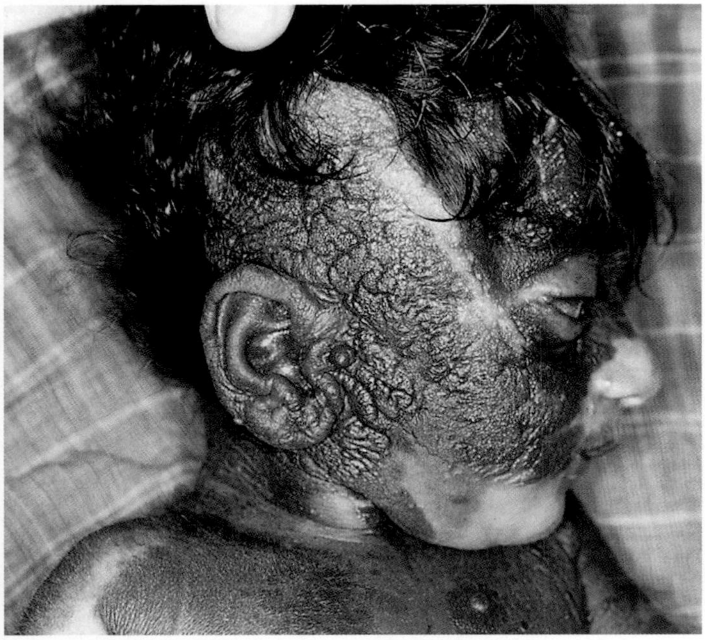

■ **Fig. 1.120** Giant naevus. (Courtesy of U. Raina.)

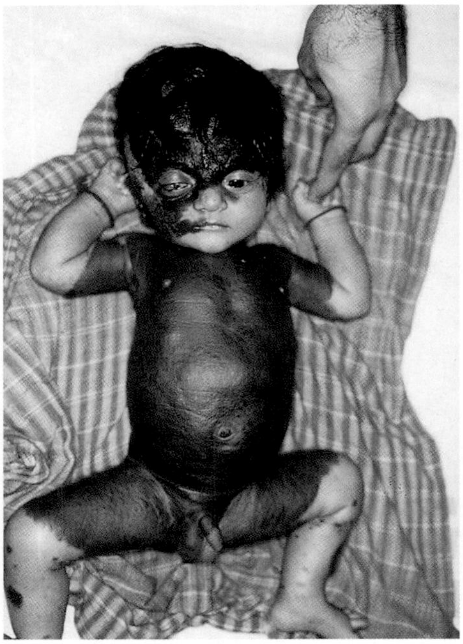

■ **Fig. 1.121** Giant naevus. (Courtesy of U. Raina.)

Strawberry naevus (capillary haemangioma)

Strawberry naevus presents shortly after birth.

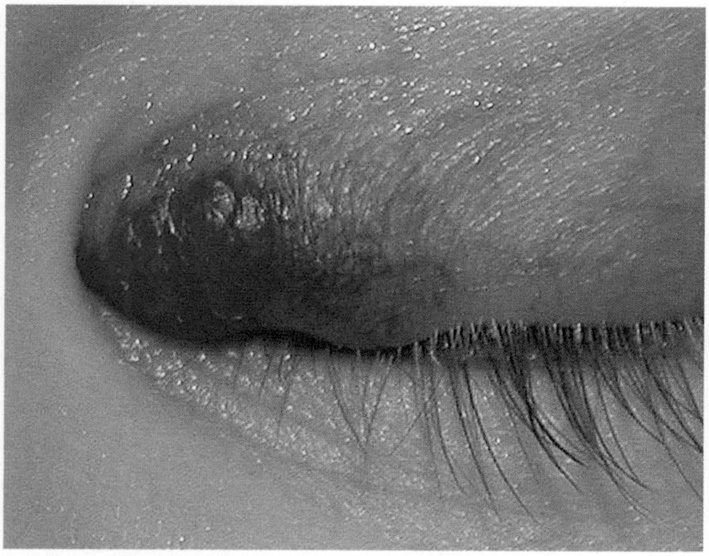

Fig. 1.122 A raised, red nodule, often on the upper lid which blanches with pressure and may swell on crying. (Courtesy of A. Pearson.)

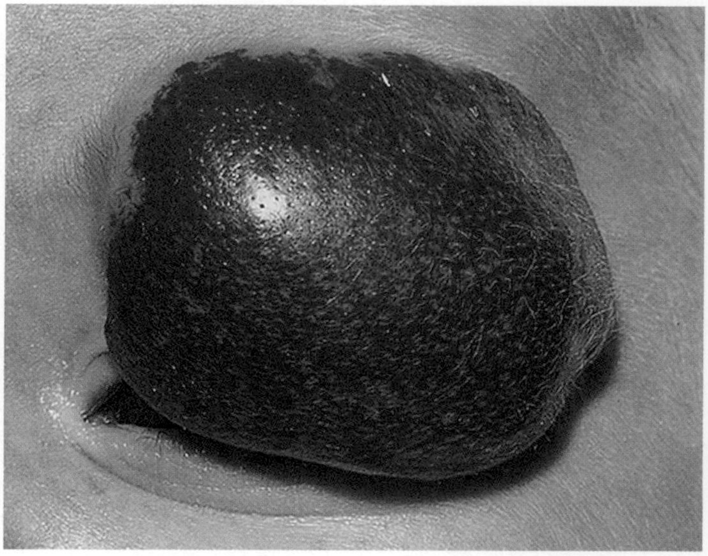

Fig. 1.123 A large tumour causing ptosis. (Courtesy of K. Nischal.)

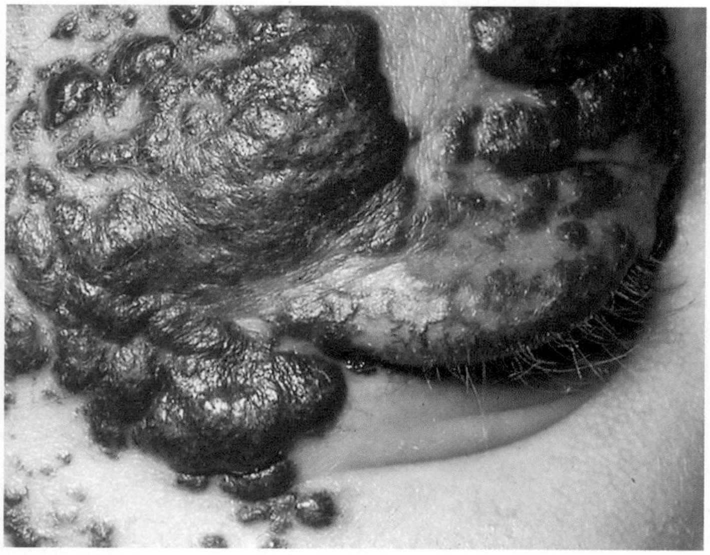

Fig. 1.124 Adjacent facial skin is occasionally involved.

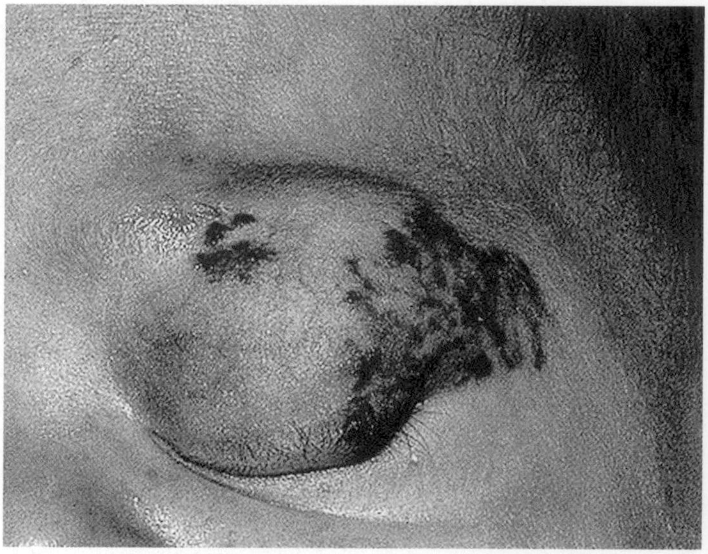

Fig. 1.125 A small lid haemangioma associated with an extensive orbital component. (Courtesy of M. Szreter.)

Systemic associations

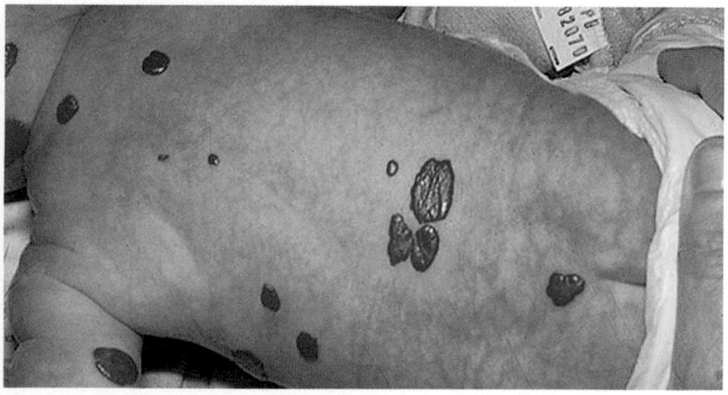

Fig. 1.126 Patients with extensive haemangiomas may have: (1) Kasabach–Merritt syndrome, which is characterised by thrombocytopenia, anaemia and low levels of coagulant factors; (2) Maffucci syndrome, which is characterised by enchondromata of hands, feet and long bones as well as bowing of long bones; (3) high-output heart failure.

Port-wine stain (naevus flammeus)

Port-wine stain is a rare congenital, subcutaneous cavernous haemangioma that most frequently occurs on the face. The lesion is usually unilateral and segmental.

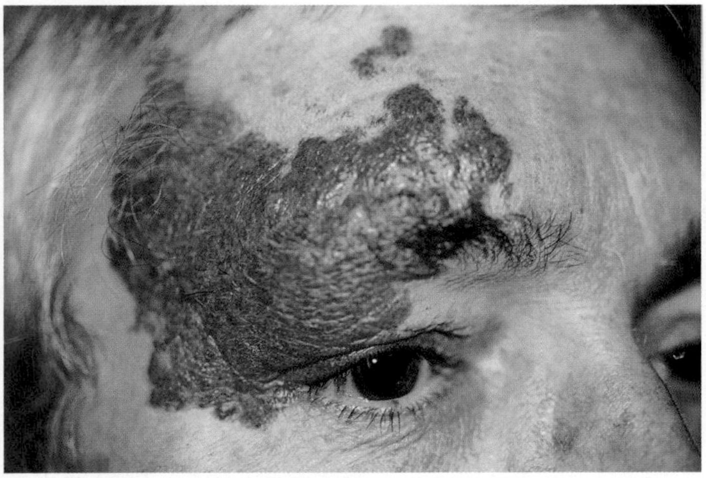

Fig. 1.127 A sharply demarcated, soft, pink patch that does not blanch with pressure.

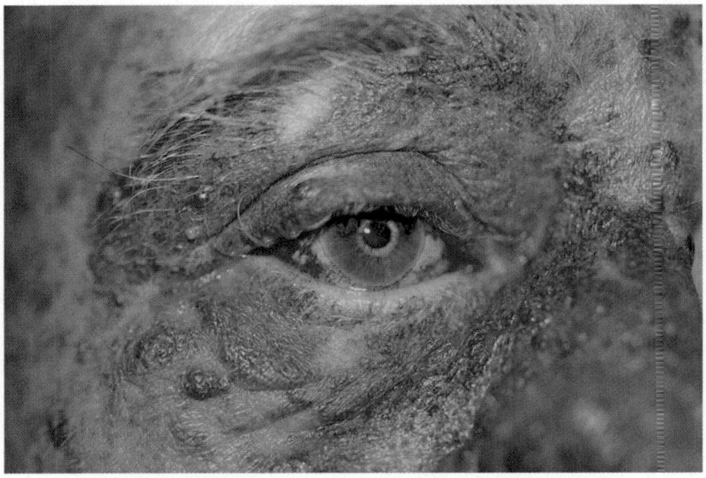

Fig. 1.128 With age the involved area may become hypertrophied, coarse and nodular.

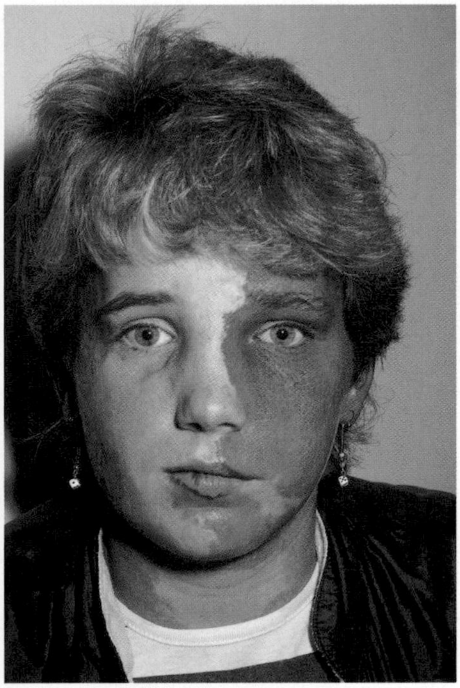

Fig. 1.129 Extensive port-wine stain with mild hypertrophy.

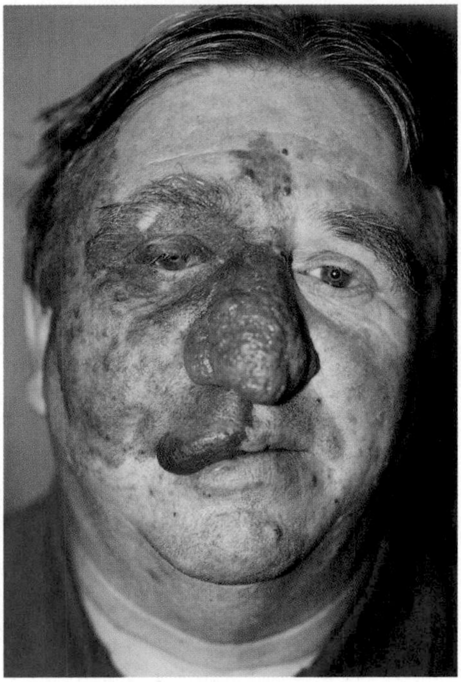

Fig. 1.130 Extensive port-wine stain with severe hypertrophy.

Systemic associations

Sturge–Weber syndrome

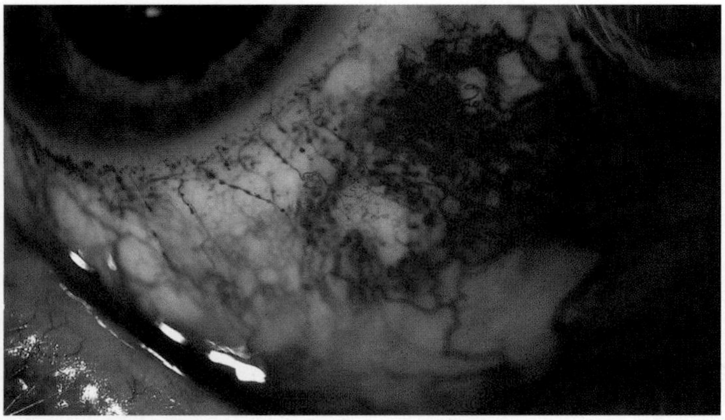

Fig. 1.131 Episcleral haemangioma ipsilateral to the port-wine stain.

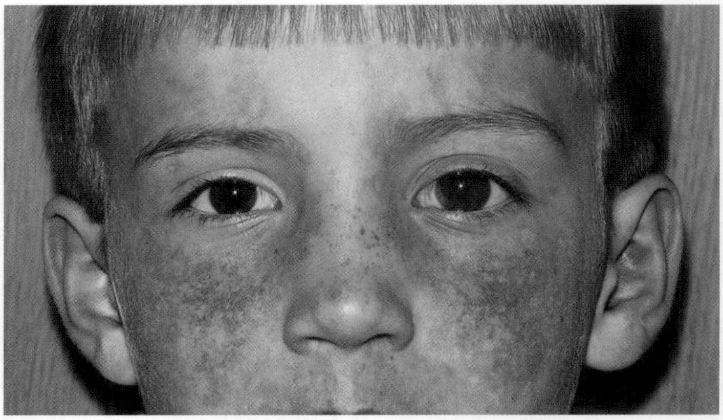

Fig. 1.132 Glaucoma, which may result in buphthalmos. (Courtesy of M. Szreter.)

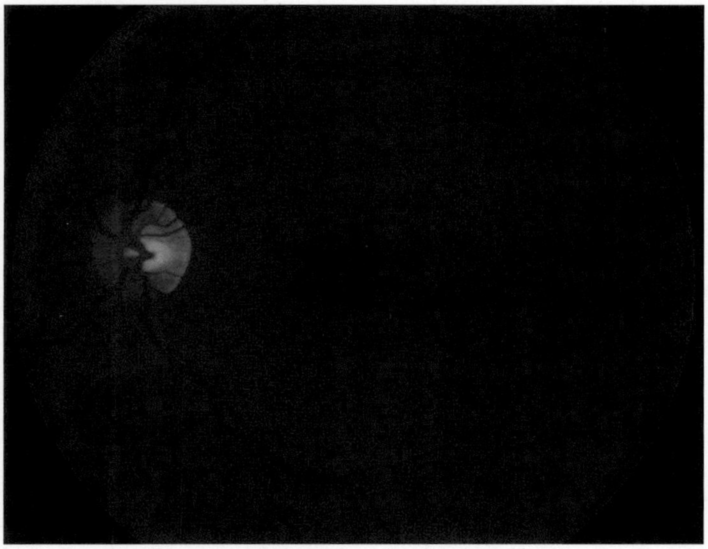

Fig. 1.133 Diffuse choroidal haemangioma.

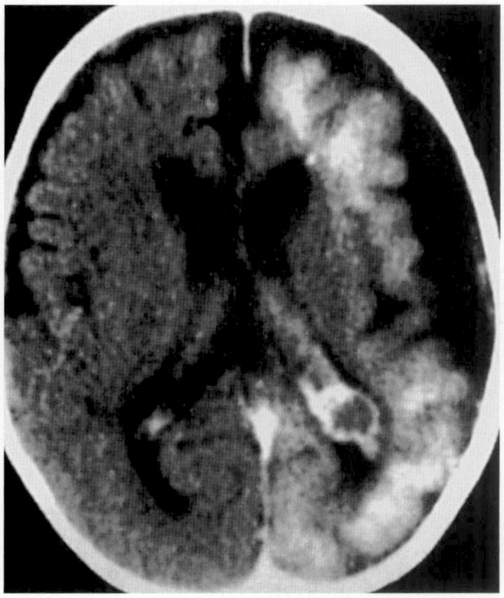

Fig. 1.134 Ipsilateral haemangioma of the pia mater and underlying cortex. (Courtesy of C. D. Forbes and W. F. Jackson.)

Klippel–Trenaunay–Weber syndrome

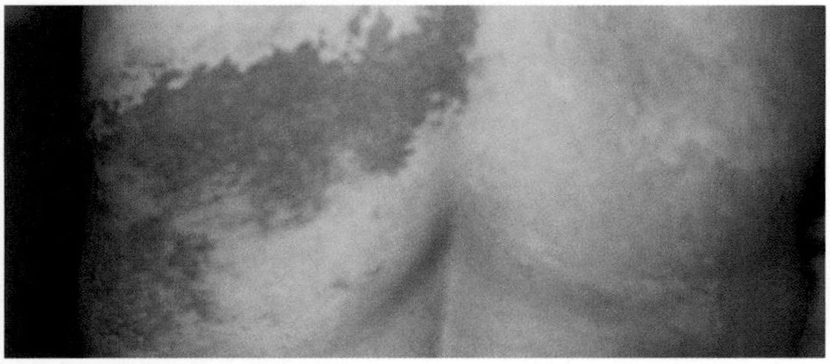

Fig. 1.135 Cutaneous haemangiomas.

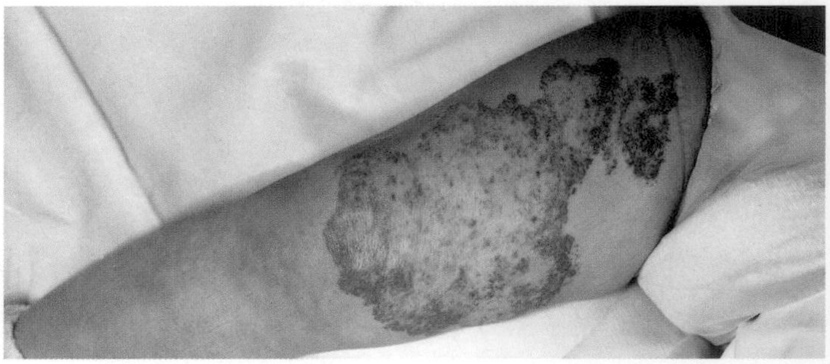

Fig. 1.136 Cutaneous haemangiomas, associated with limb hypertrophy.

Plexiform neurofibroma

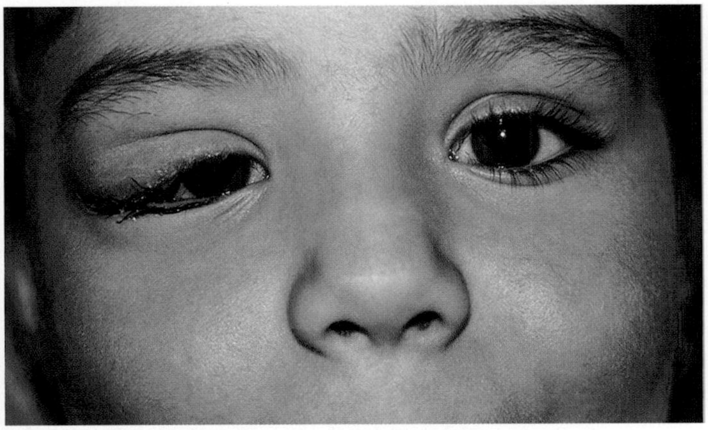

■ **Fig. 1.137** Thickening of the eyelid associated with a mechanical ptosis and a characteristic S-shaped deformity. (Courtesy of K. Nischal.)

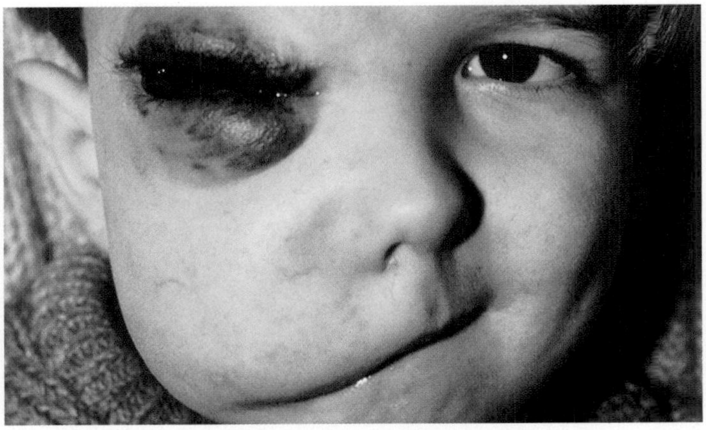

■ **Fig. 1.138** Eyelid plexiform neurofibroma associated with ipsilateral facial soft tissue hypertrophy. (Courtesy of A. Pearson.)

Systemic association

Neurofibromatosis-1

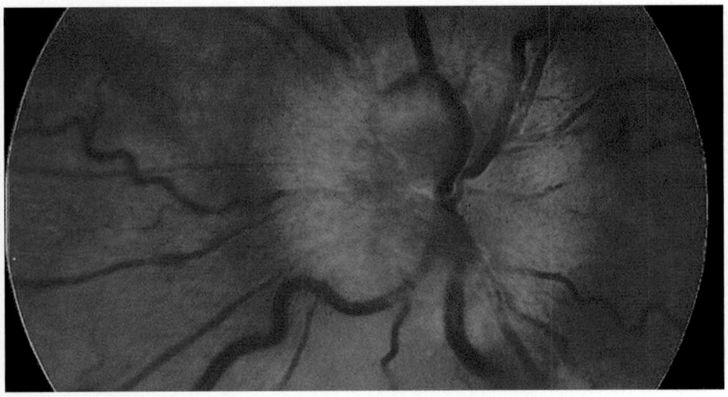

■ **Fig. 1.139** Disc oedema due to optic nerve glioma.

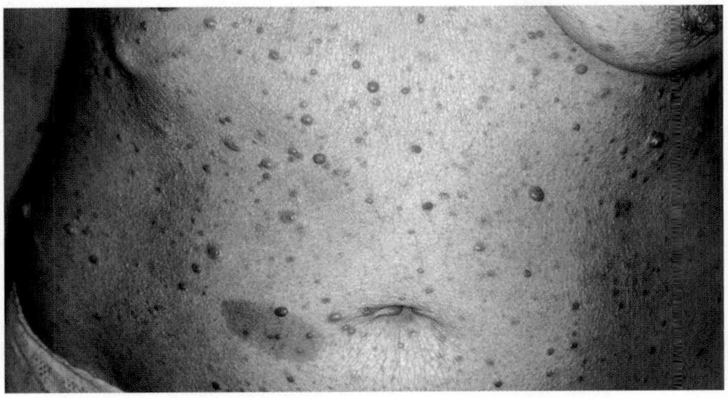

■ **Fig. 1.140** Fibroma mollusca and café-au-lait spots.

PREMALIGNANT LESIONS

Actinic (solar) keratosis

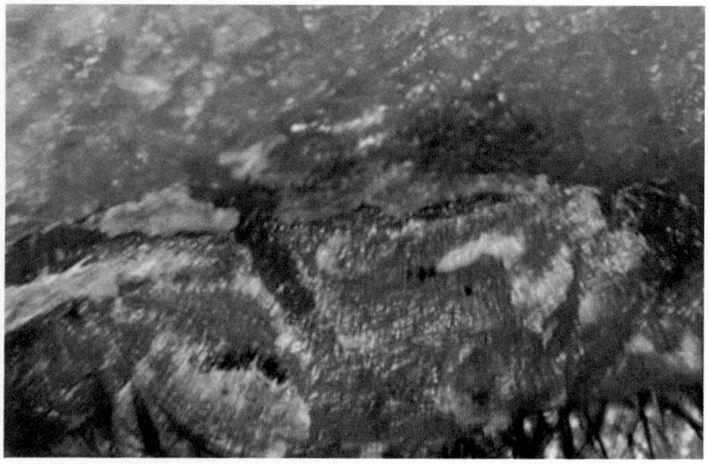

Fig. 1.141 A flat, scaly, hyperkeratotic lesion that occasionally precedes the development of basal cell or squamous cell carcinoma.

Bowen disease (intraepidermal carcinoma-in-situ)

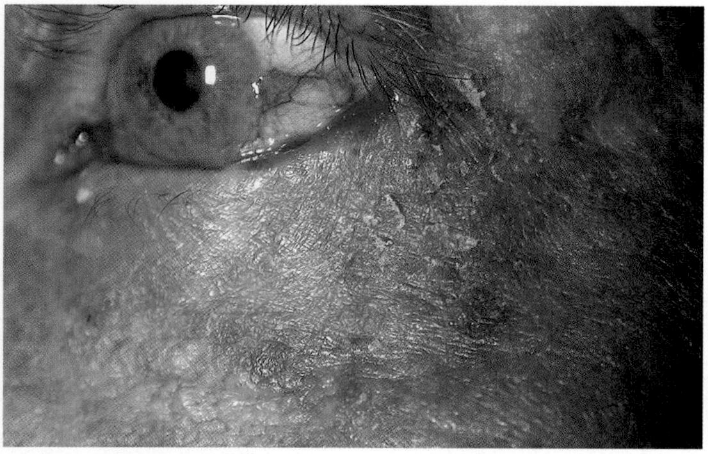

Fig. 1.142 A red scaling lesion that may be mistaken for solar keratosis or a patch of psoriasis. (Courtesy of D. Selva.)

Lentigo maligna (Hutchinson freckle)

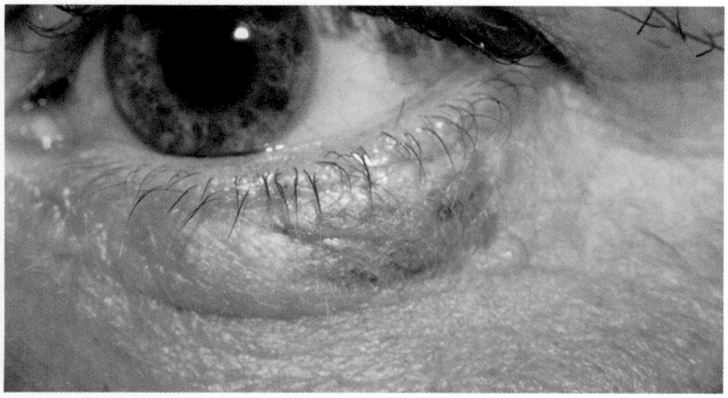

Fig. 1.143 An expanding pigmented macule that typically affects the elderly. Occasionally it antedates the development of melanoma. (Courtesy of S. Webber.)

Cutaneous horn

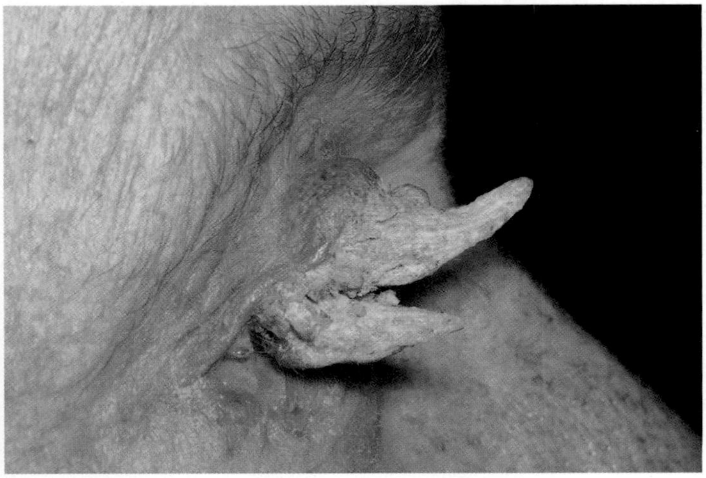

■ **Fig. 1.144** A hyperkeratotic lesion protruding through the skin. Occasionally a very large horn may be associated with underlying actinic keratosis or squamous cell carcinoma. (Courtesy of S. Ford and R. Marsh.)

Keratoacanthoma

Keratoacanthoma is an uncommon, fast-growing tumour that remains static for 2–3 months and then starts to involute spontaneously. Occasionally the lesion may precede the development of squamous cell carcinoma, particularly in immunosuppressed individuals.

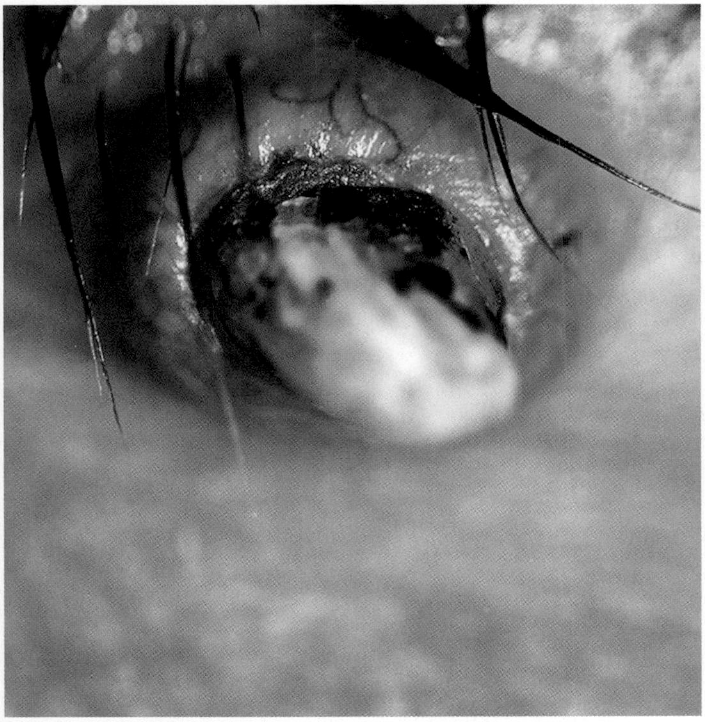

■ **Fig. 1.145** Keratoacanthoma with a keratin-filled crater.

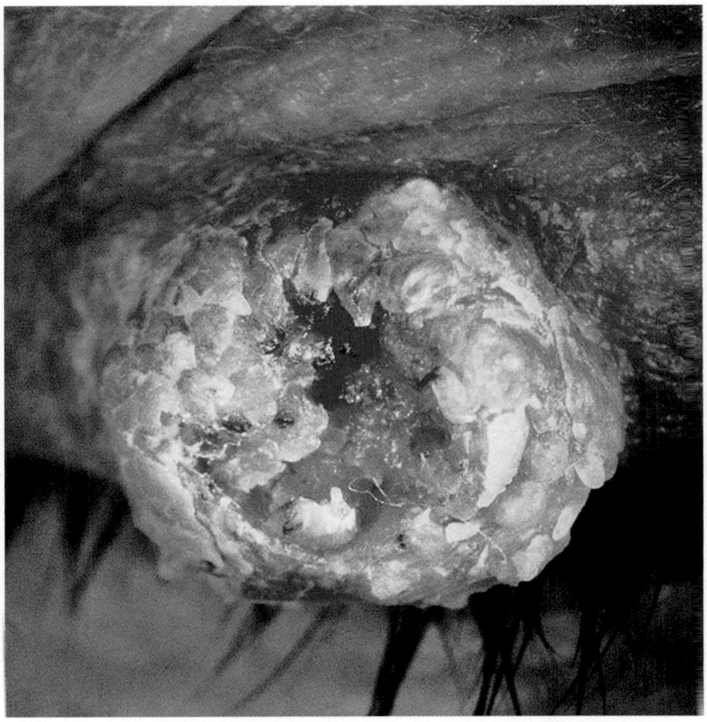

■ **Fig. 1.146** Involuting keratoacanthoma with a large crater.

Xeroderma pigmentosum

Xeroderma pigmentosum is a distressing autosomal dominant condition characterised by skin damage on exposure to natural sunlight. Patients have a great propensity for the development of cutaneous malignancies, which may be multiple. Conjunctival carcinoma may also occur.

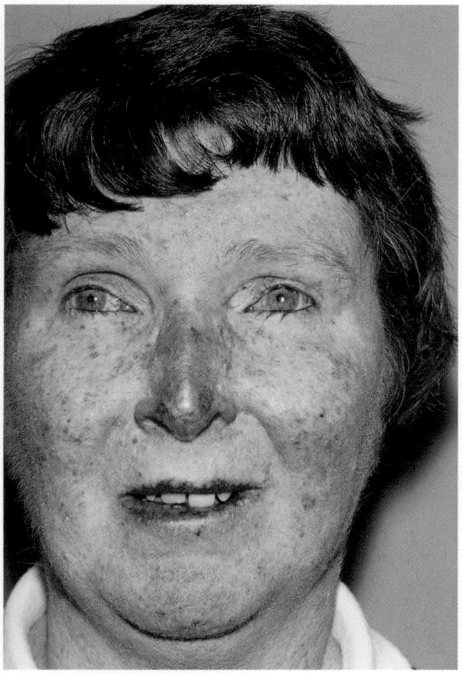

Fig. 1.147 Bird-like facies and mild pigmentary skin changes.

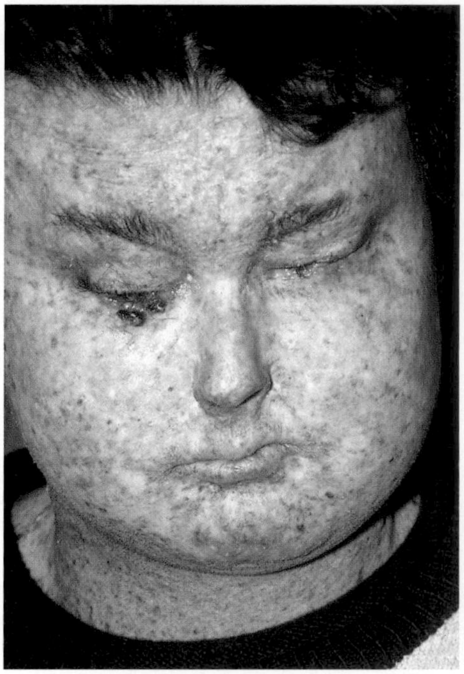

Fig. 1.148 Severe skin changes and two basal cell carcinomas on the eyelid. (Courtesy of S. Webber.)

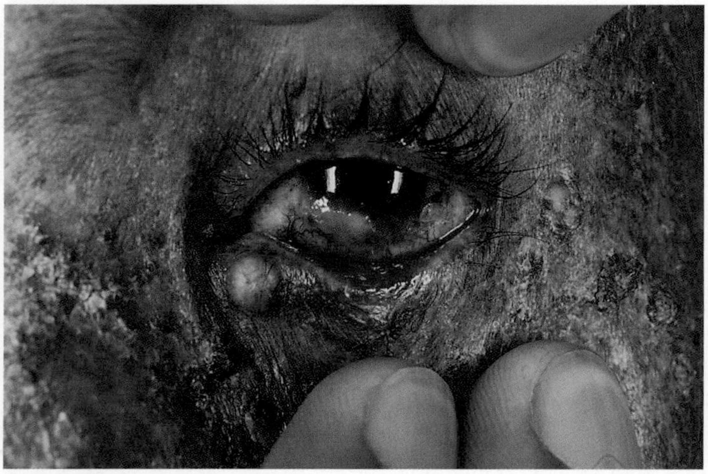

Fig. 1.149 Very severe skin changes, a small basal cell carcinoma of the eyelid and a diffuse conjunctival carcinoma. (Courtesy of U. Raina.)

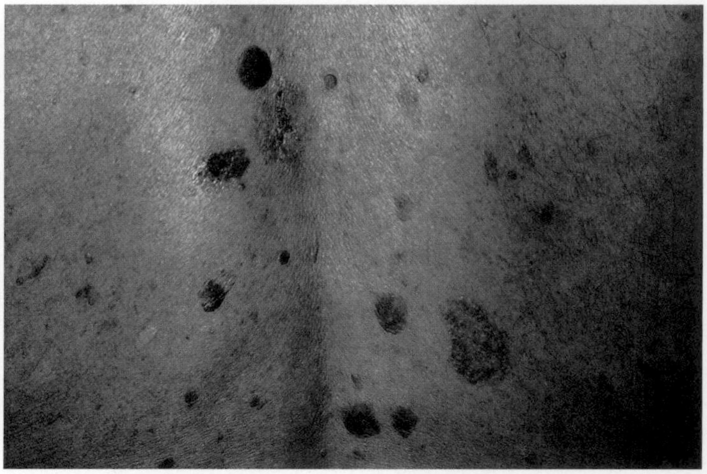

Fig. 1.150 Multiple cutaneous malignancies.

MALIGNANT TUMOURS

Basal cell carcinoma (BCC)

BCC is the most common human malignancy; 90% of tumours occur on the head and neck and, of these, about 10% involve the eyelid.

Nodular

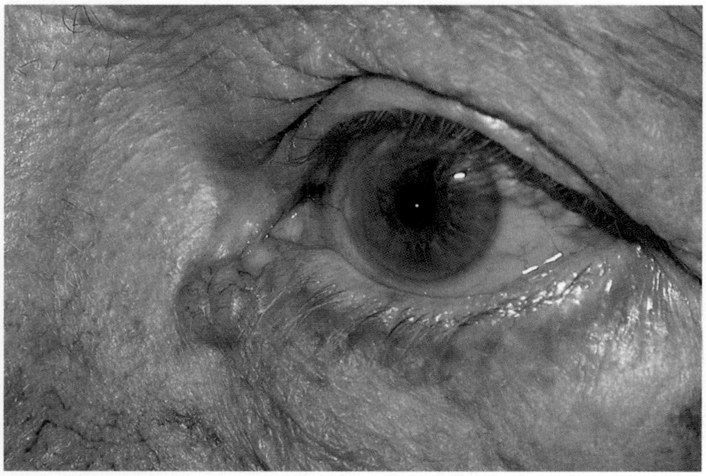

Fig. 1.151 Shiny, firm, pearly nodule with dilated surface vessels. (Courtesy of S. Ford and R. Marsh.)

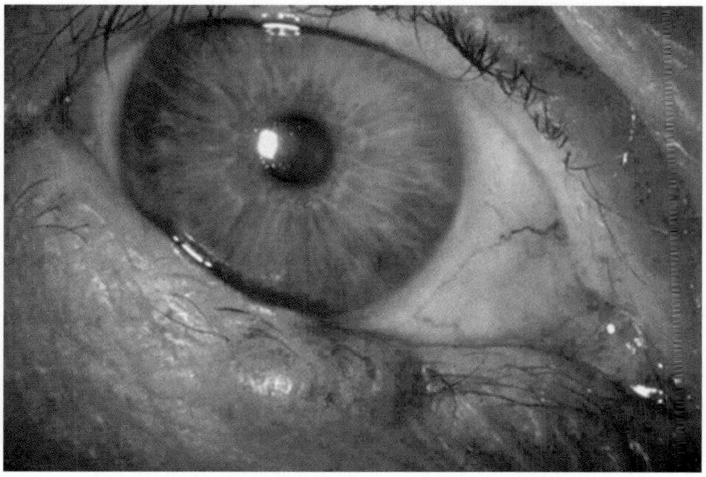

Fig. 1.152 Slightly larger nodular BCC.

Noduloulcerative

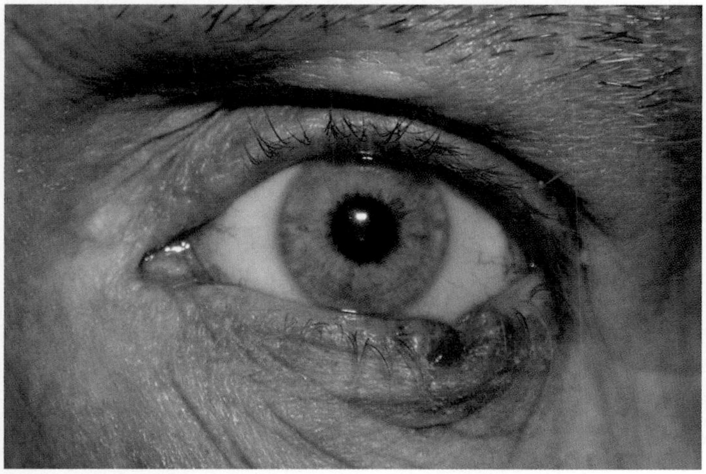

Fig. 1.153 Small nodulo-ulcerative BCC (rodent ulcer).

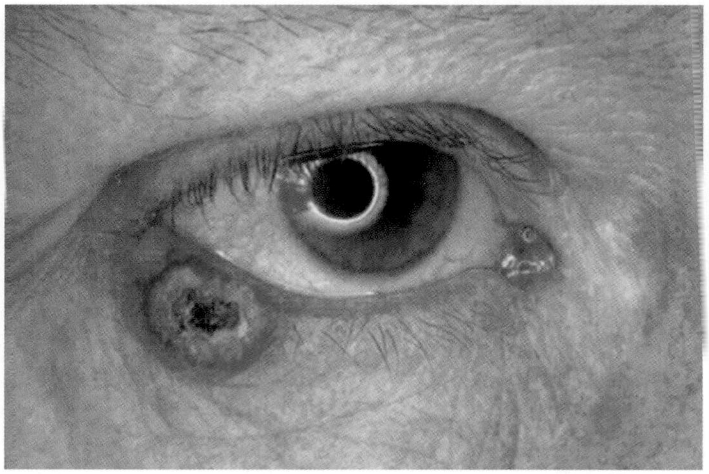

Fig. 1.154 Large rodent ulcer.

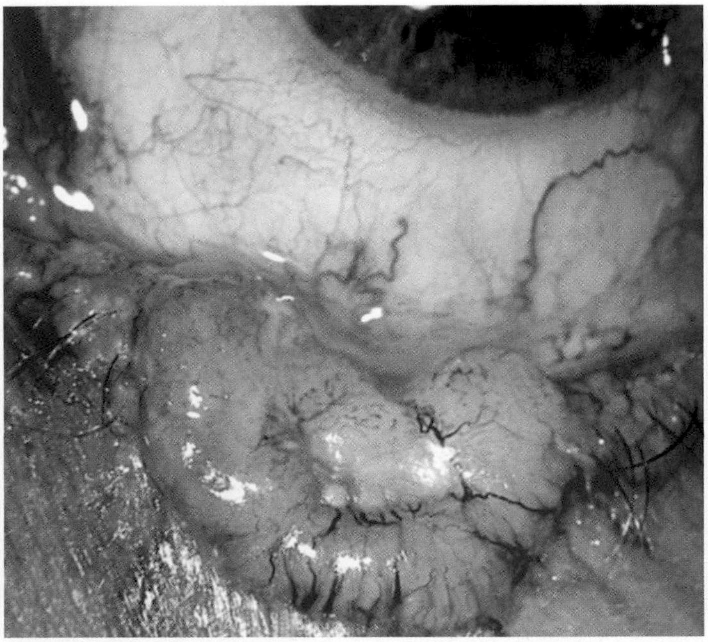

Fig. 1.155 Large rodent ulcer showing the typical raised, rolled edges and dilated surface vessels.

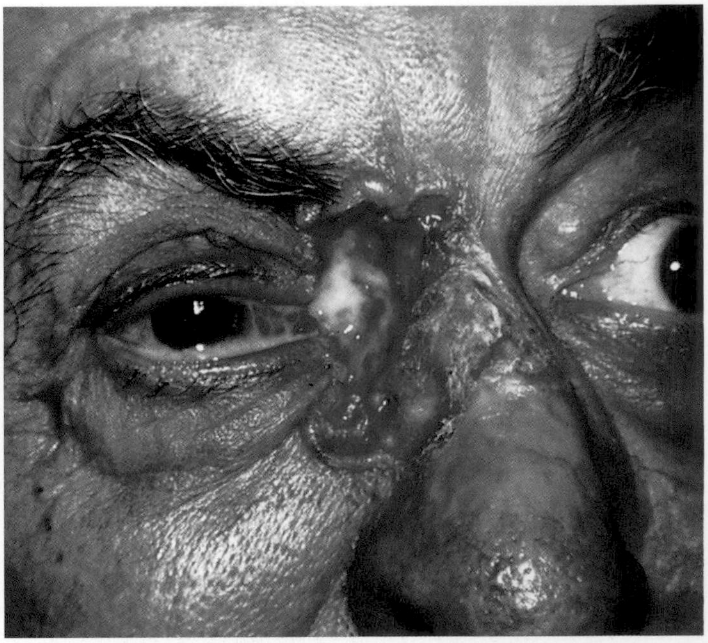

Fig. 1.156 Neglected rodent ulcer invading the lacrimal drainage system.

Sclerosing

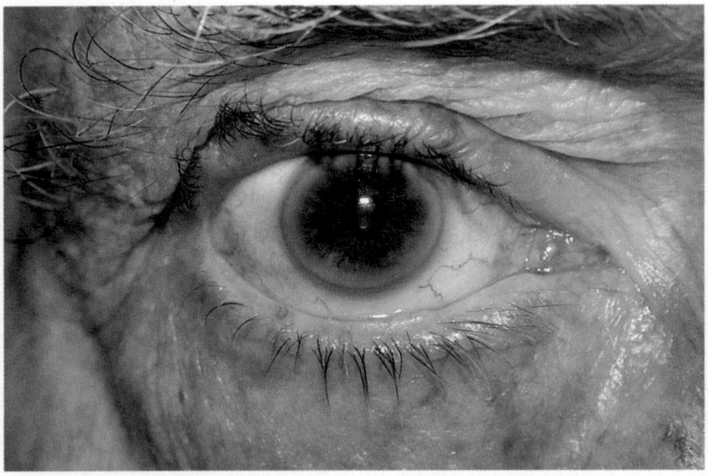

Fig. 1.157 An early sclerosing BCC causing thickening of the eyelid and a small area of madarosis. The tumor infiltrates laterally beneath the epidermis and may be more extensive than is clinically apparent. (Courtesy of A. Pearson.)

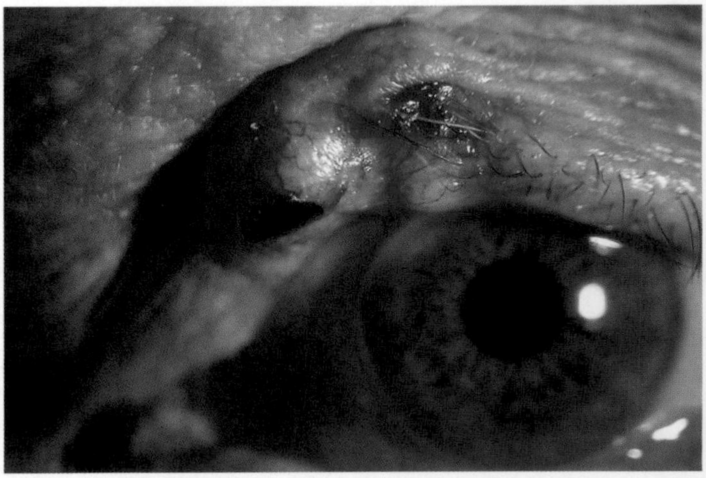

Fig. 1.158 More advanced sclerosing BCC.

Squamous cell carcinoma (SCC)

SCC is much less common than BCC but more aggressive. It may arise de novo or from a premalignant lesion.

Plaque-like

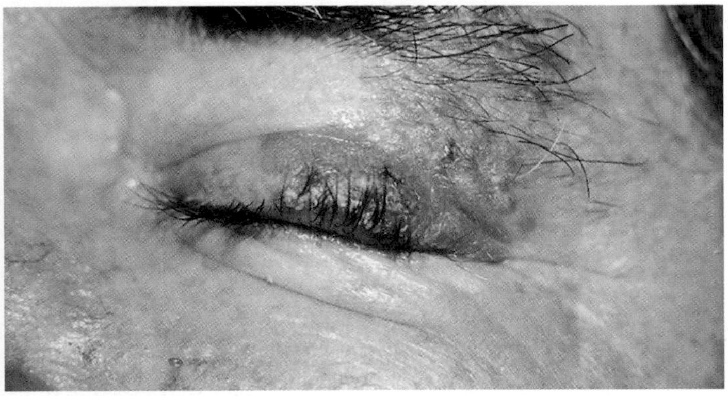

■ **Fig. 1.159** A roughened, scaly, erythematous, hyperkeratotic plaque that may arise from pre-existing actinic keratosis. (Courtesy of H. Frank.)

Nodular

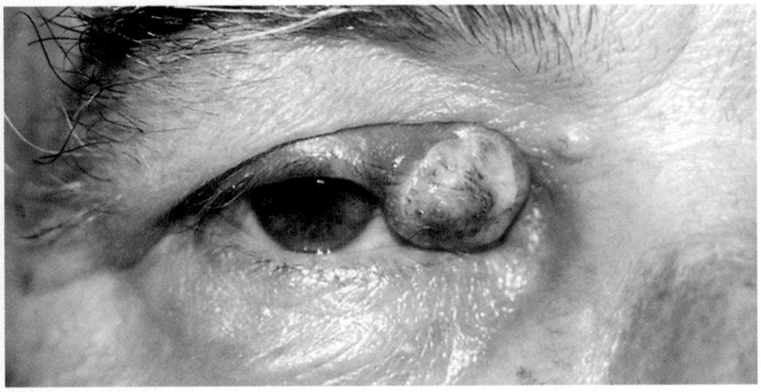

■ **Fig. 1.160** A hyperkeratotic nodule that may develop crusting erosions and fissures. (Courtesy of H. Frank.)

Ulcerative

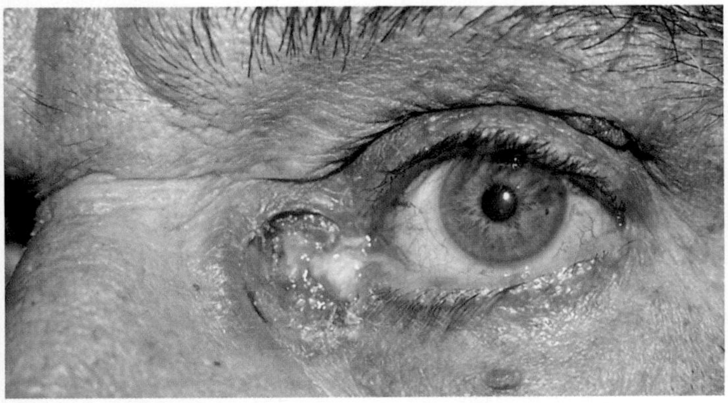

■ **Fig. 1.161** Sharply defined ulcer with a red base. (Courtesy of H. Frank.)

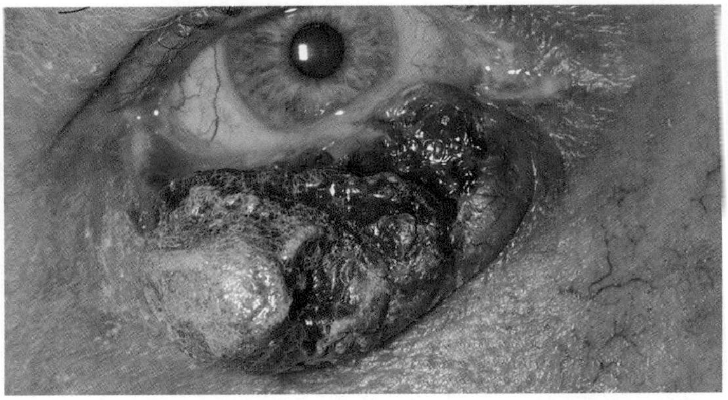

■ **Fig. 1.162** Neglected ulcerative SCC. (Courtesy of L. Merin.)

Meibomian gland carcinoma (MGC)

MGC is a rare but aggressive tumour which typically affects the upper lid of an elderly individual.

Nodular

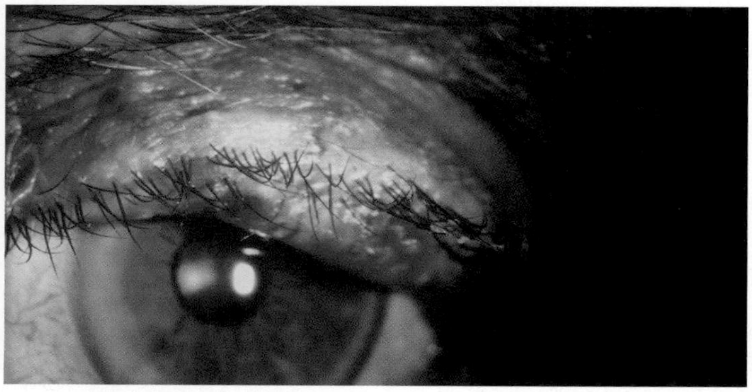

Fig. 1.163 Discrete, hard nodule most commonly within the tarsal plate. (Courtesy of S. Ford and R. Marsh.)

Noduloulcerative

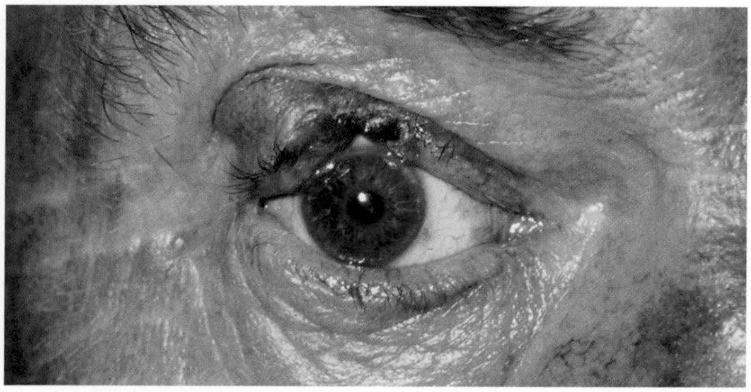

Fig. 1.164 Noduloulcerative MGC. (Courtesy of H. Frank.)

Spreading

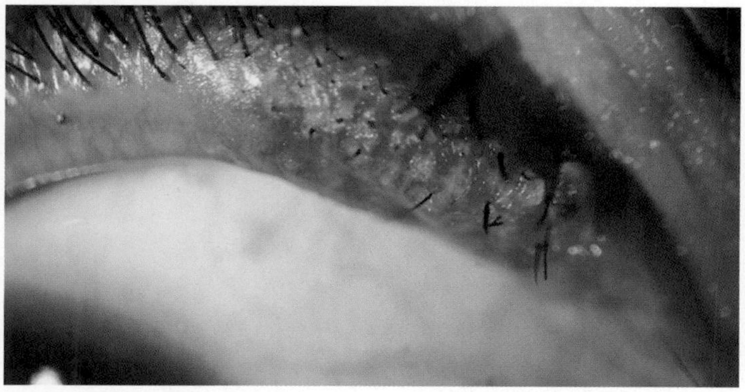

Fig. 1.165 This type infiltrates into the dermis and initially may only cause diffuse thickening of the lid margin and local madarosis.

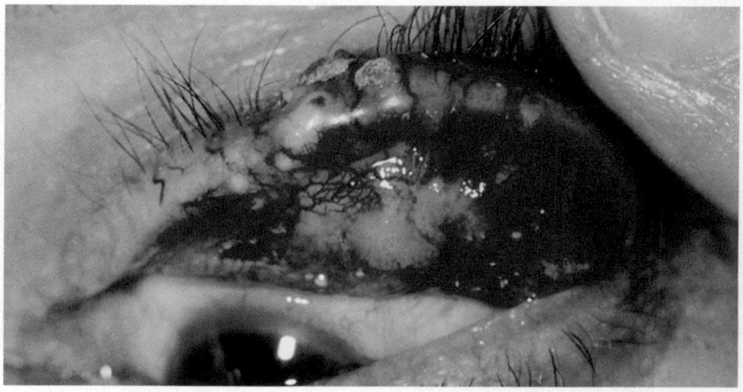

Fig. 1.166 Pagetoid spread refers to extension of the tumour within the conjunctival epithelium. (Courtesy of H. Frank.)

Gland of Zeis carcinoma

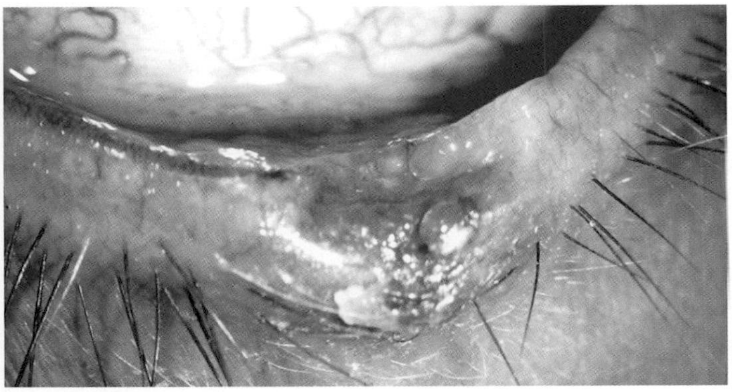

■ **Fig. 1.167** A discrete, slowly growing ulcerative lesion on the lid margin.

Melanoma

Melanoma rarely develops on the eyelids but is potentially lethal.

Nodular

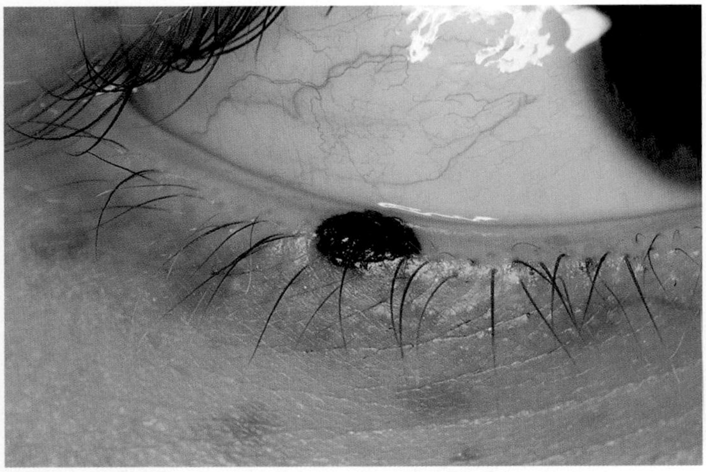

■ **Fig. 1.168** A blue-black nodule surrounded by normal skin. (Courtesy of P. Saine.)

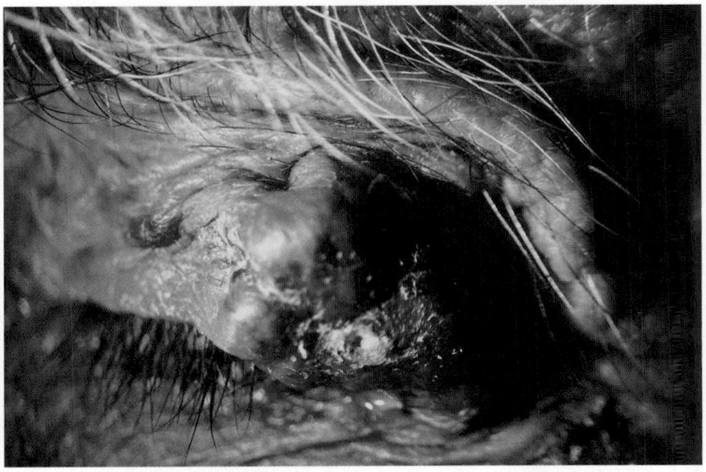

■ **Fig. 1.169** Large nodular melanoma.

Superficial spreading

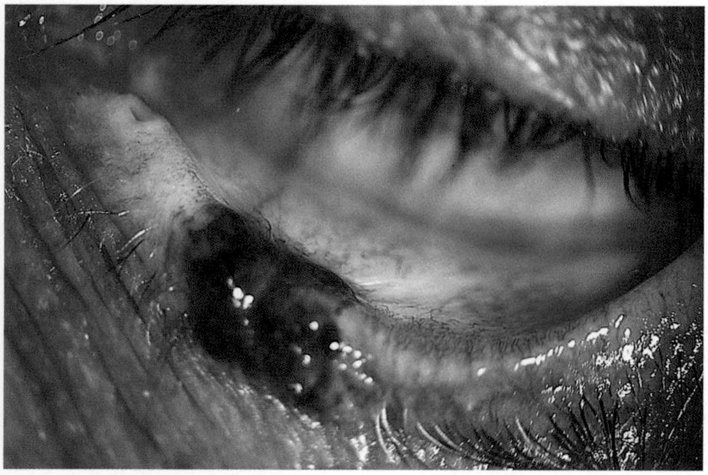

Fig. 1.170 A plaque with an irregular outline and variable pigmentation.

Arising from lentigo maligna

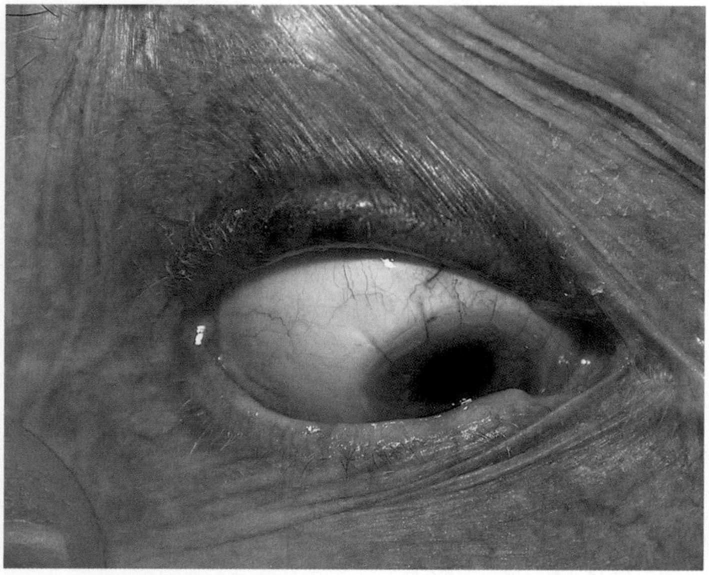

Fig. 1.171 Diffuse pigmentation associated with localised areas of thickening. (Courtesy of D. Selva.)

Kaposi sarcoma

Kaposi sarcoma is a vascular tumour that typically affects patients with the AIDS.

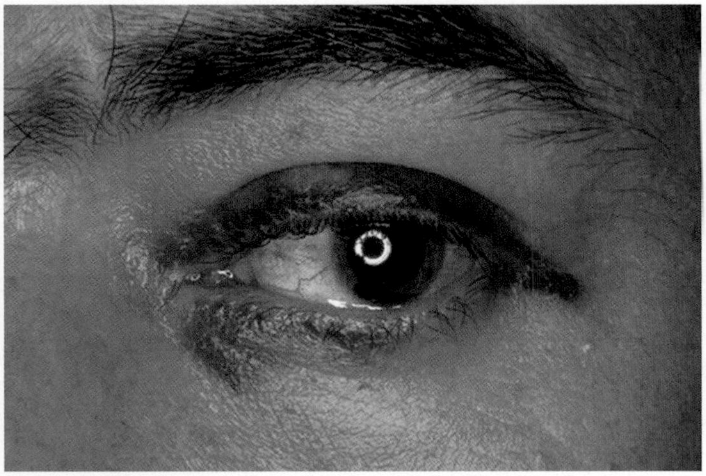

Fig. 1.172 Diffuse Kaposi sarcoma. (Courtesy of S. Ford and R. Marsh.)

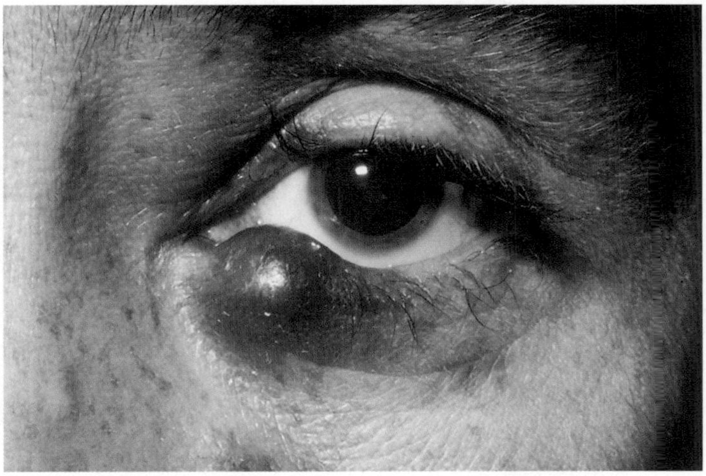

Fig. 1.173 Nodular Kaposi sarcoma. (Courtesy of S. Ford and R. Marsh.)

Merkel cell carcinoma

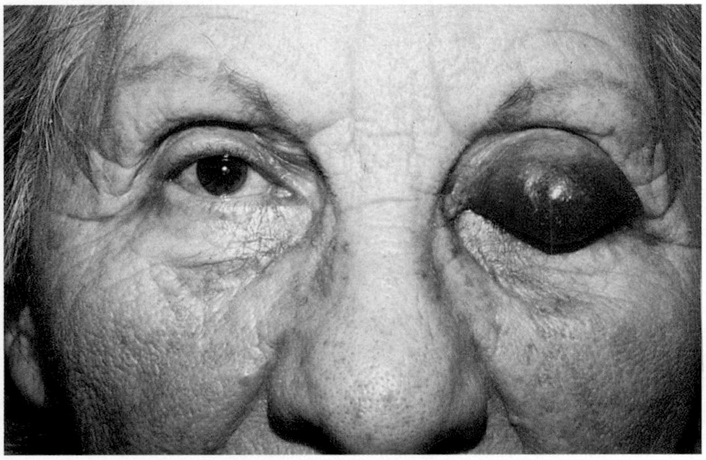

Fig. 1.174 A fast-growing, life-threatening tumour characterised by a violaceous, well-demarcated nodule with intact overlying skin, most frequently involving the upper eyelid. (Courtesy of S. Webber.)

ECTROPION

Involutional ectropion

Involutional (age-related) ectropion typically involves the lower lid of an elderly patient.

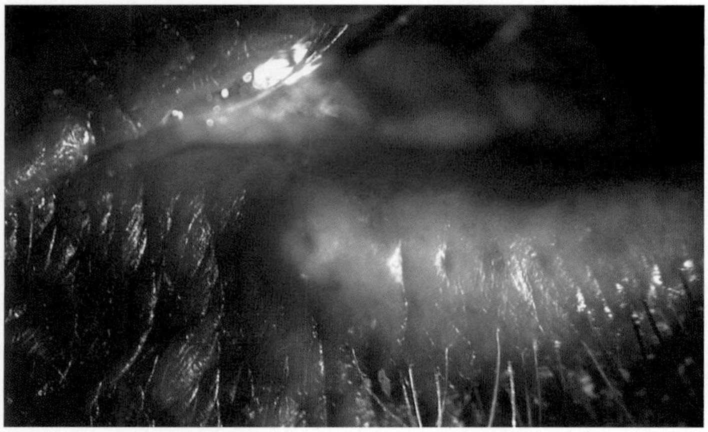

Fig. 1.175 Mild medial ectropion with punctal eversion.

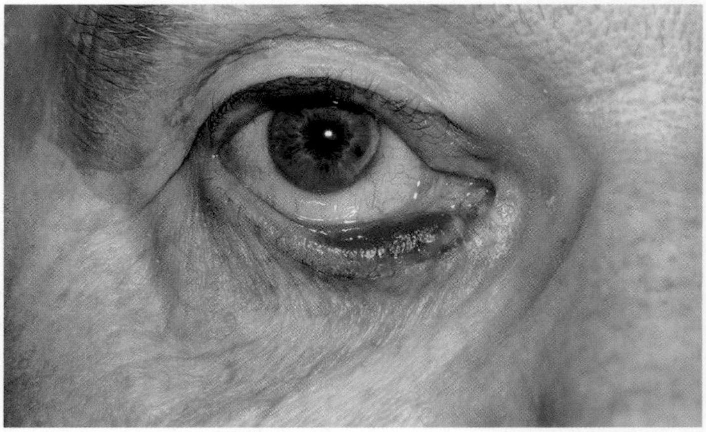

Fig. 1.176 Severe medial ectropion.

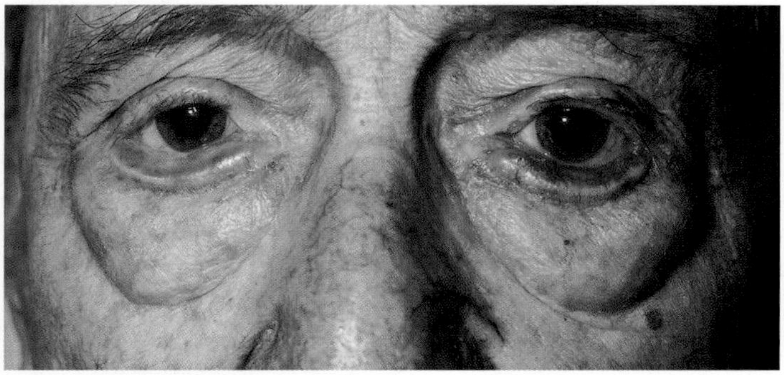

Fig. 1.177 Severe bilateral ectropion and conjunctival keratinisation.

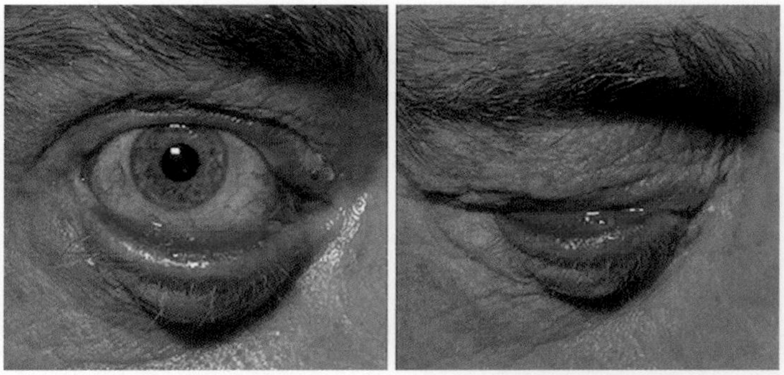

Fig. 1.178 Very severe ectropion with overriding of the upper lid over the lower lid on attempted closure. (Courtesy of S. Ford and R. Marsh.)

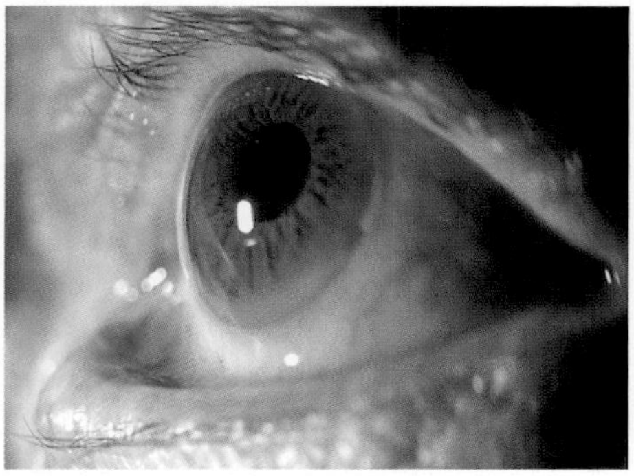

Fig. 1.179 Horizontal lid laxity is demonstrated by pulling the central part of the lid 8 mm or more away from the globe and its failure to snap back to its normal position on release without the patient first blinking.

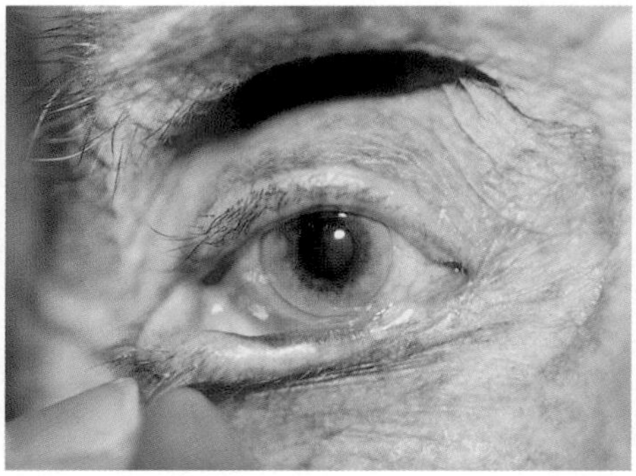

Fig. 1.180 Medial canthal tendon laxity is demonstrated by pulling the lower lid laterally and observing the position of the inferior punctum.

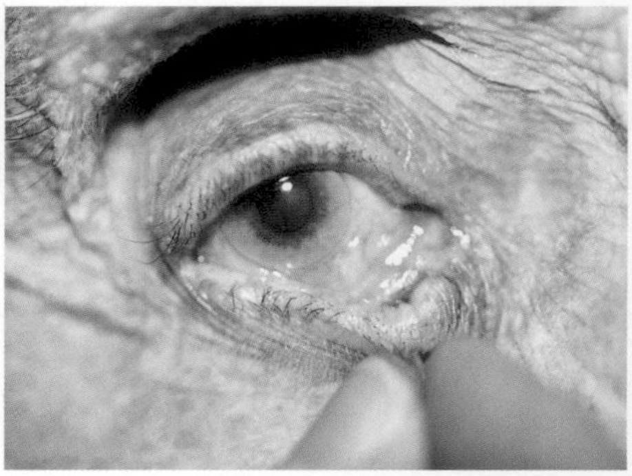

Fig. 1.181 Lateral canthal tendon laxity is characterised by a rounded appearance of the lateral canthus and the ability to pull the lower lid medially more than 2 mm.

Cicatricial ectropion

Cicatricial ectropion is caused by scarring or contracture of the skin and underlying tissues which pulls the lid away from the globe.

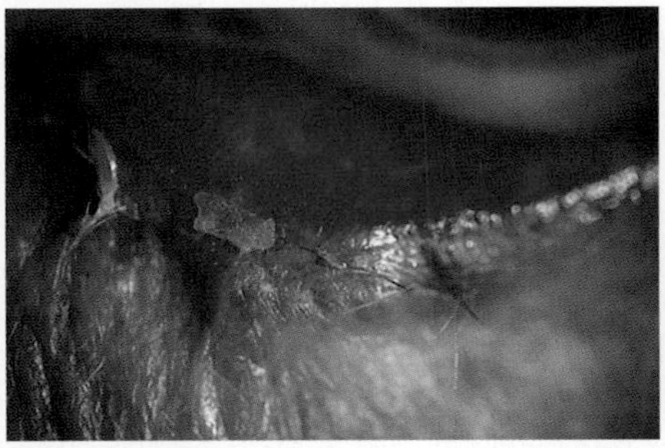

Fig. 1.182 Cicatricial ectropion caused by a sclerosing BCC.

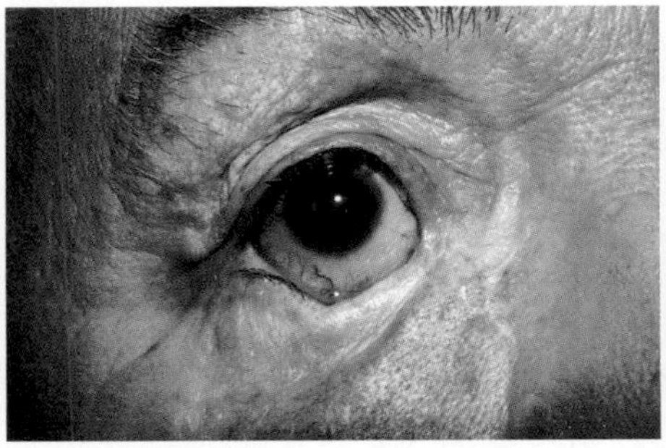

Fig. 1.183 Cicatricial ectropion and madarosis following radiotherapy of a BCC.

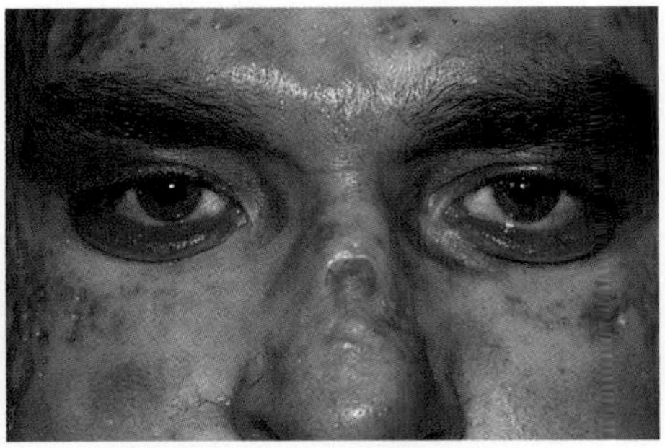

Fig. 1.184 Bilateral cicatricial ectropion due to scarring of facial skin in porphyria cutanea tarda.

Paralytic ectropion

Paralytic ectropion is caused by facial nerve palsy.

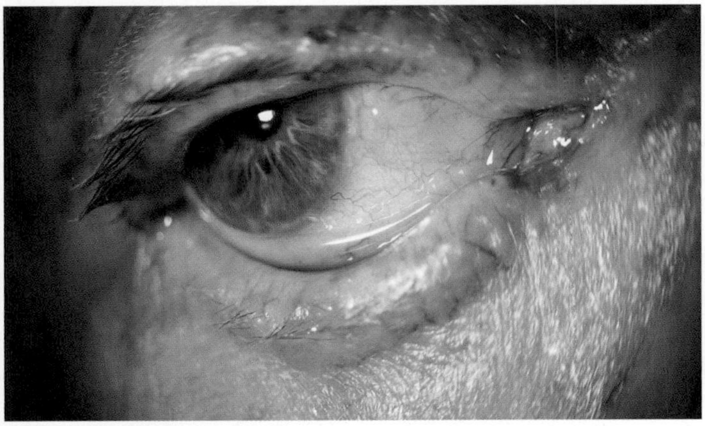

Fig. 1.185 Mild paralytic ectropion with increased tear meniscus due to failure of the lacrimal pump mechanism.

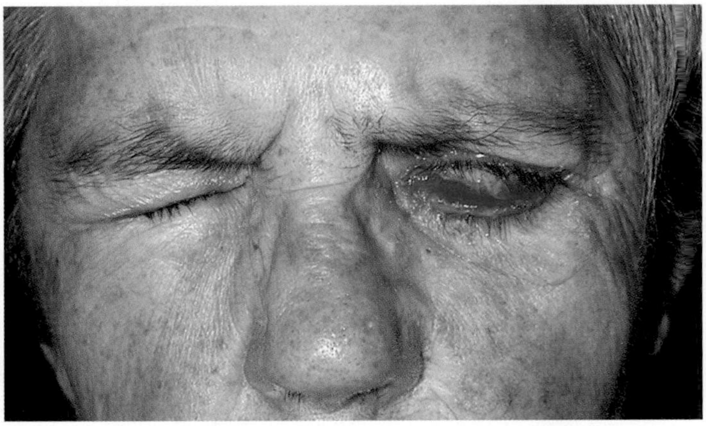

Fig. 1.186 Severe paralytic ectropion and conjunctival keratinisation.

Mechanical ectropion

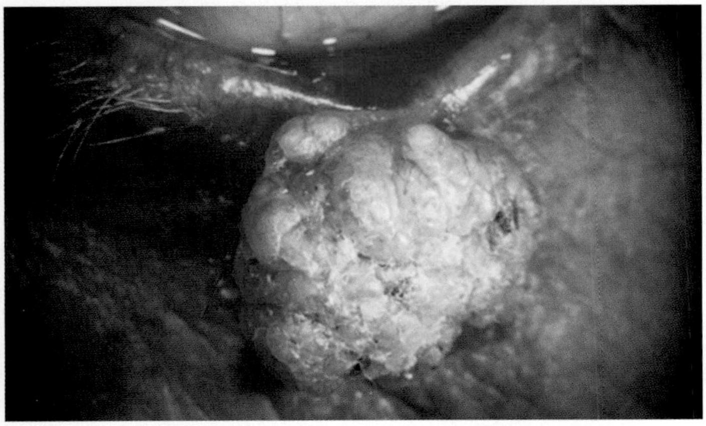

Fig. 1.187 Mechanical ectropion is caused by tumours on or near the lid margin that evert the lid.

ENTROPION

Involutional entropion

Involutional (age-related) entropion affects mainly the lower lid because the upper has a broader tarsus and is more stable.

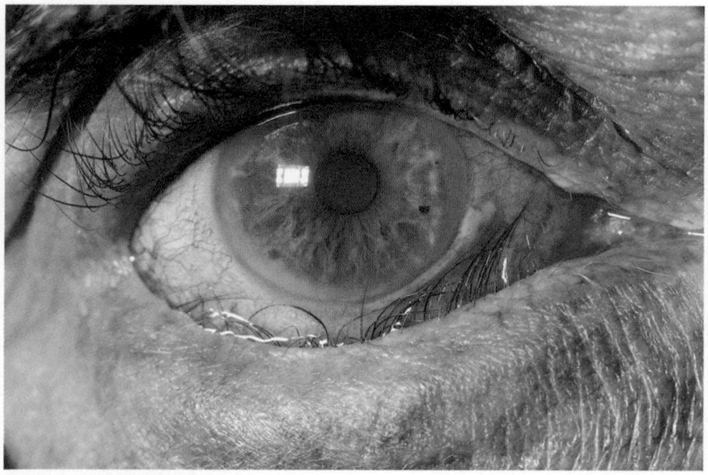

Fig. 1.188 Involutional entropion.

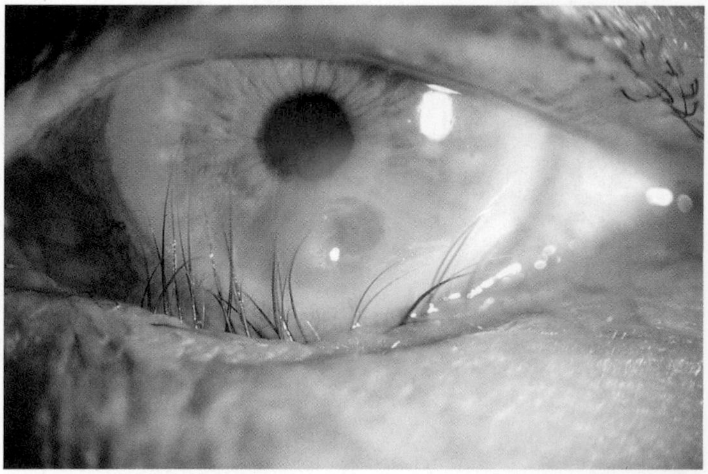

Fig. 1.189 The constant rubbing of the lashes on the cornea in long-standing entropion (pseudotrichiasis) has caused corneal ulceration.

Cicatricial entropion

Cicatricial entropion is caused by severe scarring of the palpebral conjunctiva, which pulls the lid margin towards the globe.

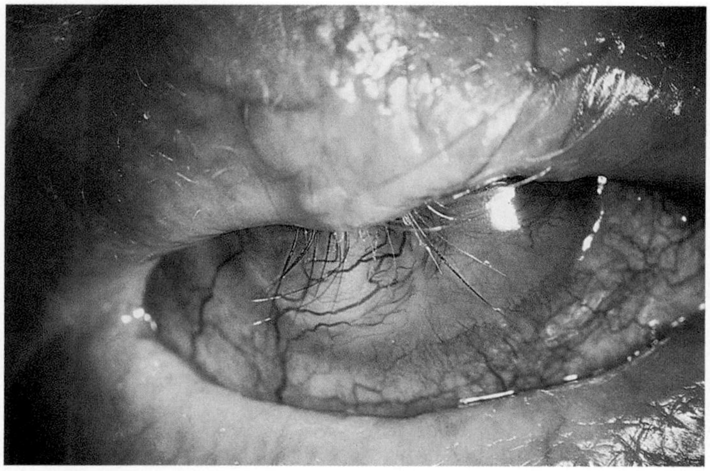

Fig. 1.190 Cicatricial entropion and corneal vascularisation due to chemical burns.

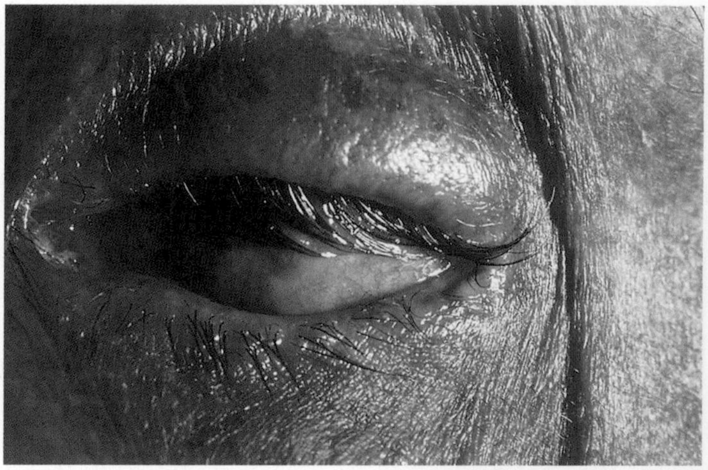

Fig. 1.191 Cicatricial entropion due to trachoma.

PTOSIS

Ptosis is an abnormally low position of the upper lid.

Neurogenic ptosis

Neurogenic ptosis may be caused by one of the following innervational defects:

Horner syndrome (oculosympathetic palsy)

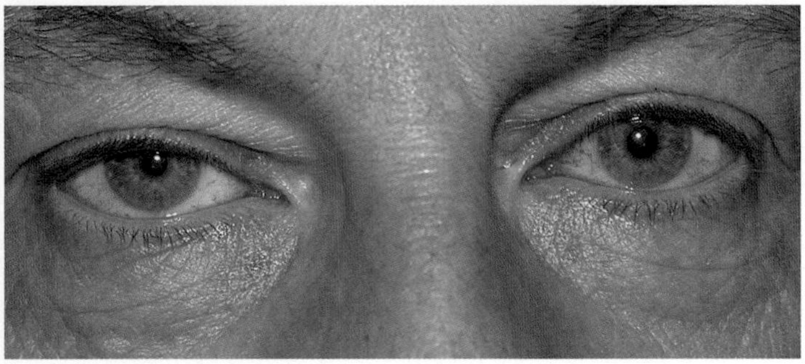

Fig. 1.192 Slight right ptosis and ipsilateral miosis.

Third nerve palsy

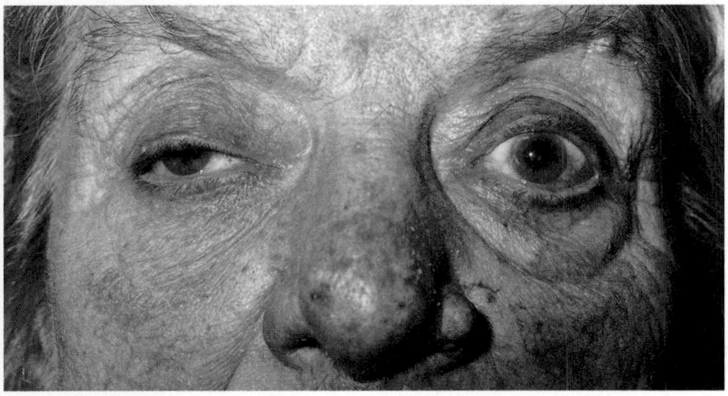

Fig. 1.193 Severe right ptosis and slight divergence of the eye due to the unopposed action of the lateral rectus.

Third nerve misdirection

Third nerve misdirection may be congenital or may follow an acquired third nerve palsy.

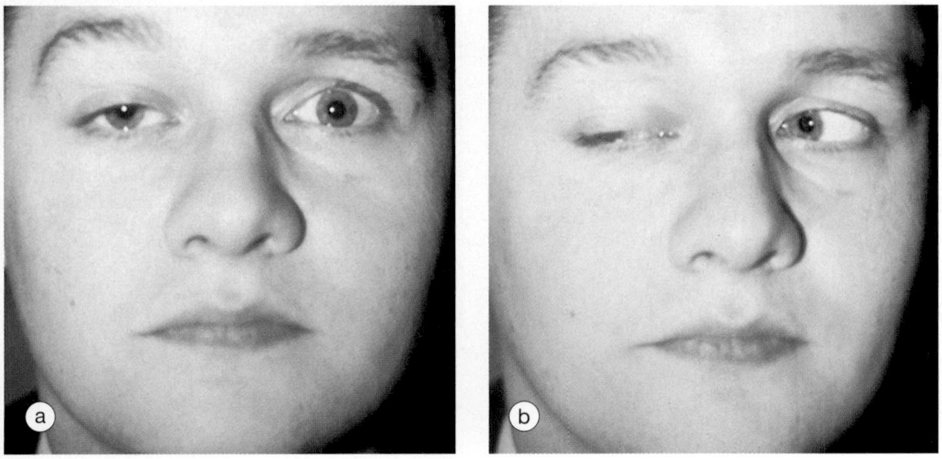

Fig. 1.194 **(a)** Right ptosis in the primary position. **(b)** Worsening of ptosis on right gaze. (Courtesy of S. Vardy.)

Myogenic ptosis

Myogenic ptosis is caused by a myopathy of the levator muscle itself, or by impairment of transmission of impulses at the neuromuscular junction (neuromyopathic). Causes of acquired myogenic ptosis are:

Myasthenia gravis

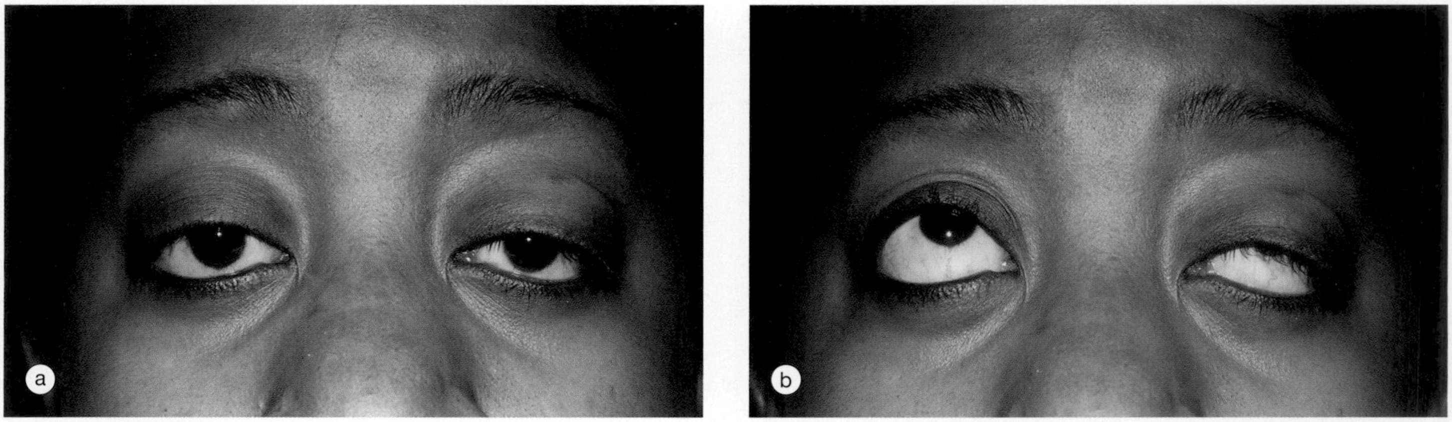

Fig. 1.195 **(a)** Ptosis is usually insidious, bilateral but frequently asymmetrical. **(b)** It worsens on upgaze and with fatigue.

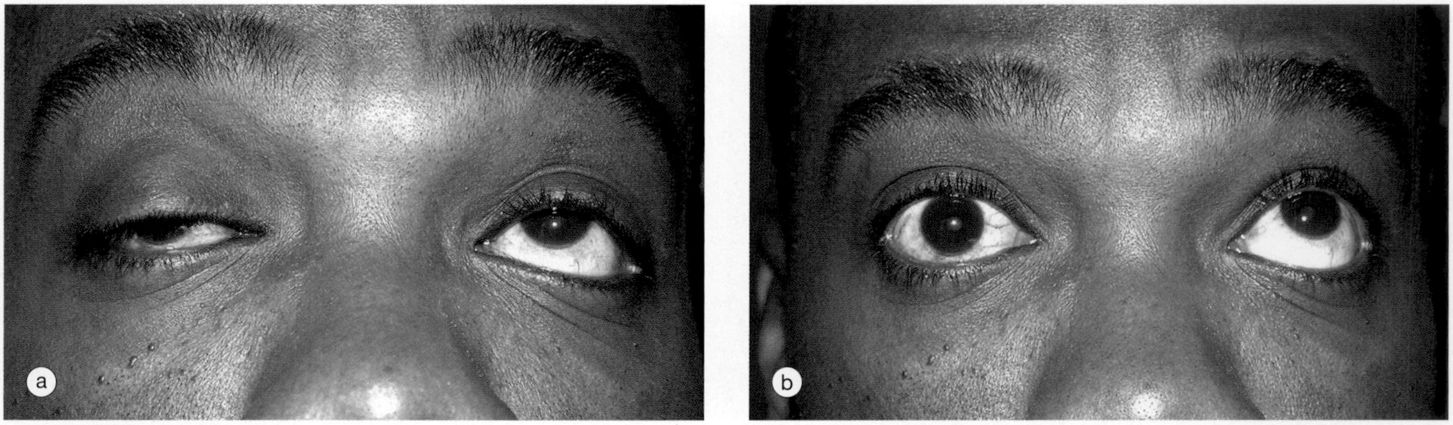

Fig. 1.196 Tensilon test. **(a)** Bilateral asymmetrical ptosis and defective upgaze. **(b)** Improvement of ptosis and left upgaze following intravenous injection of Tensilon.

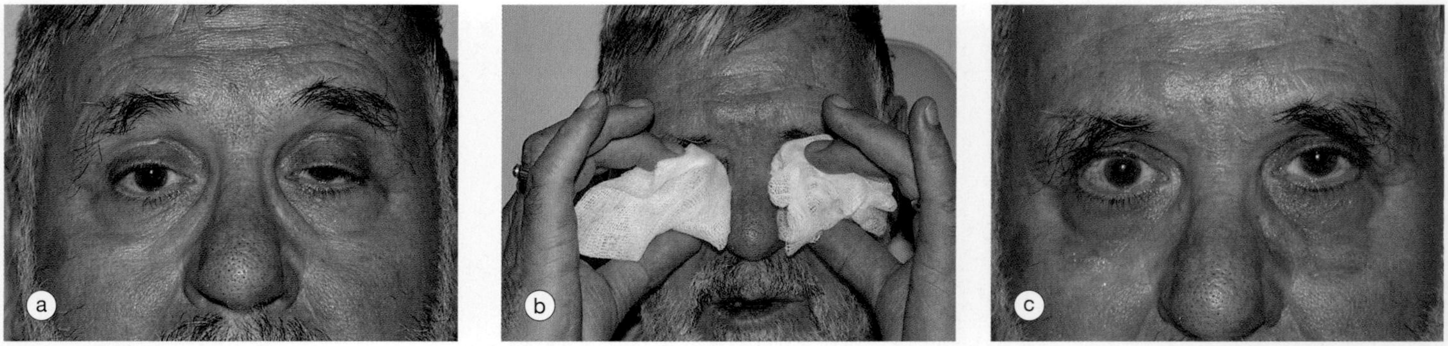

Fig. 1.197 Ice test. **(a)** Asymmetrical ptosis. **(b)** Application of ice to the eyelids. **(c)** Improvement of ptosis. (Courtesy of J. Yangüela.)

Myotonic dystrophy

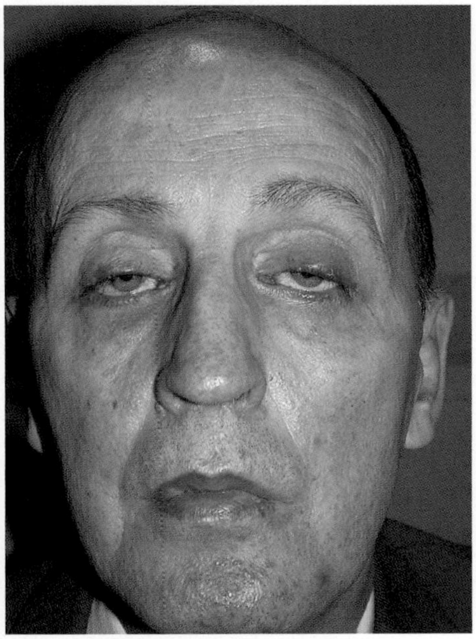

Fig. 1.198 Bilateral, symmetrical ptosis, frontal balding and a mournful facial expression.

Other manifestations

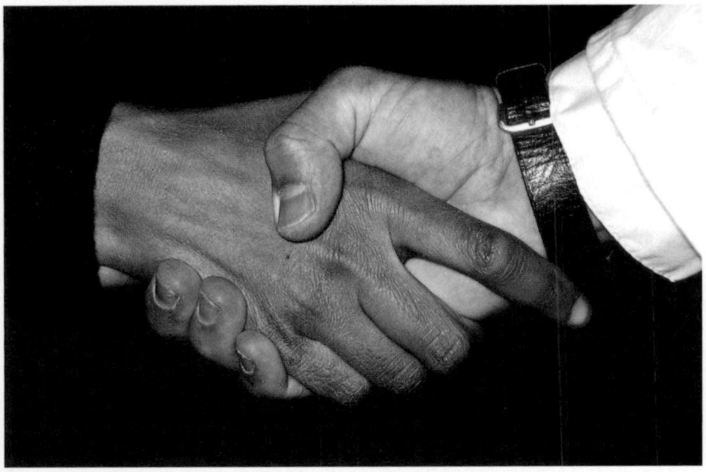

Fig. 1.199 Difficulty in relaxation of grip.

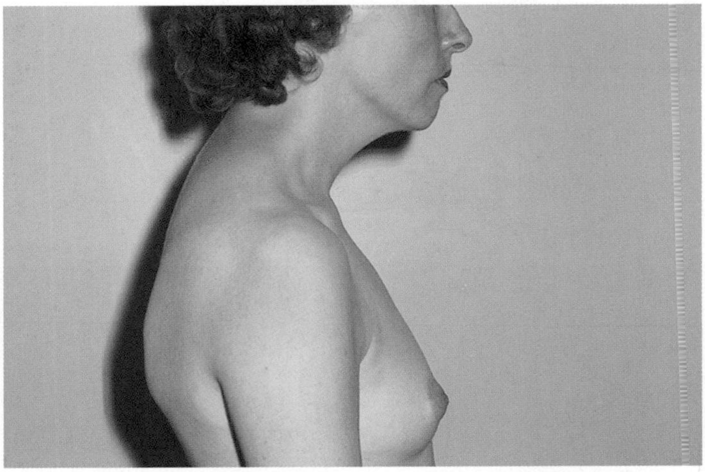

Fig. 1.200 Weakness of sternomastoids and neck extensors.

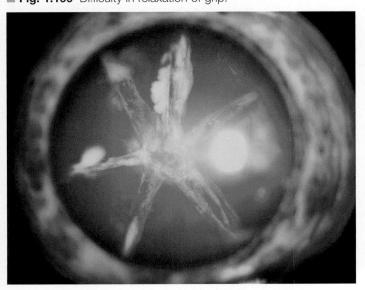

Fig. 1.201 Early-onset posterior stellate lens opacities. (Courtesy of S. Ford and R. Marsh.)

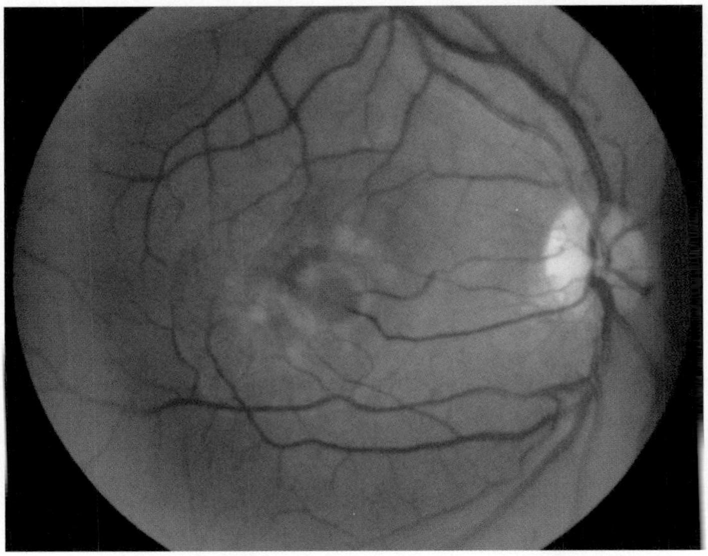

Fig. 1.202 Macular dystrophy is uncommon and relatively innocuous. (Courtesy of A. Packer.)

Kearns–Sayre syndrome

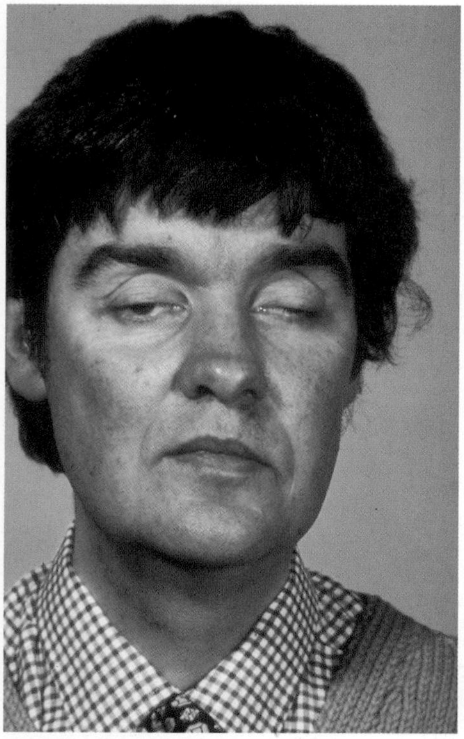

Fig. 1.203 Progressive, bilateral, symmetrical ptosis and external ophthalmoplegia starting in childhood.

Other manifestations

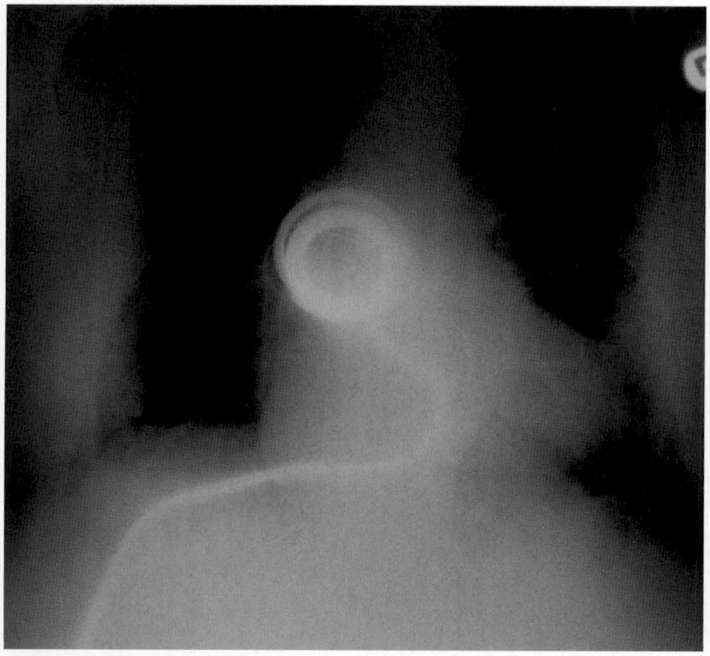

Fig. 1.204 Heart block that may require a pacemaker (shown here).

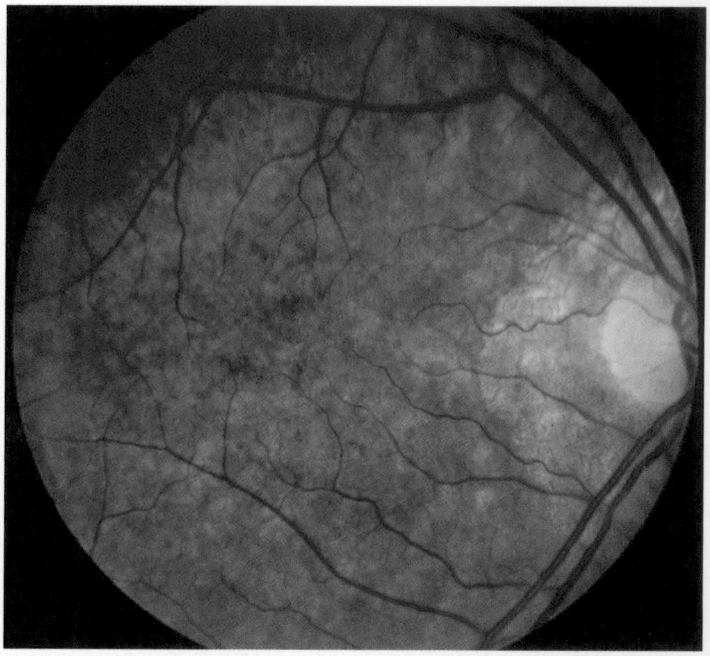

Fig. 1.205 Atypical pigmentary retinopathy characterised by salt-and-pepper mottling most pronounced at the posterior pole, and peripapillary depigmentation.

Aponeurotic ptosis

Aponeurotic ptosis is caused by dehiscence, disinsertion or stretching of the levator aponeurosis, which restricts transmission of force from a normal levator muscle to the upper lid. It is most frequently caused by involutional age-related degenerative changes.

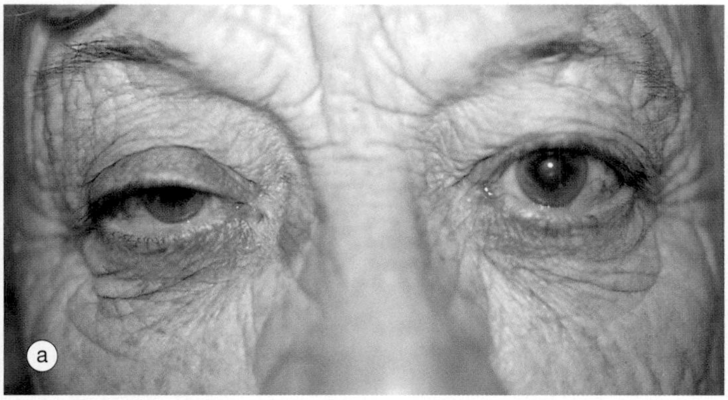

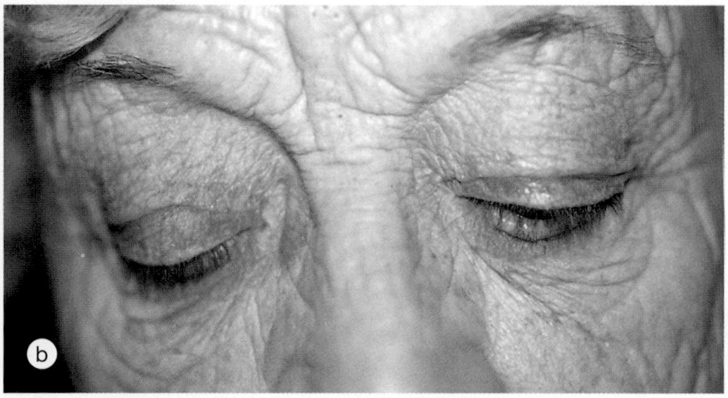

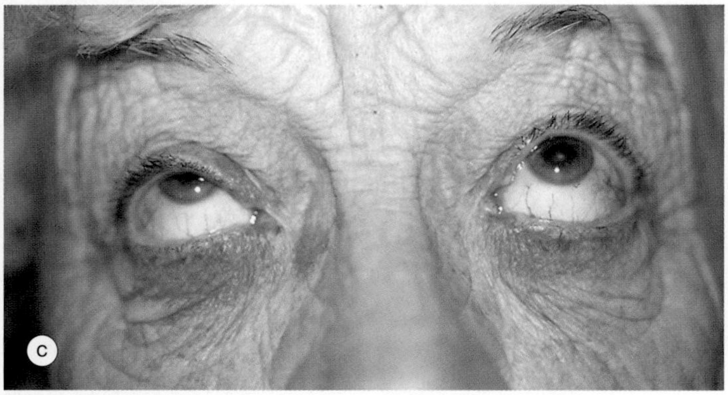

■ **Fig. 1.206** Moderate right involutional ptosis. **(a)** Brow overaction. **(b)** High upper lid crease as compared with the left. **(c)** Good levator function.

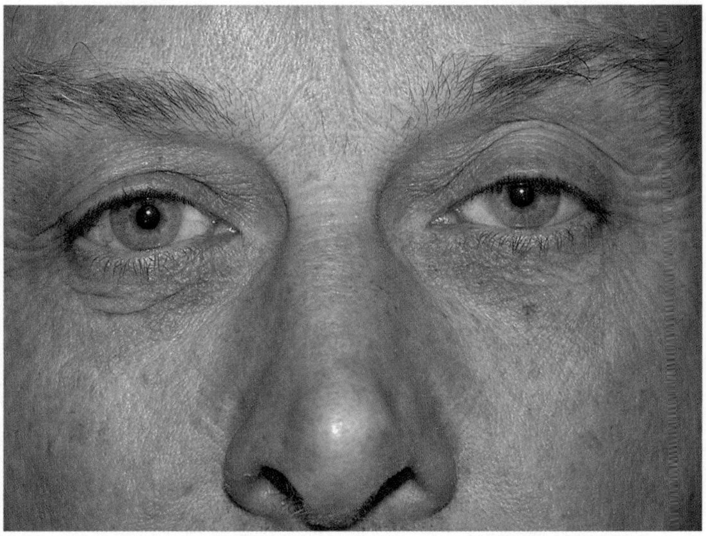

■ **Fig. 1.207** Mild left involutional ptosis with a high upper lid crease.

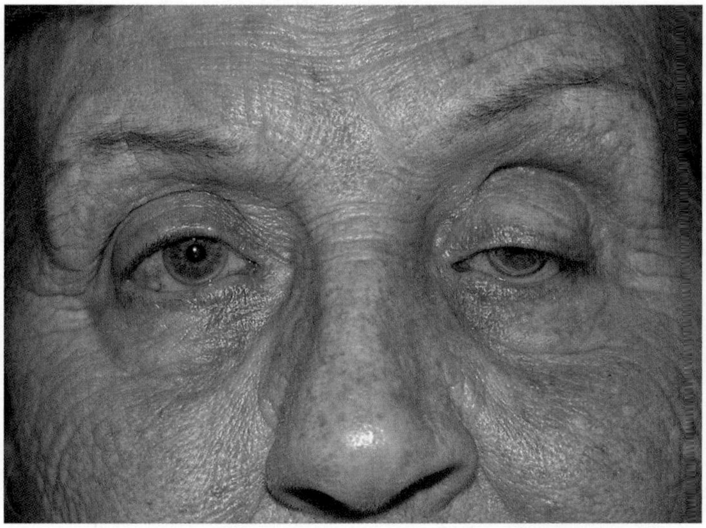

■ **Fig. 1.208** Severe left involutional ptosis with absent upper lid crease and a deep upper sulcus.

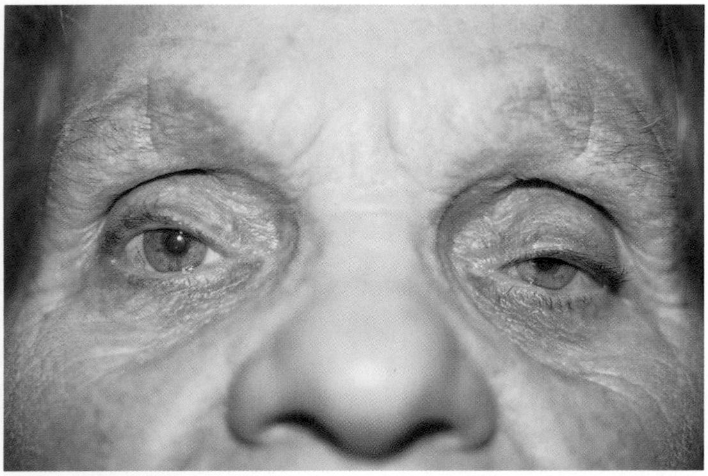

■ **Fig. 1.209** Severe bilateral involutional ptosis with absence of the upper lid creases, very thin eyelids above the tarsal plates and deep upper sulci.

Mechanical ptosis

Mechanical ptosis is caused by the gravitational effect of scarring, an eyelid mass or an anterior orbital lesion.

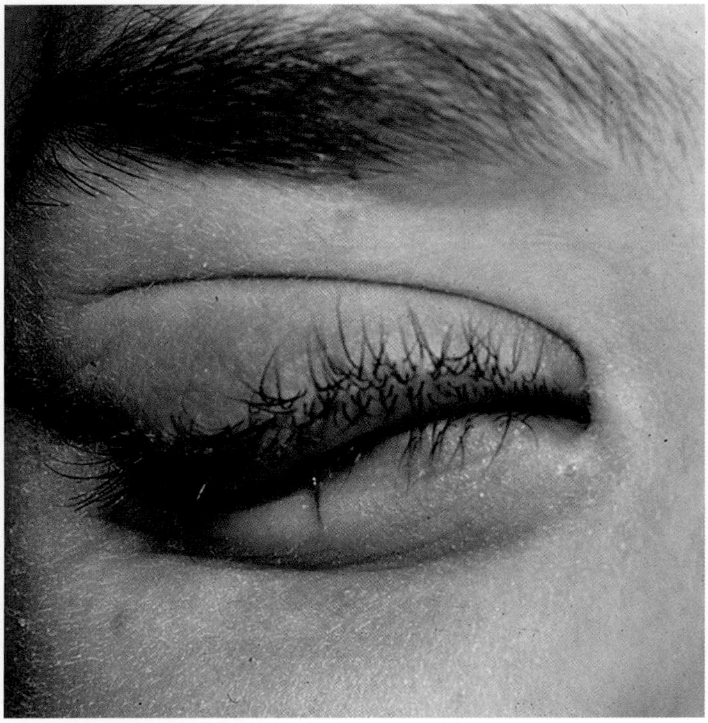

■ **Fig. 1.210** Severe ptosis due to a plexiform neurofibroma associated with neurofibromatosis-1.

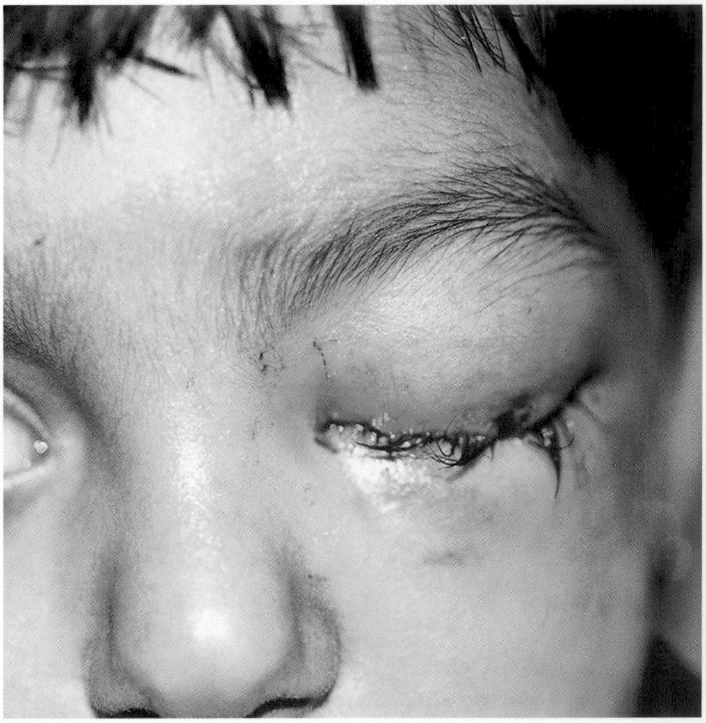

■ **Fig. 1.211** Complete ptosis due to lid oedema associated with orbital cellulitis.

Simple congenital ptosis

Simple congenital ptosis may be unilateral or bilateral.

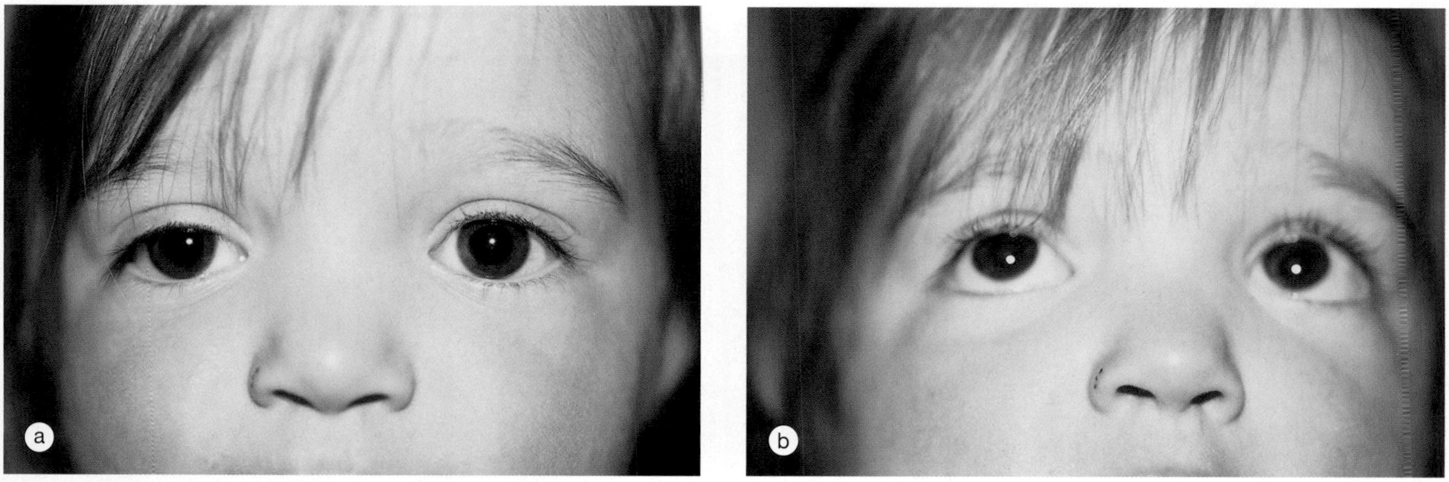

■ **Fig. 1.212** **(a)** Mild right ptosis. **(b)** Good levator function.

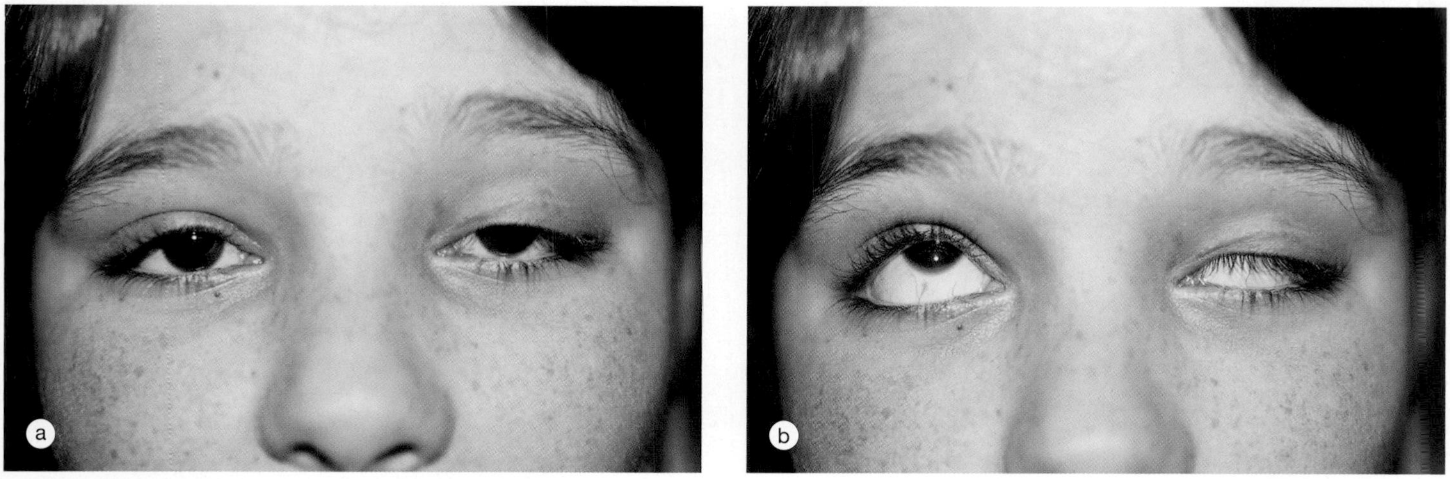

■ **Fig. 1.213** **(a)** Moderate left ptosis with absent upper lid crease. **(b)** Poor levator function, which may be associated with superior rectus weakness.

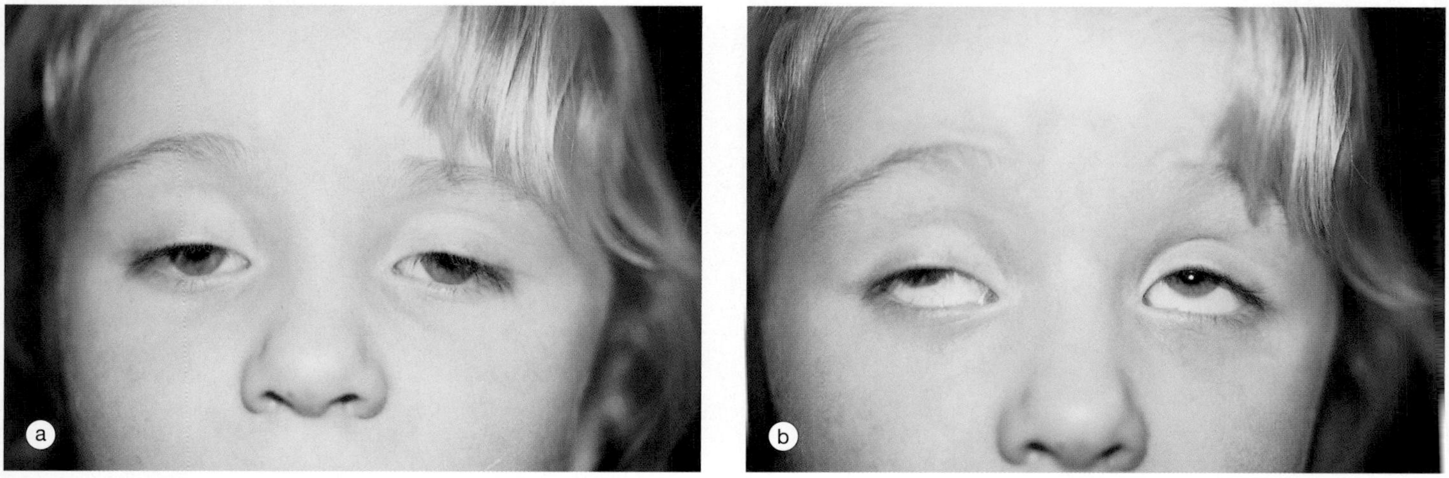

■ **Fig. 1.214** **(a)** Severe bilateral ptosis. **(b)** Very poor levator function.

Marcus Gunn jaw–winking syndrome

The Marcus Gunn jaw–winking syndrome is a congenital condition characterised by retraction of the ptotic lid in conjunction with stimulation of the ipsilateral pterygoid muscles.

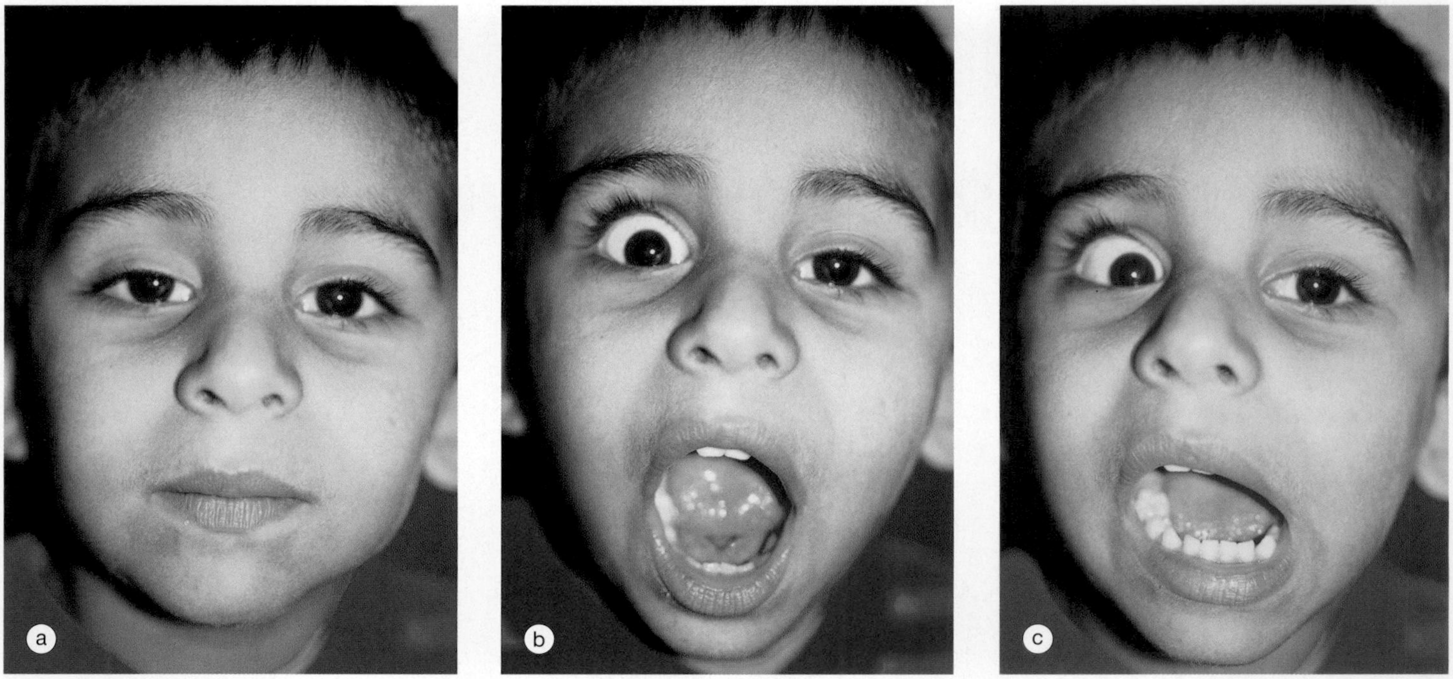

Fig. 1.215 **(a)** Mild right ptosis. **(b)** Retraction of the right eyelid on opening the mouth. **(c)** Retraction of the right eyelid on contralateral jaw movement.

Blepharophimosis syndrome

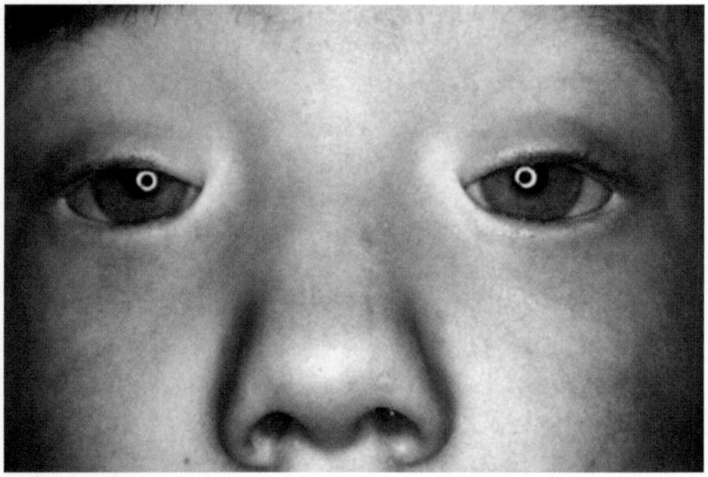

Fig. 1.216 Bilateral symmetrical ptosis; short horizontal palpebral aperture; telecanthus and epicanthus inversus; lateral ectropion of lower lids; poorly developed nasal bridge and hypoplasia of the superior orbital rims.

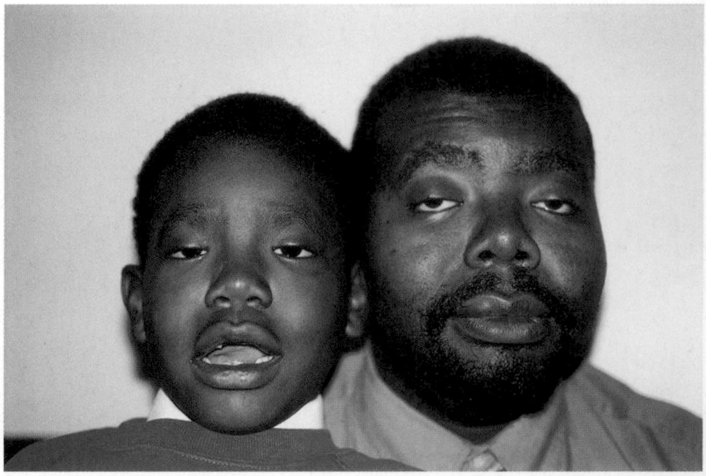

Fig. 1.217 The condition is inherited as an autosomal dominant trait.

MISCELLANEOUS ACQUIRED DISORDERS

Pseudoptosis

A false appearance of ptosis may be caused by the following conditions:

Lack of support

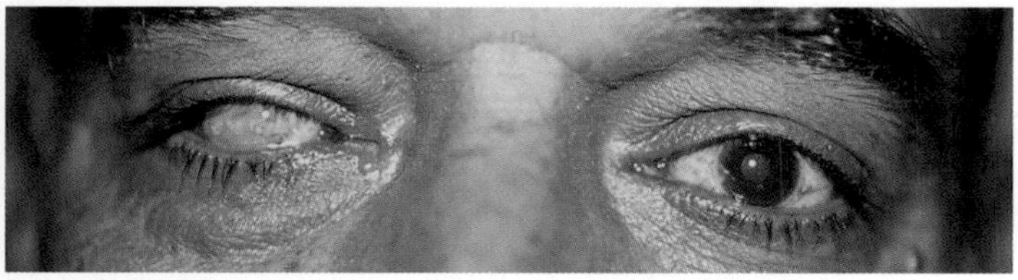

Fig. 1.218 Lack of support of the lids by the globe may be due to an orbital volume deficit associated with an artificial eye, microphthalmos, phthisis bulbi or enophthalmos.

Contralateral lid retraction

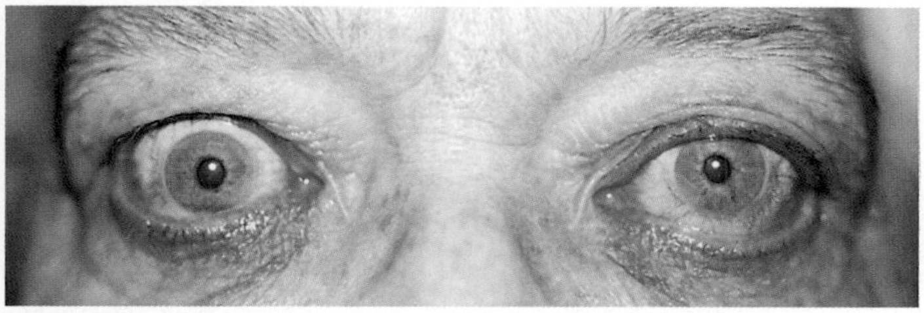

Fig. 1.219 Contralateral lid retraction, which is detected by comparing the levels of the upper lids, remembering that the margin of the upper lid normally covers the superior 2 mm of the cornea.

Ipsilateral hypotropia

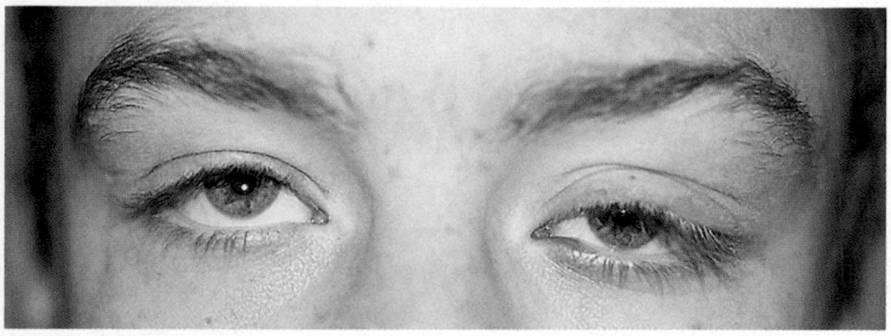

Fig. 1.220 Because the upper lid follows the globe the pseudoptosis will disappear when the hypotropic eye assumes fixation on covering the normal eye.

Brow ptosis

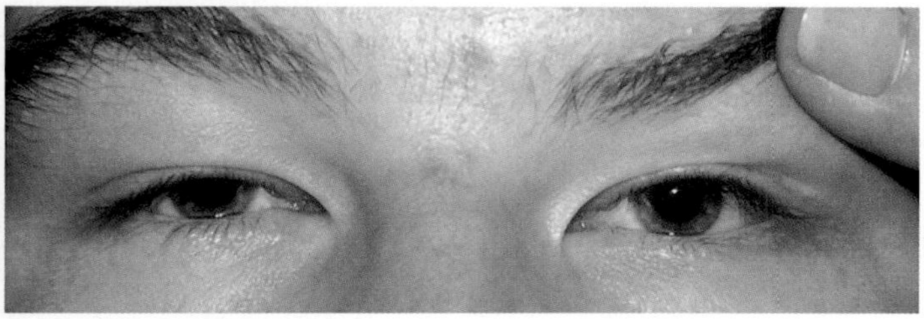

Fig. 1.221 This is due to excessive skin on the brow or seventh nerve palsy. It is diagnosed by manually elevating the eyebrow and finding the eyelid in its normal position.

Lash ptosis

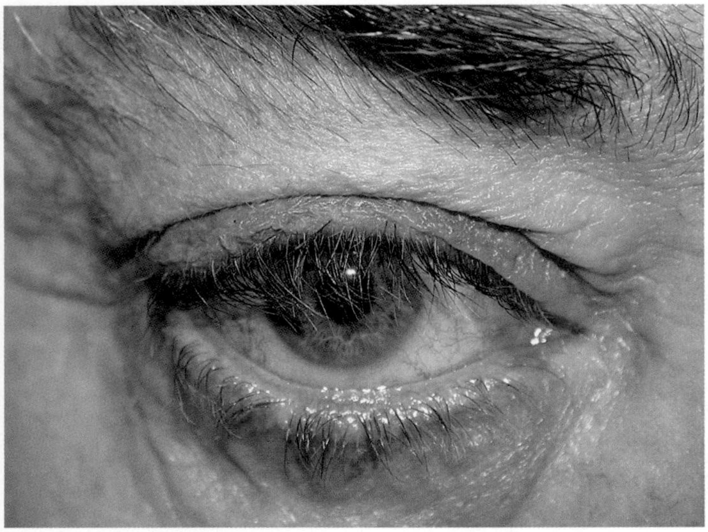

Fig. 1.222 The lid is in the correct position but the lashes point downwards. (Courtesy of A. Pearson.)

Dermatochalasis

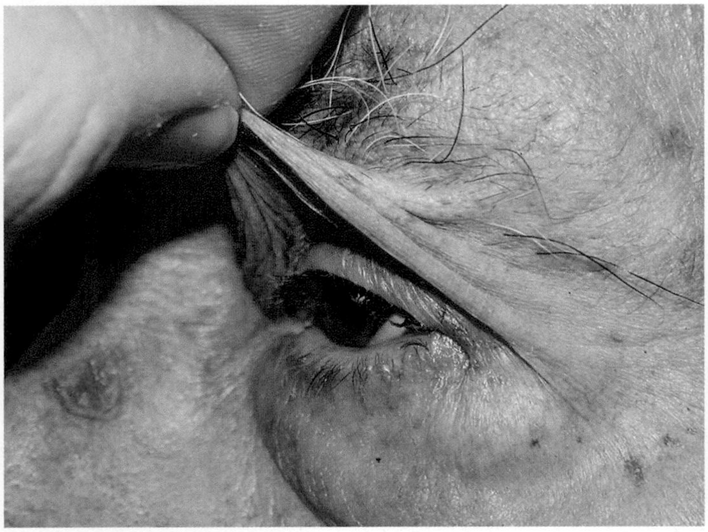

Fig. 1.223 Redundant upper lid skin.

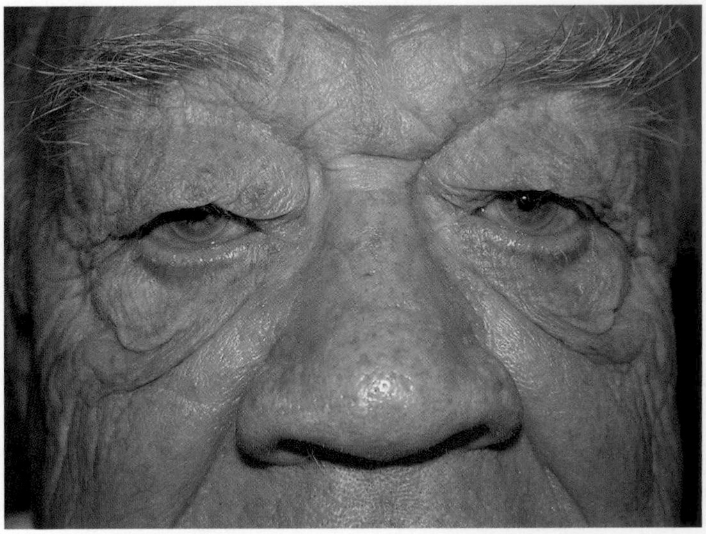

Fig. 1.224 The lids have a baggy appearance with indistinct creases.

Blepharochalasis

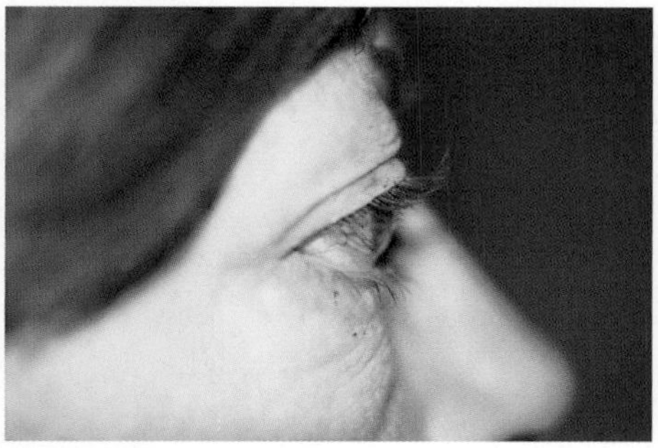

Fig. 1.225 Recurrent episodes of painless, non-pitting lid oedema of the upper lids that resolves spontaneously after a few days.

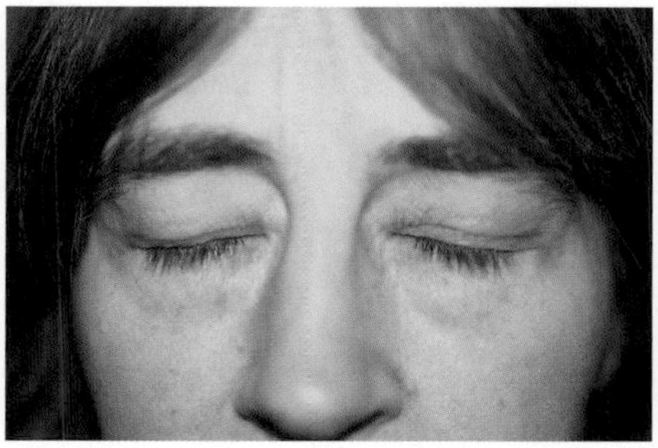

Fig. 1.226 Severe cases may cause stretching of upper lid skin so that it becomes redundant and may acquire the appearance of wrinkled cigarette paper.

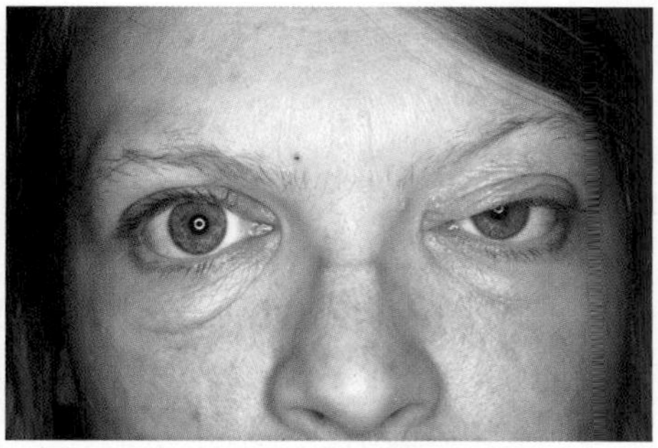

Fig.1.227 In severe cases recurrent stretching of the levator aponeurosis may also give rise to ptosis.

Floppy eyelid syndrome

A unilateral or bilateral condition which principally affects very obese men.

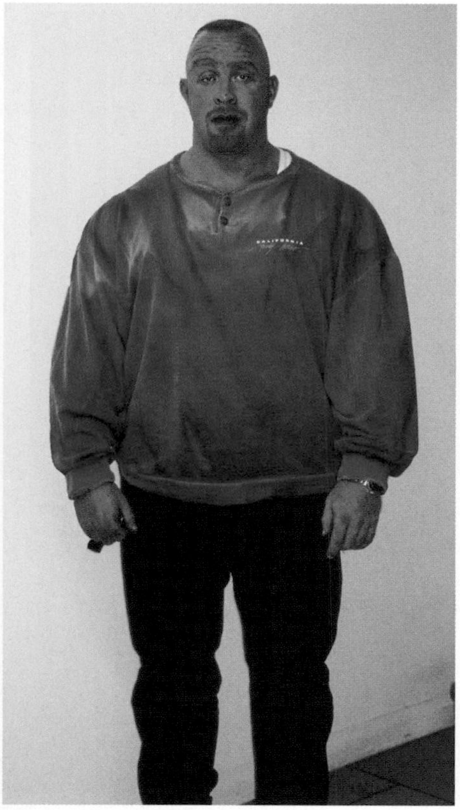

Fig. 1.228 A typical patient with floppy eyelid syndrome.

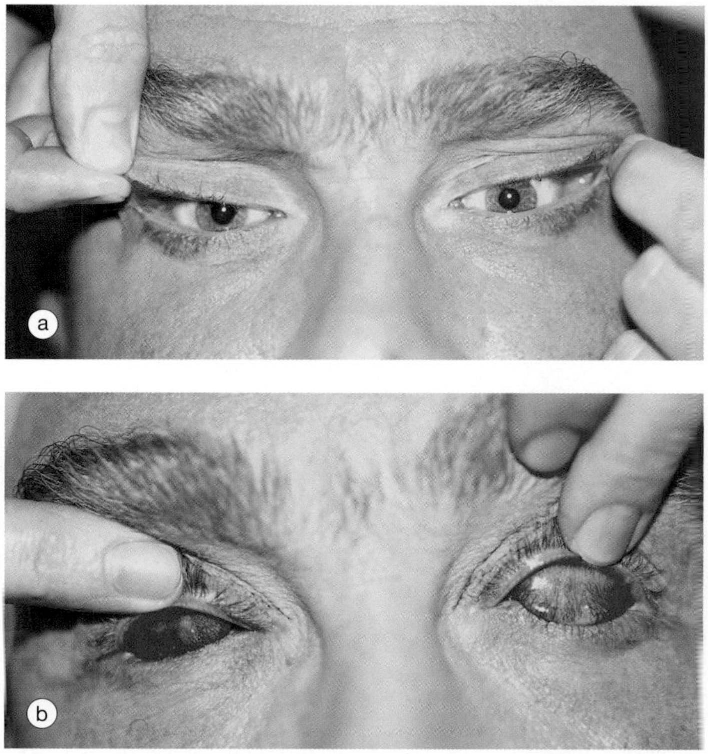

Fig. 1.229 **(a)** Rubbery and loose upper tarsal plates. **(b)** Chronic papillary conjunctivitis resulting from trauma to the everted lids during sleep.

Blepharospasm

Protective

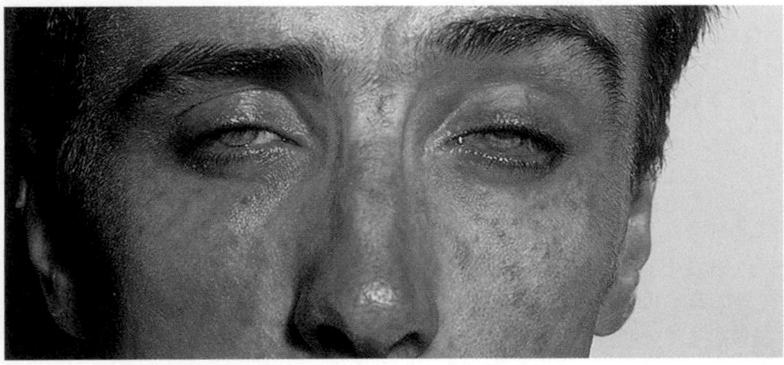

Fig. 1.230 This is caused by irritation to the corneal epithelium such as that caused by an abrasion.

Facial hemispasm

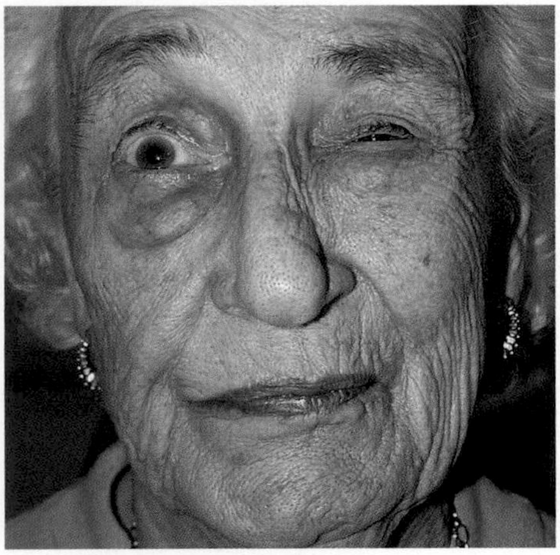

Fig. 1.231 Recurrent involuntary unilateral spasm of the face and eyelids.

Essential

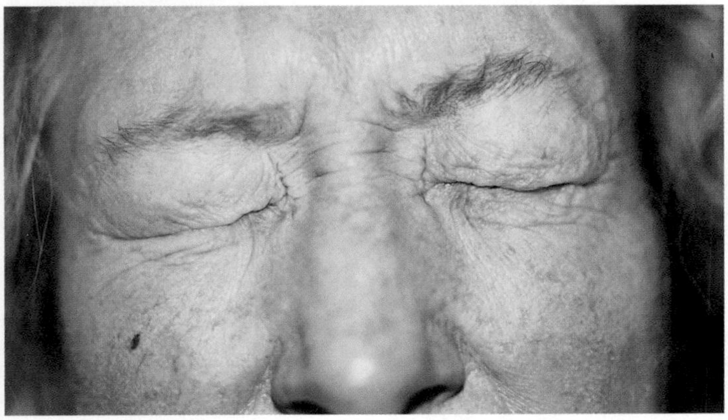

Fig. 1.232 Progressive, recurrent, involuntary bilateral spasm of the eyelids and upper facial muscles.

Lid retraction

Lid retraction is suspected when the upper lid margin is either level with or above the superior limbus. Causes include:

Thyroid eye disease

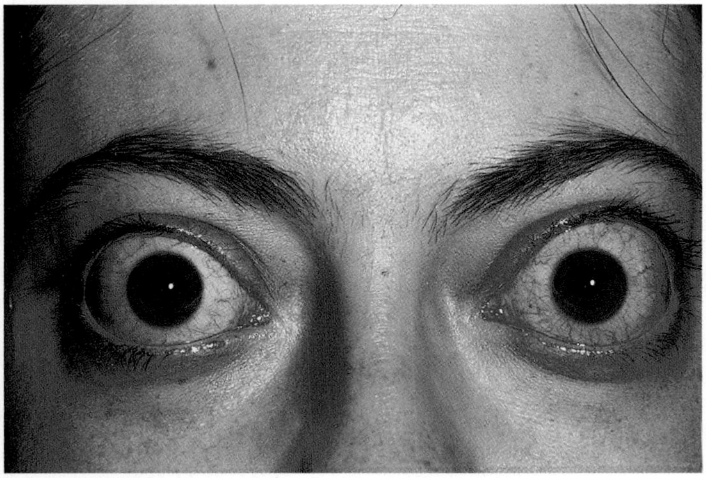

■ **Fig. 1.233** This is by far the most common cause of lid retraction, which is often associated with lid lag on downgaze.

Parinaud syndrome (Collier sign)

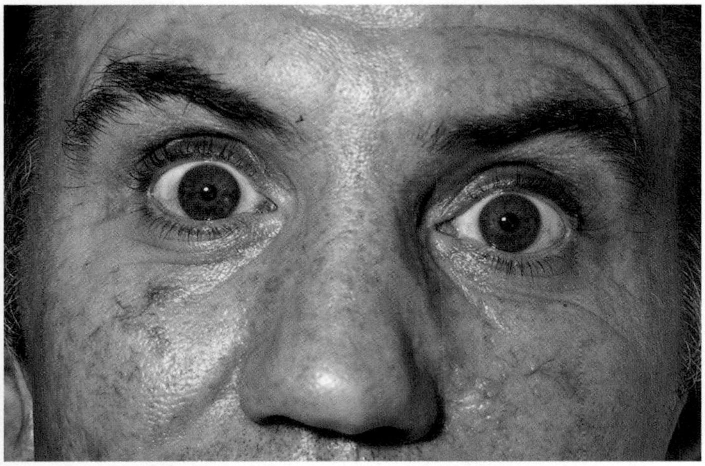

■ **Fig. 1.234** Lid retraction, paralysis of convergence, supranuclear upgaze palsy, convergence–retraction nystagmus and light–near dissociation of pupillary reactions.

Unilateral ptosis

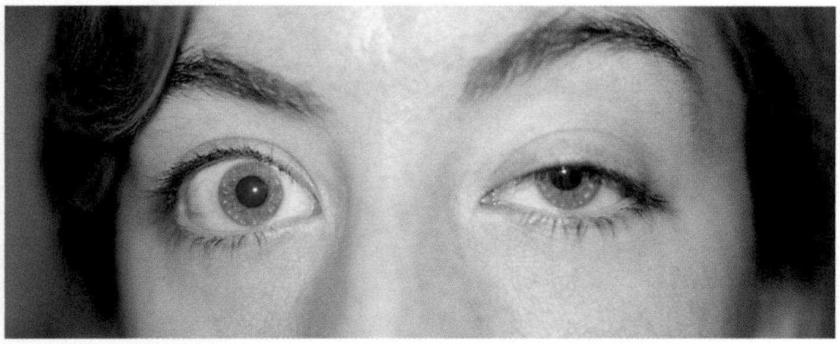

■ **Fig. 1.235** Unilateral myasthenic ptosis causing increased innervation to the contralateral levator, resulting in lid retraction.

Parkinson's disease

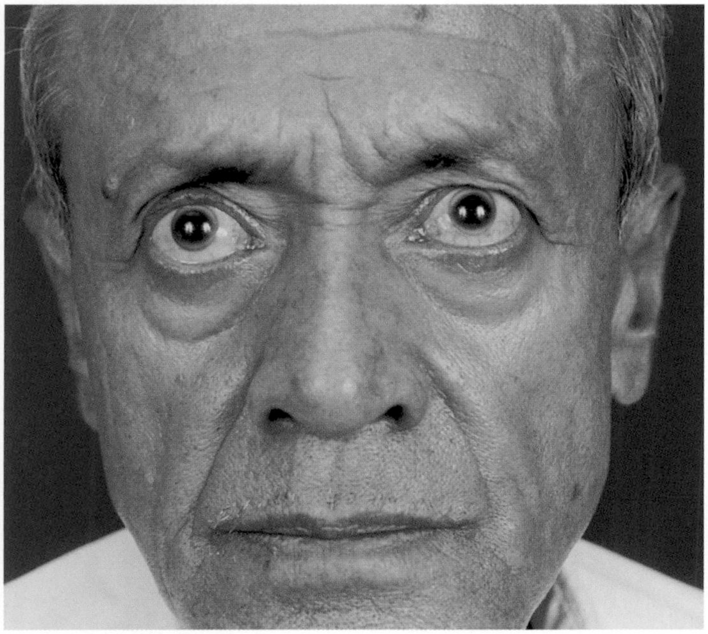

■ **Fig. 1.236** Bilateral lid retraction in Parkinson's disease; note lack of facial expression.

Infantile hydrocephalus

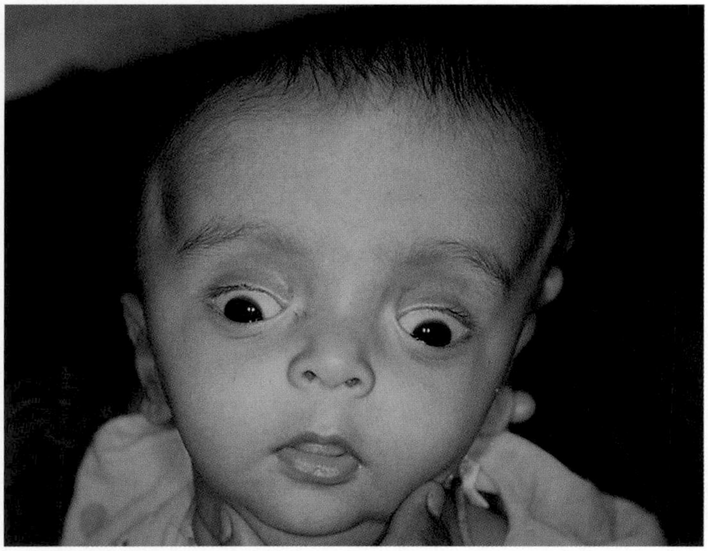

■ **Fig. 1.237** Bilateral lid retraction and 'sunset' eye position associated with failure of upgaze. (Courtesy of U. Raina.)

Marcus Gunn jaw–winking syndrome

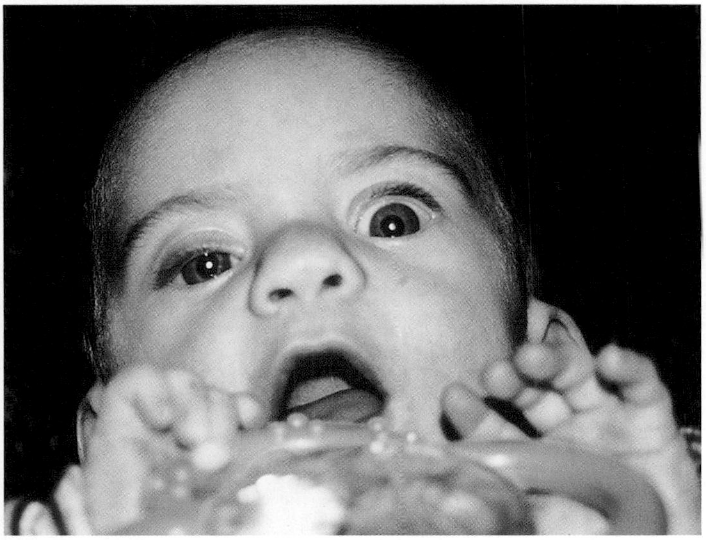

Fig. 1.238 Transient unilateral lid retraction on opening the mouth. (Courtesy of K. Nischal.)

Duane retraction syndrome

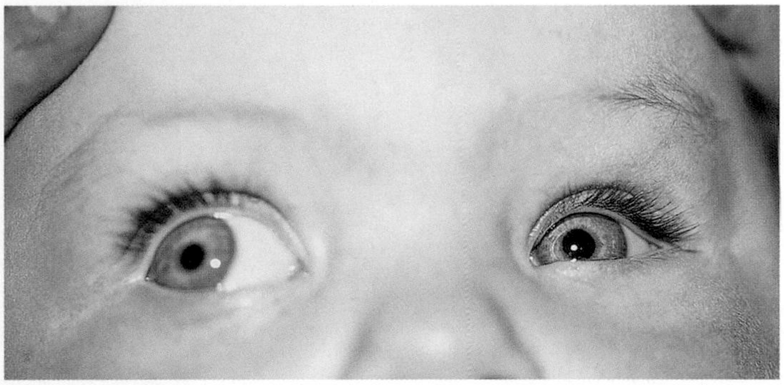

Fig. 1.239 Transient unilateral lid retraction of the abduction eye. (Courtesy of K. Nischal.)

Congenital

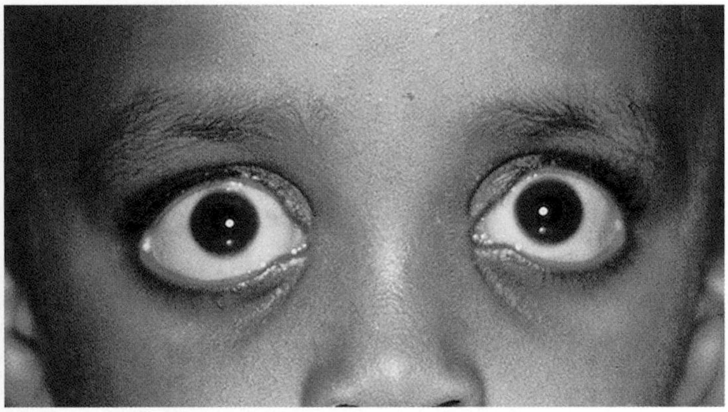

Fig. 1.240 Isolated congenital bilateral lid retraction is rare. (Courtesy of S. Ford and R. Marsh.)

EYELID MANIFESTATIONS OF SYSTEMIC DISEASES

Hypercholesterolaemia

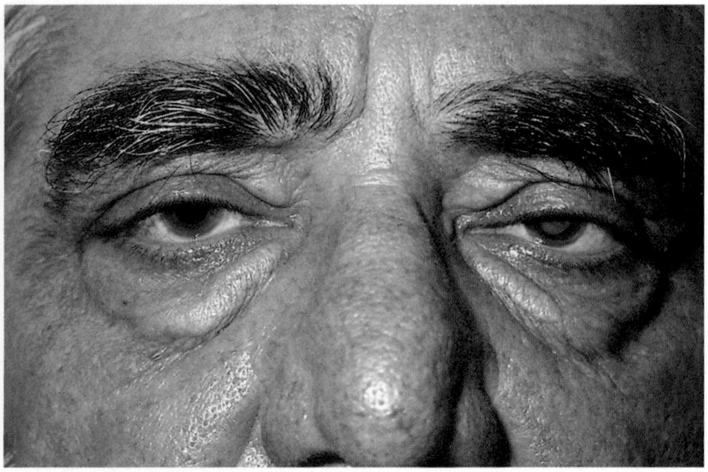

Fig. 1.241 Xanthelasma, which are bilateral, flat, yellowish soft plaques at the inner canthi.

Other manifestations

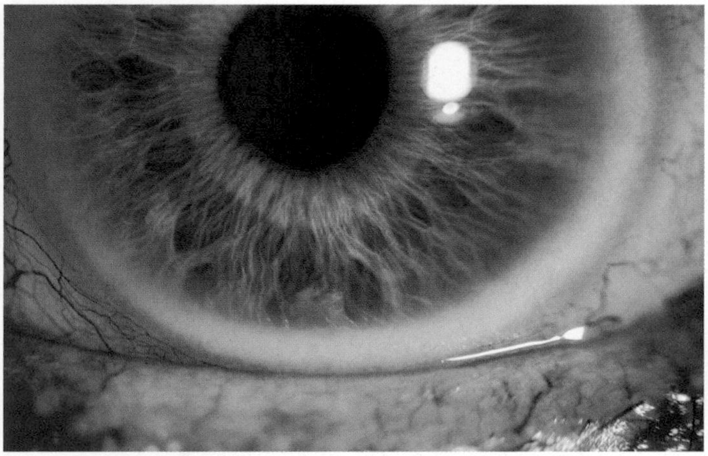

Fig. 1.242 Corneal arcus, particularly in a young patient.

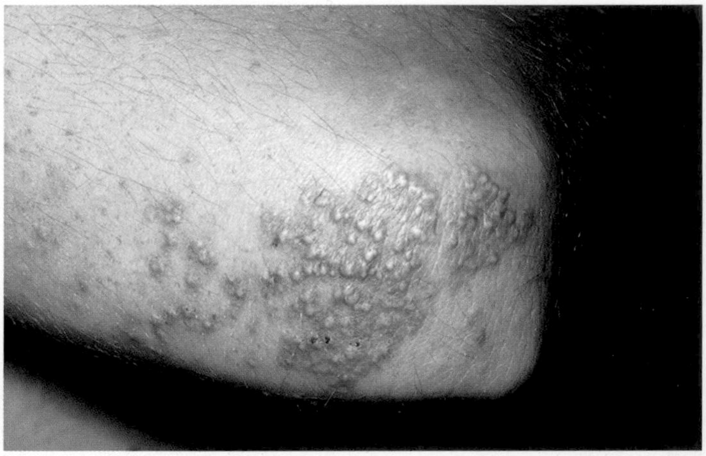

Fig. 1.243 Cutaneous xanthomata.

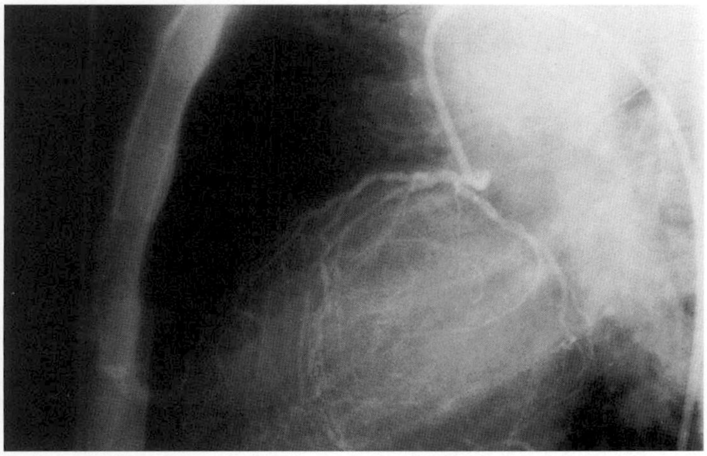

Fig. 1.244 Coronary artery disease, which may require coronary angiography to ascertain severity.

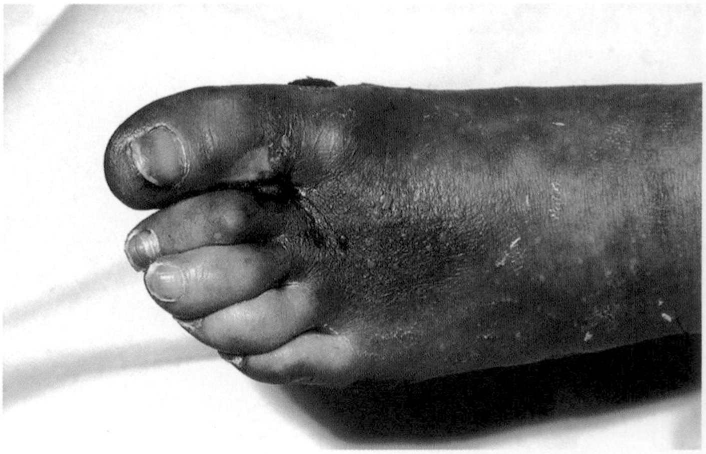

Fig. 1.245 Peripheral vascular disease, which may lead to gangrene.

Dermatomyositis

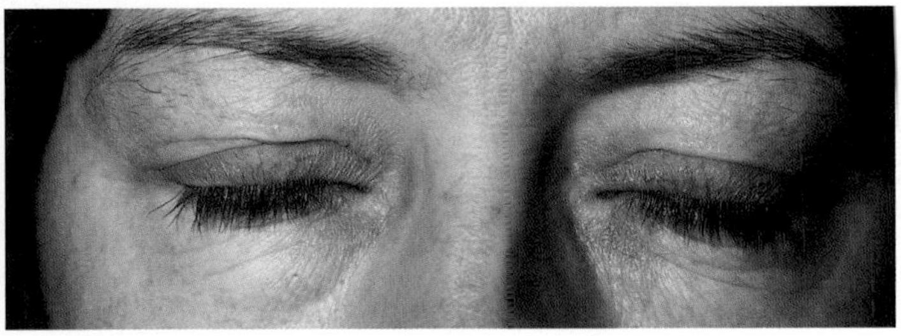

Fig. 1.246 Heliotrope (light purple) discoloration of the upper lids.

Other manifestations

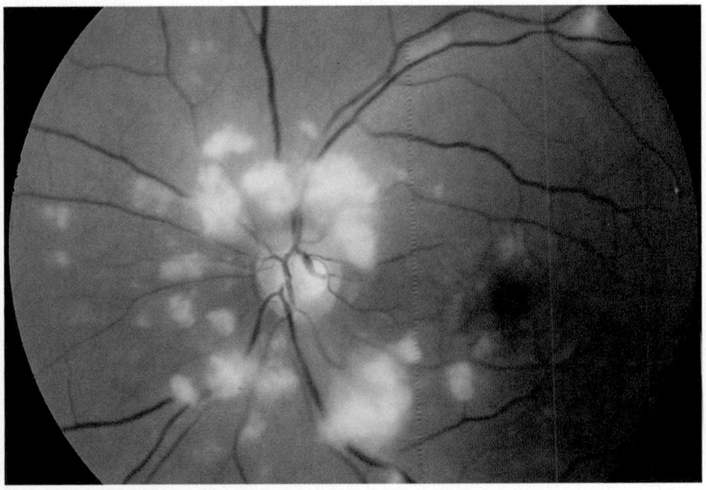

Fig. 1.247 Cotton-wool spots.

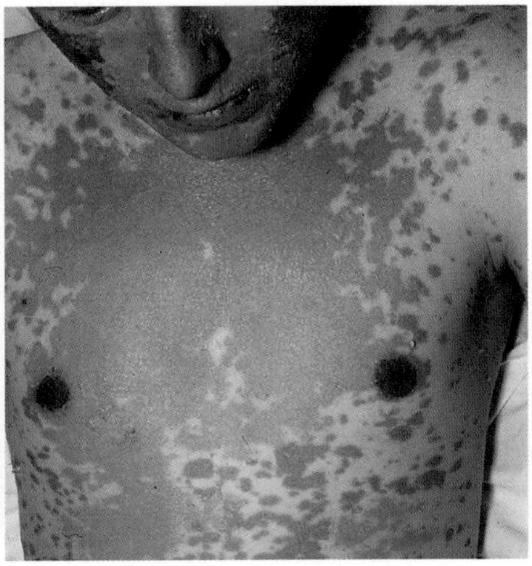

Fig. 1.248 Widespread erythematous rash.

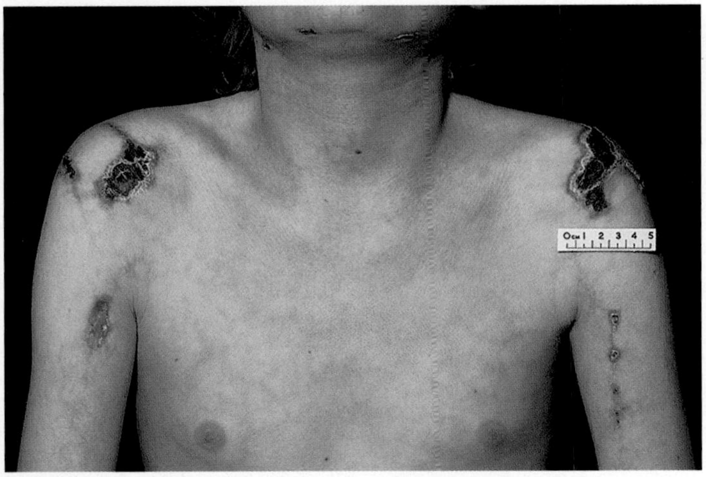

Fig. 1.249 Subcutaneous calcification and ulceration over bony prominences.

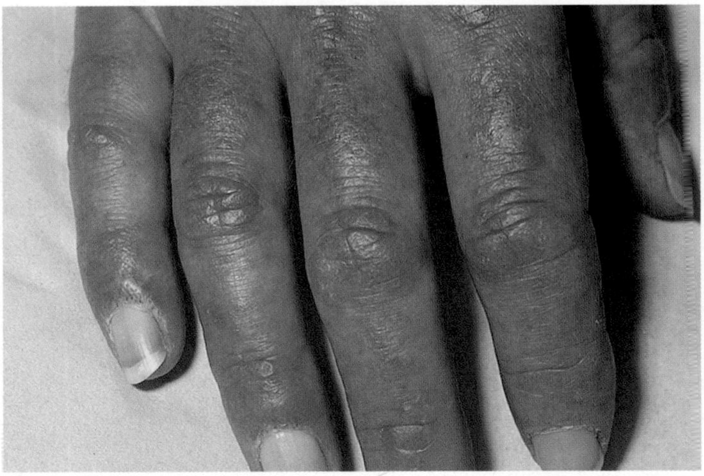

Fig. 1.250 Erythematous (colloidin) papules over finger joints.

Scleroderma

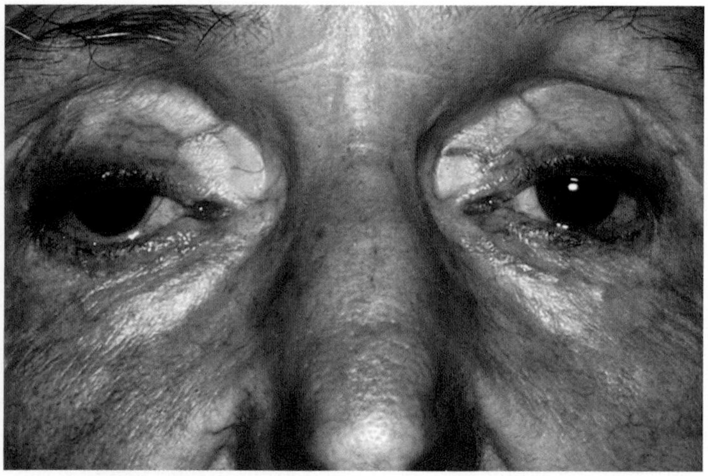

■ **Fig. 1.251** Firm, immobile eyelids.

Other manifestations

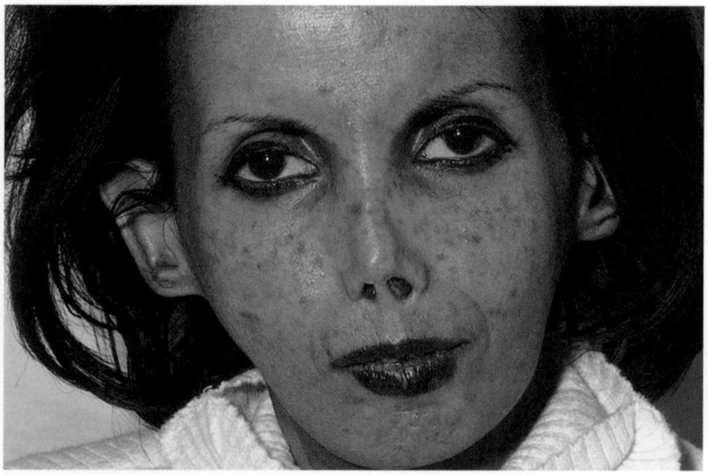

■ **Fig. 1.252** Fixed facial expression with restricted movements of the lips and a 'beaked' nose.

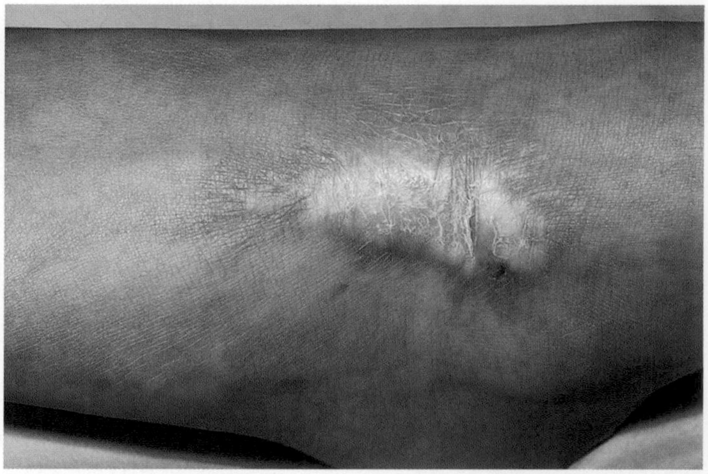

■ **Fig. 1.253** Waxy-appearing skin due to tightening and thickening.

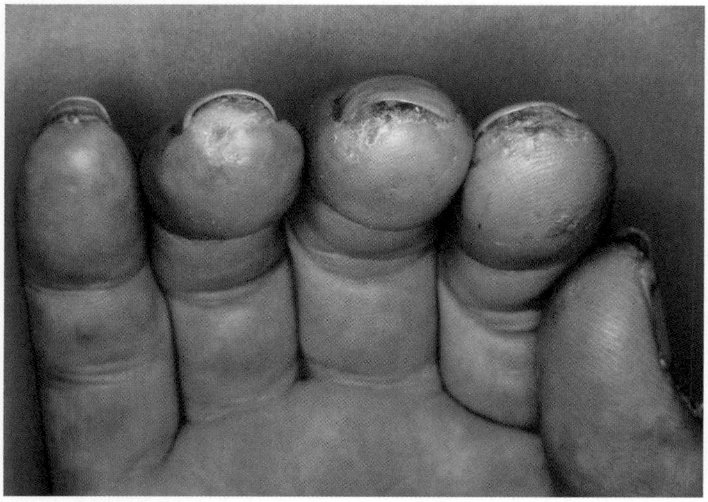

■ **Fig. 1.254** Tapering of the fingers with loss of pulps (sclerodactyly).

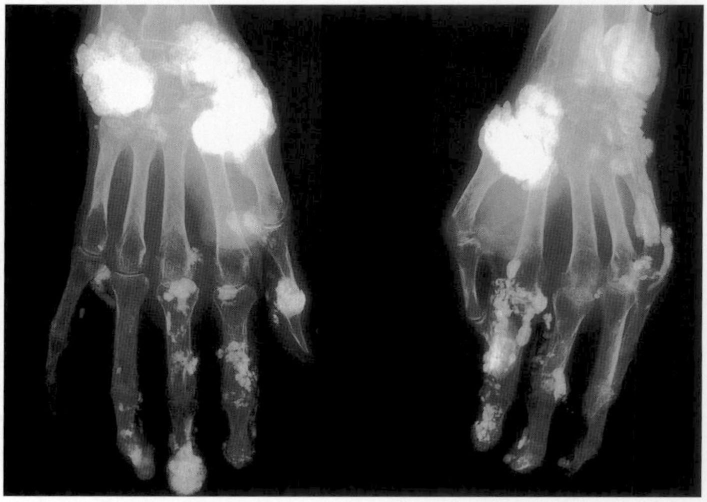

■ **Fig. 1.255** Subcutaneous calcinosis detectable on plain radiographs.

Myxoedema

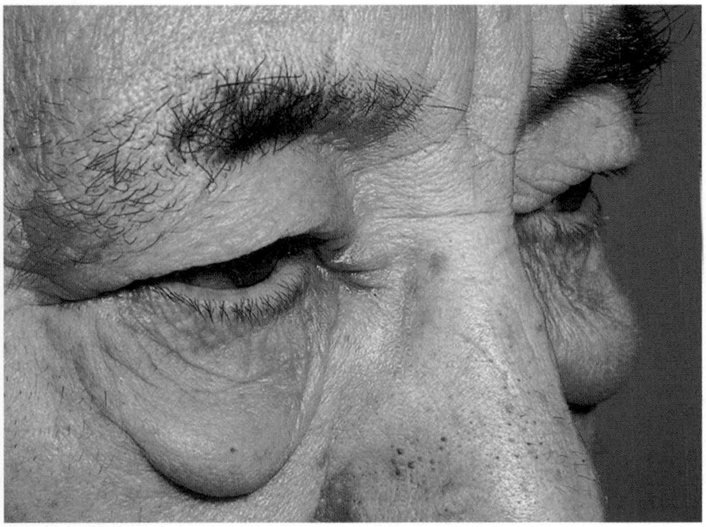

Fig. 1.256 Madarosis with puffy eyelids and face.

Other manifestations

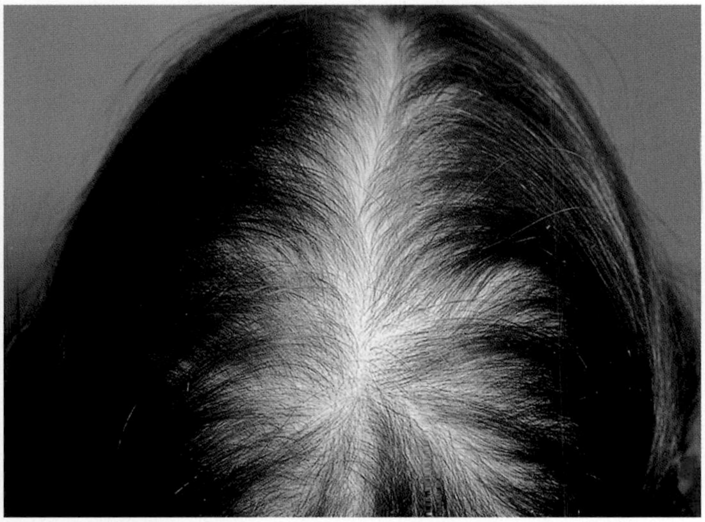

Fig. 1.257 Alopecia.

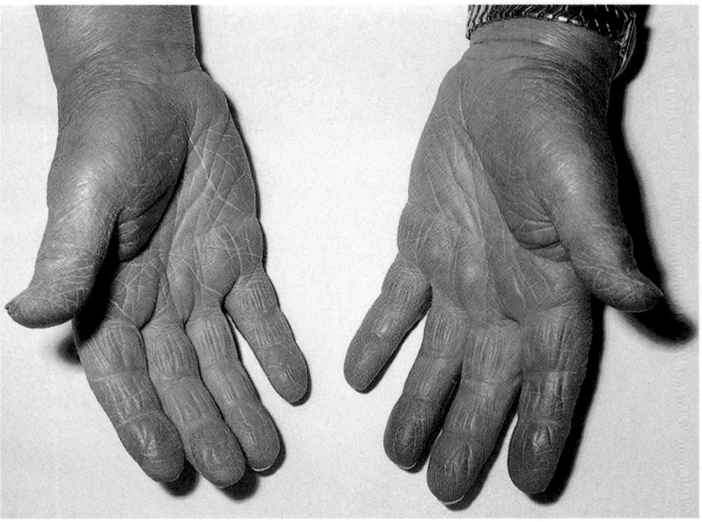

Fig. 1.258 Cold, dry skin.

Renal failure

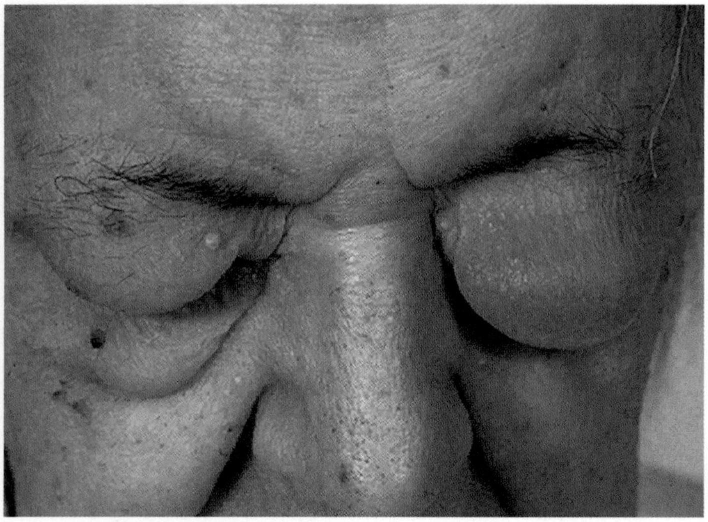

Fig. 1.259 Bilateral eyelid oedema. (Courtesy of S. Ford and R. Marsh.)

Other manifestations

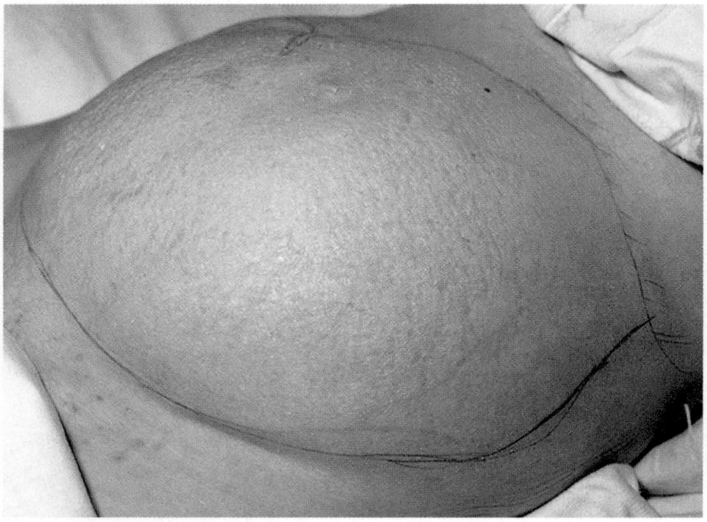

Fig. 1.260 Ascites and oedema.

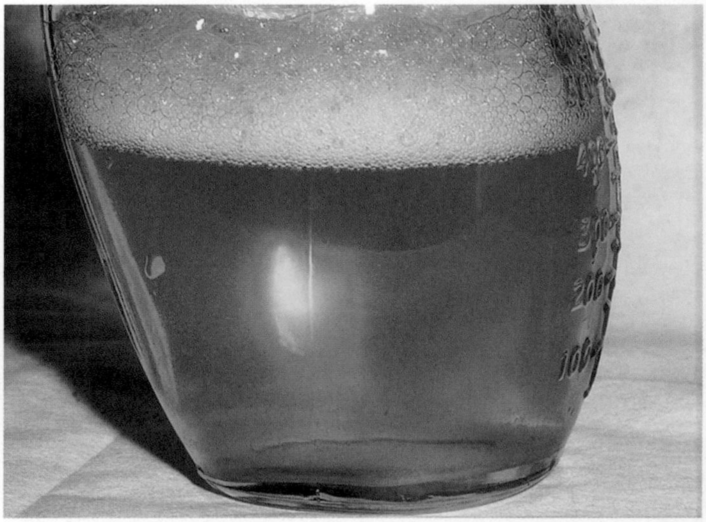

Fig. 1.261 Proteinuria and frothy urine.

MISCELLANEOUS CONGENITAL MALFORMATIONS

Epicanthic folds

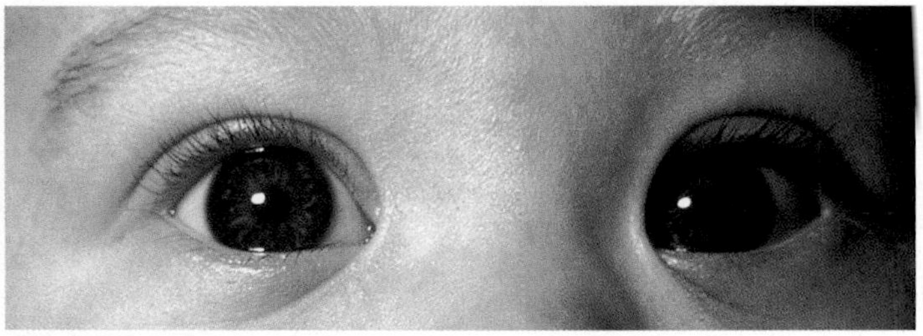

■ **Fig. 1.262** Bilateral vertical folds of skin that extend from the upper or lower lids towards the medial canthi.

Telecanthus

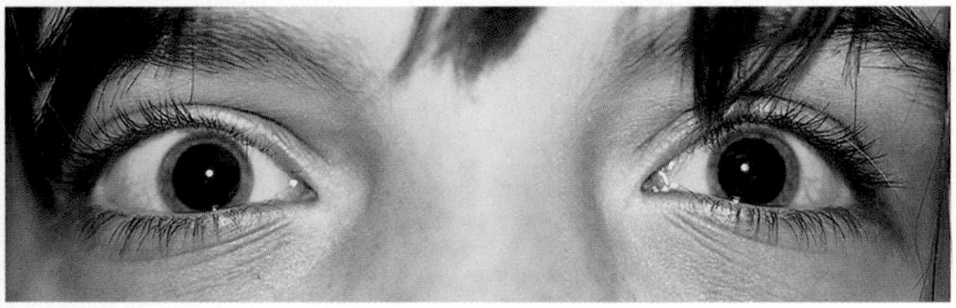

■ **Fig. 1.263** Increased distance between the medial canthi as a result of abnormally long medial canthal tendons. Telecanthus should not be confused with hypertelorism, in which there is wide separation of the orbits.

Epiblepharon

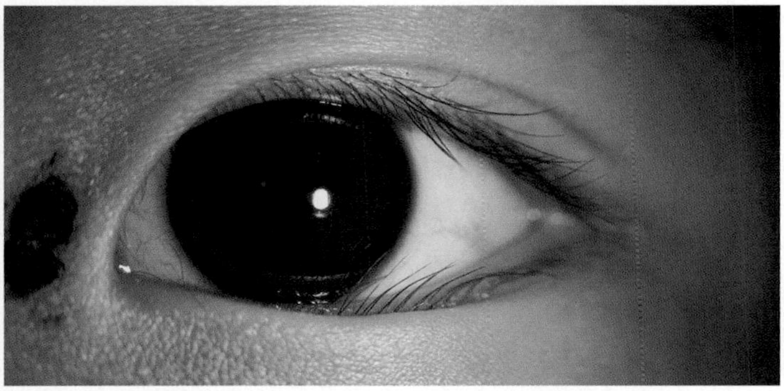

■ **Fig. 1.264** An extra horizontal fold of skin stretches across the anterior lid margin and the lashes are directed vertically, especially in the medial part of the lid.

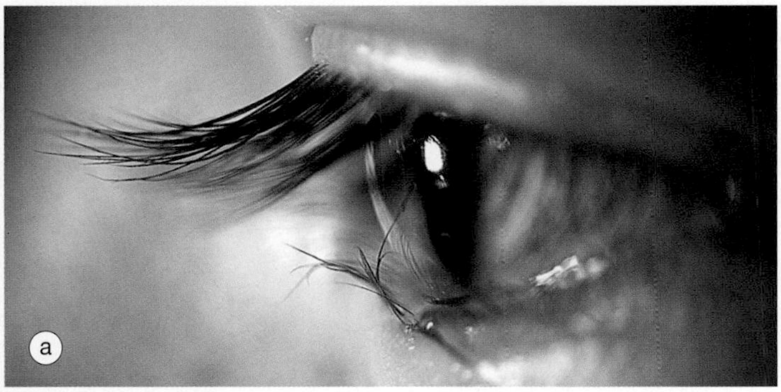

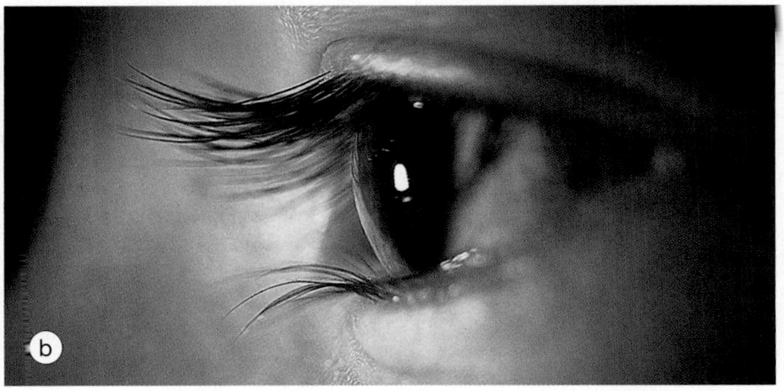

■ **Fig. 1.265** **(a)** Vertically pointing lashes. **(b)** When the fold of skin is pulled down the lashes turn out and the normal location of the lid becomes apparent. In congenital ectropion, however, the entire eyelid pulls away from the globe.

Coloboma

A coloboma is a congenital, unilateral or bilateral, partial or full-thickness eyelid defect.

Upper

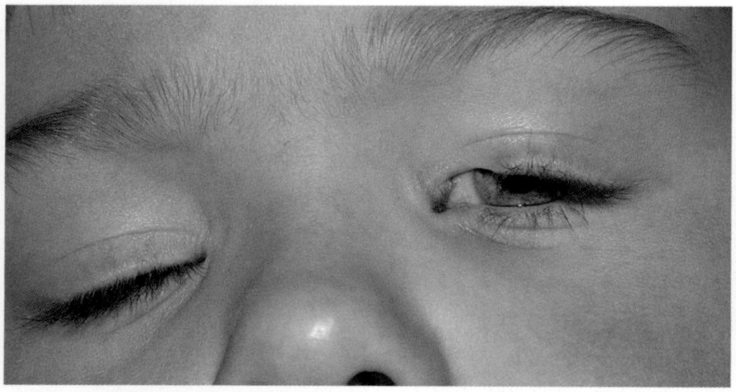

Fig. 1.266 This occurs at the junction of the middle and inner thirds of the eyelid and is not associated with systemic anomalies.

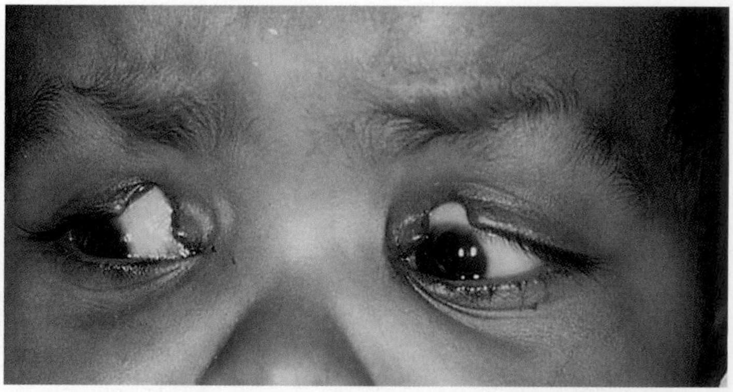

Fig. 1.267 Severe bilateral upper lid colobomas. (Courtesy of U. Raina.)

Lower

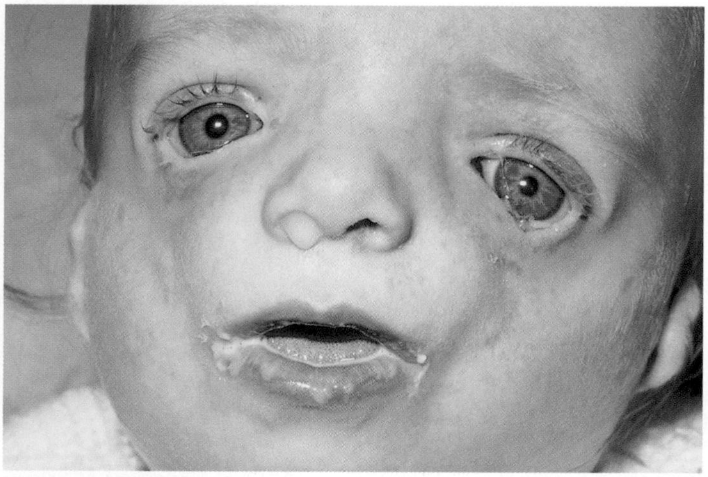

Fig. 1.268 This is bilateral, occurs at the junction of the middle and outer thirds of the eyelid and is frequently associated with systemic conditions, most notably Treacher Collins syndrome (shown here).

Euryblepharon

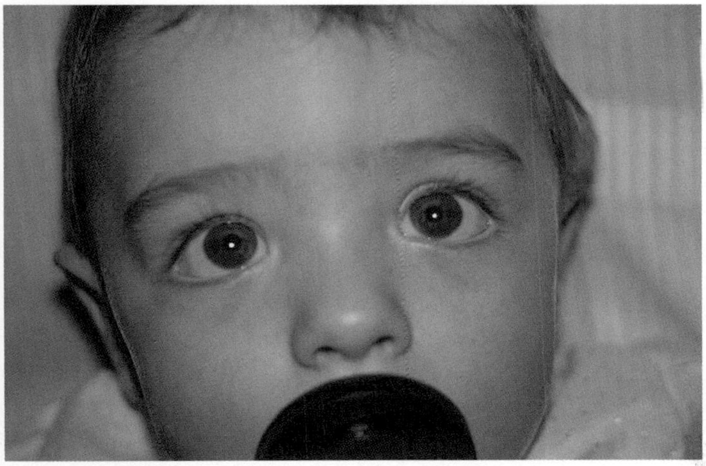

Fig. 1.269 Bilateral symmetrical enlargement of the palpebral fissures with downward displacement of the lower lids associated with downward and outward displacement of the lateral canthi. (Courtesy of J. Yangüela.)

Ankyloblepharon filiforme adnatum

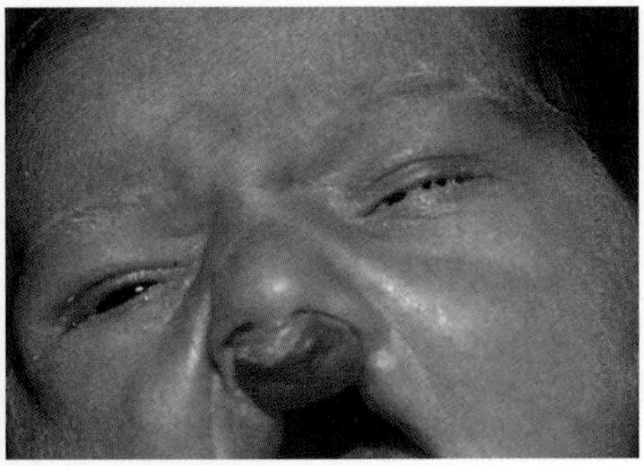

Fig. 1.270 Strands of tissue bridging the lid margins. (Courtesy of D. M. Albert and F. A. Jakobiec.)

Cryptophthalmos

Complete

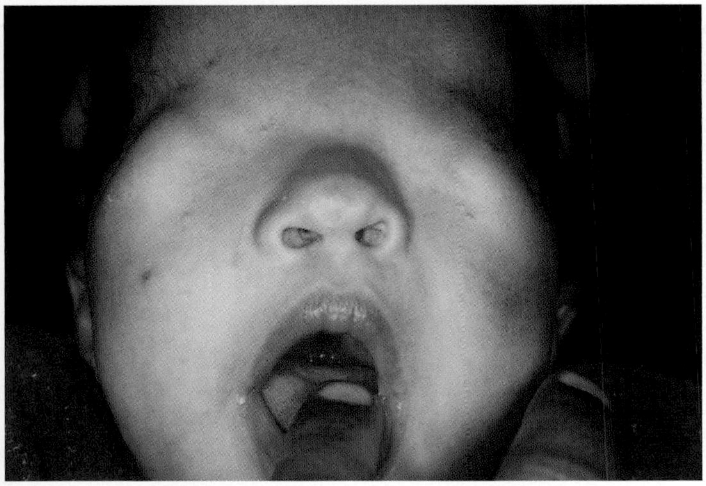

Fig. 1.271 Replacement of the lids by a layer of skin that is fused with a microphthalmic eye. (Courtesy of U. Raina).

Incomplete

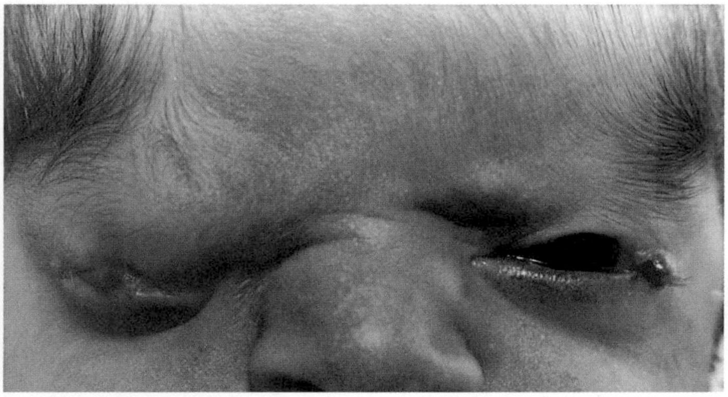

Fig. 1.272 Microphthalmos, rudimentary lids and a small conjunctival sac. It is often associated with Fraser syndrome, which is characterised by anomalies of the ears, genitalia and kidneys, syndactyly and mental handicap.

Microblepharon

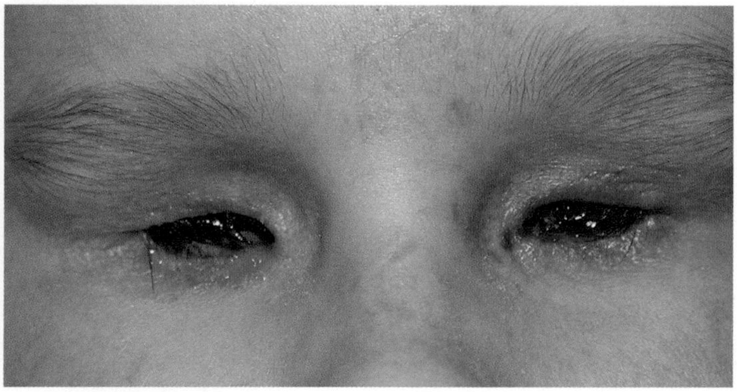

Fig. 1.273 Small eyelids, often associated with anophthalmos.

Ablepharon

Ablepharon is caused by deficiency of the anterior lamellae of the eyelids.

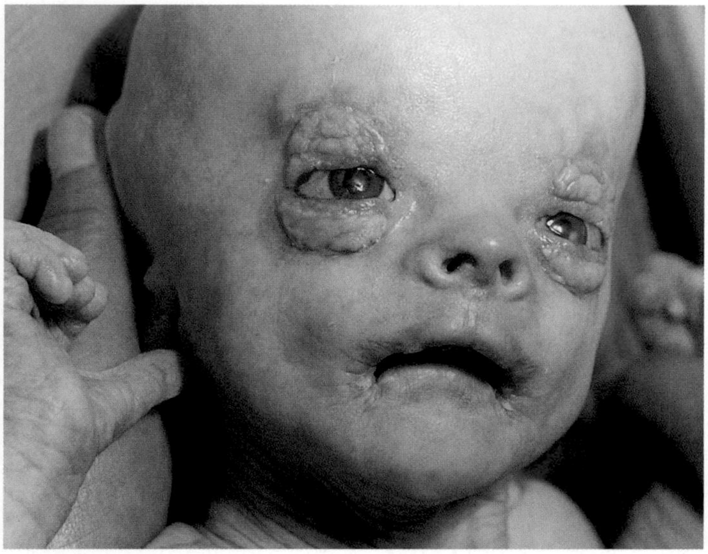

Fig. 1.274 A patient following reconstructive surgery who has the ablepharon–macrostomia syndrome characterised by an enlarged, fish-like mouth, ear and genital anomalies, and redundant skin (Courtesy of H. Mroczkowska.)

CHAPTER 2

ORBIT

GENERAL SIGNS

Proptosis

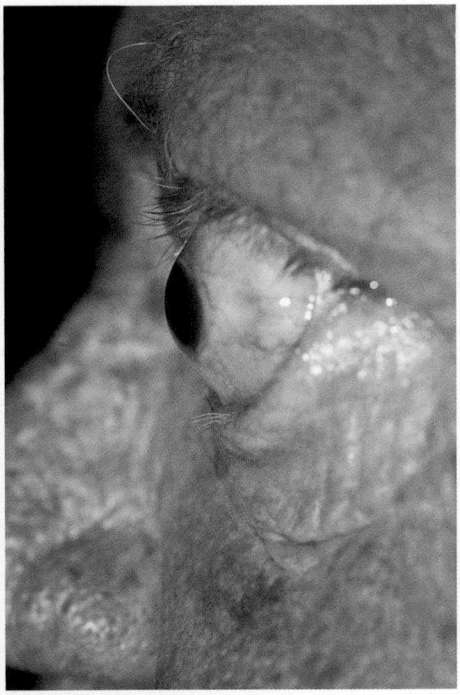

■ **Fig. 2.1** Proptosis is an abnormal protrusion of the globe. The two main causes are a retrobulbar mass and, less frequently, a shallow orbit.

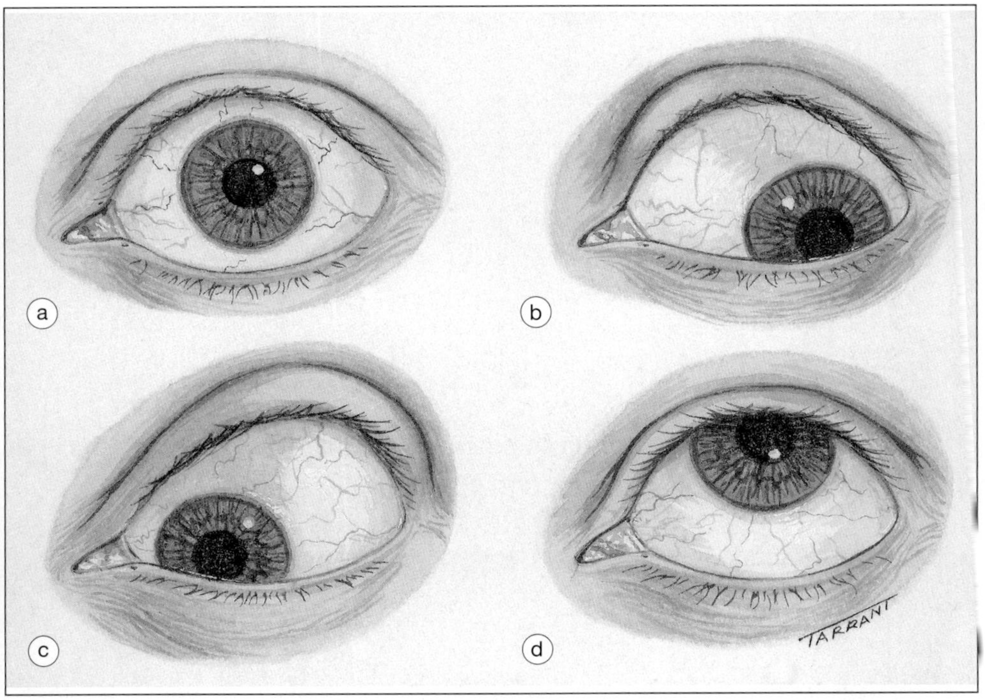

■ **Fig. 2.2** The direction of proptosis and/or displacement of the globe may indicate the possible pathology. For example: **(a)** space-occupying lesions within the muscle cone, such as cavernous haemangiomas and optic nerve tumours, will cause axial proptosis; **(b)** an anterior extraconal orbital lesion typically causes eccentric proptosis with displacement of the globe away from the location of the lesion; a superonasal mass will result in down and out displacement; **(c)** a superotemporal mass, such as a lacrimal gland tumour, will cause down and nasal displacement; **(d)** an inferior orbital mass will displace the globe upwards.

Pseudoproptosis

Pseudoproptosis is a false impression of proptosis which may be caused by the following:

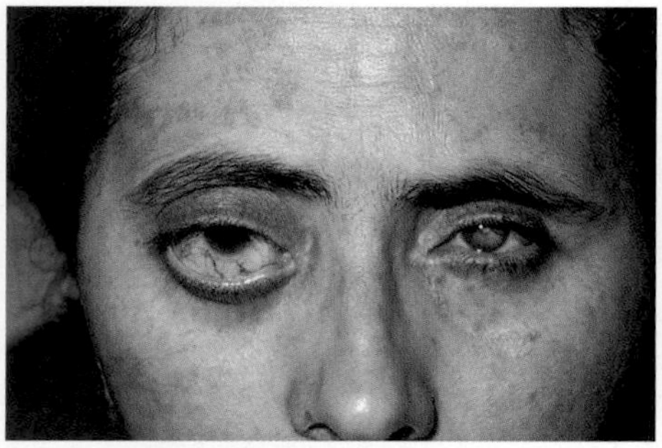

Fig. 2.3 Severe ipsilateral enlargement of the globe (e.g. high myopia or buphthalmos). This patient manifests right pseudoproptosis caused by a combination of a large globe due to myopia and phthisis of the left eye.

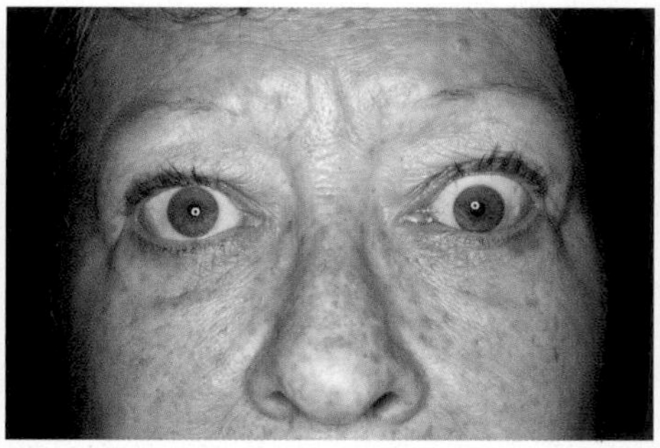

Fig. 2.4 Unilateral or asymmetrical lid retraction.

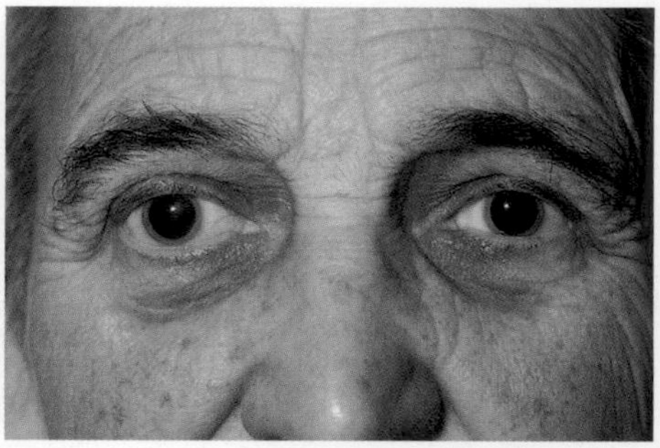

Fig. 2.5 Contralateral (left) enophthalmos.

Enophthalmos

Enophthalmos implies backward displacement of a normal globe within the orbit. Often subtle, it may be caused by the following:

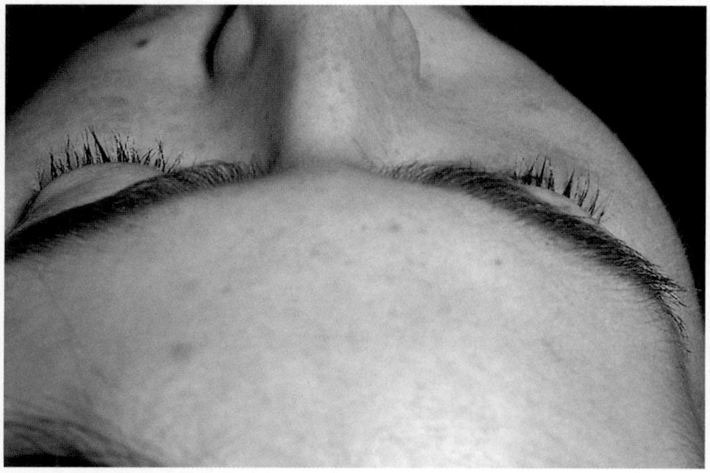

Fig. 2.6 Structural abnormalities of the orbital walls may be post-traumatic, such as blowout fractures of the orbital floor (shown here), or congenital.

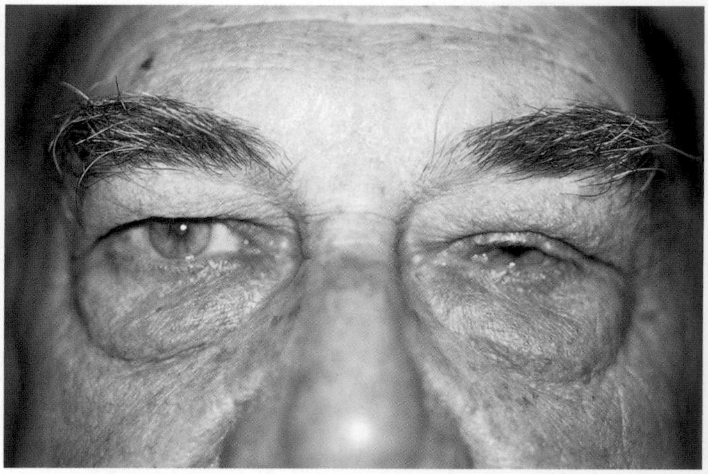

Fig. 2.7 Cicatrising orbital lesions such as metastatic schirrous carcinoma and chronic sclerosing inflammatory orbital disease.

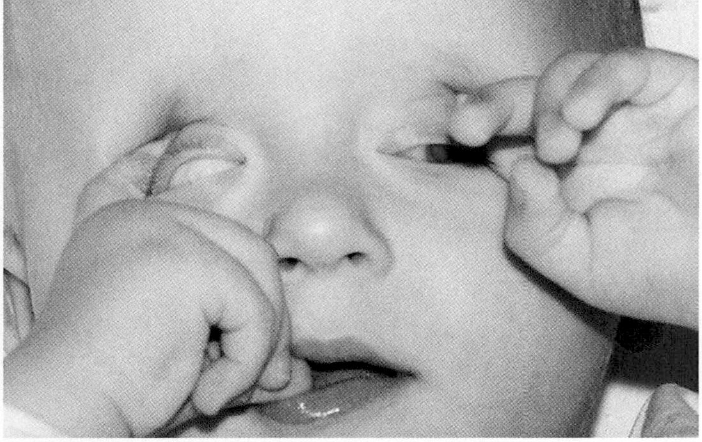

Fig. 2.8 Atrophy of orbital contents may be secondary to radiotherapy, scleroderma or eye poking (oculodigital sign) in a blind infant. (Courtesy of M. Szreter.)

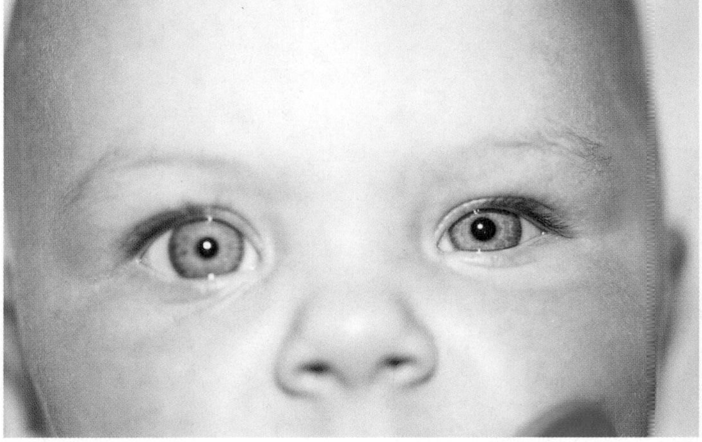

Fig. 2.9 Duane retraction syndrome manifests retraction of the globe on adduction. Occasionally there is also true enophthalmos in the primary position of gaze. (Courtesy of K. Nischal.)

Pseudo-enophthalmos

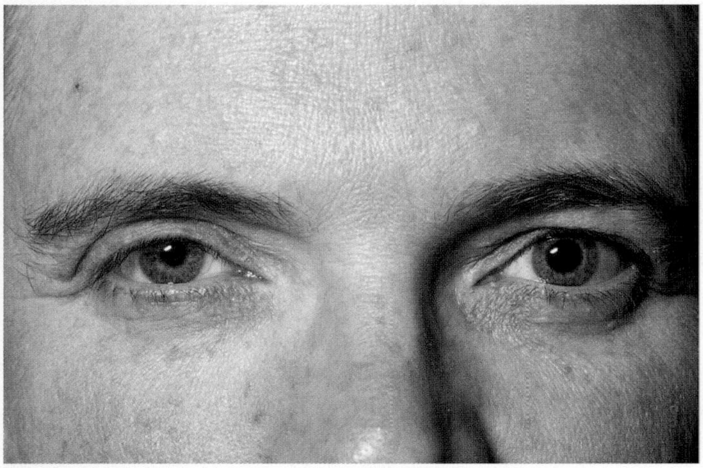

Fig. 2.10 Horner syndrome, in which ptosis combined with elevation of the lower lid gives rise to apparent enophthalmos.

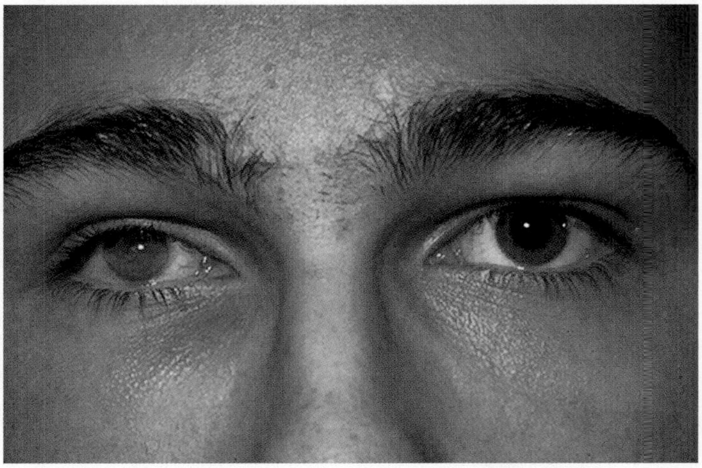

Fig. 2.11 A small or shrunken globe that cannot support the eyelids. (Courtesy of S. Ford and R. Marsh.)

THYROID DISEASE

Thyroid disease may involve the intraorbital contents, eyelids, conjunctiva and periorbital soft tissues.

Eye signs

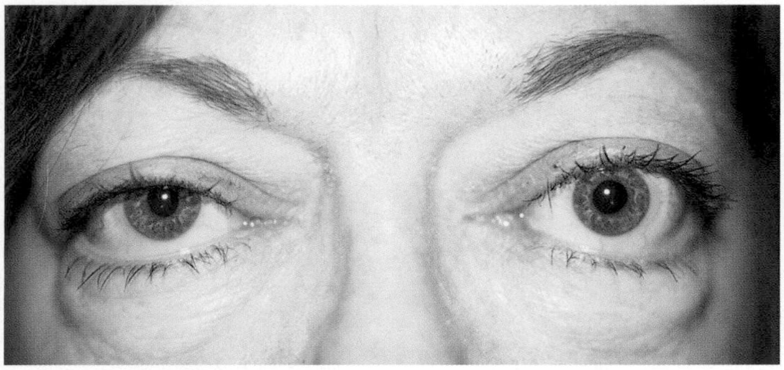

■ **Fig. 2.12** Mild, unilateral lid retraction and mild bilateral periorbital swelling.

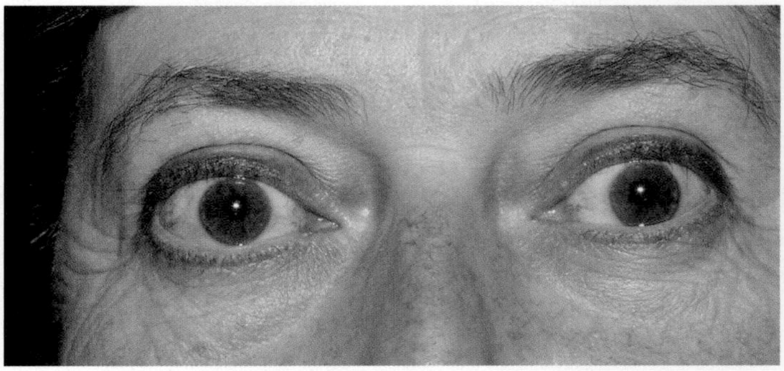

■ **Fig. 2.13** Mild, symmetrical lid retraction. (Courtesy of G. Rose.)

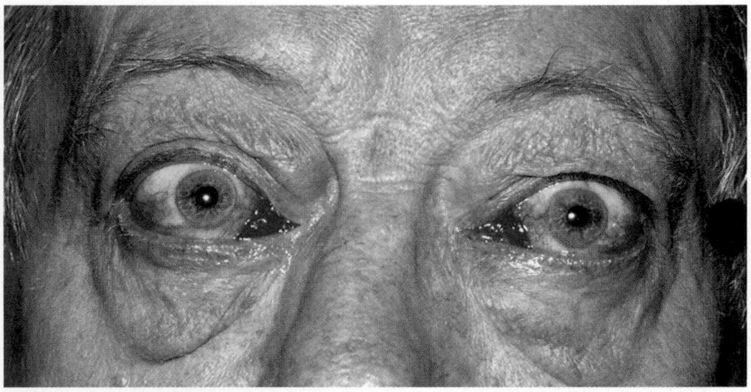

■ **Fig. 2.14** Moderate, symmetrical lid retraction and moderate periorbital swelling. (Courtesy of G. Rose.)

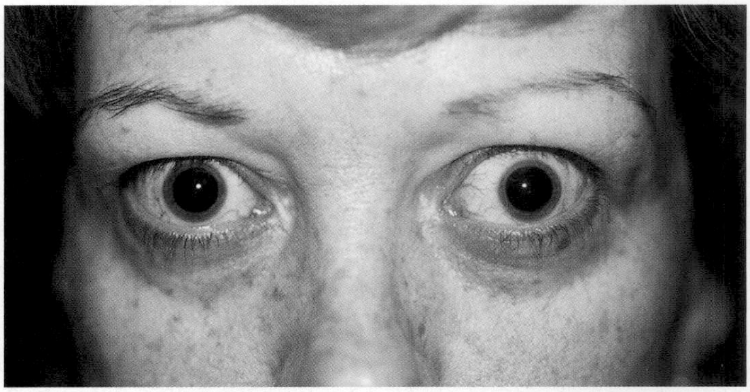

■ **Fig. 2.15** Asymmetrical lid retraction: mild right and moderate left.

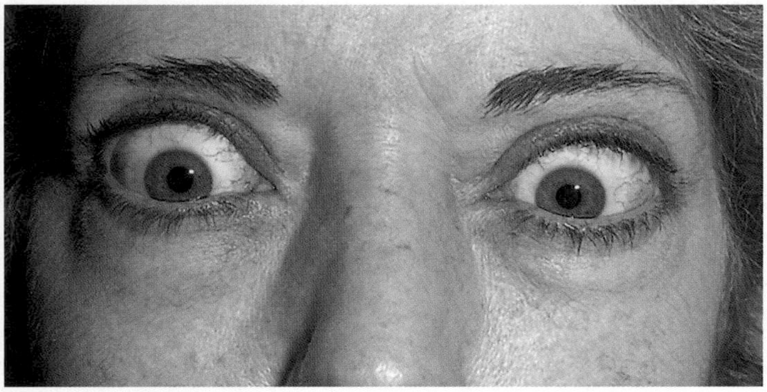

■ **Fig. 2.16** Severe, symmetrical lid retraction giving rise to frightened appearance (Kocher sign).

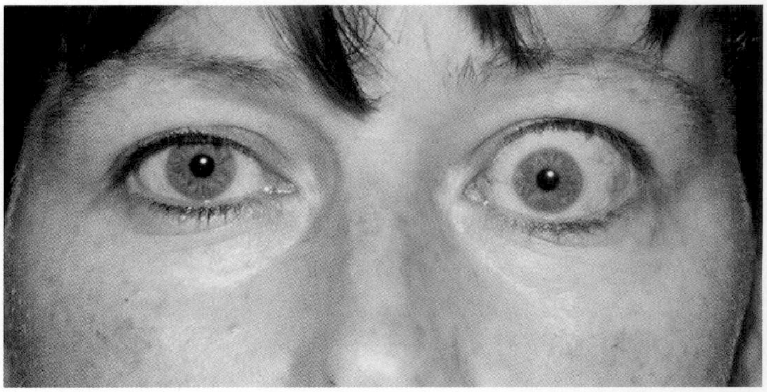

■ **Fig. 2.17** Severe, unilateral lid retraction. (Courtesy of G. Rose.)

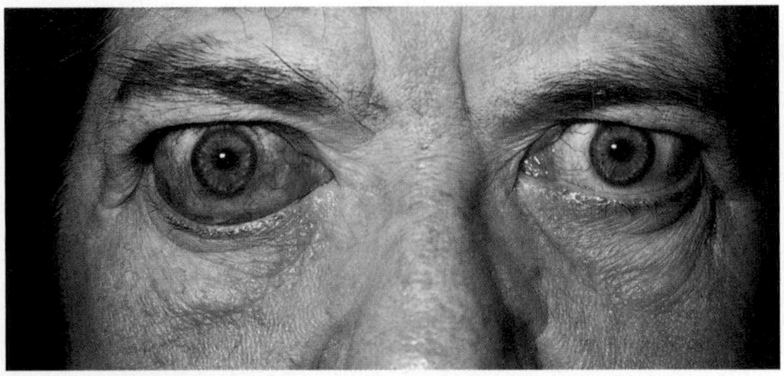

■ **Fig. 2.18** Moderate, unilateral lid retraction, proptosis and conjunctival hyperaemia.

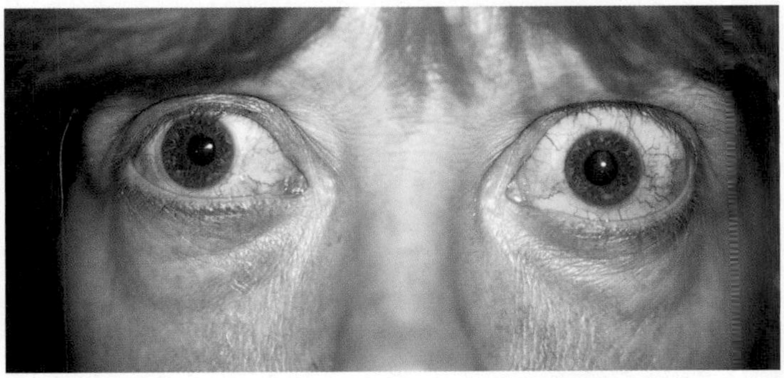

■ **Fig. 2.19** Asymmetrical lid retraction and proptosis.

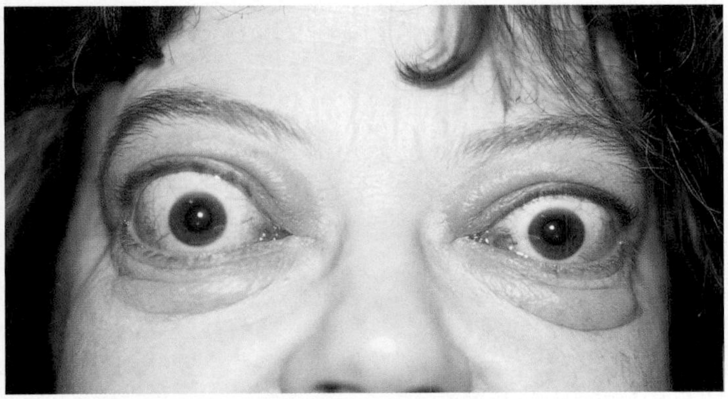

■ **Fig. 2.20** Moderate, symmetrical lid retraction, proptosis and periorbital oedema.

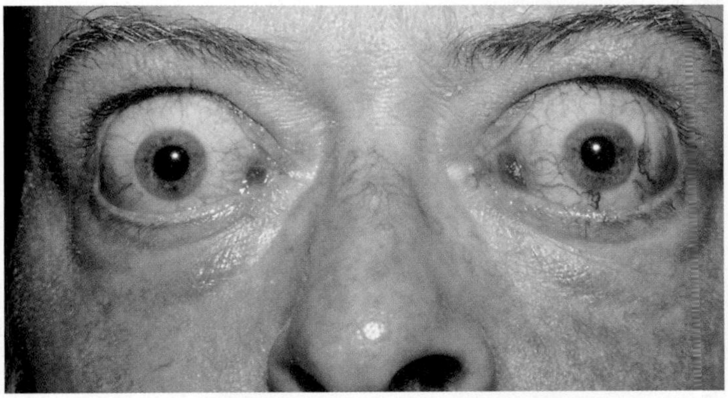

■ **Fig. 2.21** Very severe, symmetrical, lid retraction and proptosis; conjunctival injection is worse in the left eye. (Courtesy of G. Rose.)

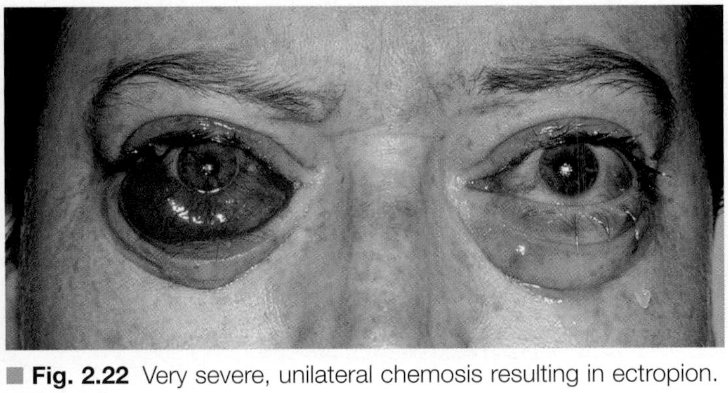

■ **Fig. 2.22** Very severe, unilateral chemosis resulting in ectropion.

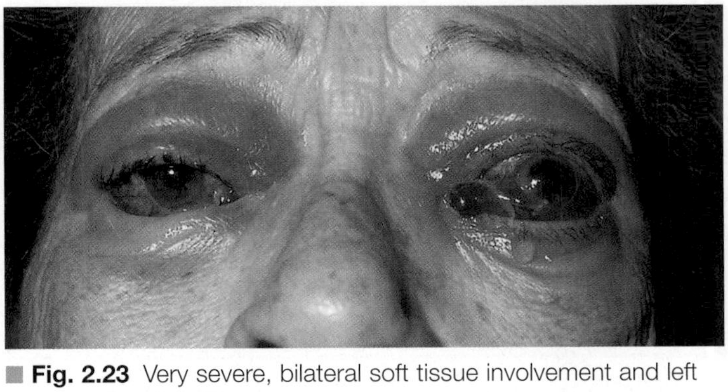

■ **Fig. 2.23** Very severe, bilateral soft tissue involvement and left exposure keratopathy.

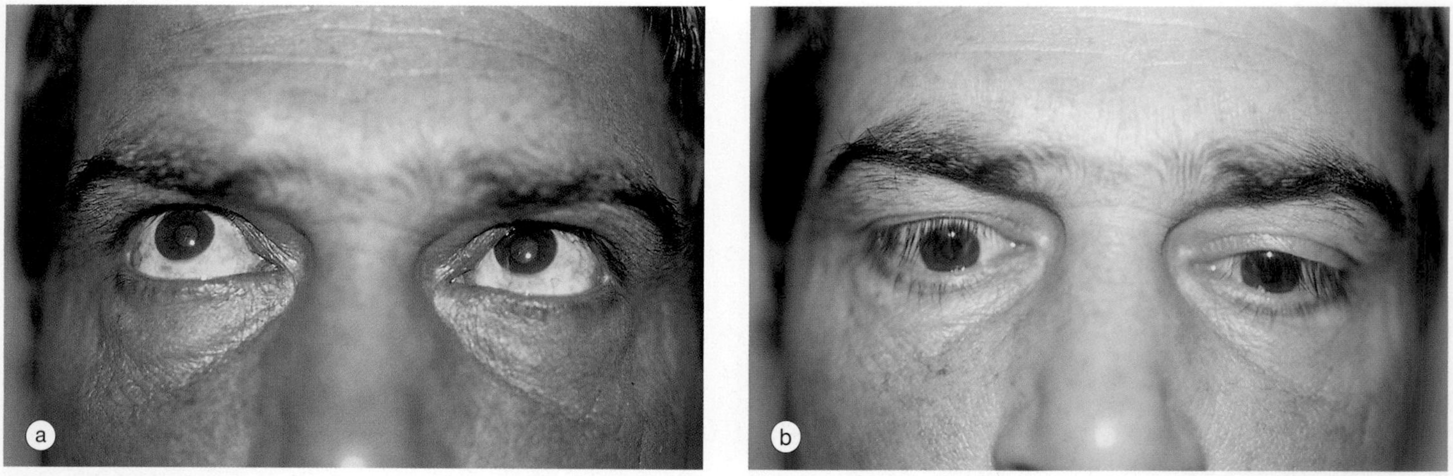

Fig. 2.24 Retarded descent of the right upper lid on downgaze (von Graefe sign).

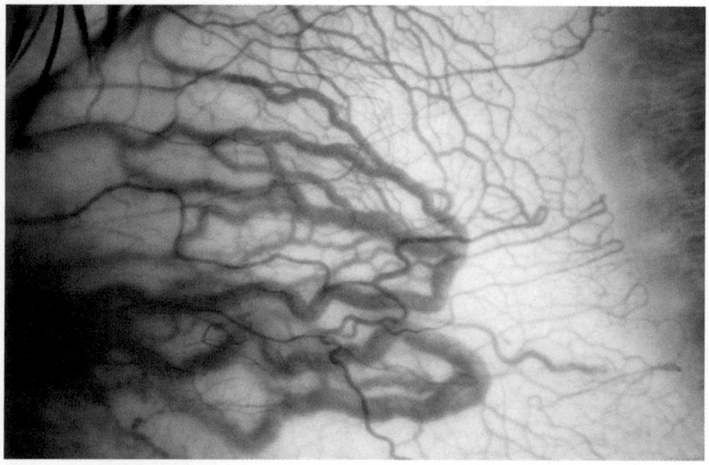

Fig. 2.25 Conjunctival and episcleral hyperaemia over a lateral rectus muscle in active disease.

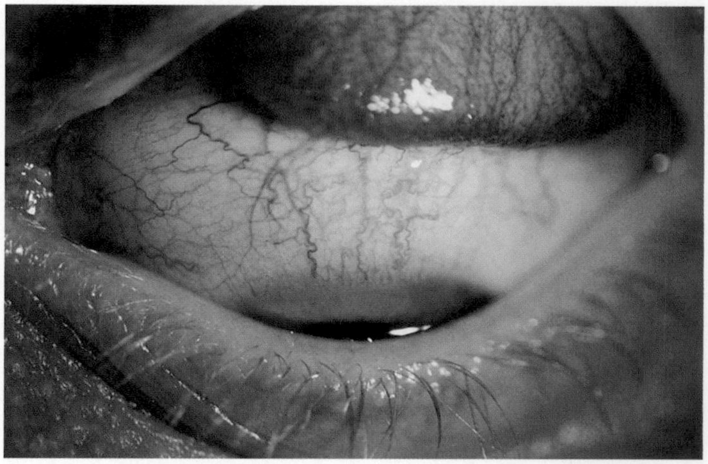

Fig. 2.26 Superior limbic keratoconjunctivitis is common in active disease.

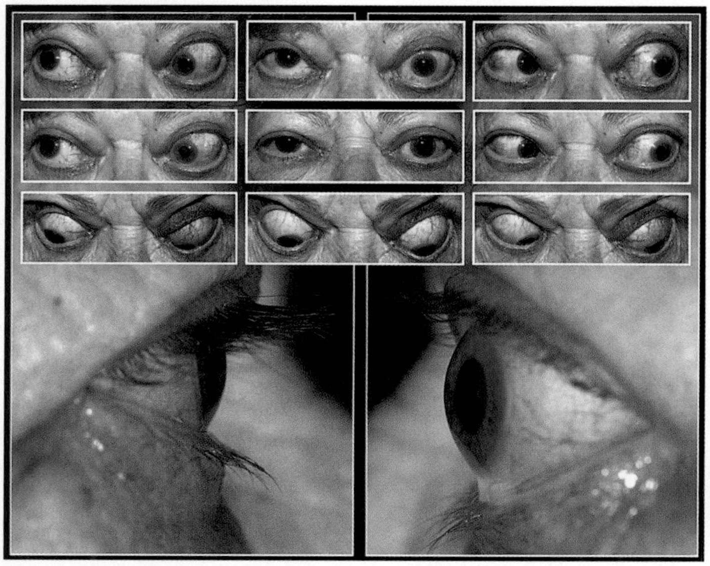

Fig. 2.27 Restrictive myopathy resulting mainly in defective elevation of both eyes; also note left superior limbic keratoconjunctivitis. (Courtesy of C. Barry.)

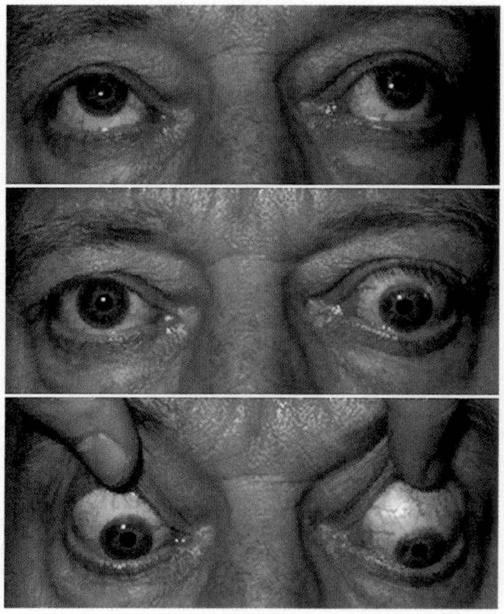

Fig. 2.28 Restrictive myopathy resulting in defective elevation and depression mainly involving the right eye. (Courtesy of S. Ford and R. Marsh.)

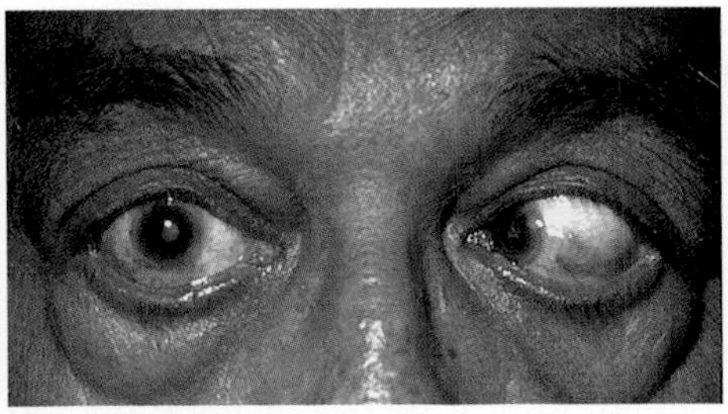

Fig. 2.29 Restricted right abduction due to fibrosis of the right medial rectus. (Courtesy of S. Ford and R. Marsh.)

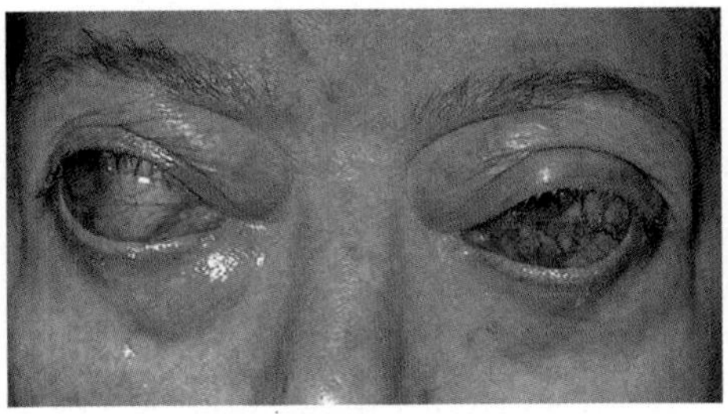

Fig. 2.30 Restricted left adduction due to fibrosis of the left lateral rectus. (Courtesy of S. Ford and R. Marsh.)

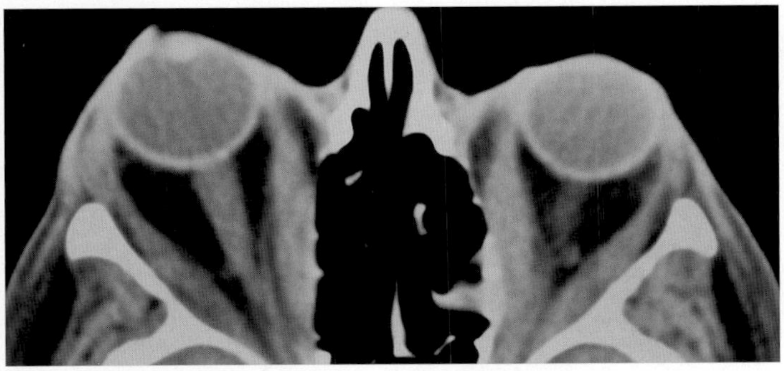

Fig. 2.31 Axial CT shows muscle enlargement and right proptosis in thyroid eye disease. (Courtesy of A. Pearson.)

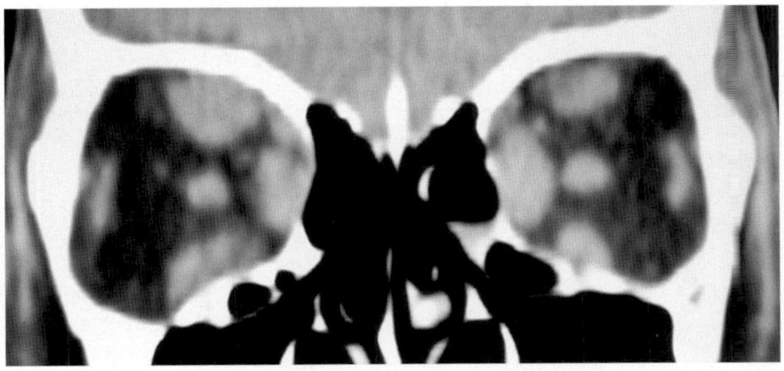

Fig. 2.32 Coronal CT shows muscle enlargement in thyroid eye disease. (Courtesy of A. Pearson.)

Systemic signs

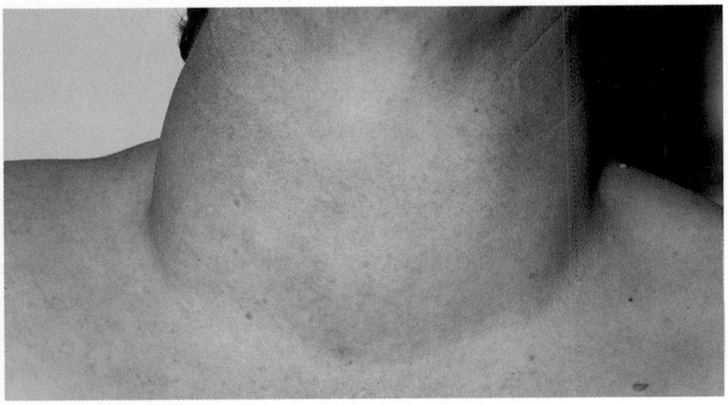

Fig. 2.33 Severe diffuse thyroid enlargement.

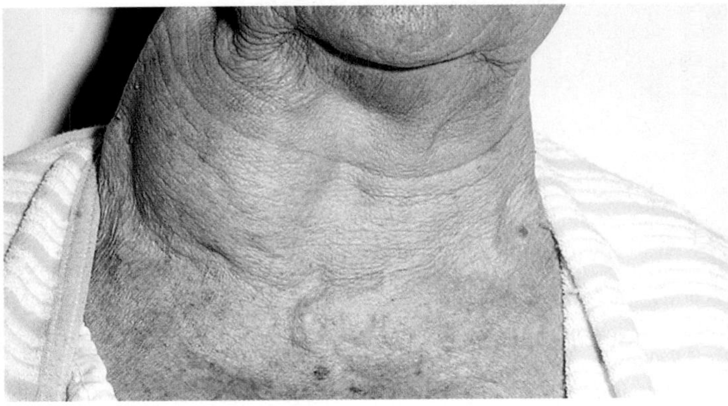

Fig. 2.34 Severe nodular thyroid enlargement suggestive of malignancy.

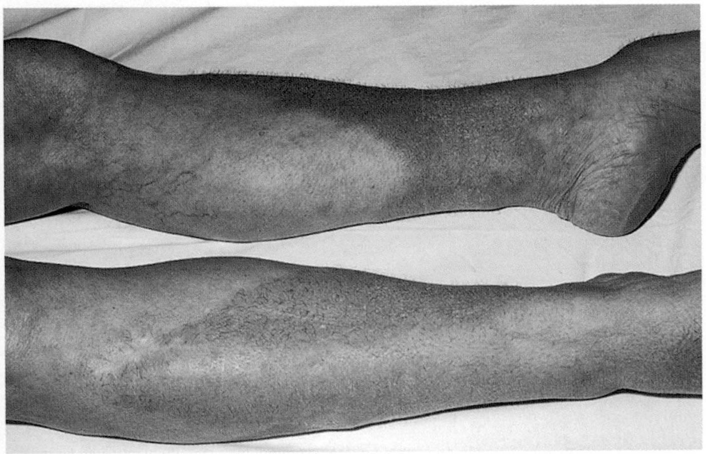

Fig. 2.35 Pretibial myxoedema is characterised by bilateral, raised lesions over the shins; the overlying skin is shiny and has an orange peel appearance.

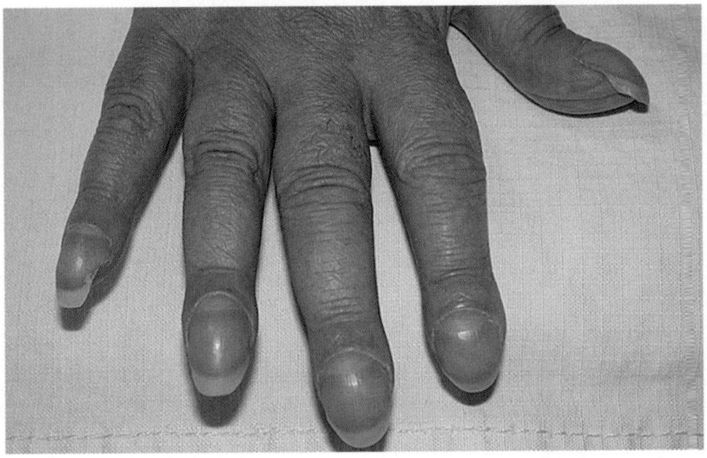

Fig. 2.36 Thyroid acropachy is characterised by increased in nail curvature and swelling of the terminal phalanges.

INFECTIONS

Preseptal cellulitis

Preseptal cellulitis is an infection of the subcutaneous tissues anterior to the orbital septum. It must be differentiated from the much less common but potentially more serious orbital cellulitis.

Pyogenic

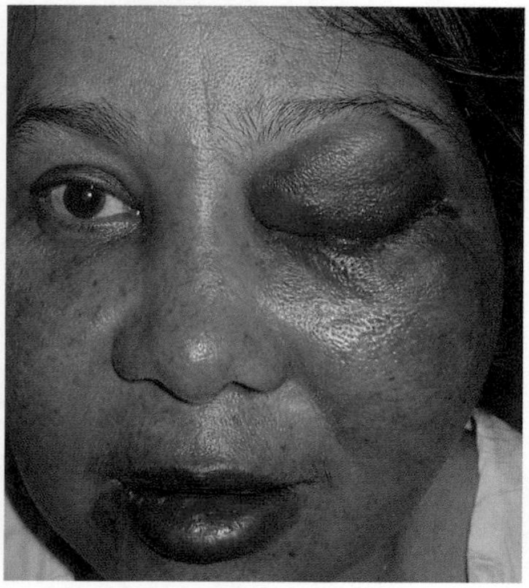

Fig. 2.37 Unilateral, tender, red periorbital oedema. Unlike orbital cellulitis proptosis is absent; visual acuity, pupillary reactions and ocular motility are unimpaired. (Courtesy of A. Pearson.)

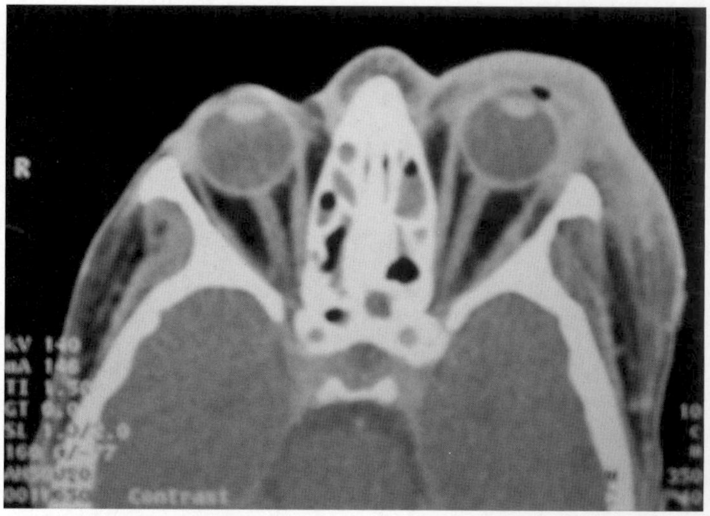

Fig. 2.38 Axial CT shows opacification anterior to the orbital septum. (Courtesy of A. Pearson.)

Tubercular

Preseptal cellulitis can be the presenting feature of tuberculosis and a marker for an underlying systemic focus in children.

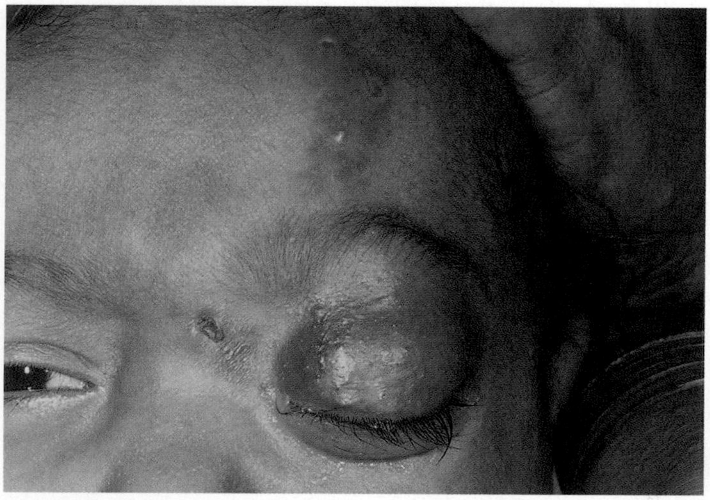

Fig. 2.39 Swelling of the upper lid and multiple discharging sinuses on the forehead and root of the nose. (Courtesy of U. Raina.)

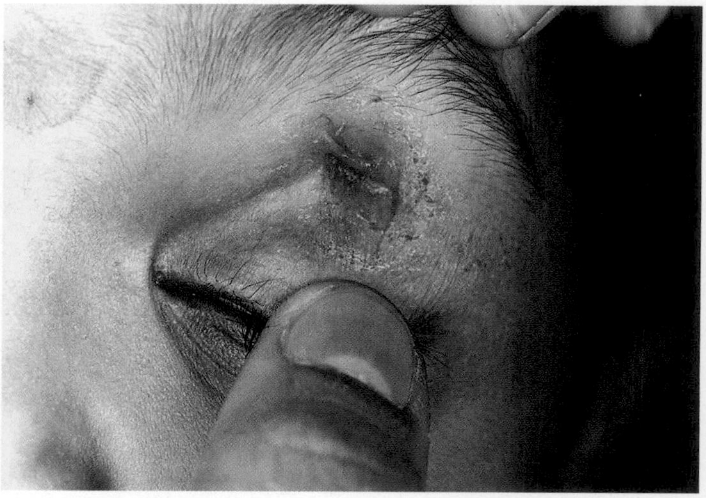

Fig. 2.40 Discharging sinus of the upper lid and tethering of the overlying skin. (Courtesy of U. Raina.)

Bacterial orbital cellulitis

Bacterial orbital cellulitis is a life-threatening infection of the soft tissues behind the orbital septum. The most common causative organisms are *Streptococcus pneumoniae*, *Staphylococcus aureus*, *Streptococcus pyogenes* and *Haemophilus influenzae*.

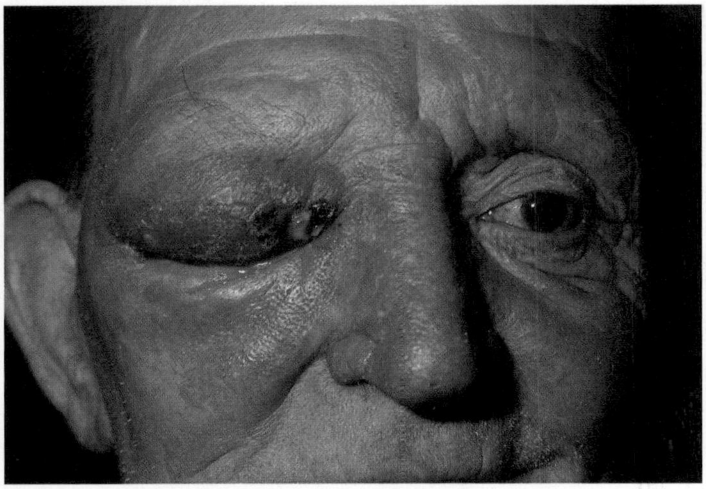

Fig. 2.41 Severe, unilateral, tender, warm and red periorbital swelling.

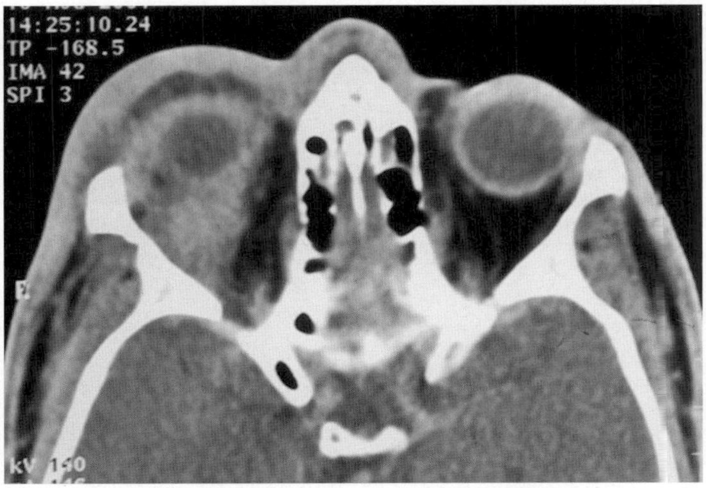

Fig. 2.42 Axial CT shows orbital involvement. (Courtesy of A. Pearson.)

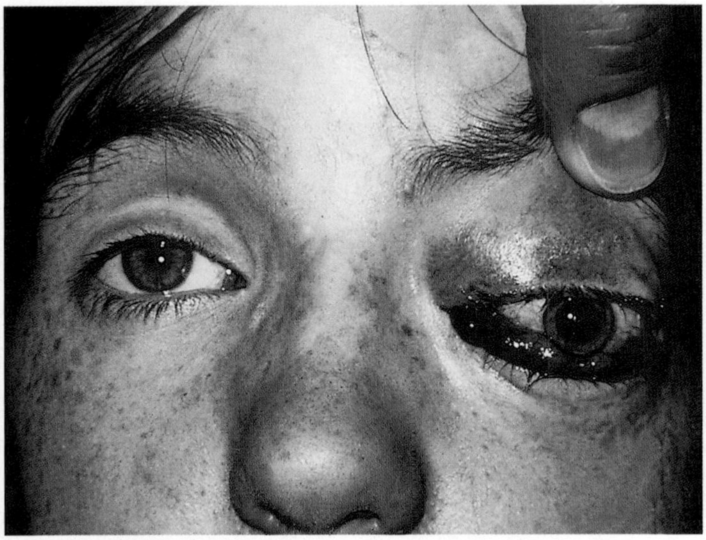

Fig. 2.43 Proptosis, often obscured by lid swelling, is most frequently out and down.

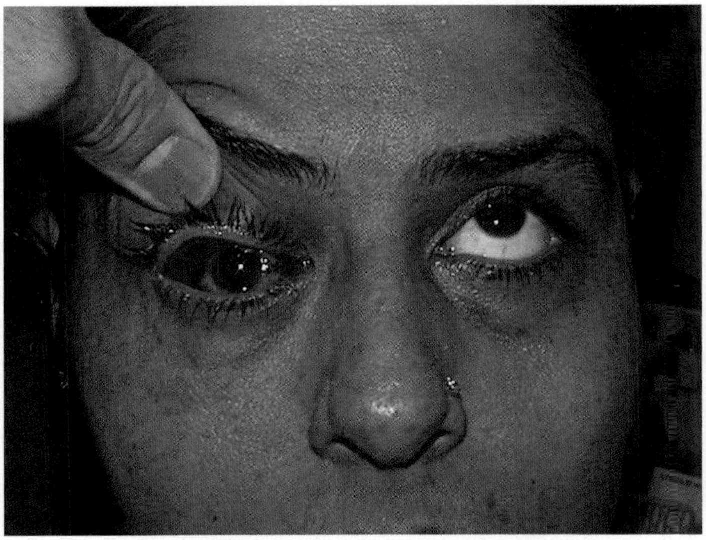

Fig. 2.44 Painful ophthalmoplegia. (Courtesy of U. Raina.)

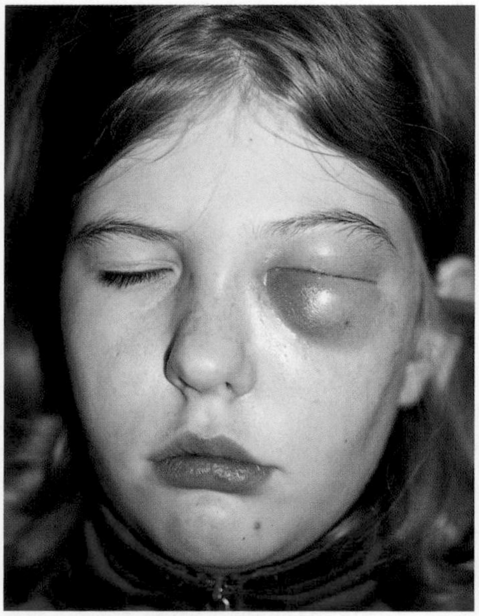

Fig. 2.45 In children orbital cellulitis is often secondary to ethmoidal sinusitis.

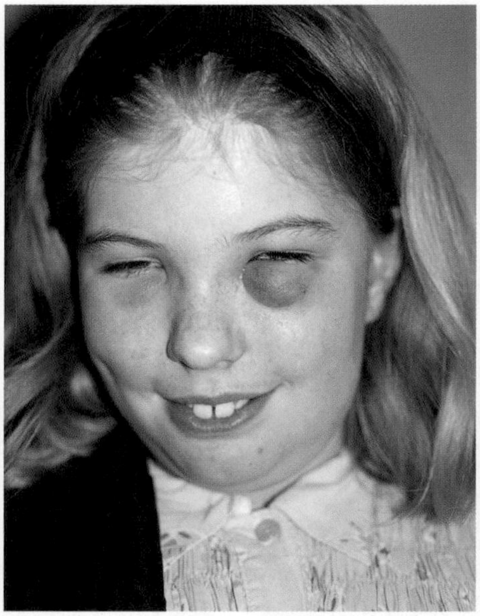

Fig. 2.46 Appearance 4 days later following a good response to treatment.

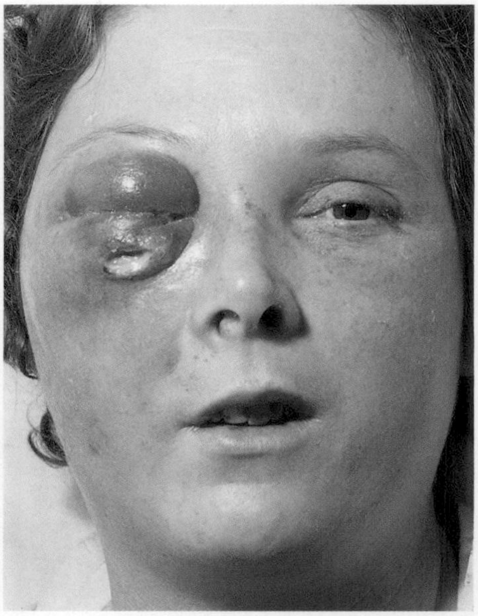

Fig. 2.47 Orbital abscess is uncommon in sinus-related orbital cellulitis but may occur in post-traumatic or postoperative cases.

Rhino-orbital mucormycosis

Mucormycosis is a very rare opportunistic infection caused by fungi of the family *Mucoraceae*, which typically affects patients with diabetic ketoacidosis or immunosuppression.

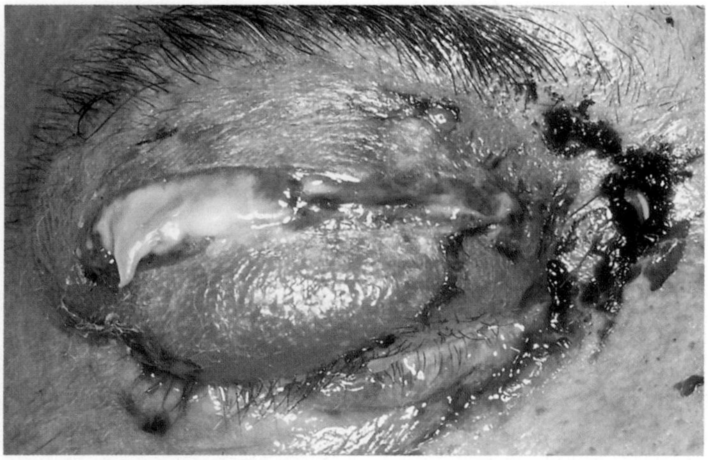

Fig. 2.48 Ischaemic infarction superimposed on septic necrosis is responsible for the black eschar that may develop on the palate, turbinates, nasal septum, skin and eyelids.

ORBITAL INFLAMMATORY DISEASE

Idiopathic orbital inflammatory disease

Idiopathic orbital inflammatory disease (IOID), previously referred to as orbital pseudotumour, is an uncommon disorder characterised by non-neoplastic, non-infectious, space-occupying orbital lesions.

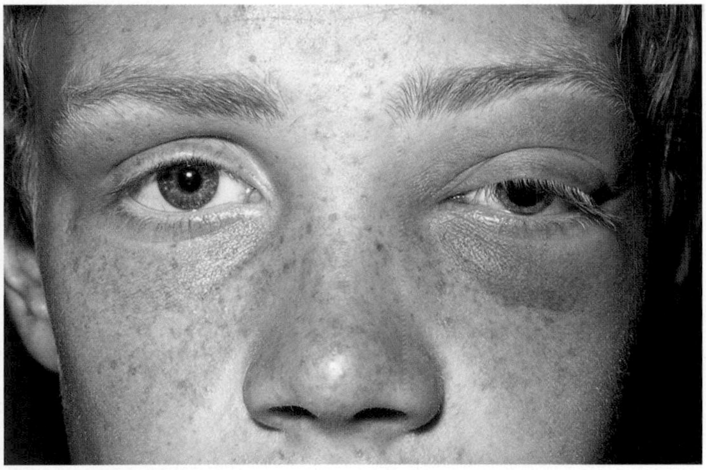

Fig. 2.49 Presentation is in the third to sixth decade with acute redness, swelling and pain, which is usually unilateral.

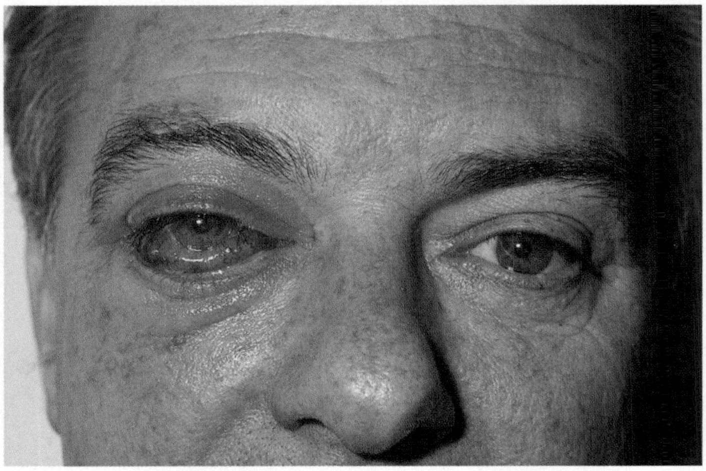

Fig. 2.50 More severe involvement with chemosis.

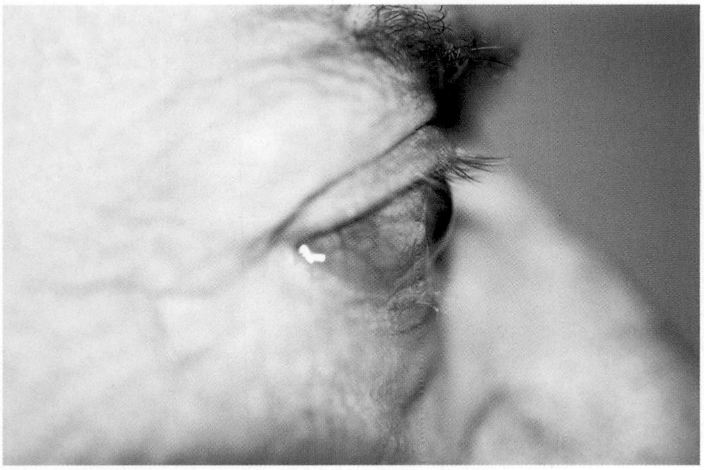

Fig. 2.51 Congestive axial proptosis and ophthalmoplegia may occur.

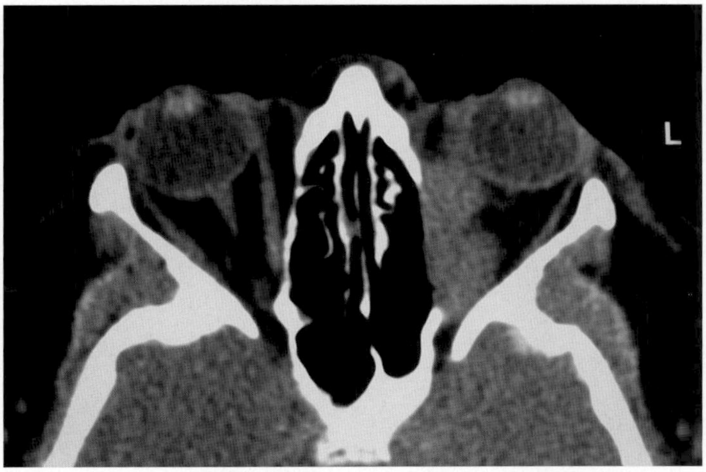

Fig. 2.52 Axial CT shows an ill-defined opacity and loss of definition of orbital contents. (Courtesy of A. Pearson.)

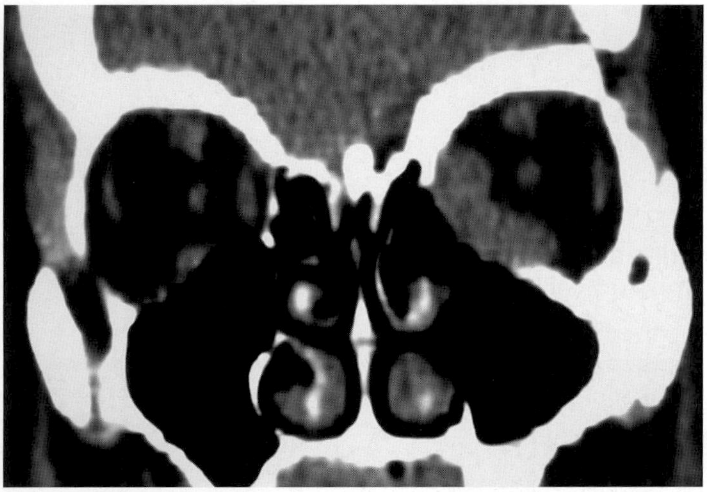

Fig. 2.53 Coronal CT of the same patient. (Courtesy of A. Pearson.)

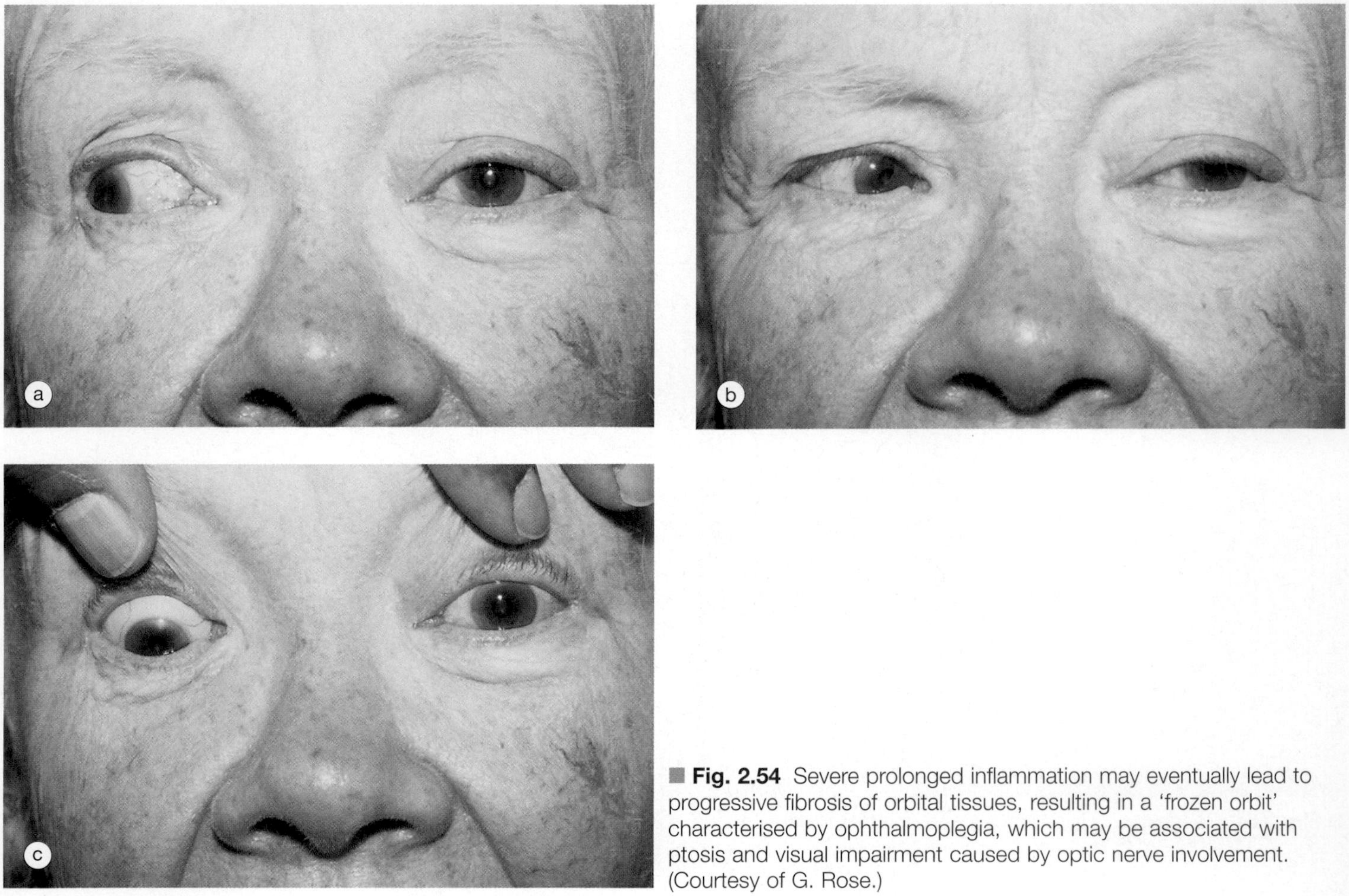

Fig. 2.54 Severe prolonged inflammation may eventually lead to progressive fibrosis of orbital tissues, resulting in a 'frozen orbit' characterised by ophthalmoplegia, which may be associated with ptosis and visual impairment caused by optic nerve involvement. (Courtesy of G. Rose.)

Acute dacryoadenitis

Lacrimal gland involvement occurs in about 25% of patients with IOID. More commonly, however, dacryoadenitis occurs in isolation, resolves spontaneously and does not require treatment. Presentation is with acute discomfort in the region of the lacrimal gland.

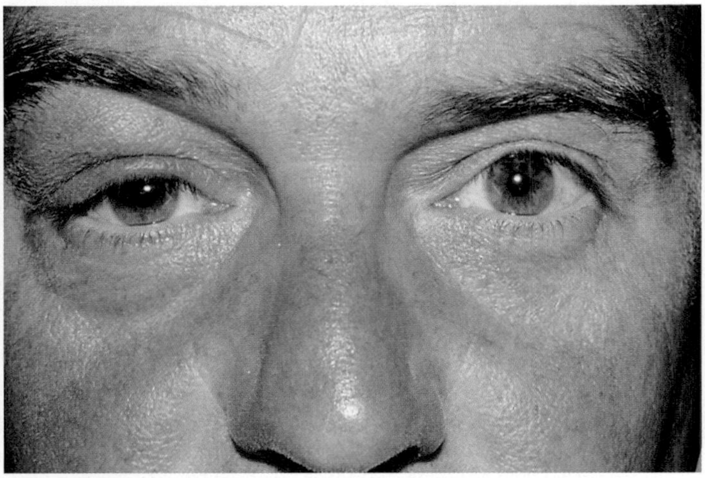

■ **Fig. 2.55** Swelling of the lateral aspect of the eyelid giving rise to a characteristic S-shaped ptosis and mild down and in displacement of the globe.

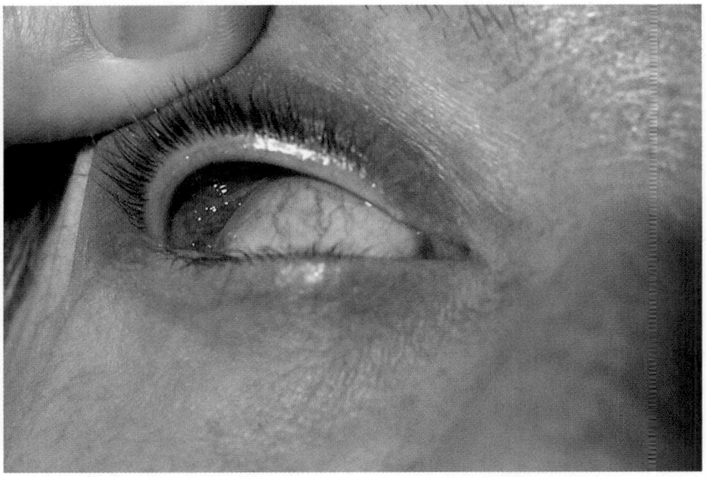

■ **Fig. 2.56** Injection of the palpebral portion of the lacrimal gland and adjacent conjunctiva; lacrimal secretion may be reduced.

Orbital myositis

Orbital myositis is an idiopathic, non-specific inflammation of one or more extraocular muscles and is considered a subtype of IOID. It typically affects young women. Presentation is sudden onset of ocular pain, worse on eye movements, and diplopia.

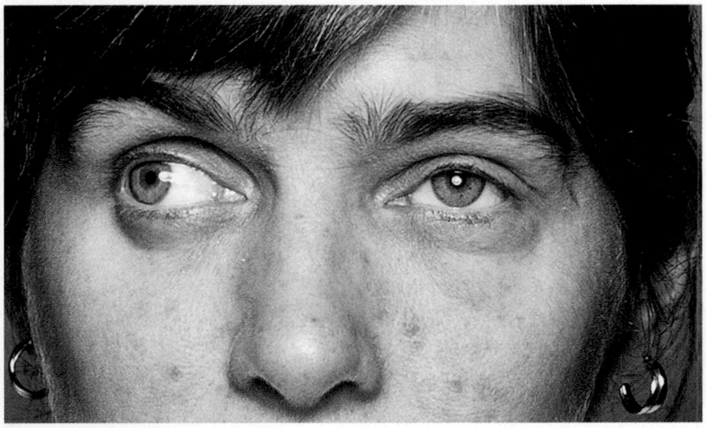

■ **Fig. 2.57** Restricted adduction and narrowing of the left palpebral fissure on right gaze due to fibrosis of the left lateral rectus muscle in chronic orbital myositis.

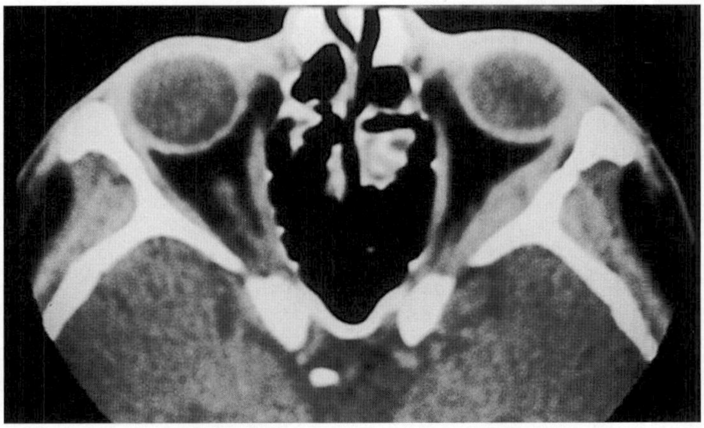

■ **Fig. 2.58** Axial CT showing fusiform enlargement of the left lateral rectus muscle.

VASCULAR MALFORMATIONS

Primary varices

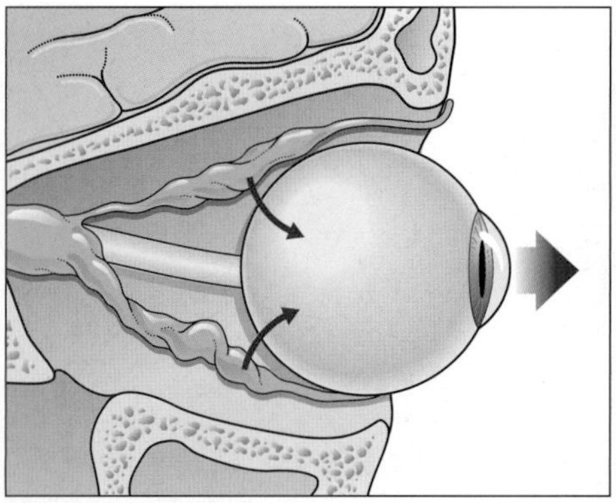

■ **Fig. 2.59** Primary varices consist of weakened segments of the orbital venous system, of variable length and complexity. Presentation ranges from early childhood to late middle age.

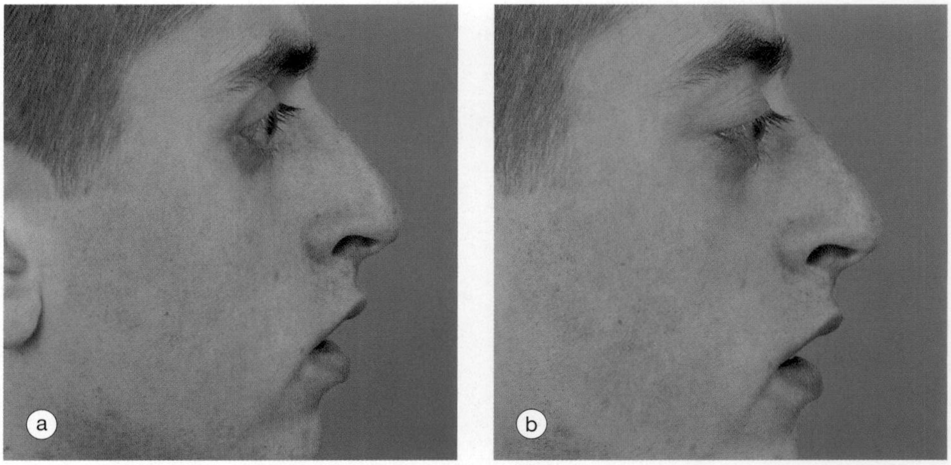

■ **Fig. 2.60** Intermittent proptosis precipitated or accentuated by the Valsalva manoeuvre. **(a)** Before Valsalva. **(b)** With Valsalva.

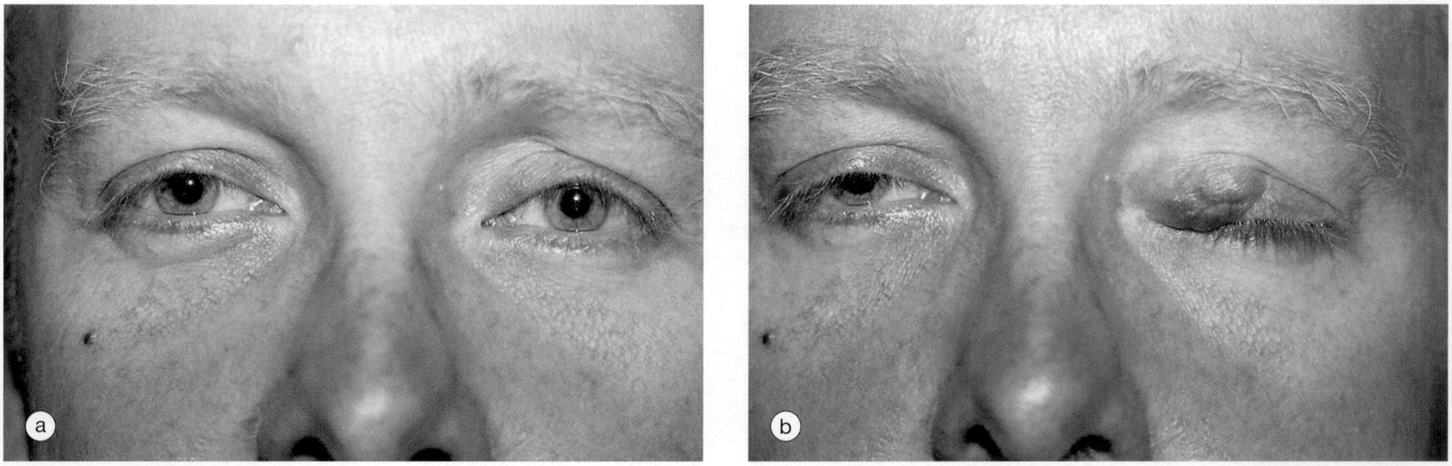

■ **Fig. 2.61** Eyelid varices may also be enhanced by performing the Valsalva manoeuvre. **(a)** Before Valsalva. **(b)** With Valsalva. (Courtesy of G. Rose.)

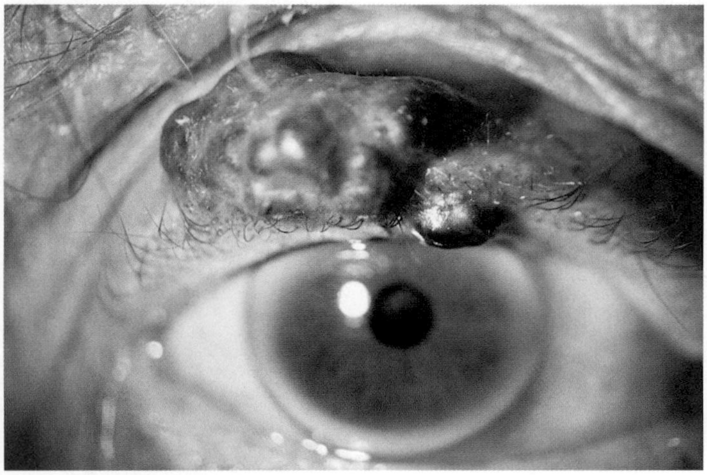

■ **Fig. 2.62** Severe eyelid varices.

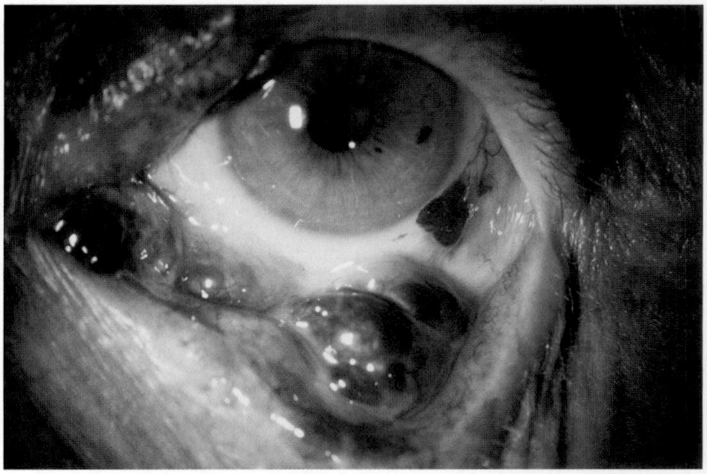

■ **Fig. 2.63** Conjunctival varices.

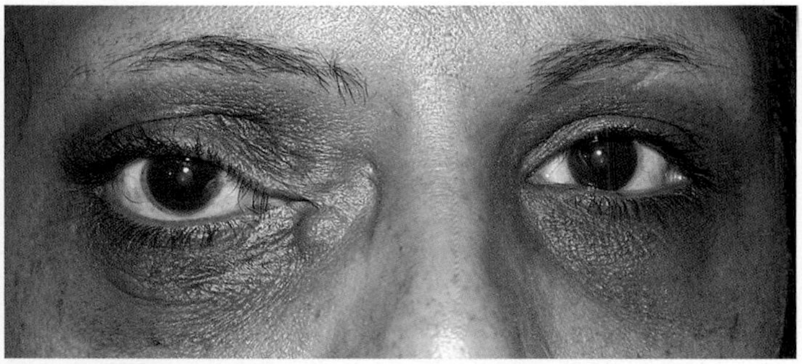

■ **Fig. 2.64** Patients with long-standing lesions may develop atrophy of surrounding fat and enophthalmos associated with a deepened superior sulcus.

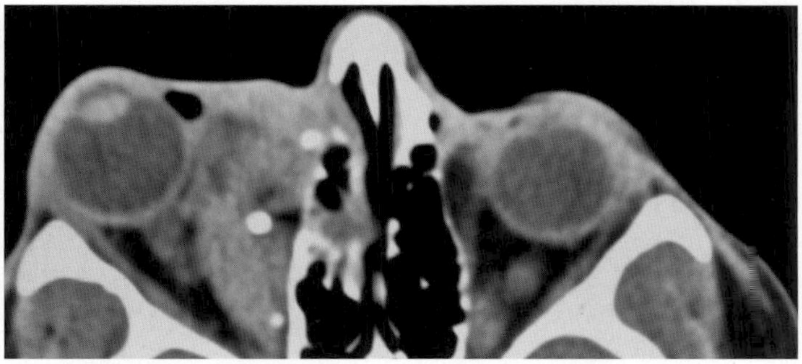

■ **Fig. 2.65** Axial CT shows right orbital varices with phleboliths and proptosis. (Courtesy of A. Pearson.)

Lymphangioma

Lymphangiomas are abortive, non-functional, benign vascular malformations that arborise through the orbit and may also involve the oropharynx. Presentation is usually in early childhood.

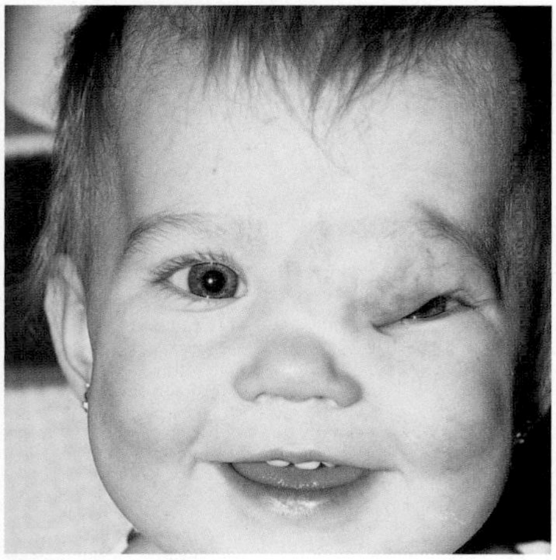

■ **Fig. 2.66** Anterior lesions typically manifest several soft bluish masses in the upper nasal quadrant with an associated cystic conjunctival component.

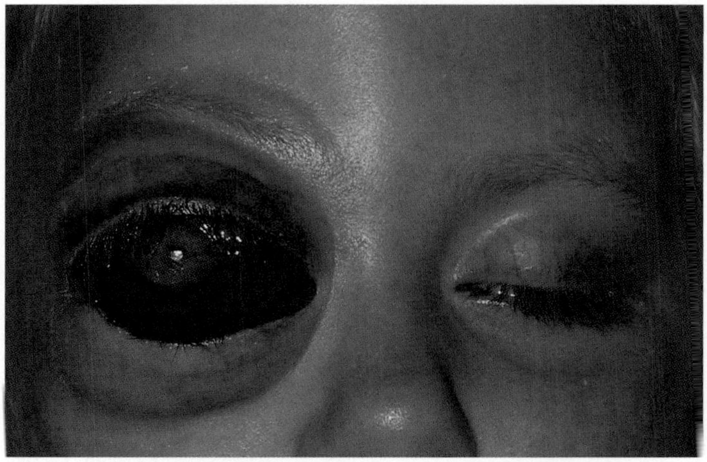

■ **Fig. 2.67** Posterior lesions may present with sudden onset of painful proptosis secondary to spontaneous haemorrhage. The blood subsequently becomes encysted with the formation of 'chocolate cysts', which may regress spontaneously with time. (Courtesy of A. Pearson.)

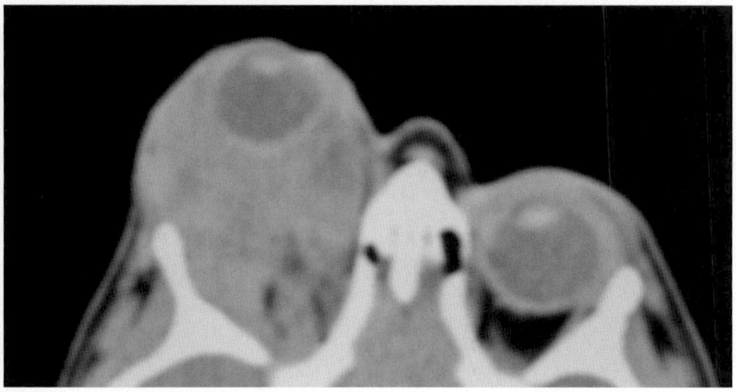

■ **Fig. 2.68** Axial CT of the same patient shows gross proptosis and orbital opacification due to blood. (Courtesy of A. Pearson.)

Arteriovenous fistula

An arteriovenous fistula is an abnormal communication between an artery and a vein. The blood within the affected vein becomes 'arterialised', the venous pressure rises and venous drainage may be altered in both rate and direction.

Low-flow

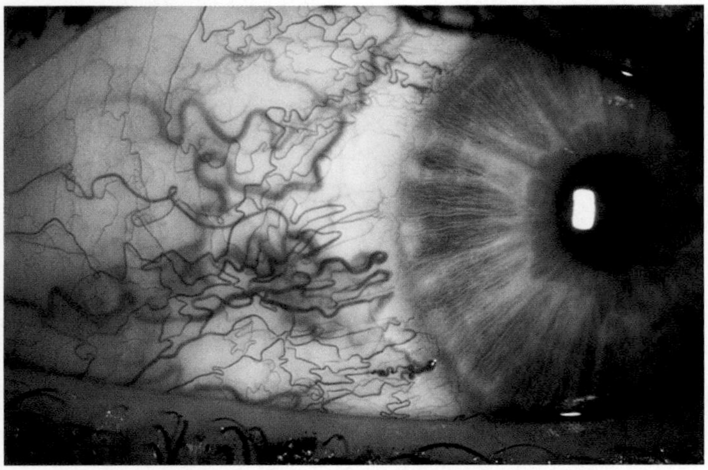

Fig. 2.69 Presentation is with gradual onset of redness of one or both eyes caused by conjunctival and episcleral vascular engorgement.

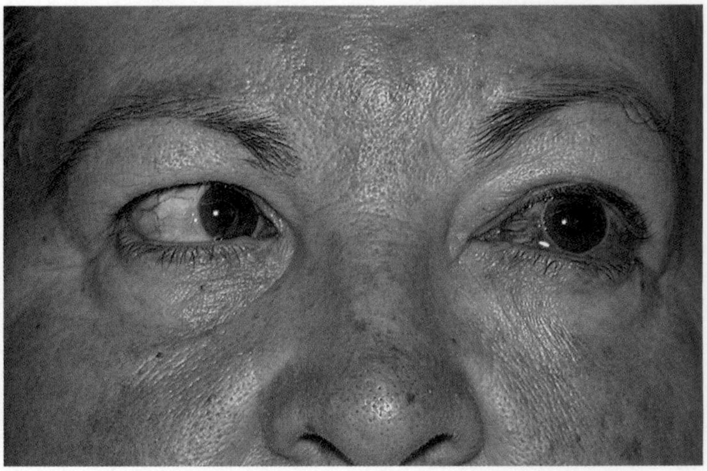

Fig. 2.70 Ophthalmoplegia is most frequently caused by sixth nerve palsy. Mild proptosis, exaggerated ocular pulse best detected on applanation tonometry and raised intraocular pressure may also be present. (Courtesy of J. Yangüela.)

High-flow

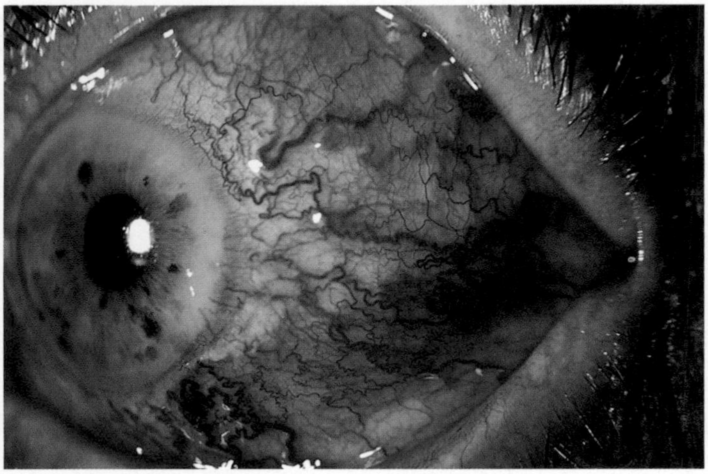

Fig. 2.71 Severe conjunctival and episcleral vascular engorgement.

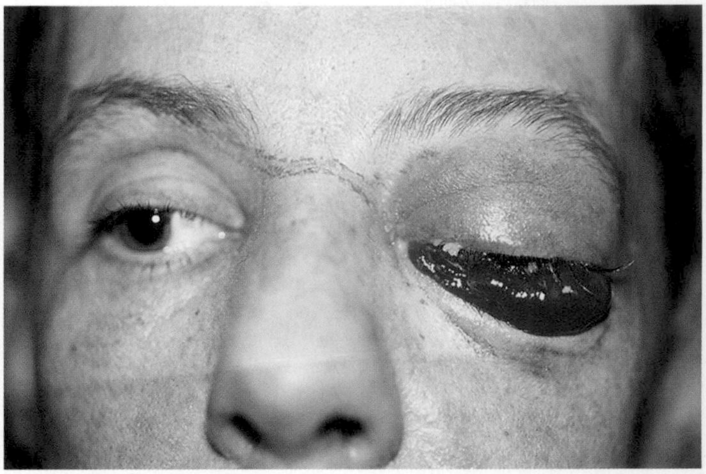

Fig. 2.72 Haemorrhagic chemosis and proptosis associated with a bruit and a thrill, both of which can be abolished by ipsilateral carotid compression in the neck.

CYSTIC LESIONS

Dacryops

A dacryops is a ductal cyst of the lacrimal gland which is frequently bilateral.

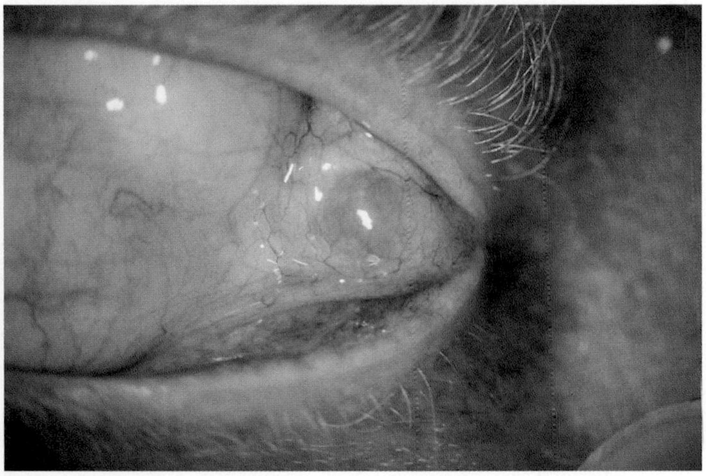

■ **Fig. 2.73** A round, cystic lesion originating from the palpebral portion of the lacrimal gland that protrudes into the superior fornix. Occasionally, the cyst extends into the orbital portion of the lacrimal gland.

Dermoid cyst

A dermoid cyst is a benign cystic teratoma (choristoma) derived from displacement of ectoderm to a subcutaneous location along embryonic lines of closure.

Superficial dermoid

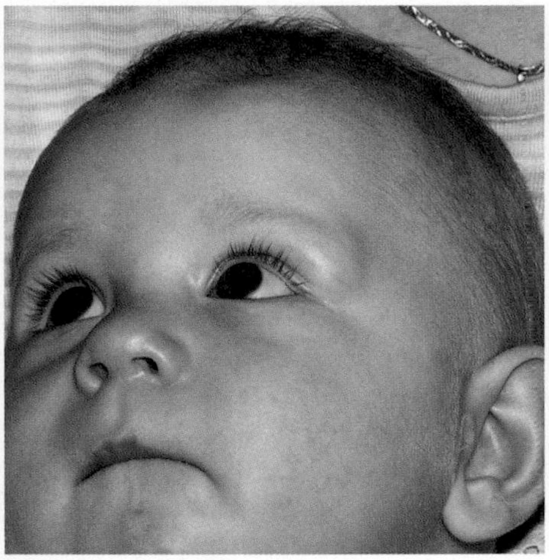

■ **Fig. 2.74** Presentation is in infancy with a painless, smooth, round, freely mobile nodule, most commonly located superotemporally. The posterior margins are easily palpable, denoting lack of deeper origin or extension.

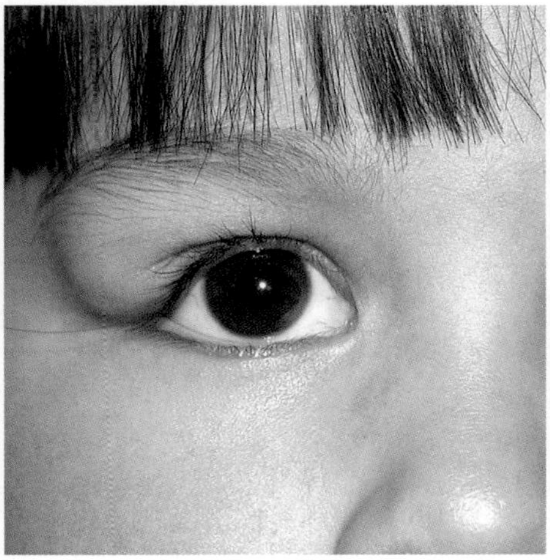

■ **Fig. 2.75** Larger dermoid in an older child. (Courtesy of G. Rose.)

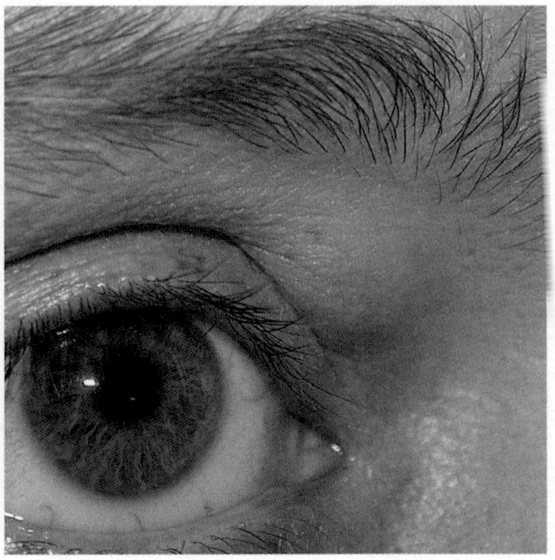

■ **Fig. 2.76** Occasionally the dermoid is located superonasally. (Courtesy of A. Pearson.)

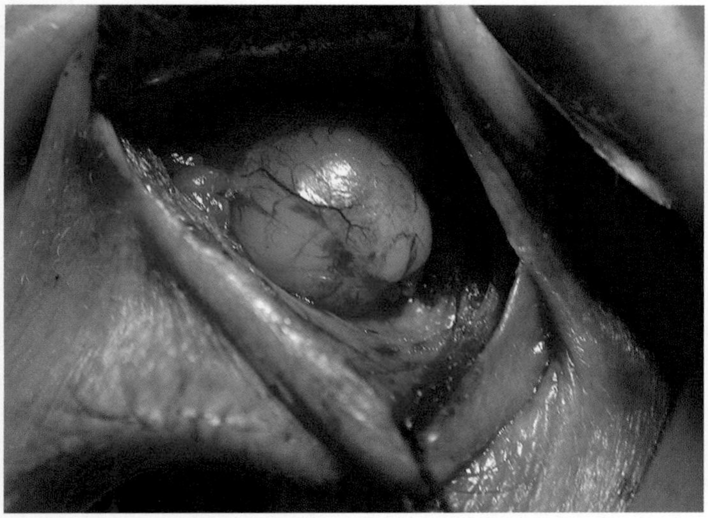

■ **Fig. 2.77** Appearance of the same cyst at surgery. (Courtesy of A. Pearson.)

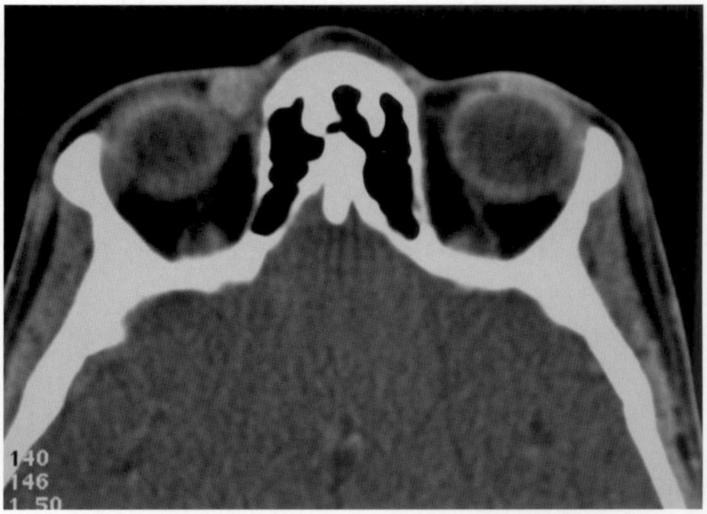

■ **Fig. 2.78** Axial CT shows a right anterior orbital heterogenous, well-circumscribed lesion. (Courtesy of A. Pearson.)

Deep dermoid

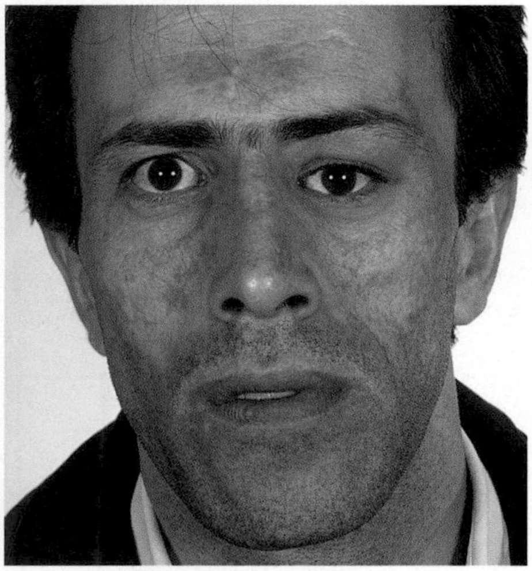

■ **Fig. 2.79** This presents in adolescence or adult life with proptosis, globe displacement or a mass lesion with indistinct posterior margins. (Courtesy of A. Pearson.)

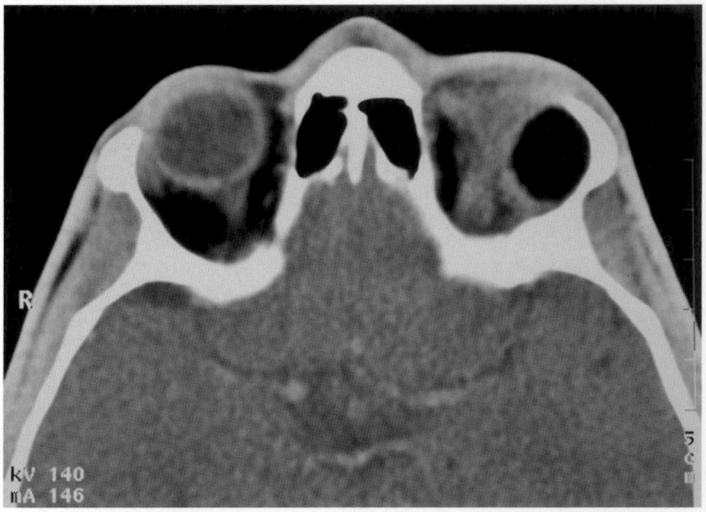

■ **Fig. 2.80** Axial CT shows a well-circumscribed cystic lesion in the left superotemporal orbit. (Courtesy of A. Pearson.)

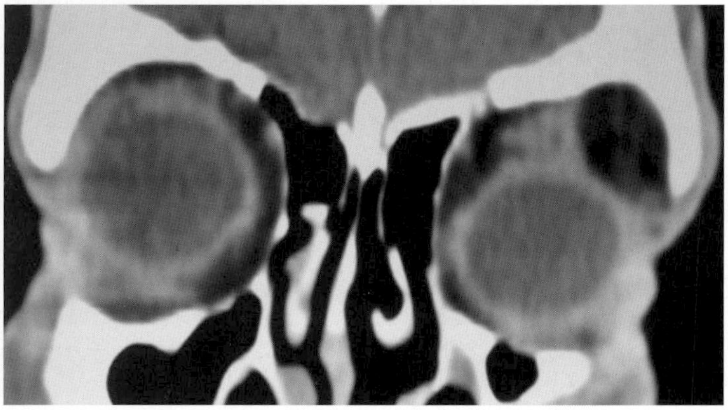

■ **Fig. 2.81** Coronal CT of the same patient. (Courtesy of A. Pearson.)

Mucocele

A mucocele develops when the drainage of normal paranasal sinus secretions is obstructed. Orbital invasion occurs most frequently from a frontal or ethmoidal mucocele.

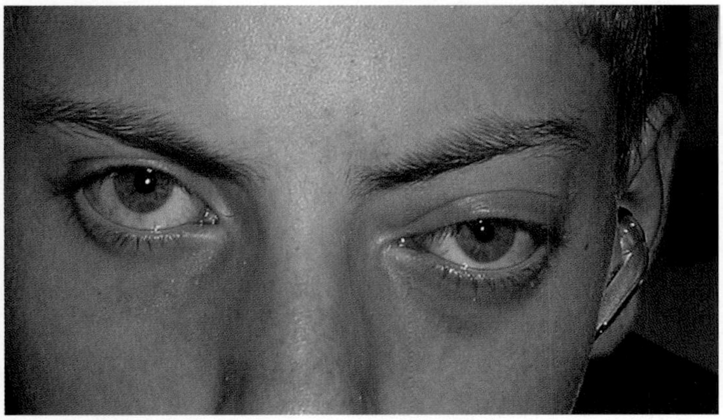

Fig. 2.82 Frontal mucocele causing a superior anterior orbital swelling, proptosis and inferior displacement of the globe. (Courtesy of A. Pearson.)

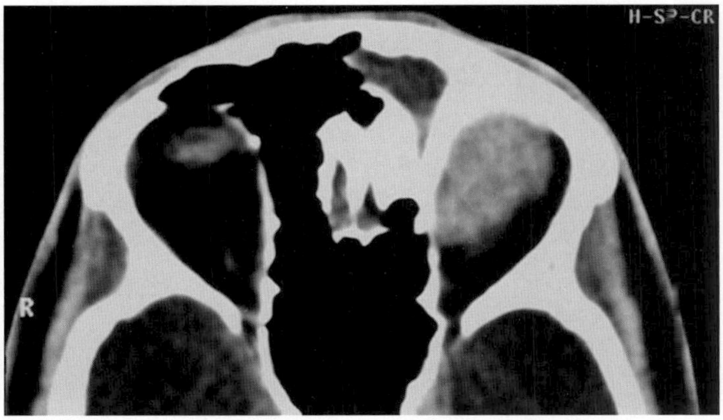

Fig. 2.83 Axial CT of the same patient shows a left soft tissue mass. (Courtesy of A. Pearson.)

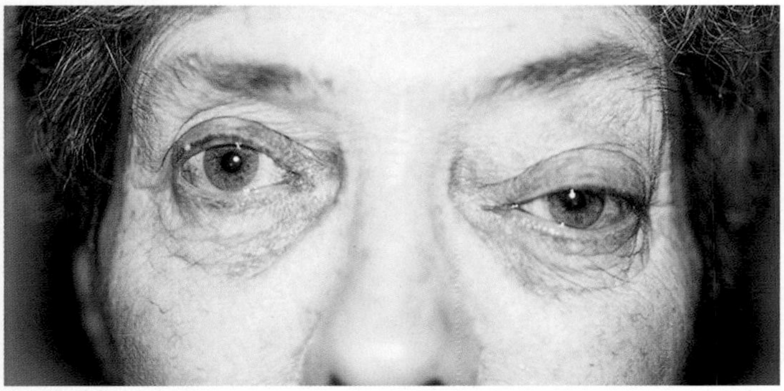

Fig. 2.84 Lateral displacement of the globe by an ethmoidal mucocele.

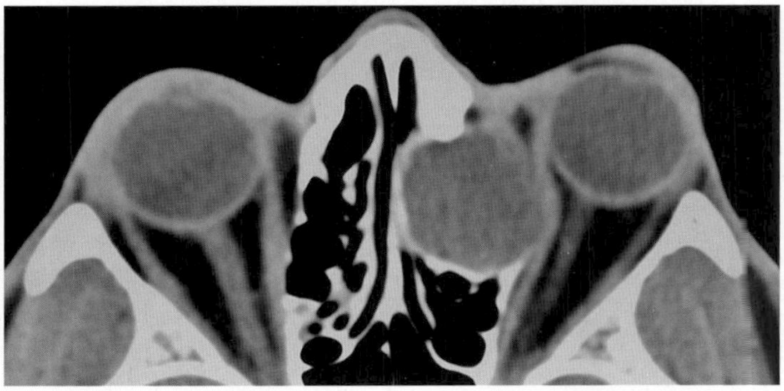

Fig. 2.85 Axial CT shows orbital invasion by a left ethmoidal mucocele. (Courtesy of A. Pearson.)

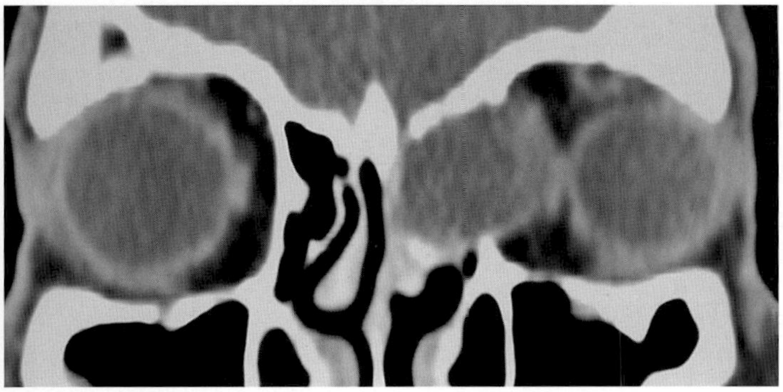

Fig. 2.86 Coronal CT of the same patient. (Courtesy of A. Pearson.)

Encephalocele

An encephalocele is formed by herniation of the intracranial contents through a congenital defect of the base of the skull.

Anterior

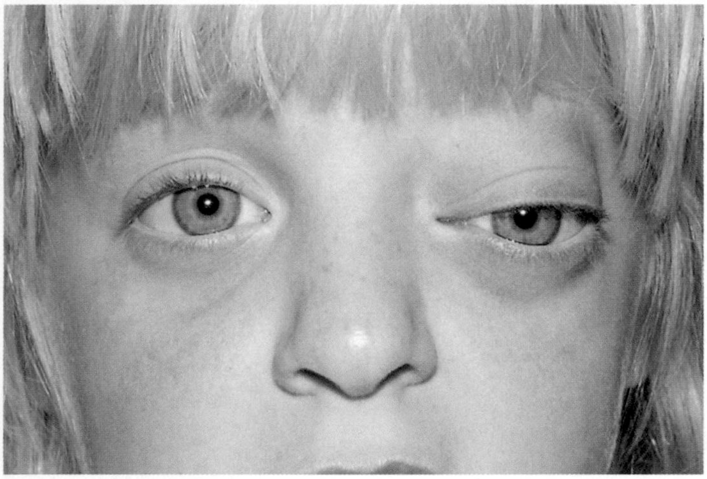

■ **Fig. 2.87** This involves the superomedial part of the orbit and displaces the globe down and out.

Posterior

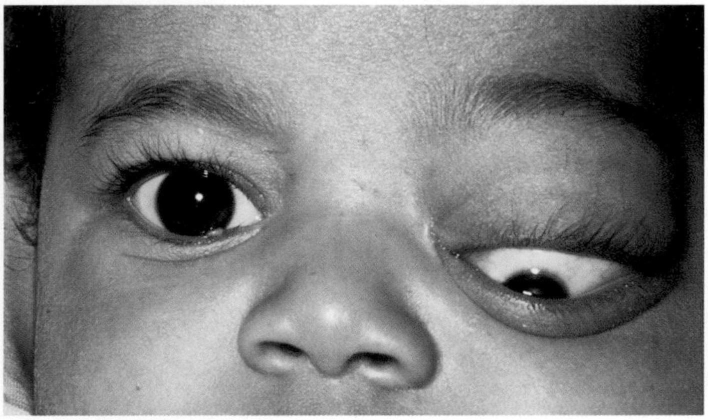

■ **Fig. 2.88** This displaces the globe downwards. The cyst increases in size on straining or crying and may be reduced by manual pressure. (Courtesy of G. Rose.)

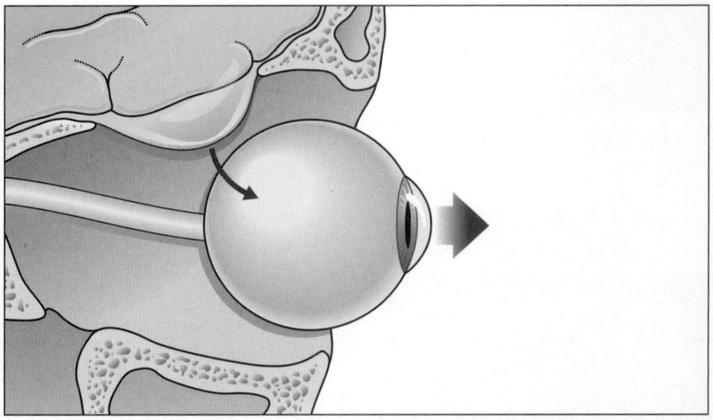

■ **Fig. 2.89** Pulsating proptosis may occur as a result of communication with the subarachnoid space but, because the communication is not vascular, there is neither a thrill nor a bruit.

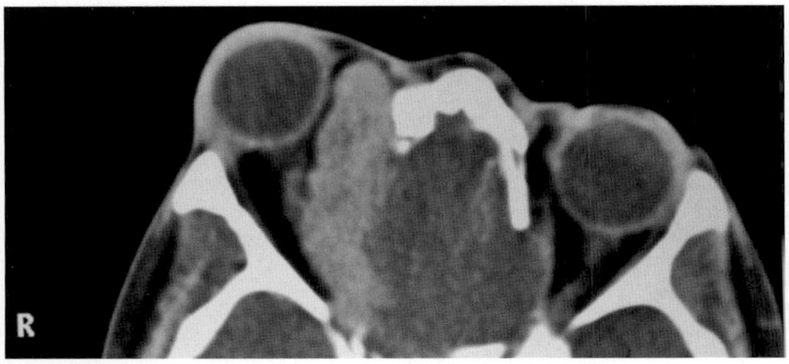

■ **Fig. 2.90** Axial CT of an anterior encephalocele showing the bony defect responsible for the herniation. (Courtesy of A. Pearson.)

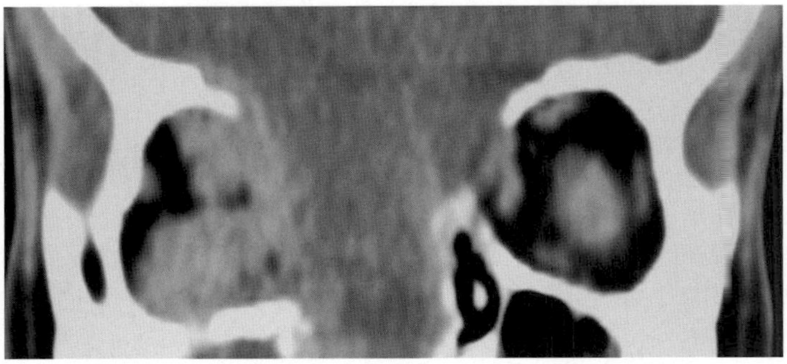

■ **Fig. 2.91** Coronal CT of the same patient. (Courtesy of A. Pearson.)

Associations

Bony

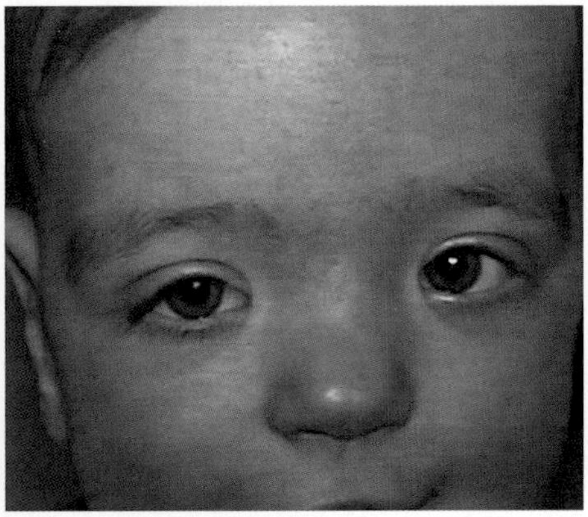

■ **Fig. 2.92** Hypertelorism and broad nasal bridge.

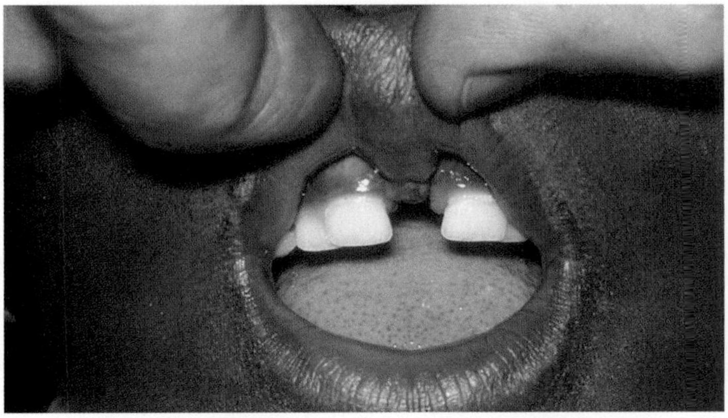

■ **Fig. 2.93** Cleft palate. (Courtesy of Moorfields Eye Hospital.)

Ocular

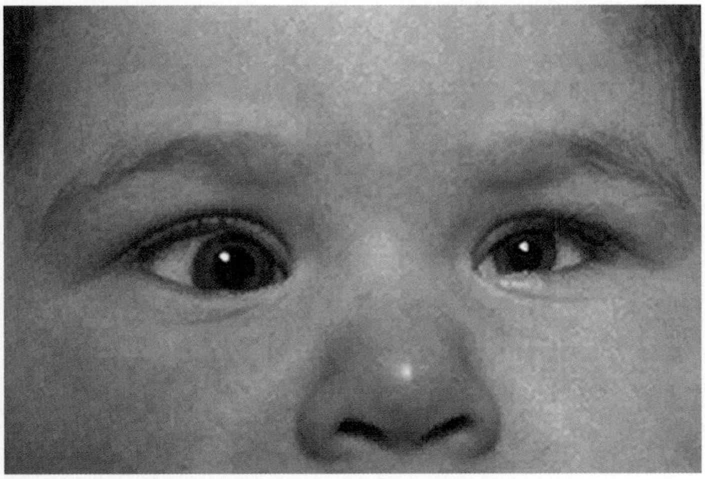

■ **Fig. 2.94** Microphthalmos. (Courtesy of S. Ford and R. Marsh.)

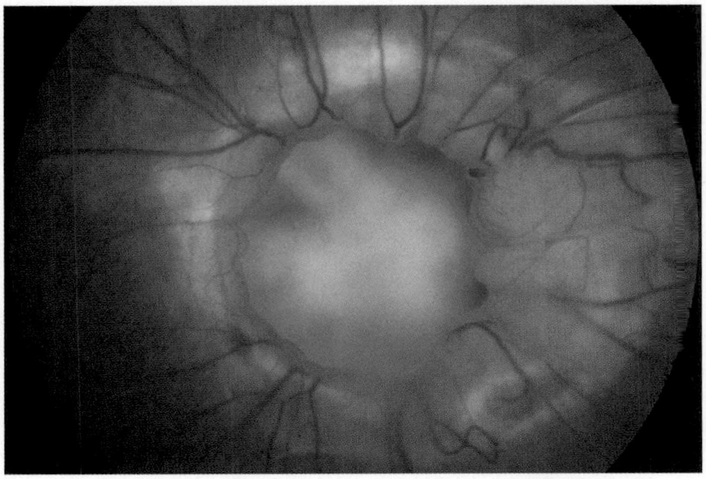

■ **Fig. 2.95** Morning glory syndrome. (Courtesy of Moorfields Eye Hospital.)

Microphthalmos with cyst

Microphthalmos with cyst is caused by incomplete closure of the fetal fissure, leading to prolapse of cystic tissue into the orbit.

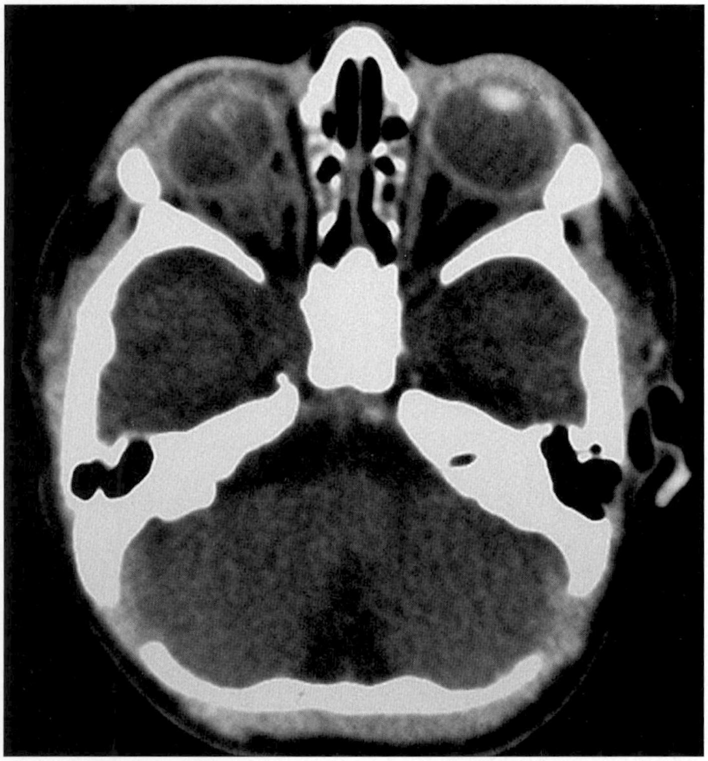

■ **Fig. 2.96** Axial CT shows a right cystic lesion behind a small globe. (Courtesy of L. MacKeen.)

Anophthalmos with cyst (congenital cystic eyeball)

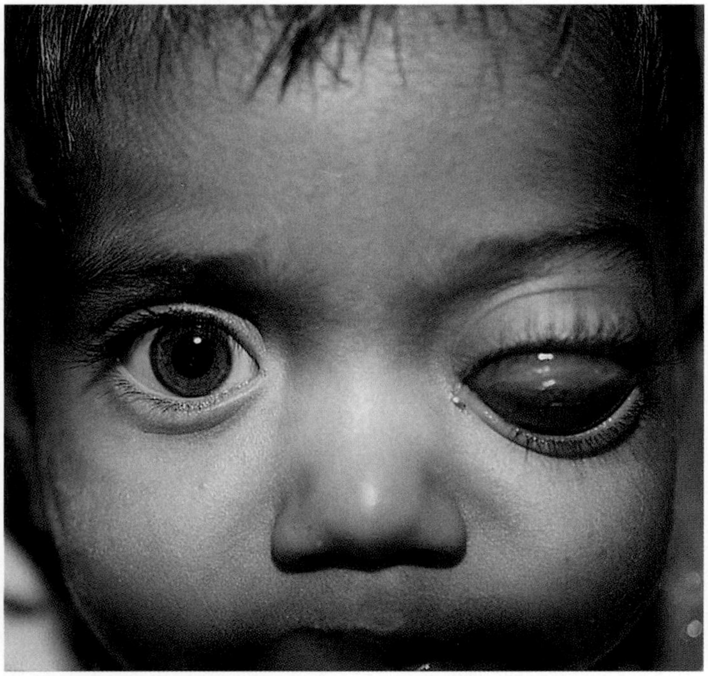

■ **Fig. 2.97** The globe is replaced by a large cyst. (Courtesy of U. Raina.)

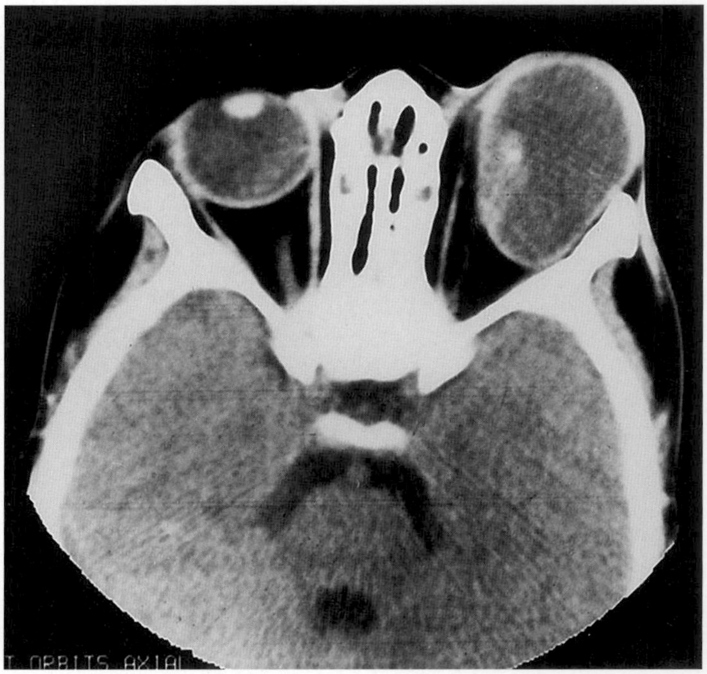

■ **Fig. 2.98** Axial CT of the same patient. (Courtesy of U. Raina.)

BENIGN TUMOURS

Capillary haemangioma

Capillary haemangioma is the most common tumour of the orbit and periorbital area in childhood. Presentation is usually in the perinatal period, but never at birth.

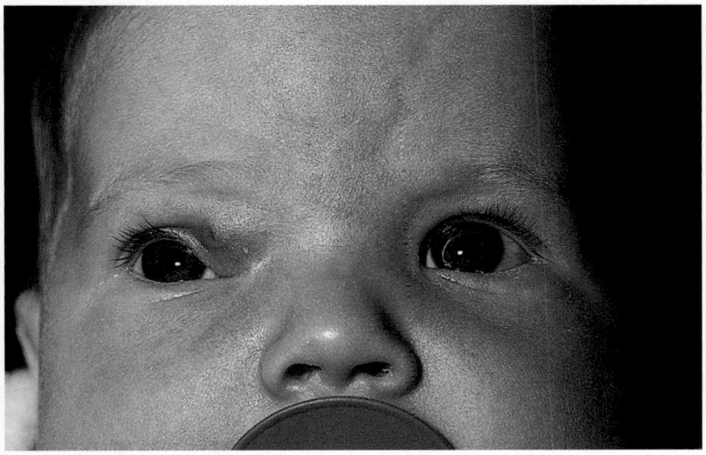

Fig. 2.99 The superior anterior orbit is most commonly involved and the tumour may cause lateral displacement of the globe.

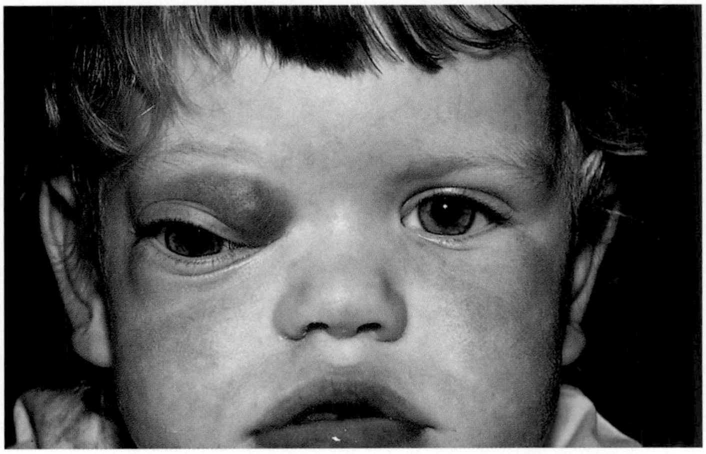

Fig. 2.100 The tumour grows till the age of about 1 year and then starts to spontaneously involute at about the age of 2 years

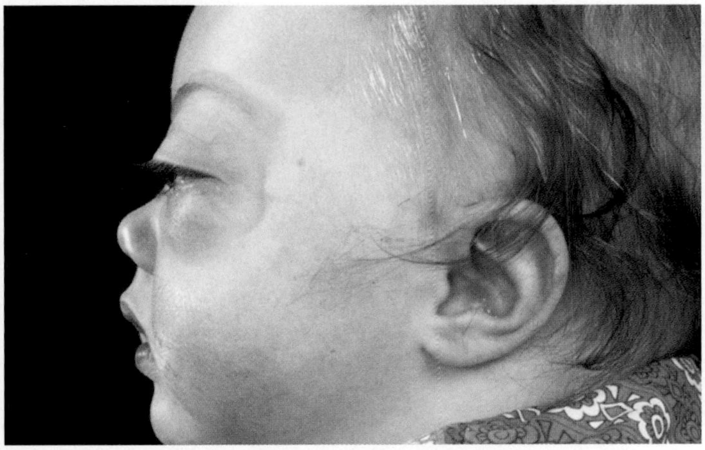

Fig. 2.101 A deep orbital tumour causing proptosis.

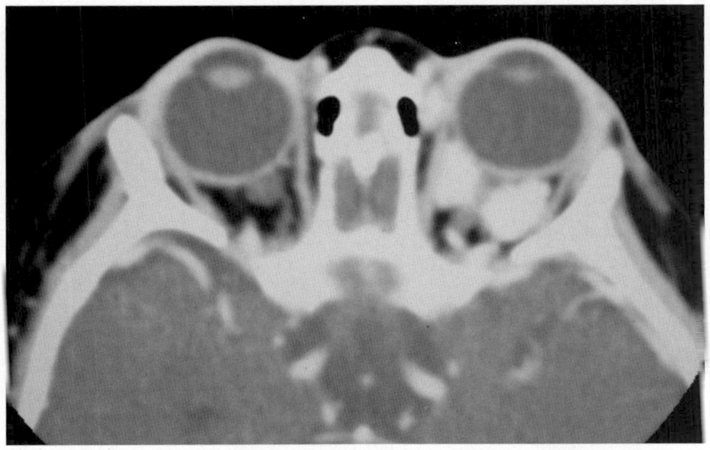

Fig. 2.102 Axial CT shows a left homogeneous soft tissue mass. (Courtesy of A. Pearson.)

Cavernous haemangioma

Cavernous haemangioma is the most common benign orbital tumour in adults.

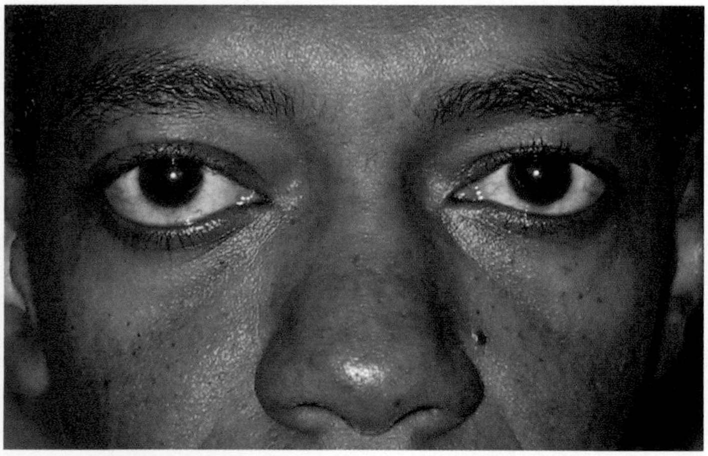

Fig. 2.103 Presentation is in the fourth to fifth decade with slowly progressive unilateral axial proptosis. (Courtesy of A. Pearson.)

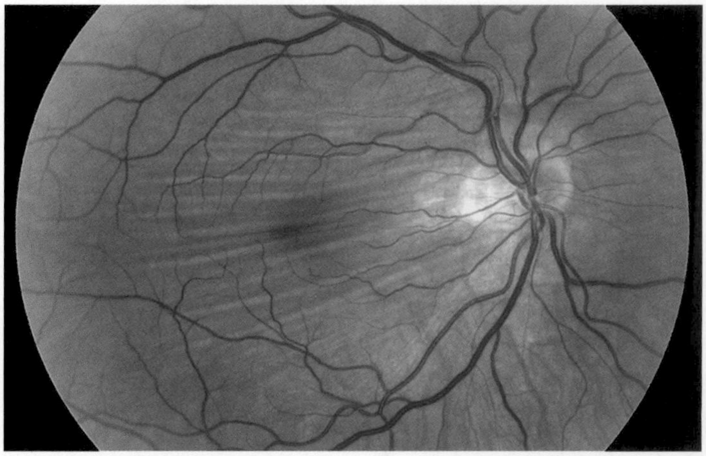

Fig. 2.104 Choroidal folds may be present.

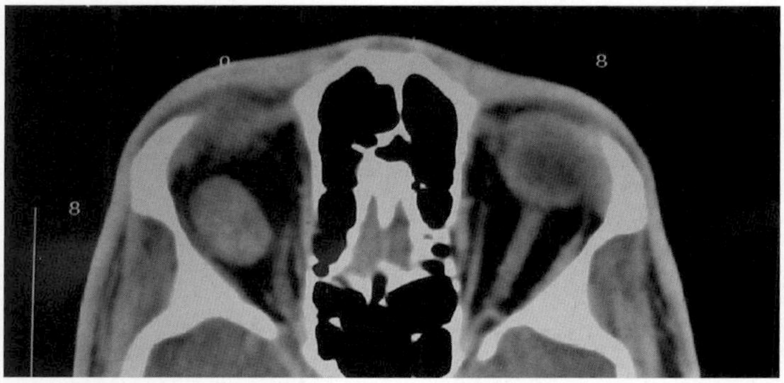

Fig. 2.105 Axial CT shows a right well-circumscribed oval lesion. (Courtesy of A. Pearson.)

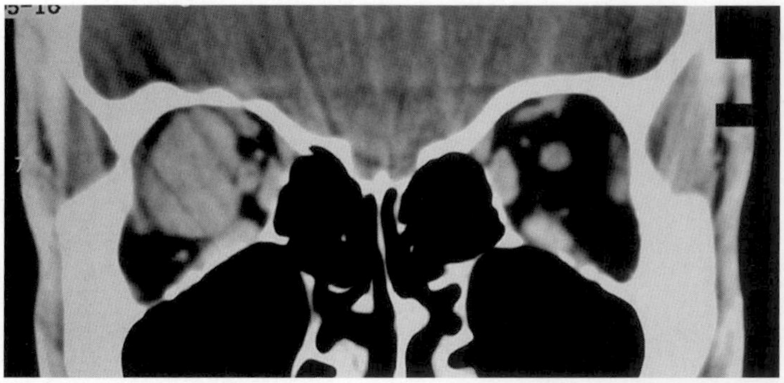

Fig. 2.106 Coronal CT of the same patient. (Courtesy of A. Pearson.)

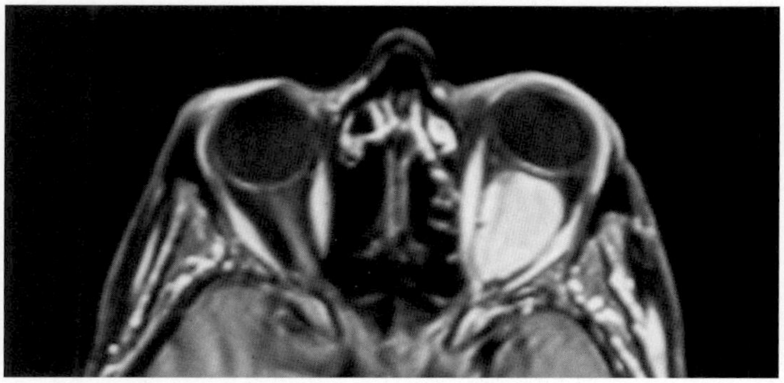

Fig. 2.107 Axial T2-weighted MRI in another patient shows a hyperintense mass. (Courtesy of A. Pearson.)

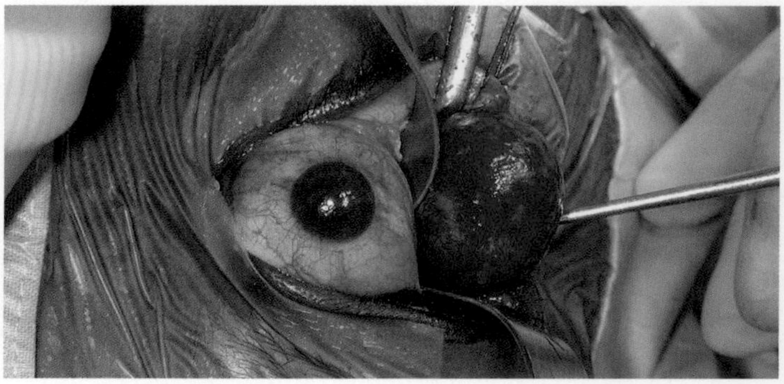

Fig. 2.108 The tumour is circumscribed and easy to remove. (Courtesy of A. Pearson.)

Pleomorphic lacrimal gland adenoma

Pleomorphic lacrimal gland adenoma (benign mixed-cell tumour) is the most common epithelial tumour of the lacrimal gland.

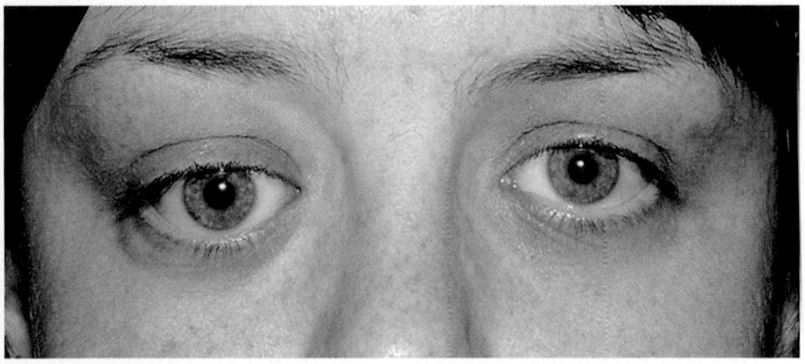

Fig. 2.109 A tumour arising from the orbital lobe gives rise to a painless, smooth, firm, non-tender mass in the lacrimal gland fossa with down and in displacement of the globe. (Courtesy of G. Rose.)

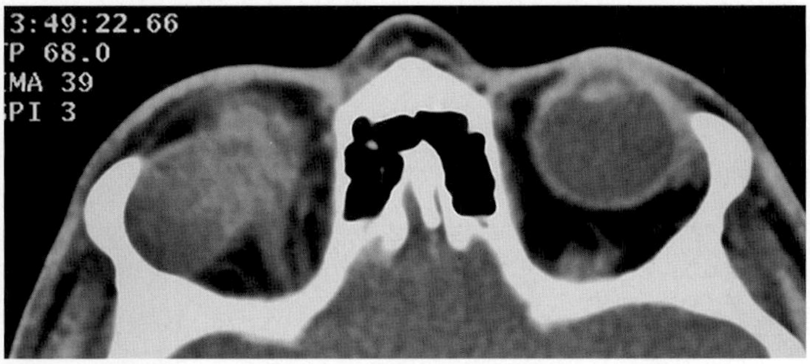

Fig. 2.110 Axial CT shows a right oval mass that indents but does not destroy the lacrimal gland fossa. The lesion may also indent the globe. (Courtesy of A. Pearson.)

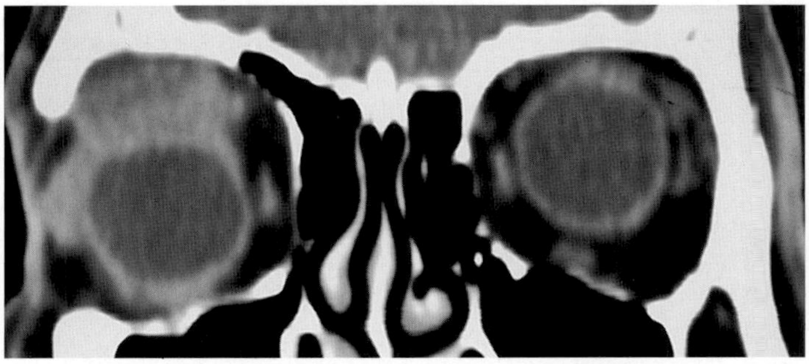

Fig. 2.111 Coronal CT of the same patient. (Courtesy of A. Pearson.)

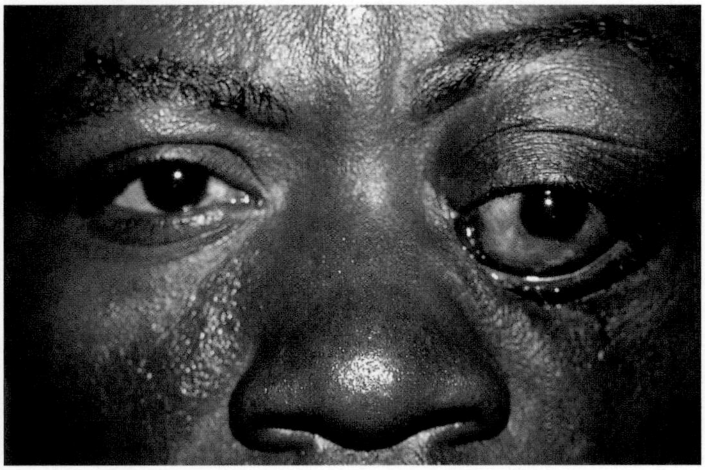

Fig. 2.112 Posterior extension causing proptosis. (Courtesy of G. Rose.)

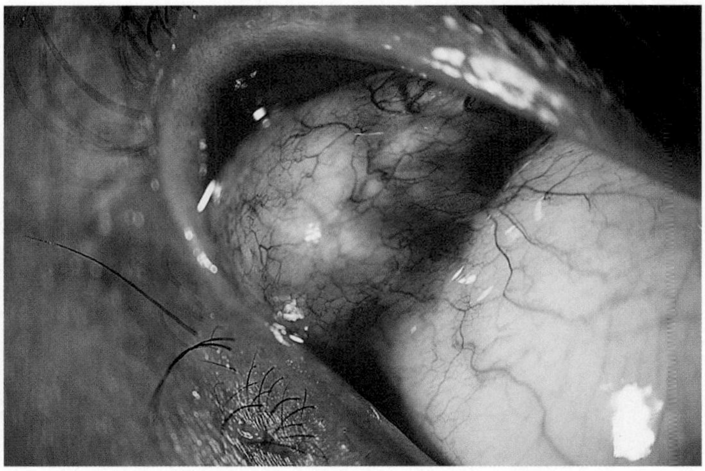

Fig. 2.113 A tumour arising from the palpebral lobe tends to grow anteriorly and causes upper lid swelling.

Optic nerve glioma

Optic nerve glioma is a slow-growing astrocytoma.

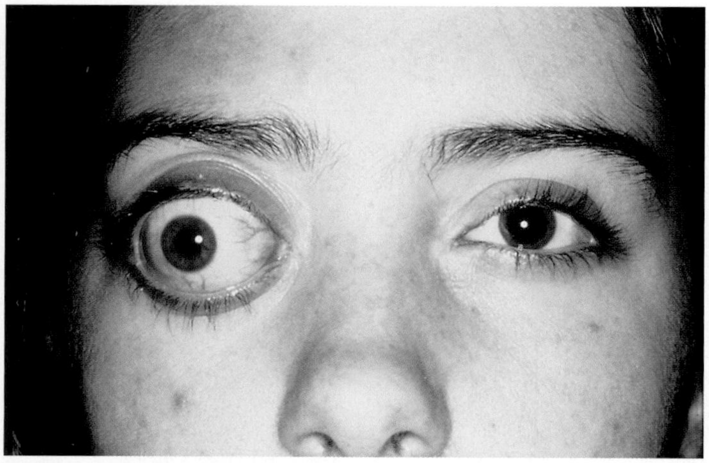

■ **Fig. 2.114** Presentation is often towards the end of the first decade with slowly progressive visual loss followed later by proptosis, although this sequence may occasionally be reversed. (Courtesy of G. Rose.)

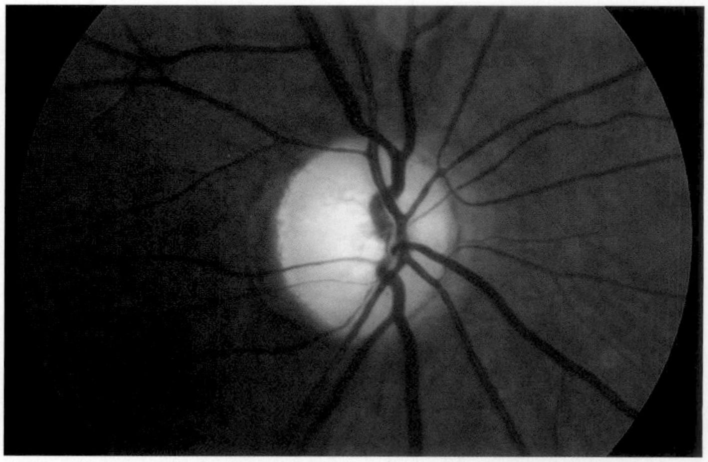

■ **Fig. 2.115** The optic nerve head, initially swollen, later becomes atrophic.

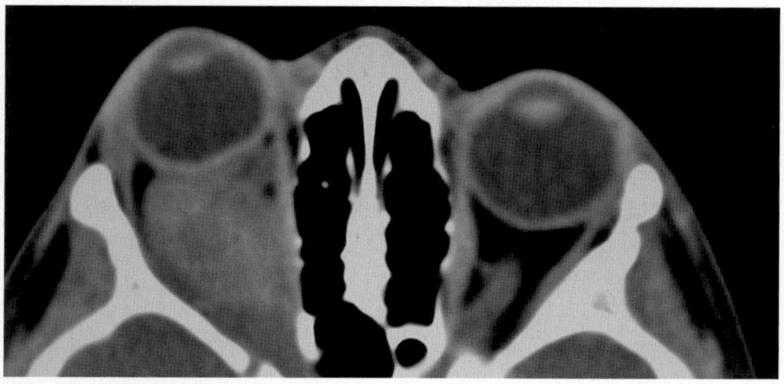

■ **Fig. 2.116** Axial CT shows fusiform enlargement of the right optic nerve. (Courtesy of A. Pearson.)

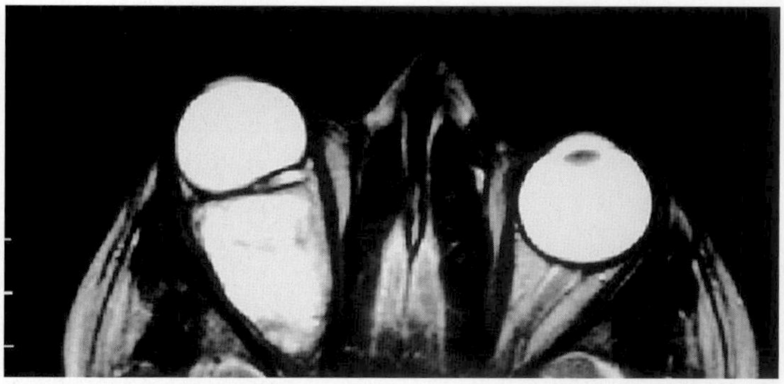

■ **Fig. 2.117** Axial T2-weighted MRI shows a hyperintense mass. (Courtesy of A. Pearson.)

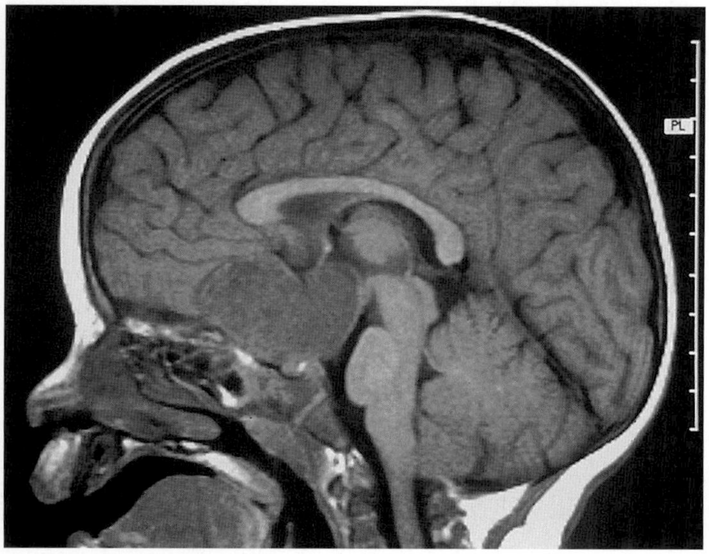

■ **Fig. 2.118** Sagittal T1-weighted MRI shows intracranial extension of an optic nerve glioma with invasion of the hypothalamus; the tumour is hypointense. (Courtesy of D. Armstrong.)

Association

Neurofibromatosis-1 is a common association of optic nerve glioma in young individuals.

Ocular signs

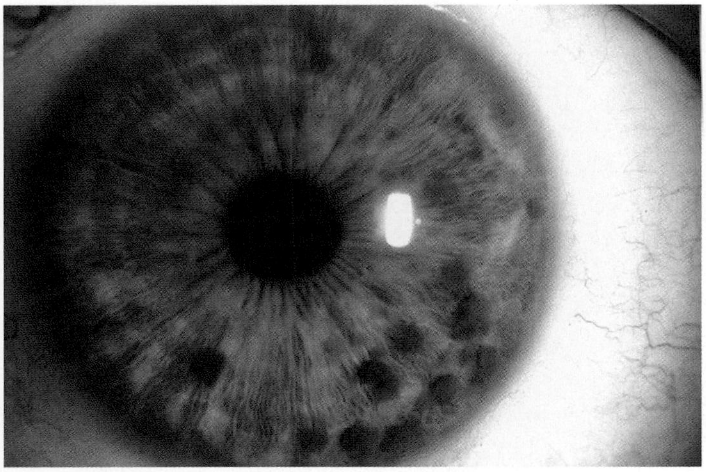

Fig. 2.119 Lisch nodules are universal after the age of about 16 years. (Courtesy of R. Curtis.)

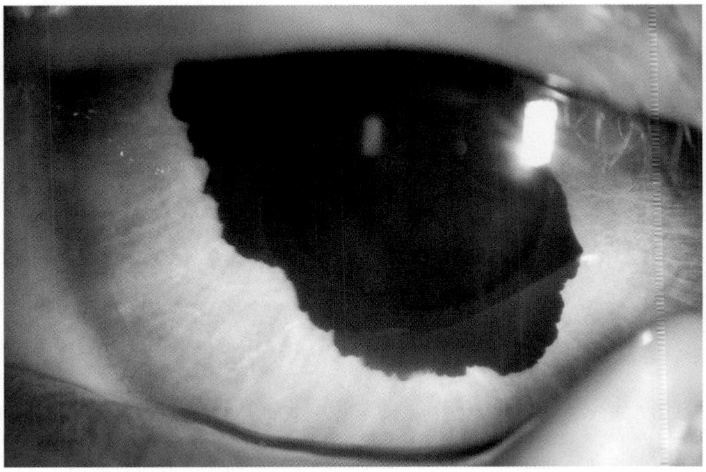

Fig. 2.120 Congenital ectropion uveae is uncommon but may be associated with glaucoma.

Café-au-lait spots

These appear during the first year of life and subsequently increase in size and number throughout childhood.

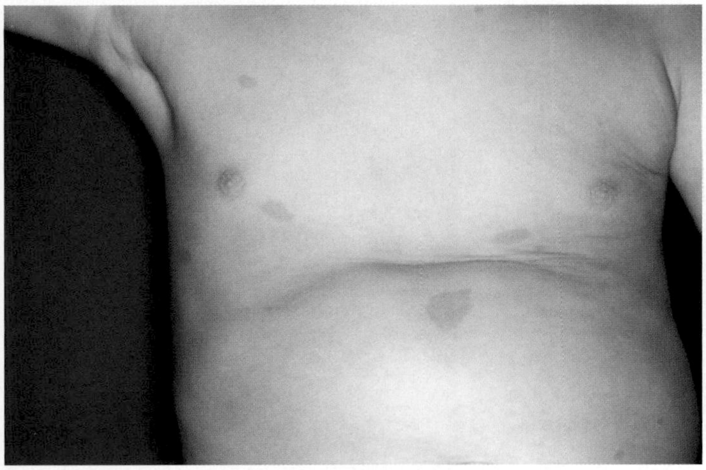

Fig. 2.121 Large but sparse café-au-lait spots.

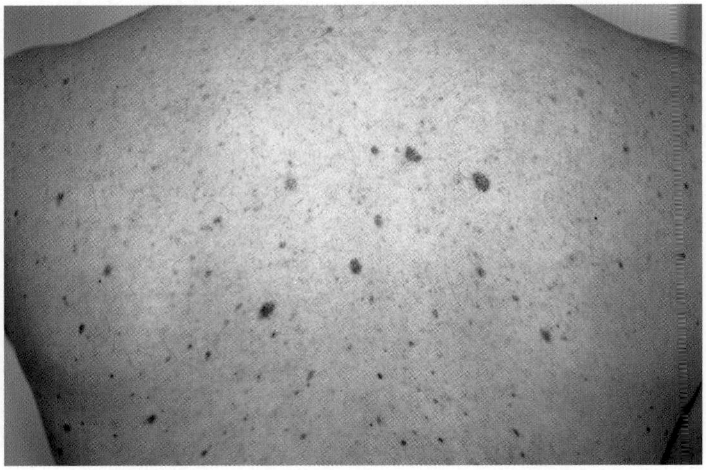

Fig. 2.122 Numerous small café-au-lait spots.

Fibroma mollusca

These appear at puberty and increase in number throughout life.

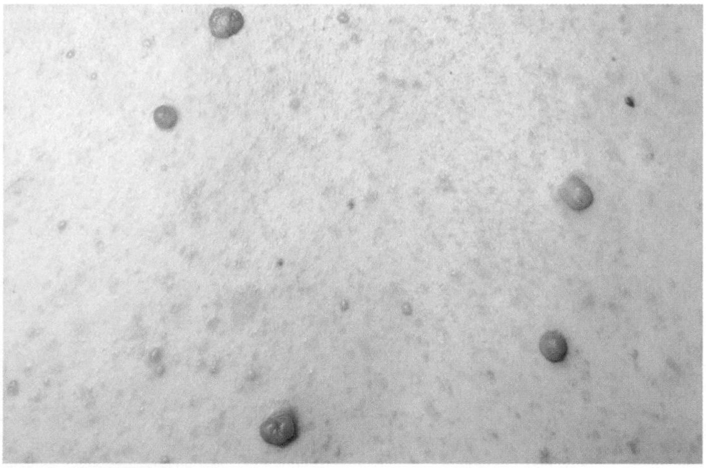

Fig. 2.123 Small fibroma mollusca on the back.

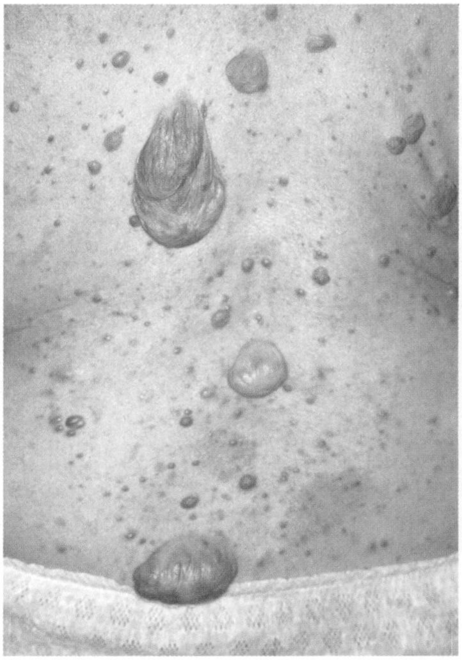

Fig. 2.124 Many small and a few large pedunculated fibroma mollusca on the chest and abdomen.

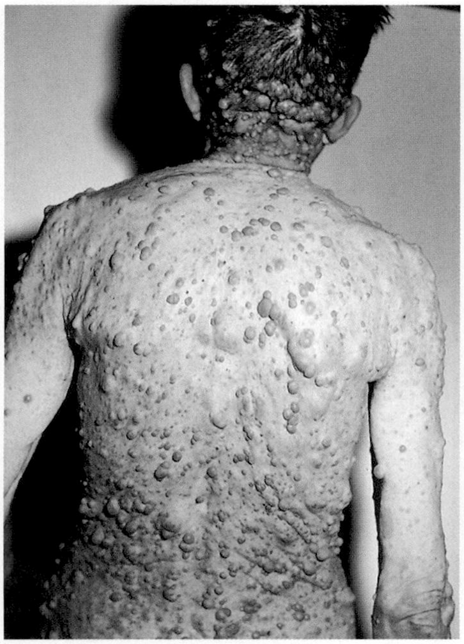

Fig. 2.125 Extensive involvement of the back by pedunculated fibroma mollusca.

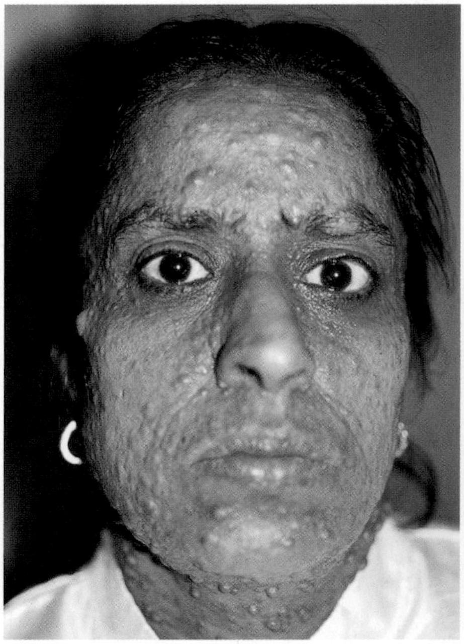

Fig. 2.126 Facial involvement by fibroma mollusca.

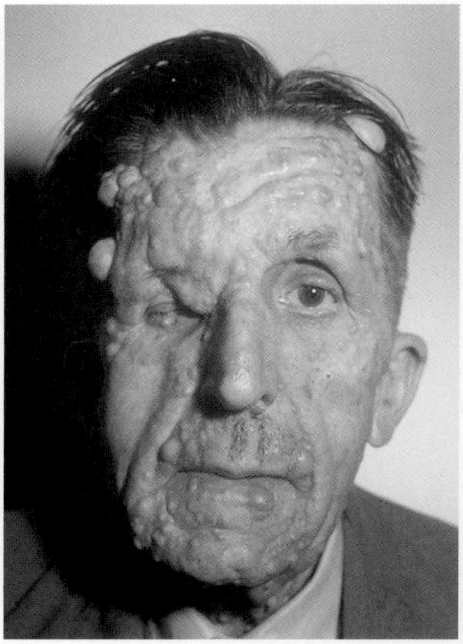

Fig. 2.127 Facial hemiatrophy and fibroma mollusca.

Plexiform neurofibroma

This may be present at birth or appear during childhood and may involve any part of the body.

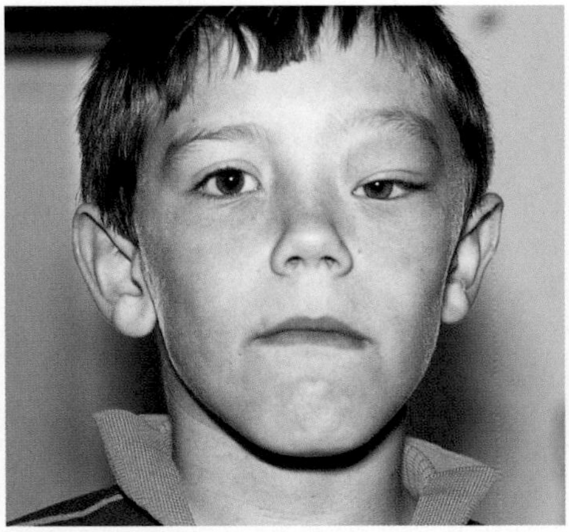

Fig. 2.128 Small eyelid plexiform neurofibroma giving rise to mild ptosis.

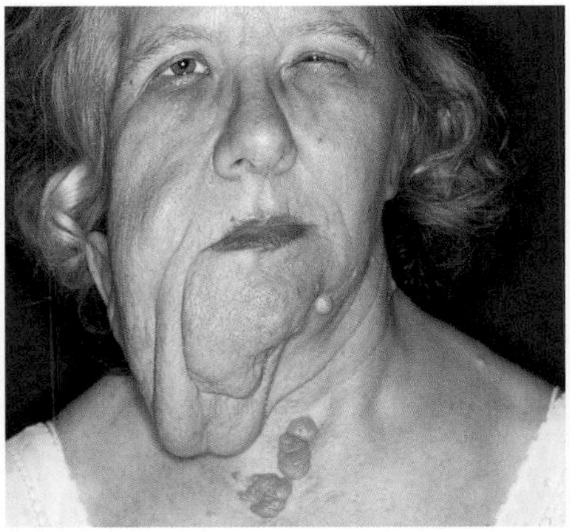

Fig. 2.129 Hypertrophy of facial soft tissues associated with an underlying diffuse plexiform neurofibroma.

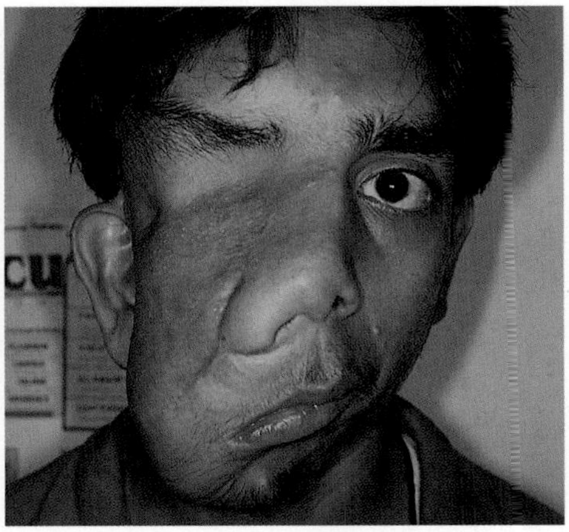

Fig. 2.130 Gross facial disfigurement associated with a diffuse plexiform neurofibroma (Courtesy of U. Raina.)

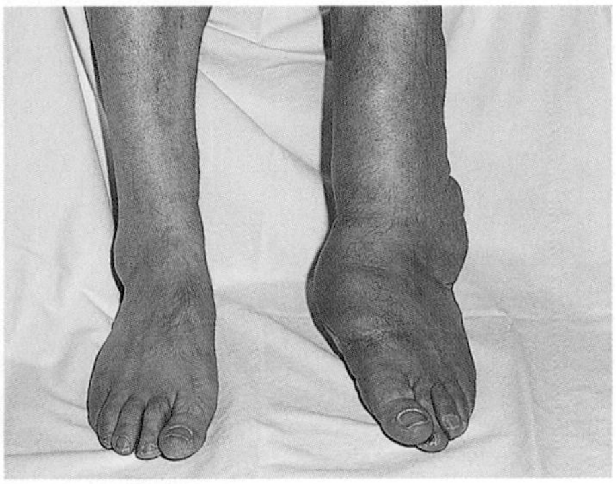

Fig. 2.131 Soft tissue hypertrophy of the foot associated with a plexiform neurofibroma.

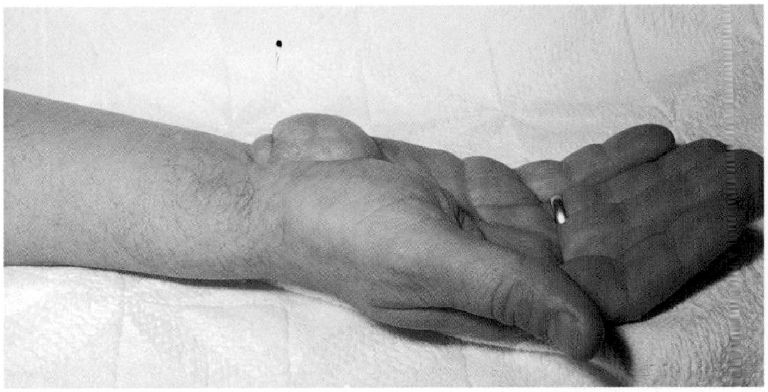

Fig. 2.132 Plexiform neurofibroma on the hand.

Skeletal anomalies

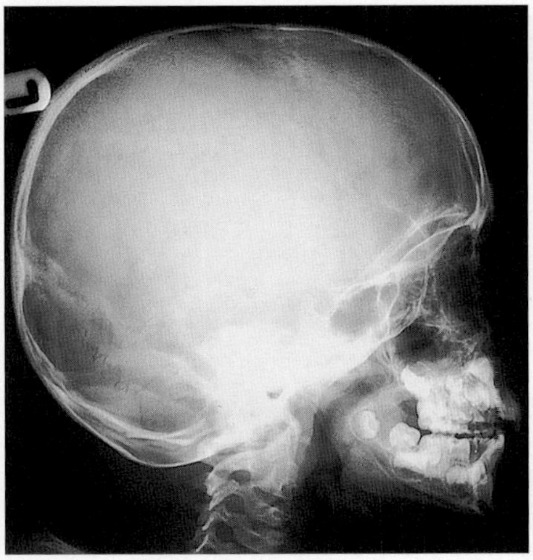

Fig. 2.133 Enlargement of the skull (macrocephaly).

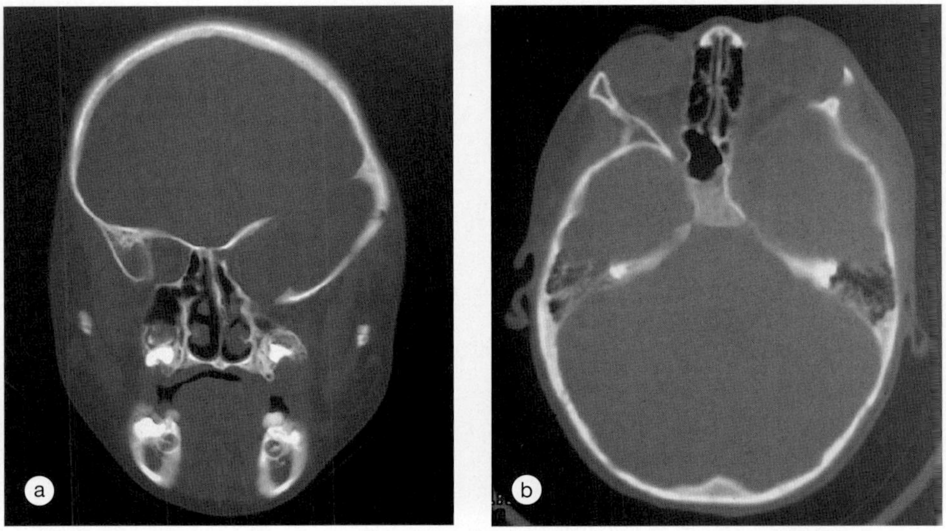

Fig. 2.134 CT shows absence of the greater wing of the left sphenoid bone. **(a)** Coronal view. **(b)** Axial view. (Courtesy of K. Nischal.)

Optic nerve sheath meningioma

Optic nerve sheath meningioma is a very rare tumour that arises from meningothelial cells of the arachnoid villi.

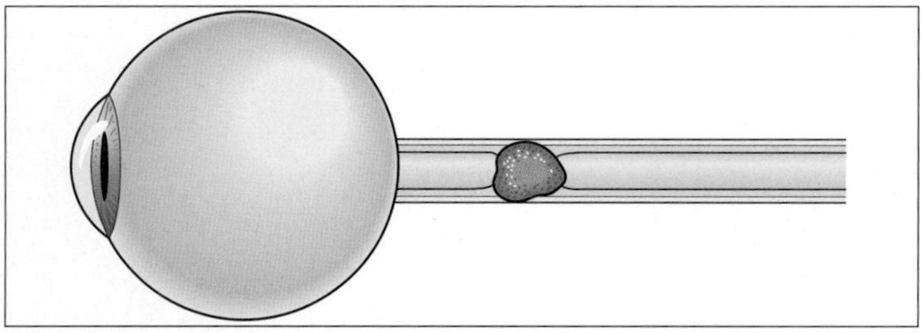

Fig. 2.135 Presentation is in middle age with unilateral gradual visual impairment due to optic nerve compression.

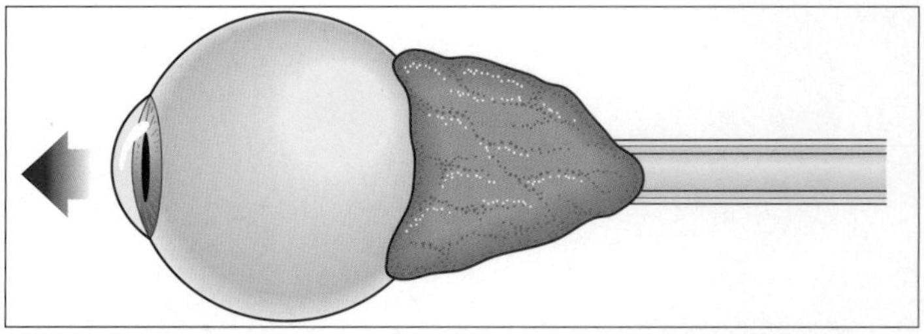

Fig. 2.136 Proptosis, caused by intraconal spread, usually develops after the onset of visual loss.

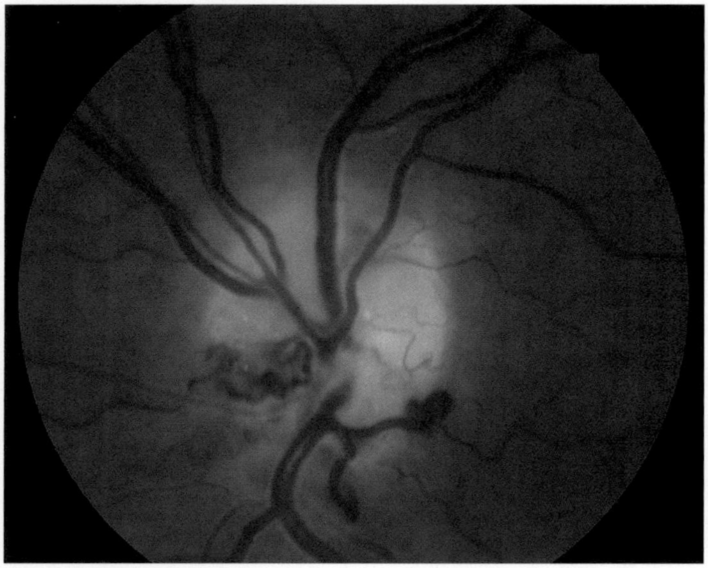

Fig. 2.137 Opticociliary shunt vessels, found in about 30% of cases, regress as optic atrophy supervenes.

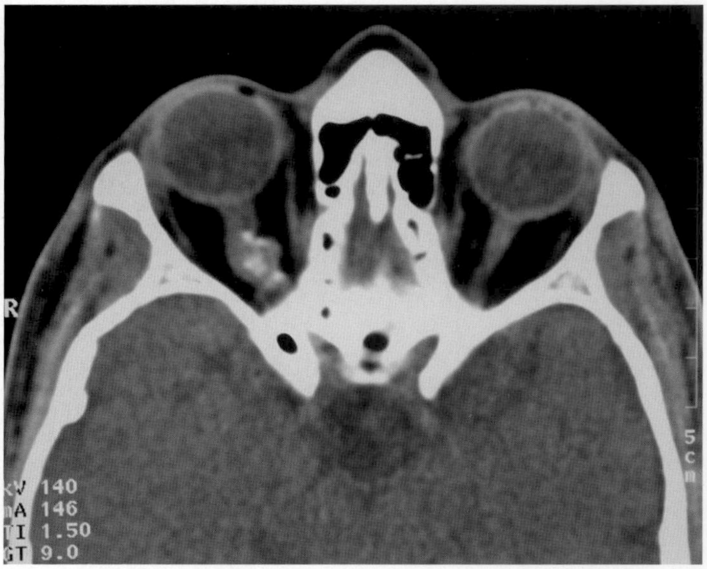

Fig. 2.138 Axial CT shows thickening and calcification of the right optic nerve. (Courtesy of A. Pearson.)

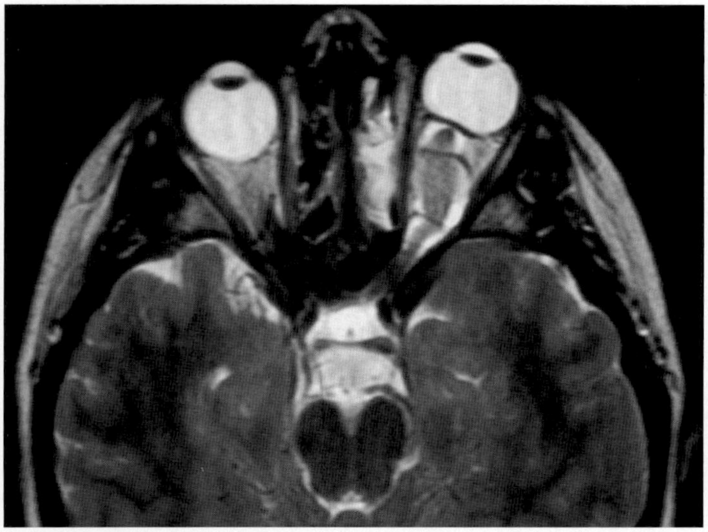

Fig. 2.139 Axial T2-weighted MRI shows fusiform enlargement of the left optic nerve and proptosis. (Courtesy of A. Pearson.)

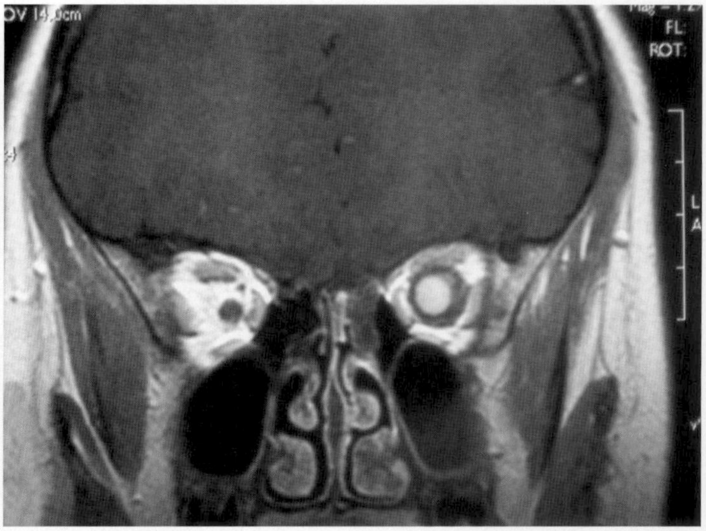

Fig. 2.140 Coronal MRI shows a hyperintense signal from a left optic nerve sheath meningioma. (Courtesy of A. Pearson.)

Sphenoidal ridge meningioma

Sphenoidal ridge meningioma is a very slow-growing intracranial tumour that may invade the orbit.

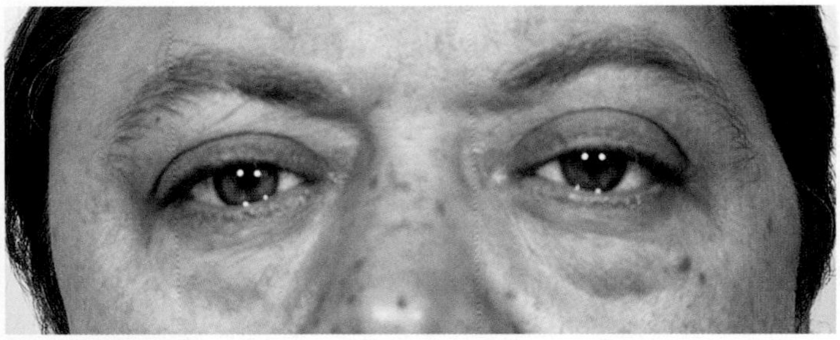

Fig. 2.141 Mild reactive hyperostosis causing fullness in the left temporal fossa.

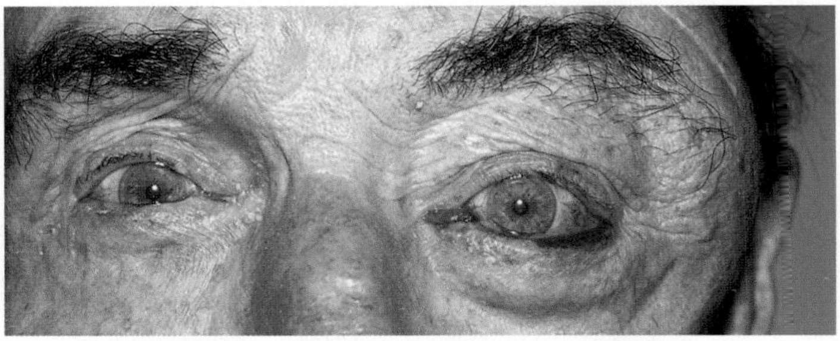

Fig. 2.142 More advanced reactive hyperostosis in the left temporal fossa and proptosis.

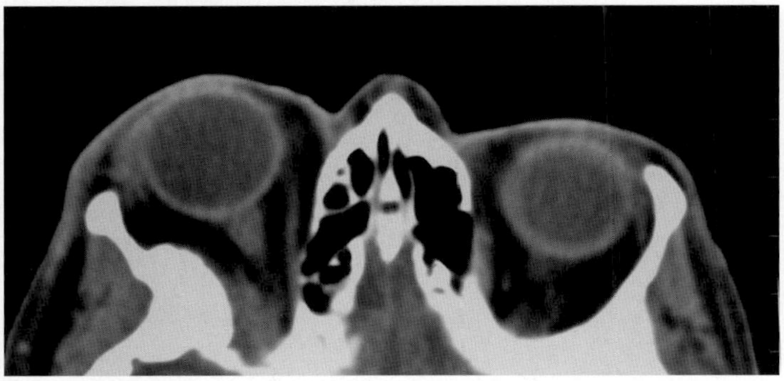

Fig. 2.143 Axial CT shows hyperostosis and a soft tissue mass due to a right sphenoidal wing meningioma. (Courtesy of A. Pearson.)

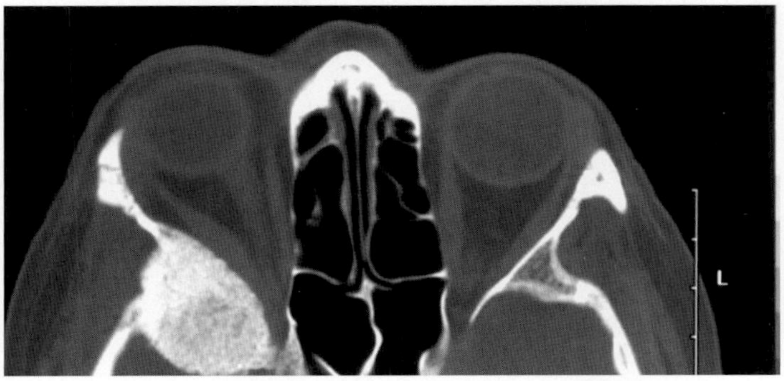

Fig. 2.144 Axial CT of a large right sphenoidal wing meningioma. (Courtesy of A. Pearson.)

Neurolemmoma (Schwannoma)

The presentation and CT appearance of this rare tumour are similar to a capillary haemangioma.

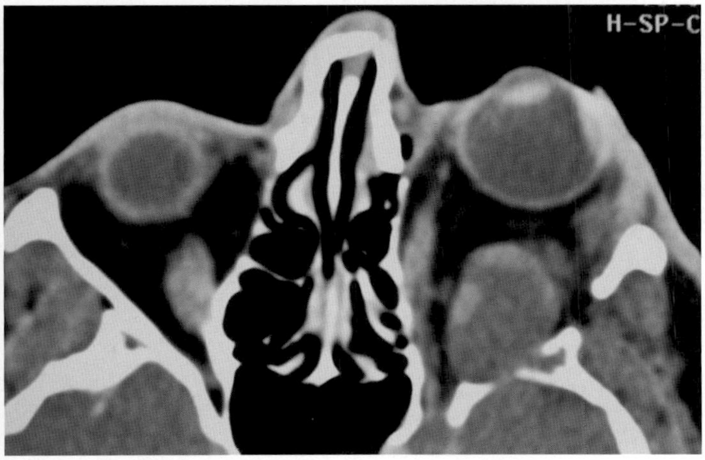

Fig. 2.145 Axial CT of a left neurolemmoma. (Courtesy of A. Pearson.)

MALIGNANT TUMOURS

Lacrimal gland carcinoma

Lacrimal gland carcinoma is a rare but very aggressive tumour. Presentation is in the fourth to sixth decade with a history shorter than that of a benign tumour.

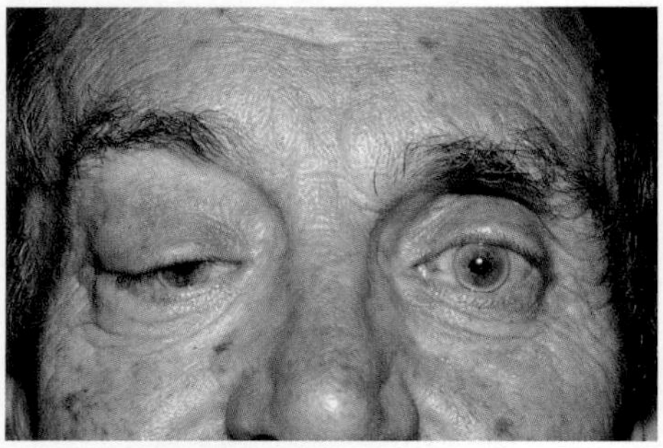

Fig. 2.146 A mass in the lacrimal area with down and in displacement of the globe. (Courtesy of G. Rose.)

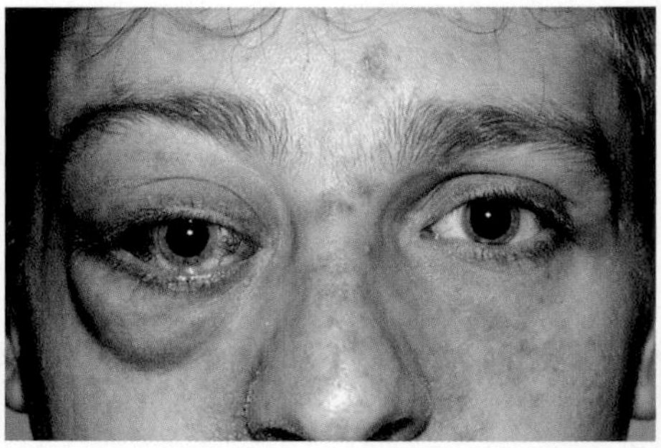

Fig. 2.147 Posterior extension involving the superior orbital fissure, causing conjunctival and episcleral congestion, and ophthalmoplegia. (Courtesy of G. Rose.)

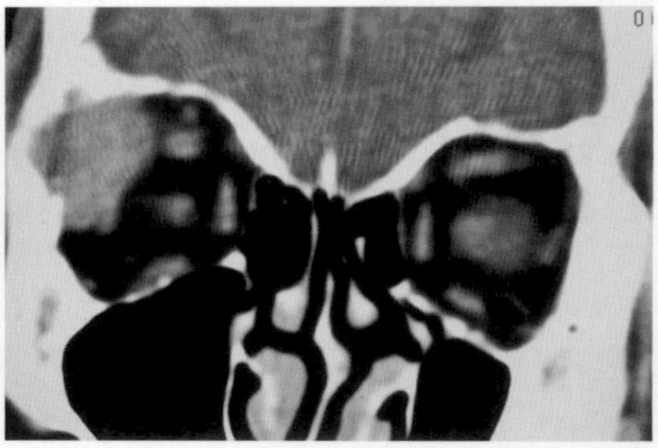

Fig. 2.148 Coronal CT shows contiguous erosion of bone and spotty calcification in the tumour. (Courtesy of A. Pearson.)

Lymphoma

Lymphoma of the ocular adnexa may involve any part of the orbit. Presentation is insidious and usually in old age.

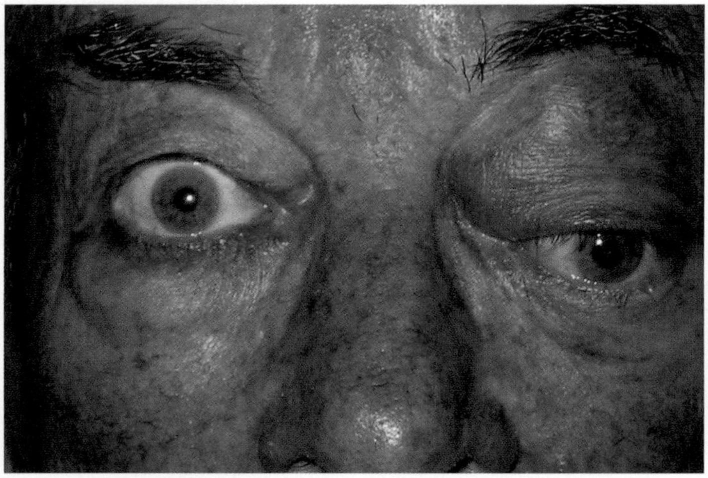

Fig. 2.149 Involvement of the superior orbit causing proptosis and down and out displacement. (Courtesy of A. Pearson.)

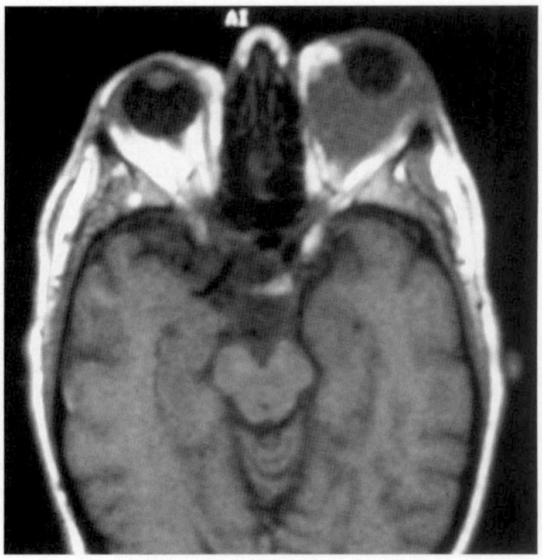

Fig. 2.150 Axial T1-weighted MRI of the same patient shows a large orbital soft tissue mass and proptosis. (Courtesy of A. Pearson.)

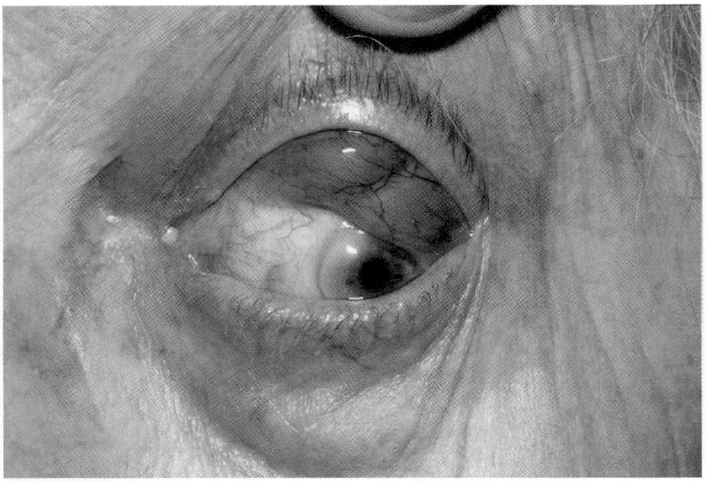

■ **Fig. 2.151** Anterior lesions have a rubbery consistency.

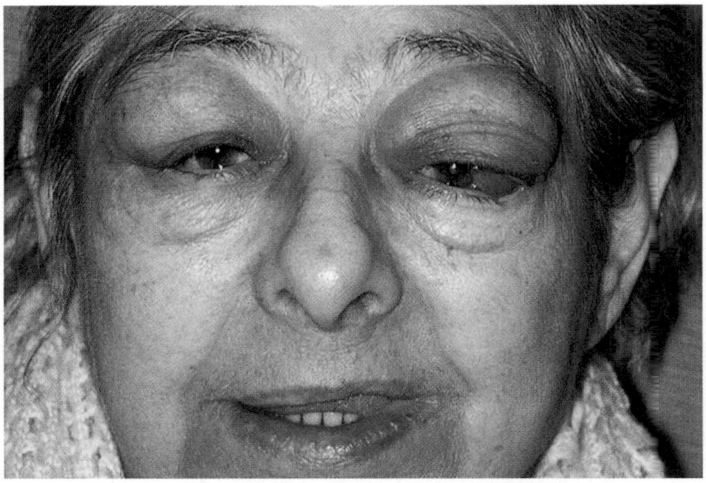

■ **Fig. 2.152** Occasionally the lymphoma may be confined to the lacrimal glands.

Rhabdomyosarcoma

Rhabdomyosarcoma is the most common childhood primary orbital malignancy.

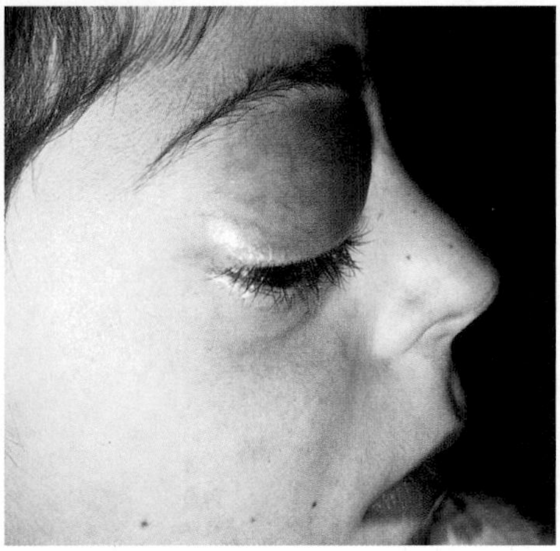

■ **Fig. 2.153** Presentation is in the first decade (average 7 years) with rapidly progressive proptosis and ptosis, which may initially mimic an inflammatory process but the skin is not warm.

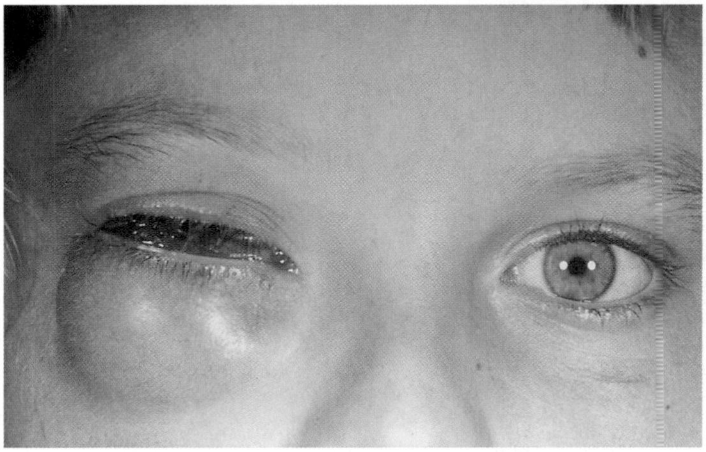

■ **Fig. 2.154** Rhabdomyosarcoma involving the inferior orbit is uncommon.

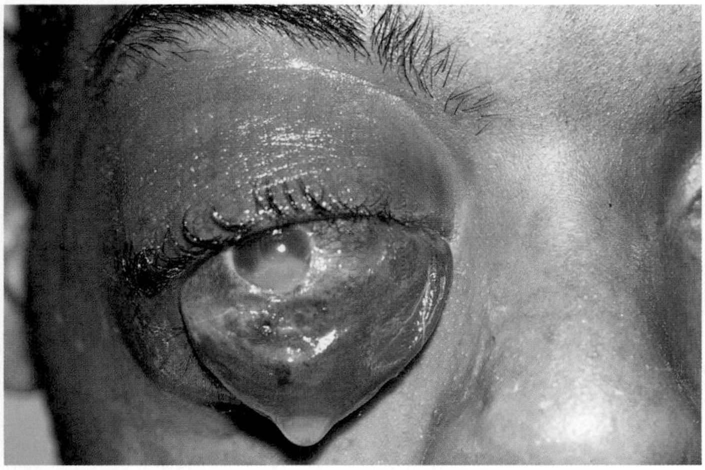

■ **Fig. 2.155** Very advanced rhabdomyosarcoma.

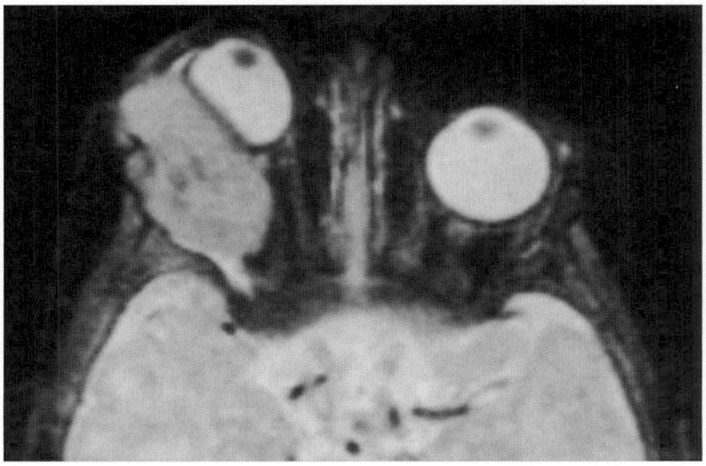

■ **Fig. 2.156** Axial T2-weighted MRI shows a poorly defined mass of homogeneous density and severe right proptosis.

SECONDARY ORBITAL TUMOURS

Langerhans cell histiocytosis

Langerhans cell histiocytosis is a paediatric condition characterised by proliferating histiocytes in the skin that may be associated with systemic disease.

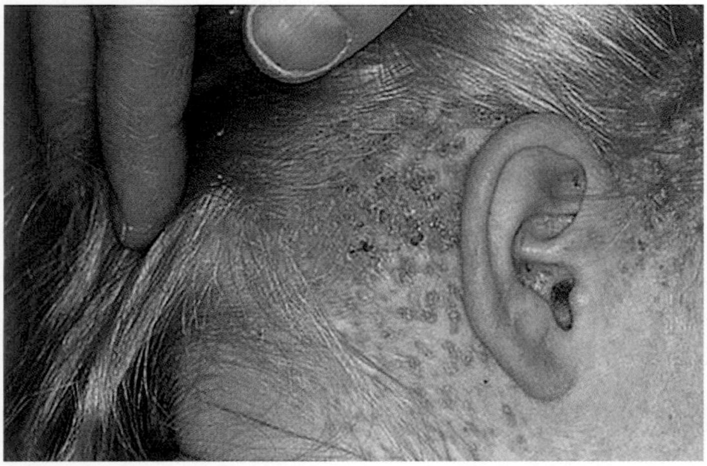

Fig. 2.157 Raised infiltrative cutaneous lesions with a scaly surface. (Courtesy of B. J. Zitelli and H. W. Davis.)

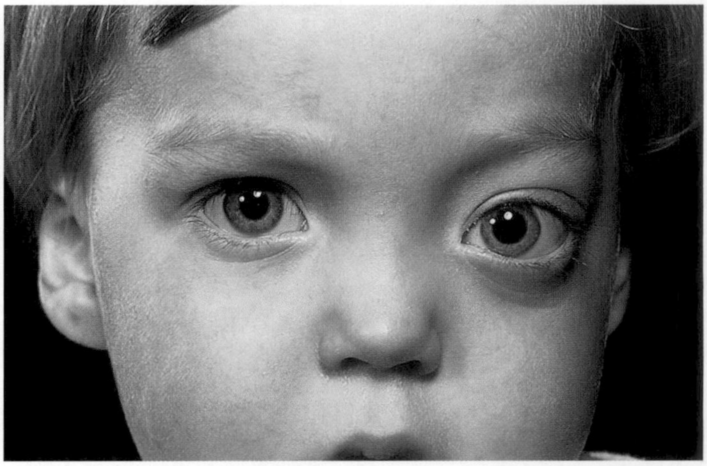

Fig. 2.158 Orbital involvement consists of unilateral or bilateral osteolytic lesions and soft tissue involvement, typically in the superotemporal quadrant. (Courtesy of D. Taylor.)

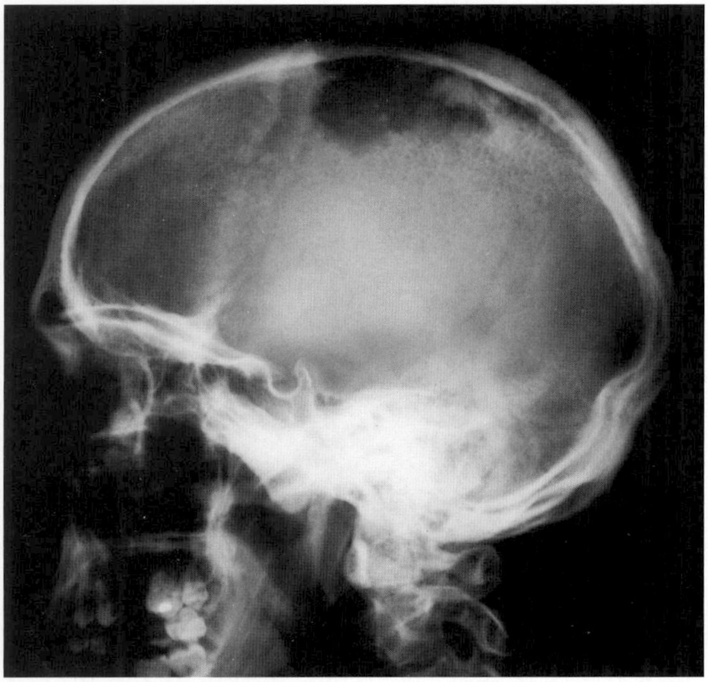

Fig. 2.159 Lytic skull lesions are uncommon.

Granulocytic sarcoma (chloroma)

Granulocytic granuloma is a localised tumour composed of malignant cells of myeloid origin that may occur as a manifestation of established myeloid leukaemia or may precede systemic disease.

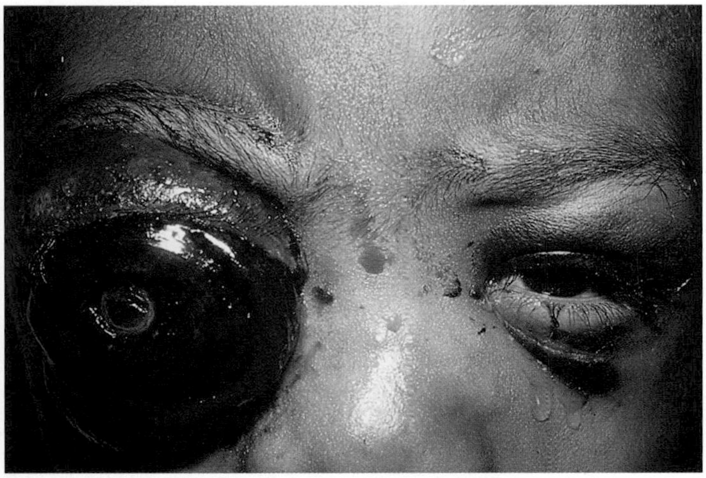

Fig. 2.160 Presentation is most frequently at about the age of 7 years with rapid onset of congestive proptosis, sometimes bilateral (Courtesy of P. Morse.)

Metastatic neuroblastoma

Neuroblastoma typically presents in early childhood and carries a poor prognosis. The tumour arises from primitive neuroblasts of the sympathetic chain, most commonly in the abdomen.

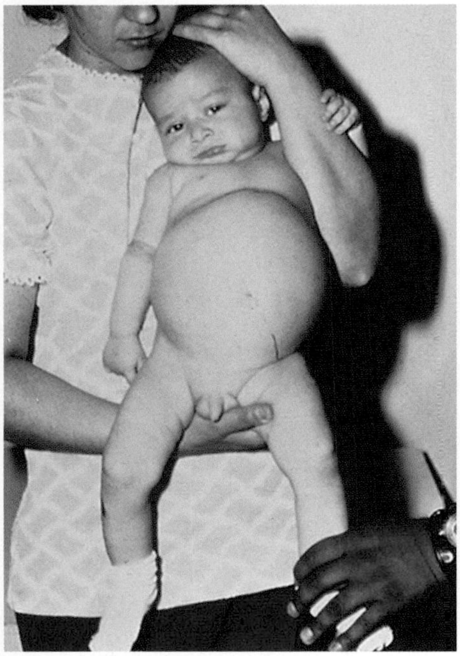

Fig. 2.161 Neuroblastoma causing abdominal swelling. (Courtesy of B. J. Zitelli and H. W. Davis.)

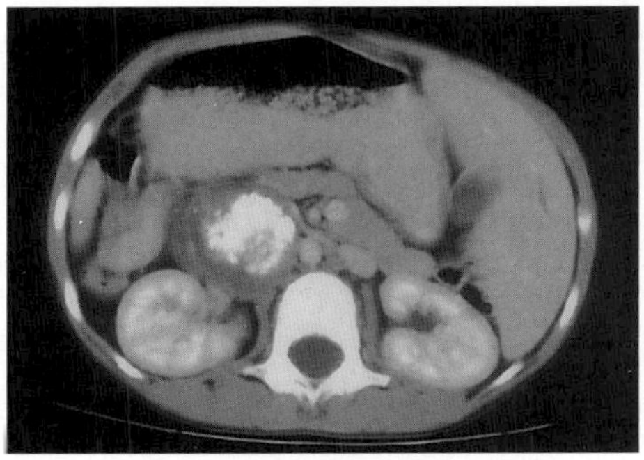

Fig. 2.162 CT scan shows calcification in an adrenal neuroblastoma. (Courtesy of B. J. Zitelli and H. W. Davis.)

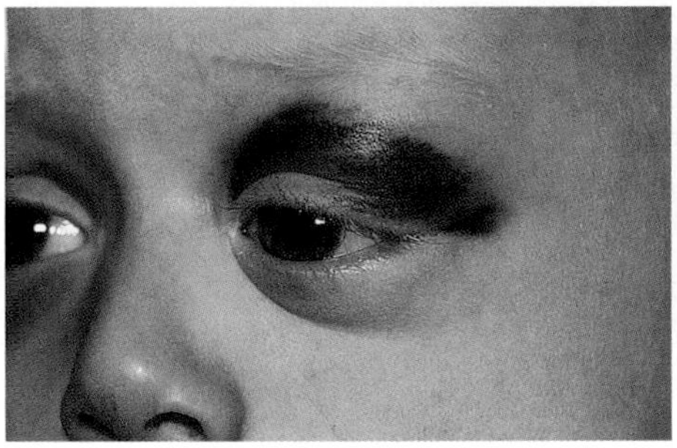

Fig. 2.163 Orbital metastases typically present with an abrupt onset of proptosis accompanied by a superior orbital mass and lid ecchymosis. (Courtesy of M. A. Mir.)

Adult metastatic tumours

Orbital metastases are an uncommon cause of adult proptosis. In order of frequency the most common primary sites are breast, bronchus, prostate, skin melanoma, gastrointestinal tract and kidney.

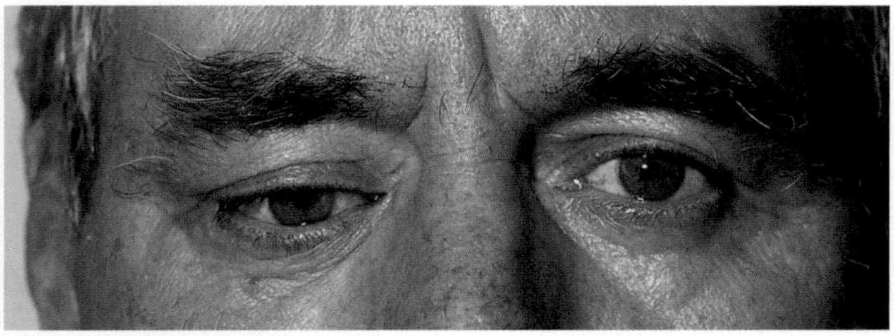

Fig. 2.164 Presentation is most frequently with rapid onset of a painful anterior orbital mass.

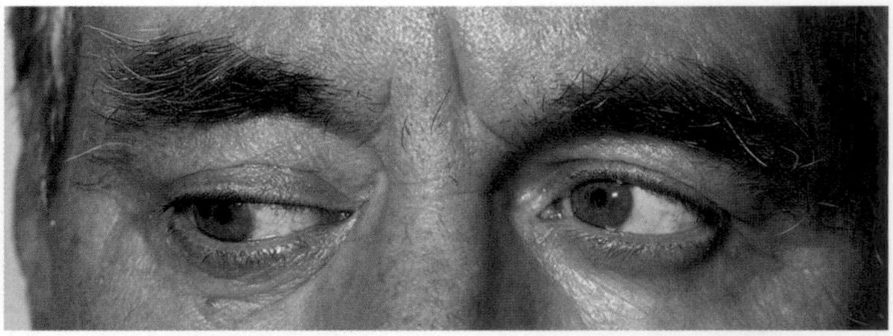

Fig. 2.165 Displacement of the globe may cause diplopia.

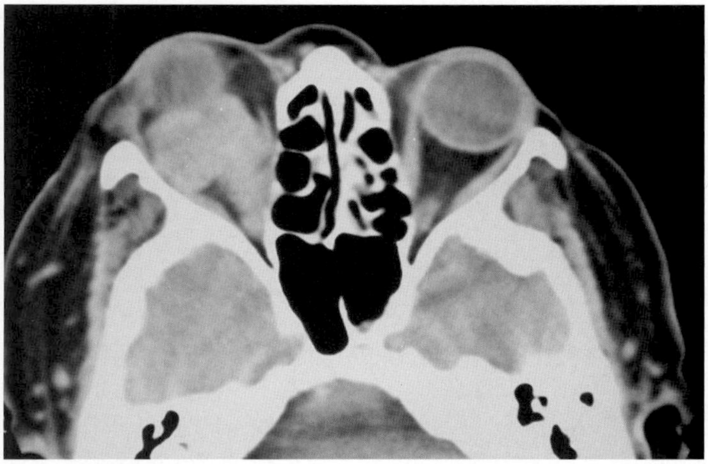

Fig. 2.166 Axial CT shows a poorly defined mass. (Courtesy of A. Pearson.)

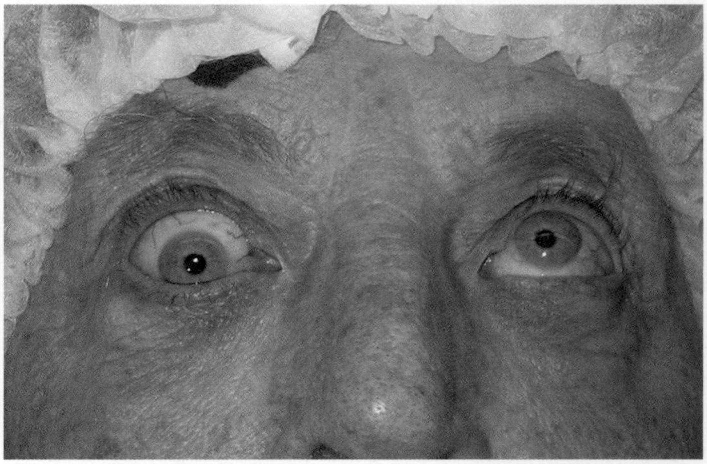

Fig. 2.167 Deposits at the orbital apex may cause cranial nerve palsies with little or no proptosis. (Courtesy of A. Pearson.)

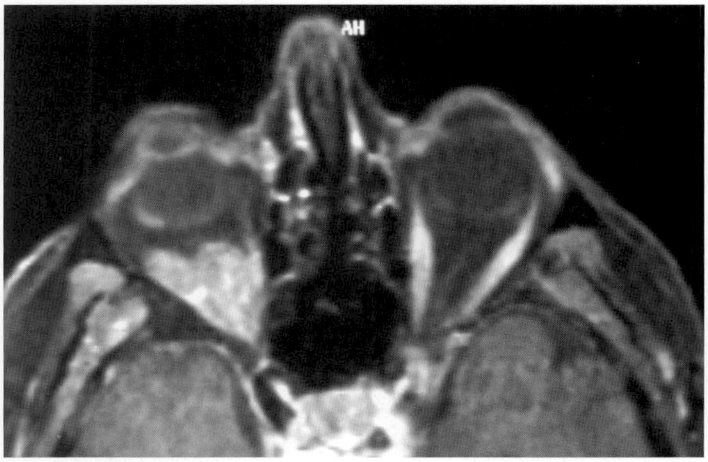

Fig. 2.168 Axial T1-weighted MRI of the same patient. (Courtesy of A. Pearson.)

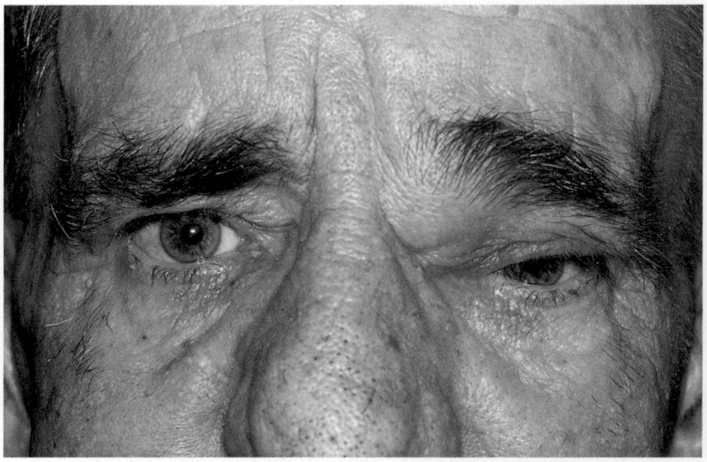

Fig. 2.169 Metastasis of a schirrous carcinoma giving rise to enophthalmos due to orbital fibrosis.

ORBITAL INVASION FROM ADJACENT SITES

Sinus tumours

Malignant tumours of the paranasal sinuses, although rare, may invade the orbit and carry a poor prognosis unless diagnosed early.

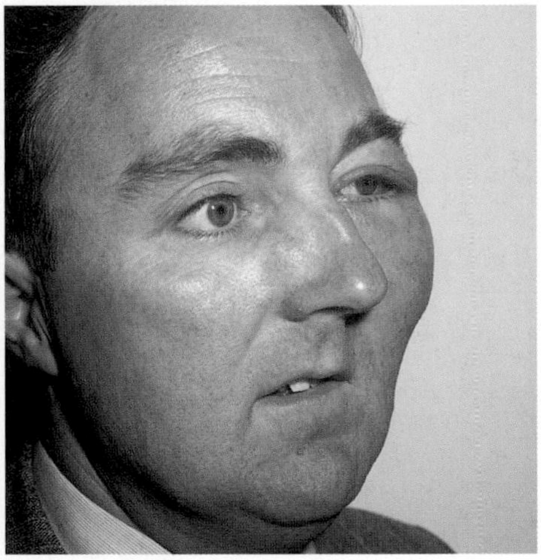

Fig. 2.170 Maxillary carcinoma typically causes facial pain, swelling, upward globe displacement, diplopia and epiphora.

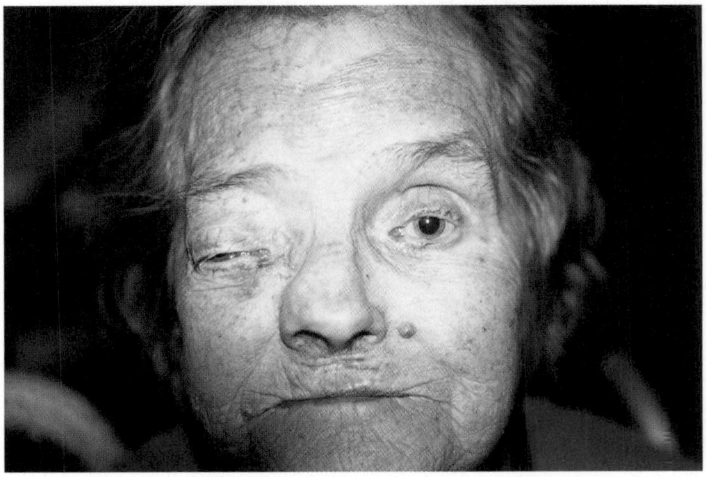

Fig. 2.171 Ethmoidal carcinoma may cause lateral globe displacement.

Eyelid tumours

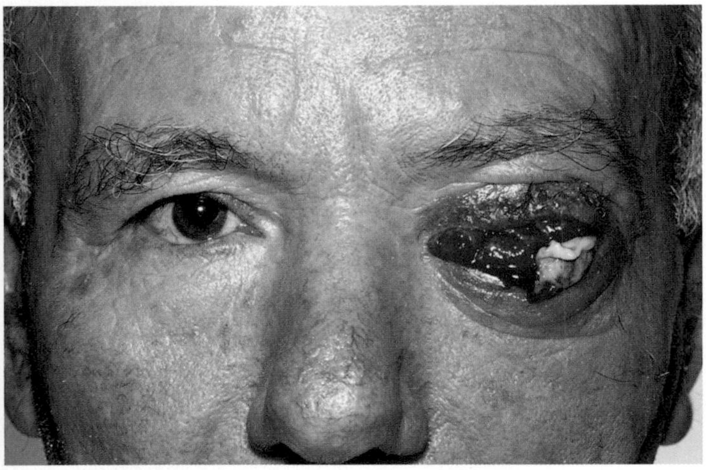

Fig. 2.172 Neglected eyelid malignancies may invade the orbit.

Ocular tumours

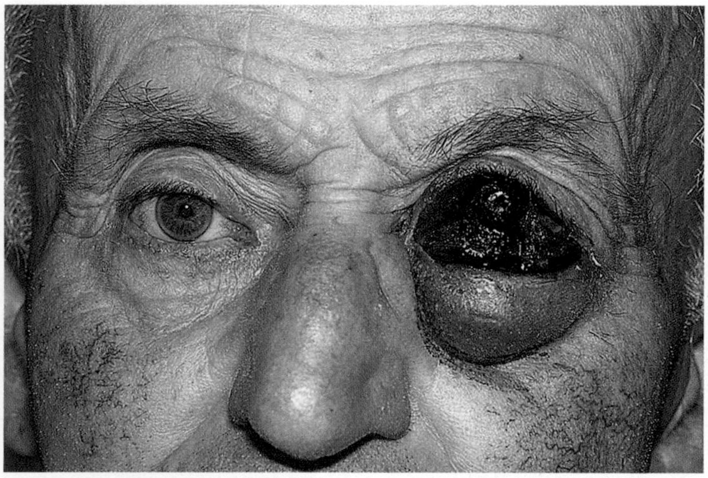

■ **Fig. 2.173** Conjunctival and choroidal melanomas may recur in the orbit following treatment.

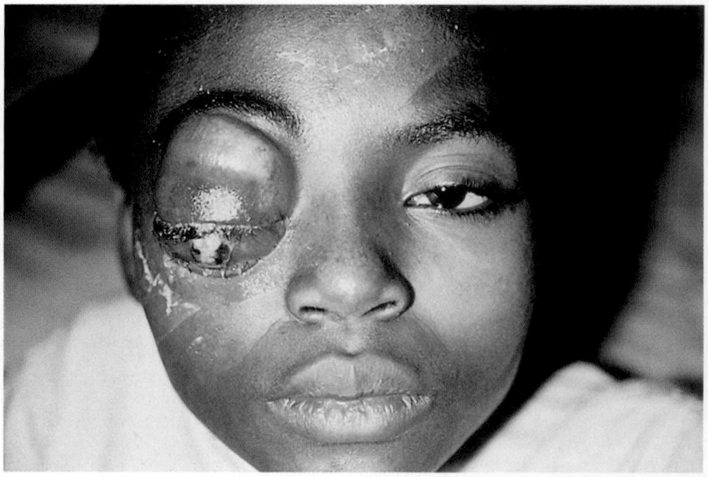

■ **Fig. 2.174** Neglected retinoblastoma may invade the orbit. A necrotic tumour may also induce an inflammatory reaction mimicking orbital or preseptal cellulitis.

Fibrous dysplasia

Fibrous dysplasia is an idiopathic disease characterised by replacement of normal bone by cellular fibrous stroma.

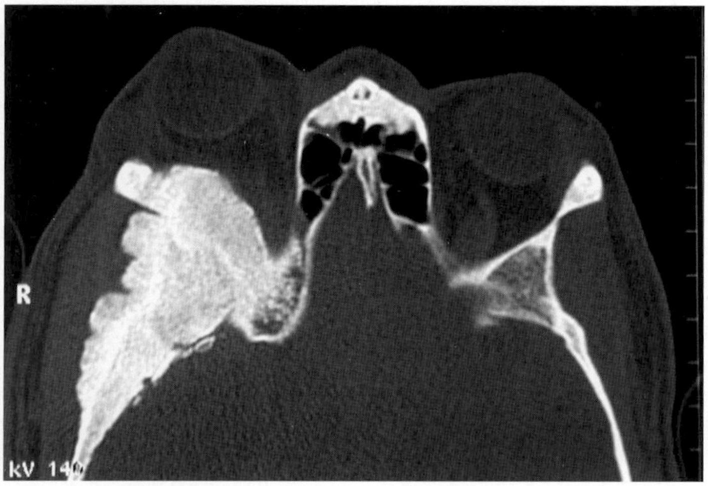

■ **Fig. 2.175** Axial CT shows thickening of bone and expansion into the orbit. (Courtesy of A. Pearson.)

CONGENITAL ANOMALIES OF THE ORBITS AND FACE

Hypertelorism

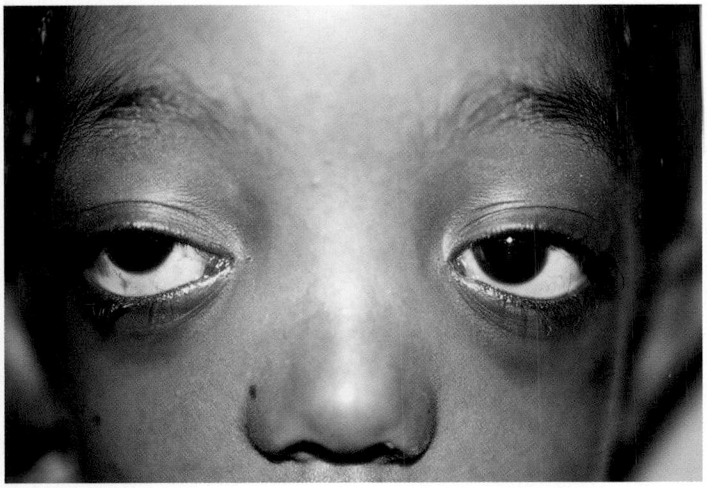

■ **Fig. 2.176** Wide separation of the orbits, which is determined by measuring the interpupillary distance. It should not be confused with telecanthus, which is due to excessive length of the medial canthal ligaments.

Shallow orbits

Shallow orbits occur in craniosynostoses, a group of rare, hereditary disorders characterised by premature fusion of the cranial sutures accompanied by severe orbital abnormalities.

Oxycephaly

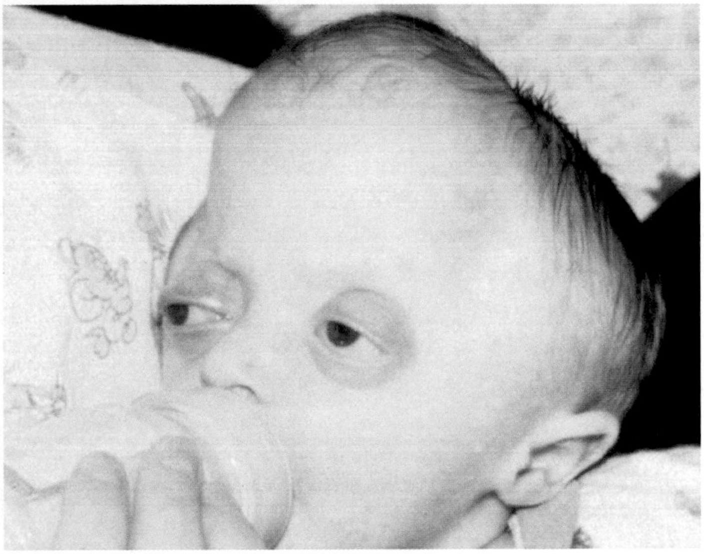

■ **Fig. 2.177** Narrow, dome-shaped skull with a high forehead.

Crouzon syndrome

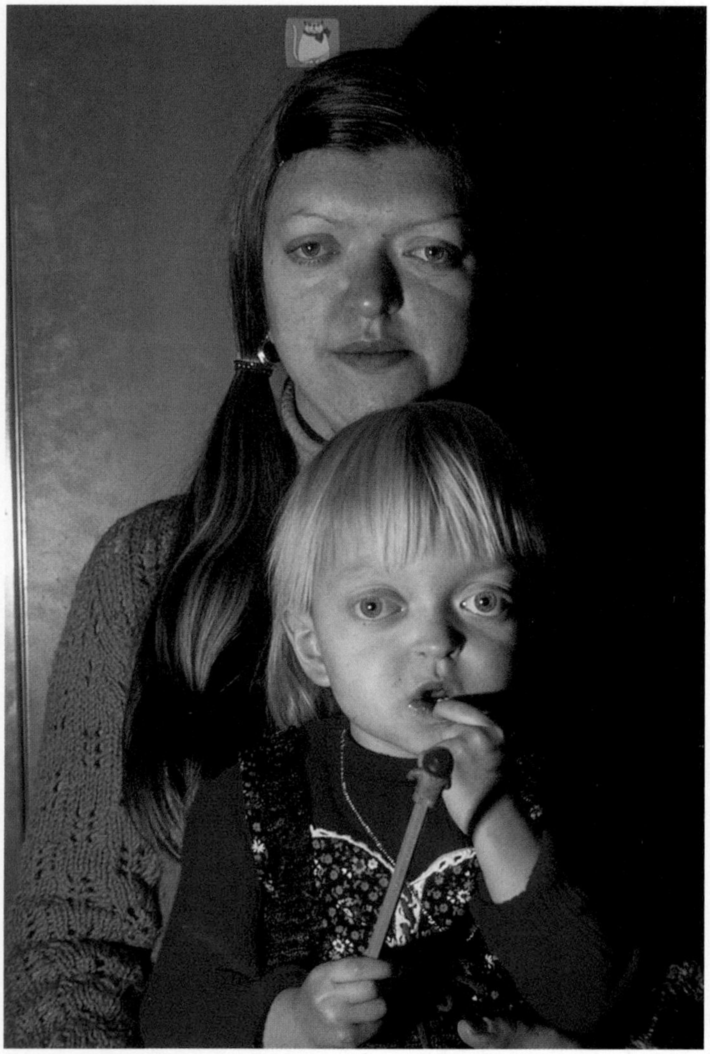

■ **Fig. 2.178** Inheritance is autosomal dominant.

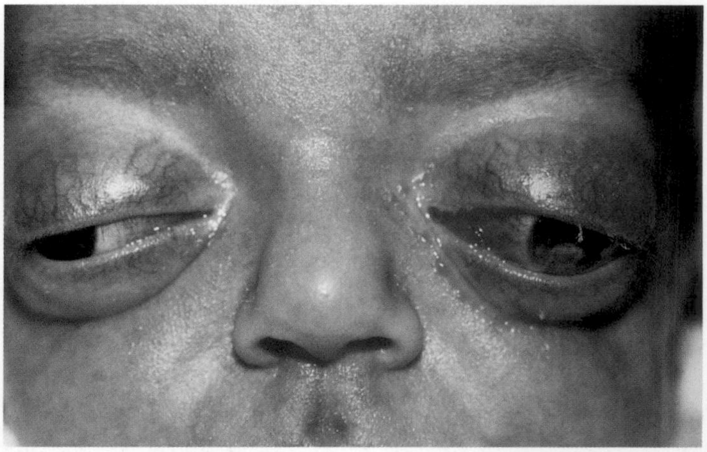

■ **Fig. 2.179** Proptosis due to shallow orbits and hypertelorism are the most conspicuous features. Midfacial hypoplasia and a curved 'parrot-beak' nose give rise to a 'frog-like' facies.

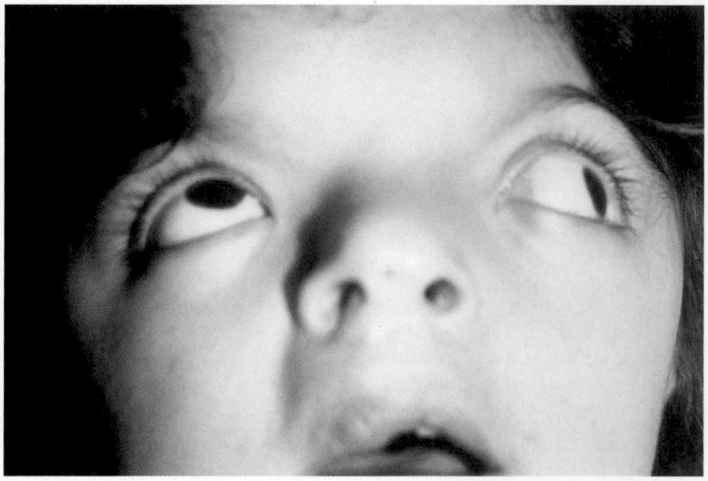

■ **Fig. 2.180** V-pattern exotropia is common.

Apert syndrome

Apert syndrome (acrocephalosyndactyly) is the most severe of the craniosynostoses and may involve all cranial sutures.

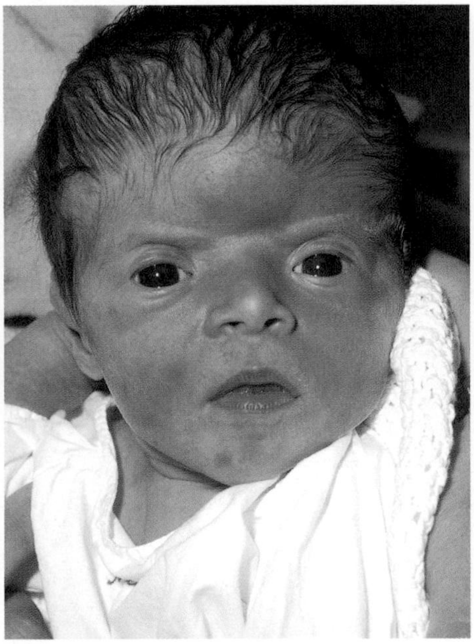

Fig. 2.181 Shallow orbits, proptosis and hypertelorism are generally less pronounced than in Crouzon syndrome. Also present are midfacial hypoplasia, a 'parrot-beak' nose and an antimongoloid slant of the palpebral apertures.

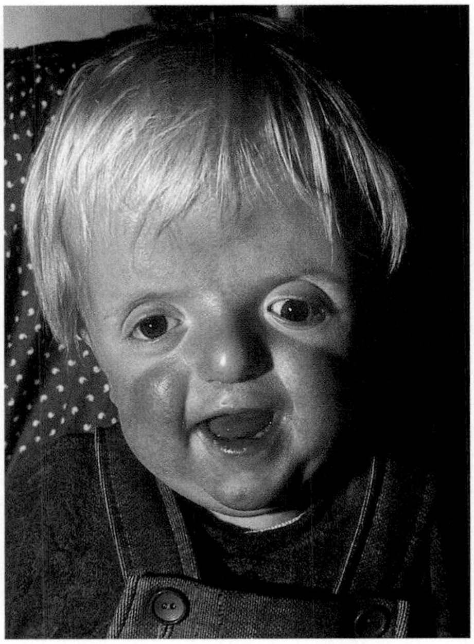

Fig. 2.182 An older child with Apert syndrome.

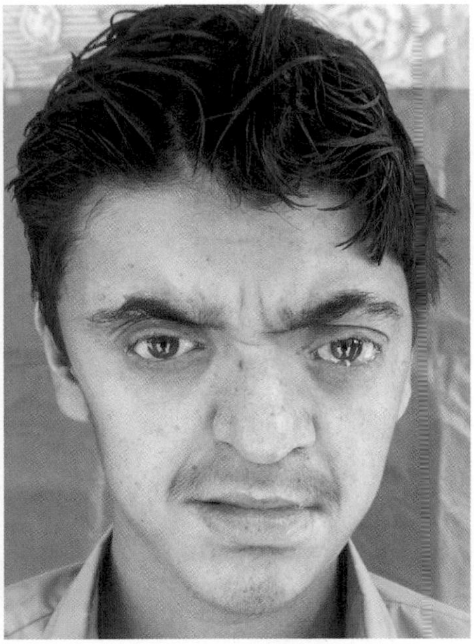

Fig. 2.183 An adult with Apert syndrome. (Courtesy of N. Raik.)

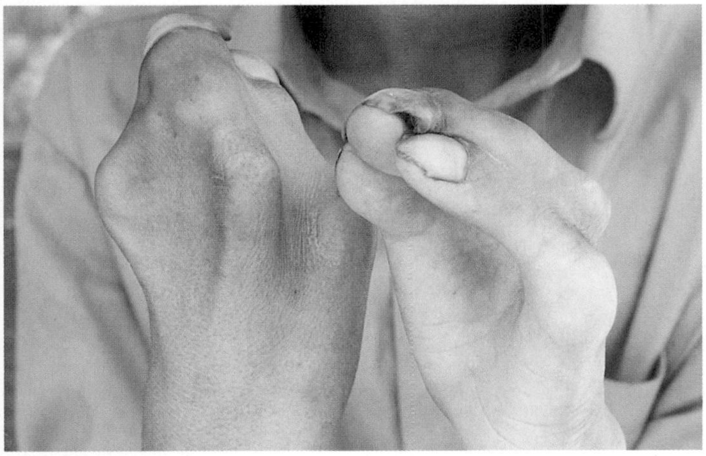

Fig. 2.184 Syndactyly of the hands in the same patient. (Courtesy of N. Raik.)

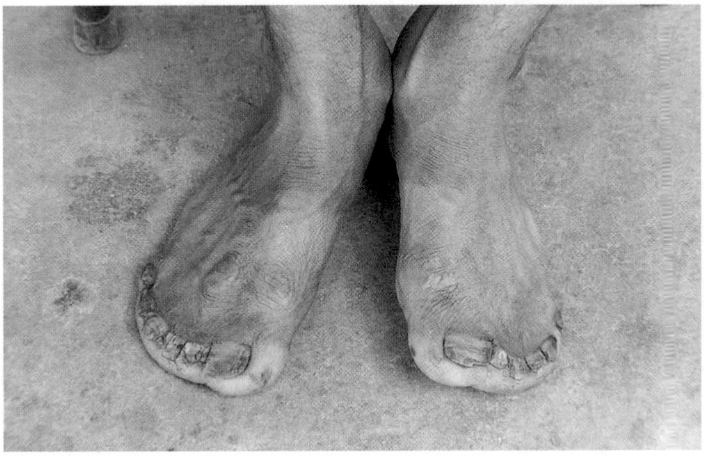

Fig. 2.185 Syndactyly of the feet. (Courtesy of N. Raik.)

Pfeiffer syndrome

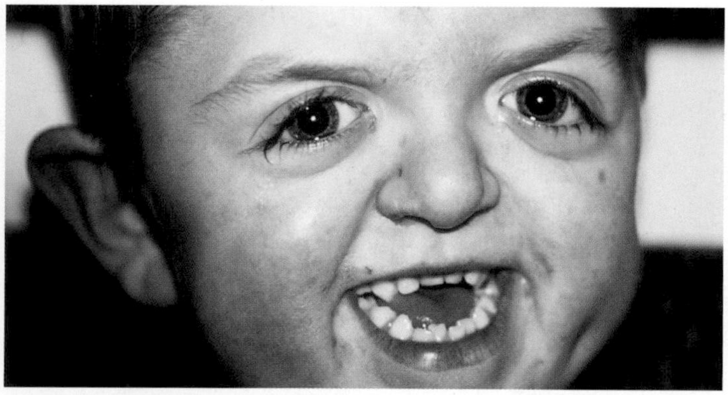

■ **Fig. 2.186** Facial features are similar to Apert syndrome. (Courtesy of K. Nischal.)

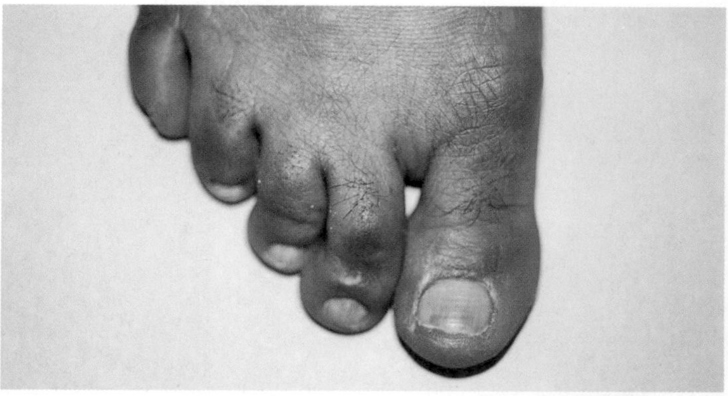

■ **Fig. 2.187** Distinctive are broad, long thumbs and great toes.

Roberts syndrome (Roberts-SC phocomelia)

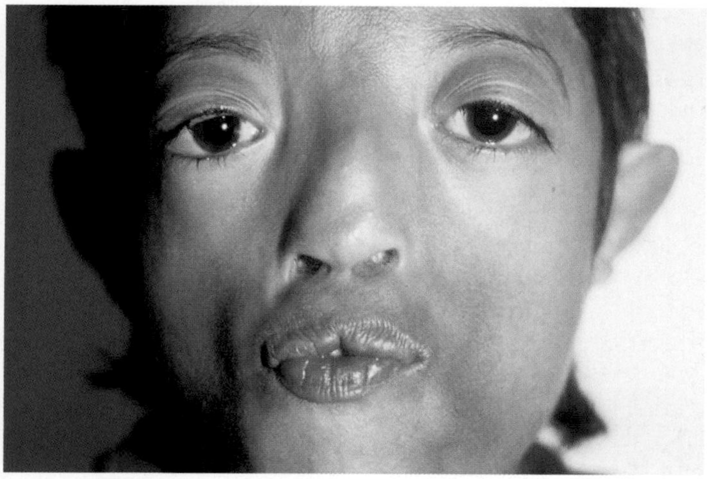

■ **Fig. 2.188** Shallow orbits, hypertelorism, corneal clouding, midfacial anomalies and phocomelia. (Courtesy of K. Nischal.)

Orbital dystopia

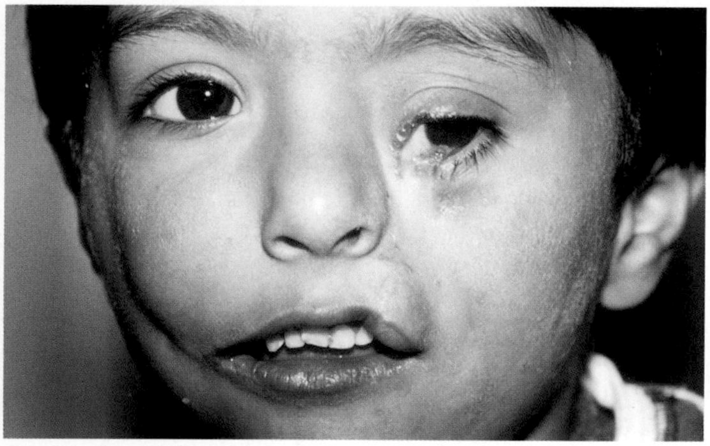

■ **Fig. 2.189** Dystopia is asymmetry of the inferior orbital margins, which may be associated with facial clefting. (Courtesy of Oxford Eye Hospital.)

Clefting syndromes

Clefting syndromes are the result of failure of fusion or defective apposition of neighbouring structures during embryonic development.

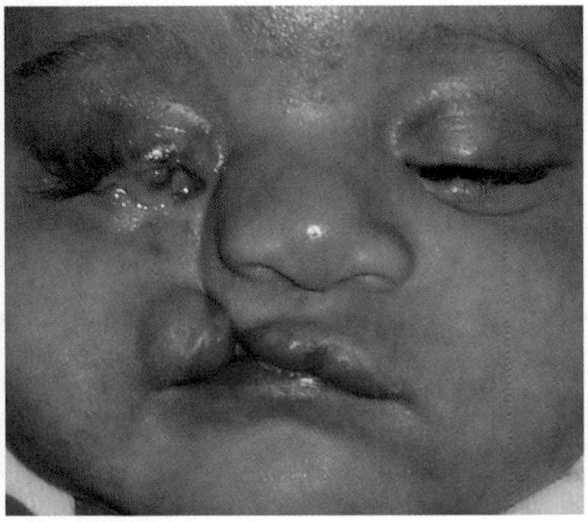

Fig. 2.190 Severe facial cleft involving the maxilla and orbit.

Treacher Collins syndrome (mandibulofacial dysostosis)

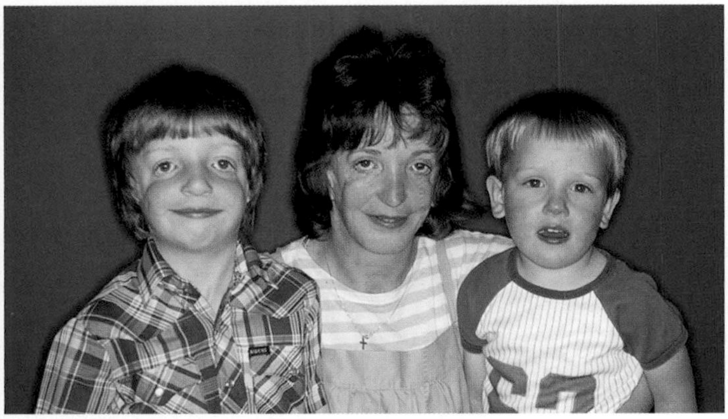

Fig. 2.191 Inheritance is autosomal dominant.

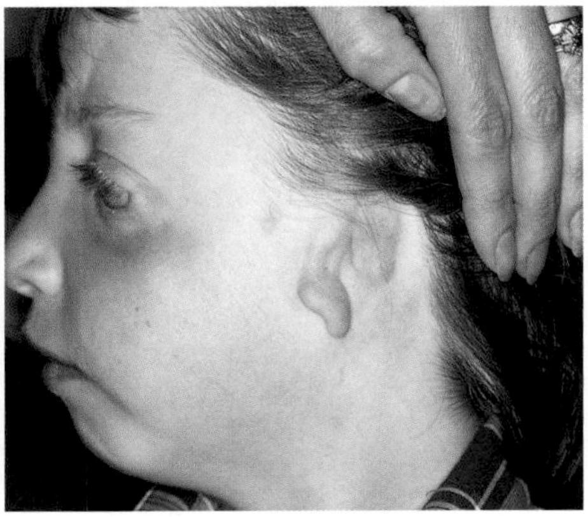

Fig. 2.192 Hypoplasia of the zygoma and mandible, and external ear malformation.

Goldenhar syndrome (oculovertebral spectrum)

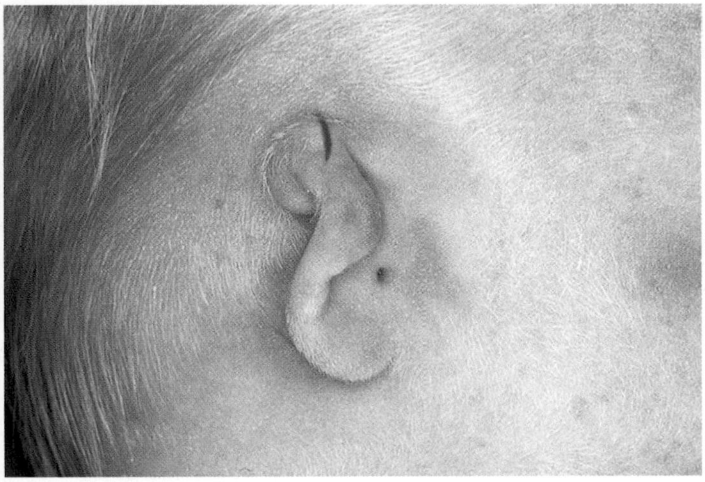

Fig. 2.193 Ear anomalies.

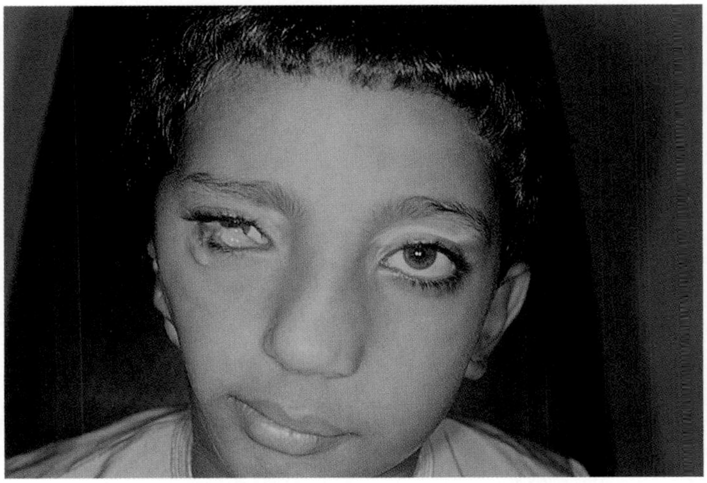

Fig. 2.194 Mandibular and malar hypoplasia, and limbal dermoids. (Courtesy of U. Raina.)

CHAPTER 3

CONJUNCTIVA

INFECTIOUS CONJUNCTIVITIS

Simple bacterial conjunctivitis

Simple bacterial conjunctivitis is a common and usually self-limiting condition. The most frequent causative organisms are *Staphylococcus epidermidis*, *Staphylococcus aureus*, *Streptococcus pneumoniae* and *Haemophilus influenzae*

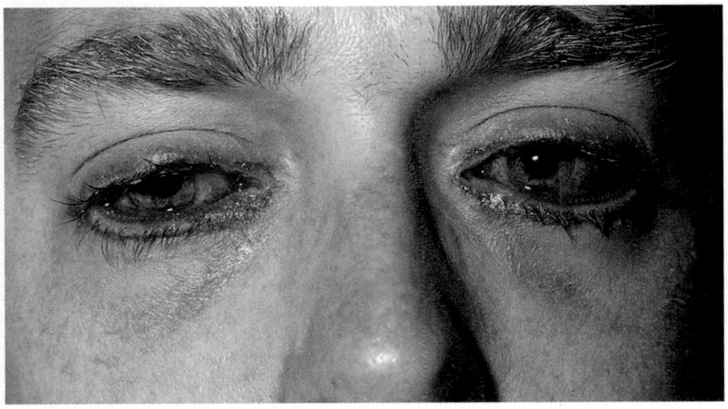

Fig. 3.1 The eyelids are crusted and may be slightly oedematous.

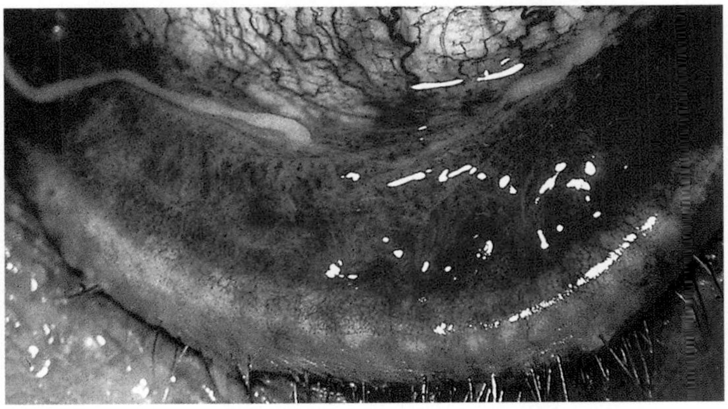

Fig. 3.2 The tarsal conjunctiva has a velvety, beefy-red appearance and mild papillary changes with mucous strands in the inferior fornix.

Gonococcal keratoconjunctivitis

Gonorrhoea is a venereal genitourinary tract infection caused by the Gram-negative diplococcus *Neisseria gonorrhoeae* which is capable of invading the intact corneal epithelium.

Conjunctivitis

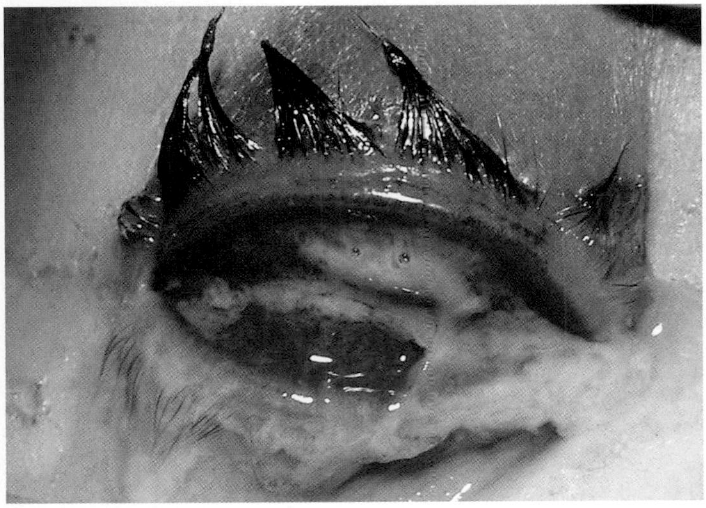

Fig. 3.3 Lid oedema and purulent discharge.

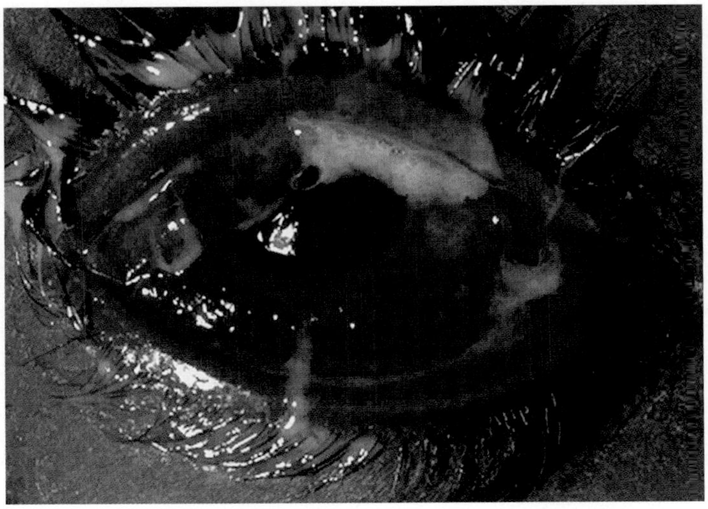

Fig. 3.4 Purulent discharge and severe chemosis. (Courtesy of S. Ford and R. Marsh.)

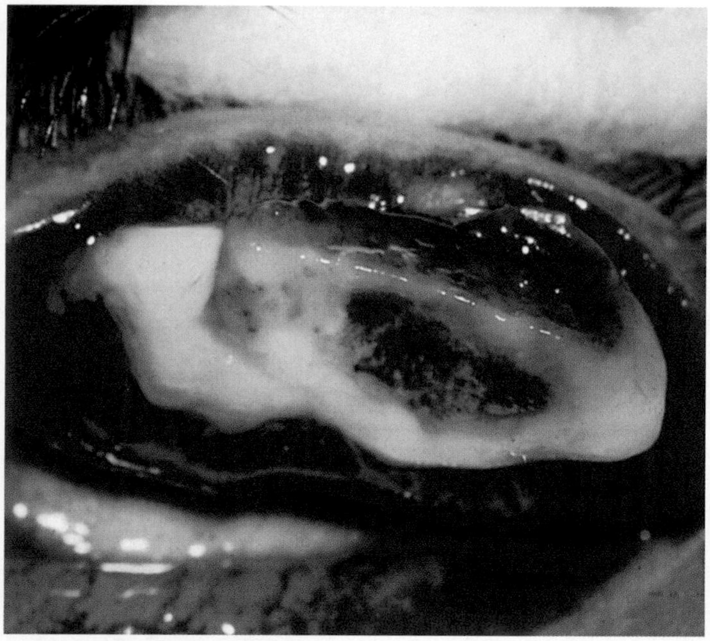

Fig. 3.5 Intense conjunctival hyperaemia, purulent discharge and pseudomembrane formation.

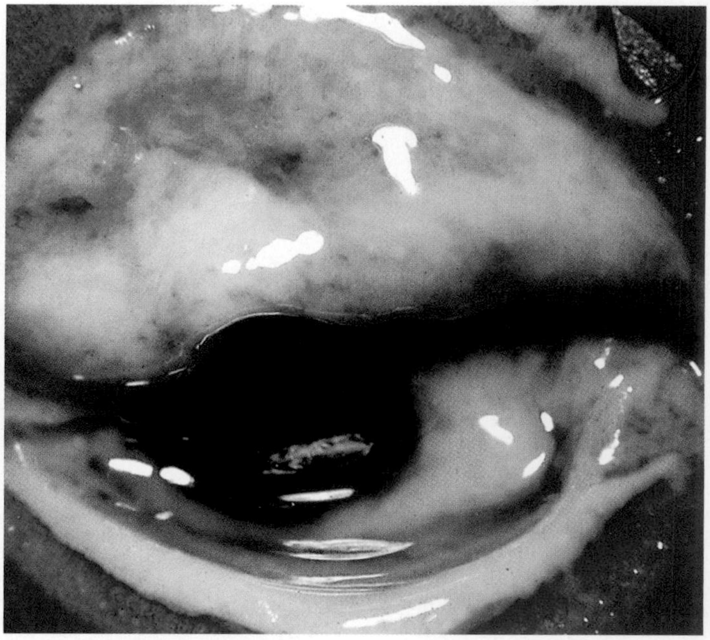

Fig. 3.6 Purulent coagulum.

Keratitis

Unless conjunctivitis is treated promptly keratitis may progress as follows:

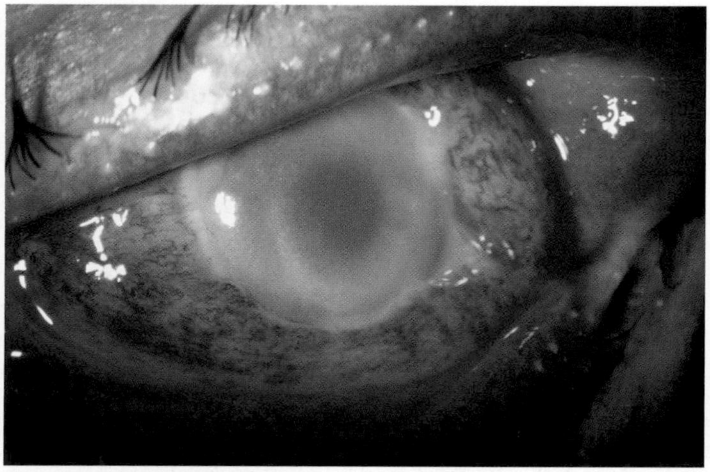

Fig. 3.7 Marginal ulceration in the pus-filled sulcus between the chemosed conjunctiva and the limbus.

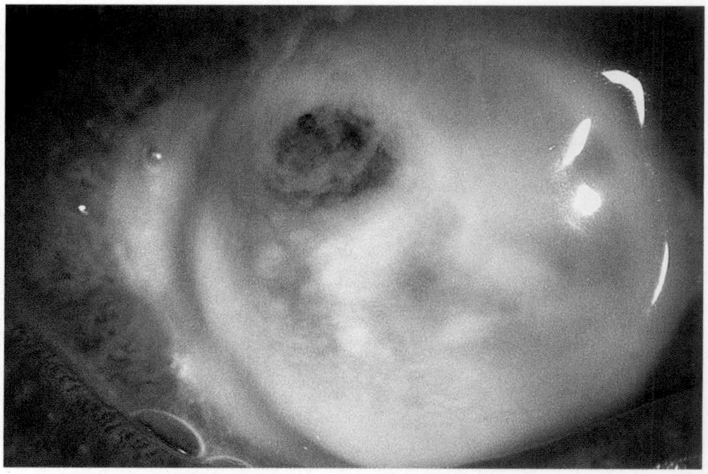

Fig. 3.8 Perforation and endophthalmitis.

Adenoviral keratoconjunctivitis

There are at least 30 distinct types of adenoviruses capable of causing a variety of clinical illnesses, some of which may have ocular involvement.

Conjunctivitis

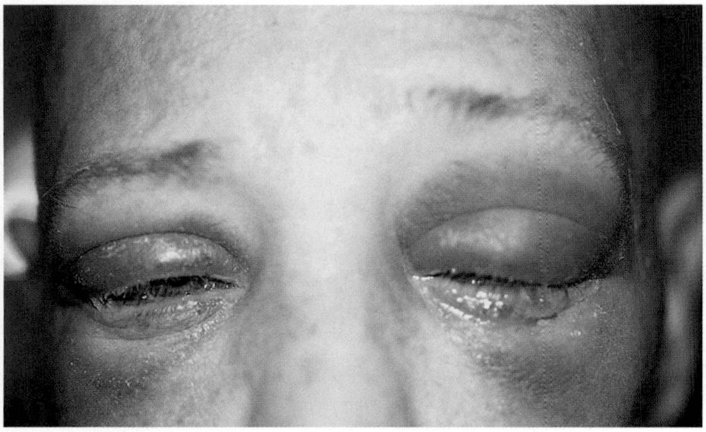

Fig. 3.9 Bilateral eyelid oedema and tender lymphadenopathy.

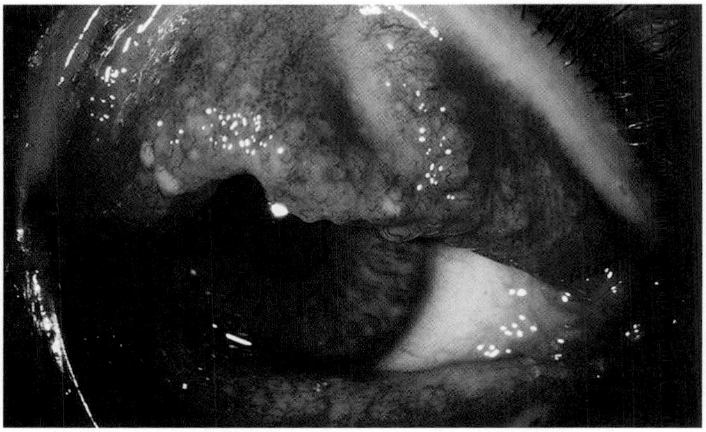

Fig. 3.10 Follicular conjunctivitis.

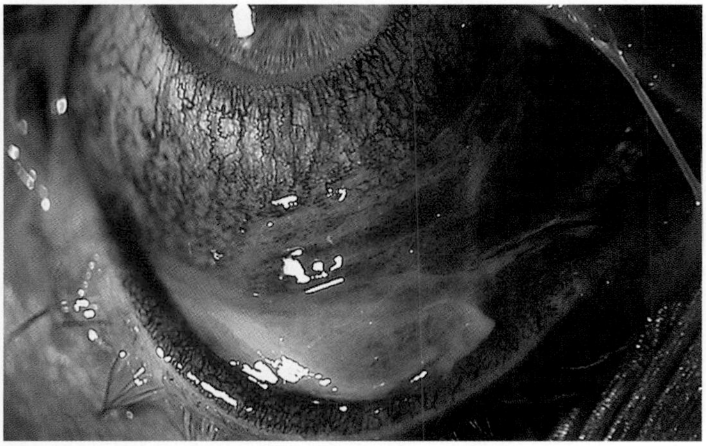

Fig. 3.11 Pseudomembranes in severe cases.

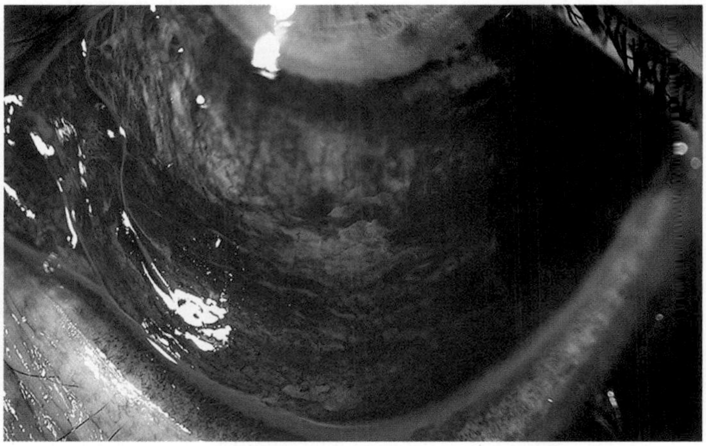

Fig. 3.12 Subconjunctival haemorrhages are uncommon.

Keratitis

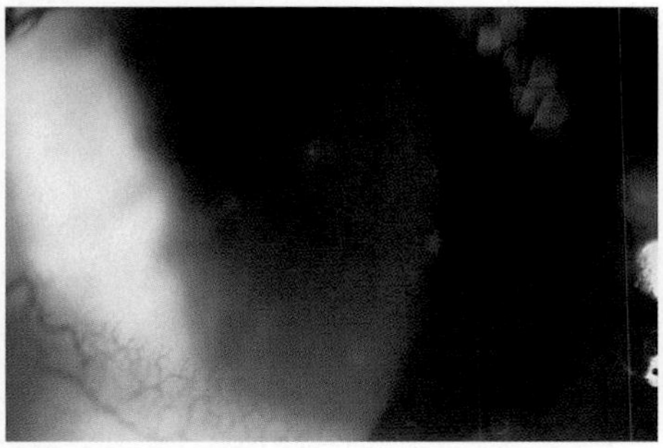

Fig. 3.13 Stage 1 occurs within 7–10 days of the onset of symptoms and is characterised by punctate epithelial lesions that resolves within 2 weeks.

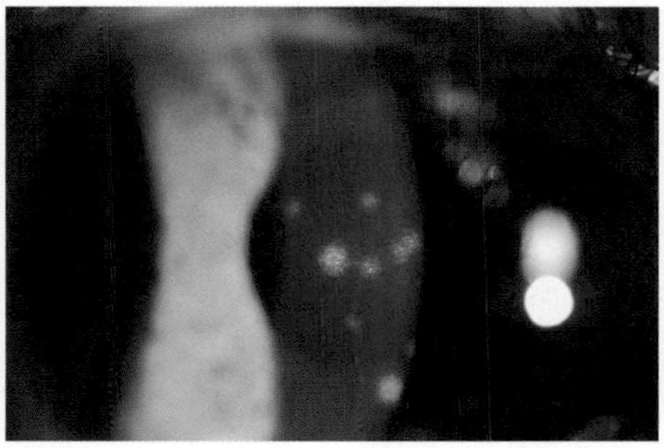

Fig. 3.14 Stage 2 is characterised by focal, white, subepithelial opacities that develop beneath the fading epithelial lesions.

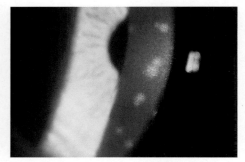

Fig. 3.15 Stage 3 is characterised by anterior stromal infiltrates, which gradually fade over months or years.

Molluscum contagiosum conjunctivitis

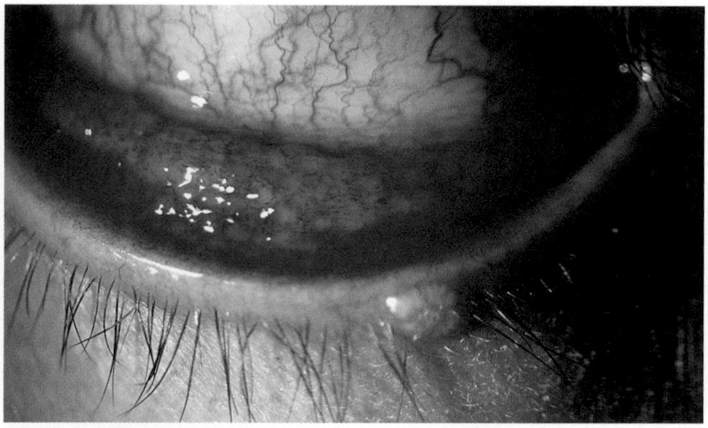

Fig. 3.16 The lid margin shows a small, pale, waxy, umbilicated nodule associated with an ipsilateral follicular conjunctivitis with a mild mucoid discharge.

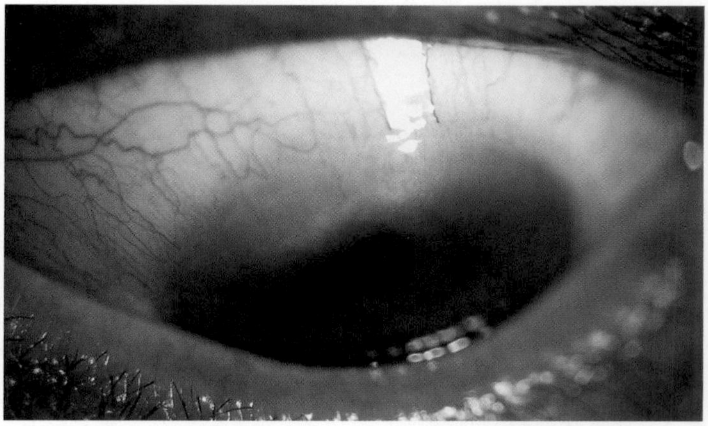

Fig. 3.17 Long-standing cases may develop fine epithelial keratitis, which may progress to superior pannus formation if untreated.

Adult chlamydial conjunctivitis

Adult chlamydial conjunctivitis is a sexually transmitted disease caused by serotypes D–K of *Chlamydia trachomatis*.

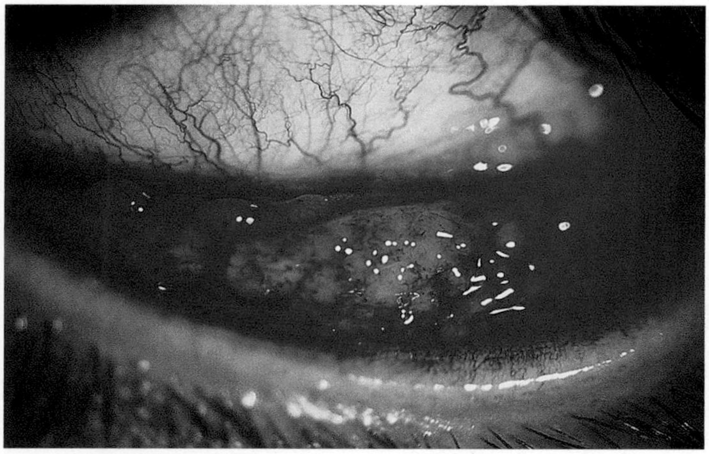

Fig. 3.18 Large follicles, most prominent in the inferior fornical conjunctiva, associated with a scant mucopurulent discharge and tender lymphadenopathy.

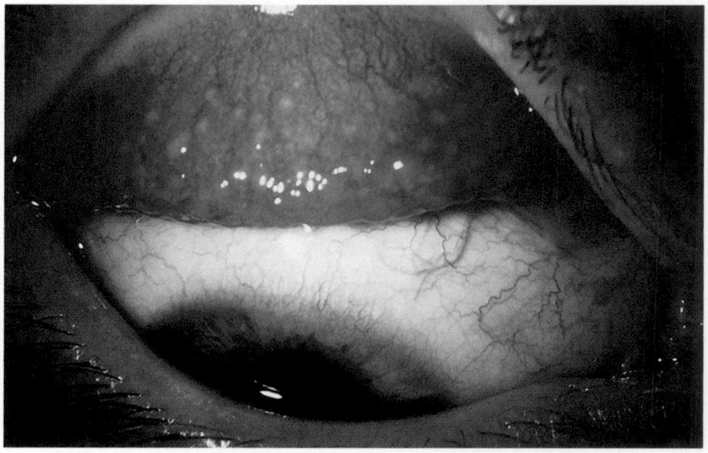

Fig. 3.19 The upper tarsal conjunctiva may also be involved.

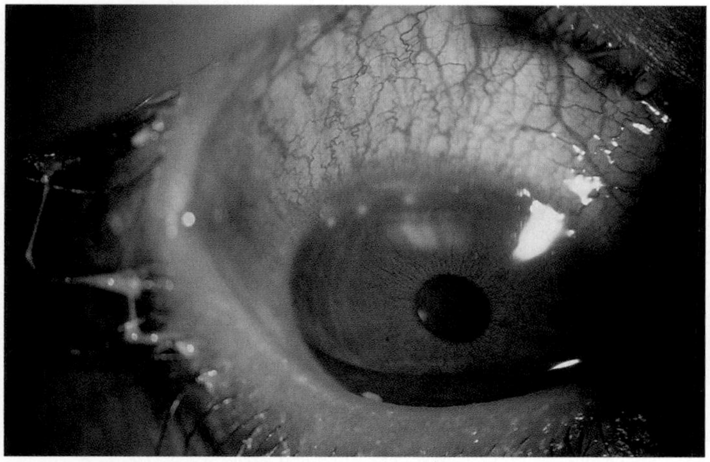

Fig. 3.20 Peripheral corneal infiltrates may appear 2–3 weeks after the onset of conjunctivitis.

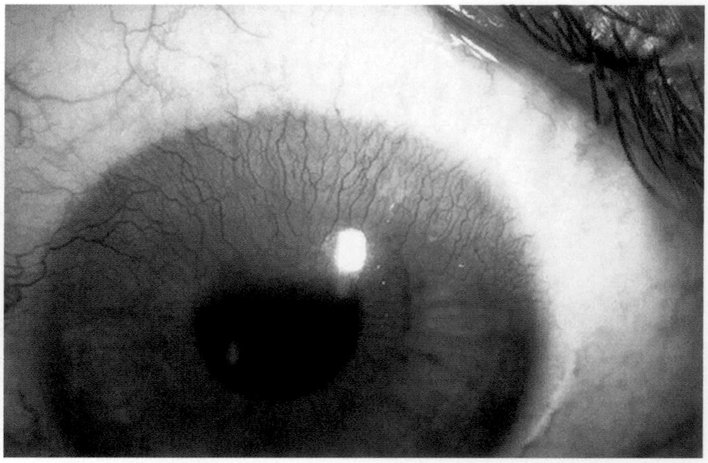

Fig. 3.21 Long-standing cases are characterised by less prominent follicles and a superior pannus. (Courtesy of S. Ford and R. Marsh.)

Neonatal chlamydial conjunctivitis

Chlamydial infection is the most common cause of neonatal conjunctivitis.

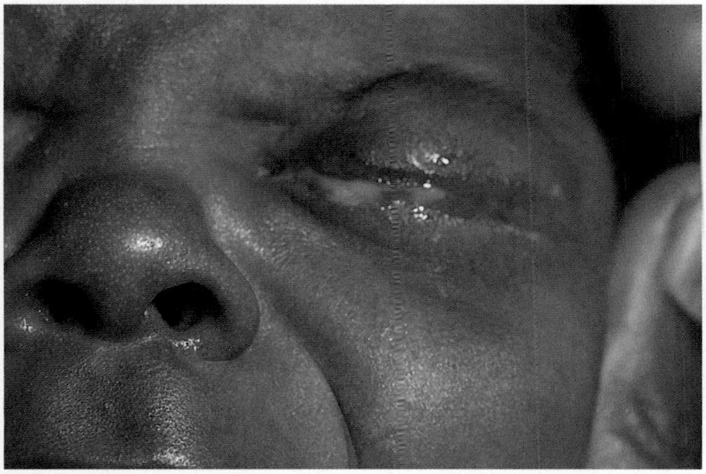

Fig. 3.22 Mucopurulent discharge developing 5–19 days after birth.

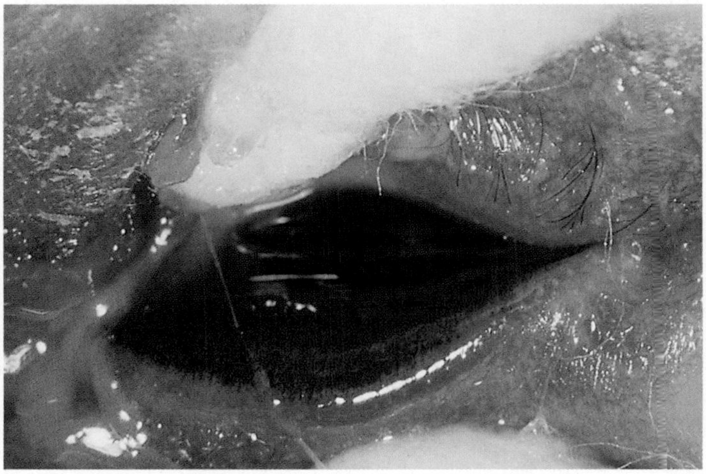

Fig. 3.23 A papillary conjunctival reaction.

Trachoma

Trachoma is caused by serotypes A, B, Ba and C of *Chlamydia trachomatis*. It is a disease of underprivileged populations with poor conditions of hygiene. The common fly is the major vector in the infection–reinfection cycle.

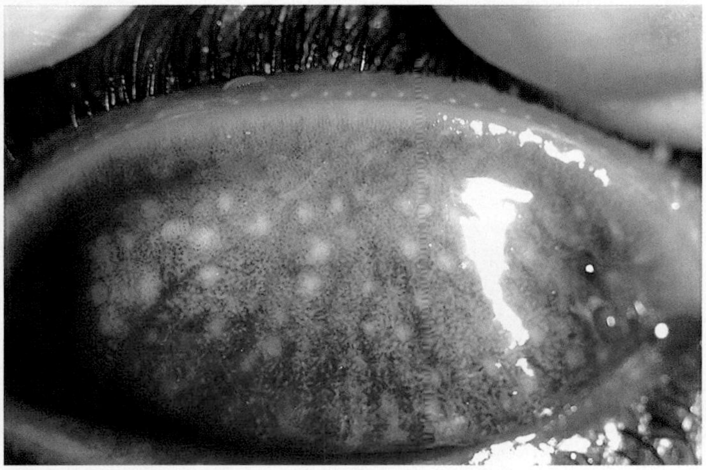

Fig. 3.24 Presentation is during childhood with a mixed follicular/papillary conjunctivitis.

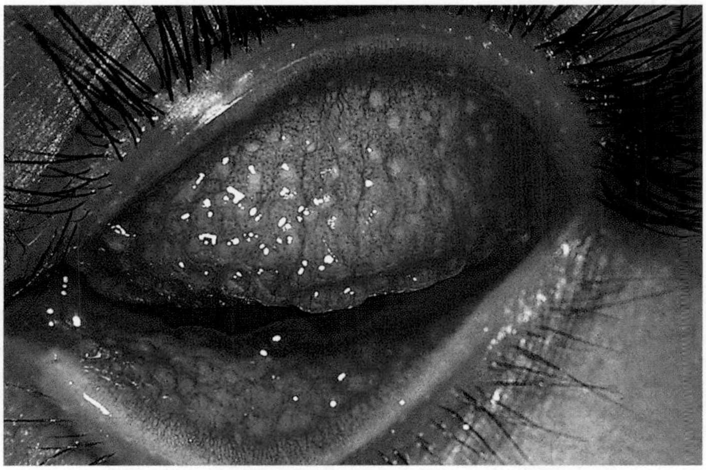

Fig. 3.25 Severe predominantly follicular conjunctivitis.

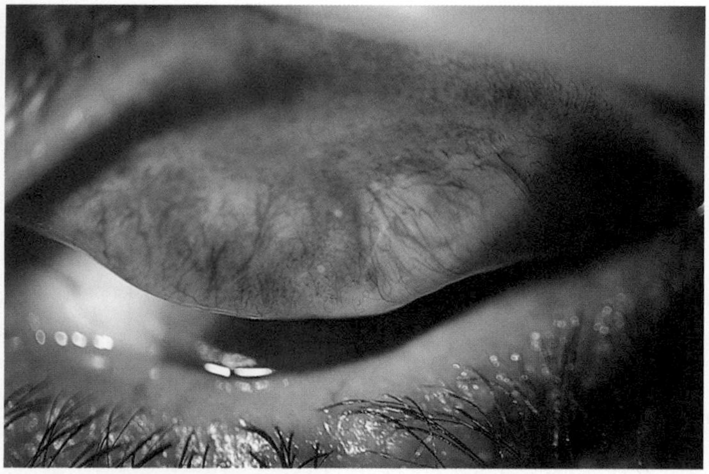

Fig. 3.26 Chronic conjunctival inflammation results in fine linear or stellate scars.

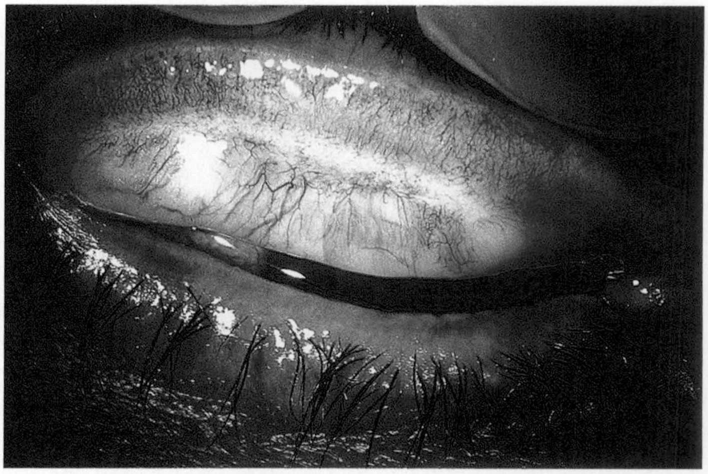

Fig. 3.27 More severe scarring (Arlt line).

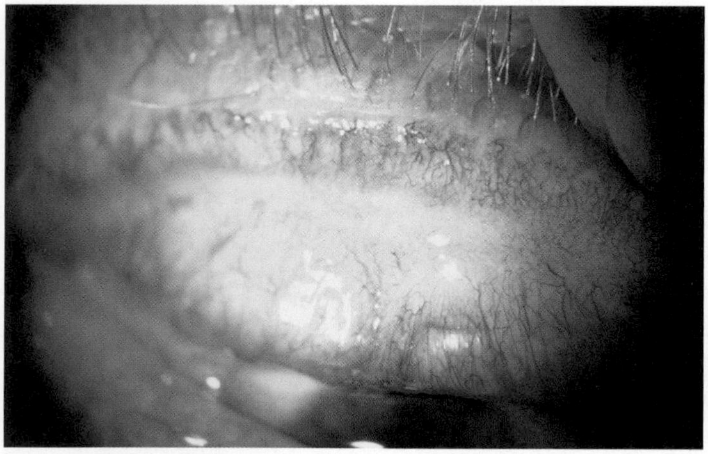

Fig. 3.28 Scarring involving the entire conjunctiva.

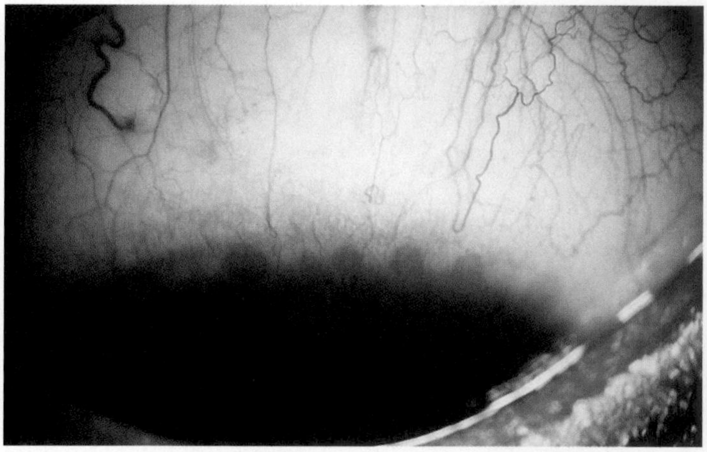

Fig. 3.29 Limbal follicles are a unique feature. They later cicatrise and become covered by epithelium, resulting in an uneven surface (Herbert pits).

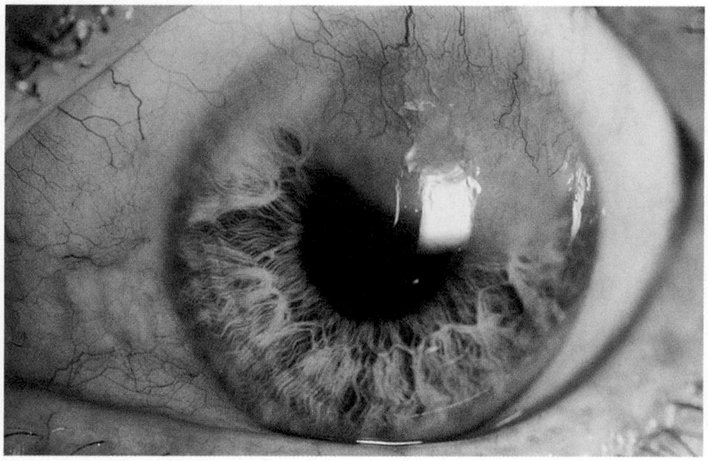

Fig. 3.30 More severe pannus formation. (Courtesy of C. Barry.)

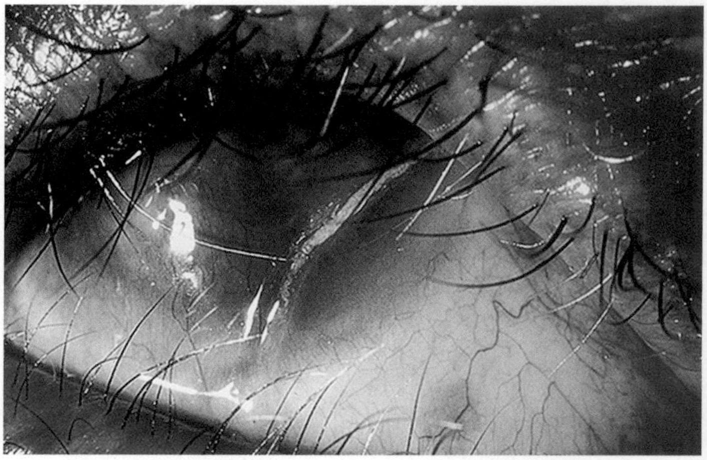

Fig. 3.31 Trichiasis, corneal scarring and early cicatricial entropion of the upper lid.

ALLERGIC CONJUNCTIVITIS

Allergic rhinoconjunctivitis

Allergic rhinoconjunctivitis is a hypersensitivity reaction to specific airborne antigens.

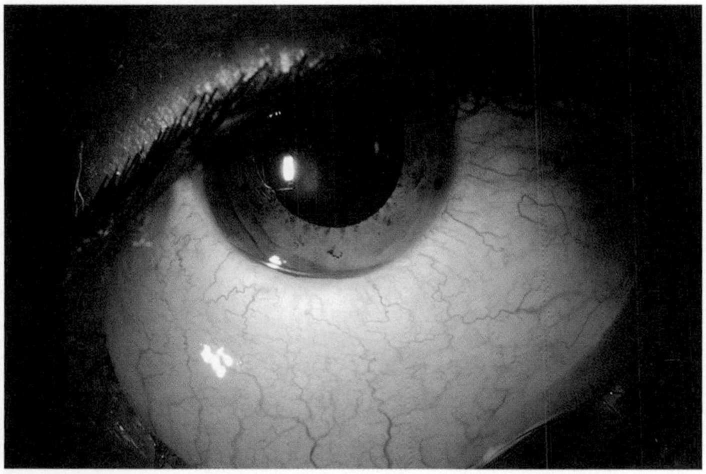

Fig. 3.32 The conjunctiva has a milky or pinkish appearance as a result of oedema and injection.

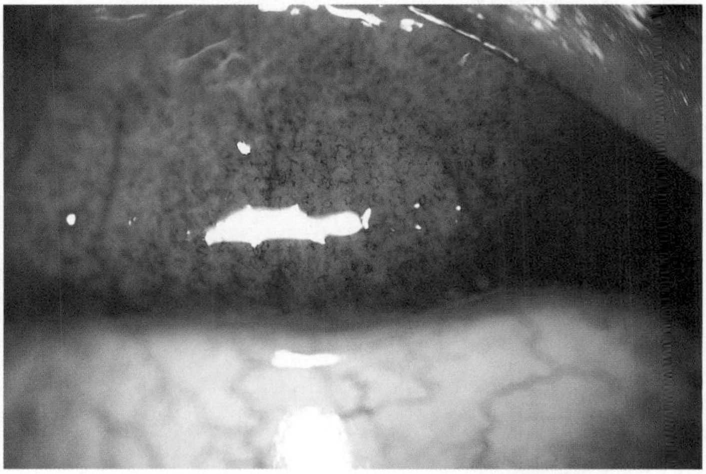

Fig. 3.33 Small papillae may occur on the upper tarsal conjunctiva.

Vernal keratoconjunctivitis

Vernal keratoconjunctivitis typically affects children and young adults who often also suffer from asthma and eczema.

Conjunctivitis

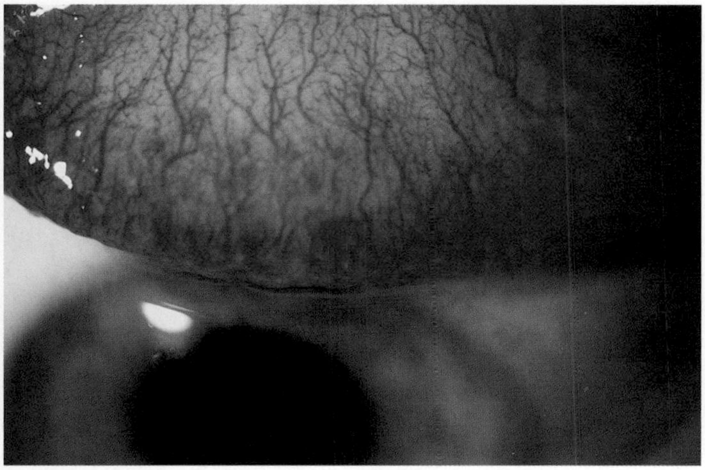

Fig. 3.34 Diffuse papillary hypertrophy.

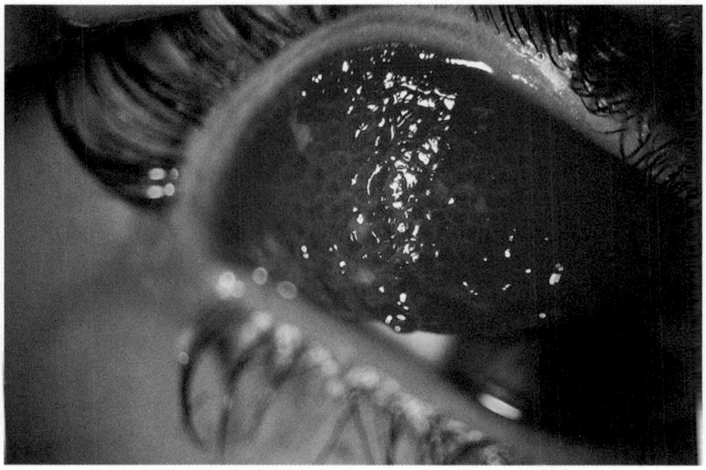

Fig. 3.35 Larger papillae.

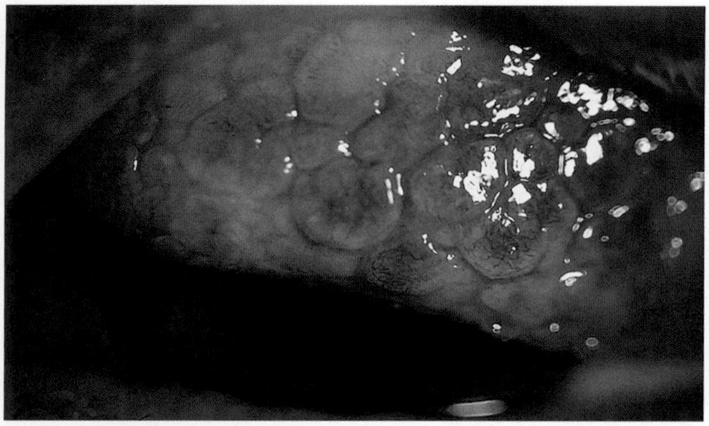

Fig. 3.36 Large papillae with a flat-topped polygonal appearance reminiscent of cobblestones.

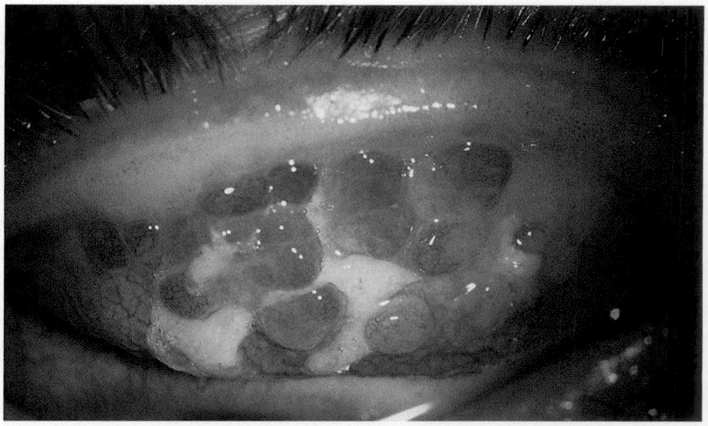

Fig. 3.37 Cobblestone papillae coated with copious mucus.

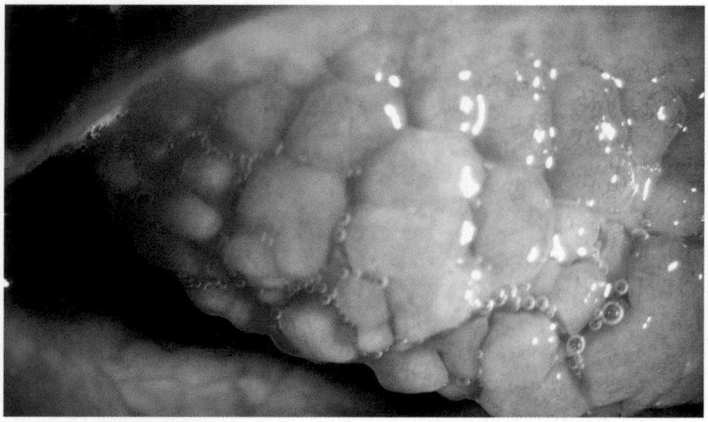

Fig. 3.38 In severe cases, the connective tissue septa rupture, giving rise to giant papillae.

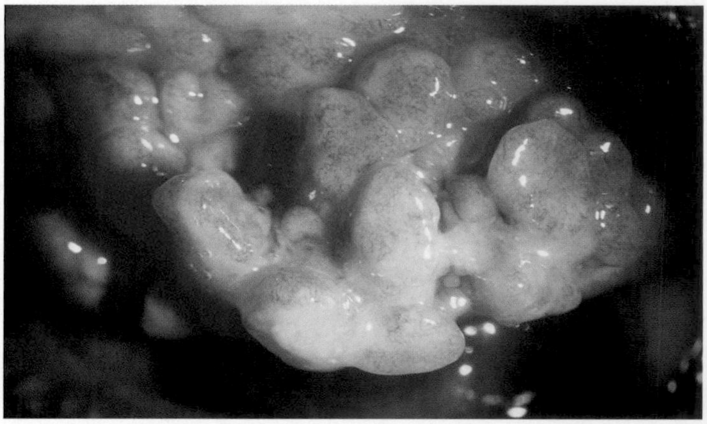

Fig. 3.39 Extremely large giant papillae, which are rarely seen.

Limbitis

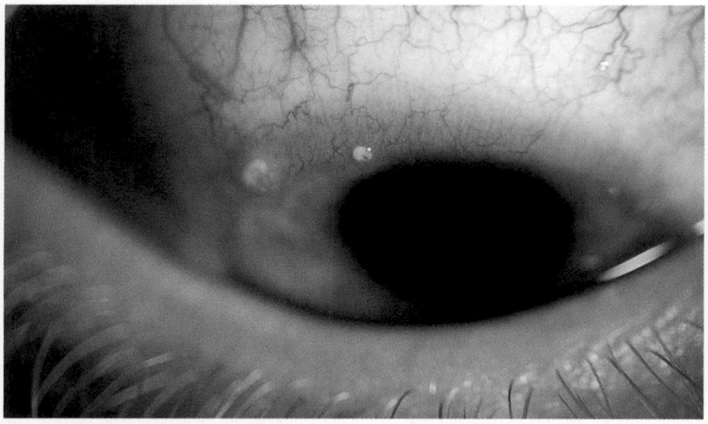

Fig. 3.40 Mucoid nodules scattered around the limbus.

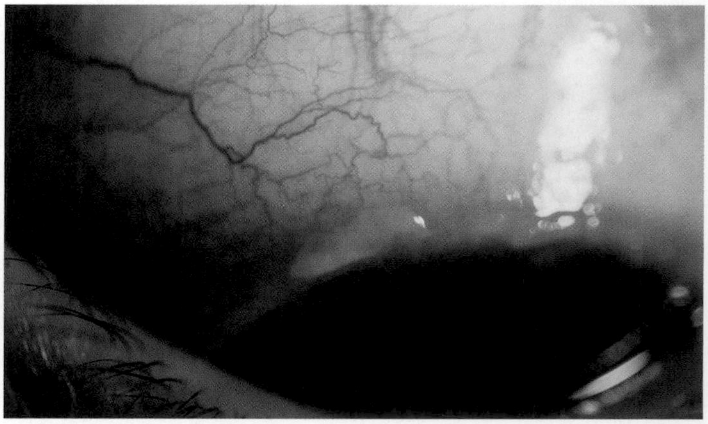

Fig. 3.41 Coalescence of mucoid nodules.

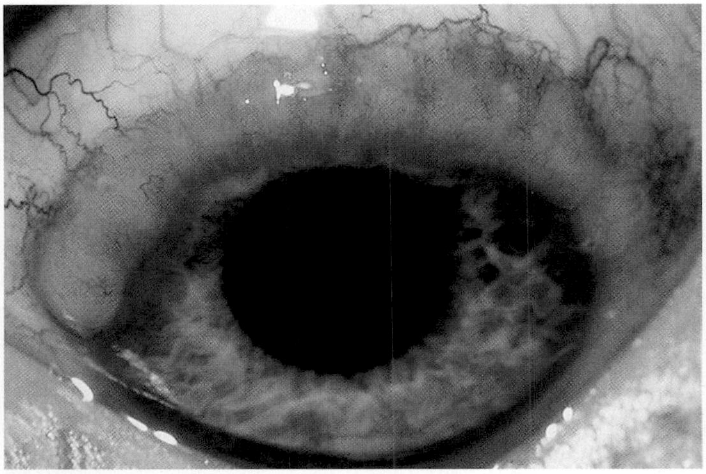

■ **Fig. 3.42** Very severe limbal involvement.

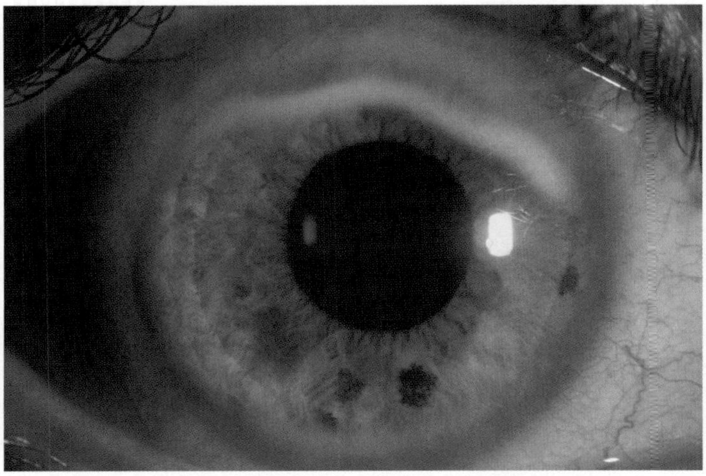

■ **Fig. 3.43** Pseudogerontoxon resembles an arcus senilis and is characterised by a 'Cupid bow' opacity in a previously inflamed segment of the limbus. (Courtesy of S. Tuft.)

Keratitis

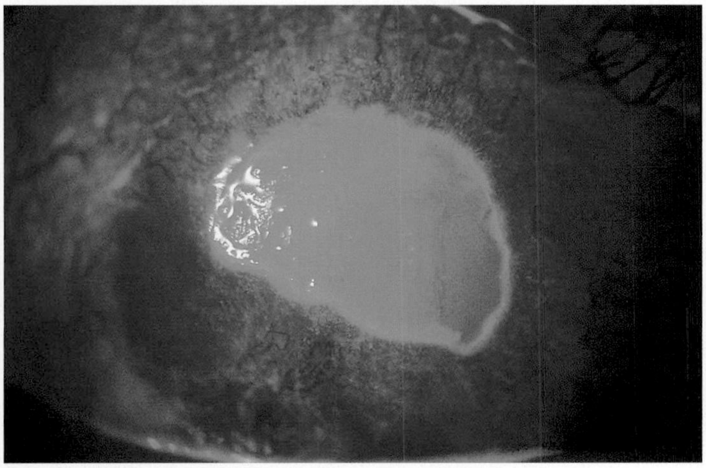

■ **Fig. 3.44** Shield-like ulceration stained with fluorescein. (Courtesy of S. Ford and R. Marsh.)

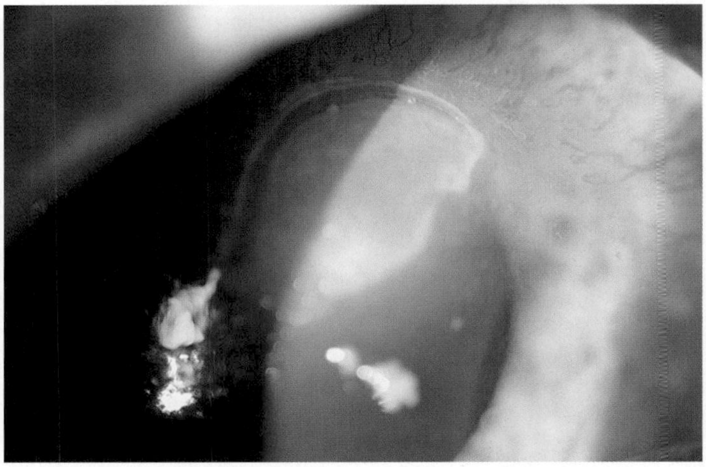

■ **Fig. 3.45** Plaque formation may occur when the base of the ulcer becomes coated with desiccated mucus.

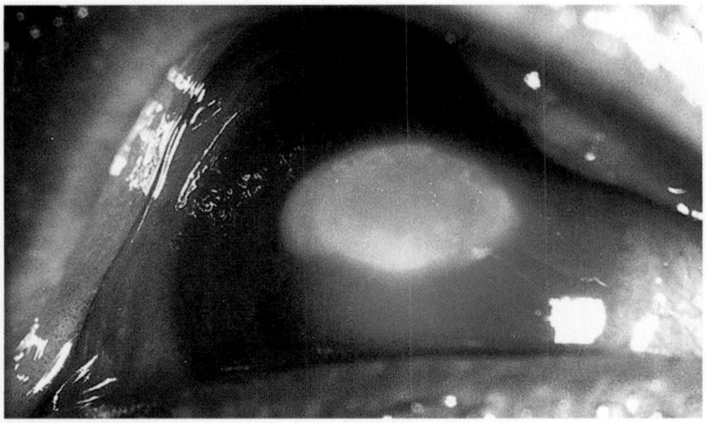

■ **Fig. 3.46** More advanced corneal plaque, which results in defective wetting by tears and prevents re-epithelialisation.

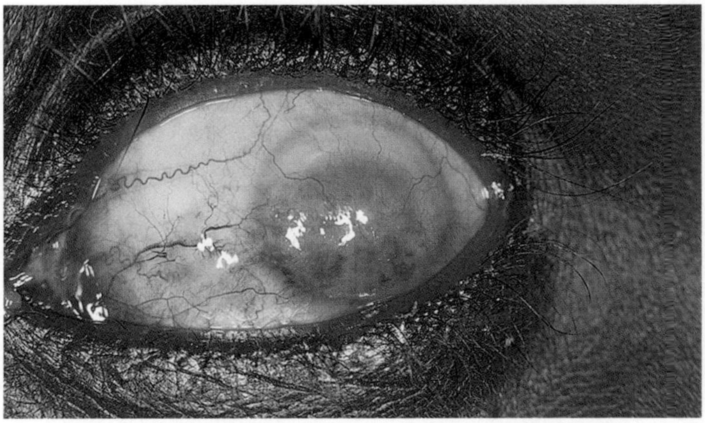

■ **Fig. 3.47** Severe scarring and vascularisation in end-stage disease.

Atopic keratoconjunctivitis

Atopic keratoconjunctivitis typically affects young men with atopic dermatitis.

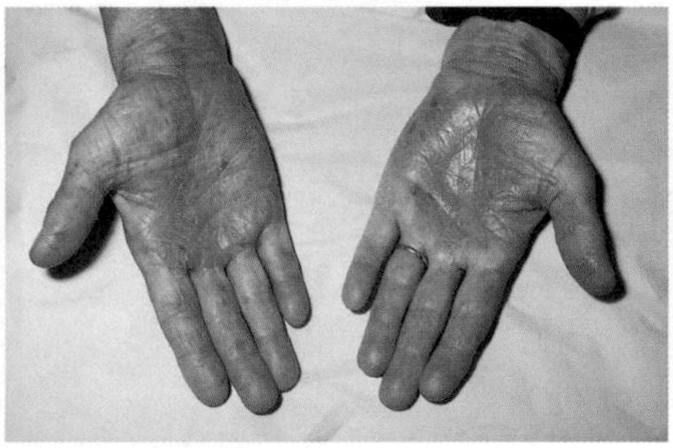

Fig. 3.48 Eczema of the hands.

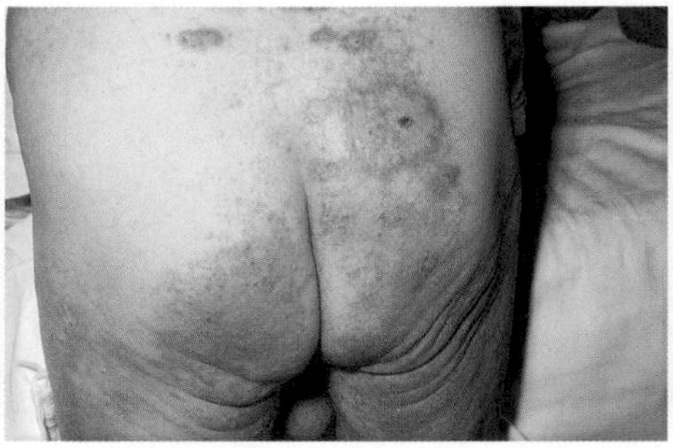

Fig. 3.49 Severe eczema of the buttocks.

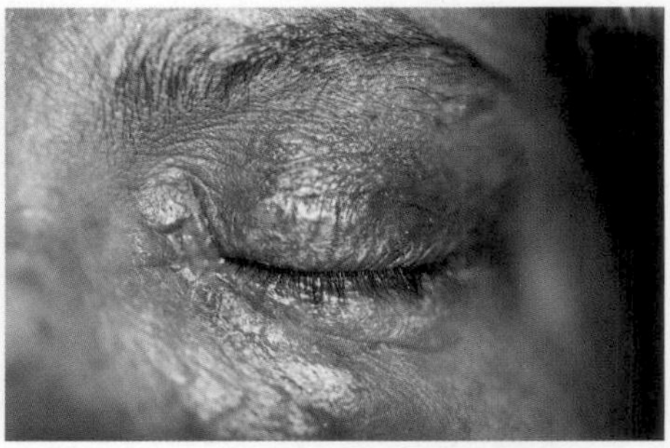

Fig. 3.50 The lids are red, thickened, macerated and fissured. Associated chronic staphylococcal and angular blepharitis are common.

Conjunctivitis

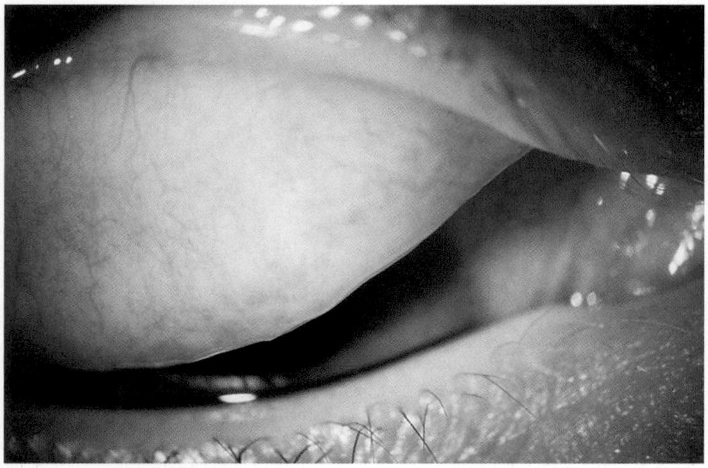

Fig. 3.51 Infiltration of the tarsal conjunctiva results in an overall pale and featureless appearance.

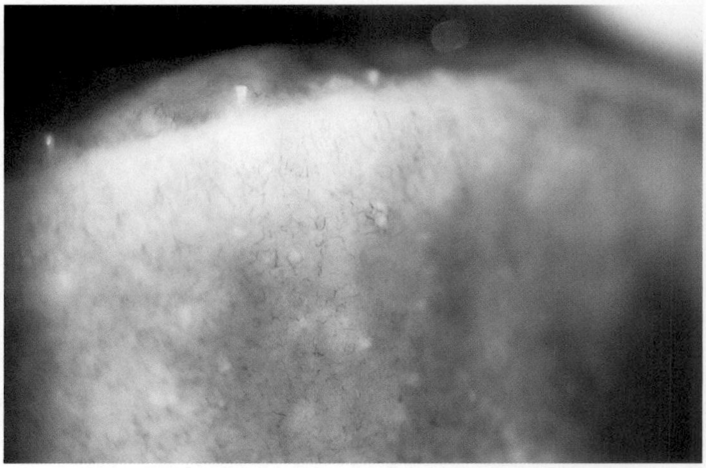

Fig. 3.52 Magnified view of the superior tarsal conjunctiva.

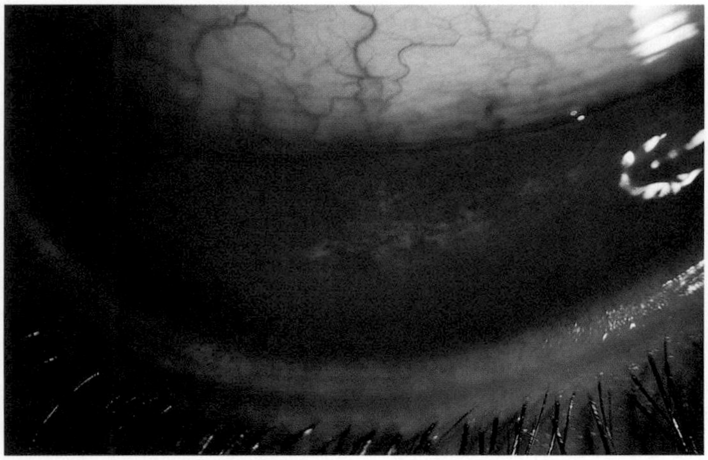

Fig. 3.53 Papillary conjunctivitis.

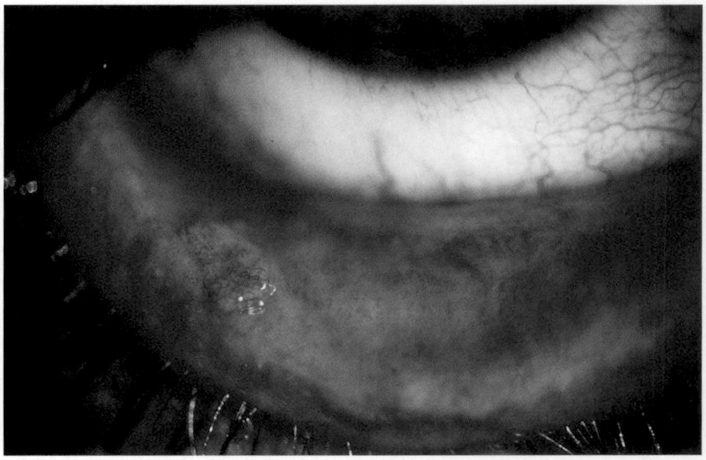

Fig. 3.54 Infiltration of the inferior palpebral conjunctiva.

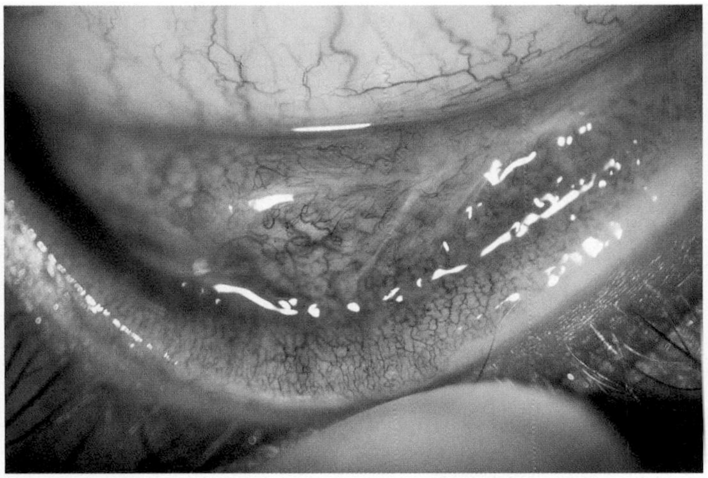

■ **Fig. 3.55** Early scarring of the inferior palpebral conjunctiva.

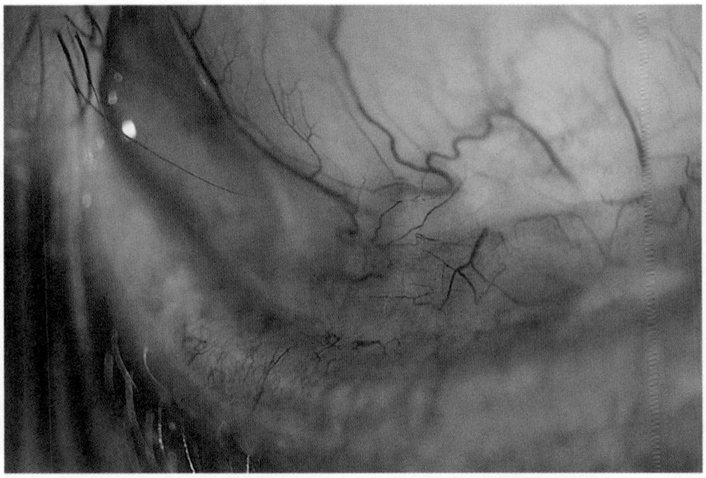

■ **Fig. 3.56** Forniceal shortening.

Keratitis

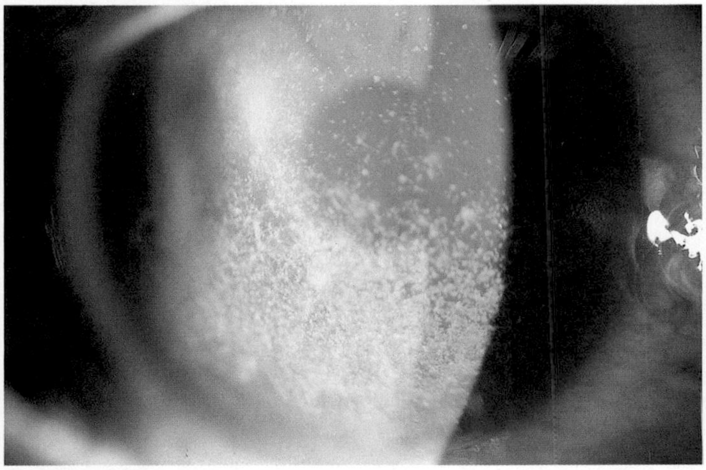

■ **Fig. 3.57** Punctate epithelial erosions.

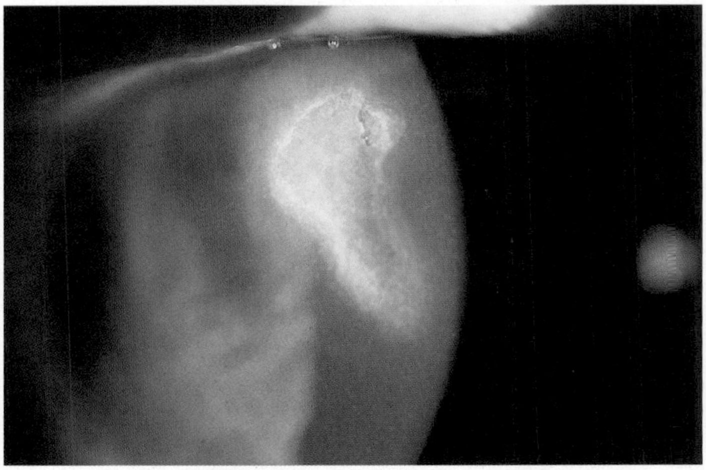

■ **Fig. 3.58** Persistent epithelial defects and shield-shaped anterior stromal scars.

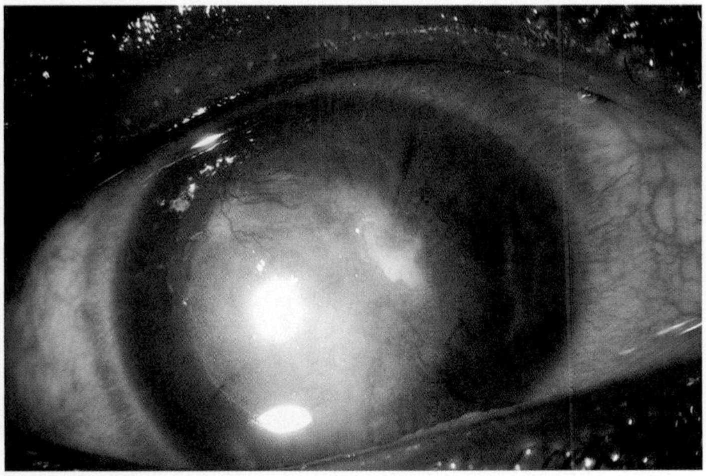

■ **Fig. 3.59** Severe scarring and vascularisation in end-stage disease.

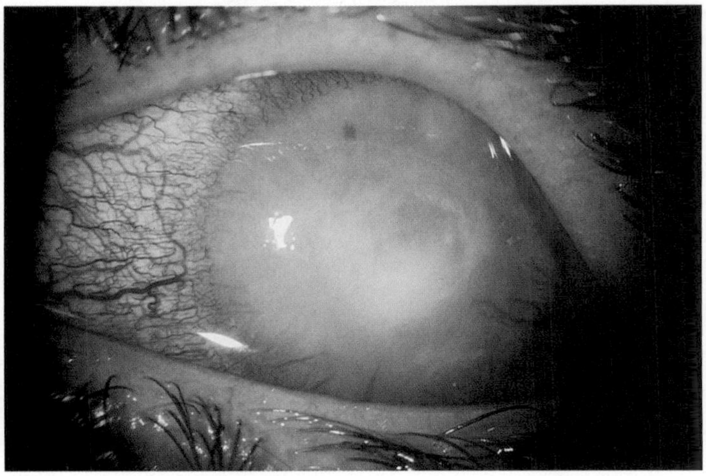

■ **Fig. 3.60** Secondary microbial keratitis.

CICATRISING CONJUNCTIVITIS

Cicatricial pemphigoid

Cicatricial pemphigoid is a rare, chronic, autoimmune disease characterised by recurrent mucocutaneous blistering.

Systemic signs

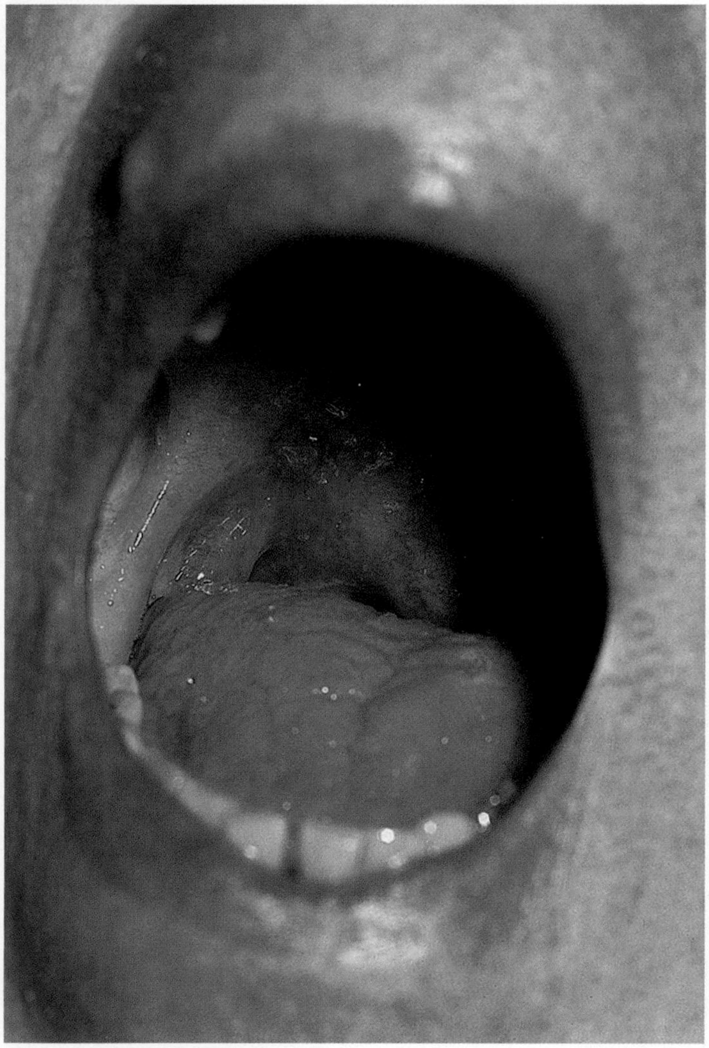

Fig. 3.61 Oral mucosal blisters.

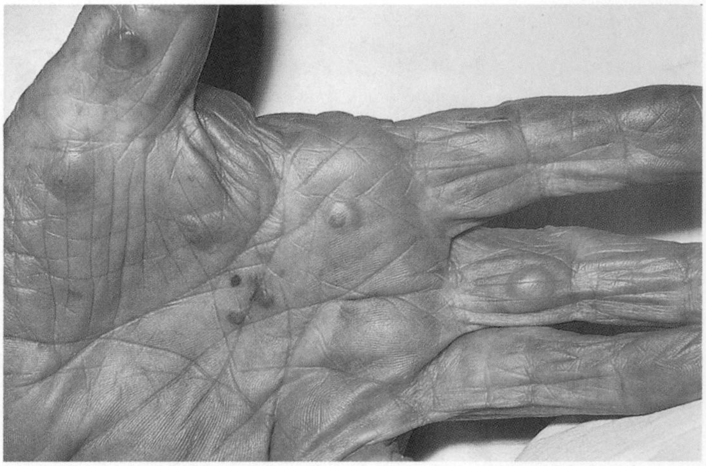

Fig. 3.62 Cutaneous, recurrent blisters, which are usually sparse and often involve the extremities.

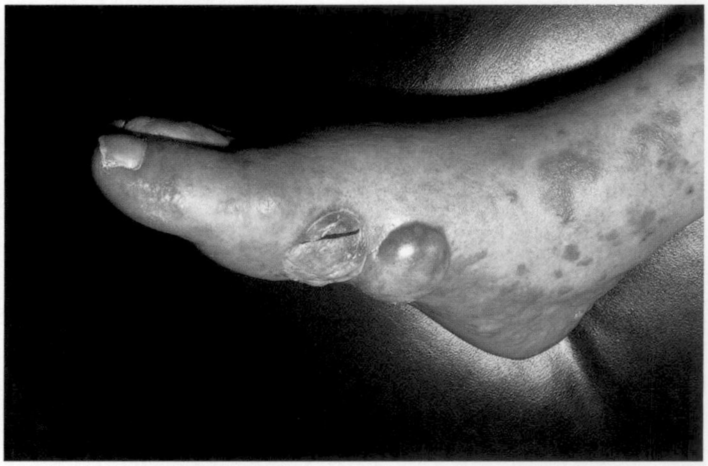

Fig. 3.63 More severe blistering.

Conjunctivitis

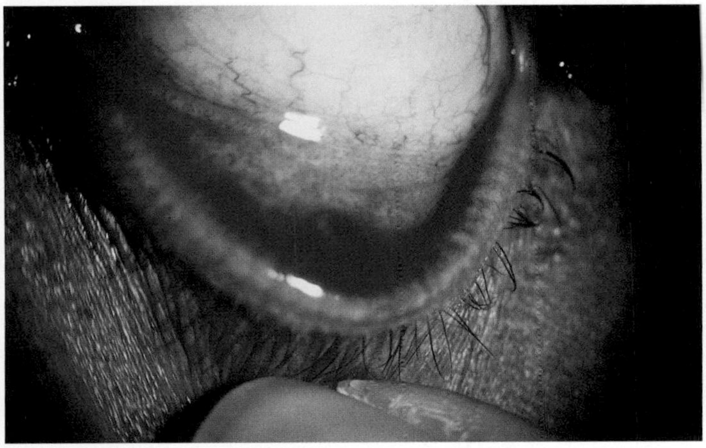

Fig. 3.64 Papillary conjunctivitis.

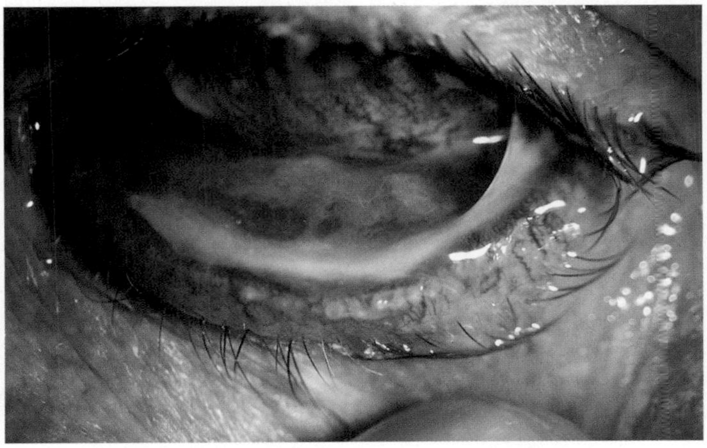

Fig. 3.65 Pseudomembrane formation.

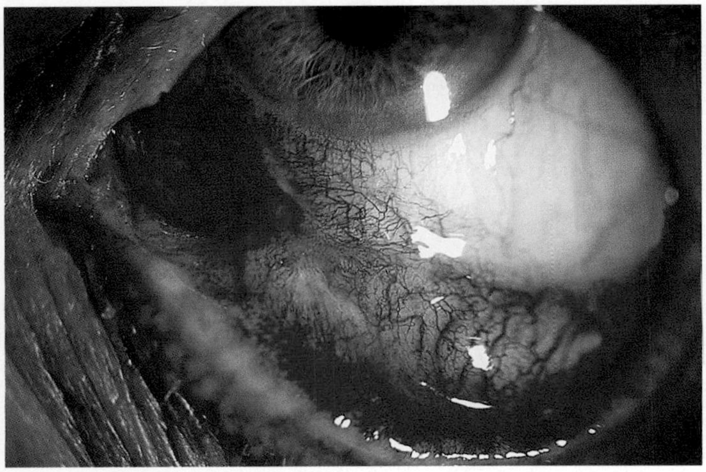

Fig. 3.66 Subepithelial fibrosis.

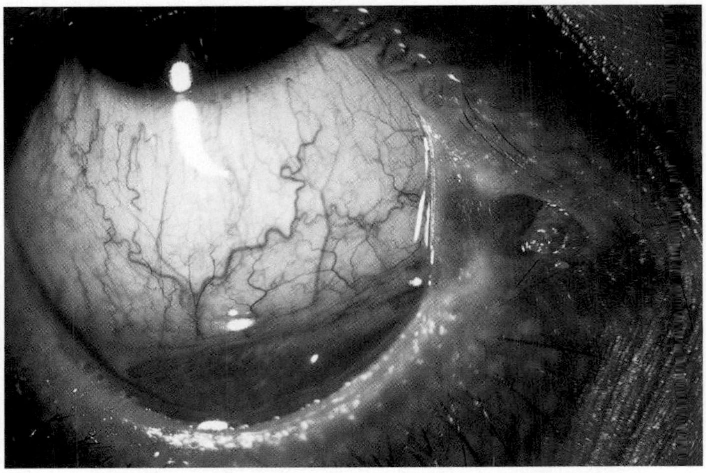

Fig. 3.67 Flattening of the contour of the plica and caruncle.

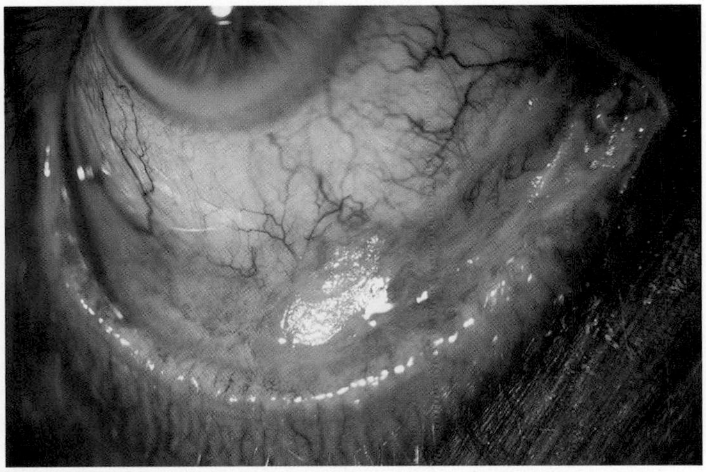

Fig. 3.68 Early obliteration of the inferior fornix.

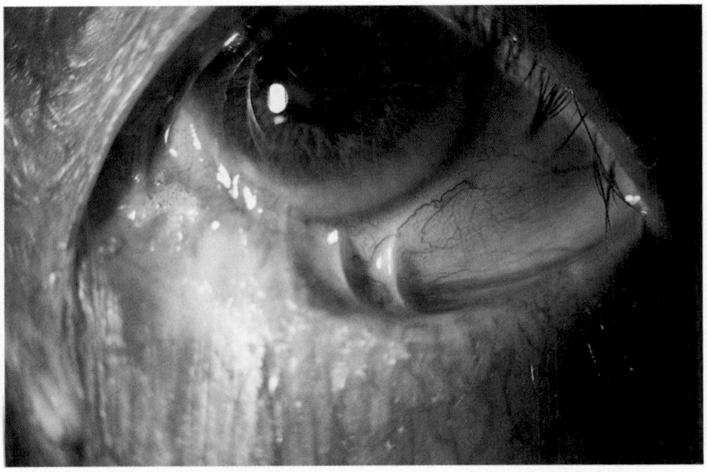

Fig. 3.69 Formation of adhesions between the palpebral and bulbar conjunctiva (symblepharon).

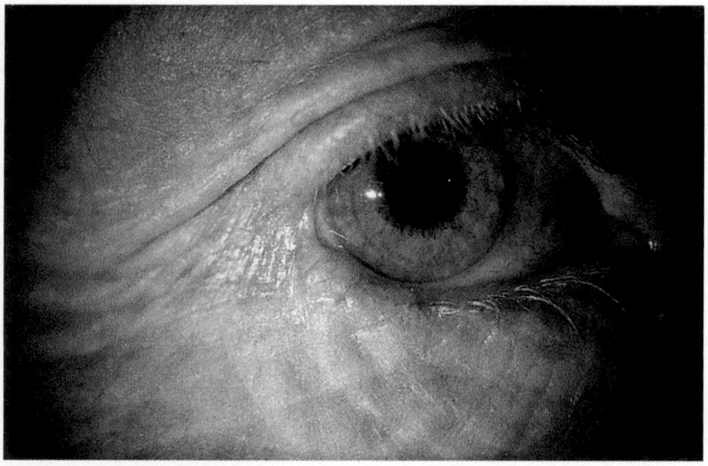

Fig. 3.70 Formation of adhesions at the outer canthi between the upper and lower eyelids (ankyloblepharon).

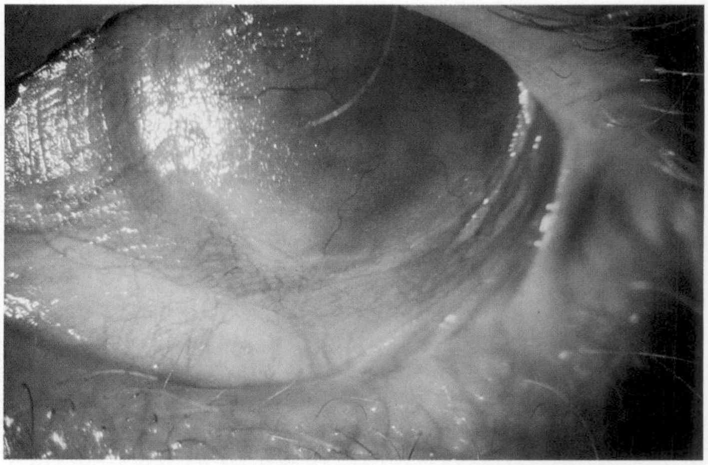

Fig. 3.71 Corneal keratinisation.

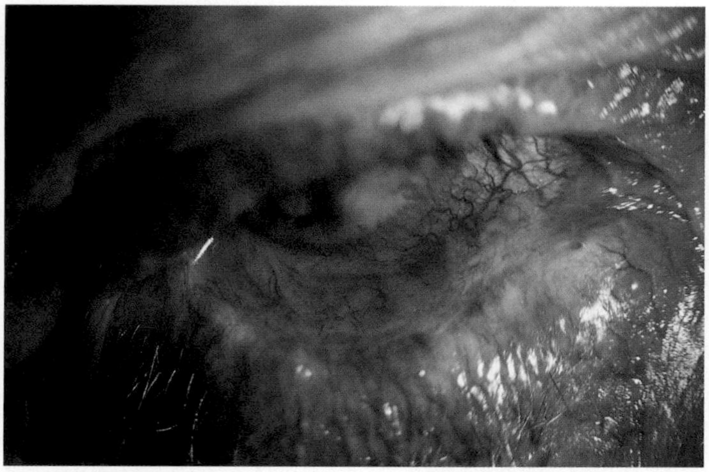

Fig. 3.72 Severe obliteration of the inferior fornix, plica and caruncle.

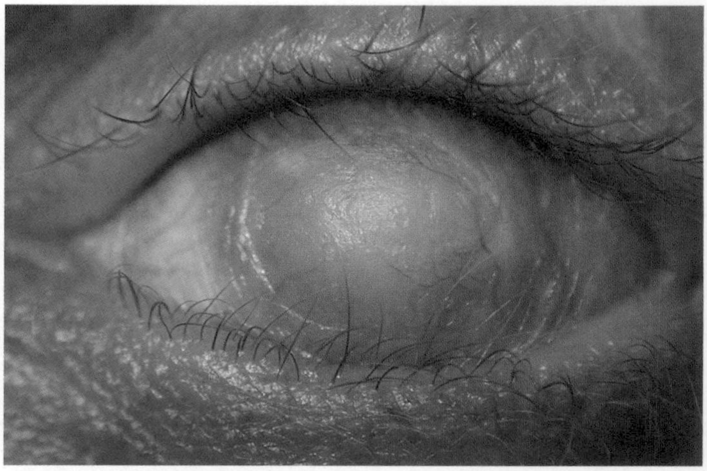

Fig. 3.73 Secondary keratopathy is caused by a combination of entropion, metaplastic lashes, lagophthalmos secondary to symblepharon, dryness and limbal stem cell depletion. (Courtesy of A. Pearson.)

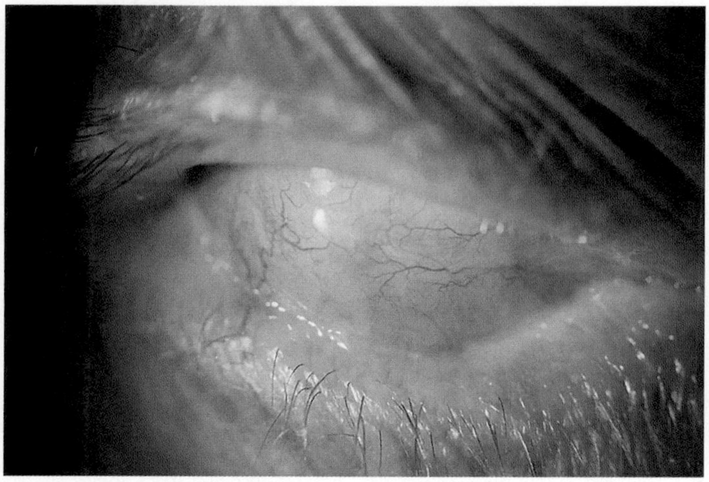

Fig. 3.74 Total obliteration of the fornices and corneal opacification.

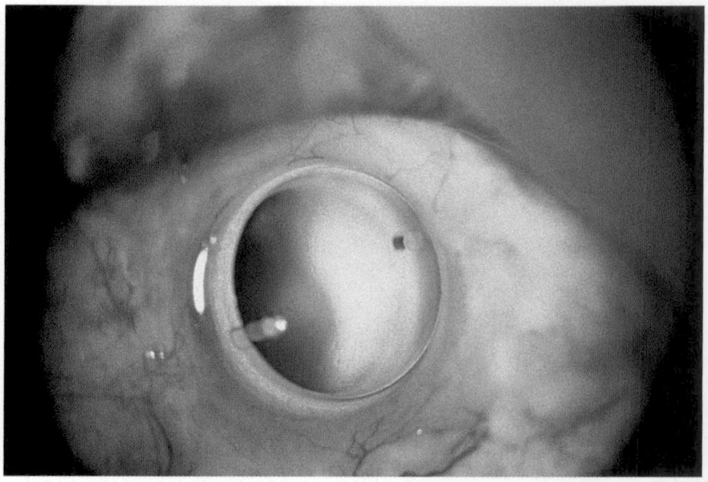

Fig. 3.75 Keratoprosthesis may be useful in end-stage disease provided optic nerve function is normal.

Stevens–Johnson syndrome

Stevens–Johnson syndrome is an acute, severe, mucocutaneous blistering disease, which primarily occurs in young, healthy individuals.

Systemic signs

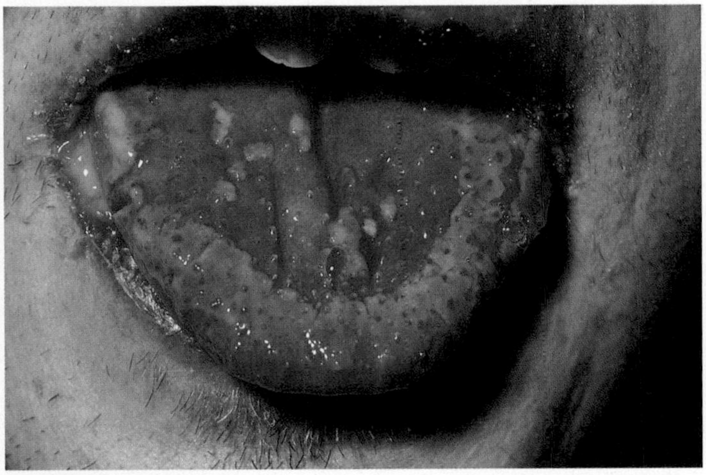

Fig. 3.76 Blisters on the tongue and oral mucosa, which rupture to form erosions.

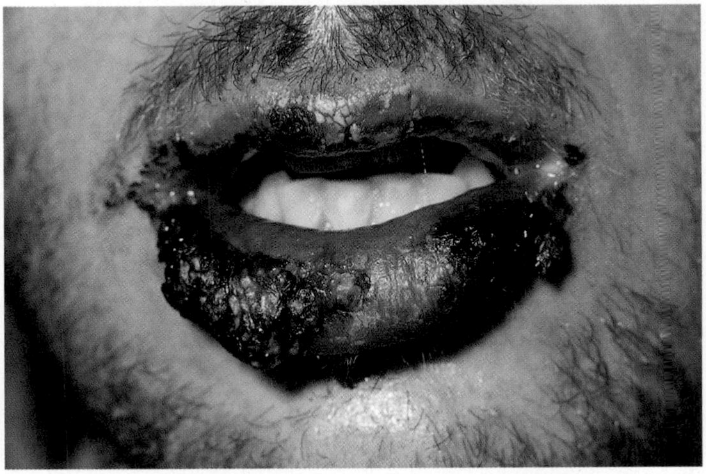

Fig. 3.77 Haemorrhagic crusting of the lips.

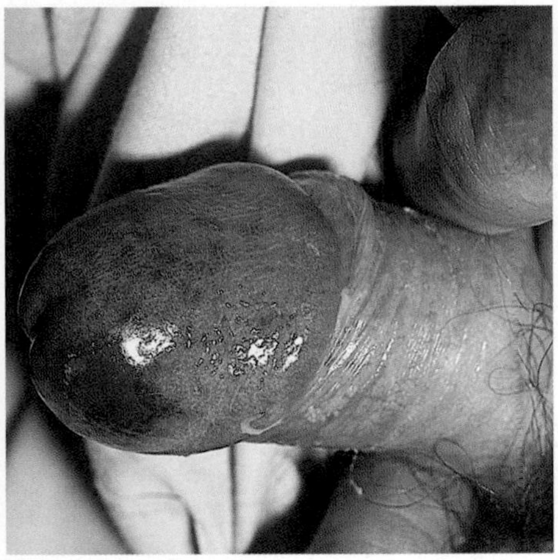

Fig. 3.78 Involvement of the glans penis is uncommon.

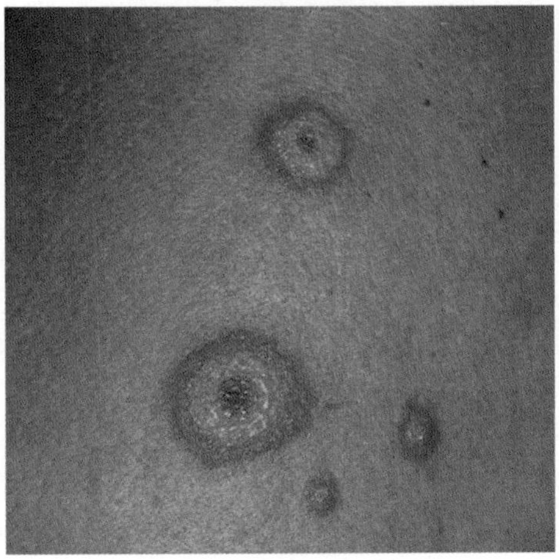

Fig. 3.79 Cutaneous 'target' lesions are characteristic. (Courtesy of R. T. D Emond, P. D. Welsby and H. A. Rowland.)

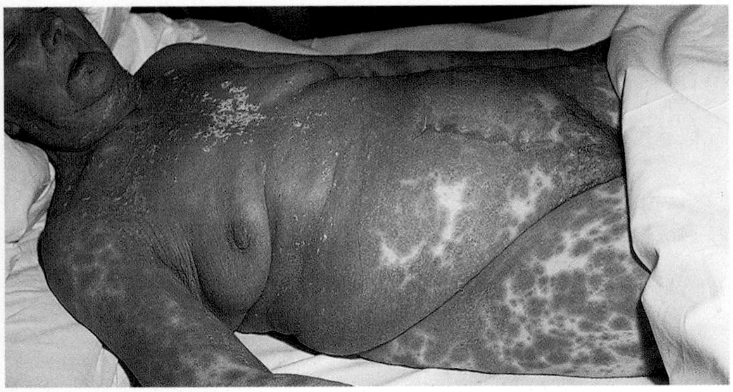

Fig. 3.80 Generalised erythematous rash in severe disease.

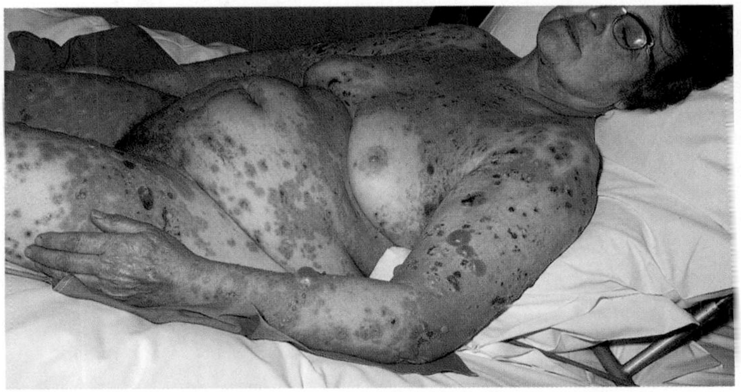

Fig. 3.81 Generalised blistering, which is usually transient.

Conjunctivitis

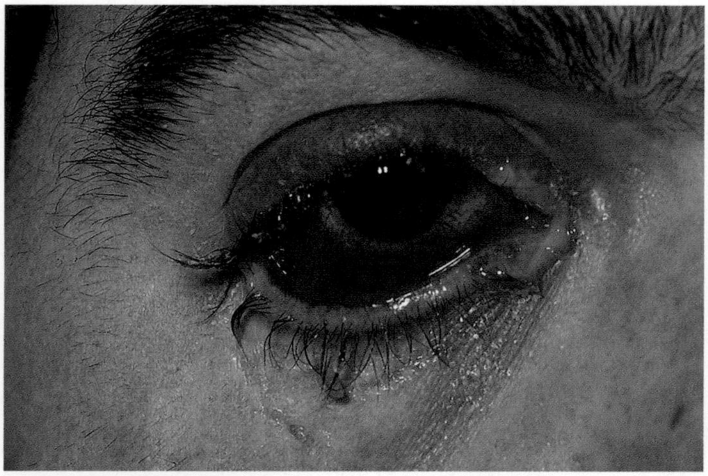

Fig. 3.82 Transient papillary conjunctivitis.

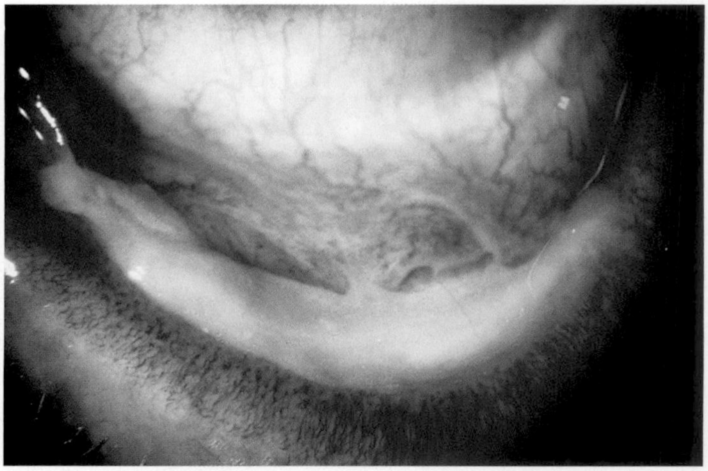

Fig. 3.83 Pseudomembranous conjunctivitis with patchy conjunctival infarction.

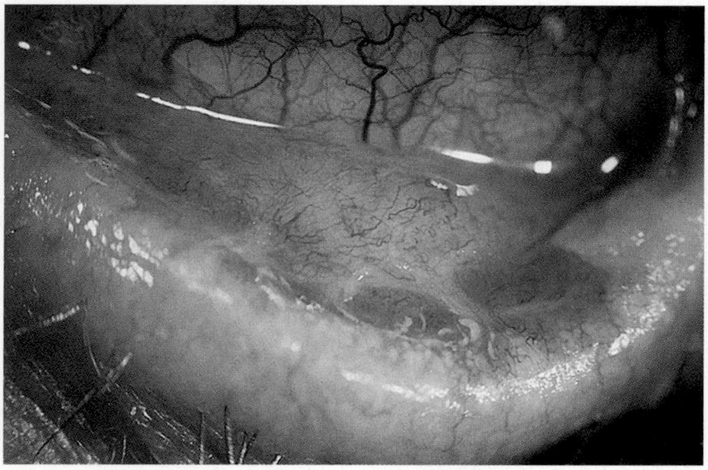

Fig. 3.84 Residual focal fibrotic areas are uncommon.

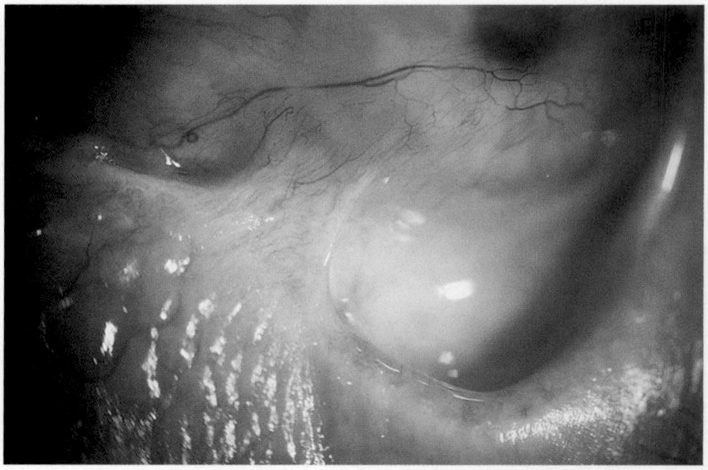

Fig. 3.85 Symblepharon formation is uncommon and the prognosis is more favourable than in cicatricial pemphigoid.

Other causes of cicatrising conjunctivitis

Epidermolysis bullosa

Epidermolysis bullosa is a hereditary condition of which there are 16 subtypes.

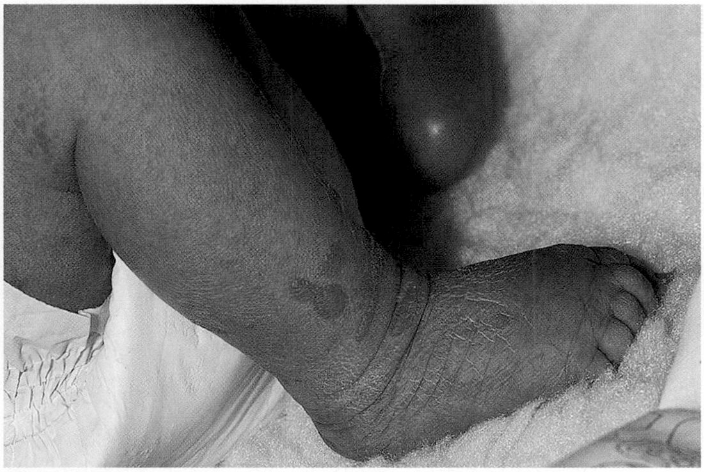

Fig. 3.86 Onset may be soon after birth with cutaneous blistering.

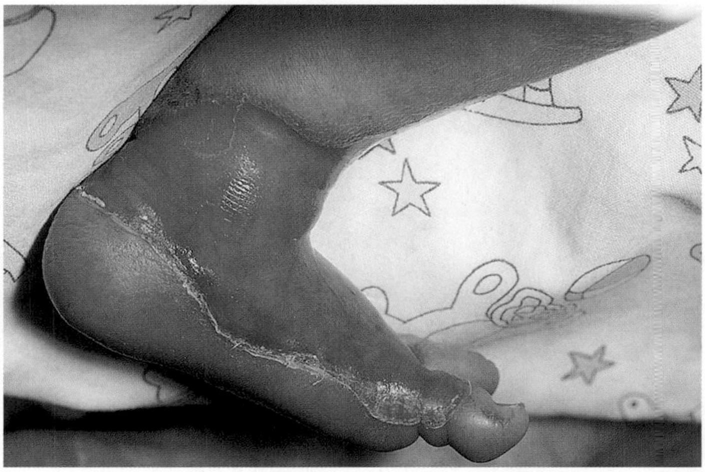

Fig. 3.87 Cutaneous erosions and sloughing following minor trauma.

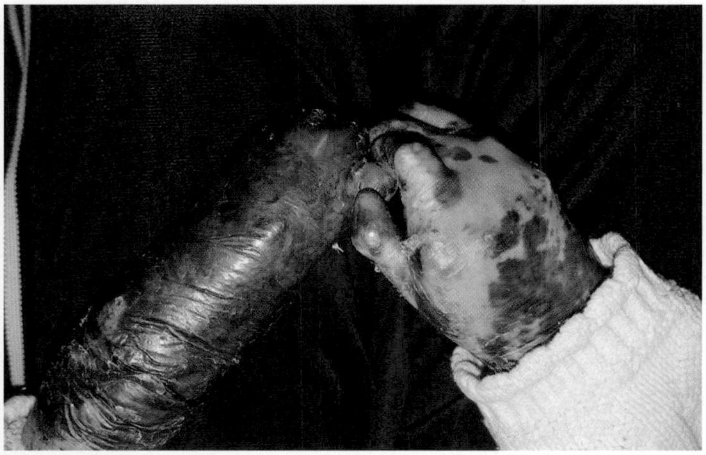

Fig. 3.88 Very severe involvement with partial fusion of the fingers. (Courtesy of K. Nischal.)

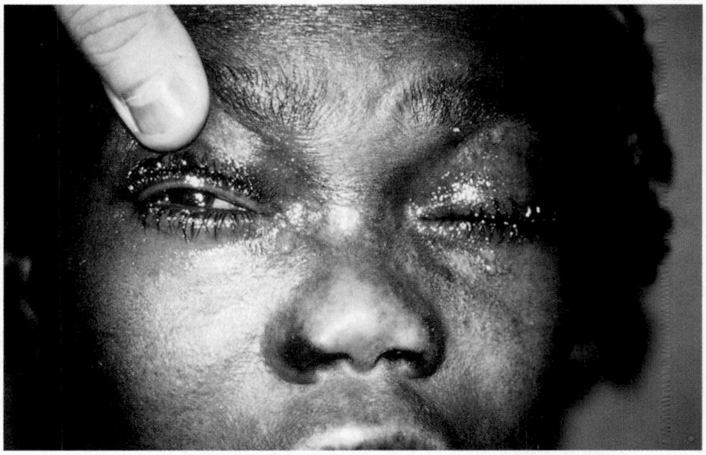

Fig. 3.89 Corneal erosions are frequent but cicatrising conjunctivitis is uncommon. (Courtesy of K. Nischal.)

Toxic epidermal necrolysis (Lyell disease)

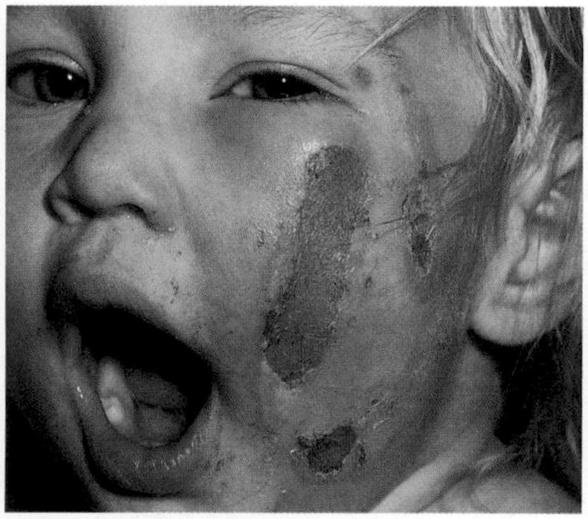

Fig. 3.90 Acute 'scalded skin' lesions.

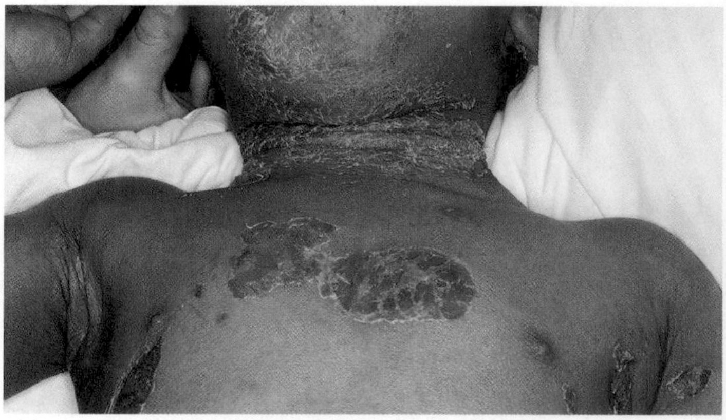

Fig. 3.91 Healing with scab formation.

Pemphigus vulgaris

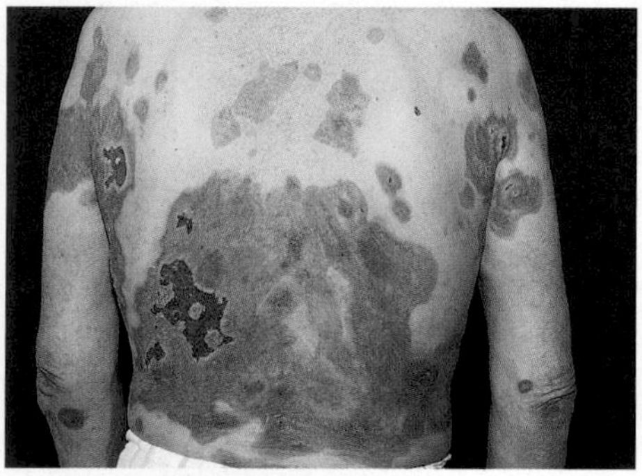

Fig. 3.92 Erosion of bullae leads to large leaking areas.

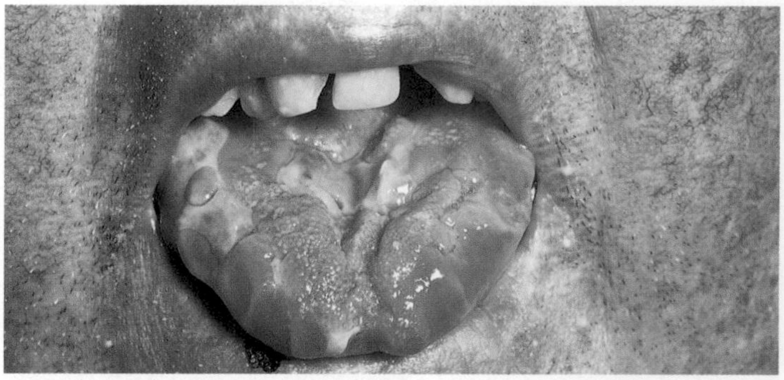

Fig. 3.93 Involvement of the oral mucosa is common.

Bullous pemphigoid

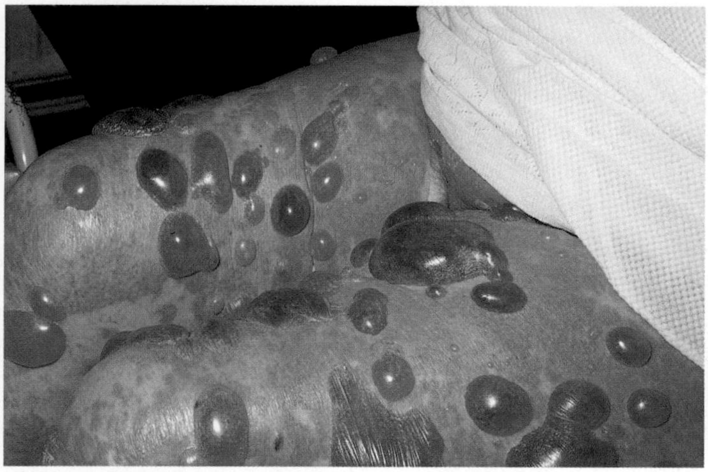

Fig. 3.94 Tense skin blisters, which may contain blood.

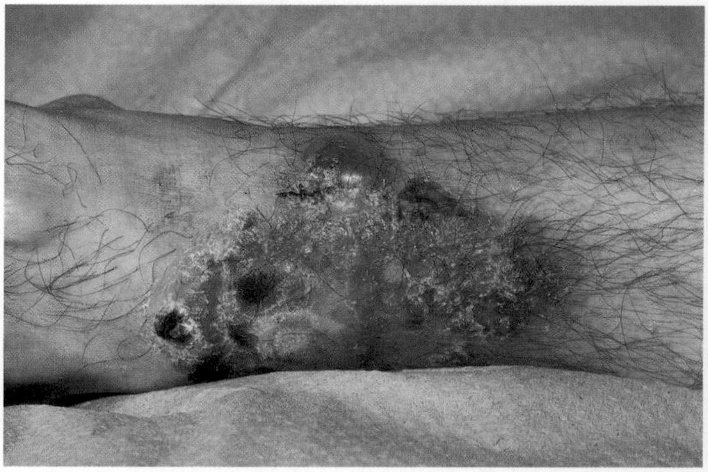

Fig. 3.95 Crusting following rupture of blisters and resolution without scarring.

Dermatitis herpetiformis

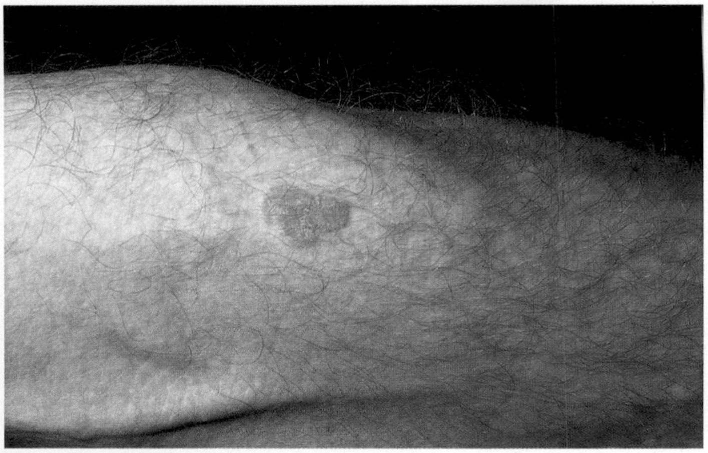

Fig. 3.96 Small annular blisters associated with urticaria, often involving the elbows.

Porphyria cutanea tarda

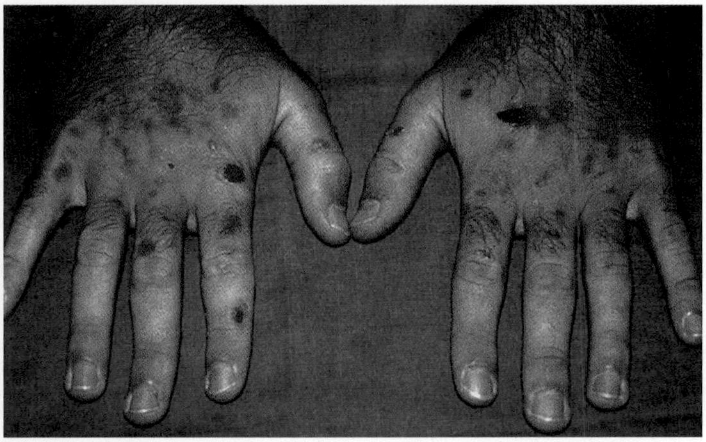

Fig. 3.97 Skin blisters and ulcers following exposure to sunlight with subsequent scarring and hyperpigmentation. (Courtesy of M. A. Mir.)

Xeroderma pigmentosum

This is an autosomal recessive condition caused by skin damage on exposure to natural sunlight and characterised by skin pigmentation, multiple cutaneous malignancies and a 'bird-like' facies.

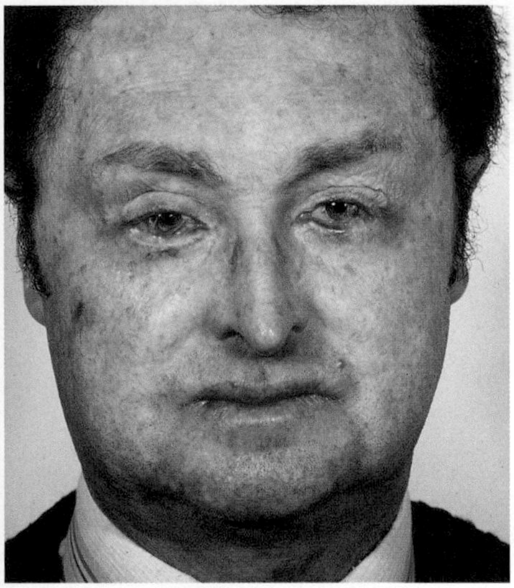

Fig. 3.98 Cicatrising conjunctivitis in xeroderma pigmentosum.

MISCELLANEOUS CONJUNCTIVAL INFLAMMATION

Superior limbic keratoconjunctivitis

Superior limbic keratoconjunctivitis of Theodore is an uncommon, chronic inflammatory disorder that typically affects middle-aged women with thyrotoxicosis.

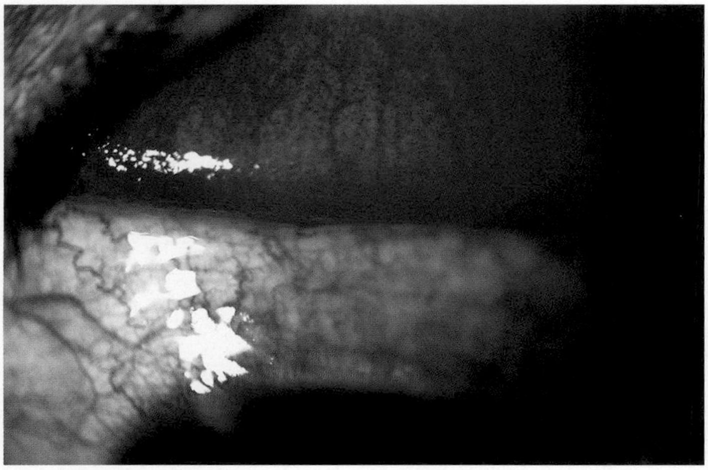

Fig. 3.99 Papillary hypertrophy of the superior tarsus, which may give rise to a diffuse velvety appearance.

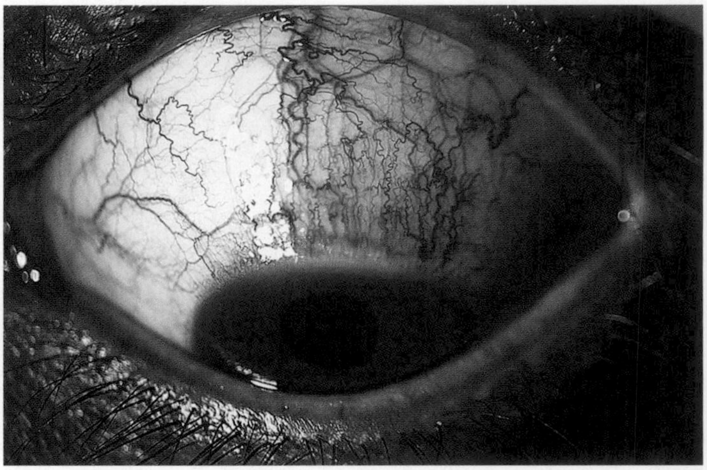

Fig. 3.100 Hyperaemia of the superior bulbar conjunctiva, most intense at the limbus, and superior limbic papillary hypertrophy.

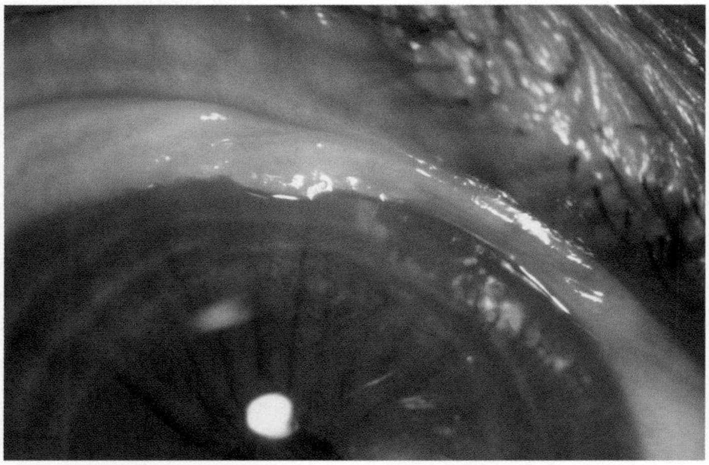

Fig. 3.101 Light pressure on the upper lid results in the formation of redundant conjunctiva crossing the upper limbus. (Courtesy of S. Tuft.)

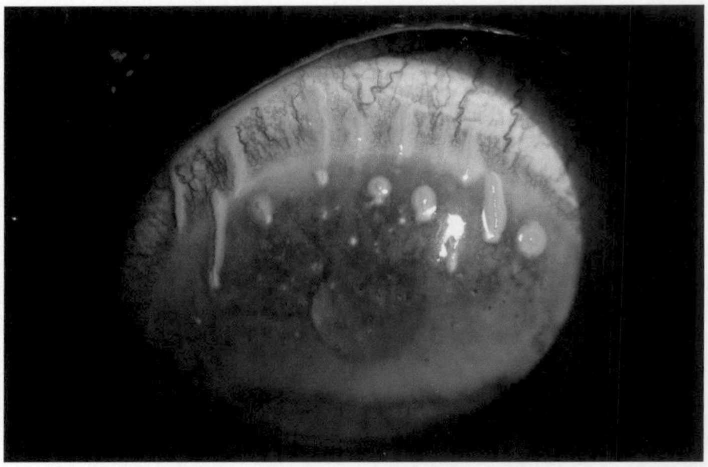

Fig. 3.102 Superior filamentary keratitis is common. (Courtesy of C. Barry.)

Parinaud oculoglandular syndrome

Parinaud oculoglandular syndrome is a rare condition that may be caused by cat-scratch fever, tularaemia, sporotrichosis, tuberculosis, syphilis, lymphogranuloma venereum and infectious mononucleosis.

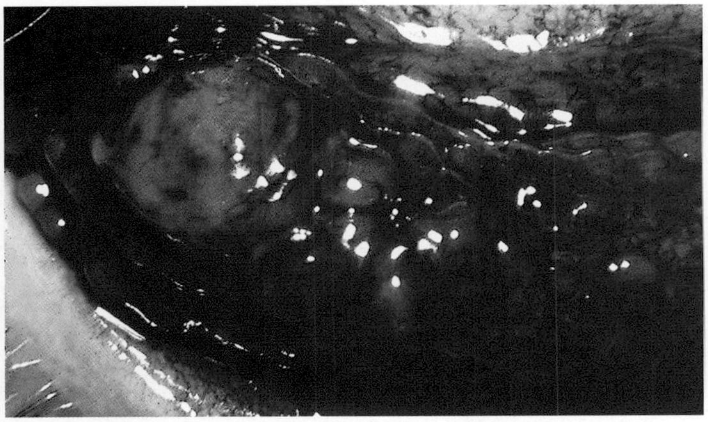

Fig. 3.103 Unilateral granulomatous conjunctivitis with nodular elevations surrounded by follicles.

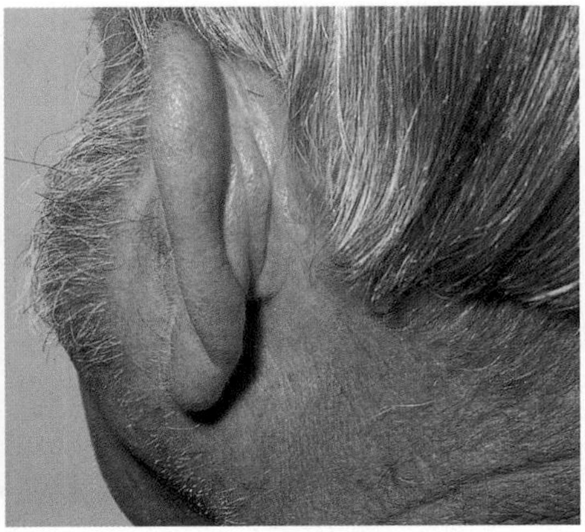

Fig. 3.104 Severe, painful, ipsilateral lymphadenopathy.

Ligneous conjunctivitis

Ligneous conjunctivitis is a rare chronic disease characterised by wood-like indurated membranes on the tarsal conjunctiva. The disease typically affects children but may occur at any age.

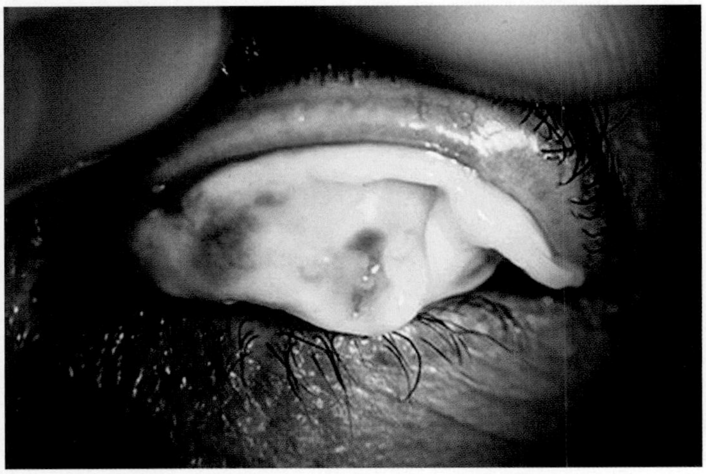

Fig. 3.105 Involvement of the superior tarsal conjunctiva. (Courtesy of S. Barabino.)

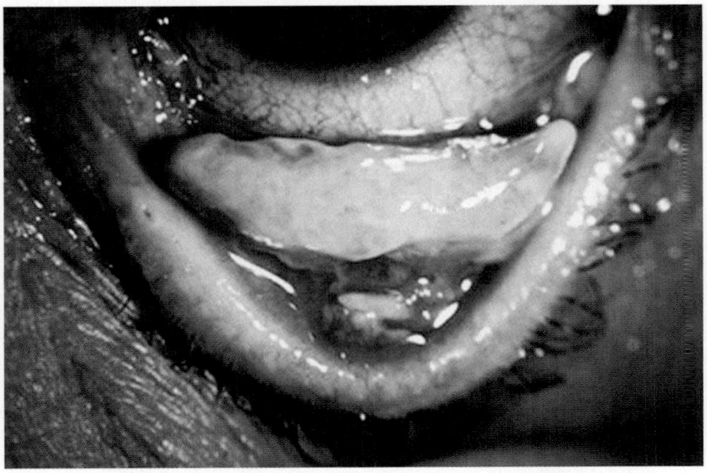

Fig. 3.106 Involvement of the inferior tarsal conjunctiva. (Courtesy of S. Barabino.)

Reiter syndrome

Reiter syndrome is a seronegative spondyloarthropathy characterised by the triad of conjunctivitis, urethritis and arthritis.

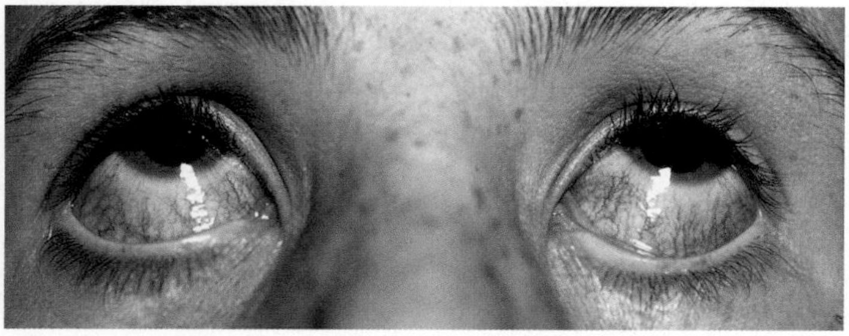

Fig. 3.107 A self-limiting, bilateral, mucopurulent conjunctivitis is universal.

Toxic conjunctivitis

Toxic conjunctivitis is caused by over-the-counter non-prescription eye decongestants used as self-medication.

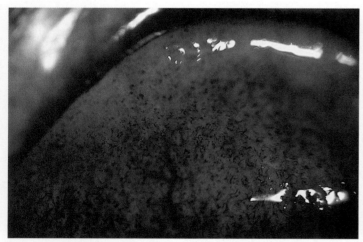

Fig. 3.108 Diffuse conjunctival hyperaemia, a rebound phenomenon associated with papillae on the upper and lower tarsal conjunctiva.

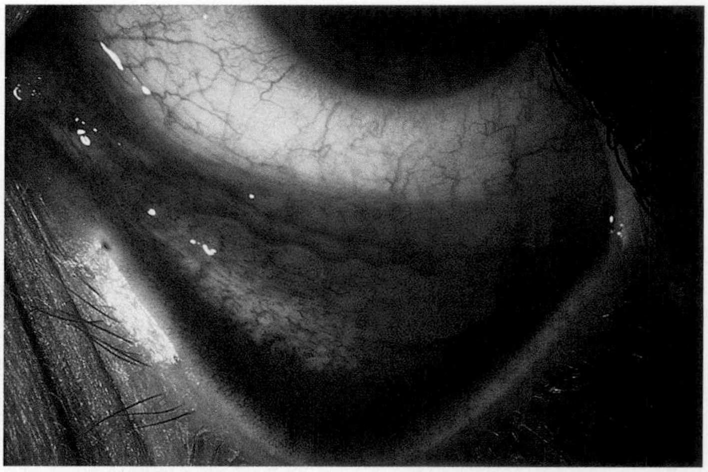

Fig. 3.109 Follicular conjunctivitis, due to a toxic effect, is less common and most prominent on the inferior fornix.

Floppy eyelid syndrome

Floppy eyelid syndrome typically affects obese men.

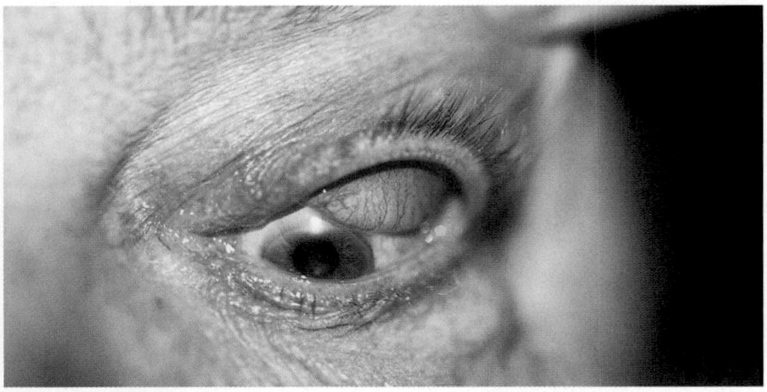

Fig. 3.110 Severe upper lid laxity with easy eversion of the tarsal plate.

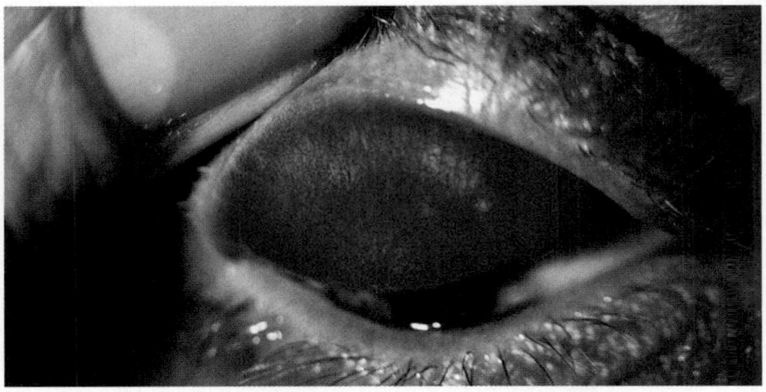

Fig. 3.111 Superior tarsal papillary conjunctivitis due to trauma of the everted lid during sleep.

Mucus fishing syndrome

Mucus fishing syndrome is the result of self-inflicted trauma when trying to remove excess mucus from the conjunctival sac. The condition should be suspected when appropriate treatment of an external ocular disease does not produce the expected result.

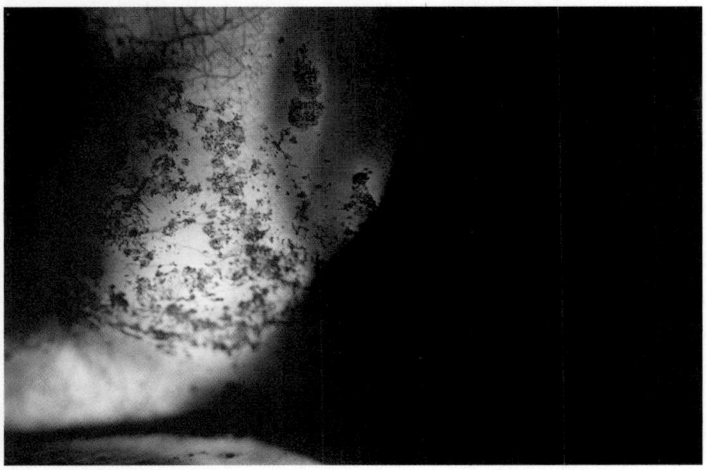

Fig. 3.112 Isolated, well-circumscribed areas that stain heavily with rose bengal.

Chronic canaliculitis

Chronic canaliculitis is frequently caused by *Actinomyces*, which are anaerobic Gram-positive bacteria.

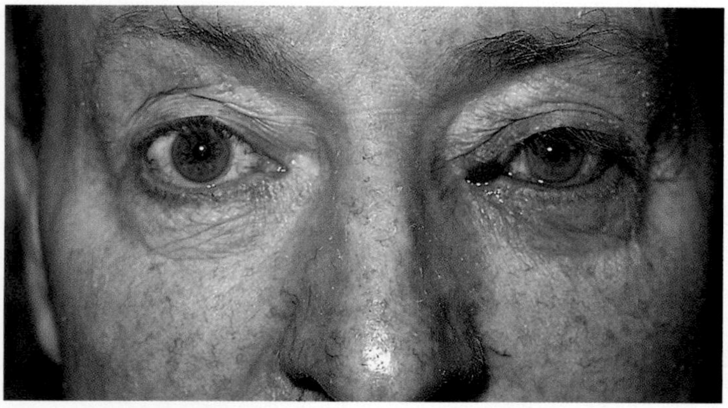

Fig. 3.113 Presentation is with unilateral epiphora and chronic mucopurulent discharge, which may be associated with oedema around the involved punctum.

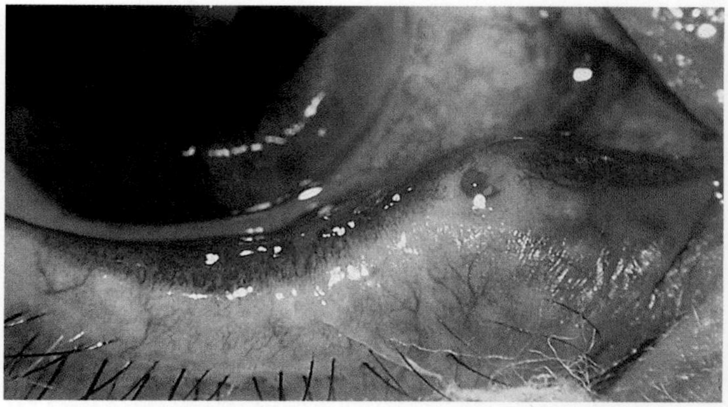

Fig. 3.114 A 'pouting' punctum is highly suggestive of canaliculitis.

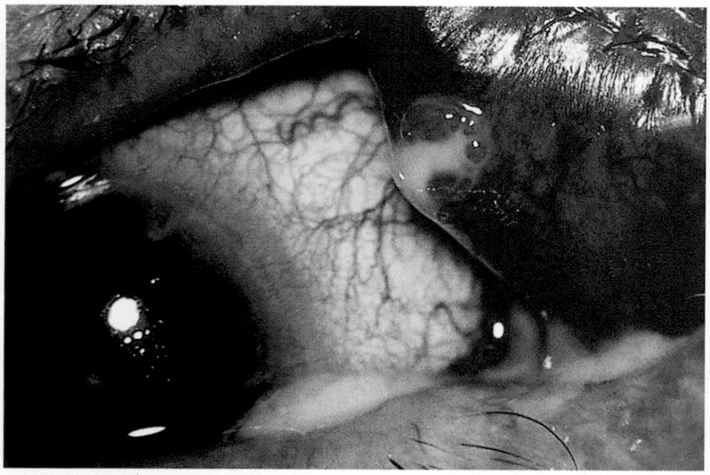

Fig. 3.115 Mucopurulent discharge on pressure over the canaliculus.

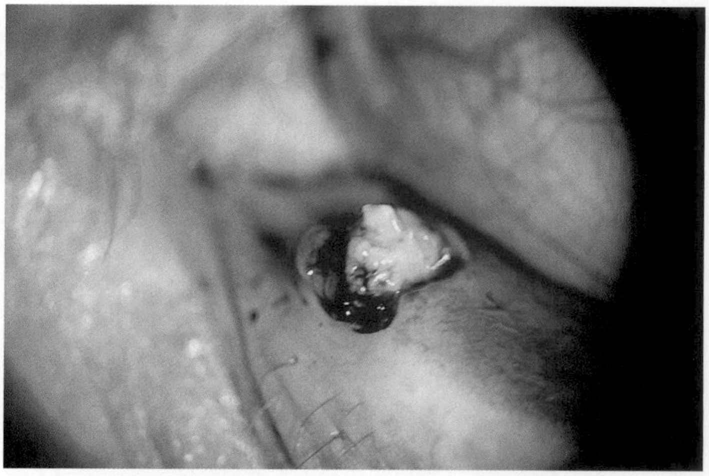

Fig. 3.116 Expressed concretions consisting of sulphur granules.

Chronic dacryocystitis

Chronic dacryocystitis presents with unilateral epiphora associated with a chronic or recurrent mucopurulent discharge.

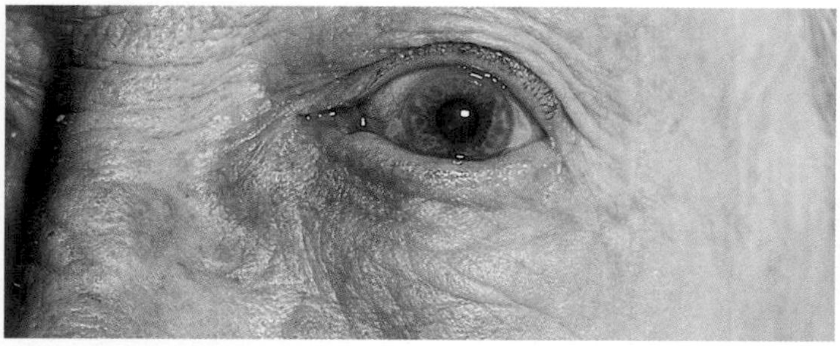

Fig. 3.117 Lacrimal sac mucocele characterised by a painless swelling at the inner canthus.

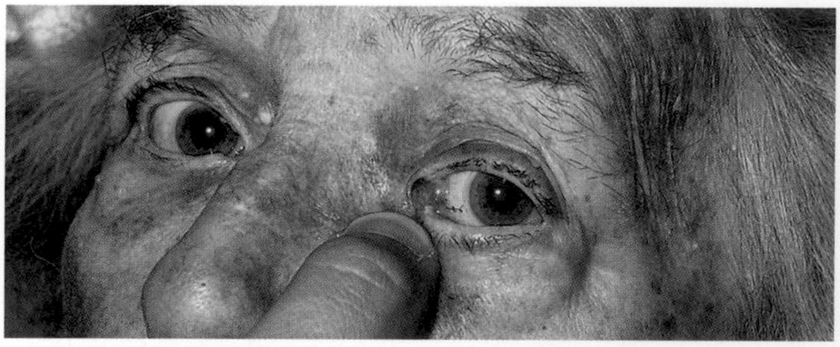

Fig. 3.118 Compression over the sac results in regurgitation of mucopurulent material through the canaliculi.

DEGENERATIONS

Pinguecula

A pinguecula is an extremely common, innocuous, usually bilateral, asymptomatic condition.

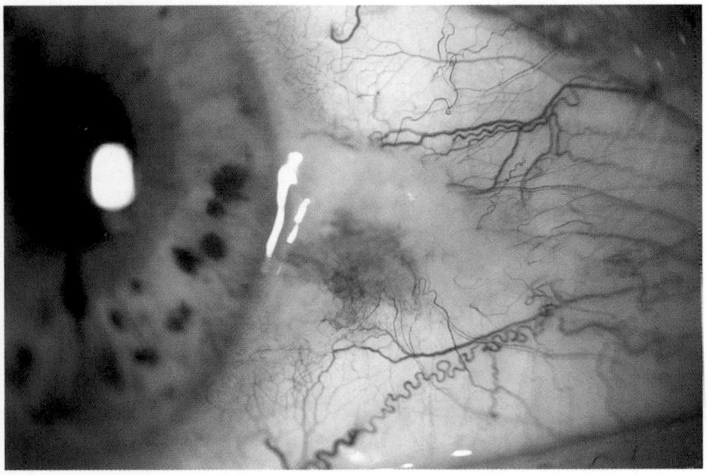

Fig. 3.119 Yellow-white deposits on the bulbar conjunctiva adjacent to the nasal or temporal limbus.

Pterygium

A pterygium is a triangular fibrovascular subepithelial ingrowth of degenerative bulbar conjunctival tissue over the limbus onto the cornea.

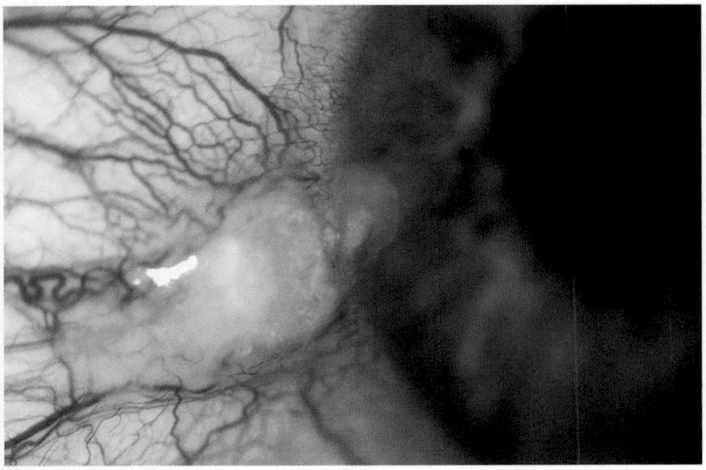

Fig. 3.120 A small, grey corneal opacity develops near the nasal limbus.

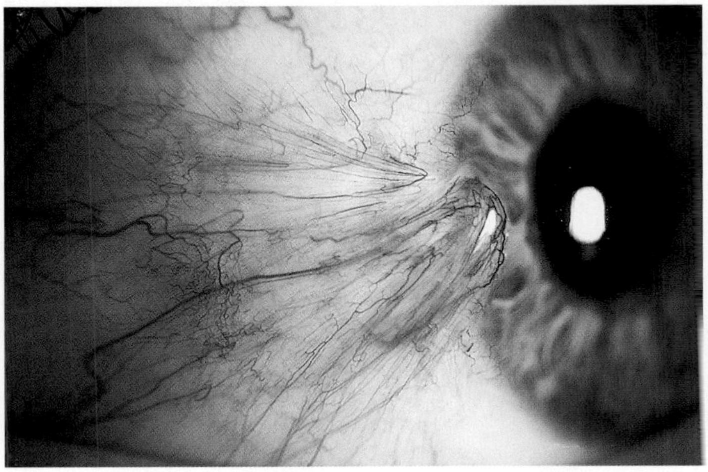

Fig. 3.121 The conjunctiva overgrows the opacity.

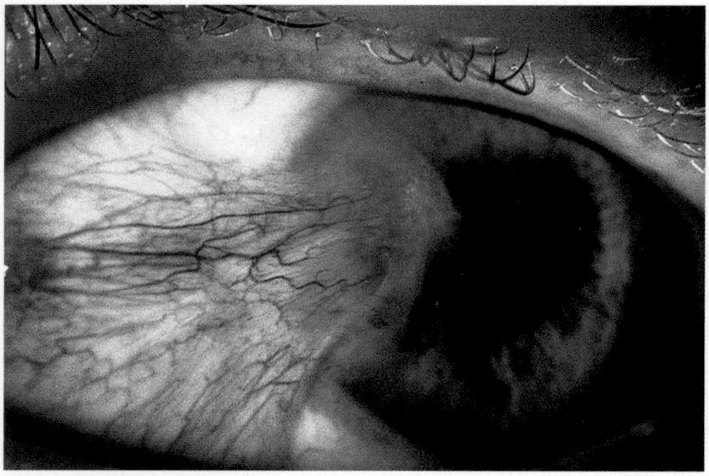

Fig. 3.122 Progressive encroachment on to the cornea in a triangular fashion.

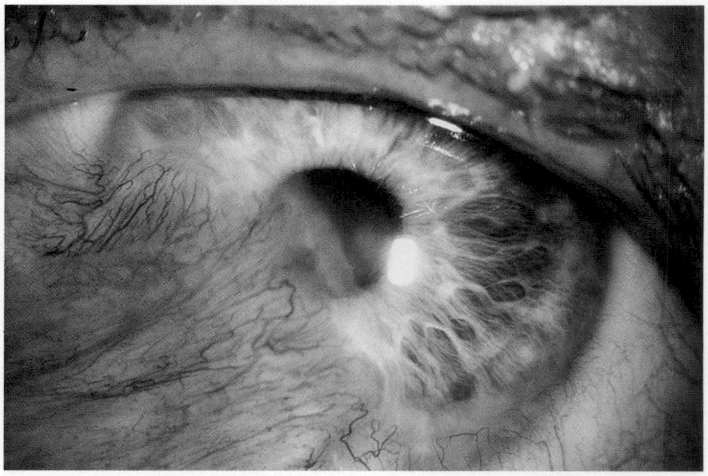

Fig. 3.123 Very advanced pterygium involving the visual axis. A deposit of iron (Stocker line) may be seen in the corneal epithelium anterior to the advancing head.

Pseudopterygium

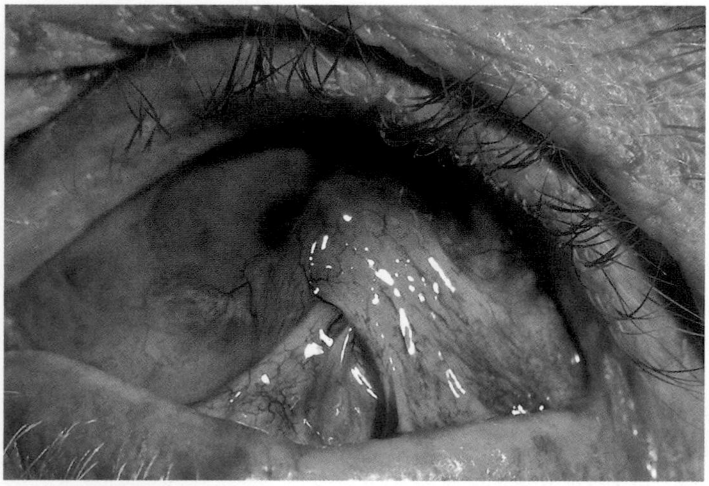

Fig. 3.124 This is caused by the adhesion of a fold of conjunctiva to a peripheral corneal ulcer or area of peripheral thinning, and is fixed only at its apex to the cornea.

Concretions

Concretions are extremely common lesions that most frequently affect elderly patients.

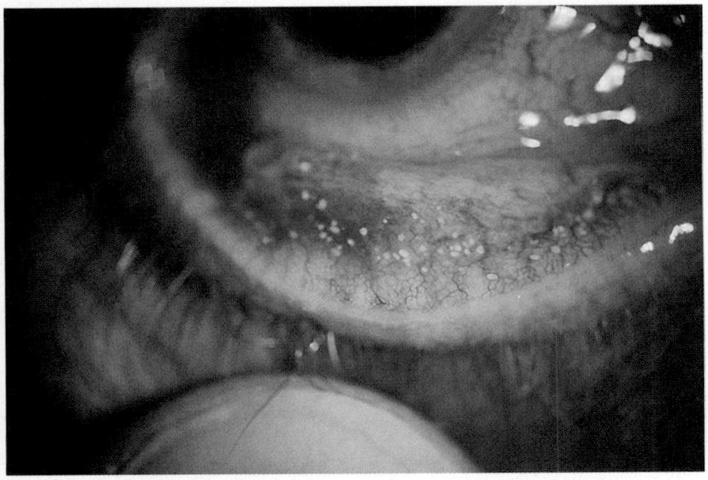

■ **Fig. 3.125** Small, often multiple, chalky, yellow-white deposits most commonly seen in the inferior conjunctiva.

Bitot spot

Bitot spot is an uncommon, usually bilateral lesion associated with vitamin A deficiency.

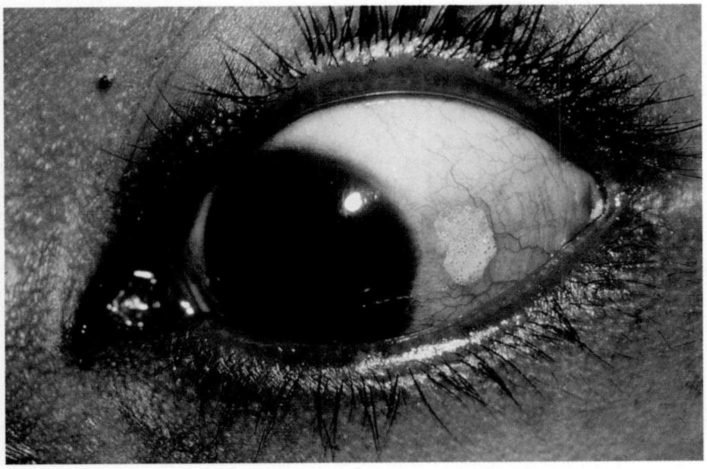

■ **Fig. 3.126** Foamy-looking plaque temporal to the limbus.

CYSTIC LESIONS

Primary retention cyst

Primary retention cysts are very common, usually asymptomatic, thin-walled lesions containing clear fluid.

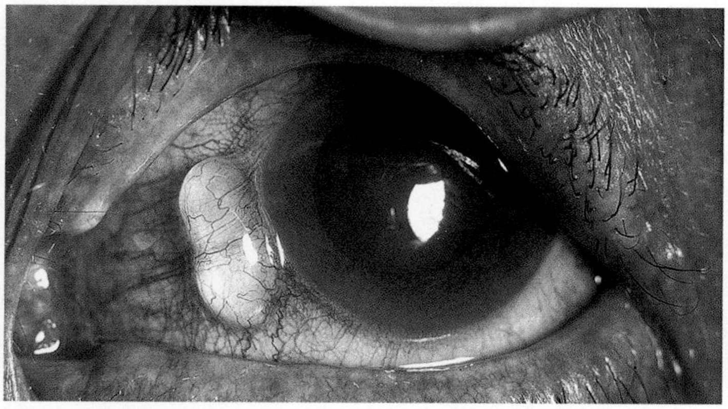

Fig. 3.127 Solitary cyst. (Courtesy of S. Ford and R. Marsh.)

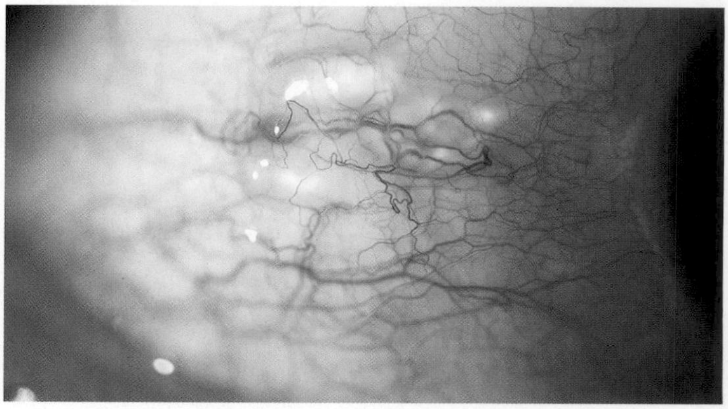

Fig. 3.128 A cluster of small retention cysts.

Secondary implantation cyst

Implantation cysts follow surgery involving a conjunctival incision.

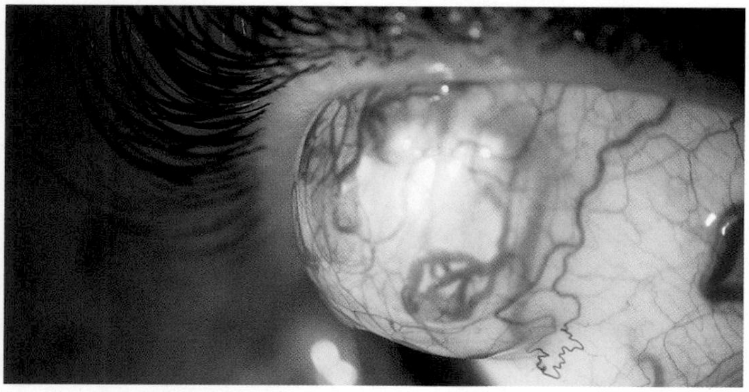

Fig. 3.129 The cyst has a thicker wall than a primary retention cyst and prominent surface vascularisation.

Cyst of a gland of Wolfring

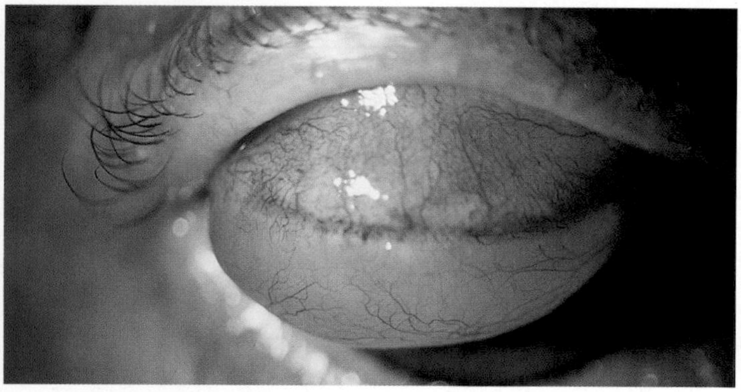

Fig. 3.130 A thin-walled cystic swelling involving the lower or upper tarsus.

NON-NEOPLASTIC INFILTRATION

Sarcoid

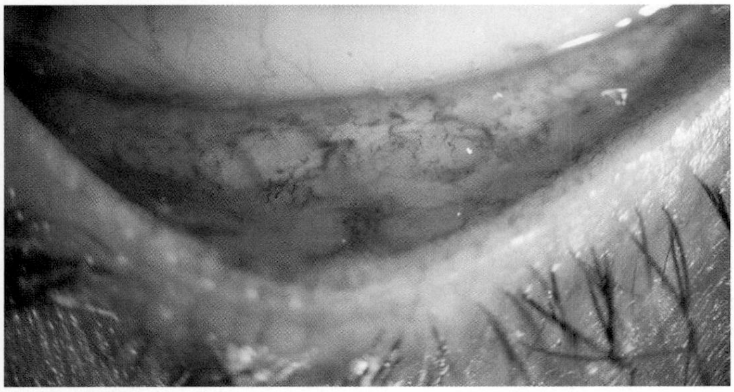

■ **Fig. 3.131** Small conjunctival granulomas are relatively common and may be used for diagnostic biopsy.

Tuberculosis

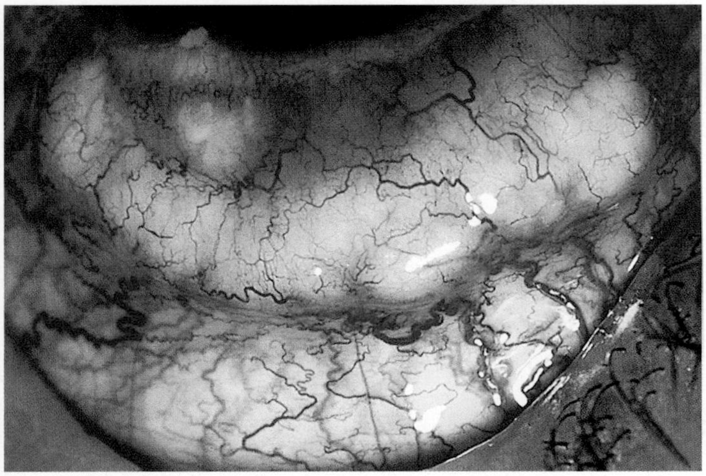

■ **Fig. 3.132** Conjunctival tuberculomas may rarely occur in both primary and reactive disease.

Amyloid

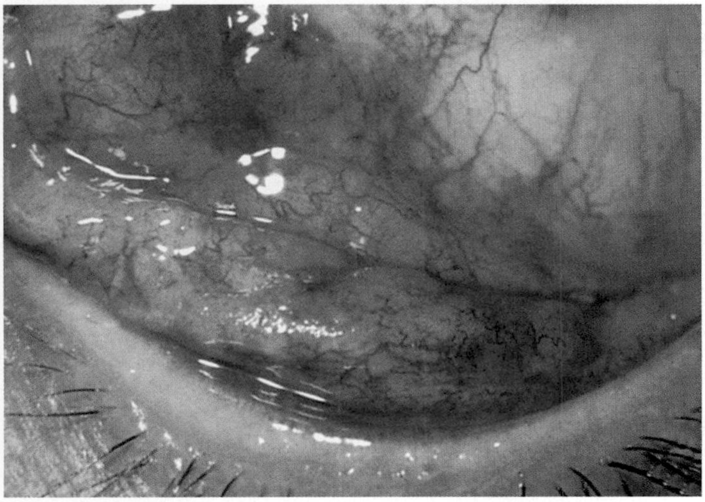

■ **Fig. 3.133** Rubbery, nodular deposits with a waxy appearance that are usually primary and localised, having no systemic implications.

NON-NEOPLASTIC PIGMENTED LESIONS

Freckle

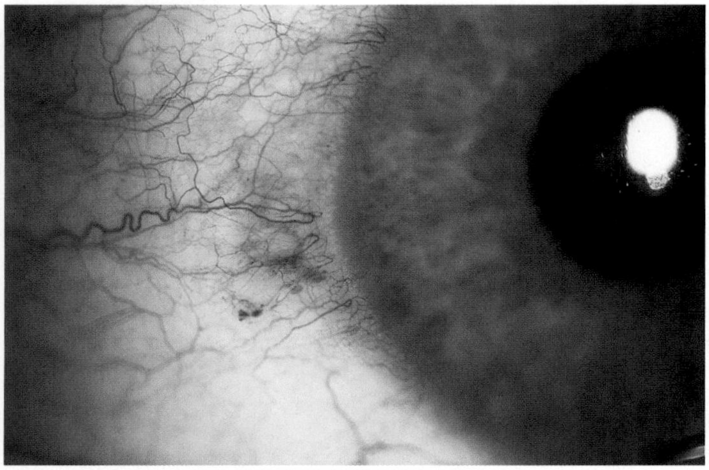

Fig. 3.134 A tiny area of epithelial pigmentation (melanosis).

Axenfeld loop

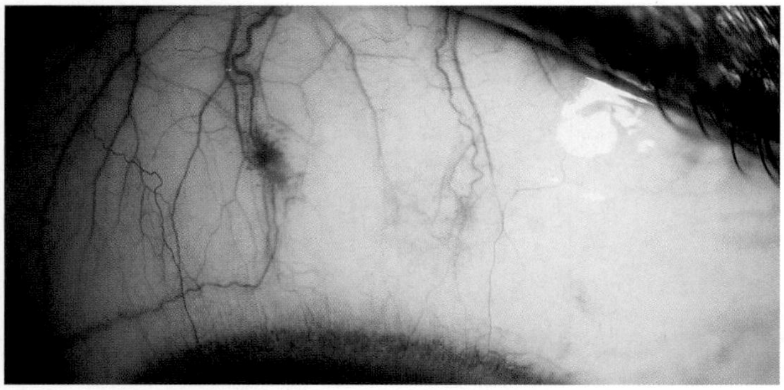

Fig. 3.135 Areas of melanosis around an intrascleral nerve or anterior ciliary vessel.

Mascara deposits

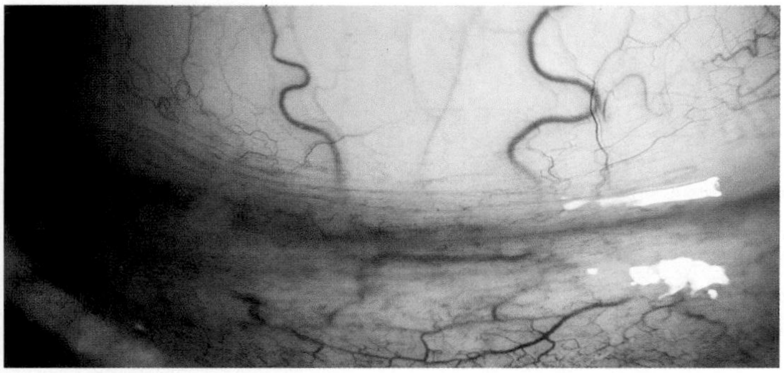

Fig. 3.136 Tiny black spots in the inferior fornix.

Adrenochrome deposits

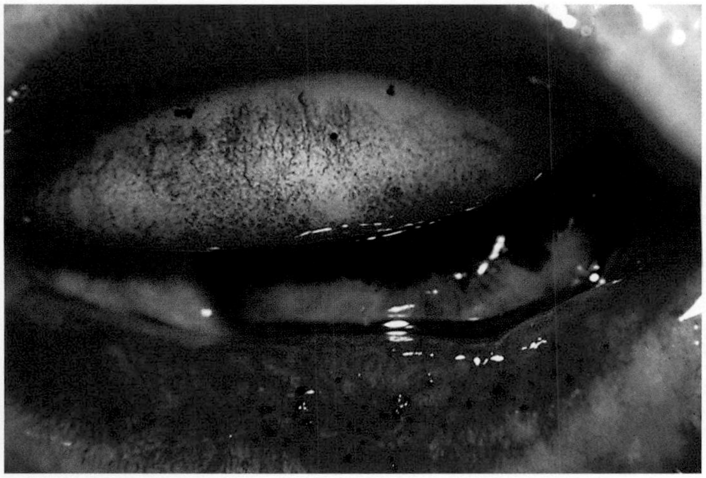

■ **Fig. 3.137** Tiny black clumps of pigment on the tarsal or forniceal conjunctiva associated with the long-term use of adrenaline (epinephrine) drops for glaucoma.

Epithelial melanosis

Conjunctival epithelial melanosis is often seen in dark-skinned individuals.

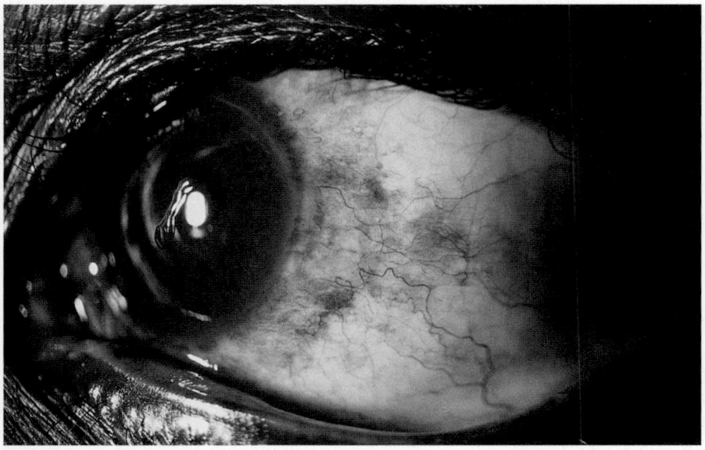

■ **Fig. 3.138** Areas of flat, patchy, brownish pigmentation scattered throughout the conjunctival epithelium that moves freely over the surface of the globe.

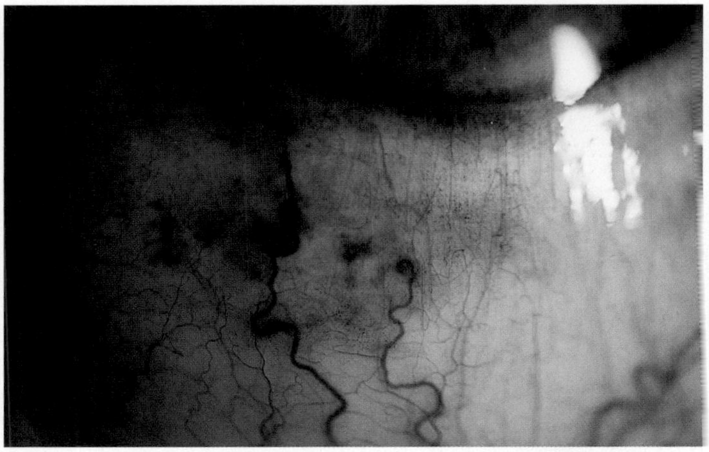

■ **Fig. 3.139** The pigmentation is more intense at the limbus and around the perforating branches of the anterior ciliary vessels.

Congenital ocular melanocytosis

Congenital melanocytosis is an uncommon melanocytic hyperplasia that occurs in the following three clinical settings:

Dermal melanocytosis

Dermal melanocytosis involves only the skin and accounts for about one-third of cases.

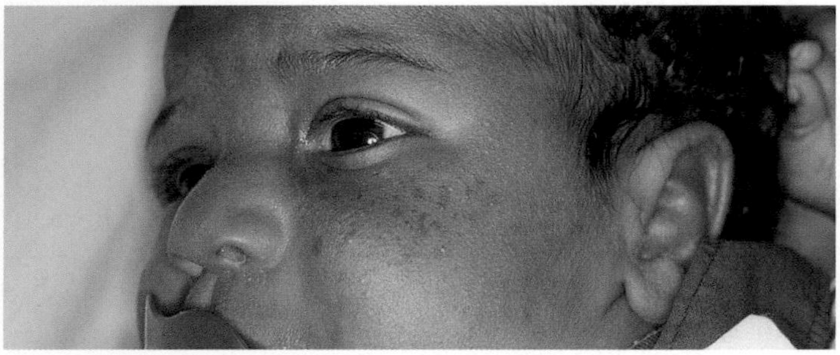

Fig. 3.140 Unilateral deep hyperpigmentation of facial skin, most frequently in the distribution of the first and second divisions of the trigeminal nerve. (Courtesy of A. Singh.)

Ocular melanocytosis

Ocular melanocytosis involves only the eye and is the least common.

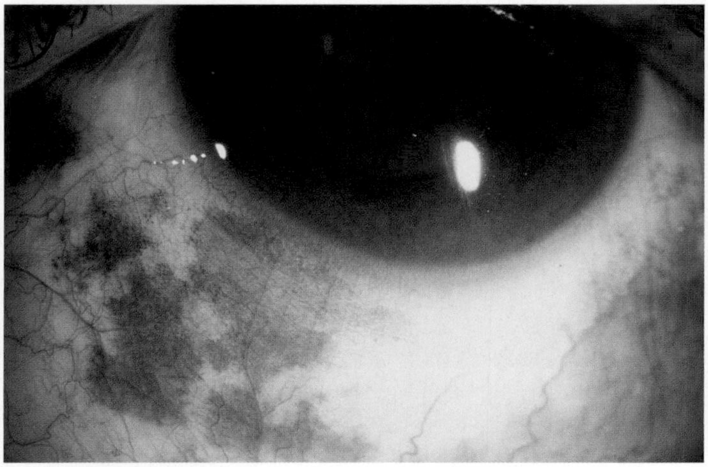

Fig. 3.141 Multifocal, slate-grey subconjunctival pigmentation that cannot be moved over the globe.

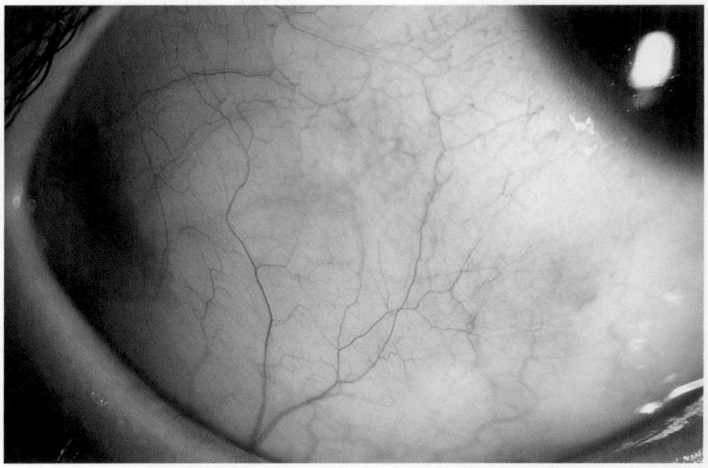

Fig. 3.142 Subtle diffuse involvement.

Oculodermal melanocytosis (Naevus of Ota)

Naevus of Ota involves both skin and eye and is the most frequently encountered type.

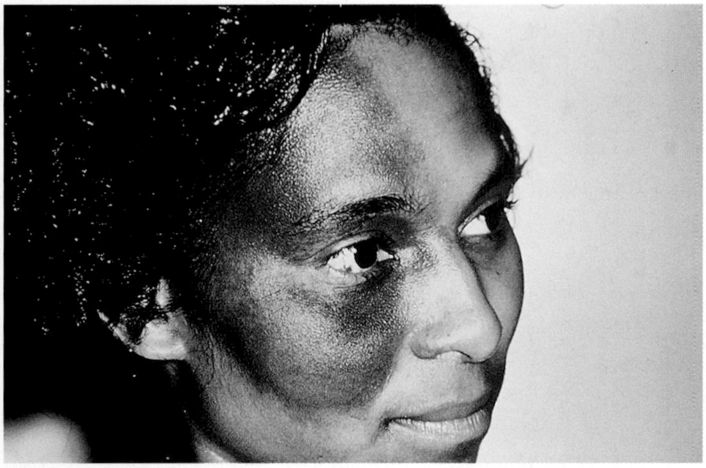

Fig. 3.143 Naevus of Ota. (Courtesy of P. G. Watson, B. L. Hazelman, C. E. Parvesio and W. R. Green.)

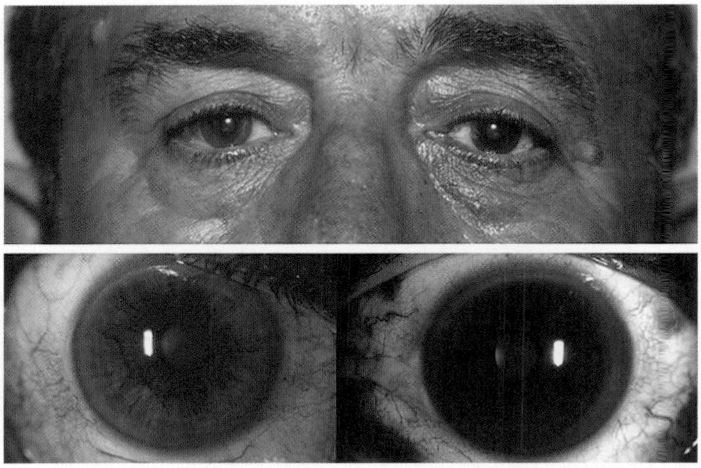

Fig. 3.144 Unilateral involvement with ipsilateral iris hyperpigmentation is common. (Courtesy of P. Gili.)

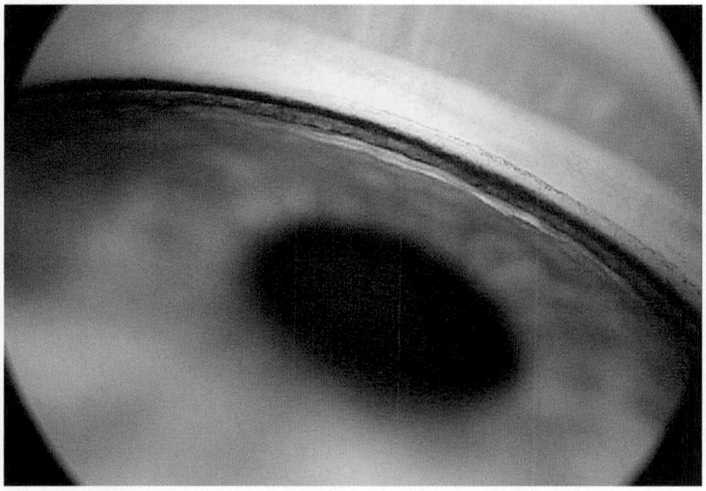

Fig. 3.145 Trabecular hyperpigmentation, which may be associated with glaucoma, is uncommon. (Courtesy of L. MacKeen.)

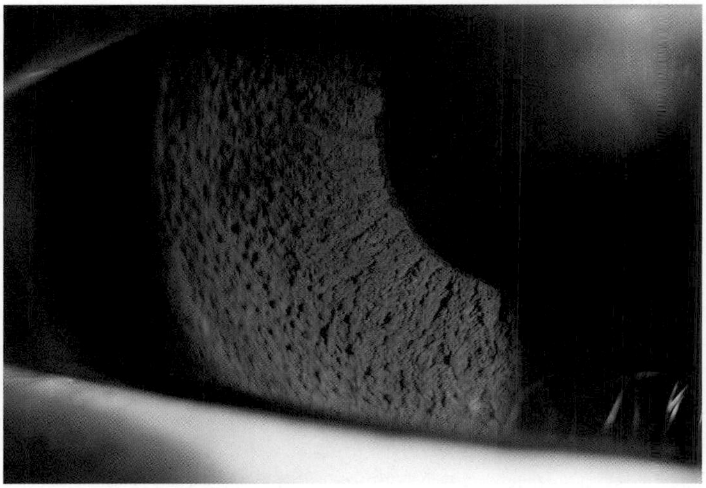

Fig. 3.146 Iris mammillations, which are tiny, regularly spaced, villiform lesions, are uncommon.

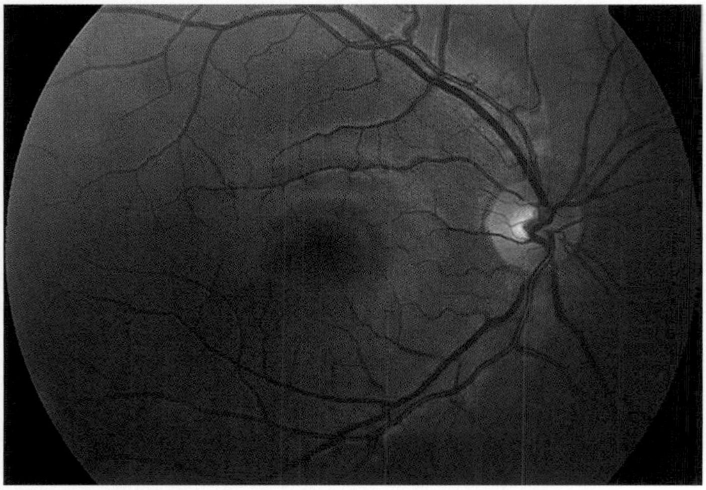

Fig. 3.147 Ipsilateral fundus hyperpigmentation is rare.

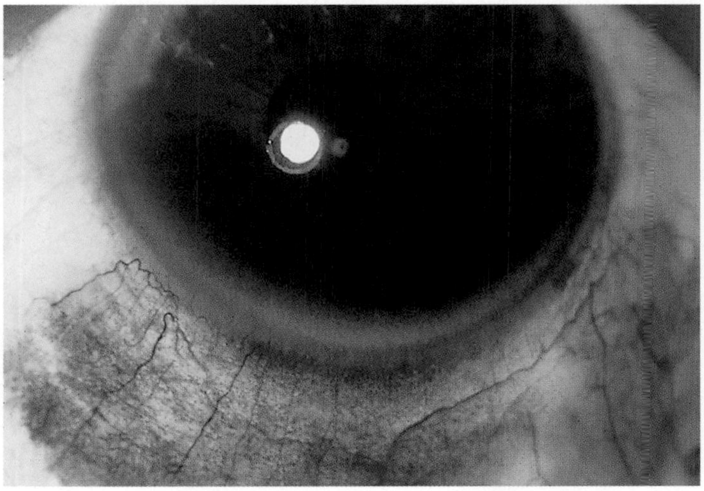

Fig. 3.148 Diffuse melanoma of the inferior iris in naevus of Ota.

BENIGN TUMOURS

Melanocytic tumours

Naevus

A conjunctival naevus is a solitary, sharply demarcated, flat or slightly elevated lesion that can be moved over the sclera. The most frequent location is juxtalimbal.

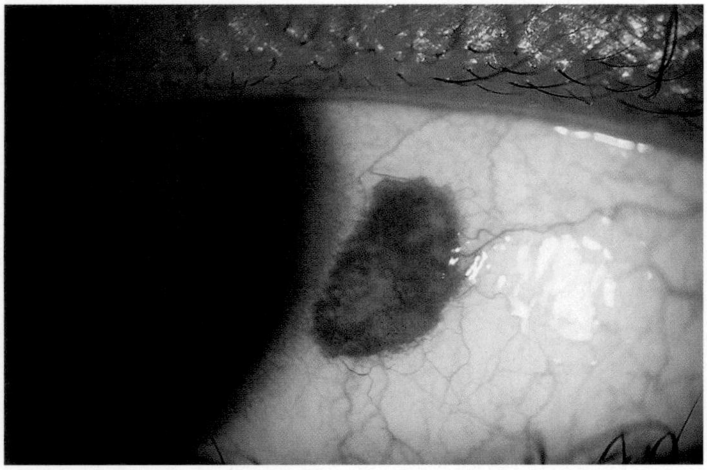

Fig. 3.149 A pigmented juxtalimbal naevus.

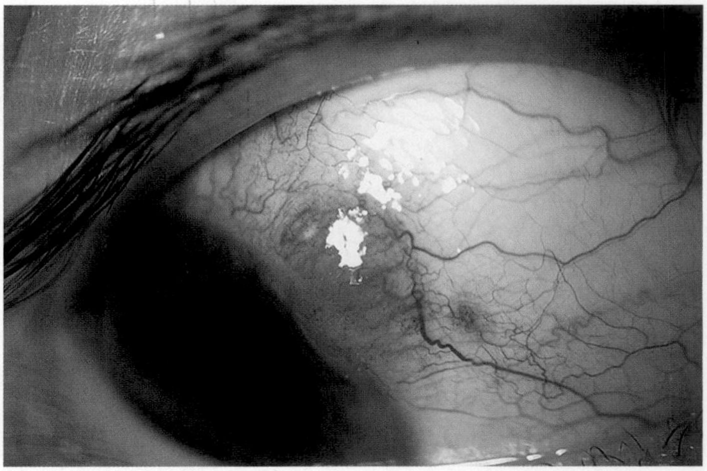

Fig. 3.150 A hypopigmented juxtalimbal naevus.

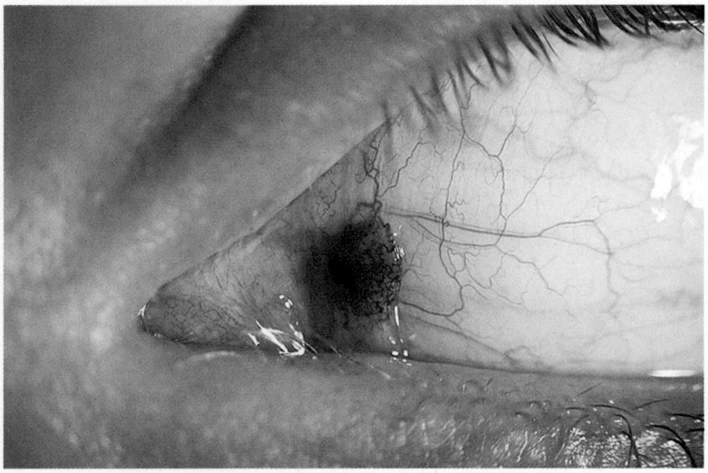

Fig. 3.151 Involvement of the plica is relatively common.

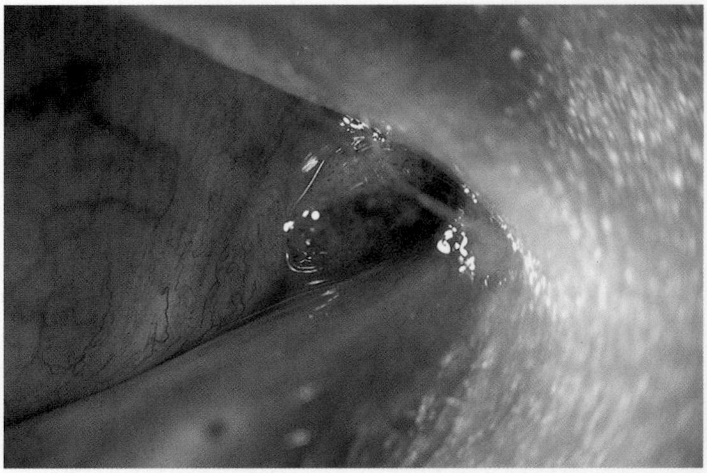

Fig. 3.152 Involvement of the caruncle is uncommon.

Melanocytoma

A melanocytoma is a rare condition which may be mistaken for a naevus but is present at birth.

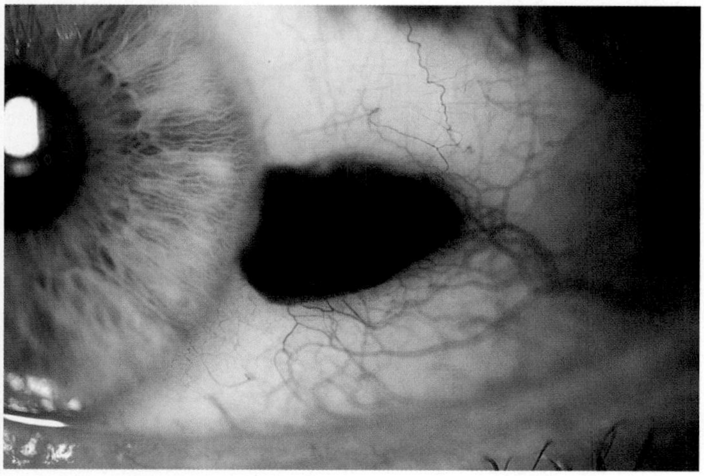

Fig. 3.153 A heavily pigmented, slow-growing lesion that cannot be moved over the sclera.

Epithelial tumours

Pedunculated papilloma

Pedunculated papillomas are caused by infection with human papillomavirus (types 6 and 11) and may occasionally be multiple and bilateral.

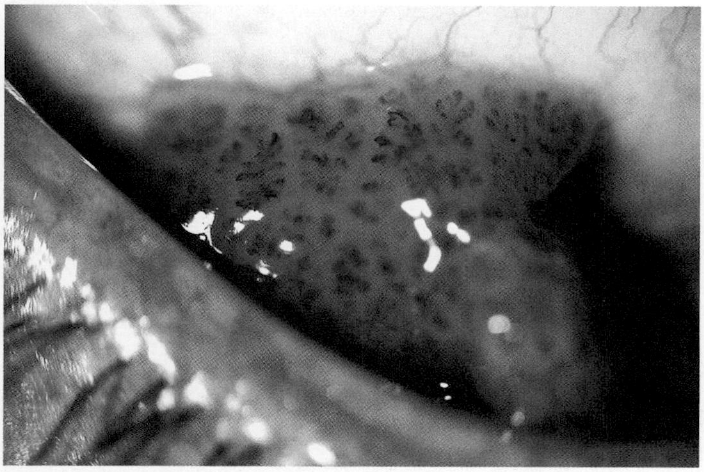

Fig. 3.154 The lesion has a raspberry-like surface and frequently arises in the fornix.

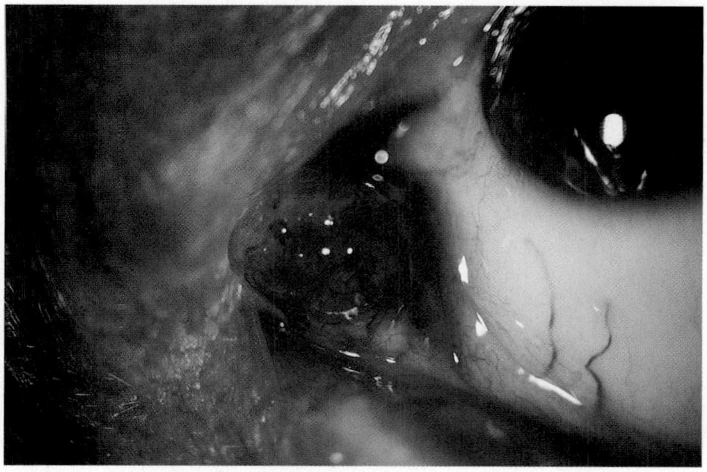

Fig. 3.155 Papilloma at the caruncle.

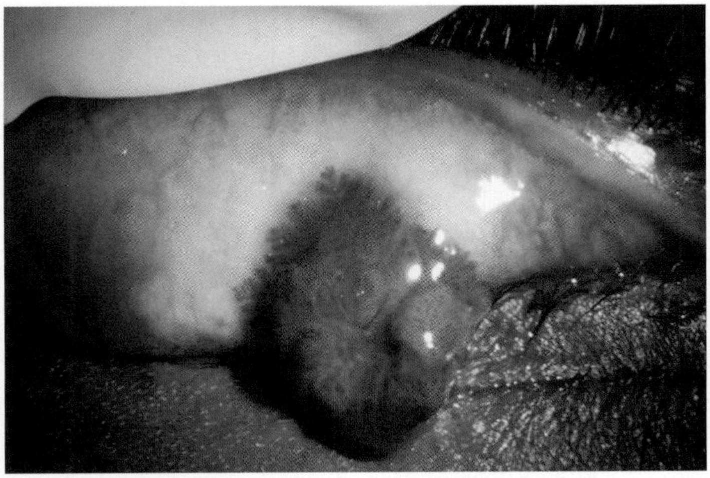

■ **Fig. 3.156** Pigmented papilloma arising from the tarsal conjunctiva. (Courtesy of R. Curtis.)

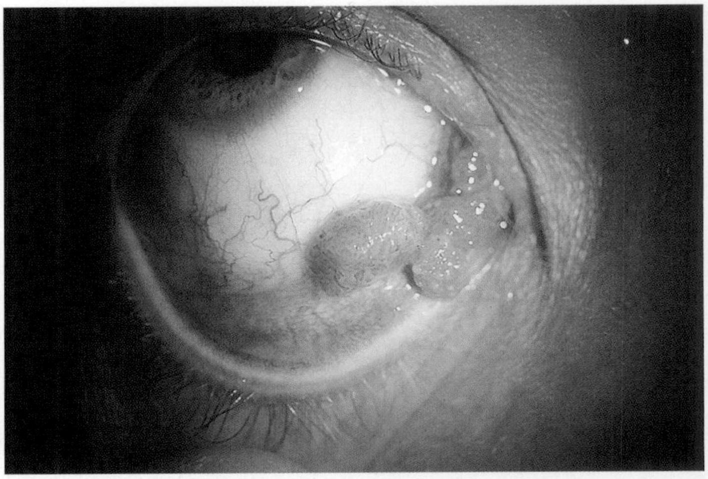

■ **Fig. 3.157** Multiple papillomas.

Sessile papilloma

Sessile (neoplastic) papillomas are not infectious, invariably unilateral, most frequently located on the bulbar conjunctiva and associated with feeding vessels.

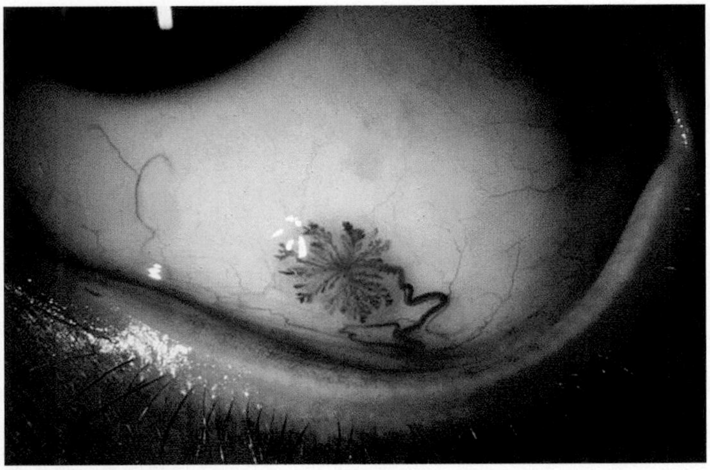

■ **Fig. 3.158** A very small papilloma. (Courtesy of R. Curtis.)

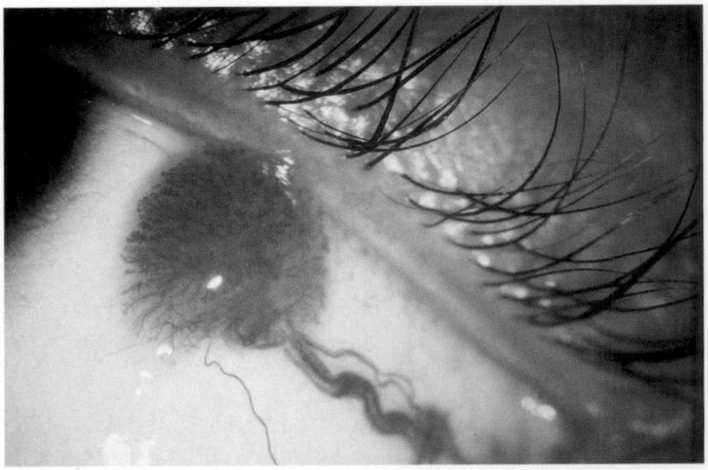

■ **Fig. 3.159** A larger papilloma. (Courtesy of S. Ford and R. Marsh.)

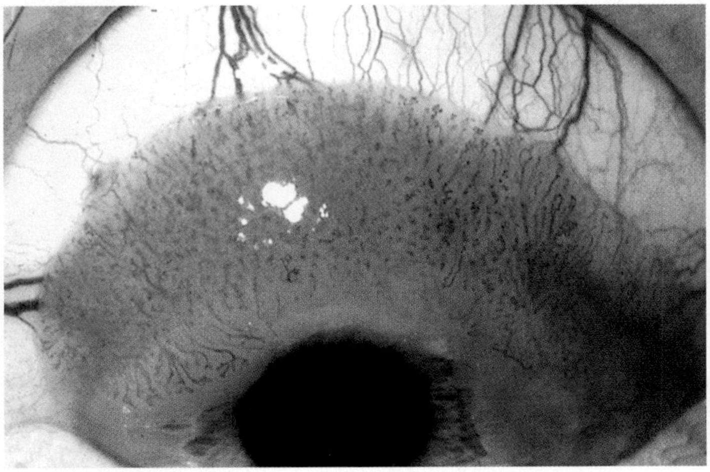

■ **Fig. 3.160** Large, diffuse, limbal papilloma encroaching on to the cornea.

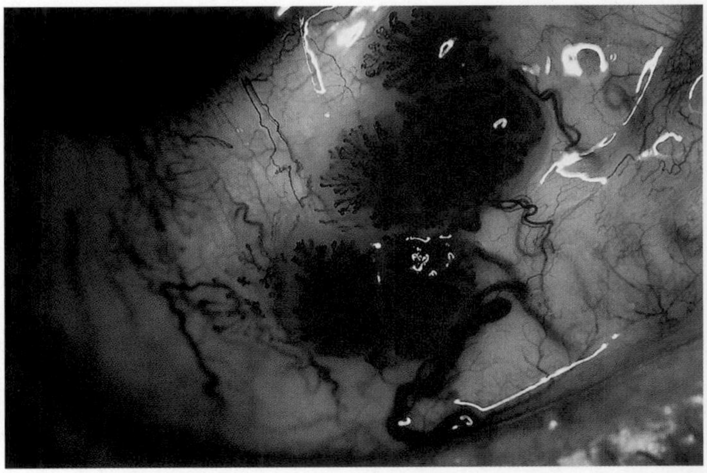

■ **Fig. 3.161** Multiple papillomas.

Conjunctival intraepithelial neoplasia

Conjunctival intraepithelial neoplasia is an uncommon, slowly progressive unilateral disease with low malignant potential.

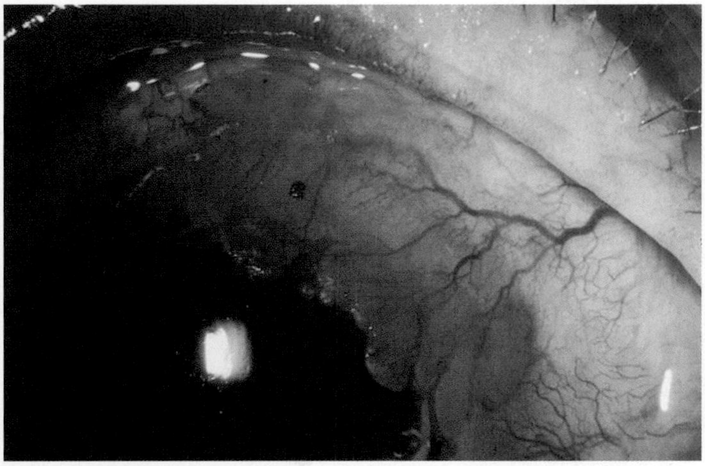

Fig. 3.162 A flat, gelatinous, plaque-like lesion with tufts of superficial blood vessels at the limbus within the interpalpebral fissure. (Courtesy of R. Curtis.)

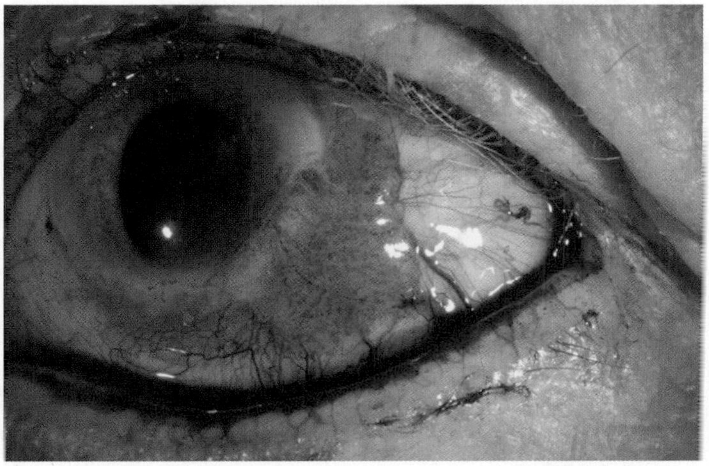

Fig. 3.163 A raised, discrete, papillomatous lesion with surface corkscrew-like blood vessels. (Courtesy of L. Merin.)

Pseudoepitheliomatous hyperplasia

Pseudoepitheliomatous hyperplasia is a reactive epithelial proliferation secondary to irritation.

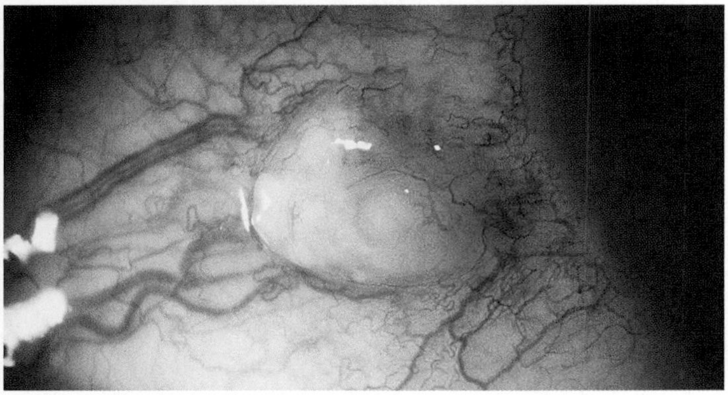

Fig. 3.164 A rapidly growing, white, hyperkeratotic, juxtalimbal nodule.

Hereditary benign intraepithelial dyskeratosis

Hereditary benign intraepithelial dyskeratosis is a rare, bilateral hereditary condition.

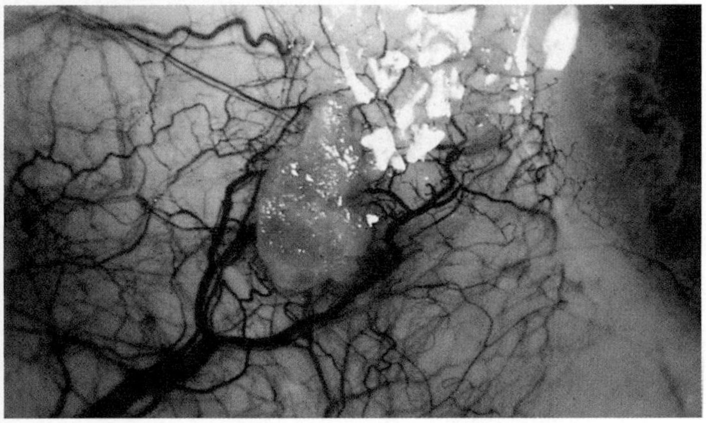

Fig. 3.165 Bilateral elevated perilimbal hyperplastic plaques associated with vascular dilatation.

Vascular tumours and malformations

Capillary haemangioma

Capillary haemangioma typically presents in infancy and may be associated with 'strawberry naevi' on the eyelids and skin. Just like its cutaneous counterpart it initially enlarges and then spontaneously involutes.

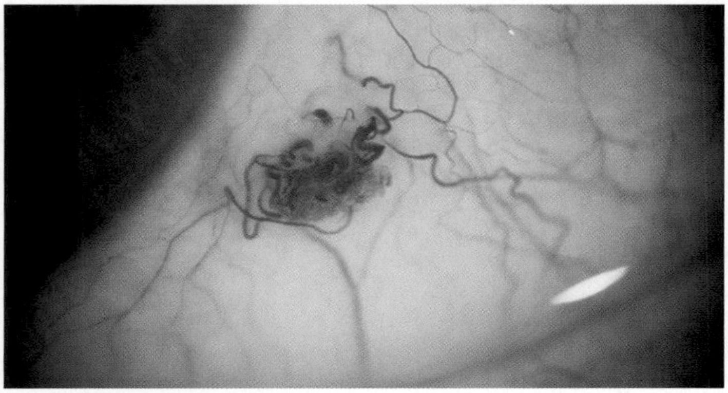

Fig. 3.166 A small capillary haemangioma.

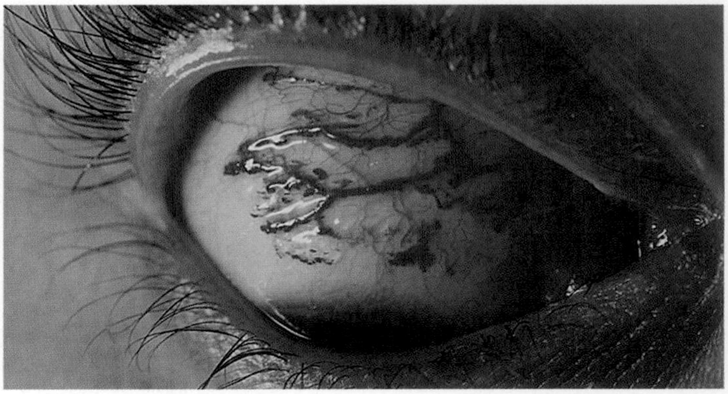

Fig. 3.167 Larger capillary haemangioma. (Courtesy of U. Raina.)

Cavernous haemangioma

Cavernous haemangioma is very rare and typically occurs in young children.

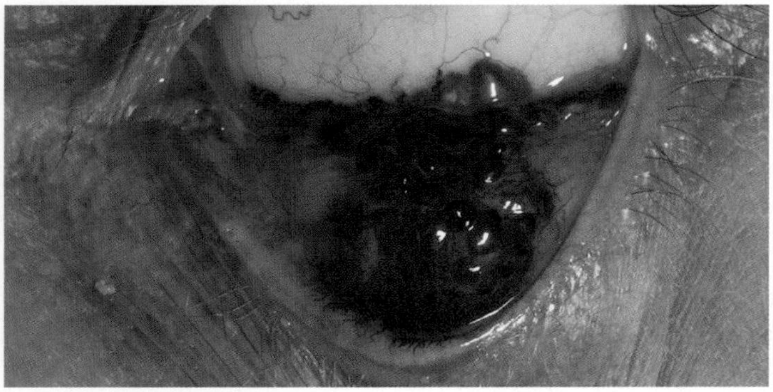

Fig. 3.168 A red or blue loculated lesion in the deep stroma. (Courtesy of L. Merin.)

Lymphangioma

Conjunctival lymphangiomas may occur in isolation or in association with orbital lymphangiomas.

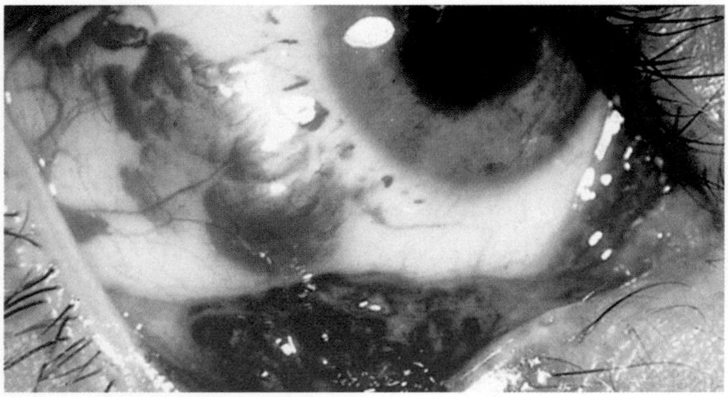

Fig. 3.169 A multilobular lesion containing cystic channels, which are often filled with blood.

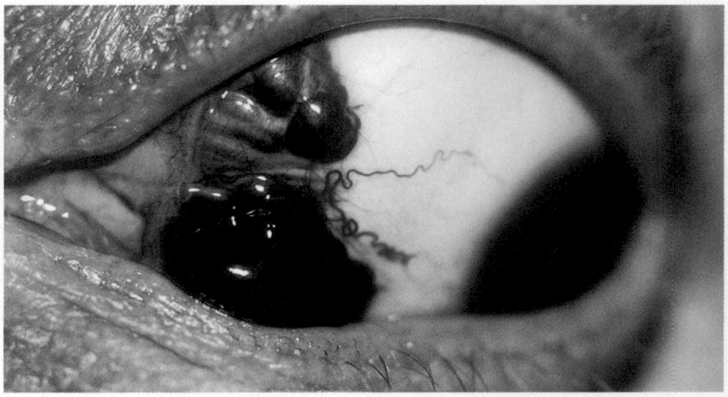

Fig. 3.170 Lymphangioma at the inner canthus. (Courtesy of C. Barry.)

Lymphangiectasia

Lymphangiectasia is an uncommon condition which may be associated with vascular malformations of the eyelid and parotid gland.

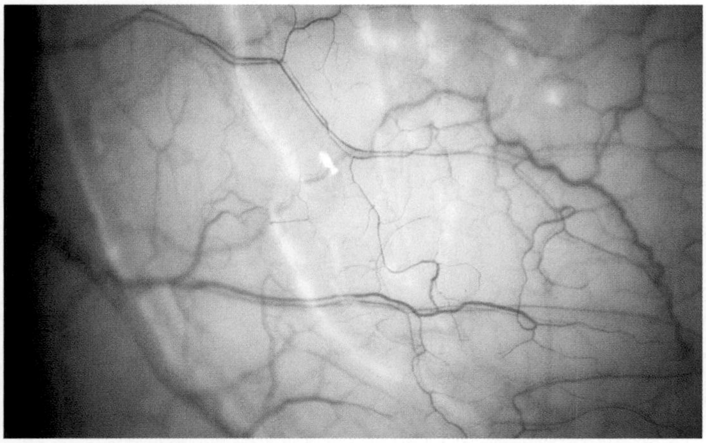

Fig. 3.171 Dilated and tortuous bulbar lymphatic channels.

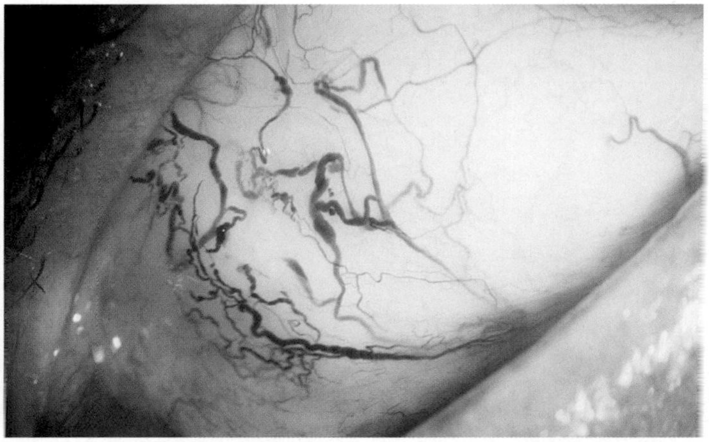

Fig. 3.172 Occasionally the channels become filled with blood if they communicate with conjunctival veins.

Varices

Conjunctival varices are invariably associated with orbital varices.

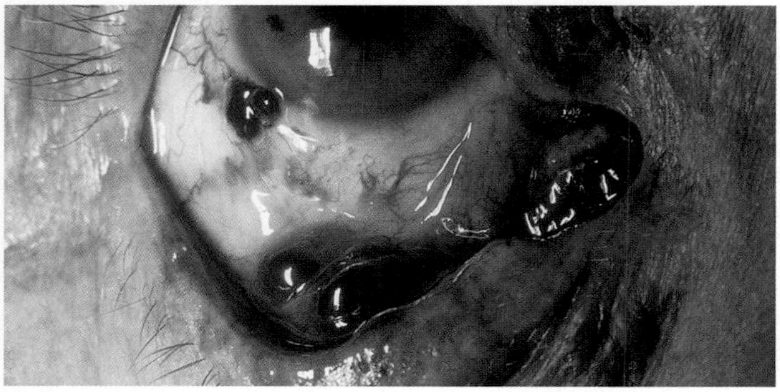

Fig. 3.173 Saccular, venous dilatation accentuated on performing the Valsalva manoeuvre.

Pyogenic granuloma

Pyogenic granuloma is a vascularised proliferation of granulomatous tissue that typically develops a few weeks following surgery involving the conjunctiva.

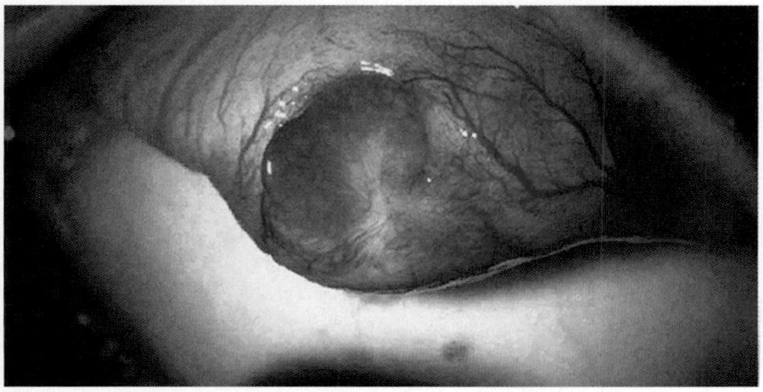

Fig. 3.174 Pyogenic granuloma following excision of a chalazion.

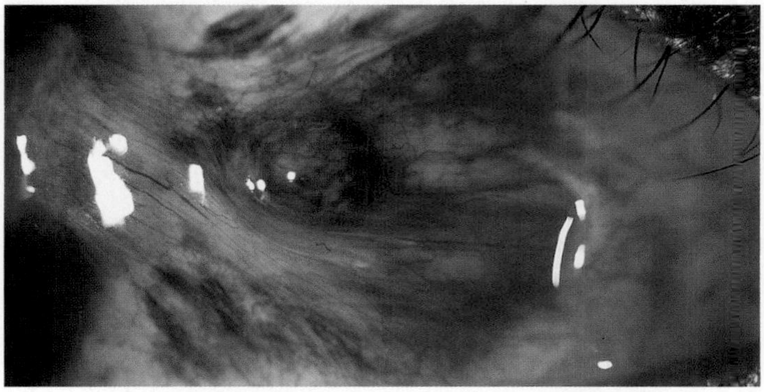

Fig. 3.175 Small pyogenic granuloma following pterygium surgery.

Choristomas

A choristoma is a congenital overgrowth of normal tissue in an abnormal location containing a variety of tissues such as cartilage, fat, muscle, hair follicles and sebaceous glands.

Dermoid

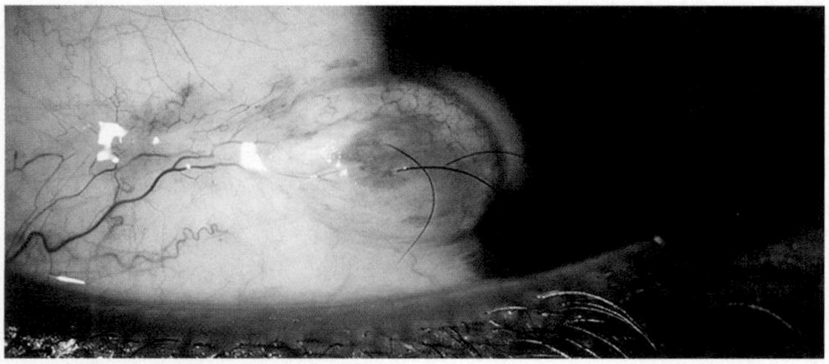

Fig. 3.176 Smooth, yellowish mass often at the inferotemporal limbus that may show protruding hair.

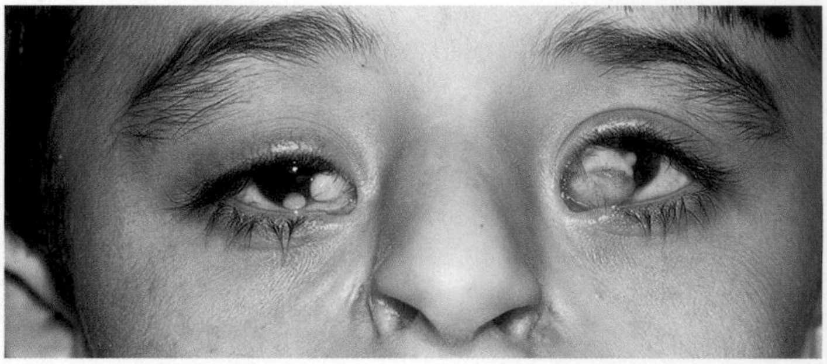

Fig. 3.177 Bilateral and multiple dermoids are rare.

Association

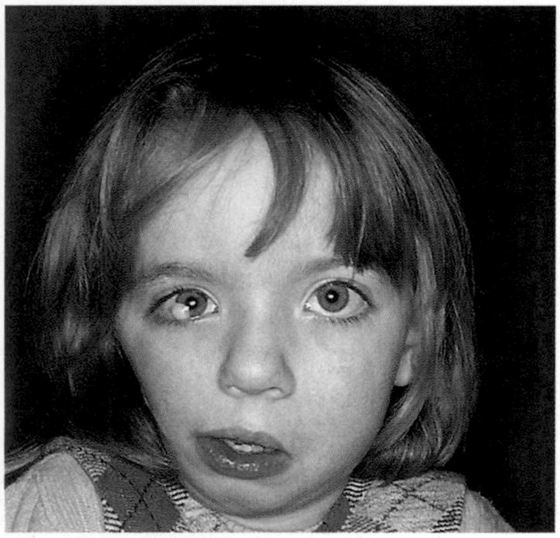

Fig. 3.178 Mandibular hypolasia and a limbal dermoid in Goldenhar syndrome.

Complex choristoma

A complex choristoma contains a greater variety of abnormal tissue than a dermoid and has a more fleshy appearance.

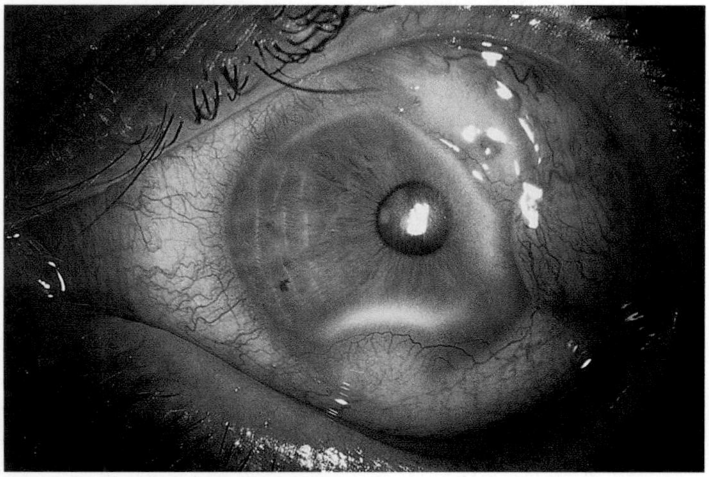

Fig. 3.179 The lesion covers much of the epibulbar surface and extends circumferentially around the limbus and deeply into the cornea.

Association

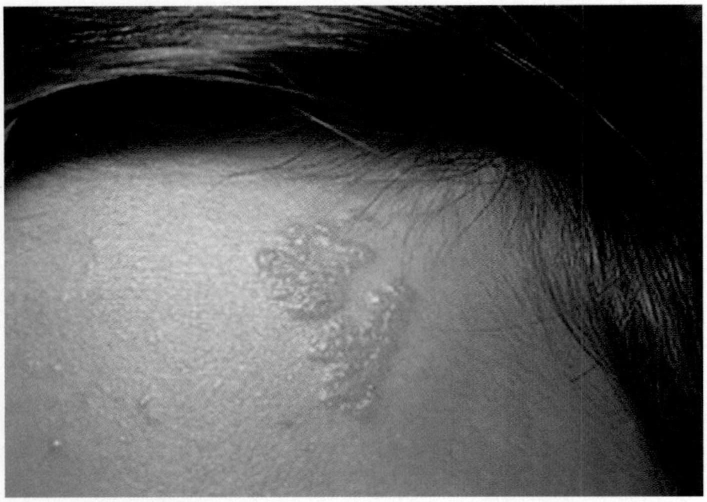

Fig. 3.180 Yellowish, waxy skin lesion in a patient with seizures and mental retardation associated with naevus sebaceus of Jadassohn. (Courtesy of B. J. Zitelli and H. W. Davis.)

Dermolipoma

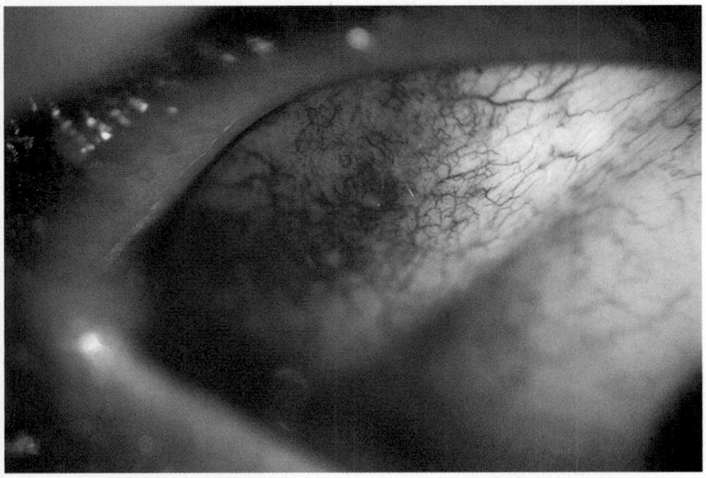

Fig. 3.181 A soft, pale yellow, fluctuant, fusiform mass below the palpebral lobe of the lacrimal gland.

MALIGNANT TUMOURS

Primary acquired melanosis (PAM)

PAM is characterised by irregular, unifocal or multifocal areas of flat, brown pigmentation that may involve any part of the conjunctiva. Histologically, PAM without atypia is benign whereas PAM with atypia predisposes to melanoma.

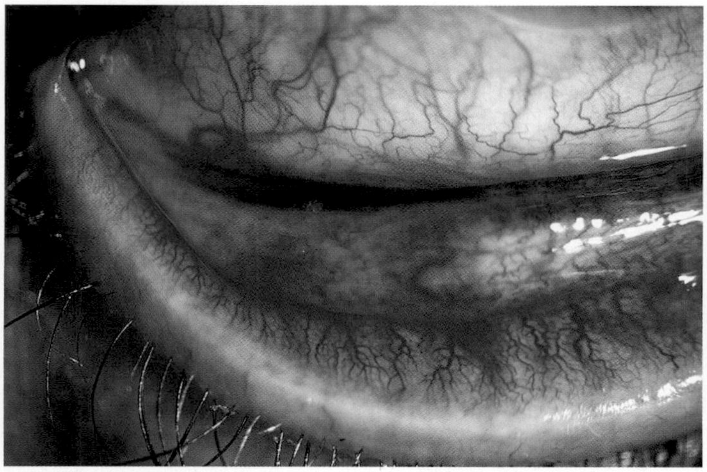

Fig. 3.182 Small patch of PAM in the inferior fornix, which may be easily overlooked.

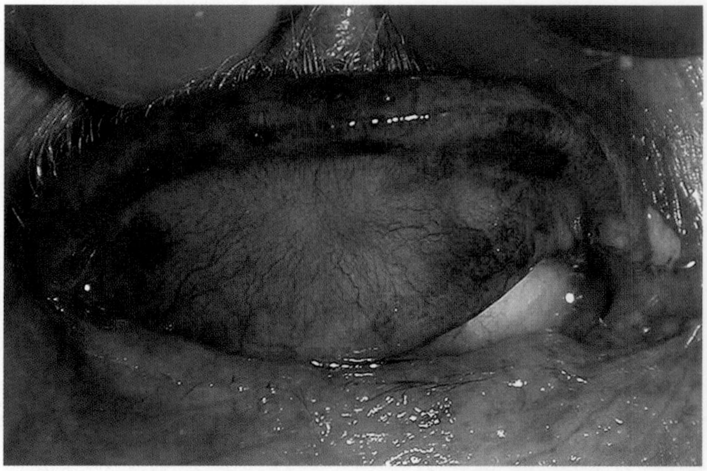

Fig. 3.183 PAM and lentigo maligna on the lid margin. (Courtesy of D. Selva.)

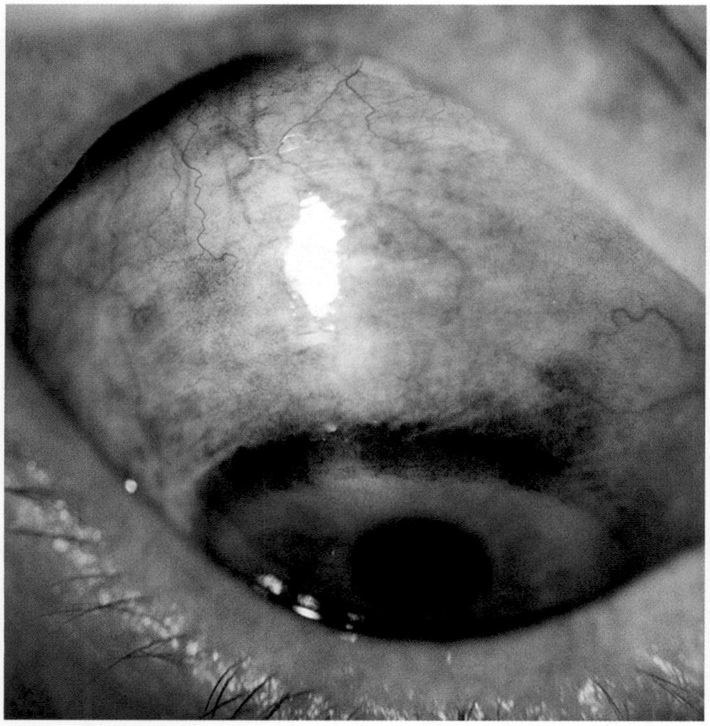

Fig. 3.184 Diffuse PAM.

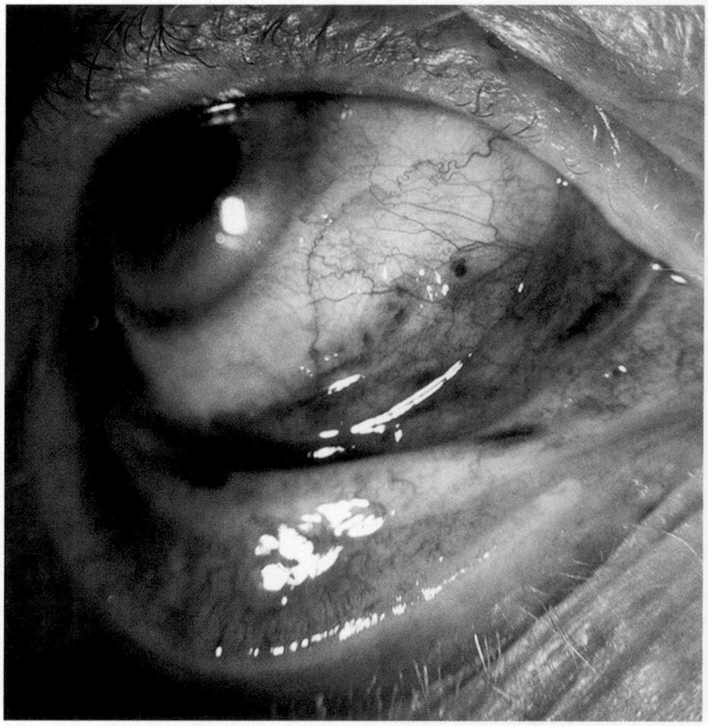

Fig. 3.185 PAM with focal areas of increased thickening and pigmentation suggestive of malignant transformation.

Melanoma

Arising from PAM

Seventy-five percent of conjunctival melanomas arise from PAM with atypia.

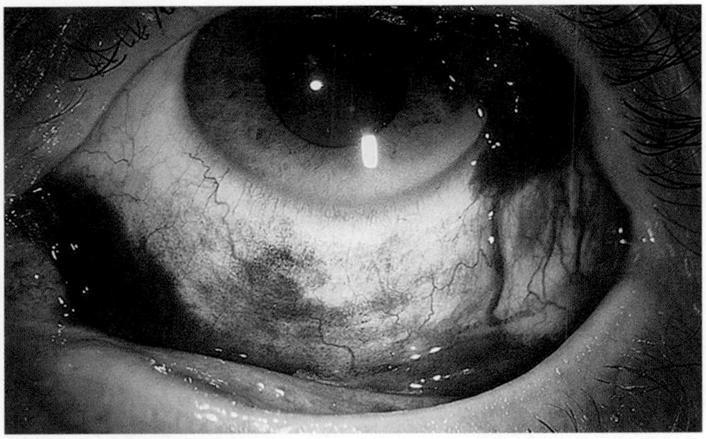

Fig. 3.186 Multifocal melanoma arising from PAM.

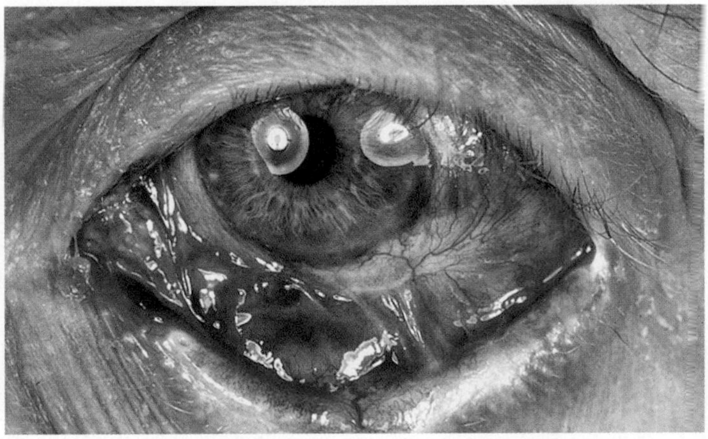

Fig. 3.187 Advanced melanoma arising from PAM.

Primary

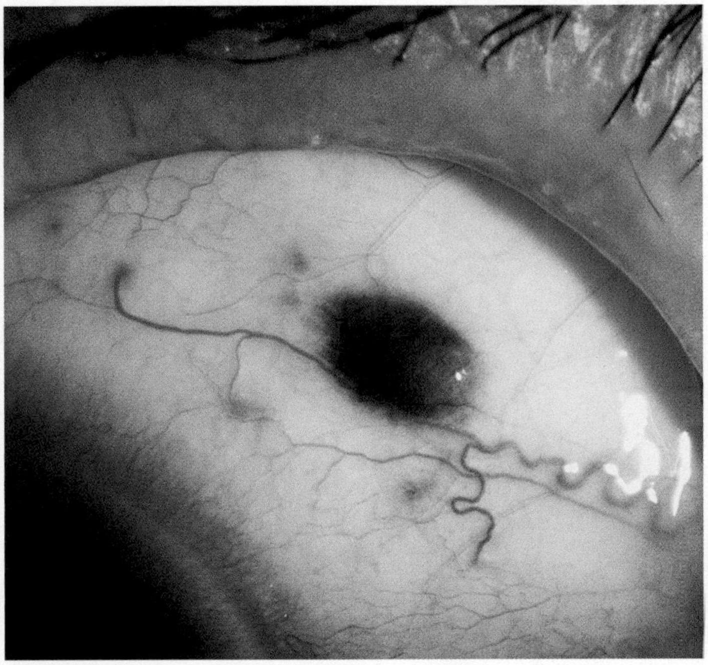

Fig. 3.188 A solitary, black or grey nodule containing dilated feeder vessels, which may become fixed to episclera.

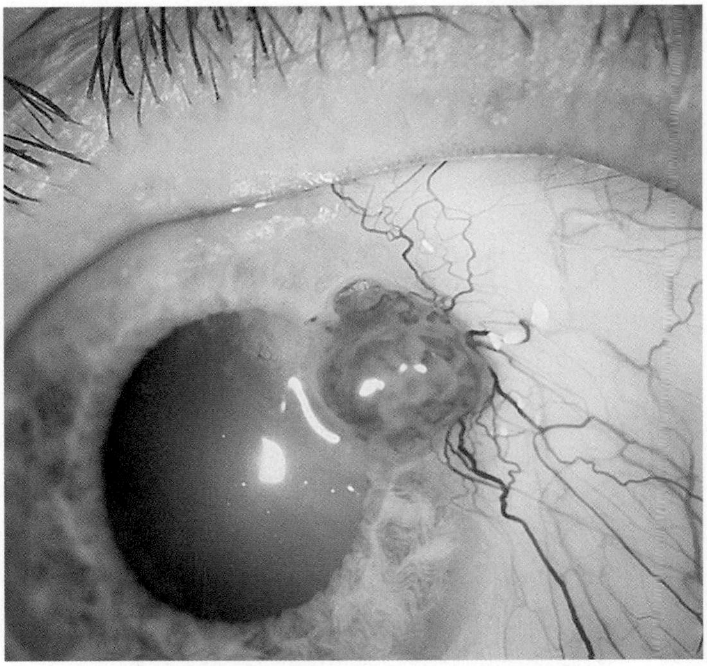

Fig. 3.189 Juxtalimbal amelanotic melanoma, which has a characteristic pink, smooth, fish-flesh appearance.

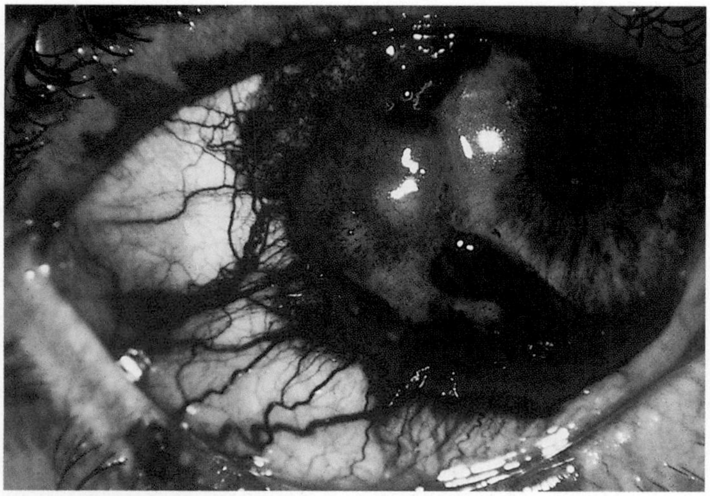

Fig. 3.190 Advanced juxtalimbal melanoma.

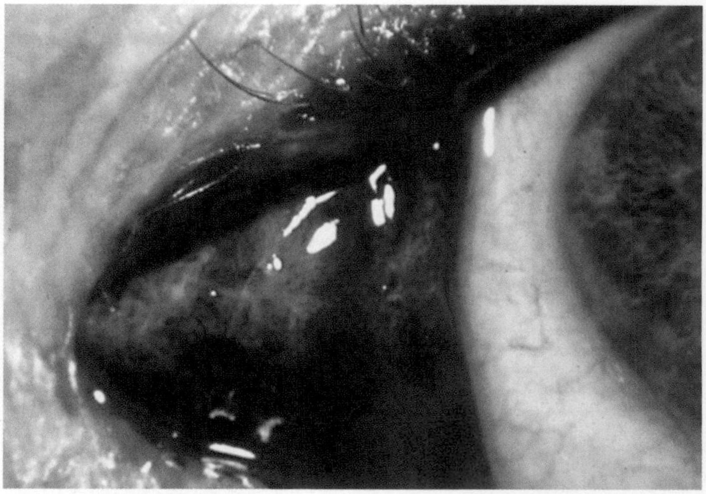

Fig. 3.191 Melanoma involving the medial canthus.

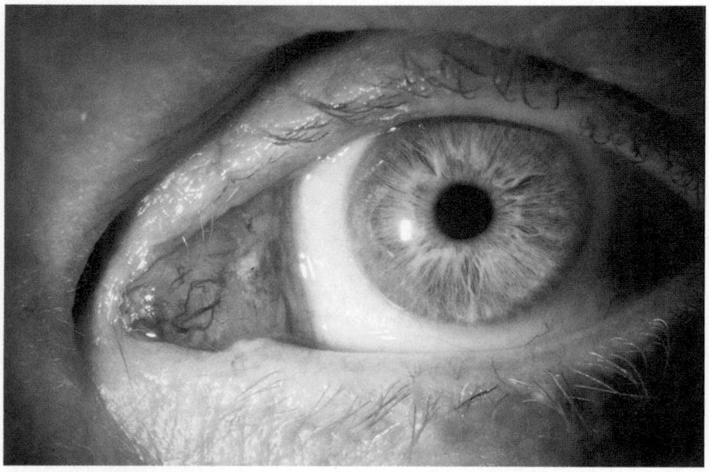

Fig. 3.192 Amelanotic melanoma involving the medial canthus.

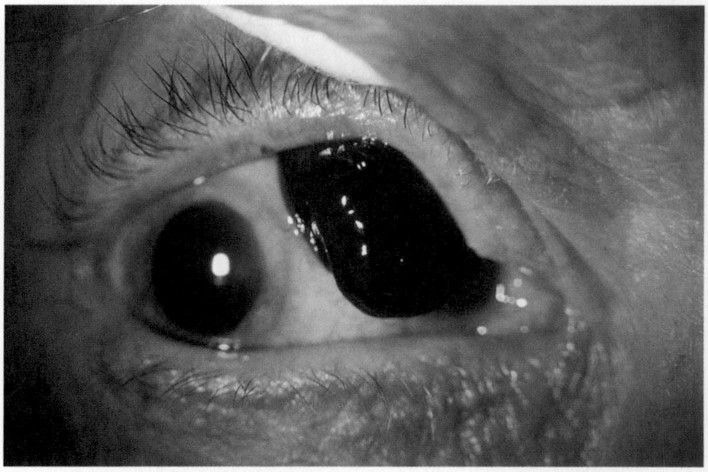

Fig. 3.193 Very large melanoma arising from the superior fornix. (Courtesy of Z. Zagorski.)

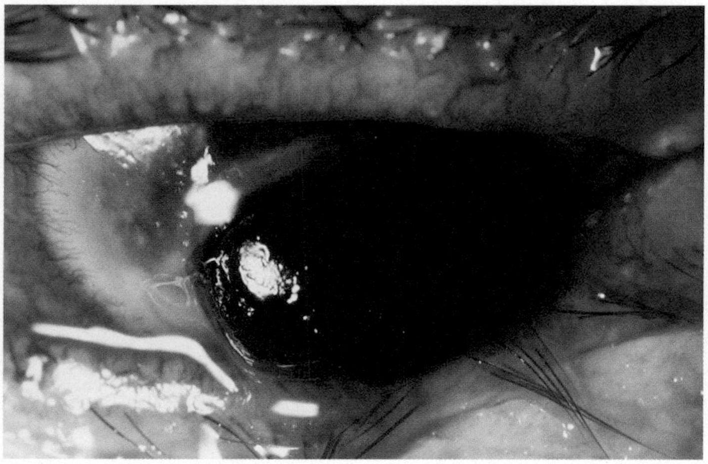

Fig. 3.194 Enormous melanoma invading the cornea. (Courtesy of C. Barry.)

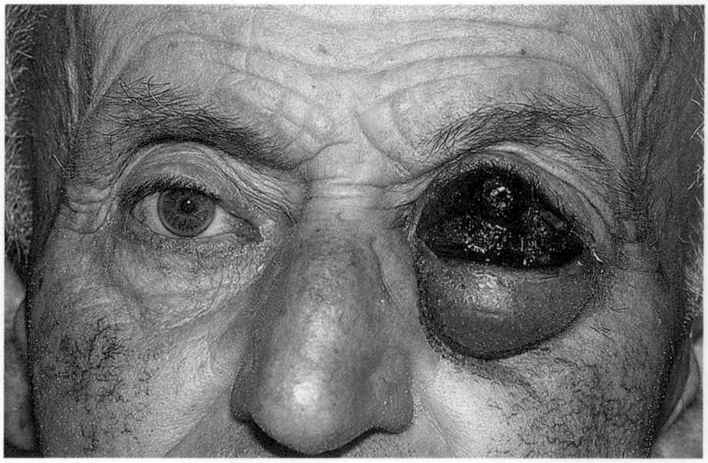

Fig. 3.195 Orbital invasion by recurrent melanoma.

Squamous cell carcinoma

Conjunctival squamous cell carcinoma is a rare, slowly growing tumour of low-grade malignancy, which may arise de novo or from pre-existing conjunctival intraepithelial neoplasia.

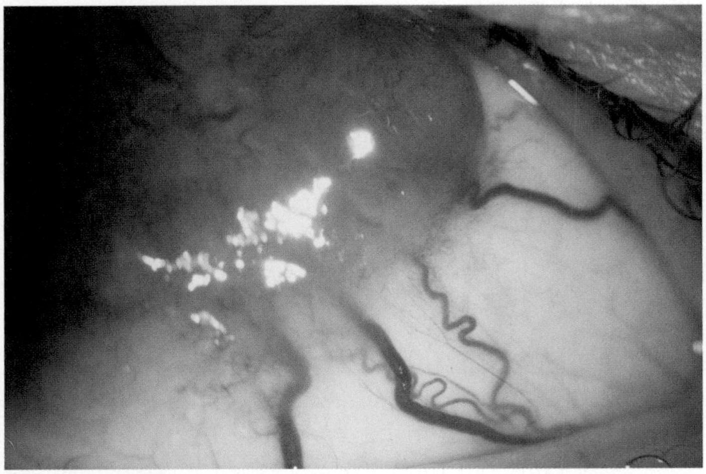

Fig. 3.196 A fleshy, pink, gelatinous mass, often associated with feeder vessels.

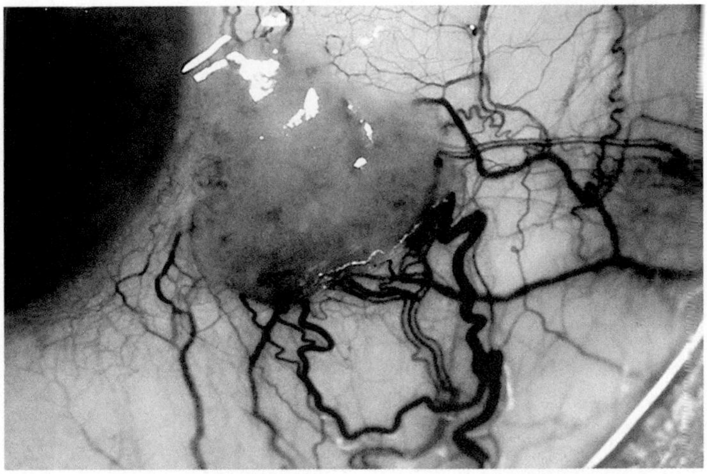

Fig. 3.197 A papillomatous mass, often associated with feeder vessels, which may sometimes be covered by plaques of keratin.

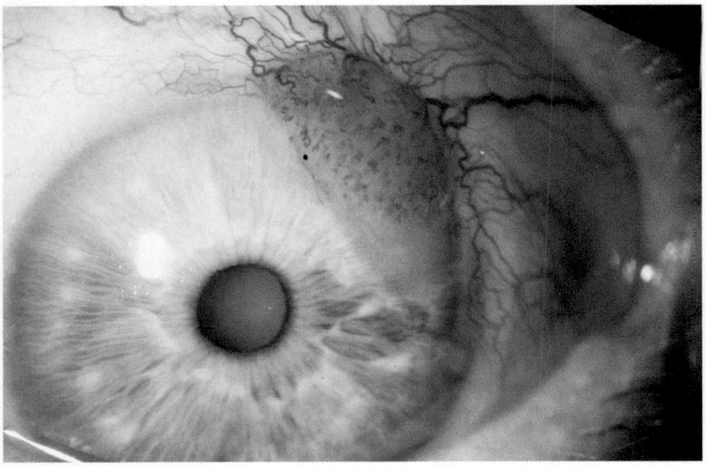

Fig. 3.198 The tumour is most frequently juxtalimbal and may involve adjacent cornea.

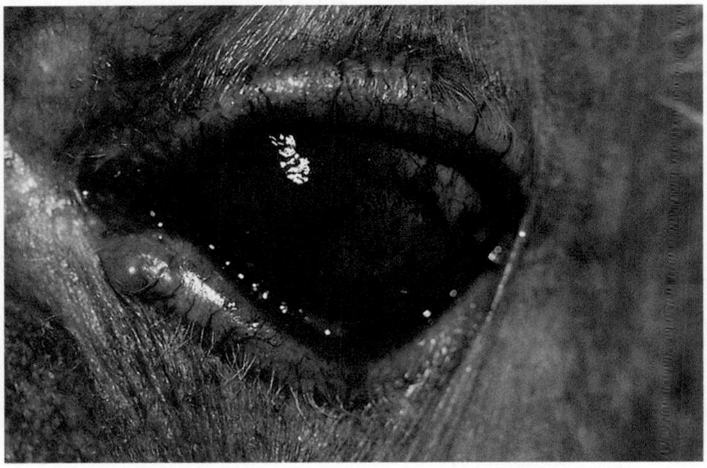

Fig. 3.199 More extensive corneal invasion.

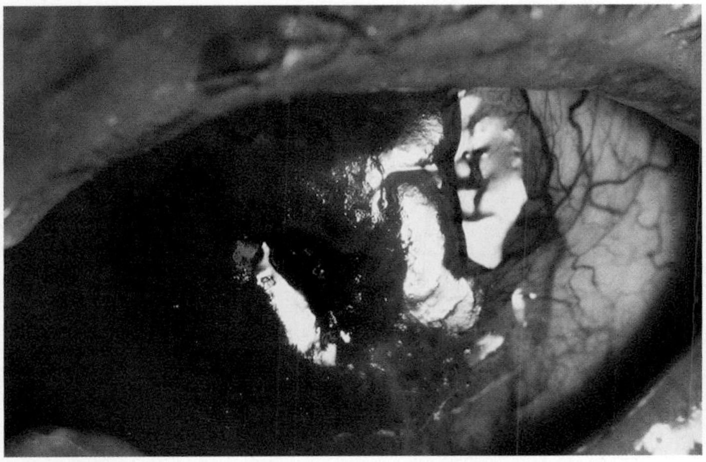

Fig. 3.200 Very extensive flat diffuse corneal invasion. (Courtesy of C. Barry.)

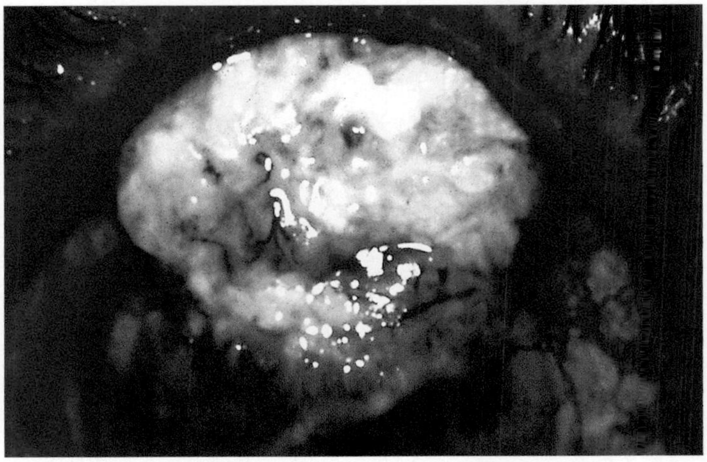

Fig. 3.201 Fungating squamous cell carcinoma.

Lymphoma

Conjunctival lymphoma may occur in isolation or as part of systemic disease.

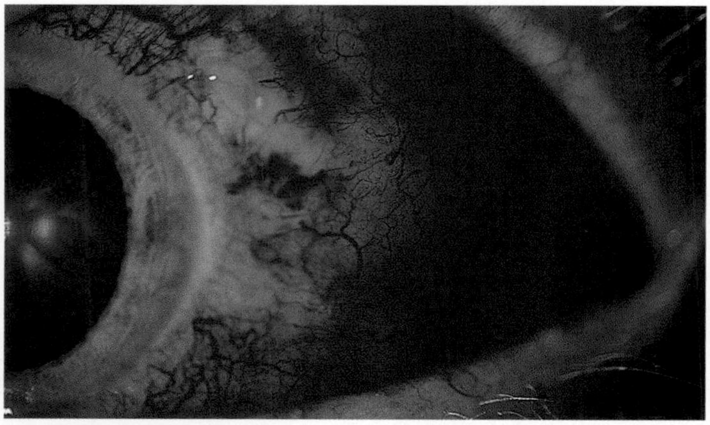

■ **Fig. 3.202** Diffuse infiltration, which may mimic chronic conjunctivitis.

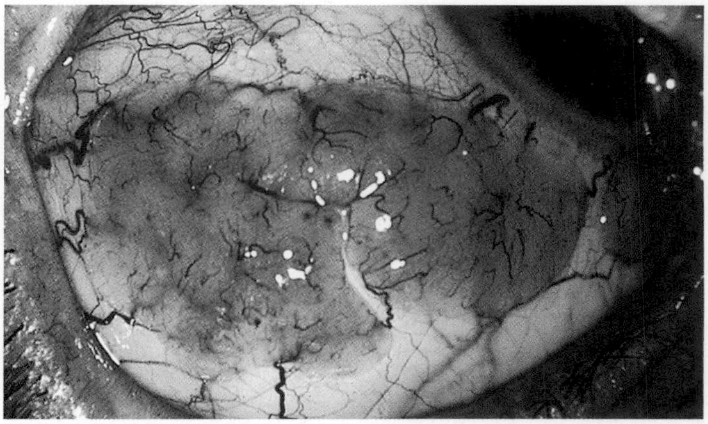

■ **Fig. 3.203** Salmon-pink or flesh-coloured elevated infiltrates, which may be bilateral.

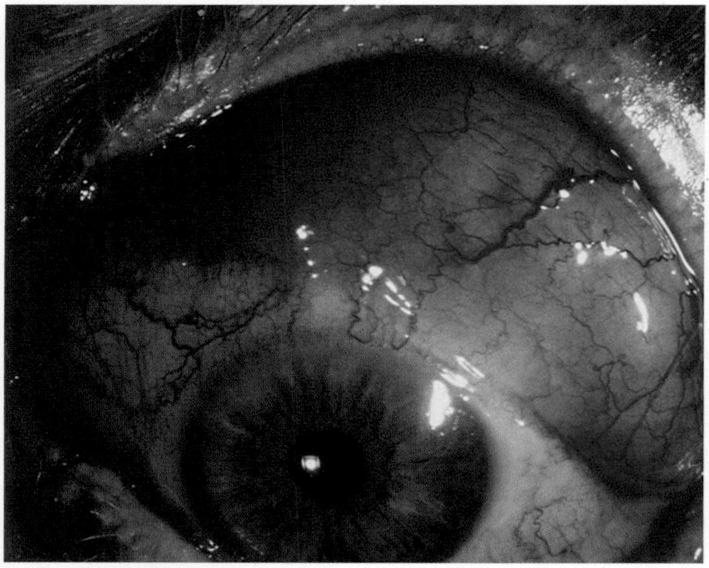

■ **Fig. 3.204** More extensive involvement. (Courtesy of P. Gili.)

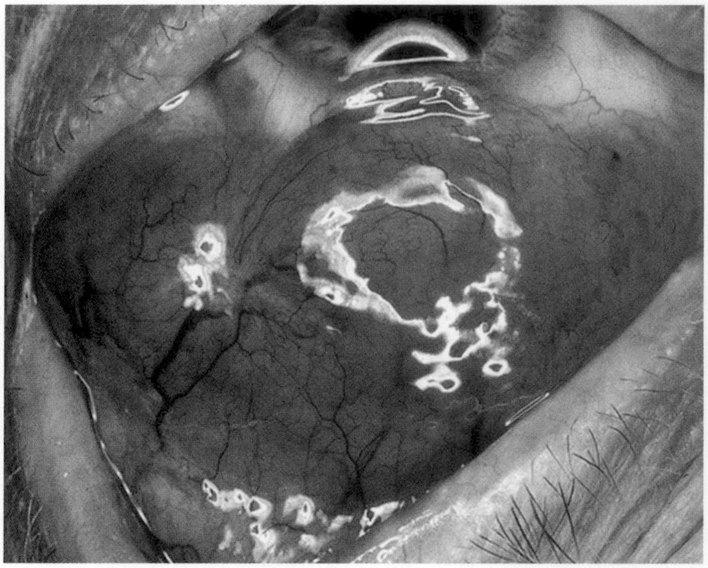

■ **Fig. 3.205** Very advanced lymphoma. (Courtesy of S. Ford and R. Marsh.)

Kaposi sarcoma

Kaposi sarcoma is a slow-growing, low-grade malignancy that occurs in AIDS.

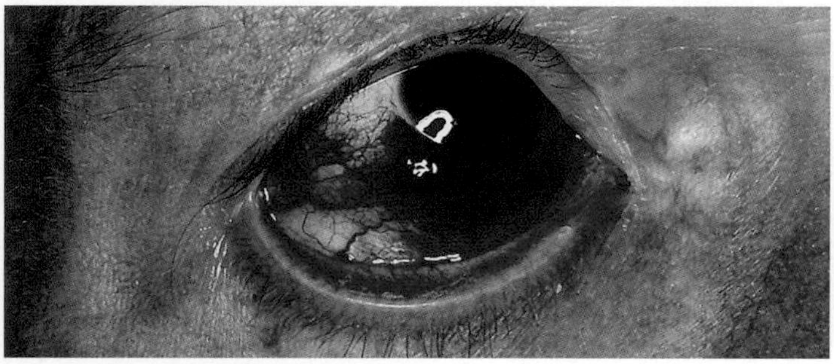

■ **Fig. 3.206** A painless, flat, bright red lesion that on cursory examination may be mistaken for a 'chronic' subconjunctival haemorrhage.

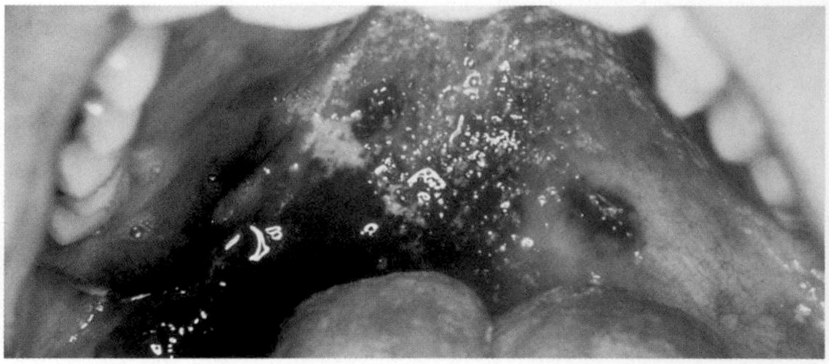

■ **Fig. 3.207** Kaposi sarcoma may be present elsewhere, for example in the mouth.

VASCULAR LESIONS ASSOCIATED WITH SYSTEMIC DISEASES

Sturge–Weber syndrome (encephalotrigeminal angiomatosis)

Sturge–Weber syndrome is a sporadic phakomatosis characterised by naevus flammeus and leptomeningeal haemangioma.

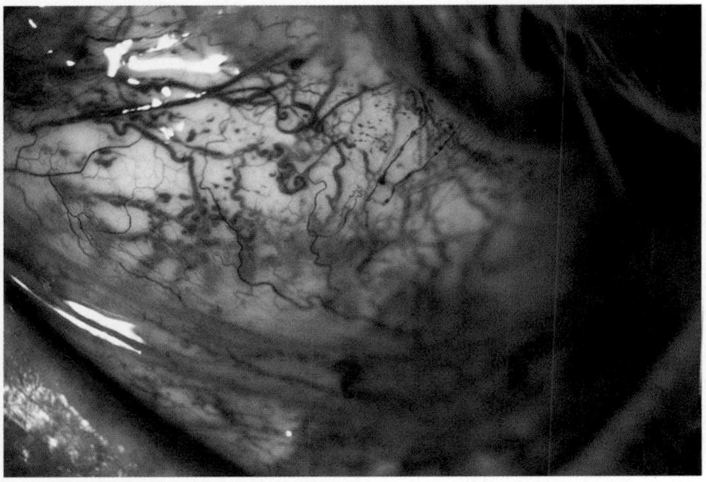

■ **Fig. 3.208** Episcleral haemangioma.

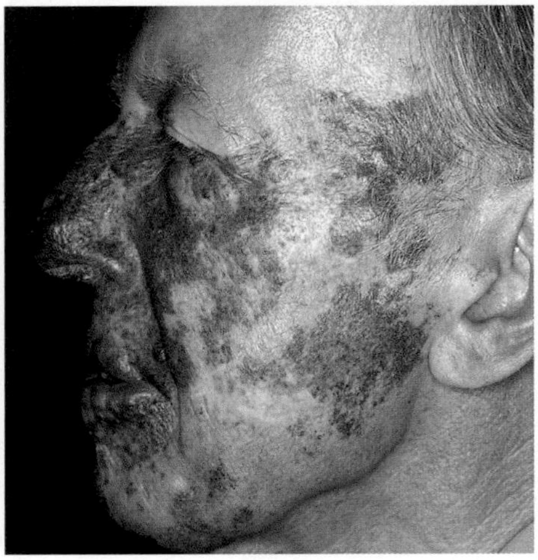

■ **Fig. 3.209** Naevus flammeus.

Louis–Bar syndrome (ataxia telangiectasia)

Louis–Bar syndrome is an autosomal dominant condition characterised by ataxia, skin telangiectasia, lymphopenia, growth retardation and mental handicap.

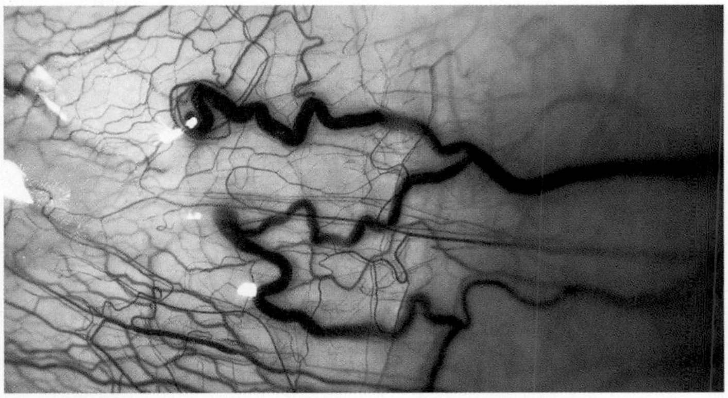

■ **Fig. 3.210** Engorged and tortuous bulbar conjunctival vessels.

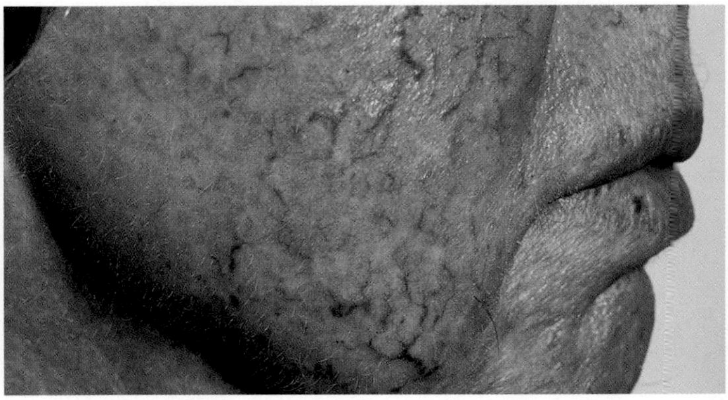

■ **Fig. 3.211** Facial telangiectasia.

Rendu–Osler–Weber syndrome (hereditary haemorrhagic telangiectasia)

Rendu–Osler–Weber syndrome is an autosomal dominant condition characterised by mucocutaneous telangiectasia.

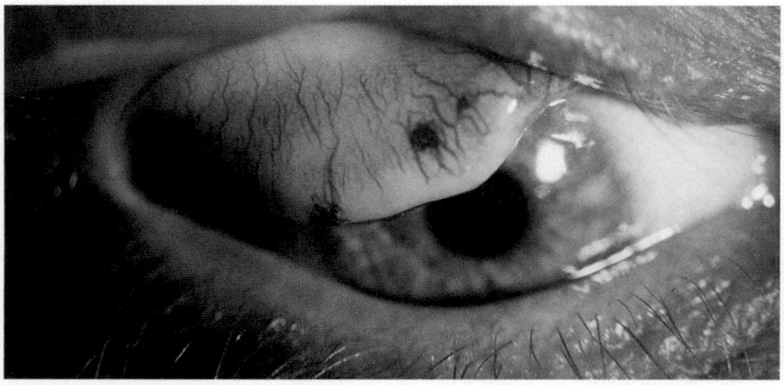

Fig. 3.212 Stellate vascular conjunctival lesions are located on the palpebral but not bulbar conjunctiva. They may cause recurrent subconjunctival haemorrhages and 'bloody' tears.

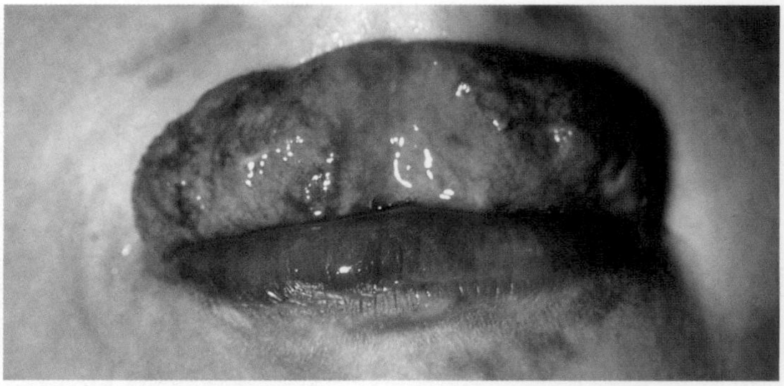

Fig. 3.213 Telangiectasia of the tongue in Rendu–Osler–Weber disease.

CHAPTER 4

EPISCLERA AND SCLERA

EPISCLERITIS

Simple

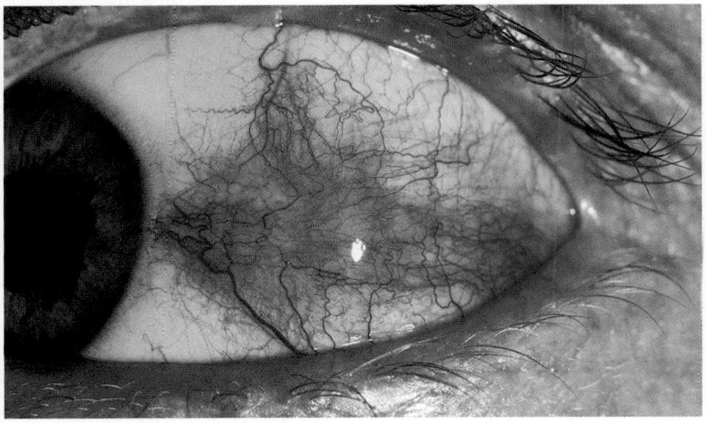

Fig. 4.1 Sectoral redness.

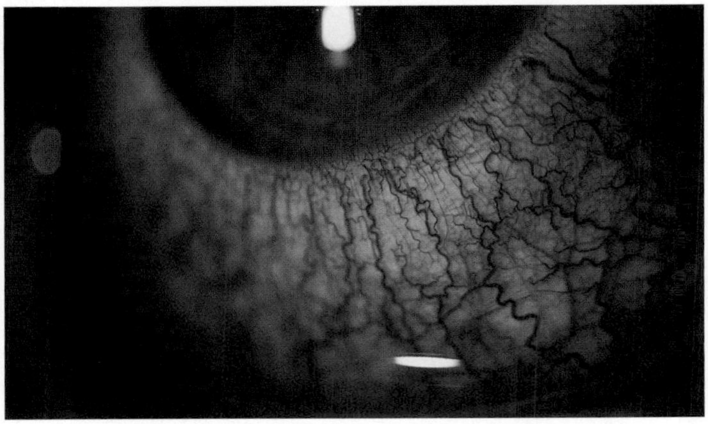

Fig. 4.2 Diffuse redness is less common.

Nodular

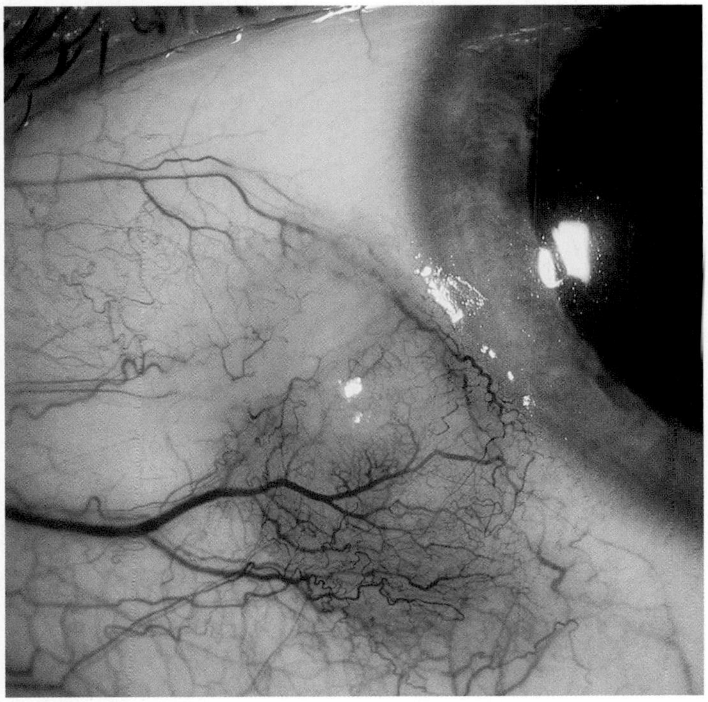

Fig. 4.3 Localised, congested nodule. (Courtesy of P. G. Watson, B. L. Hazelman, C. E. Pavesio and W. R. Green.)

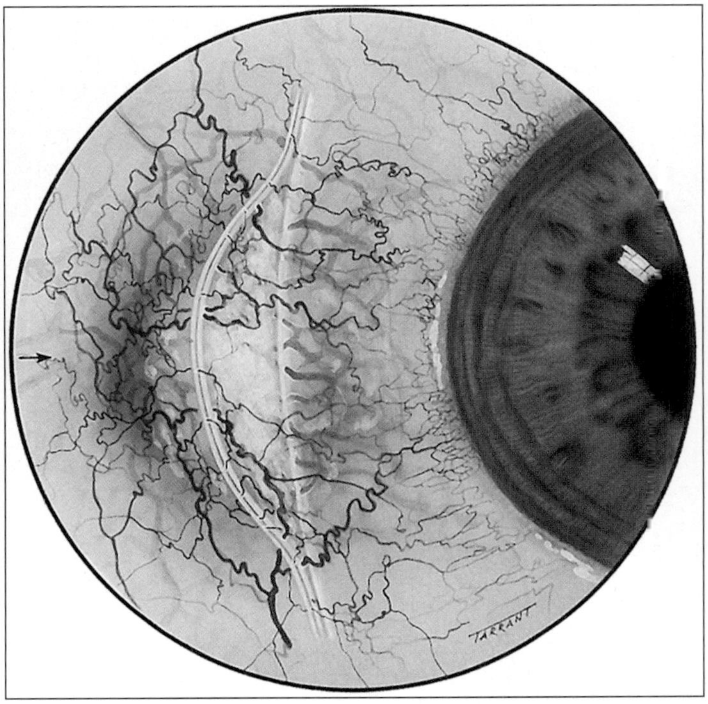

Fig. 4.4 A thin slit-lamp section shows that the scleral surface is flat, indicating that the sclera is not swollen.

SCLERITIS

Scleritis is much less common than episcleritis and covers a spectrum ranging from trivial self-limiting episodes to a serious necrotising process.

Systemic associations

The following systemic associations are present in about 50% of patients with autoimmune scleritis.

Rheumatoid arthritis

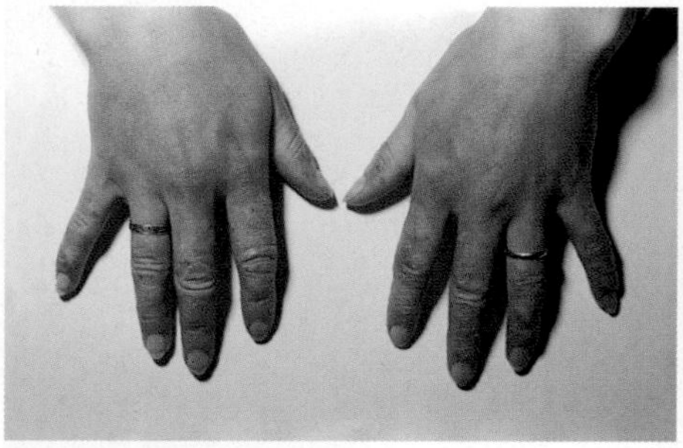

Fig. 4.5 Early involvement with 'spindling' of the fingers.

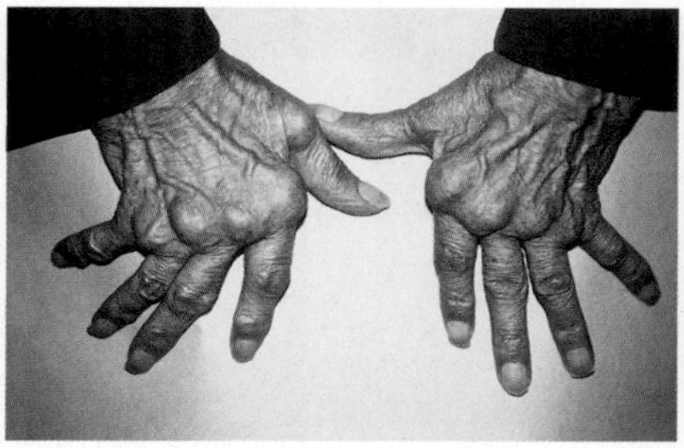

Fig. 4.6 Severe involvement with bilateral ulnar deviation of the fingers.

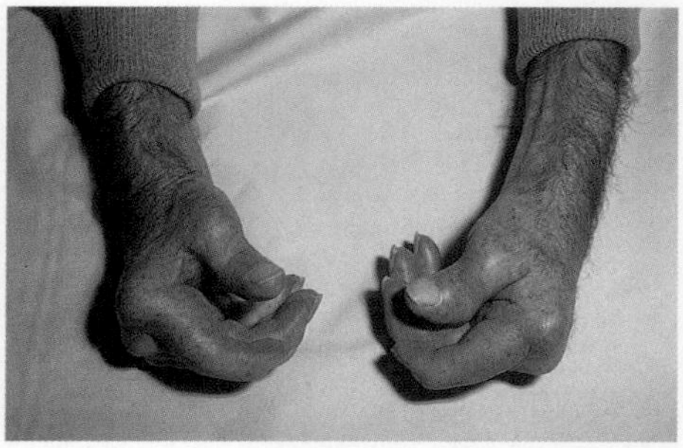

Fig. 4.7 Claw deformity in rapidly progressive disease.

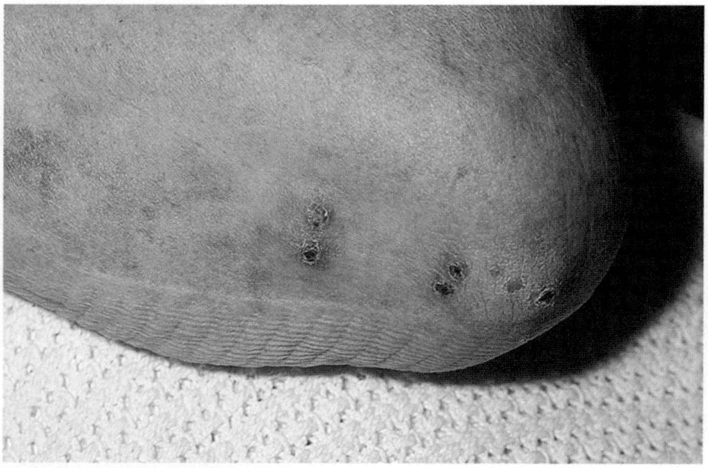

Fig. 4.8 Vasculitis causing small dermal infarcts.

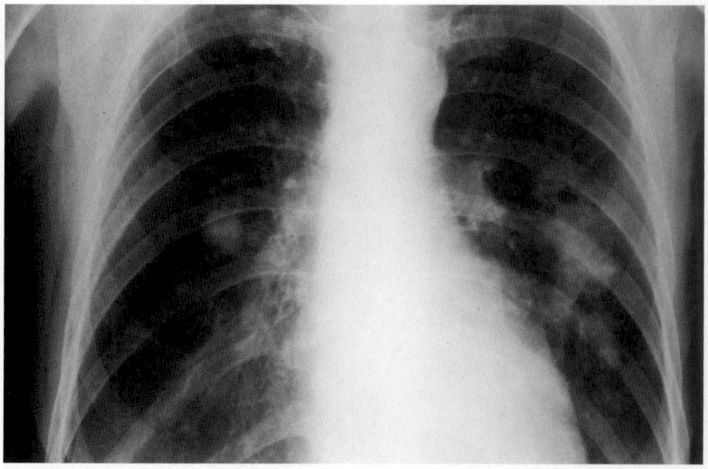

Fig. 4.9 Pulmonary nodules and fibrosis are uncommon.

Wegener granulomatosis

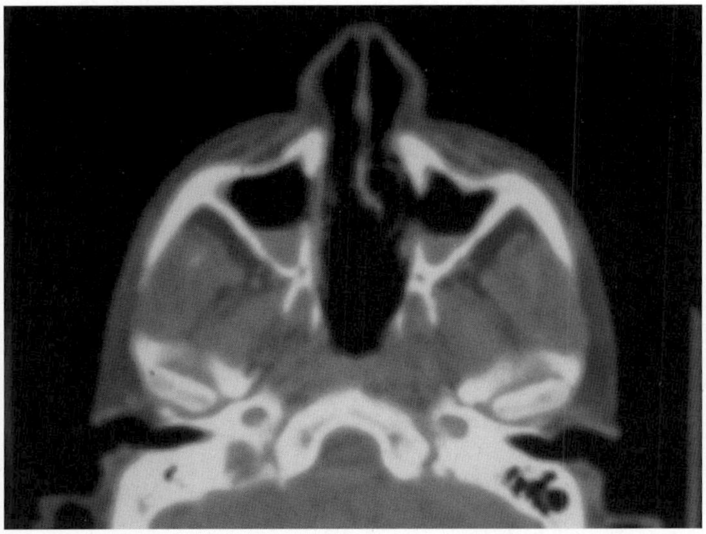

Fig. 4.10 Axial CT showing fluid levels in the maxillary sinuses.

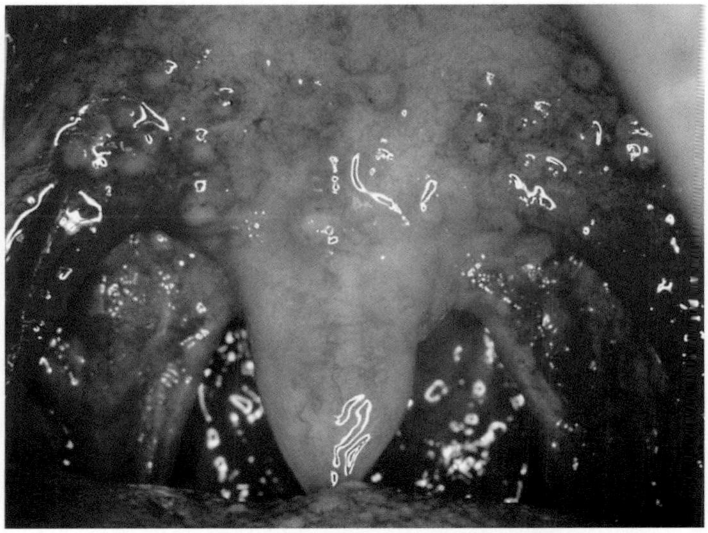

Fig. 4.11 Necrotising granulomas of the upper respiratory tract. (Courtesy of M. A. Mir.)

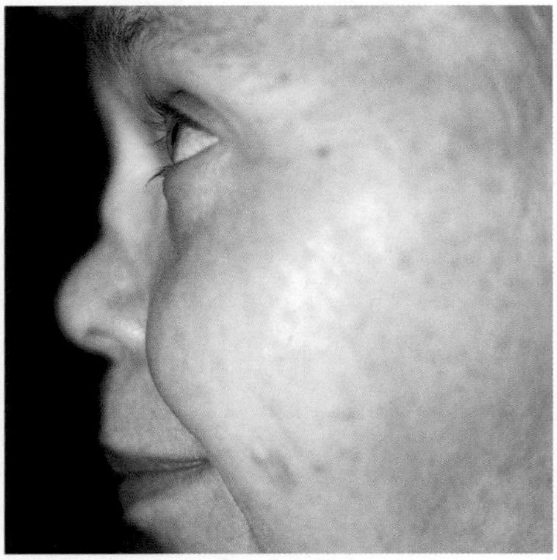

Fig. 4.12 Saddle-shaped nasal deformity.

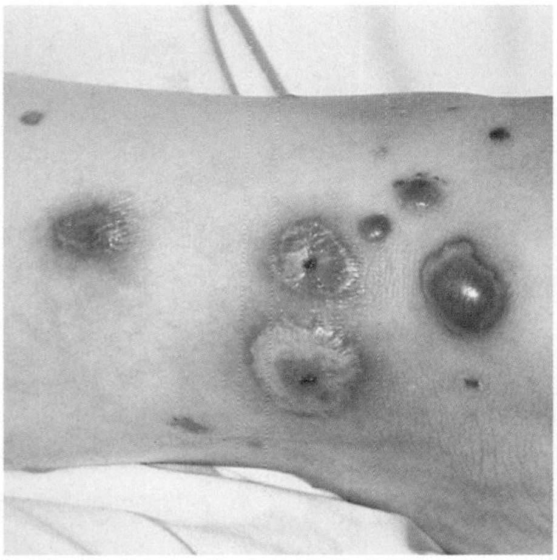

Fig. 4.13 Cutaneous vasculitis and bullae. (Courtesy of M. A. Mir.)

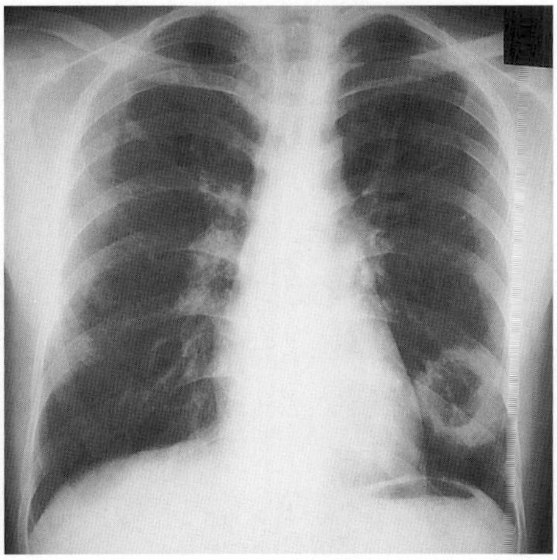

Fig. 4.14 Pulmonary cavitation with fluid levels.

Polyarteritis nodosa

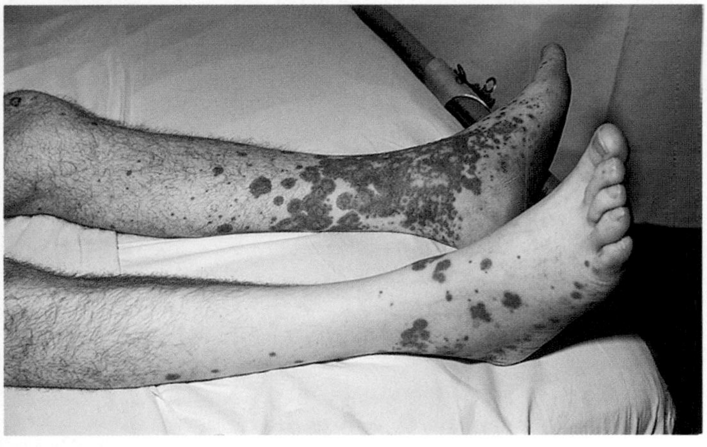

Fig. 4.15 Purpura.

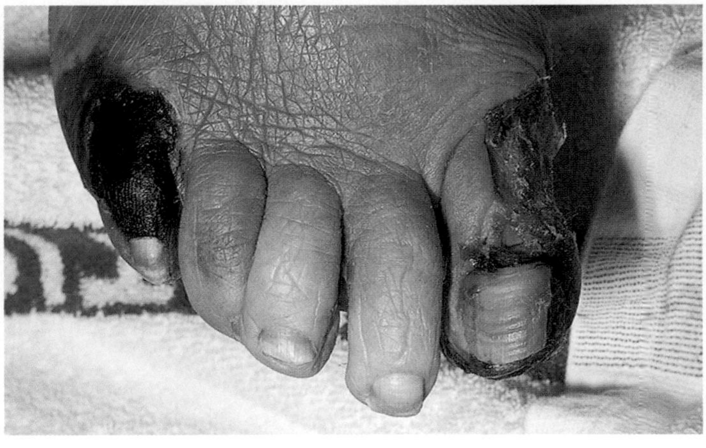

Fig. 4.16 Gangrene.

Relapsing polychondritis

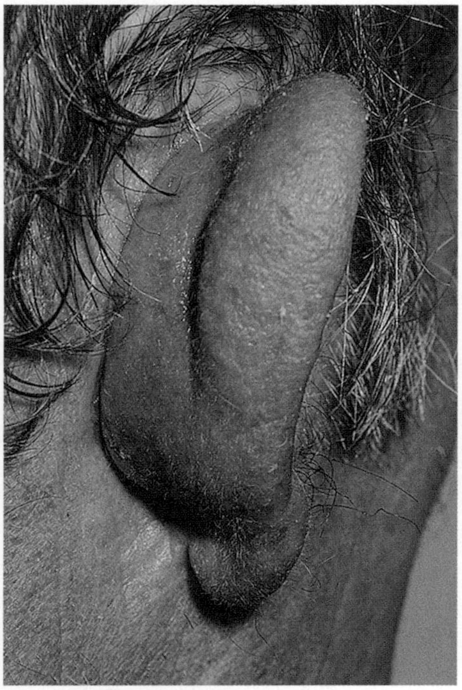

Fig. 4.17 Inflammation and swelling of cartilage such as the pinnae.

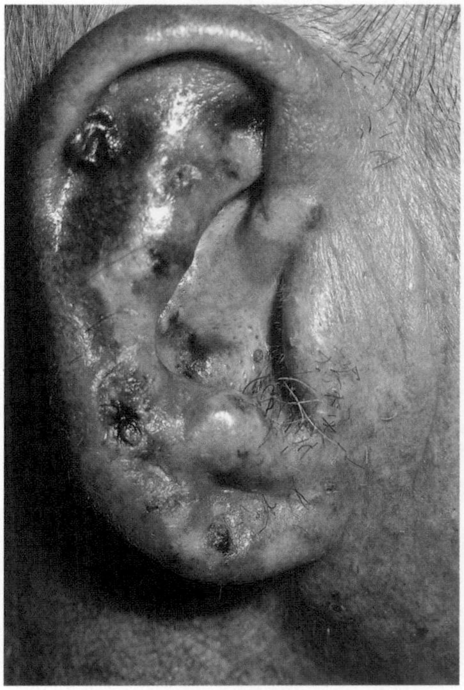

Fig. 4.18 Destruction of cartilage.

Anterior non-necrotising scleritis

Diffuse

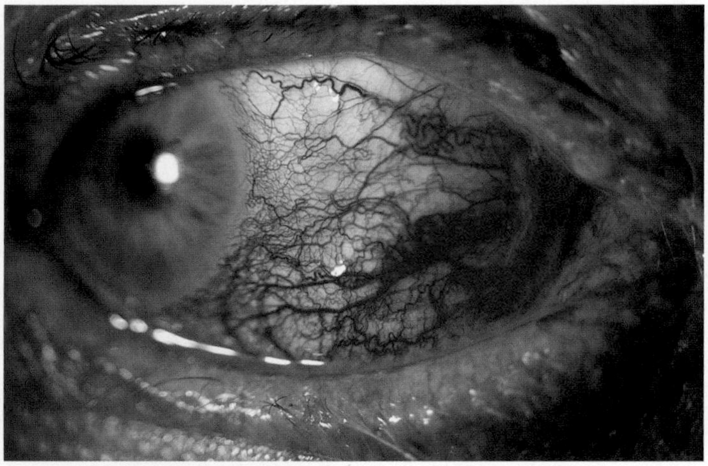

Fig. 4.19 Mild diffuse scleritis.

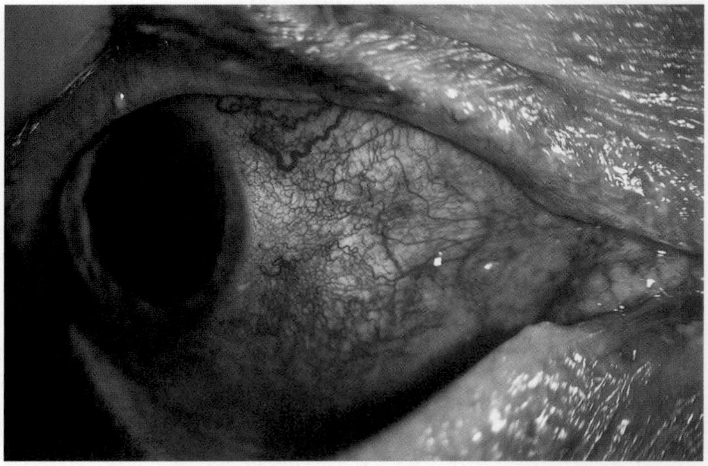

Fig. 4.20 More advanced diffuse scleritis with distortion of the normal radial vascular pattern.

Nodular

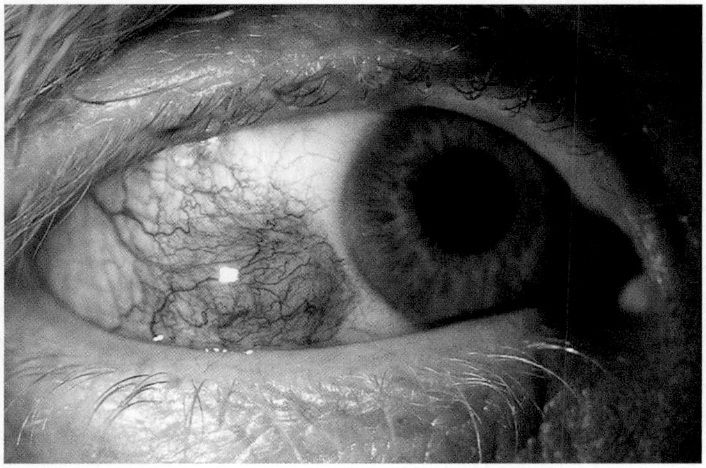

■ **Fig. 4.21** Nodular scleritis may, on cursory examination, resemble nodular episcleritis.

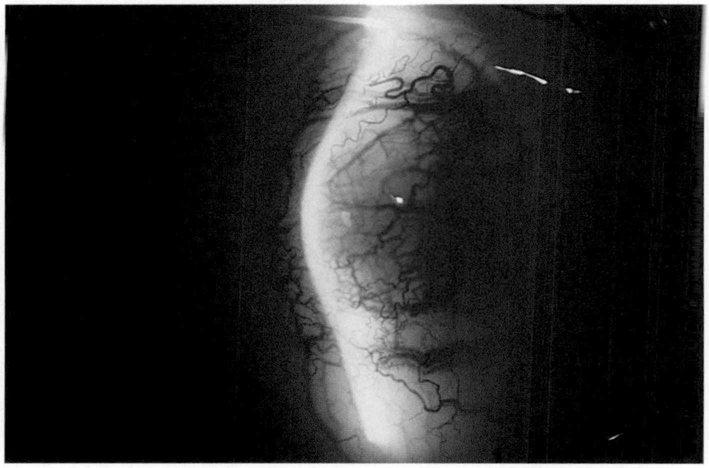

■ **Fig. 4.22** However, the scleral nodule cannot be moved over the underlying tissue and a slit-beam shows that the sclera is raised.

Anterior necrotising scleritis with inflammation

Anterior necrotising scleritis with inflammation is the most severe form. Most patients have associated systemic disease.

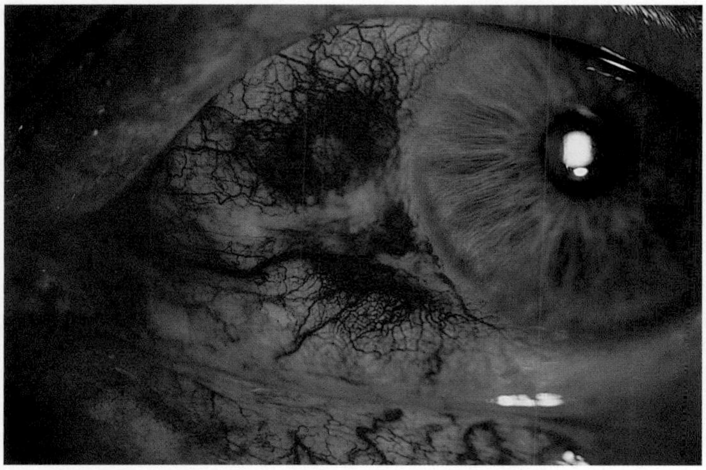

■ **Fig. 4.23** Deep vascular congestion and distortion.

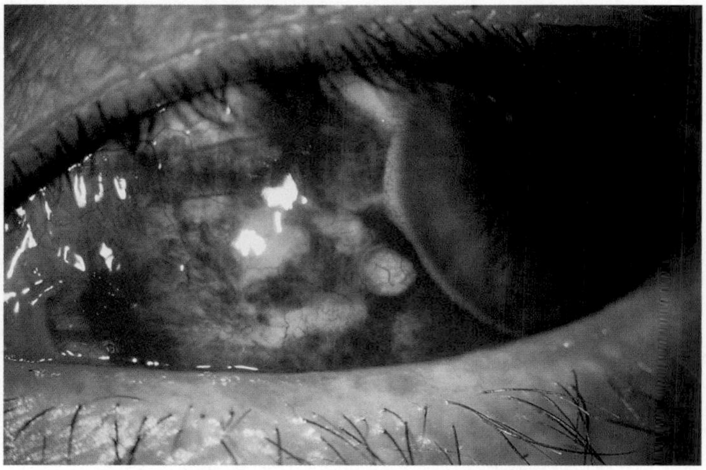

■ **Fig. 4.24** Vascular occlusion and formation of avascular patches.

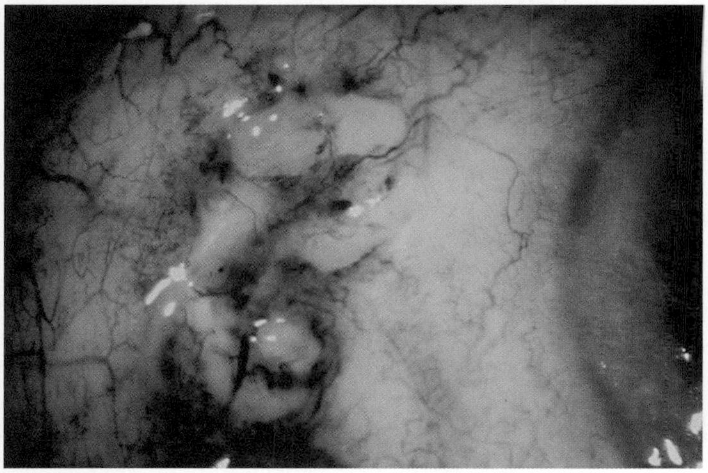

■ **Fig. 4.25** Early scleral necrosis.

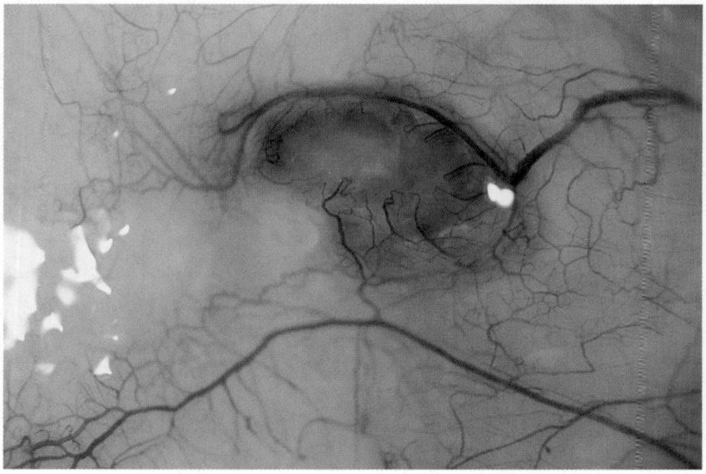

■ **Fig. 4.26** More severe scleral necrosis.

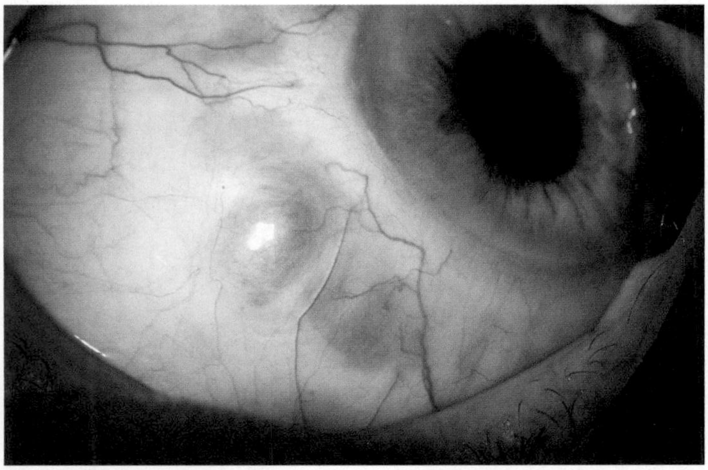

Fig. 4.27 Early staphyloma secondary to scleral thinning.

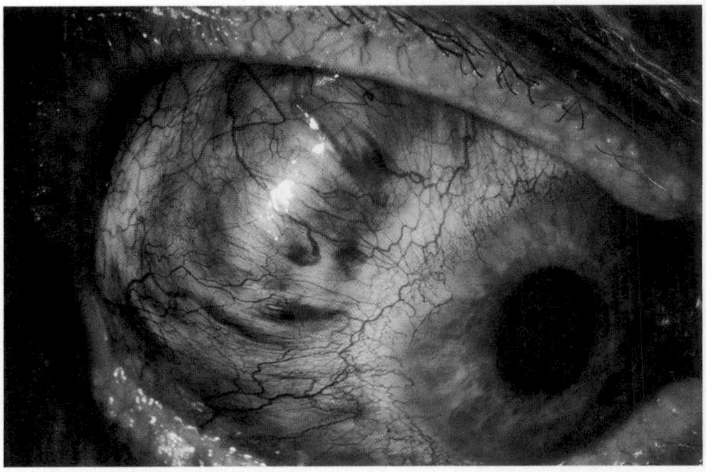

Fig. 4.28 Extensive staphyloma.

Anterior necrotising scleritis without inflammation (scleromalacia perforans)

Scleromalacia perforans typically occurs in women with long-standing rheumatoid arthritis and is usually bilateral.

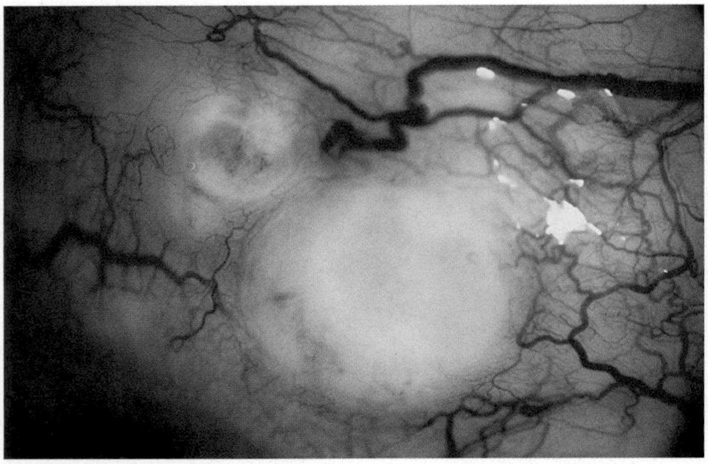

Fig. 4.29 Asymptomatic yellow, necrotic scleral patches and focal scleral thinning in uninflamed sclera. (Courtesy of P. G. Watson, B. L. Hazelman, C. E. Pavesio and W. R. Green.)

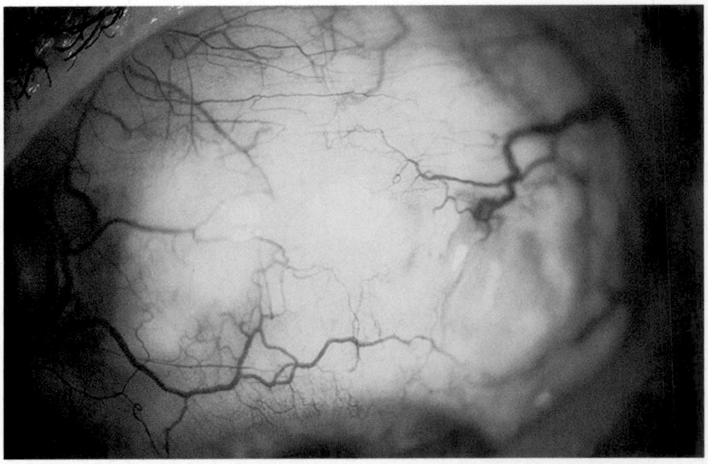

Fig. 4.30 Enlargement of necrotic patches. (Courtesy of P. G. Watson, B. L. Hazelman, C. E. Pavesio and W. R. Green.)

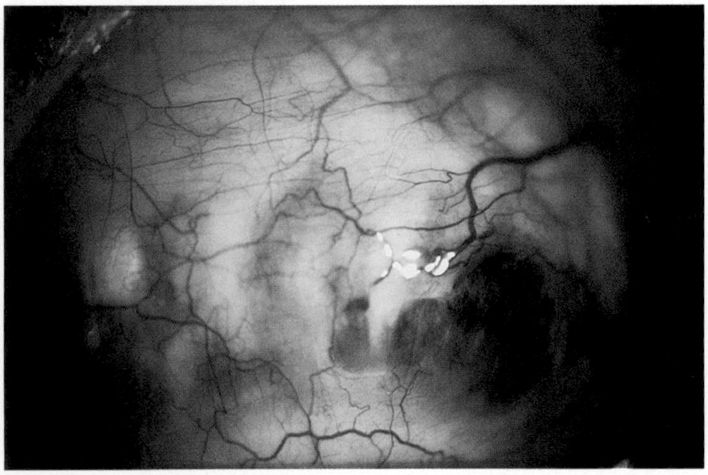

Fig. 4.31 Exposure of underlying uvea. (Courtesy of P. G. Watson, B. L. Hazelman, C. E. Pavesio and W. R. Green.)

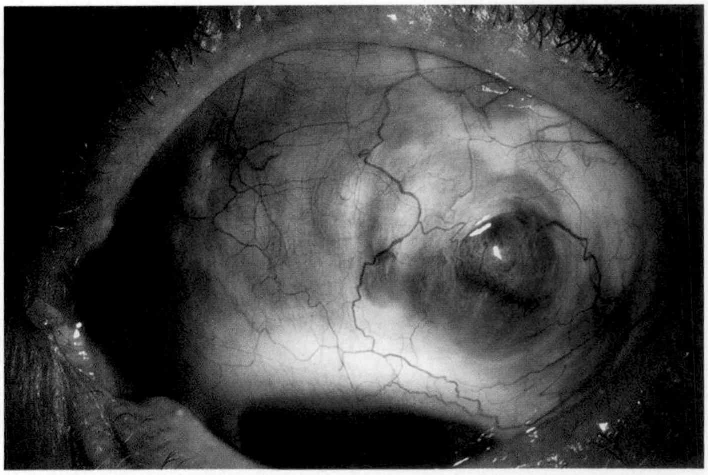

Fig. 4.32 Extensive scleromalacia perforans. (Courtesy of P. G. Watson, B. L. Hazelman, C. E. Pavesio and W. R. Green.)

Posterior scleritis

Posterior scleritis is uncommon and often misdiagnosed because it may present with a range of clinical findings.

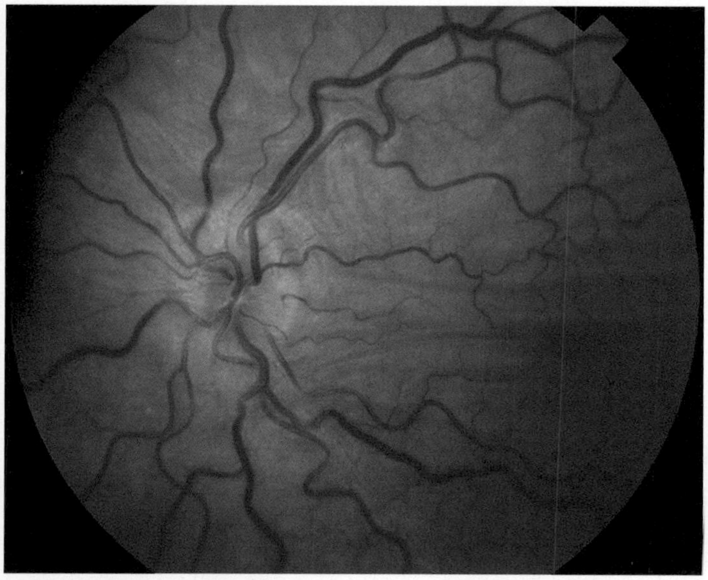

Fig. 4.33 Choroidal folds and disc oedema. (Courtesy of S. Ford and R. Marsh.)

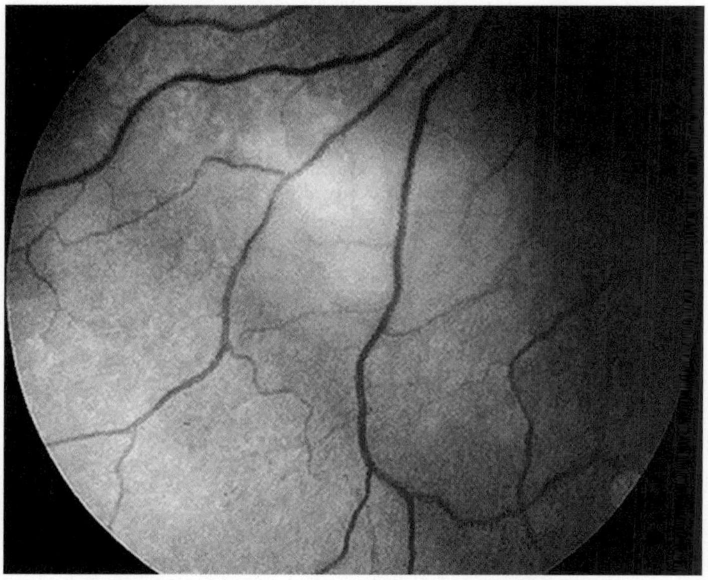

Fig. 4.34 Subretinal mass. (Courtesy of S. Ford and R. Marsh.)

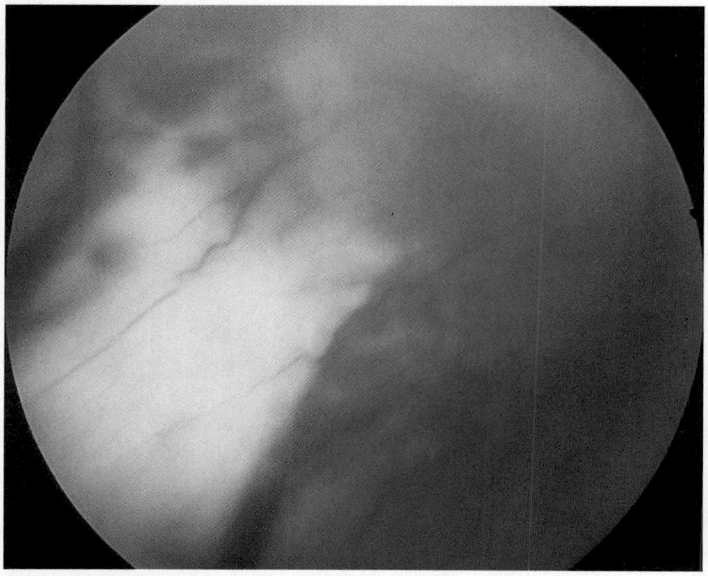

Fig. 4.35 Subretinal exudation. (Courtesy of P. Watson.)

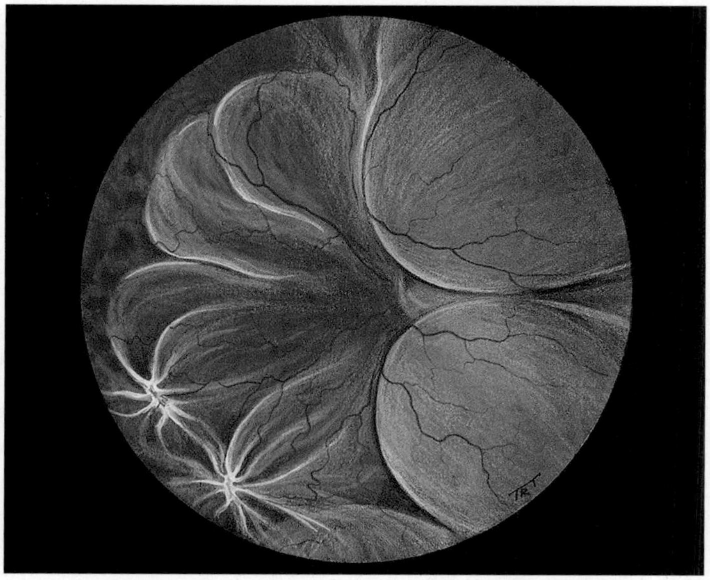

Fig. 4.36 Exudative retinal detachment. (Courtesy of P. G. Watson, B. L. Hazelman, C. E. Pavesio and W. R. Green.)

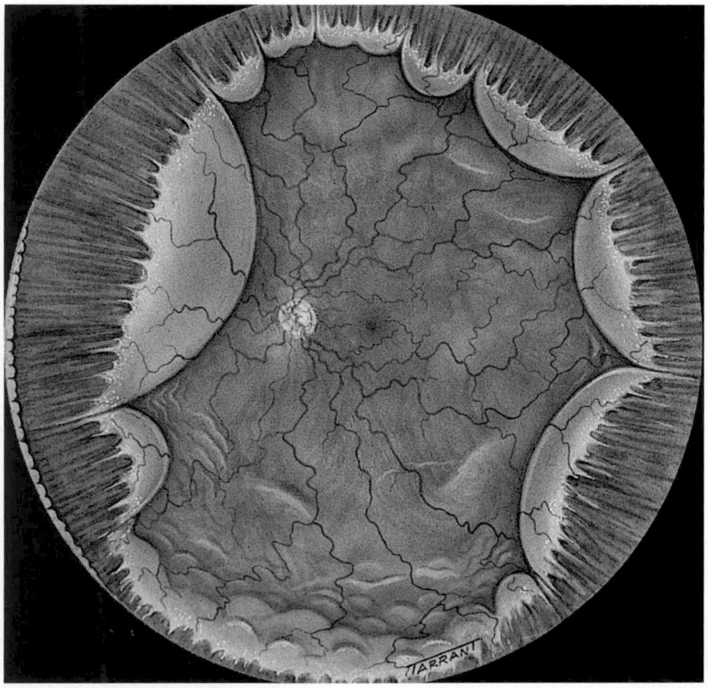

■ **Fig. 4.37** Uveal effusion syndrome characterised by exudative retinal detachment and choroidal detachment.

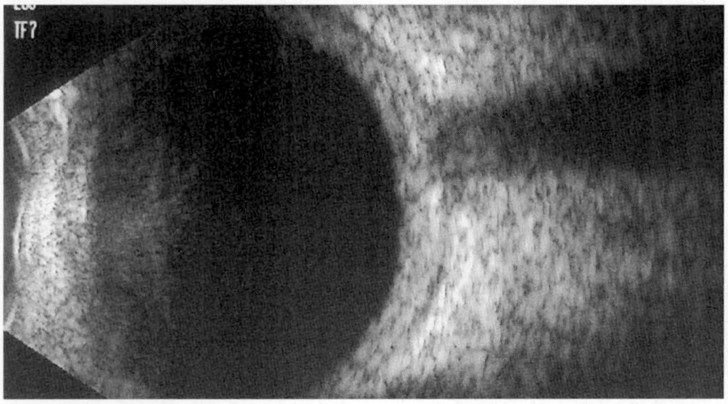

■ **Fig. 4.38** US shows thickening of the posterior sclera and fluid in Tenon space, giving rise to the characteristic 'T' sign. The stem of the T is formed by the optic nerve on its side and the cross bar by the gap containing fluid in the sub-Tenon space.

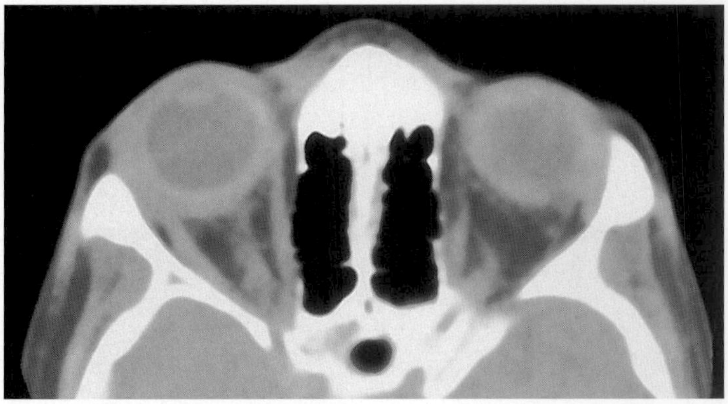

■ **Fig. 4.39** Axial CT shows right scleral thickening and slight proptosis.

Surgically induced scleritis

Surgically induced scleritis typically presents within 6 months postoperatively as a focal area of intense inflammation and necrosis adjacent to the surgical site.

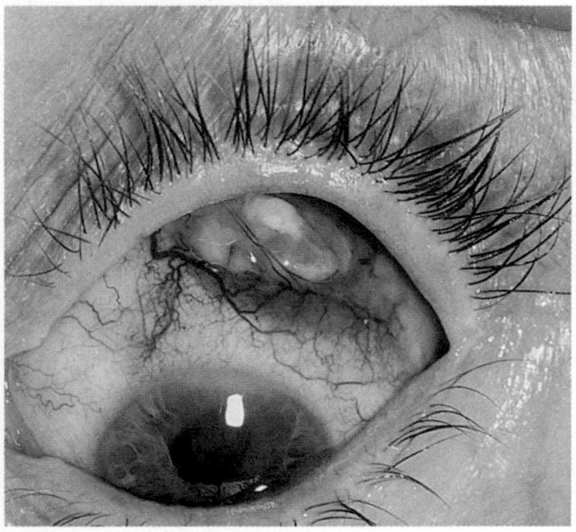

■ **Fig. 4.40** Scleritis following scleral buckling surgery for retinal detachment.

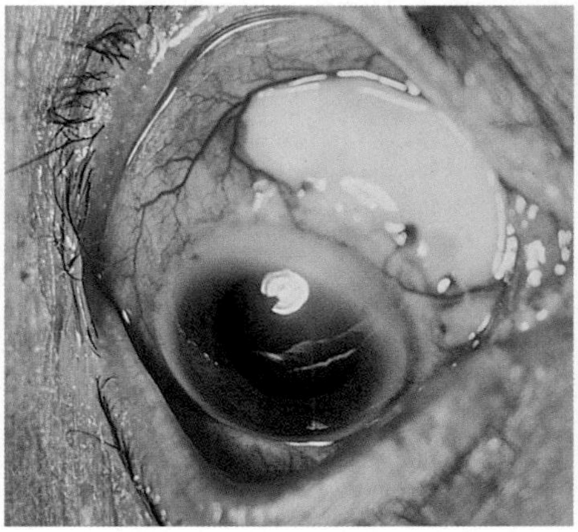

■ **Fig. 4.41** Scleritis following trabeculectomy.

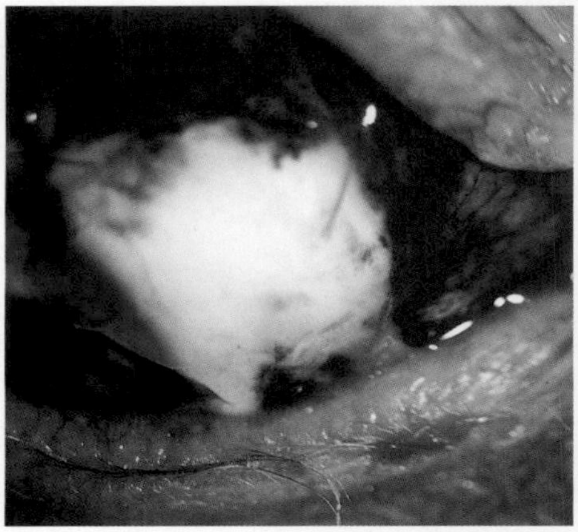

■ **Fig. 4.42** Scleral graft for scleral thinning following excision of a pterygium with adjunctive mitomycin C.

SCLERAL DISCOLORATION

Senile translucency

Senile scleral translucency is a common, often bilateral, innocuous condition.

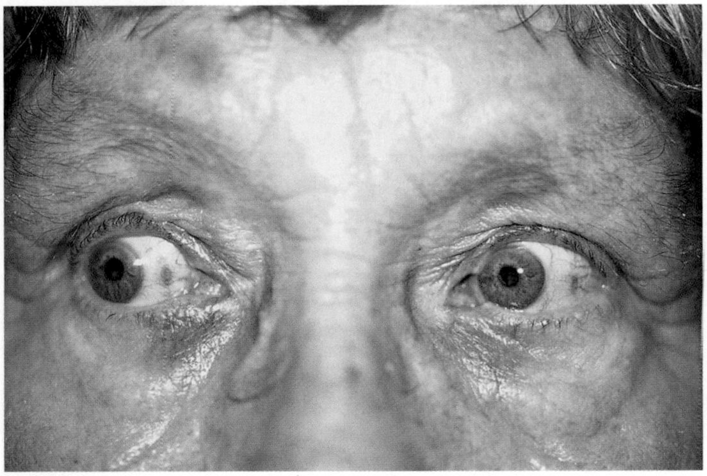

■ **Fig. 4.43** Oval, dark greyish areas anterior to the insertion of the horizontal recti.

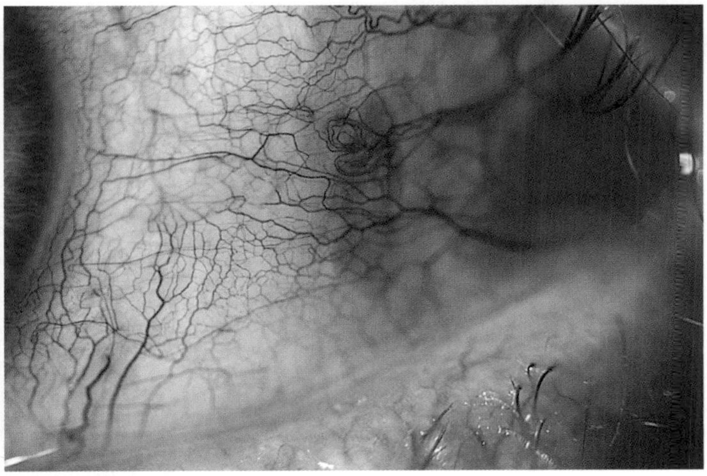

■ **Fig. 4.44** Magnified view.

Alcaptonuria

Alcaptonuria is a rare autosomal dominant metabolic disorder.

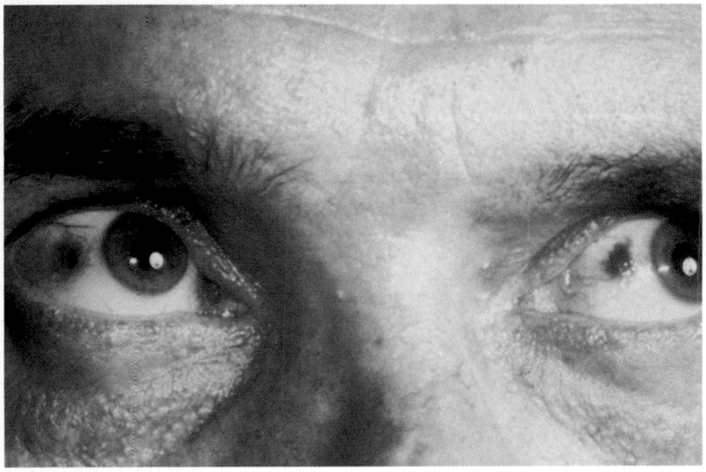

■ **Fig. 4.45** Brown-black discoloration (ochronosis) at the insertions of the horizontal recti. (Courtesy of J. M. H. Moll.)

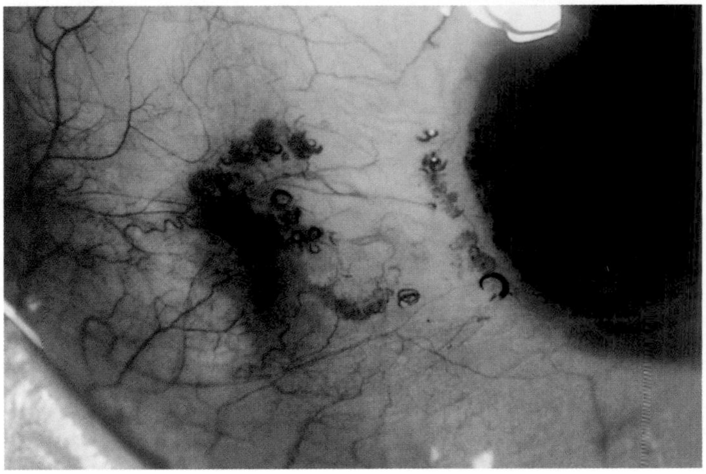

■ **Fig. 4.46** Magnified view.

Type 3

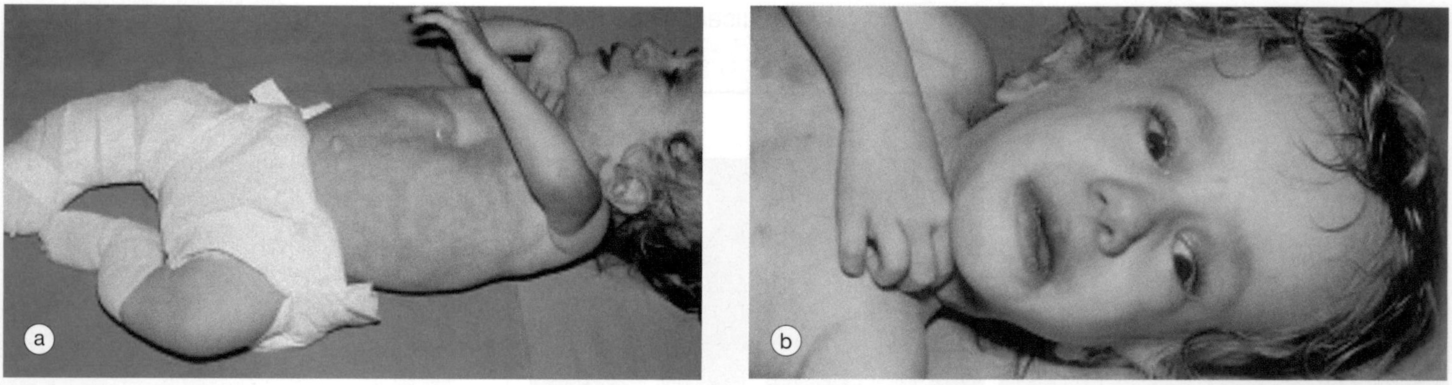

Fig. 4.53 (a) Extreme small stature of a 5-year-old child with deformity of the rib cage and legs with a recent fracture. **(b)** Triangular face, broad nose and frontal bossing. (Courtesy of B. J. Zitelli and H. W. Davis.)

CHAPTER 5

DRY EYE

CAUSES

Primary Sjögren syndrome

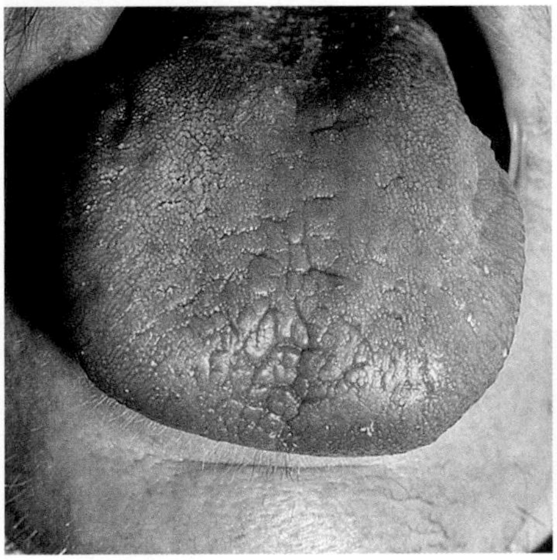

■ **Fig. 5.1** Dry mouth and a dry, fissured tongue (xerostomia).

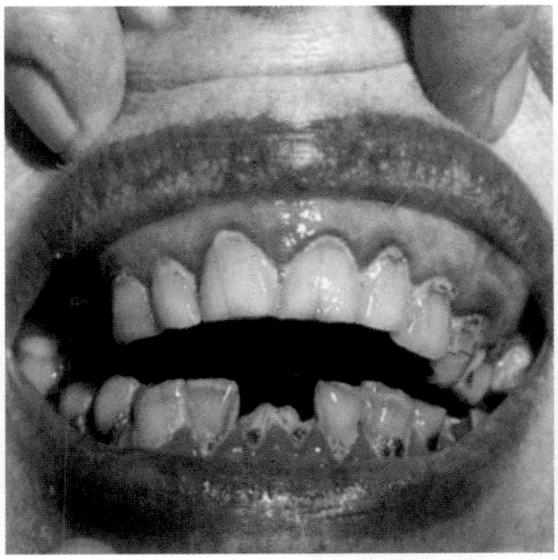

■ **Fig. 5.2** Severe dental caries and gingivitis in very severe cases. (Courtesy of J. M. H. Moll.)

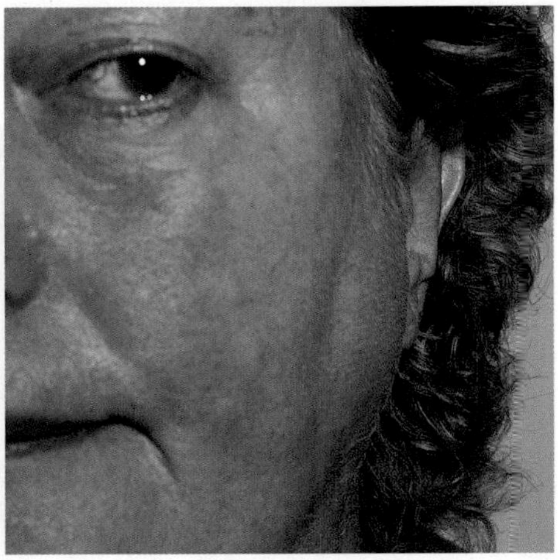

■ **Fig. 5.3** Parotid gland enlargement.

Secondary Sjögren syndrome

Secondary Sjögren syndrome is characterised by the features of primary Sjögren syndrome and a systemic autoimmune connective tissue disorder such as one of the following:

Rheumatoid arthritis

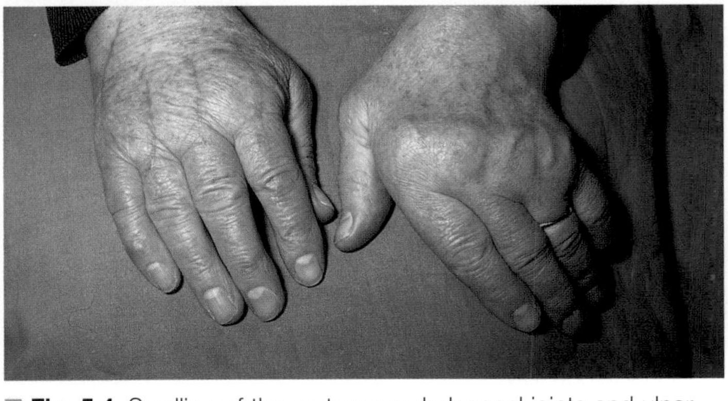

■ **Fig. 5.4** Swelling of the metacarpophalangeal joints and ulnar deviation of the fingers of the left hand; the right hand has undergone successful reconstructive surgery.

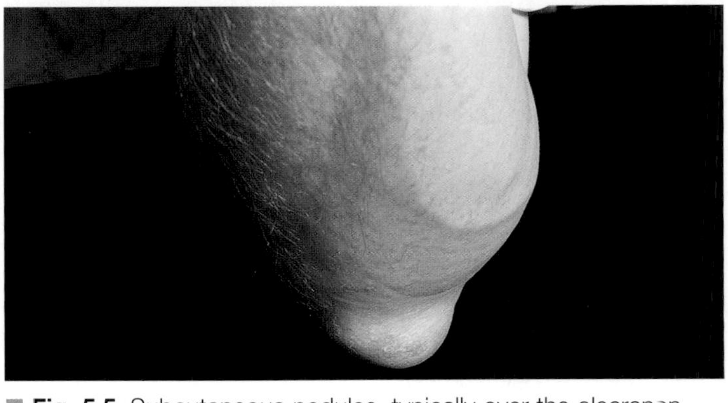

■ **Fig. 5.5** Subcutaneous nodules, typically over the olecranon.

SIGNS

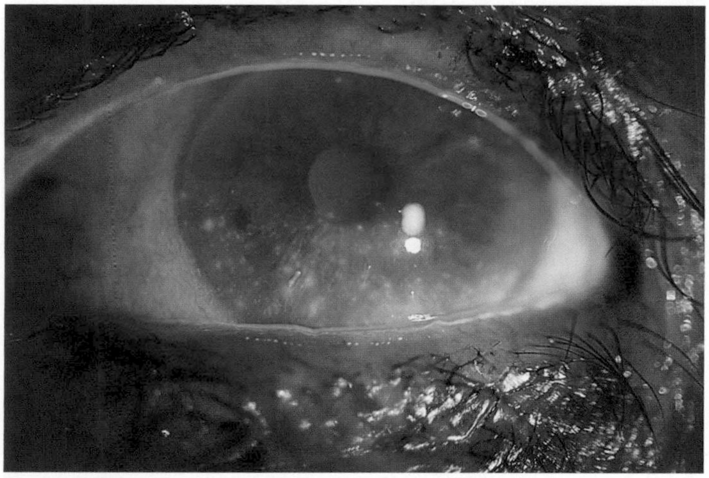

Fig. 5.17 The fluorescein-stained marginal tear meniscus is concave, irregular, thin or absent and the inferior cornea shows punctate epithelial erosions.

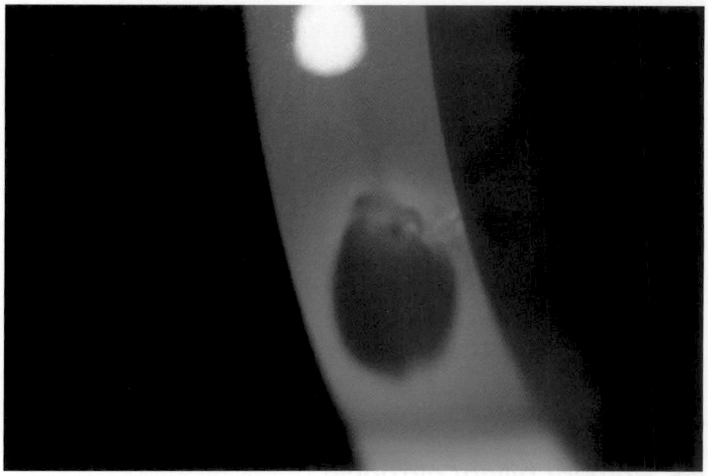

Fig. 5.18 Early break-up of the tear film stained with fluorescein following a blink.

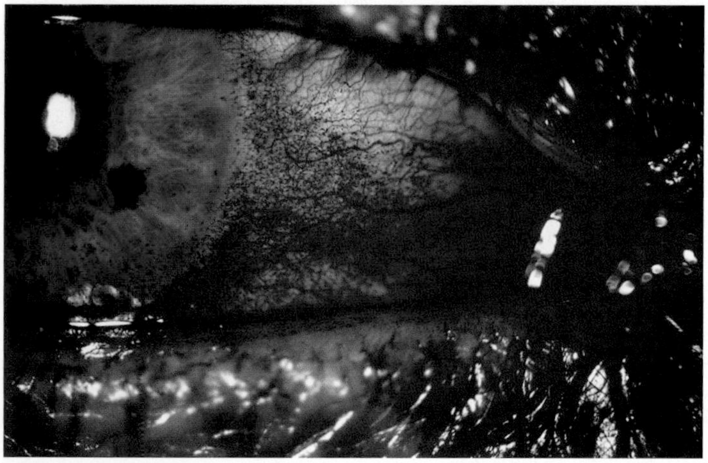

Fig. 5.19 Conjunctival staining with rose bengal.

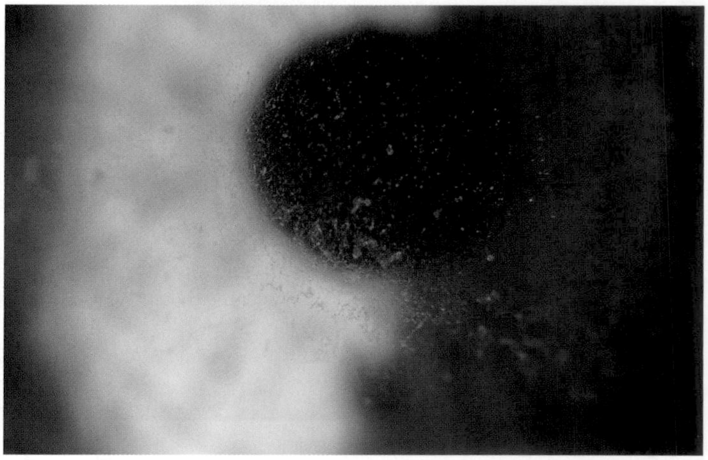

Fig. 5.20 Cobweb-like coating of the corneal epithelium with mucus.

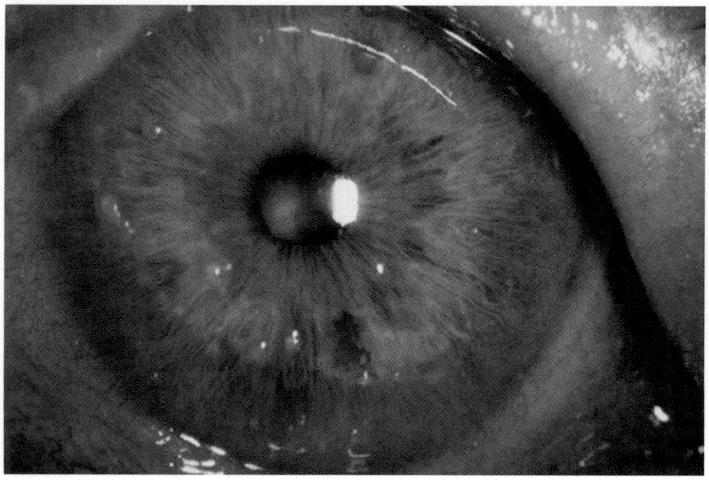

Fig. 5.21 Corneal filaments. (Courtesy of S. Ford and R. Marsh.)

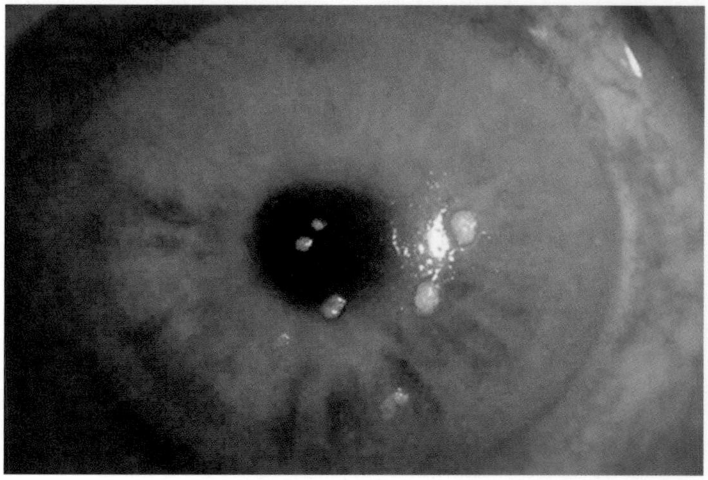

Fig. 5.22 Mucous plaques consist of semi-transparent, white to grey, slightly elevated lesions of various sizes and shapes. (Courtesy of S. Ford.)

CHAPTER 6

CORNEA

MICROBIAL KERATITIS

Bacterial keratitis

Bacterial keratitis usually only develops when ocular defences have been compromised. The most common pathogens are *Pseudomonas aeruginosa*, *Staphylococcus aureus*, *Streptococcus pyogenes* and *Streptococcus pneumoniae*.

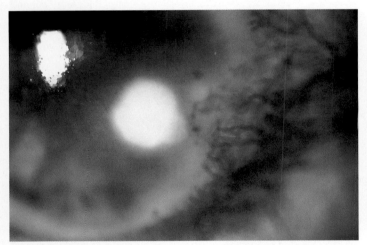

Fig. 6.1 Stromal infiltrate with epithelial breakdown.

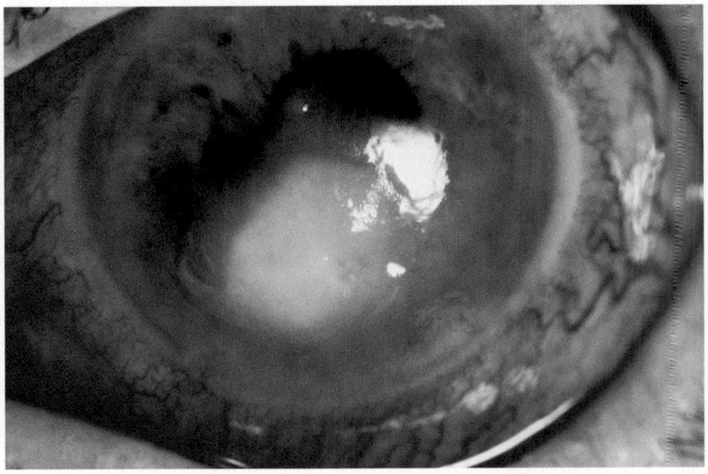

Fig. 6.2 Progressive infiltration. (Courtesy of C. Barry.)

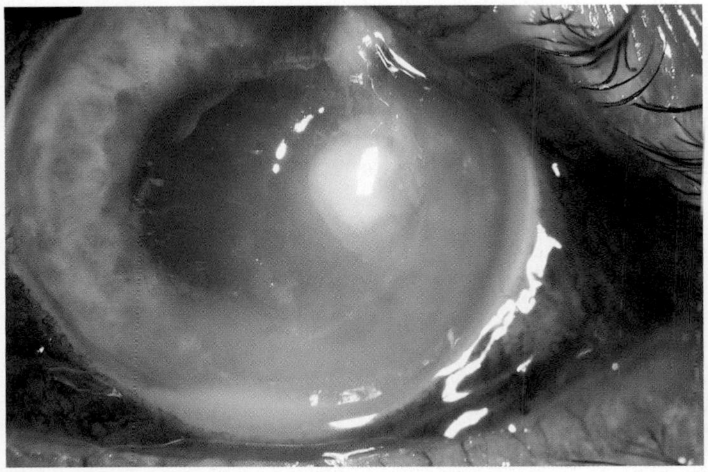

Fig. 6.3 Small hypopyon.

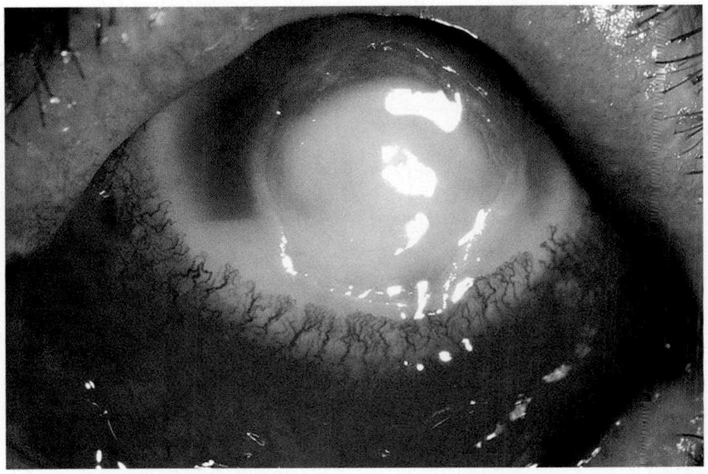

Fig. 6.4 Large hypopyon.

Fungal keratitis

Filamentous

Filamentous keratitis typically occurs following trauma, particularly involving organic matter such as plants or wood.

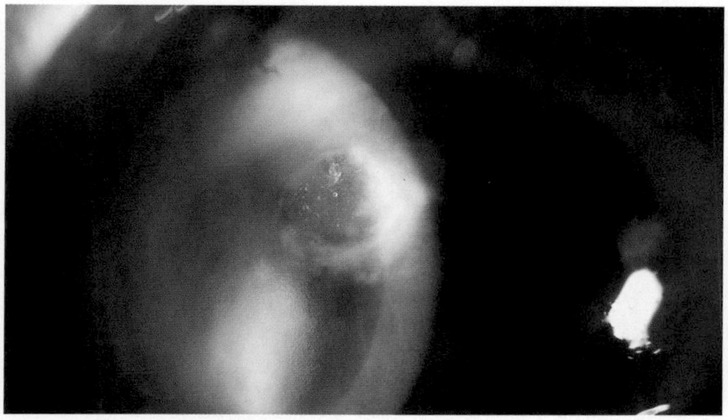

Fig. 6.5 Greyish, stromal infiltrate with a 'dry' texture and indistinct margins.

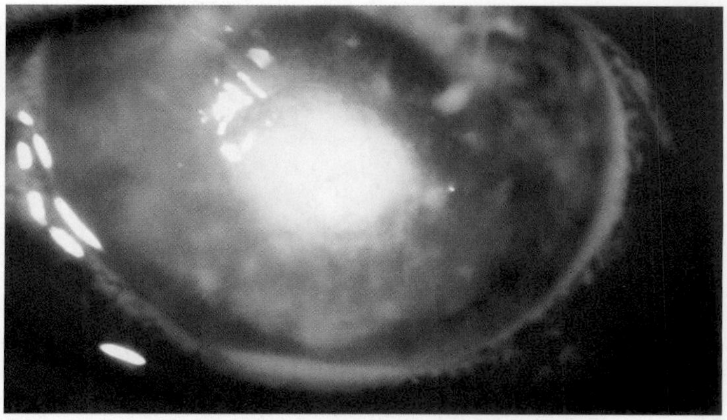

Fig. 6.6 Denser infiltrate associated with round satellite stromal lesions and a small hypopyon.

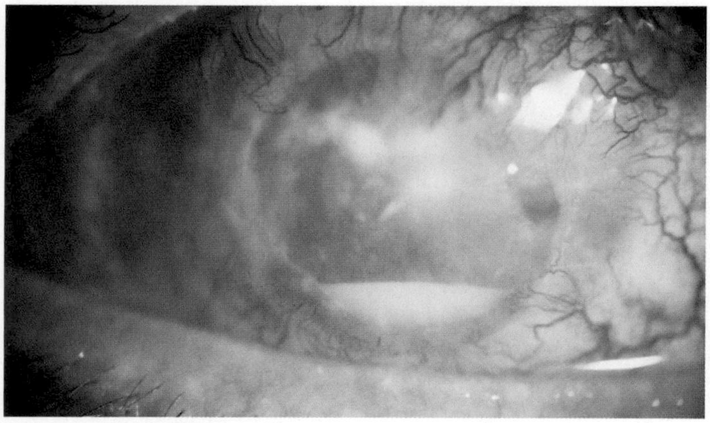

Fig. 6.7 Less dense infiltration but a larger hypopyon.

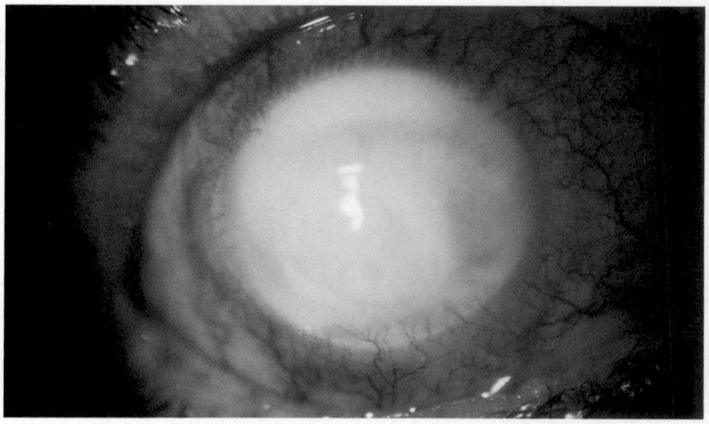

Fig. 6.8 Total corneal opacification. (Courtesy of A. Tullo.)

Candida

Candida keratitis typically occurs in association with previous corneal disease or long-term use of topical steroids.

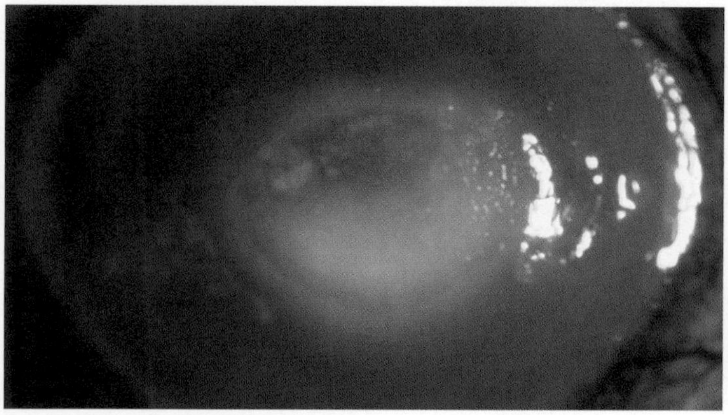

Fig. 6.9 A yellow-white ulcer associated with dense suppuration. (Courtesy of S. Tuft.)

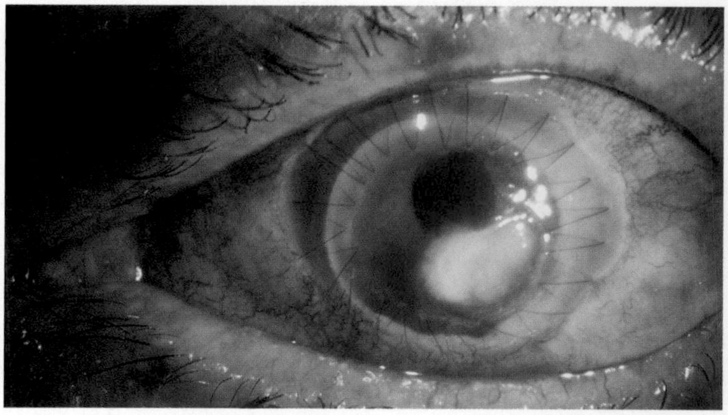

Fig. 6.10 Candida keratitis following penetrating keratoplasty and long-term use of topical steroids.

Acanthamoeba keratitis

Acanthamoeba keratitis typically affects contact lens wearers.

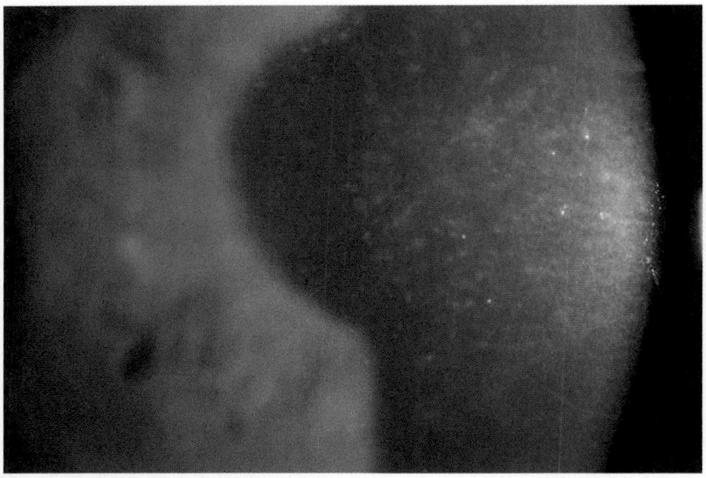

■ **Fig. 6.11** Irregular greyish epithelial keratitis and considerable pain. (Courtesy of S. Tuft.)

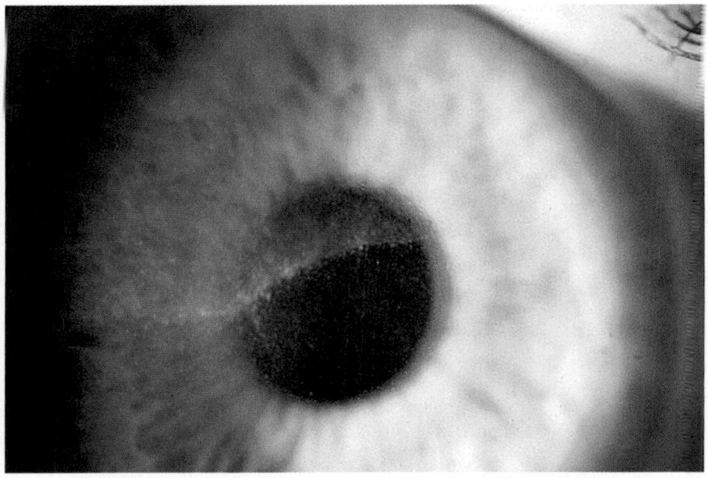

■ **Fig. 6.12** Pseudodendritic lesion. (Courtesy of R. Curtis.)

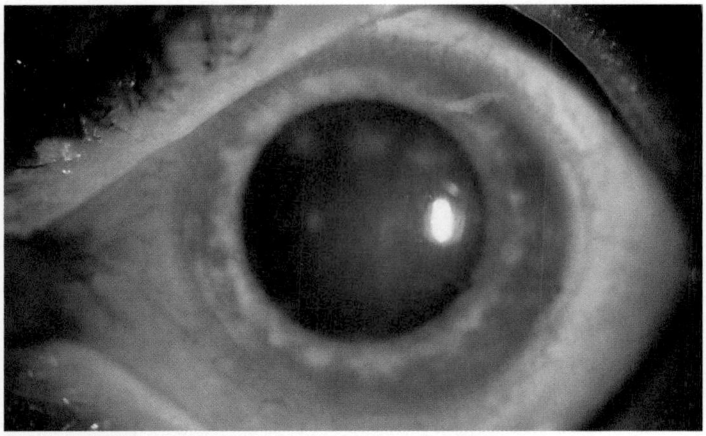

■ **Fig. 6.13** Focal anterior stromal infiltrates. (Courtesy of A. Ridgway.)

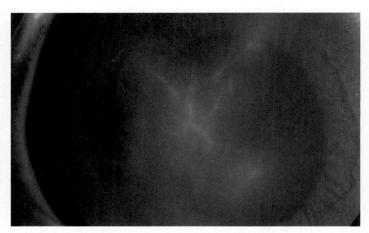

■ **Fig. 6.14** Perineural infiltrates (radial keratoneuritis). (Courtesy of S. Tuft.)

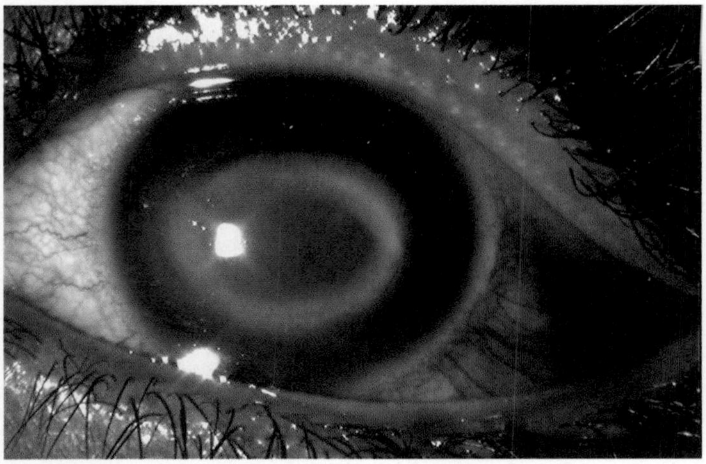

■ **Fig. 6.15** Gradual enlargement and coalescence of the infiltrates to form a central ring abscess. (Courtesy of S. Tuft.)

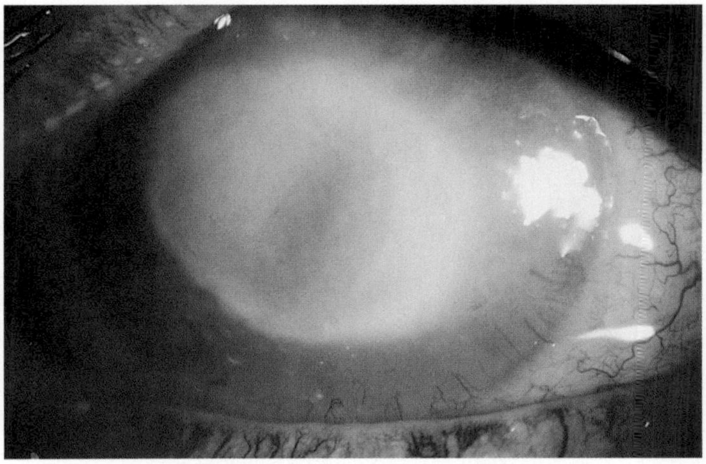

■ **Fig. 6.16** Enlargement of the abscess.

Interstitial keratitis

Interstitial keratitis is a midstromal vascularisation and non-suppurative infiltration without primary involvement of the epithelium or endothelium. Important causes are congenital syphilis and Cogan syndrome.

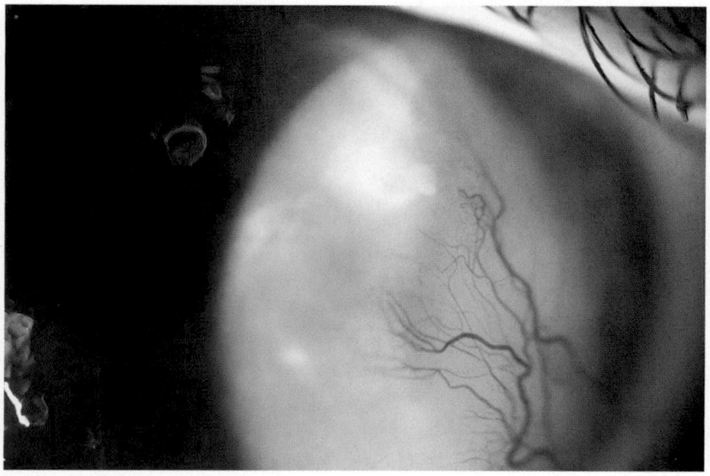

Fig. 6.17 Anterior stromal infiltrates and vascularisation with an intact epithelium.

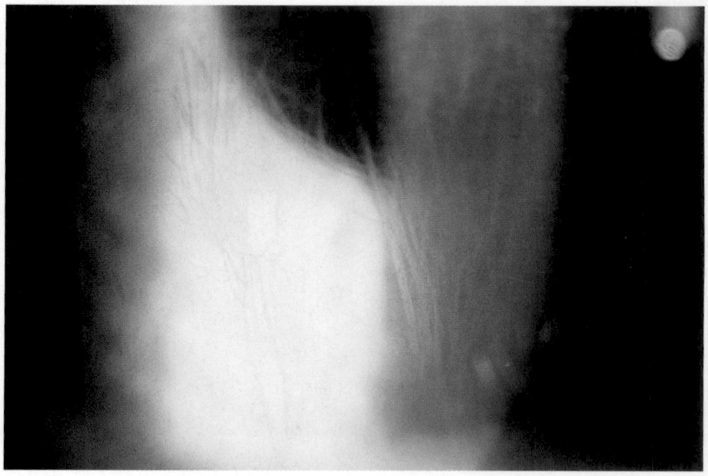

Fig. 6.18 Non-perfused (ghost) vessels in inactive disease.

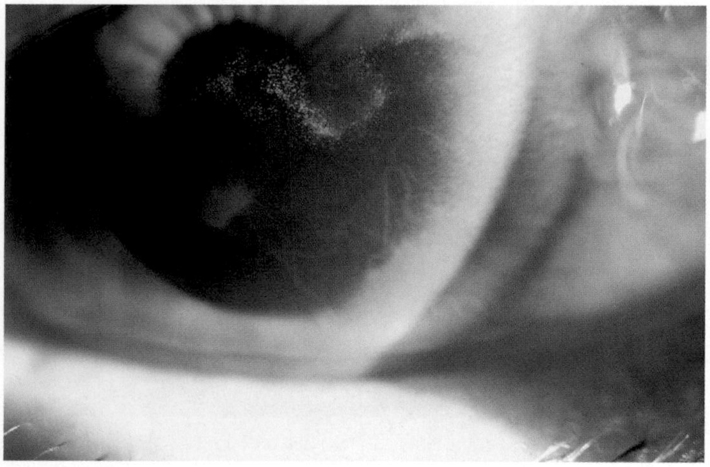

Fig. 6.19 If the keratitis reactivates the vessels may refill with blood and bleed.

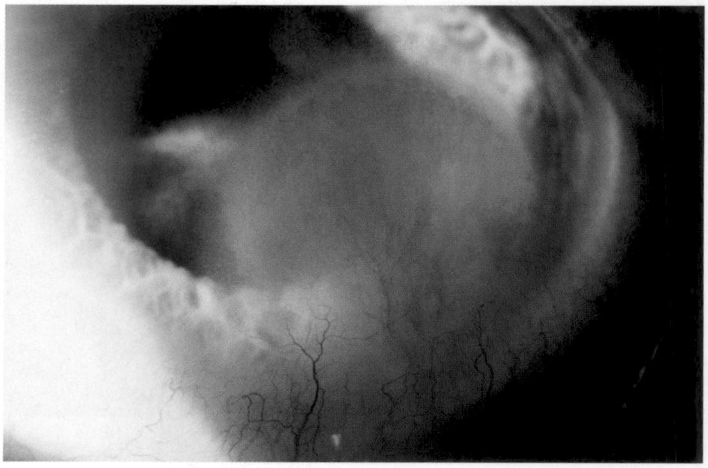

Fig. 6.20 Localised residual scarring.

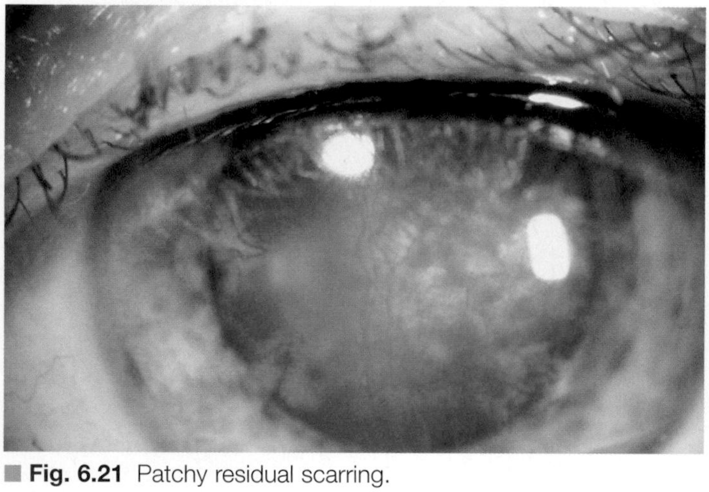

Fig. 6.21 Patchy residual scarring.

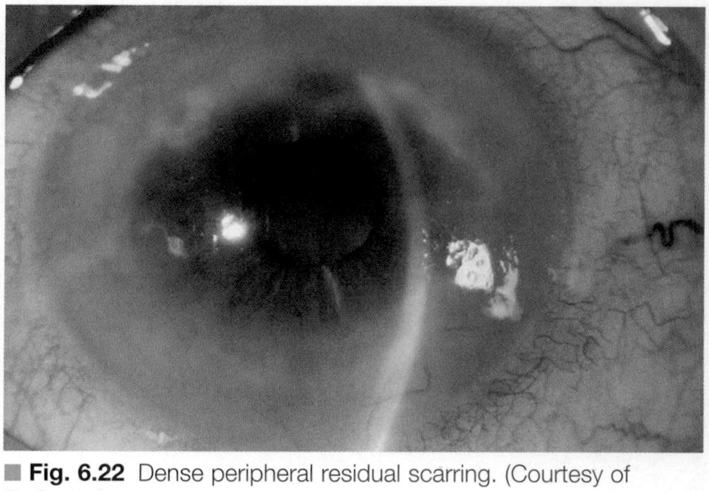

Fig. 6.22 Dense peripheral residual scarring. (Courtesy of R. Curtis.)

Signs of congenital syphilis

Early

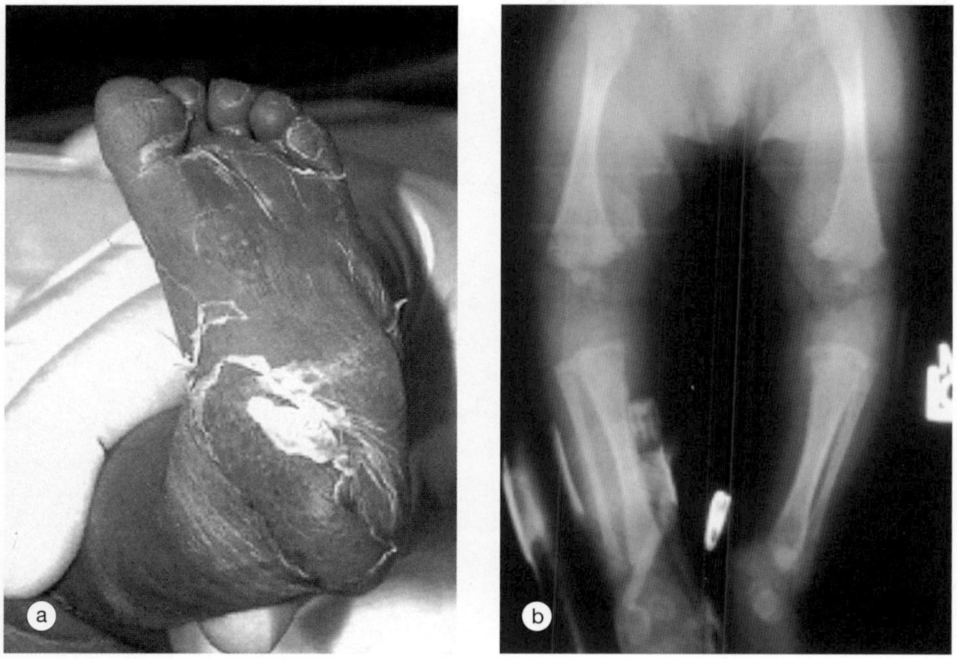

Fig. 6.23 **(a)** Desquamation of skin of the feet. **(b)** Osseous destruction of the proximal tibial metaphyses. (Courtesy of B. J. Zitelli and H. W. Davis.)

Late

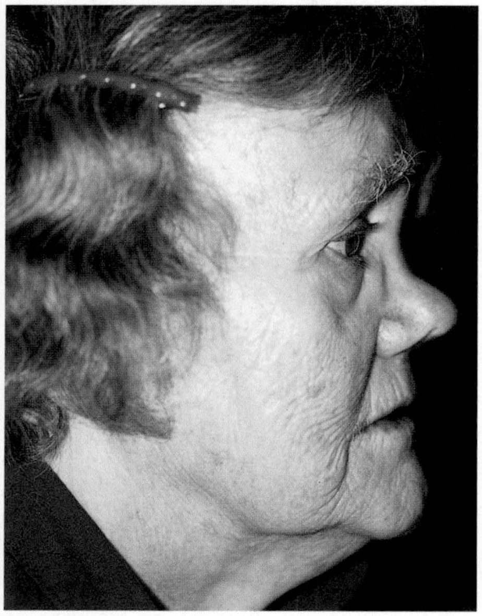

Fig. 6.24 Saddle-shaped nasal deformity.

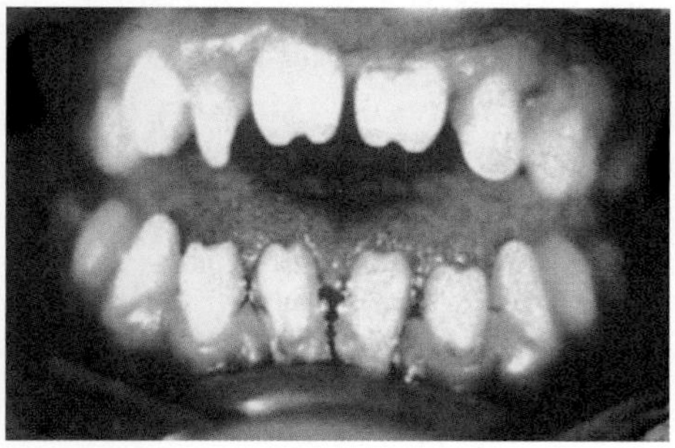

Fig. 6.25 Peg incisors with marginal notching (Hutchinson teeth). (Courtesy of C. D. Forbes and W. F. Jackson.)

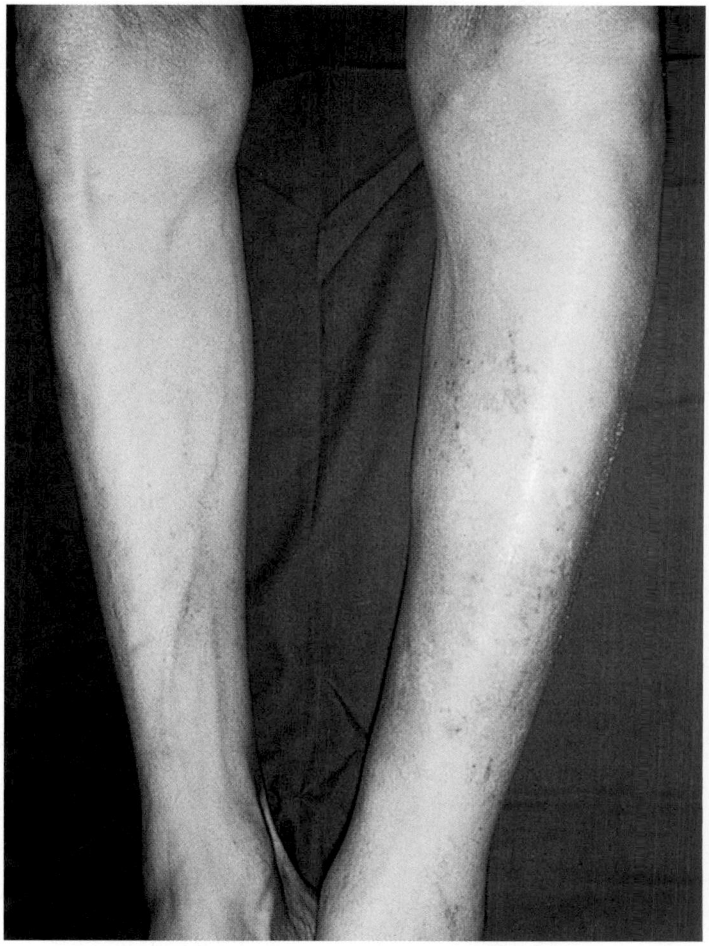

Fig. 6.26 Sabre tibiae. (Courtesy of M. A. Mir.)

Infective crystalline keratopathy

Infective crystalline keratopathy is a rare, indolent infection usually associated with long-term topical steroid therapy, particularly following penetrating keratoplasty.

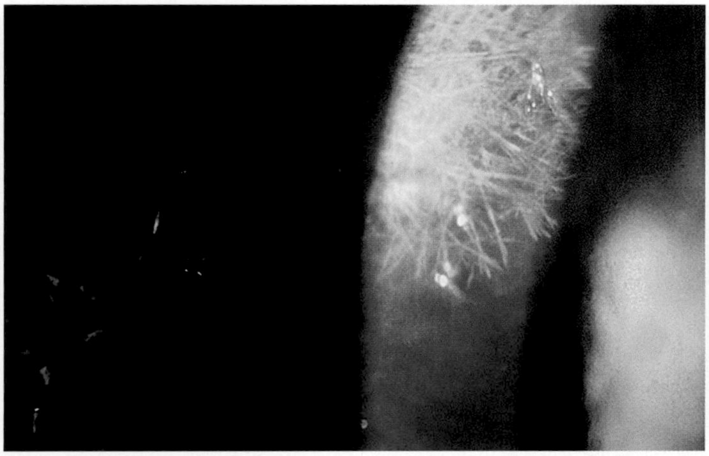

Fig. 6.27 Slowly progressive, grey-white, branching stromal opacities with minimal inflammation. (Courtesy of M. Kerr-Muir.)

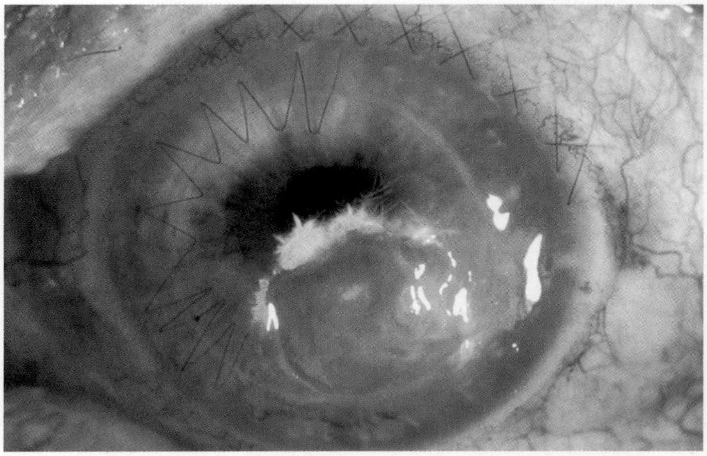

Fig. 6.28 Crystalline keratopathy following penetrating keratoplasty.

VIRAL KERATITIS

Herpes simplex

Herpes simplex keratitis is usually caused by HSV-1 which may also affect the face and mouth.

Systemic features

Primary infection

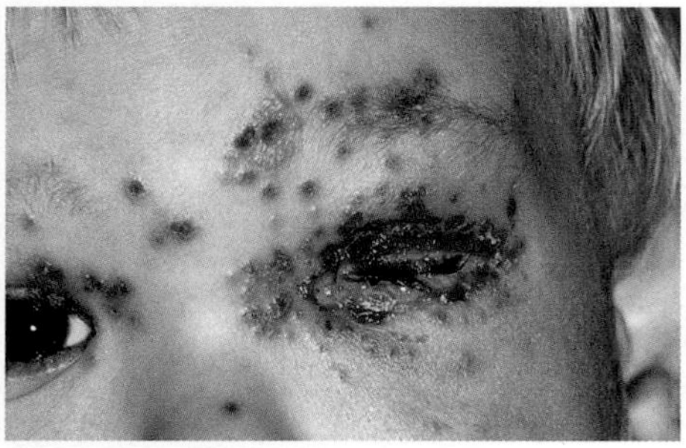

Fig. 6.29 Skin vesicles associated with blepharo-conjunctivitis.

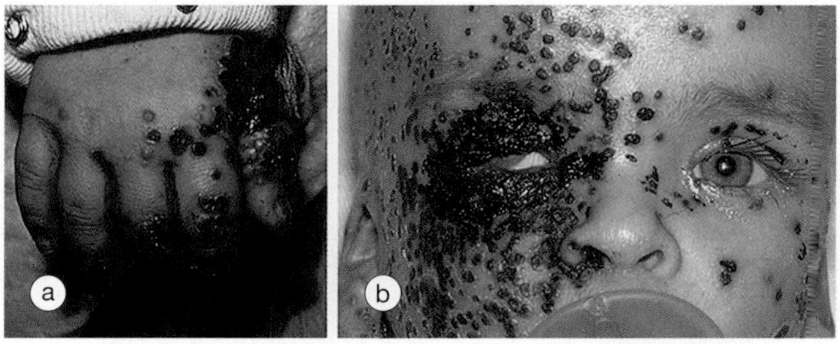

Fig. 6.30 Very severe infection in a child with underlying eczema (eczema herpeticum). (Courtesy of B. J. Zitelli and H. W. Davis.)

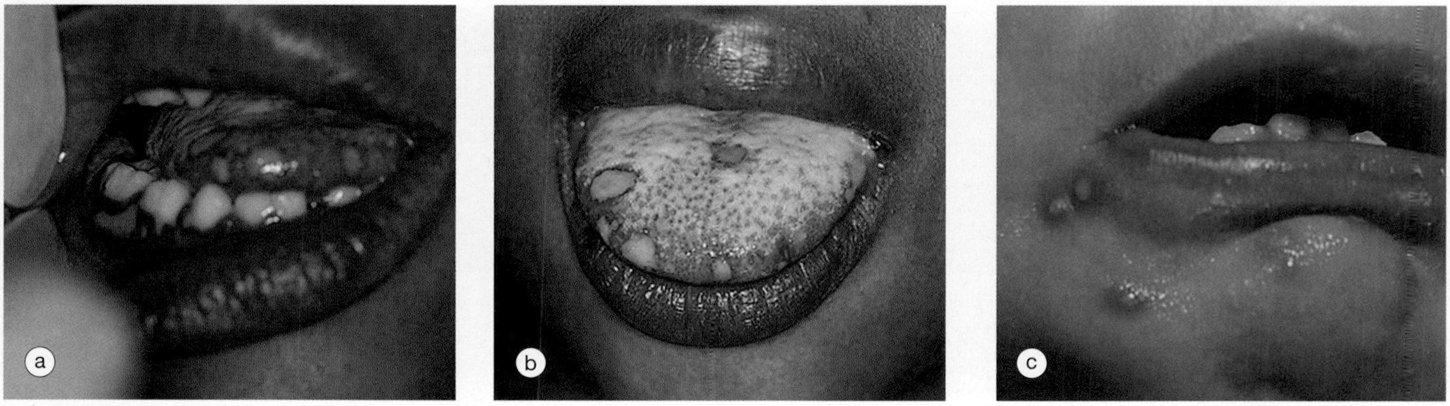

Fig. 6.31 **(a)** Gingival erythema and swelling. **(b)** Numerous yellow ulcers on the tongue. **(c)** Involvement of the lips and chin. (Courtesy of B. J. Zitelli and H. W. Davis.)

Recurrent infection

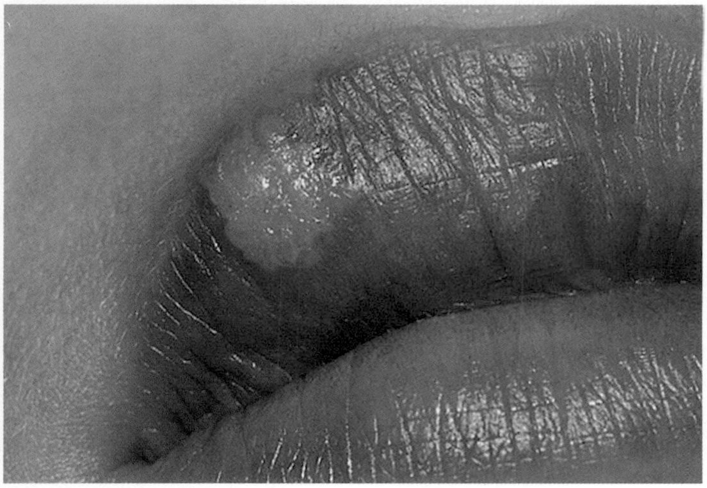

Fig. 6.32 Herpes labialis (cold sore). (Courtesy of B. J. Zitelli and H. W. Davis.)

Dendritic ulcer

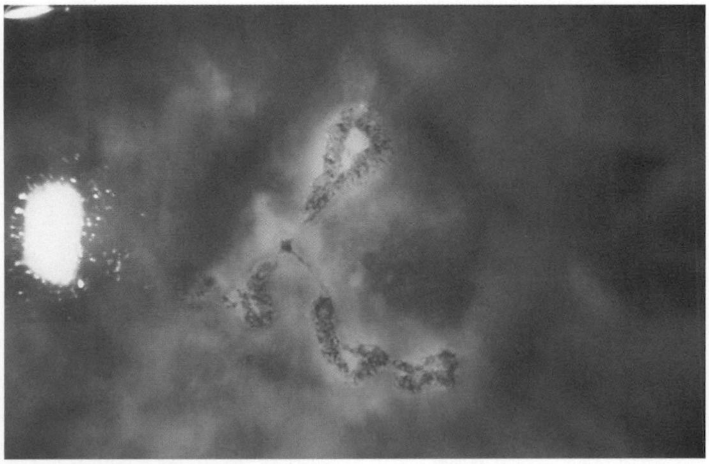

Fig. 6.33 Opaque epithelial cells arranged in a coarse punctate or stellate pattern.

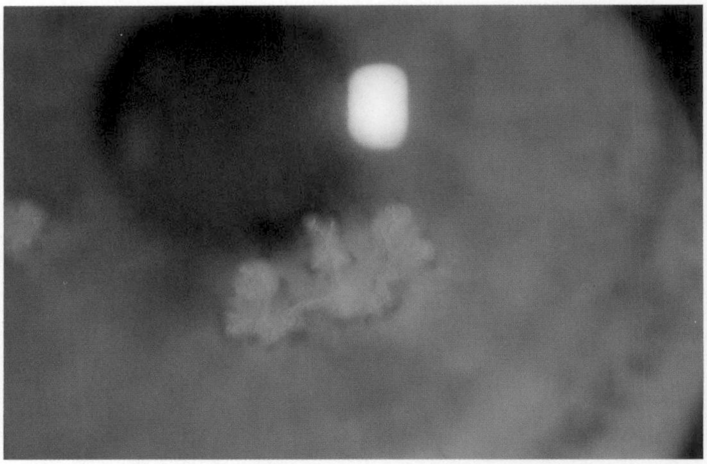

Fig. 6.34 Central desquamation results in a linear–branching (dendritic) ulcer, often located centrally.

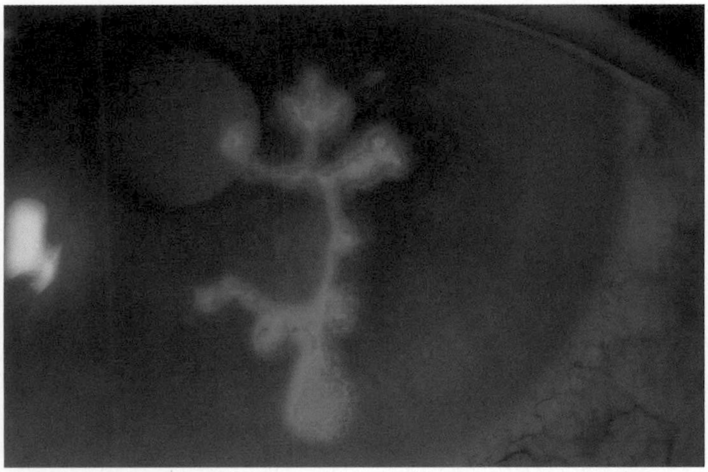

Fig. 6.35 The ends of the branches manifest a characteristically swollen appearance (terminal bulbs). The bed of the ulcer stains with fluorescein.

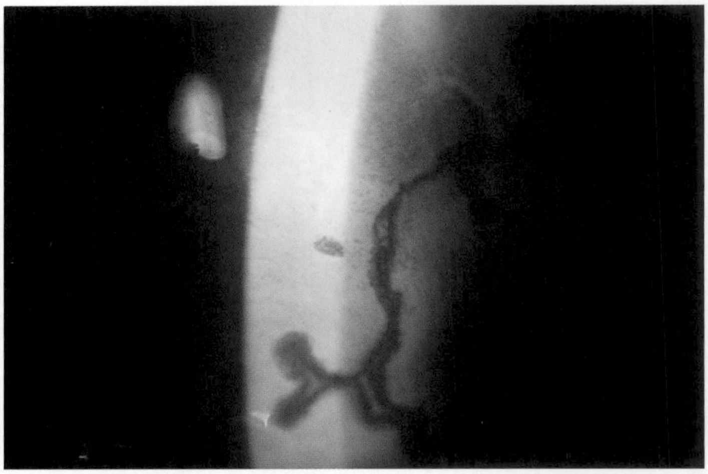

Fig. 6.36 The virus-laden cells at the margin of the ulcer stain with rose bengal.

Geographic ulcer

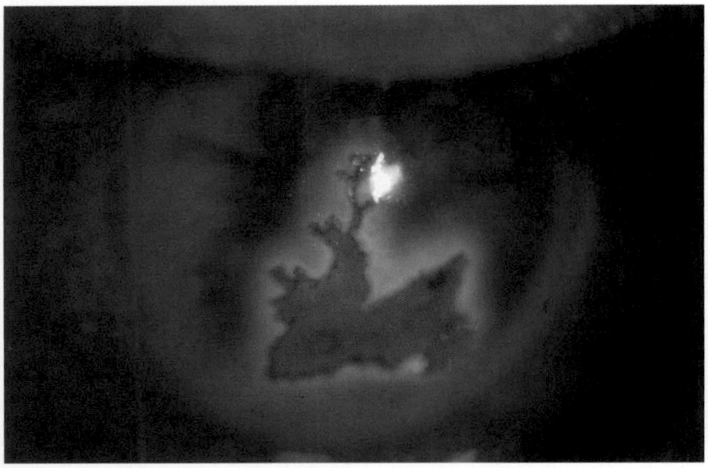

Fig. 6.37 Progressive centrifugal enlargement may result in a larger epithelial defect with a geographical or 'amoeboid' configuration.

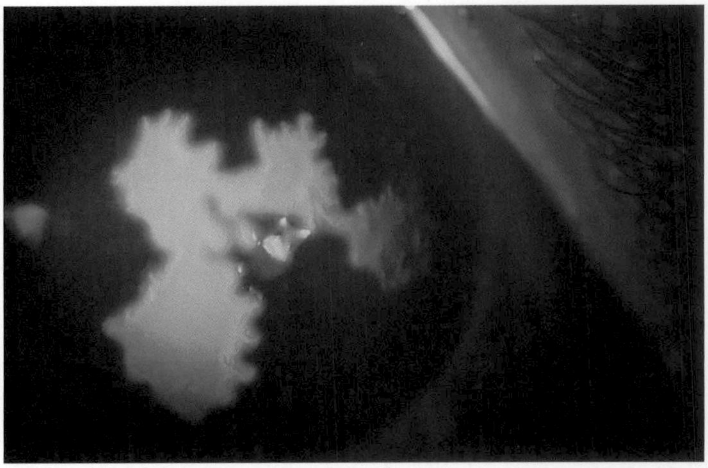

Fig. 6.38 Enormous geographic ulcer.

Disciform keratitis

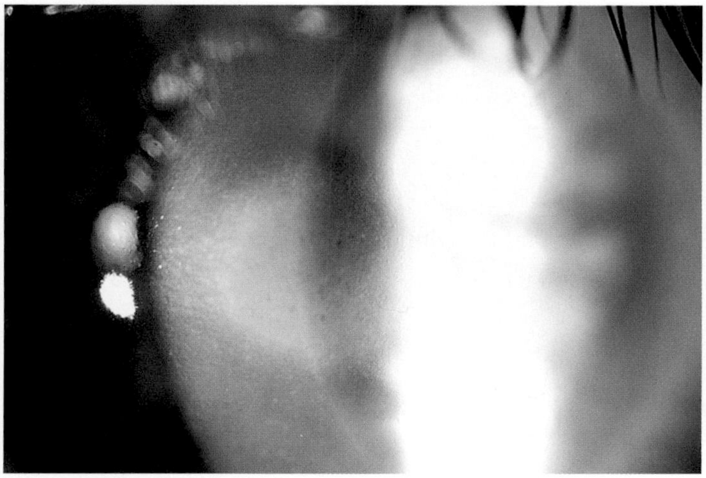

Fig. 6.39 A central zone of epithelial oedema.

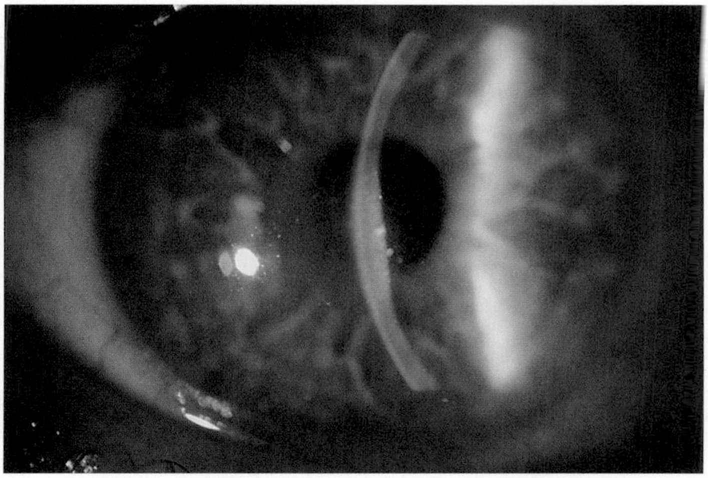

Fig. 6.40 Stromal thickening and keratic precipitates.

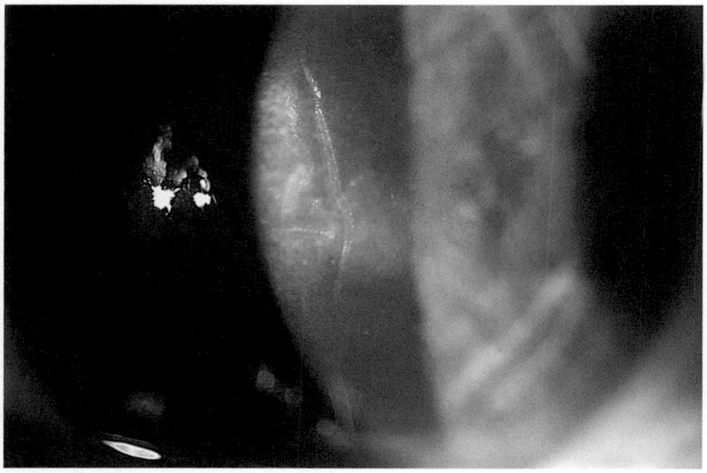

Fig. 6.41 Folds in Descemet membrane.

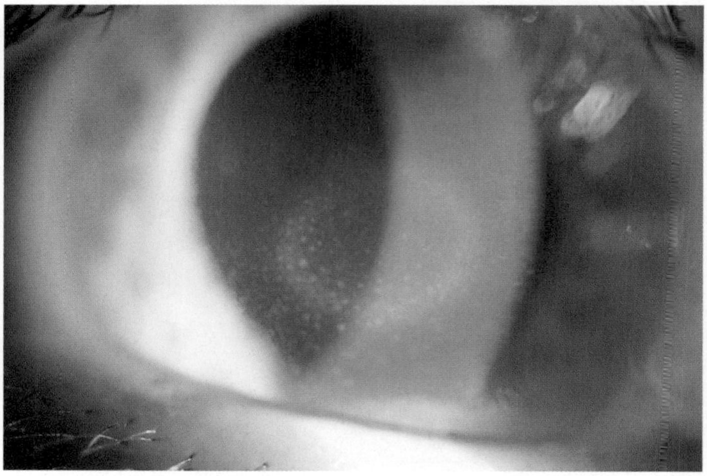

Fig. 6.42 A surrounding (Wessely) ring of stromal precipitates may be present, signifying the junction between viral antigen and host antibody.

Stromal necrotic keratitis

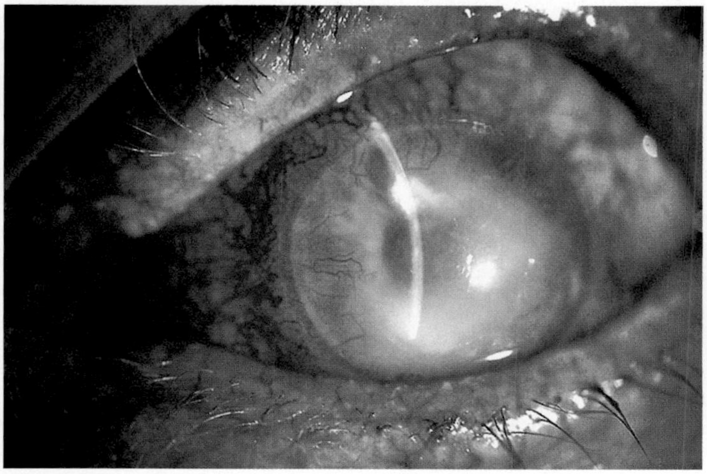

Fig. 6.43 Cheesy and necrotic stroma reminiscent of a bacterial or fungal infection.

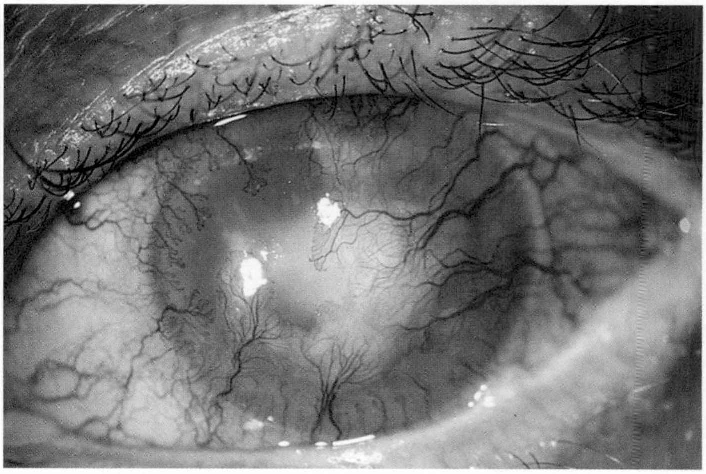

Fig. 6.44 Scarring and vascularisation.

Herpes zoster ophthalmicus

Herpes zoster (shingles) is caused by the varicella zoster virus which is morphologically identical to HSV but has different clinical manifestations.

Cutaneous lesions

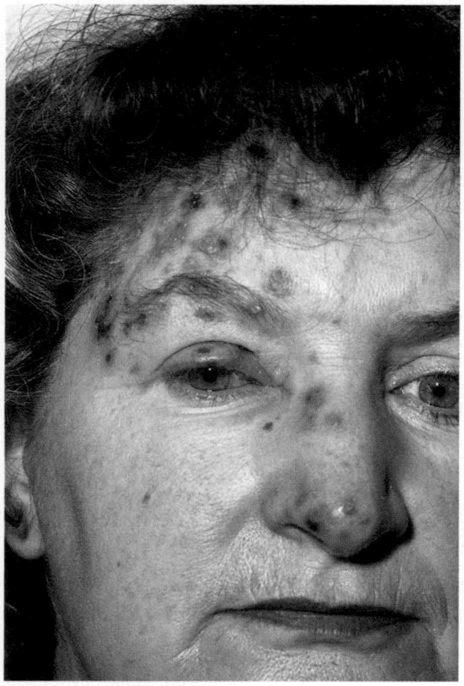

Fig. 6.45 Cutaneous lesions vary in distribution, density and severity and may involve one or more of the cutaneous branches of the ophthalmic nerve. Involvement of the tip of the nose signifies a high risk of ocular complications.

Acute epithelial keratitis

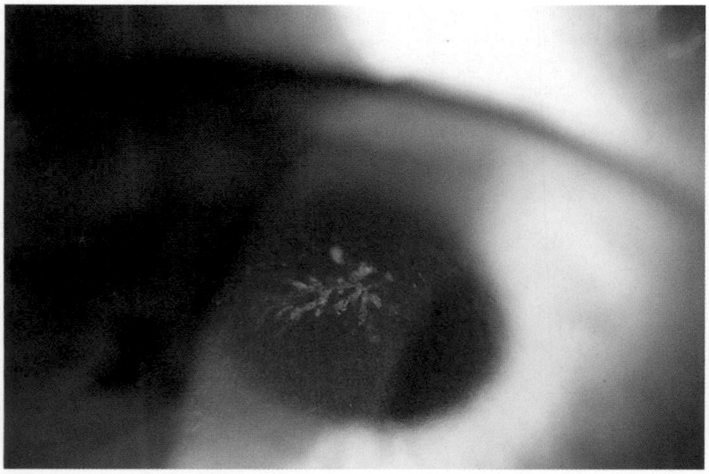

Fig. 6.46 Small, fine, dendritic or stellate 'heaped-up' epithelial lesions.

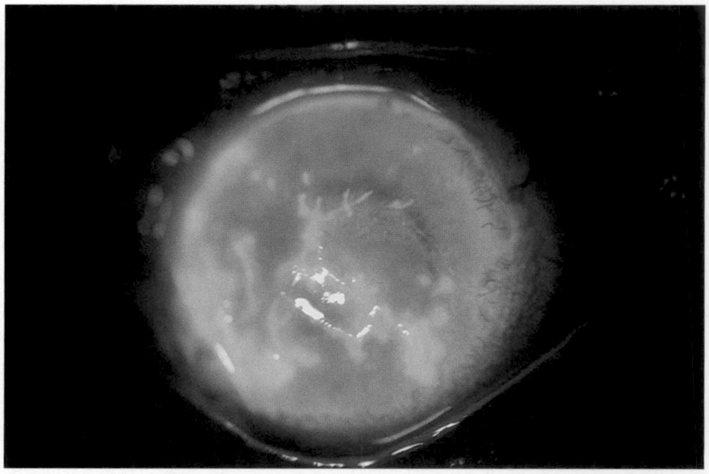

Fig. 6.47 Larger pseudodendritic epithelial lesions with tapering ends stained with fluorescein. (Courtesy of R. Marsh.)

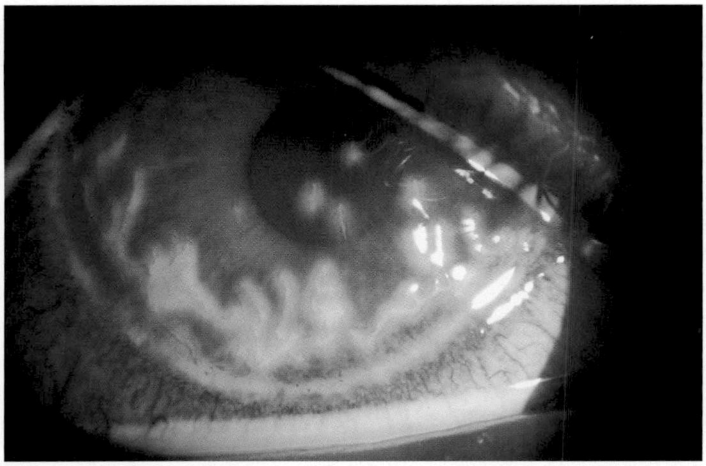

■ **Fig. 6.48** Multiple peripheral pseudodendritic lesions stained with fluorescein.

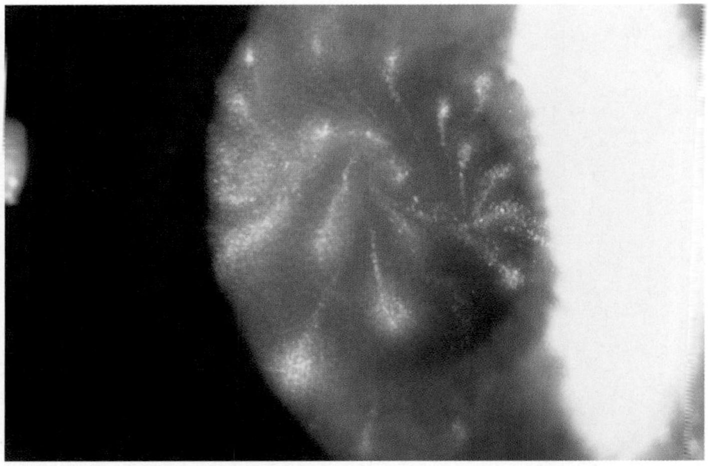

■ **Fig. 6.49** Multiple large central pseudodendritic lesions. (Courtesy of L. Merin.)

Nummular keratitis

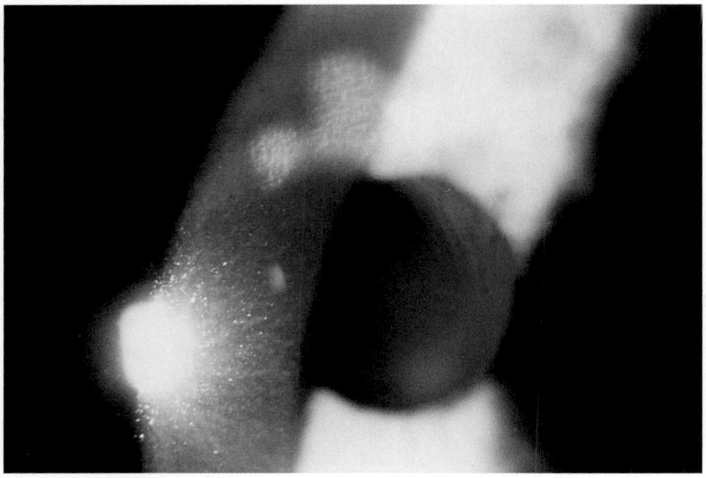

■ **Fig. 6.50** Multiple fine granular subepithelial deposits surrounded by a halo of stromal haze, which may resolve without trace.

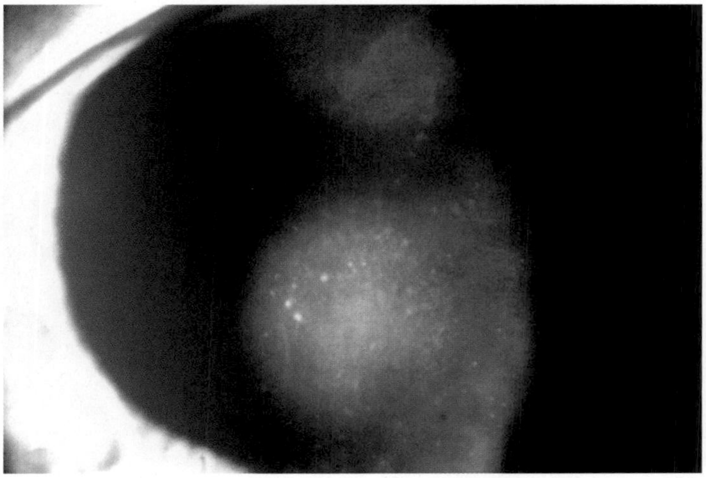

■ **Fig. 6.51** Magnified view of a nummular lesion.

Disciform keratitis

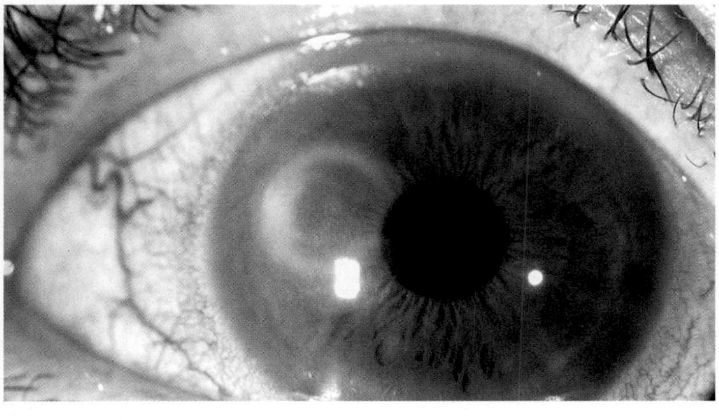

■ **Fig. 6.52** Disciform keratitis is almost always preceded by nummular keratitis. (Courtesy of R. Marsh.)

Mucous plaque keratitis

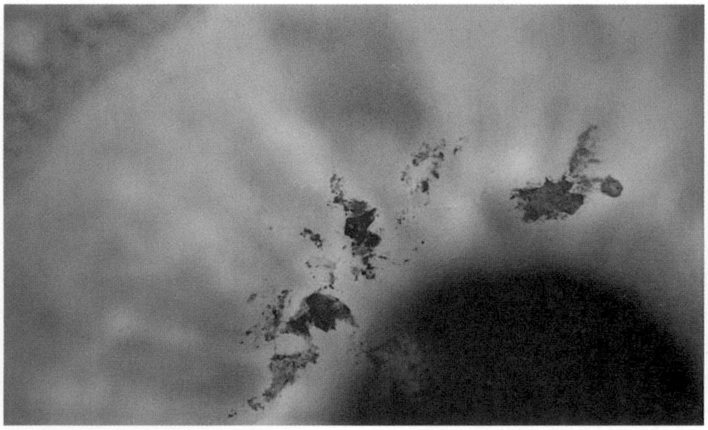

Fig. 6.53 Sudden appearance of elevated mucous plaques that stain with rose bengal. (Courtesy of R. Marsh.)

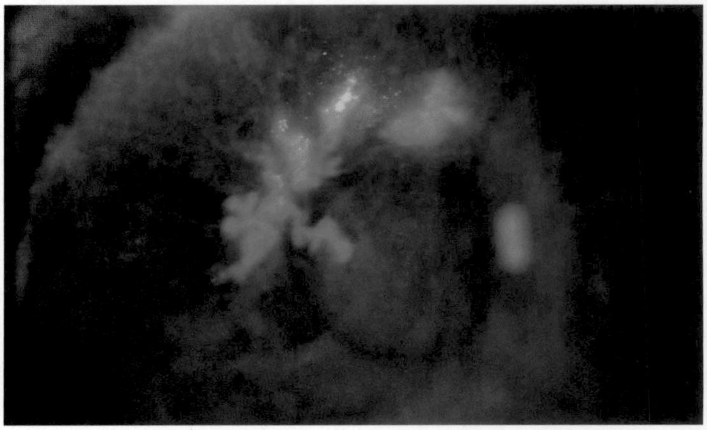

Fig. 6.54 More severe mucous plaque keratitis. (Courtesy of R. Marsh.)

Neurotrophic keratitis

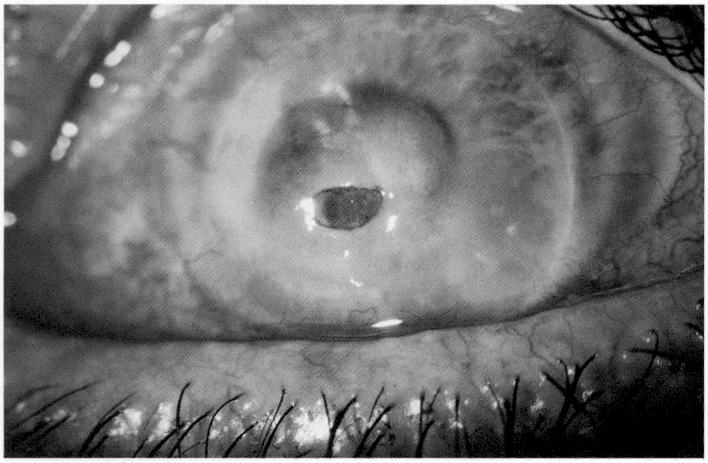

Fig. 6.55 Severe epithelial loss and ulceration.

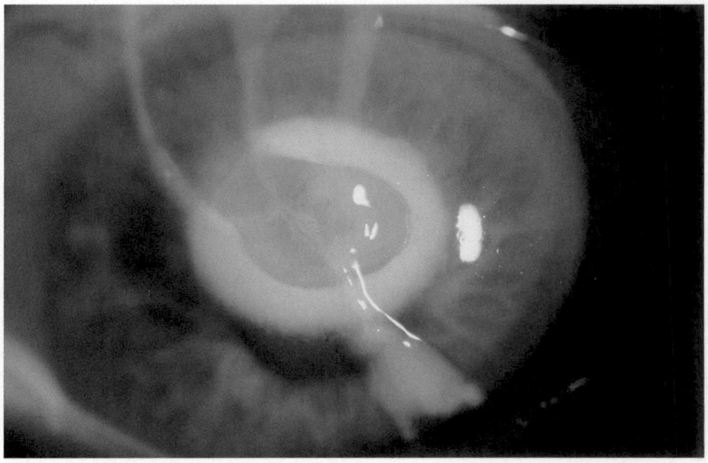

Fig. 6.56 An ulcer coated with a mucous plaque.

Lipid keratopathy

Lipid keratopathy may be the end result of chronic disciform or nummular keratitis.

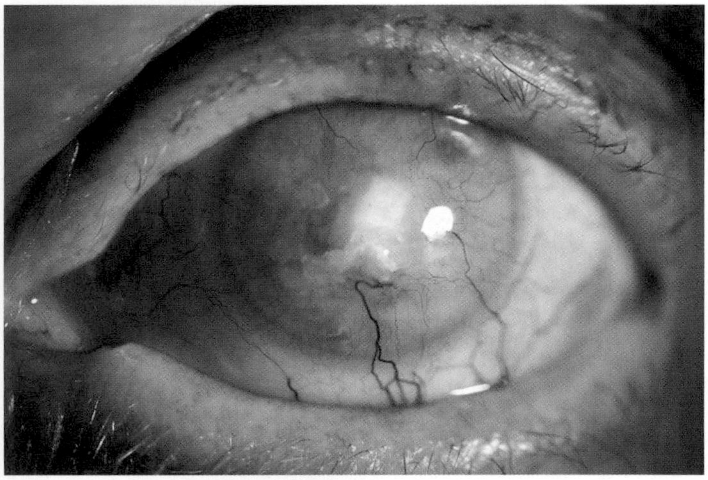

Fig. 6.57 Corneal scarring, lipid deposition and vascularisation.

Other ocular signs

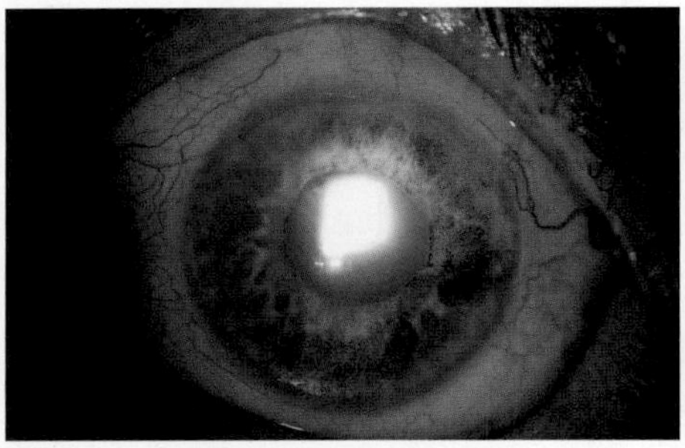

■ **Fig. 6.58** Sectoral iris atrophy caused by anterior uveitis.

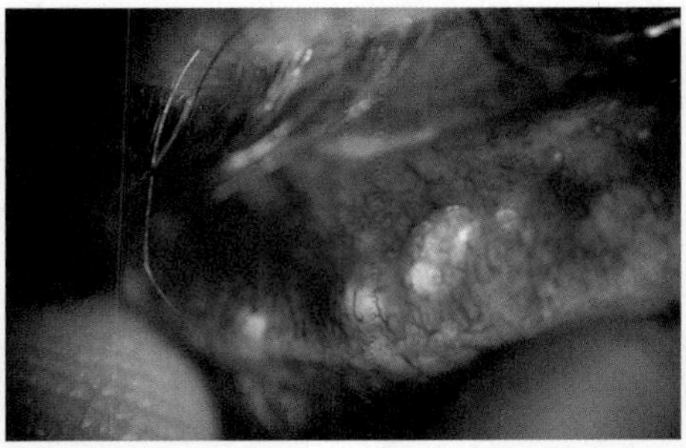

■ **Fig. 6.59** Mucus-secreting conjunctivitis characterised by lipid-filled granulomata under the tarsal conjunctiva and subconjunctival scarring.

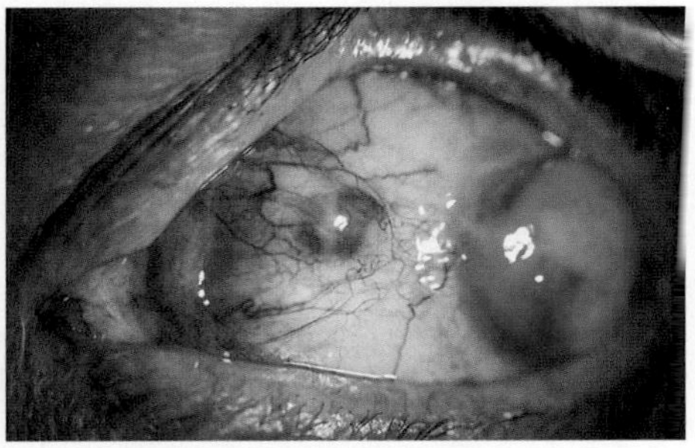

■ **Fig. 6.60** Scleritis may become chronic and lead to patchy scleral atrophy; also note severe corneal scarring.

Thygeson superficial punctate keratitis

Thygeson disease is an uncommon, bilateral, recurrent condition of unknown aetiology. Because a viral cause is suspected, it is included in this section.

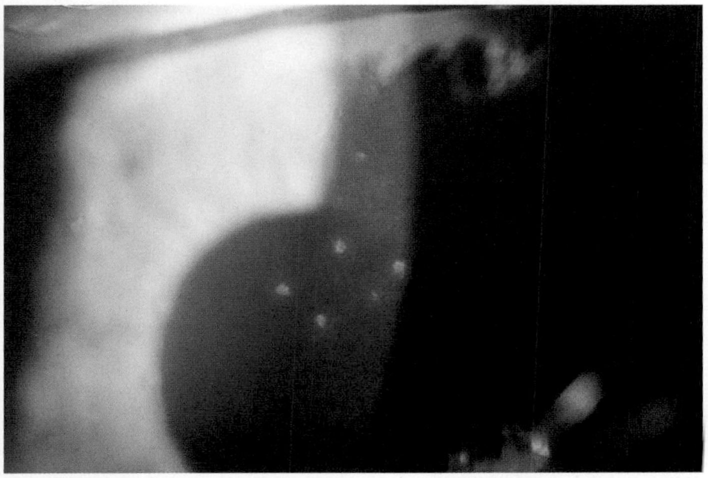

■ **Fig. 6.61** Round or oval conglomerates of distinct, granular, greyish, elevated, punctate epithelial lesions; the conjunctiva is uninvolved

PERIPHERAL CORNEAL DISORDERS

Dellen

Dellen is caused by localised tear film instability which may be idiopathic or secondary to raised limbal lesions.

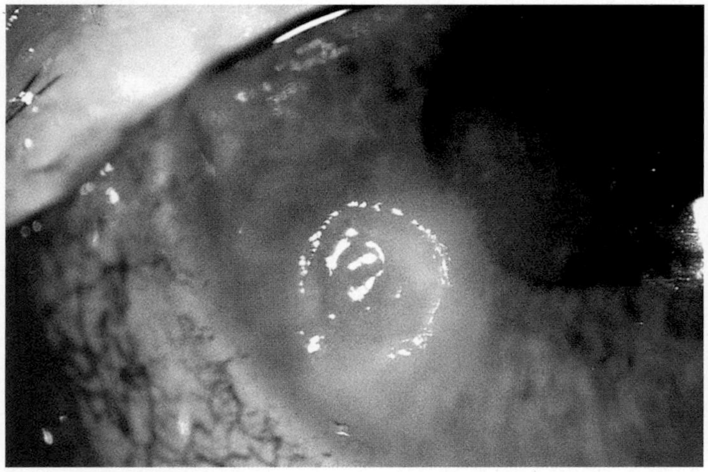

Fig. 6.62 Localised, saucer-like thinning of the peripheral cornea.

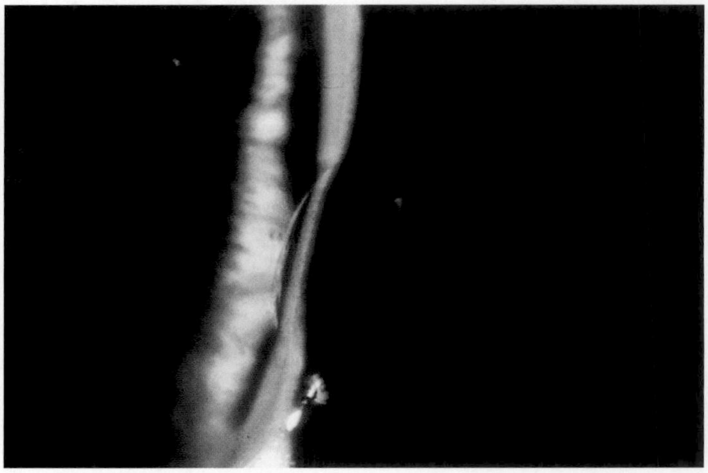

Fig. 6.63 Cross-sectional view.

Marginal keratitis

Marginal keratitis (catarrhal ulcer) is caused by hypersensitivity to staphylococcal exotoxins and is therefore frequently associated with chronic staphylococcal blepharitis.

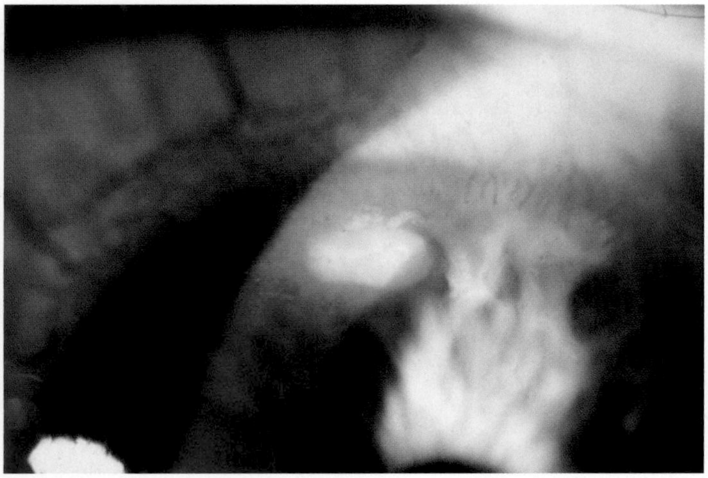

Fig. 6.64 A subepithelial marginal infiltrate separated from the limbus by a clear zone.

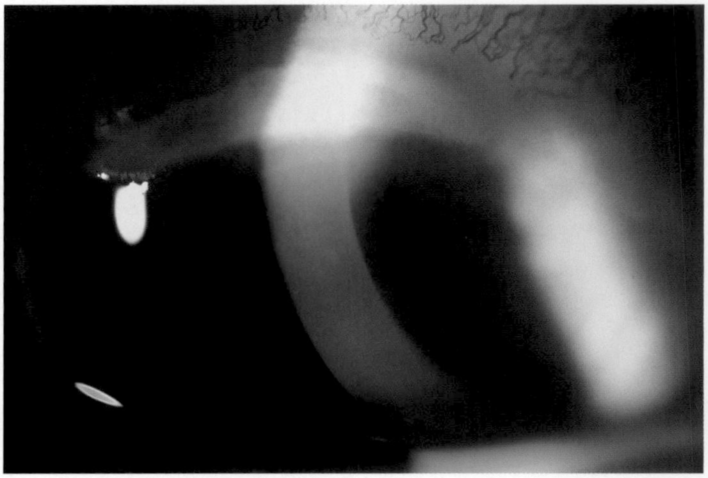

Fig. 6.65 Circumferential extension.

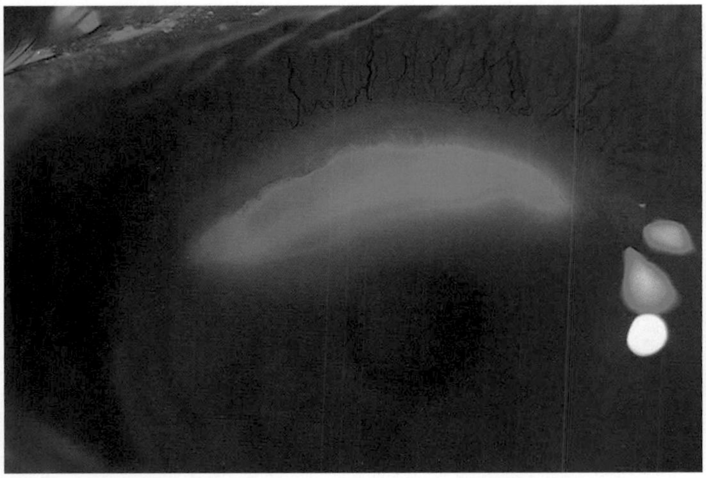

■ **Fig. 6.66** Breakdown of the overlying epithelium gives rise to a fluorescein-staining ulcer.

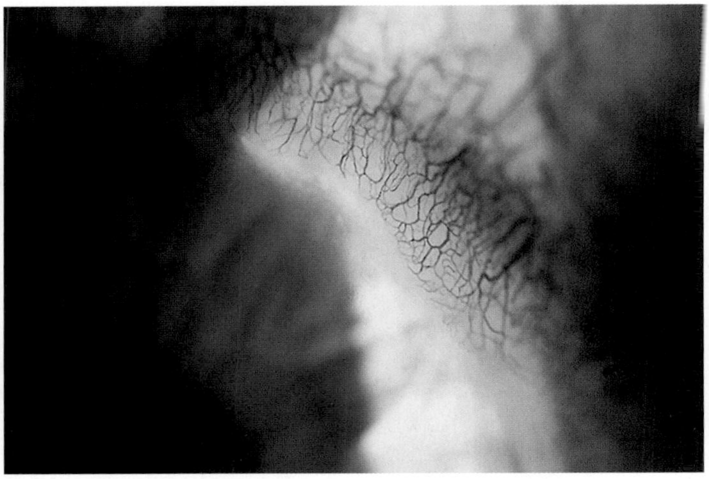

■ **Fig. 6.67** Within a few days blood vessels bridge the clear corneal zone and resolution occurs.

Rosacea keratitis

Acne rosacea is a common, chronic, progressive condition of unknown aetiology involving facial skin and the eyes.

Keratitis

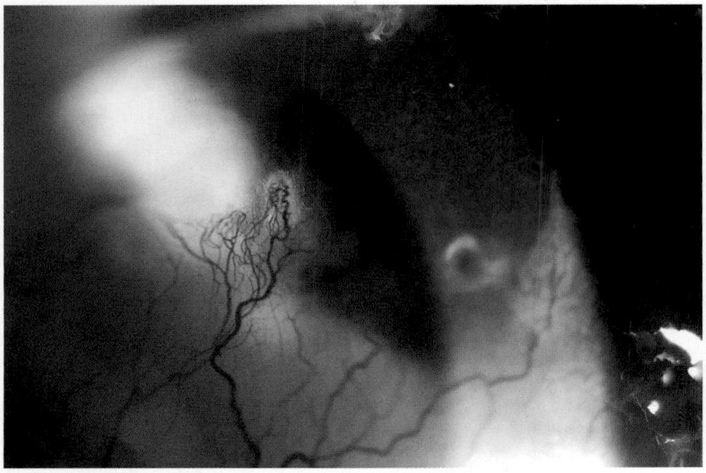

■ **Fig. 6.68** Inferior peripheral neovascularisation.

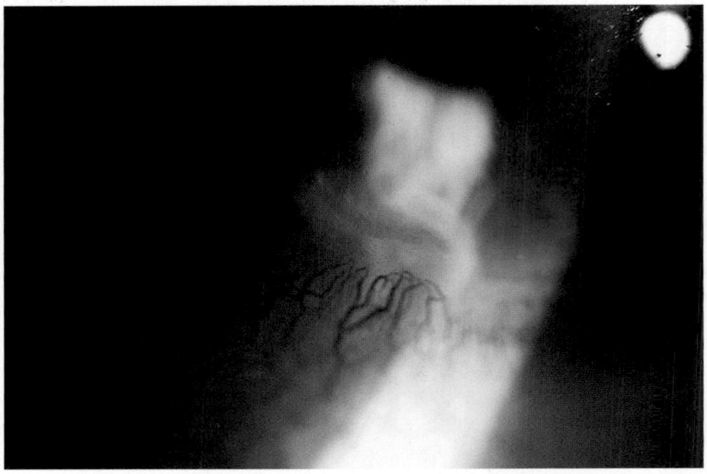

■ **Fig. 6.69** Superficial infiltration central to neovascularisation.

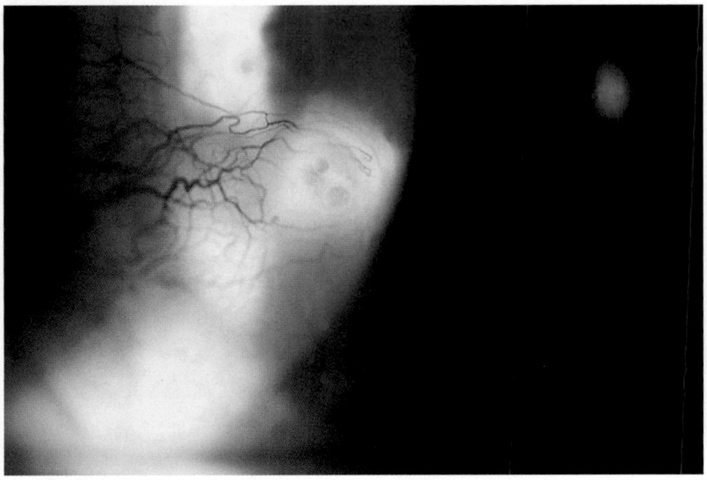

■ **Fig. 6.70** Early corneal thinning.

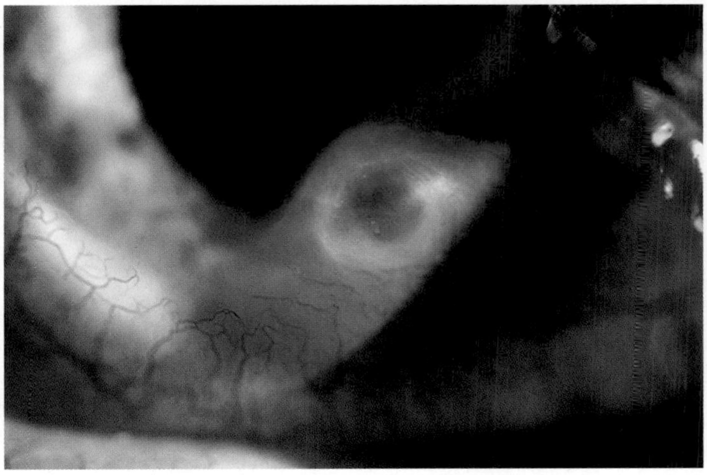

■ **Fig. 6.71** Severe corneal thinning.

Other ocular signs

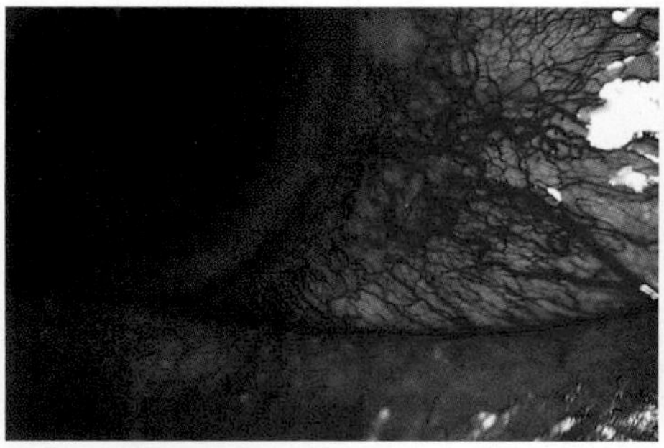

Fig. 6.72 Chronic conjunctival hyperaemia.

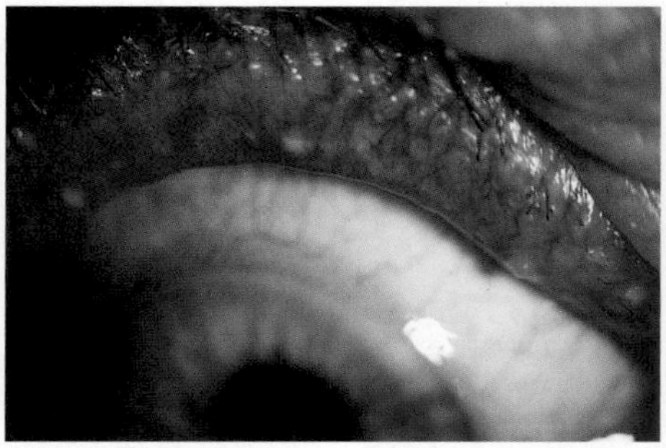

Fig. 6.73 Meibomian gland dysfunction and chronic posterior blepharitis.

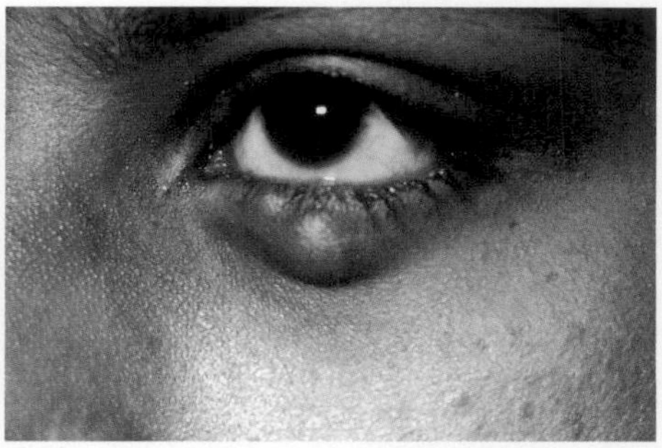

Fig. 6.74 Recurrent chalazion formation.

Cutaneous signs

Rosacea principally involves the glabella, cheeks, nose and chin.

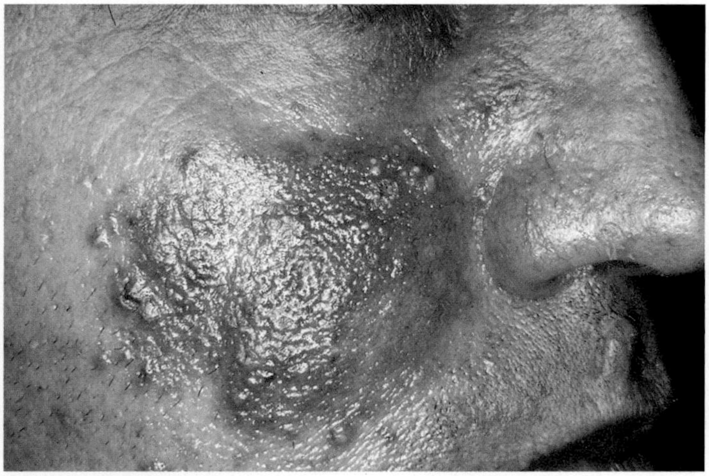

Fig. 6.75 Erythema and early telangiectasia.

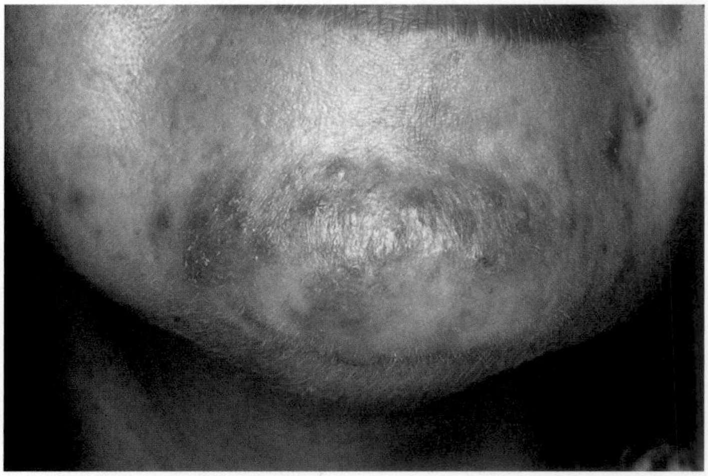

Fig. 6.76 Papules and pustules.

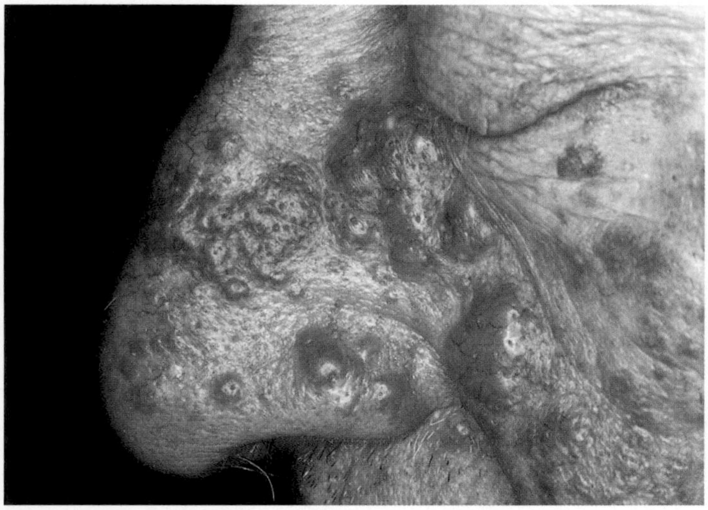

Fig. 6.77 Severe sebaceous gland hypertrophy.

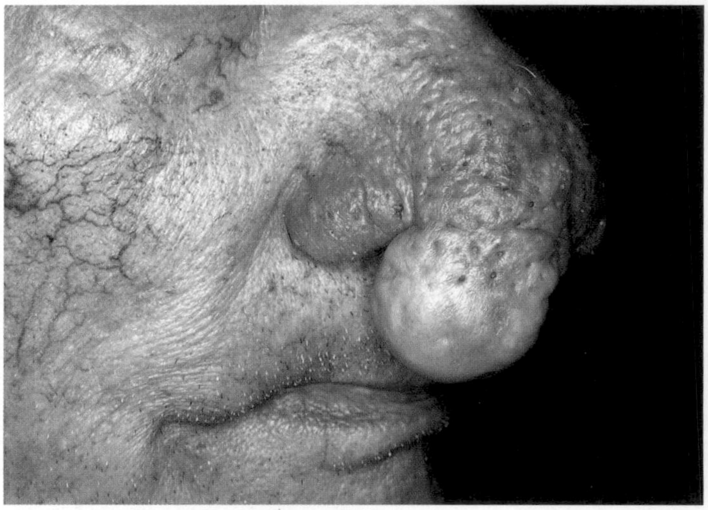

Fig. 6.78 Rhinophyma is rare.

Phlyctenulosis

Phlyctenulosis is caused by a non-specific delayed hypersensitivity reaction to bacterial antigens.

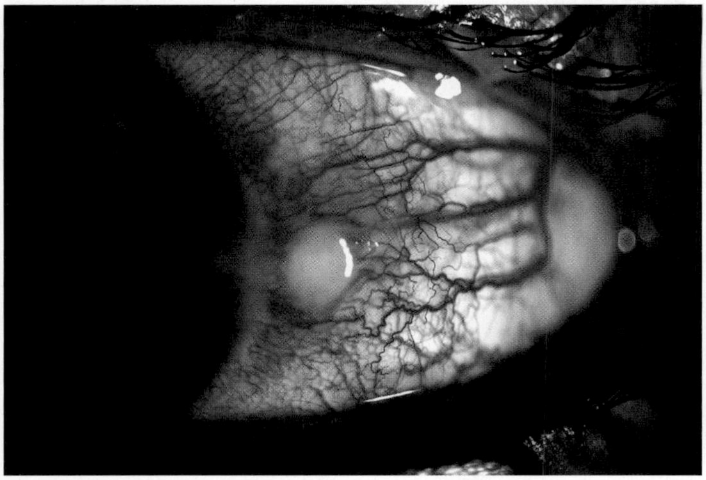

Fig. 6.79 A pinkish white conjunctival nodule associated with hyperaemia.

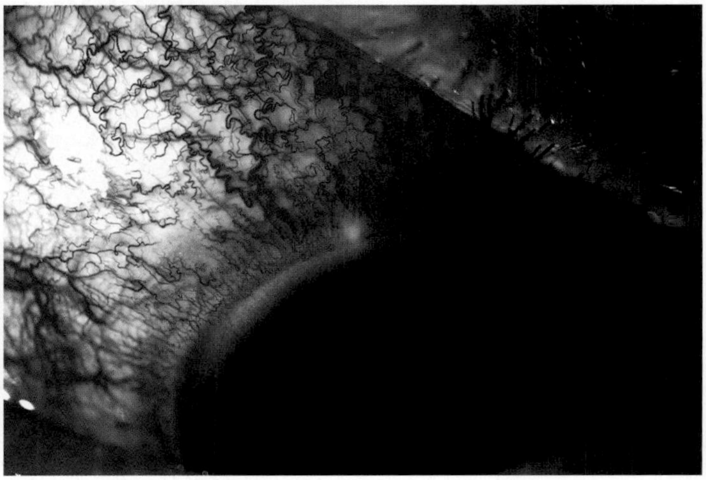

Fig. 6.80 A small limbal phlycten.

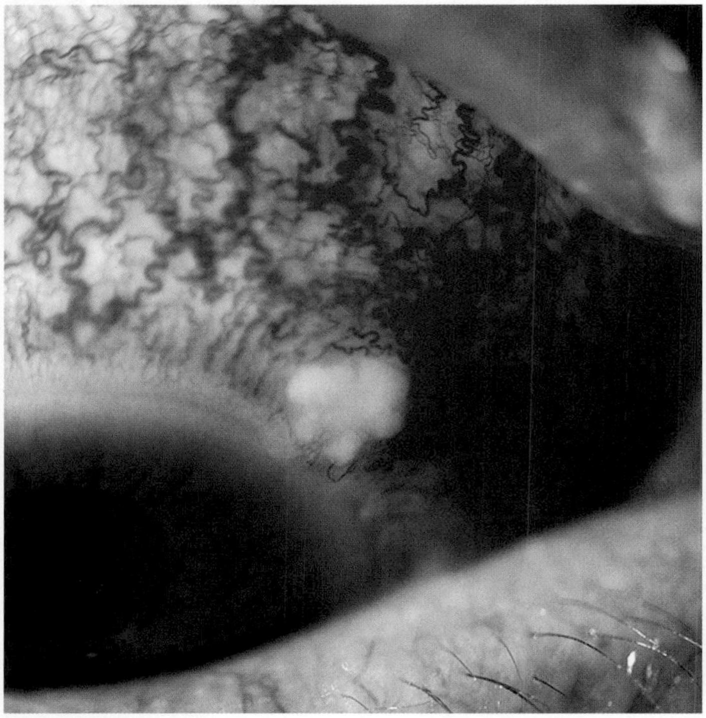

Fig. 6.81 A larger limbal phlycten.

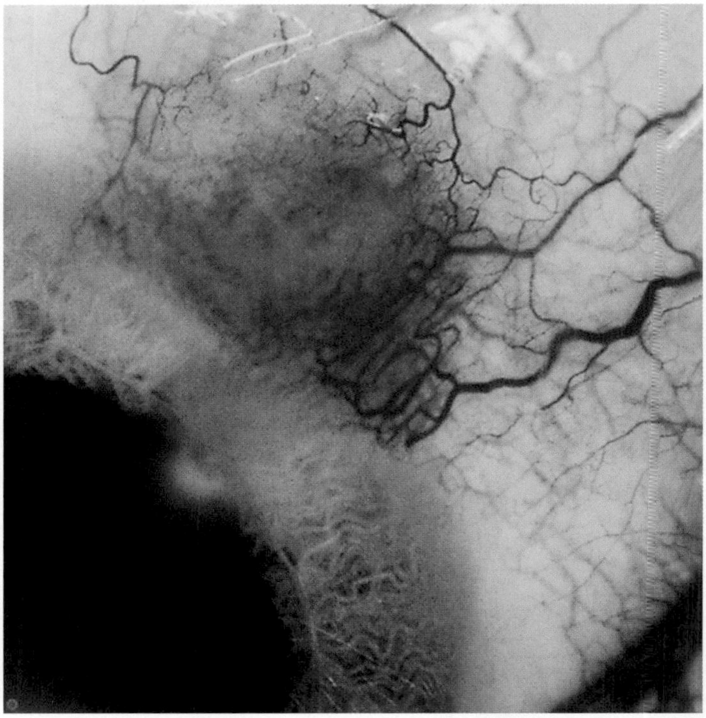

Fig. 6.82 A large phlycten with a triangular limbal-based corneal scar due to previous attacks.

Mooren ulcer

Mooren ulcer is a rare but serious condition probably caused by an autoimmune response to corneal stromal antigens.

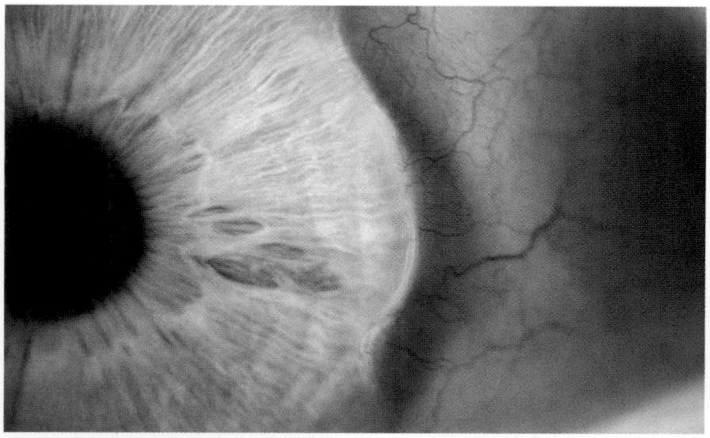

Fig. 6.83 Peripheral corneal infiltration 2–3 mm from the limbus.

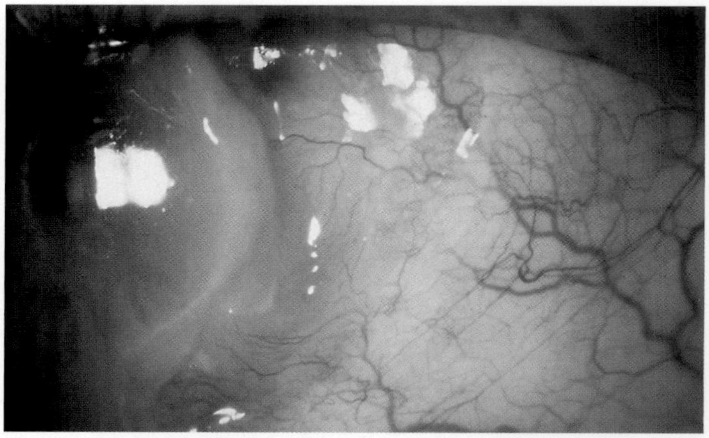

Fig. 6.84 Crescent-shaped corneal ulceration characterised by extensive undermining of the leading edge over the infiltrates.

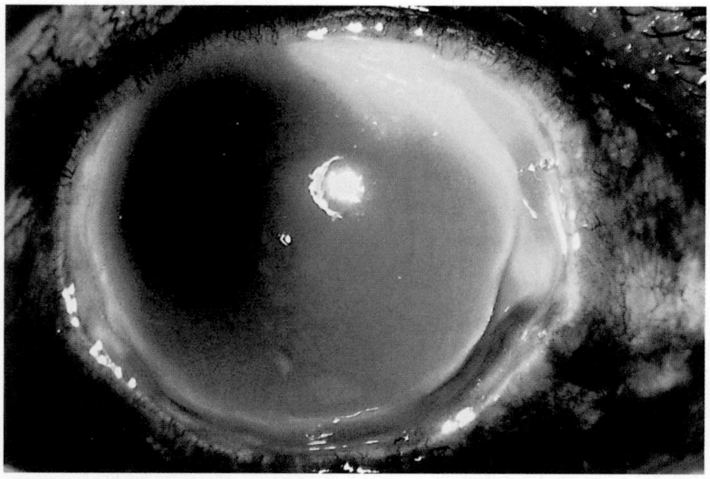

Fig. 6.85 Circumferential spread.

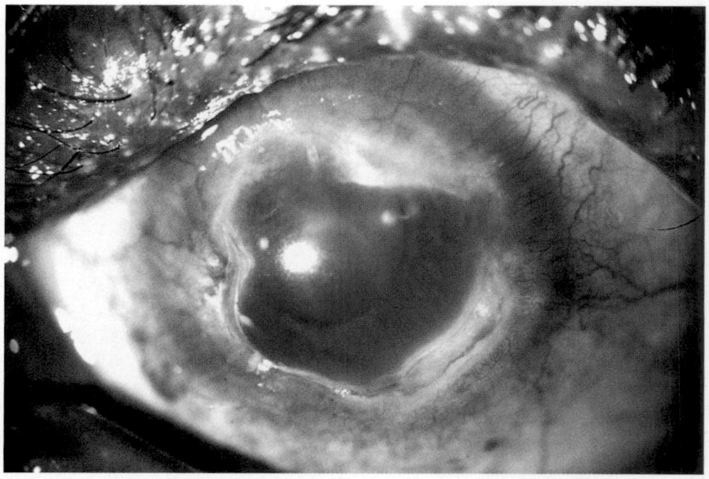

Fig. 6.86 Central spread.

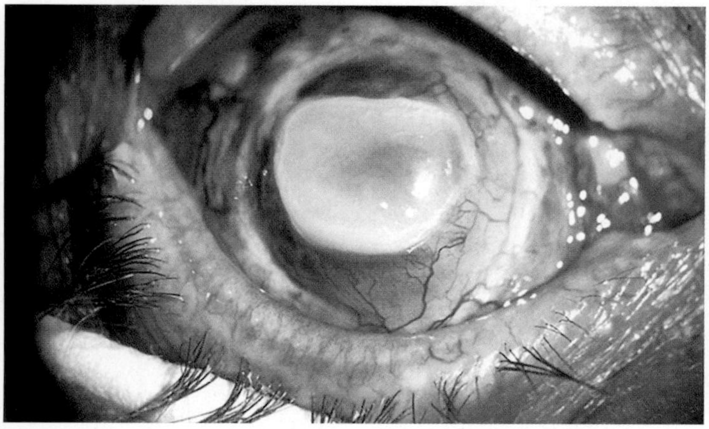

Fig. 6.87 Central opacification with peripheral vascularisation.

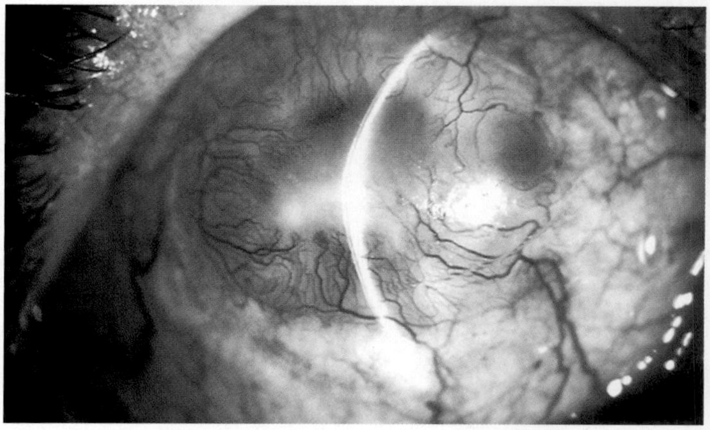

Fig. 6.88 Healing is characterised by thinning and vascularisation.

Ulcerative keratitis in rheumatoid arthritis

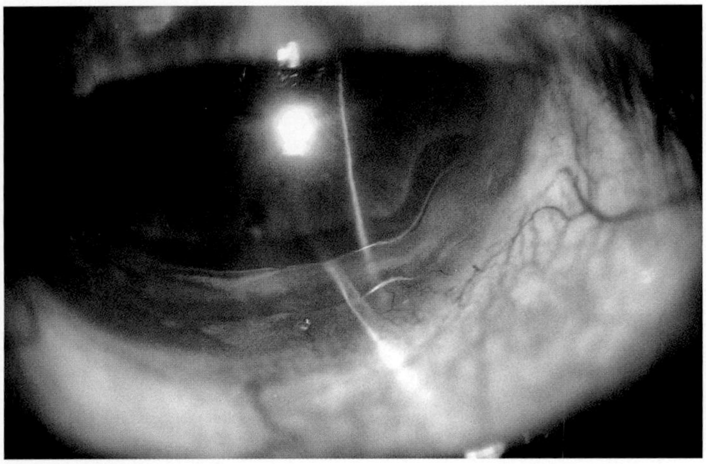

■ **Fig. 6.89** Gradual resorption of peripheral stroma leaving the epithelium intact. (Courtesy of M. Ko-Hua Chen.)

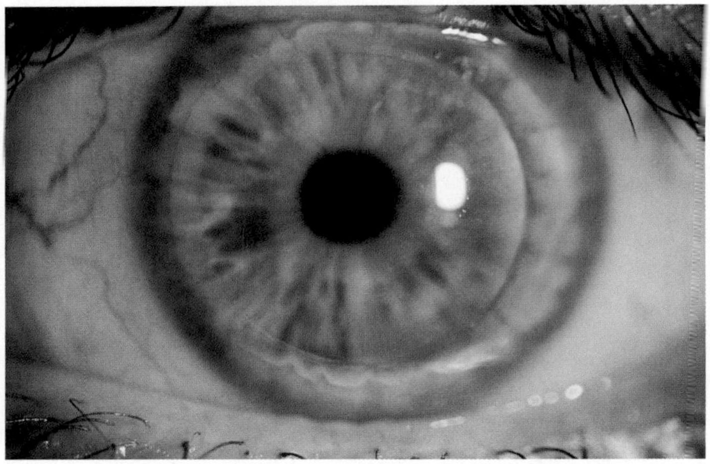

■ **Fig. 6.90** Circumferential spread in which the normal central cornea resembles a contact lens placed on the eye.

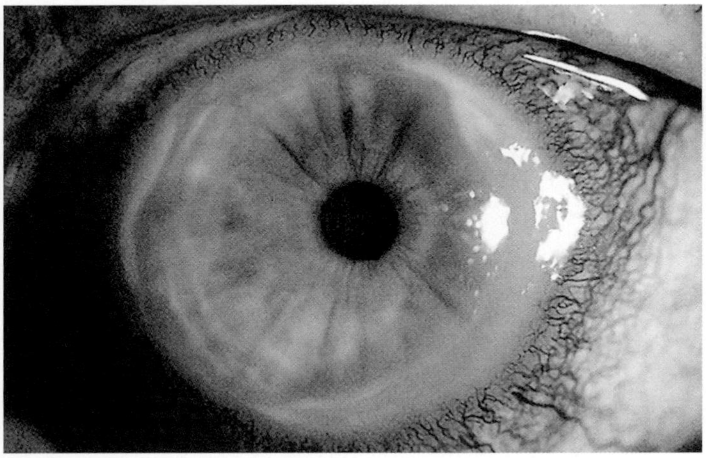

■ **Fig. 6.91** Peripheral ulceration associated with intense inflammation at the limbus.

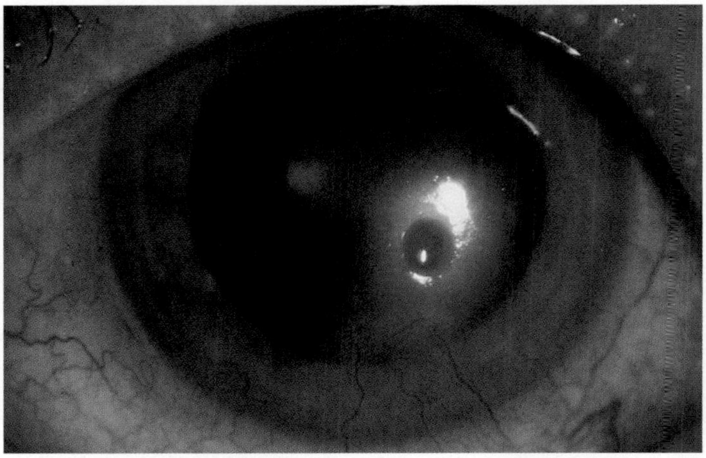

■ **Fig. 6.92** Central melting is uncommon. (Courtesy of R. Curtis.)

Ulcerative keratitis in systemic vasculitides

The two most important systemic vasculitides associated with ulcerative keratitis are Wegener granulomatosis and polyarteritis nodosa.

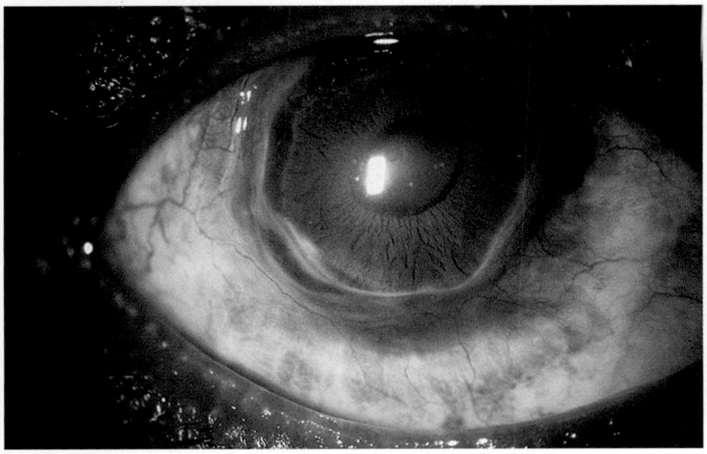

■ **Fig. 6.93** Progressive circumferential ulceration.

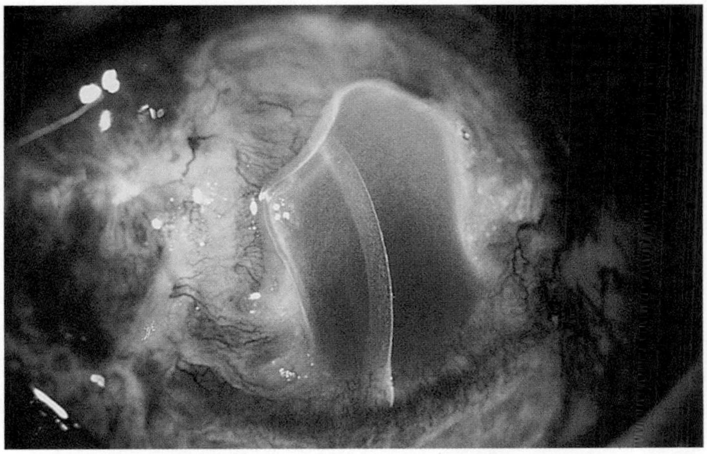

■ **Fig. 6.94** Occasionally central and peripheral spread to involve the sclera, unlike Mooren ulcer.

CORNEAL DEGENERATIONS

Corneal arcus

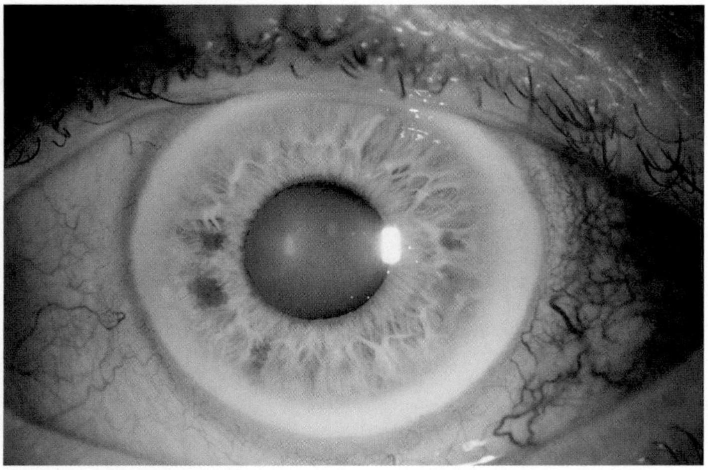

■ **Fig. 6.95** Bilateral, white circumferential band in the perilimbal cornea that is separated from the limbus by a thin clear zone.

Vogt limbal girdle

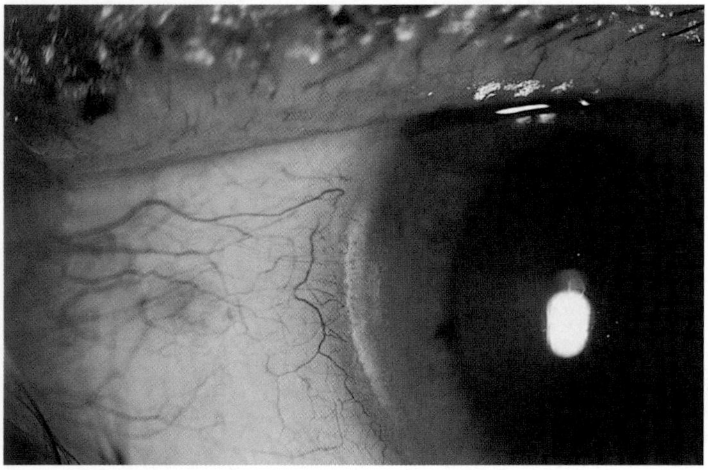

■ **Fig. 6.96** Bilateral, narrow, crescentic lines composed of chalk-like flecks running in the interpalpebral fissure along the nasal and temporal limbus. Type 1 is separated from the limbus by a clear interval but type 2 is not.

Crocodile shagreen of Vogt

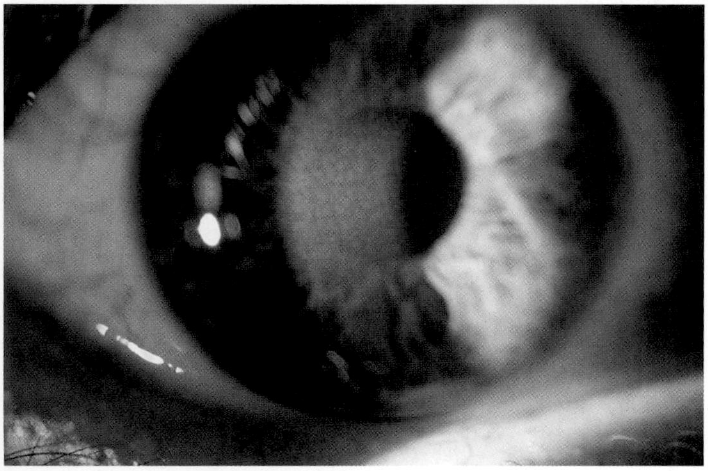

■ **Fig. 6.97** Greyish-white, polygonal opacities in the anterior third of the stroma, separated by relatively clear spaces.

Cornea guttata

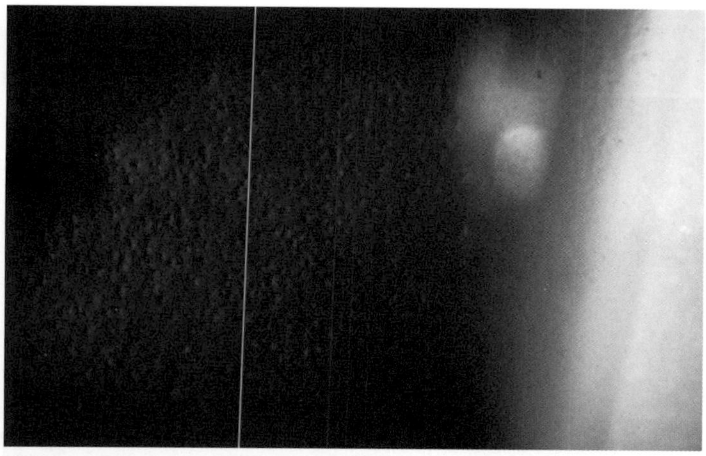

■ **Fig. 6.98** Specular reflection shows tiny dark spots caused by disruption of the regular endothelial mosaic.

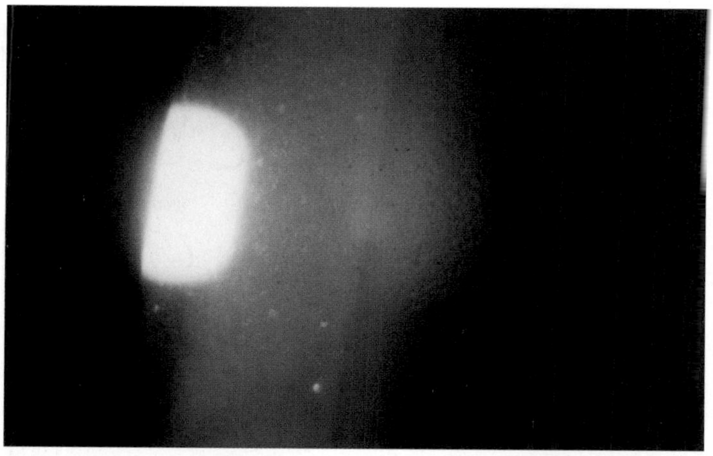

■ **Fig. 6.99** In more advanced cases, there is a 'beaten metal' appearance.

Lipid keratopathy

Primary

This is rare and occurs in the absence of previous keratitis.

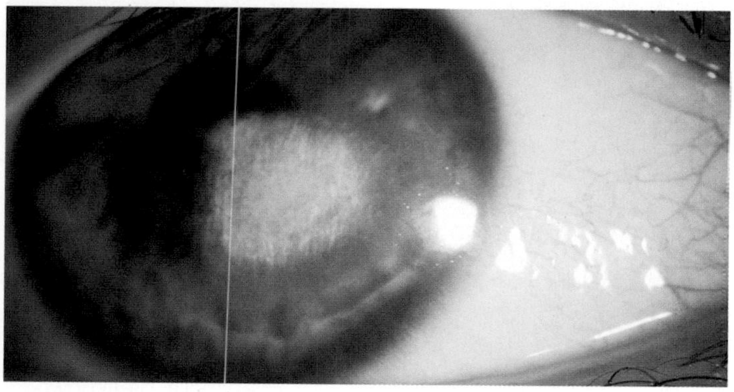

■ **Fig. 6.100** White or yellowish stromal deposits not associated with vascularisation.

Secondary

This is common and most frequently associated with previous simplex or zoster disciform keratitis.

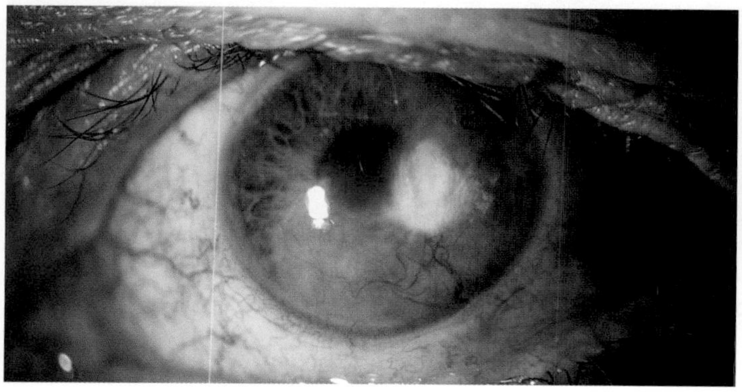

■ **Fig. 6.101** White stromal deposits associated with vascularisation.

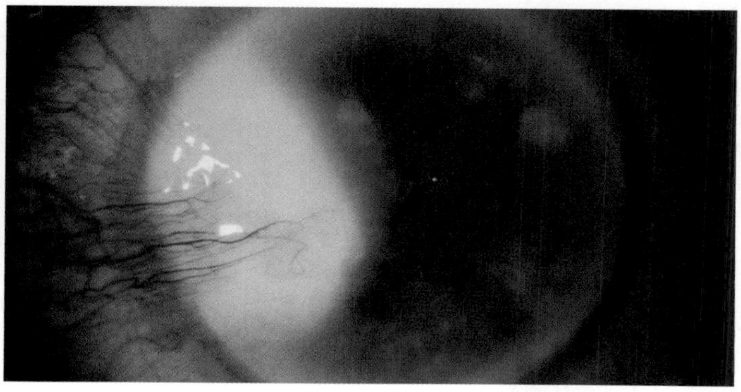

■ **Fig. 6.102** More severe secondary lipid keratopathy. (Courtesy of P. Gili.)

Terrien marginal degeneration

Terrien marginal degeneration is an uncommon, idiopathic, non-inflammatory thinning of the peripheral cornea.

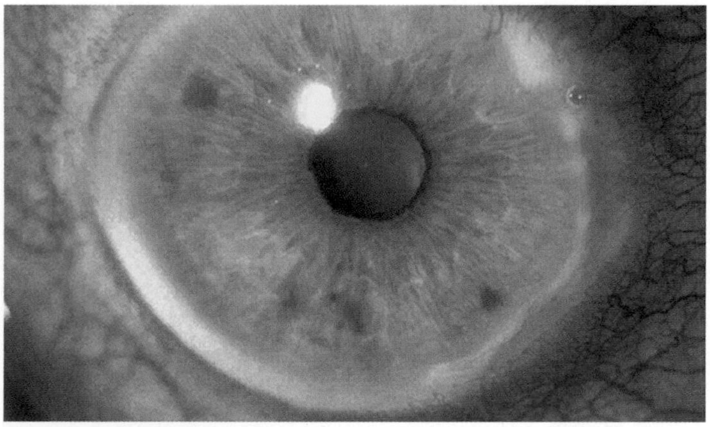

Fig. 6.114 Progressive circumferential thinning. (Courtesy of S. Ford and R. Marsh.)

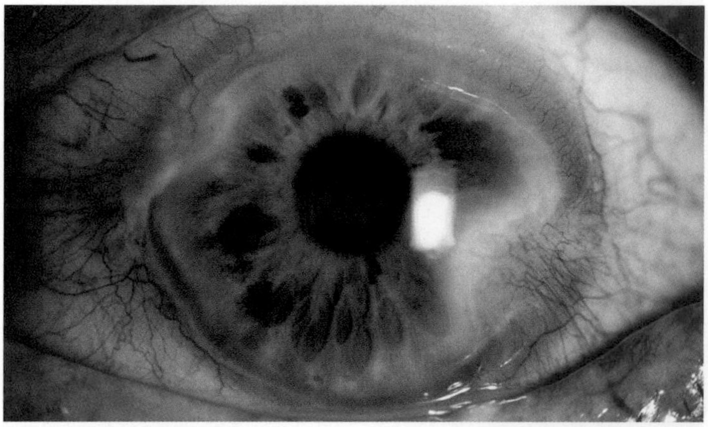

Fig. 6.115 Pseudopterygium formation. (Courtesy of P. Gili.)

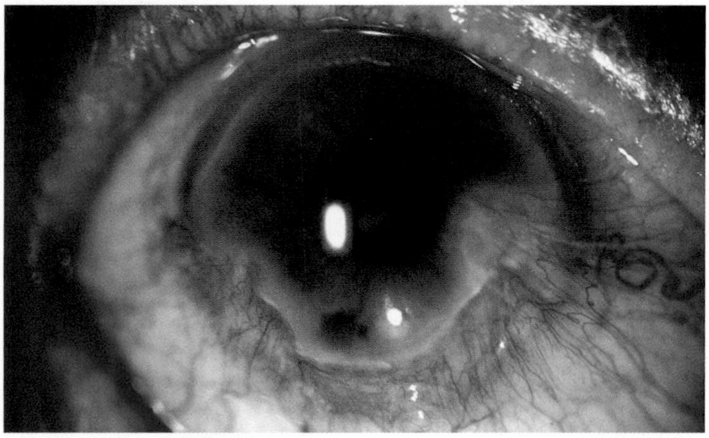

Fig. 6.116 Extensive pseudopterygium formation in long-standing cases at positions other than the 9 o'clock and 3 o'clock meridia. (Courtesy of P. Gili.)

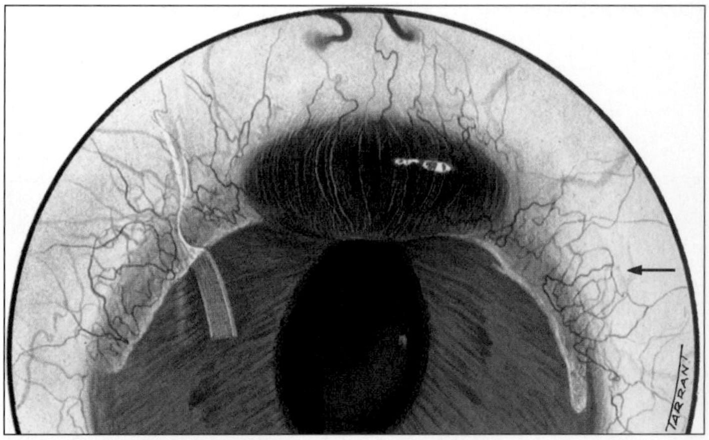

Fig. 6.117 Perforation may rarely occur either spontaneously or following blunt trauma. (Courtesy of T. A. Casey and K. W. Sharif.)

Amyloid degeneration

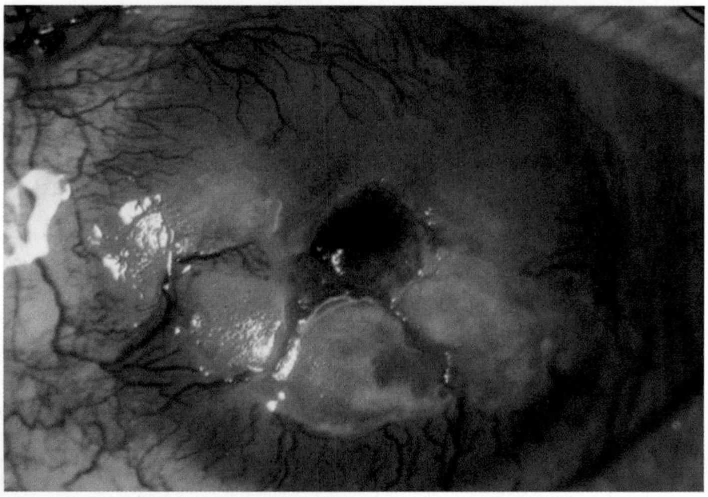

Fig. 6.118 Superficial, irregular nodular deposits associated with previous chronic keratitis.

CORNEAL DYSTROPHIES

Epithelial dystrophies

Basement membrane dystrophy

Also known as Cogan microcystic or map–dot–fingerprint dystrophy, it is neither familial nor progressive. Onset is in the second decade. About 10% of patients develop recurrent corneal erosions.

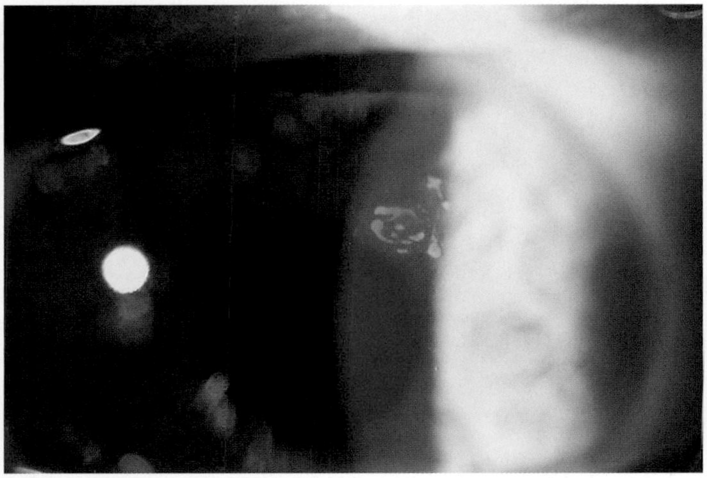

Fig. 6.119 Dot-like opacities.

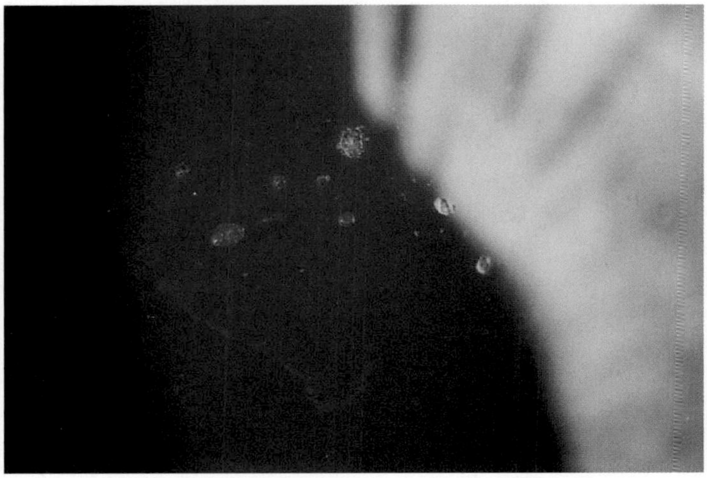

Fig. 6.120 Epithelial microcysts.

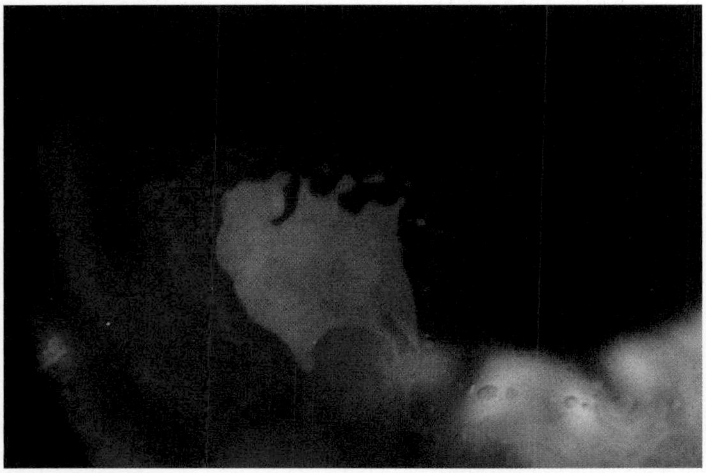

Fig. 6.121 Subepithelial map-like patterns. (Courtesy of J. Talks.)

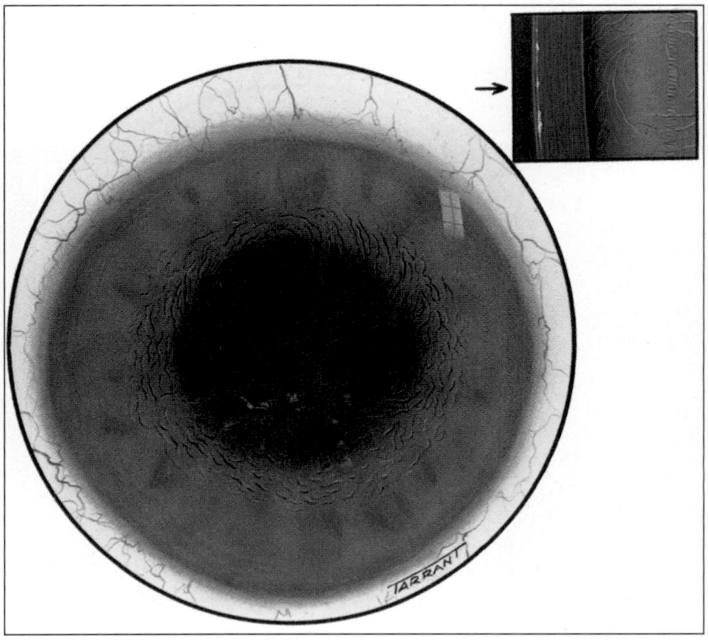

Fig. 6.122 Whorled fingerprint-like lines. (Courtesy of T. A. Casey and K. W. Sharif.)

Meesman dystrophy

Inheritance is autosomal dominant (AD) with the gene locus on 12q13 or 17q12. Onset is in the first 2 years of life with ocular irritation.

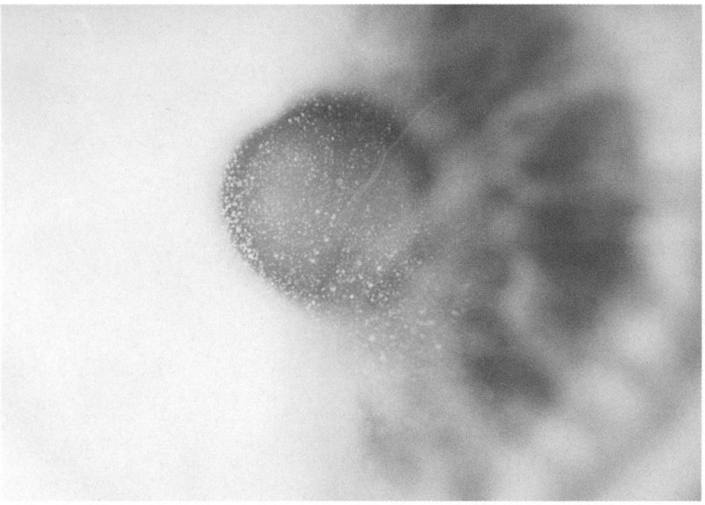

■ **Fig. 6.123** Myriads of tiny intraepithelial cysts of uniform size but variable density.

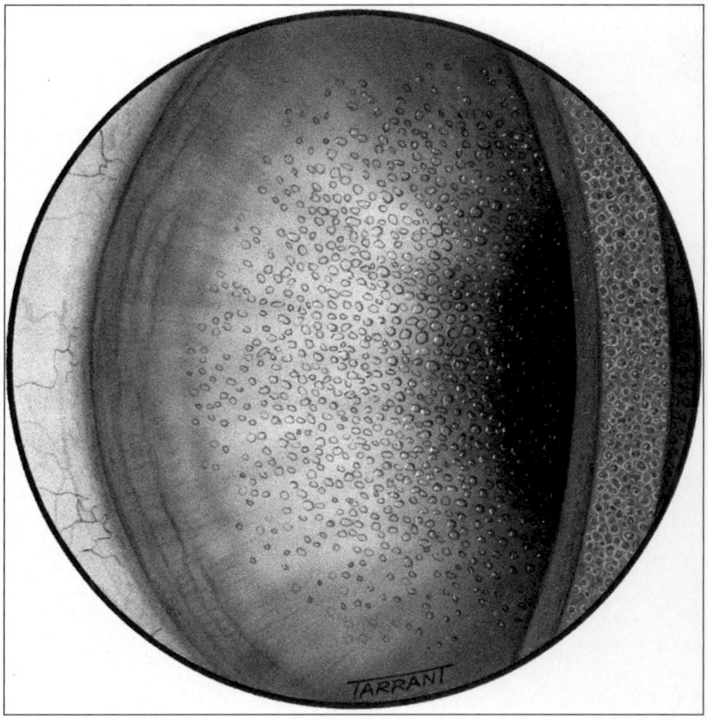

■ **Fig. 6.124** The lesions are better seen on retroillumination.

Lisch dystrophy

Inheritance is either AD or X-linked dominant with the gene locus on Xp22.3.

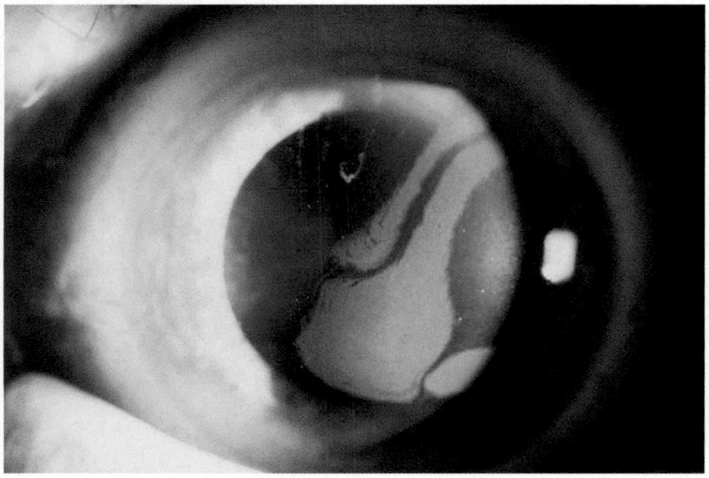

■ **Fig. 6.125** Grey, band-like stripes with a whorled or wheel-spotted pattern. (Courtesy of W. Lisch.)

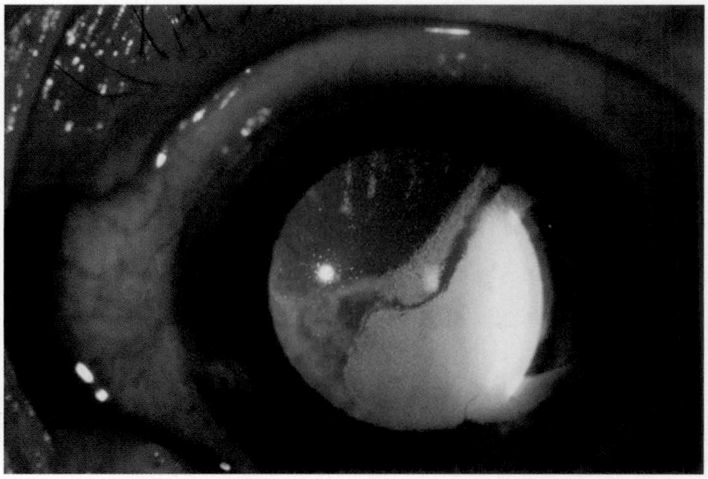

■ **Fig. 6.126** On retroillumination, the opacities consist of clear, densely crowded microcysts. (Courtesy of W. Lisch.)

Bowman layer dystrophies

Reis–Bucklers dystrophy (Bowman layer type 1)

Inheritance is AD with the gene locus on 5q31. Onset is in early childhood with recurrent erosions.

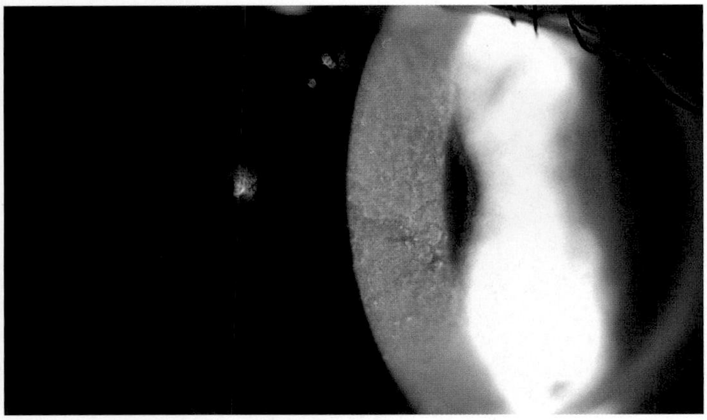

Fig. 6.127 Grey-white, fine, round and polygonal opacities in Bowman layer, most dense centrally.

Thiel–Behnke dystrophy (Bowman layer type 2)

Inheritance is AD with the gene locus on 10q24. Onset is at the end of the first decade with recurrent erosions.

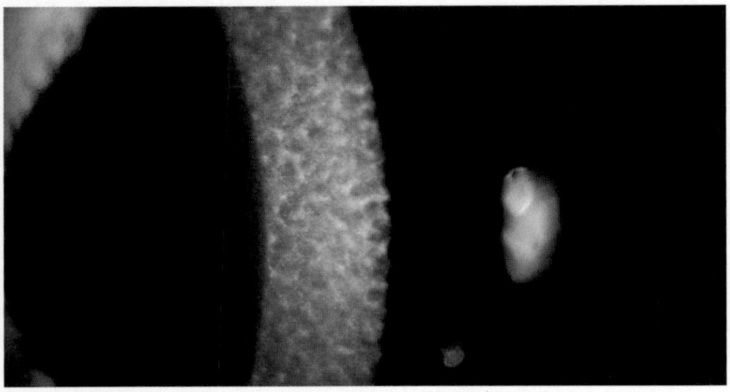

Fig. 6.128 Similar to Reis–Bucklers dystrophy except that the opacities have a more distinct honeycomb pattern.

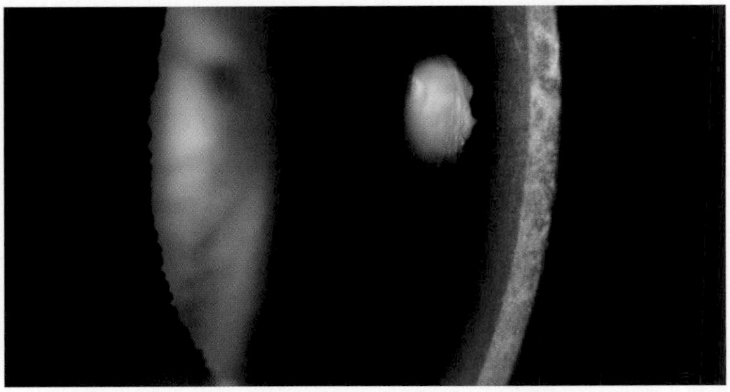

Fig. 6.129 Slit view showing the superficial location of the lesions.

Central Schnyder (crystalline) dystrophy

Inheritance is AD with the gene locus on 1p36–p34.1. Onset is in the second decade with visual impairment, and g are.

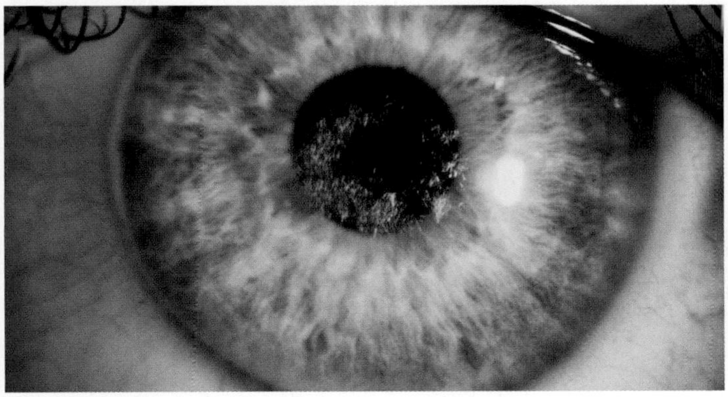

Fig. 6.130 Central, oval area of scintillating, subepithelial 'crystalline' opacity in a generally hazy cornea. (Courtesy of S. Ford and R. Marsh.)

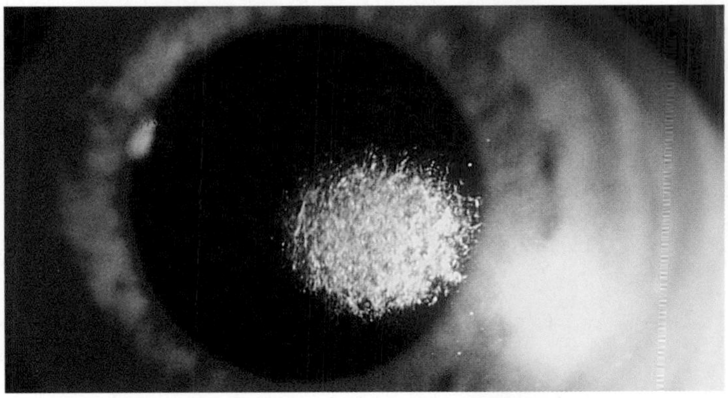

Fig. 6.131 A more compact crystalline opacity. (Courtesy of K. Nischal.)

Stromal dystrophies

Lattice dystrophy type 1 (Biber–Haab–Dimmer)

Inheritance is AD with the gene locus on 5q31. Onset is at the end of the first decade with recurrent erosions, which precede typical stromal changes.

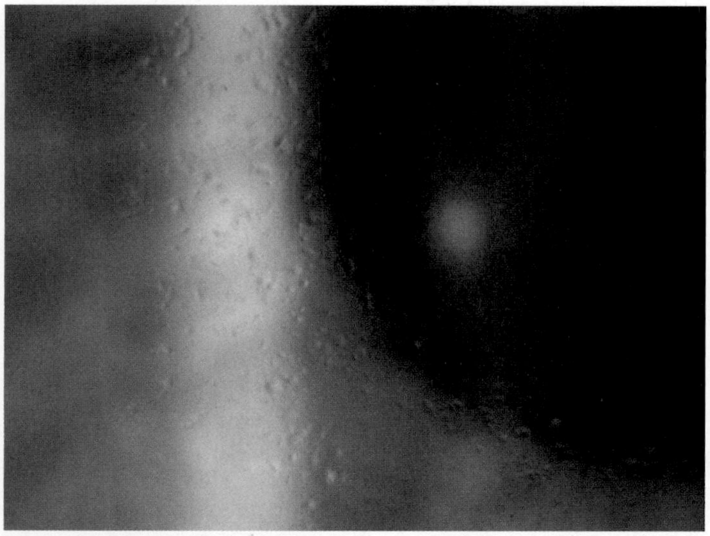

Fig. 6.132 Anterior stromal, glassy, refractile dots. (Courtesy of T. A. Casey and K. W. Sharif.)

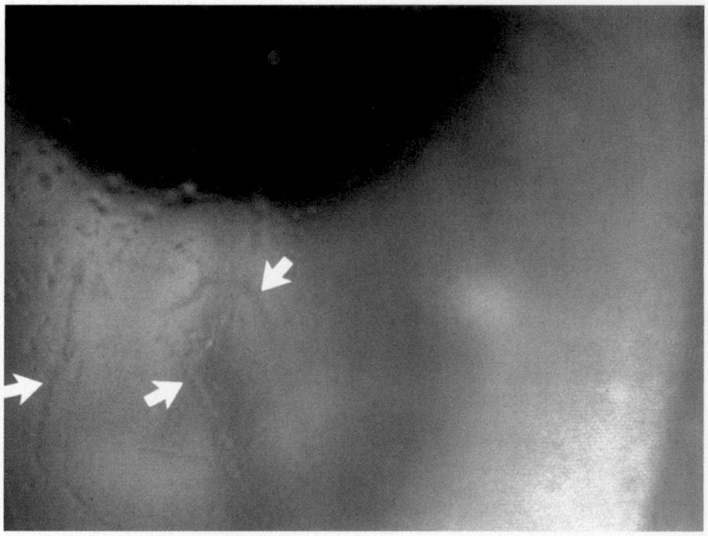

Fig. 6.133 Subtle lattice lines (arrows). (Courtesy of T. A. Casey and K. W. Sharif.)

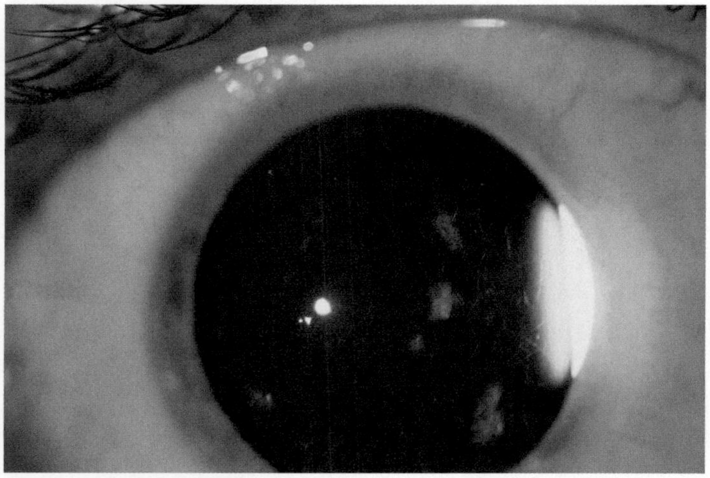

Fig. 6.134 Fine, anterior stromal, spidery, branching lattice lines, best seen on retroillumination. (Courtesy of W. Lisch.)

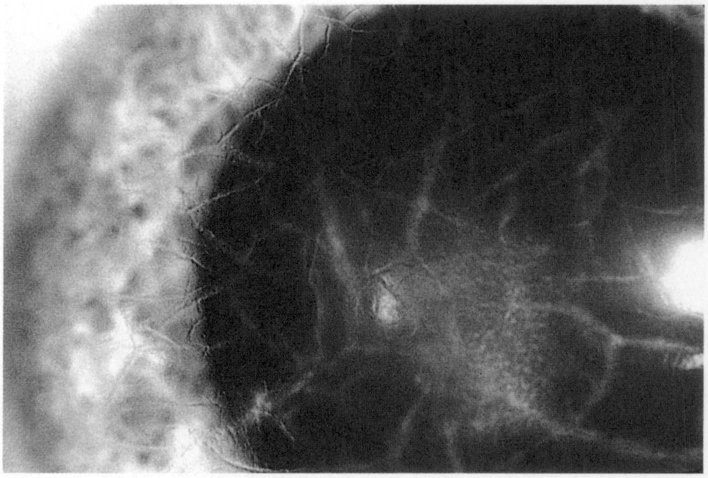

Fig. 6.135 Anterior stromal haze.

Lattice dystrophy type 2 (Meretoja syndrome)

Inheritance is AD with the gene locus on 9q34. Onset is in middle age with progressive facial palsy and cornea involvement. Recurrent erosions are less frequent than in type 1 lattice dystrophy.

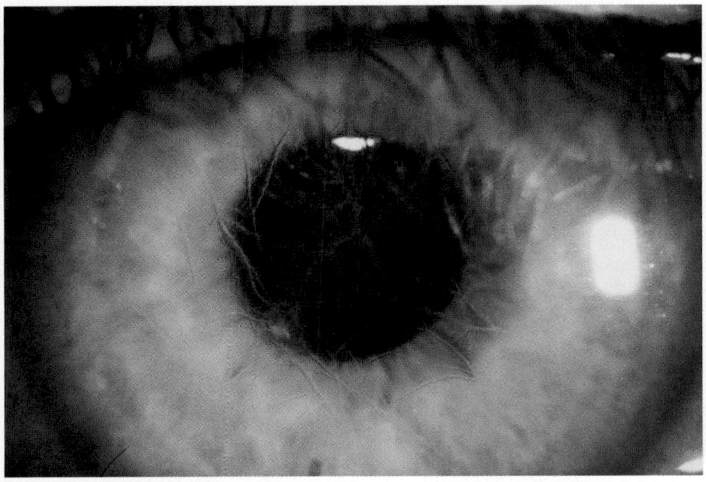

Fig. 6.136 Randomly scattered, short, fine lattice lines that are sparse, more delicate and more radially orientated than in type 1 lattice dystrophy.

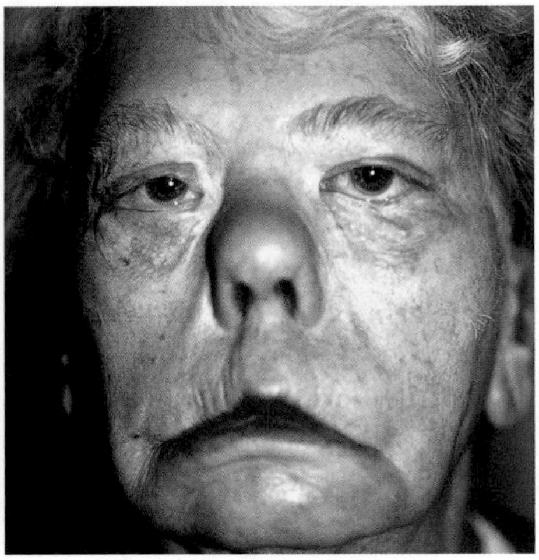

Fig. 6.137 'Mask-like' facial expression due to bilateral facial palsy.

Lattice dystrophy type 3 and 3a

Inheritance of type 3 is presumed to be autosomal recessive (AR) and that of type 3A is AD with the gene locus on 5q31 in both. Onset is between the fourth and sixth decades with visual impairment, but recurrent erosions are uncommon.

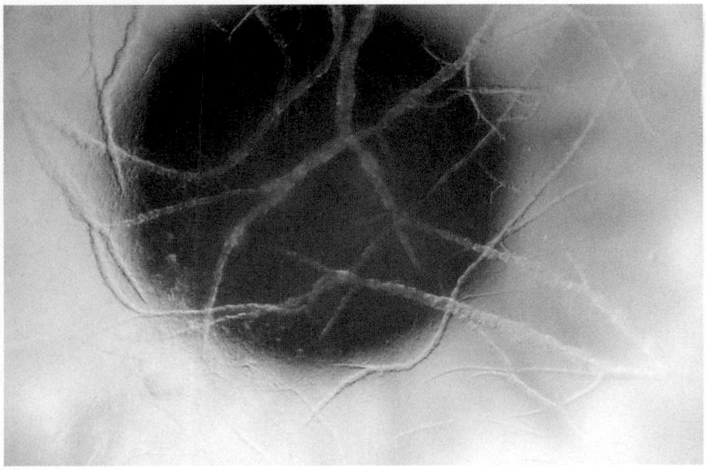

Fig. 6.138 Thick, ropy lines extending from limbus to limbus with minimal intervening haze. There may be gross asymmetry or the lesions may be unilateral for a time.

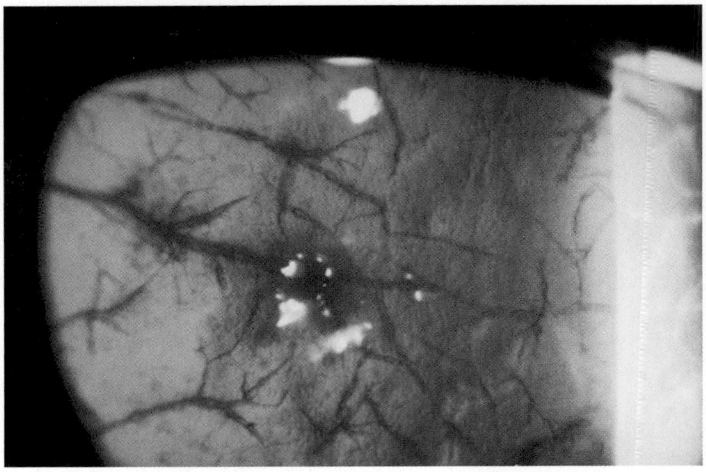

Fig. 6.139 View on retroillumination.

Granular dystrophy type 1

Inheritance is AD with the gene locus on 5q31. Onset is in the first decade with recurrent erosions.

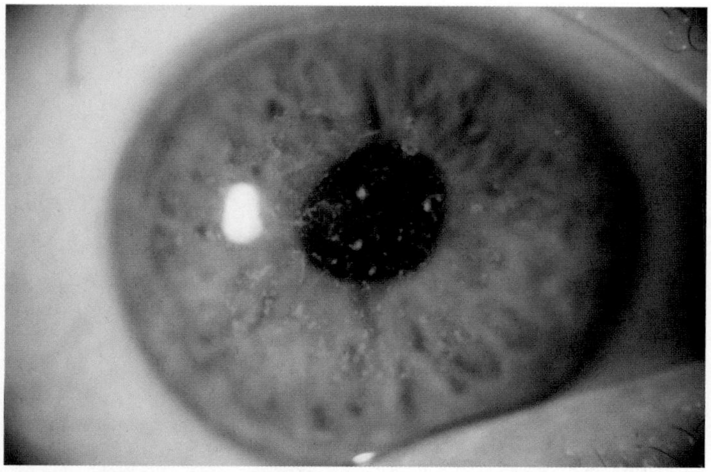

Fig. 6.140 Small, white, sharply demarcated deposits resembling crumbs or snowflakes in the central anterior stroma. (Courtesy of A. Ridgway.)

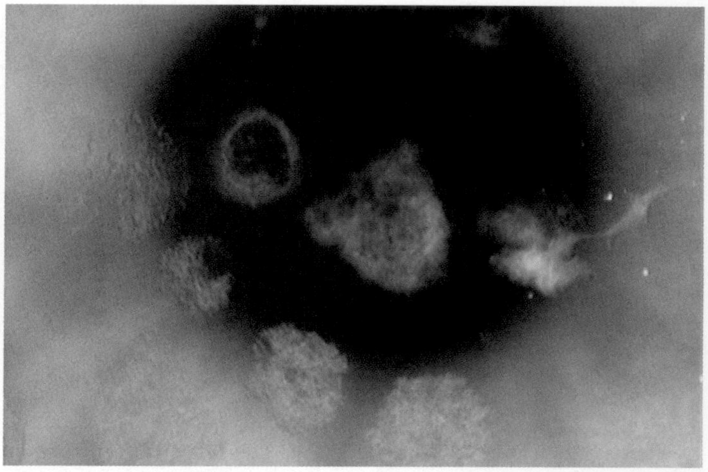

Fig. 6.141 Magnified view. (Courtesy of B. Tompkins.)

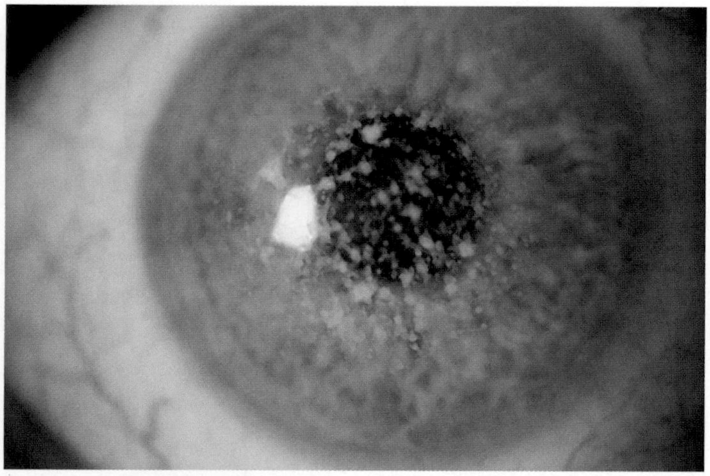

Fig. 6.142 Increase in number of lesions with deeper and outward spread but sparing the limbus. (Courtesy of A. Ridgway.)

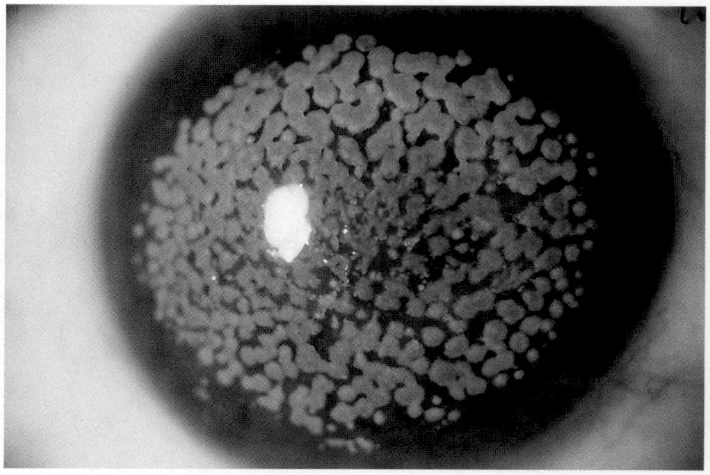

Fig. 6.143 Gradual confluence. (Courtesy of A. Ridgway.)

Granular dystrophy type 2 (Avellino)

Inheritance is AD with the gene locus on 5q31. Onset is in the first or second decade. Recurrent erosions are rare and very mild.

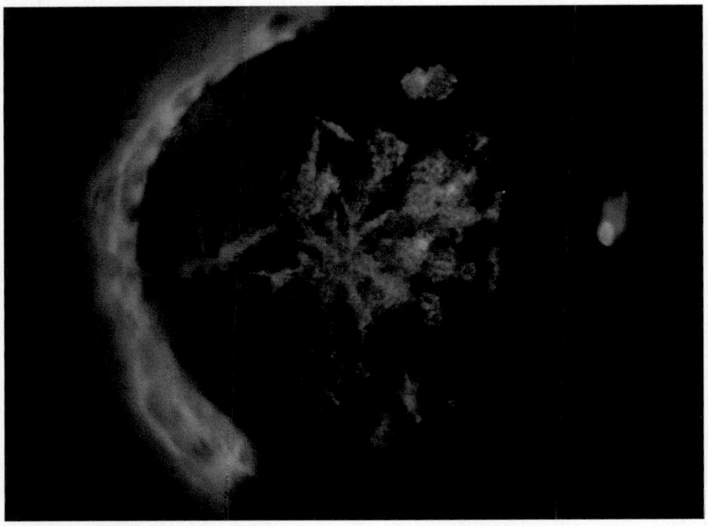

■ **Fig. 6.144** Superficial, fine opacities that resemble rings, discs, stars or snowflakes, most dense centrally, resembling those seen in granular dystrophy type 1, associated with deeper linear opacities reminiscent of lattice dystrophy. (Courtesy of W. Lisch.)

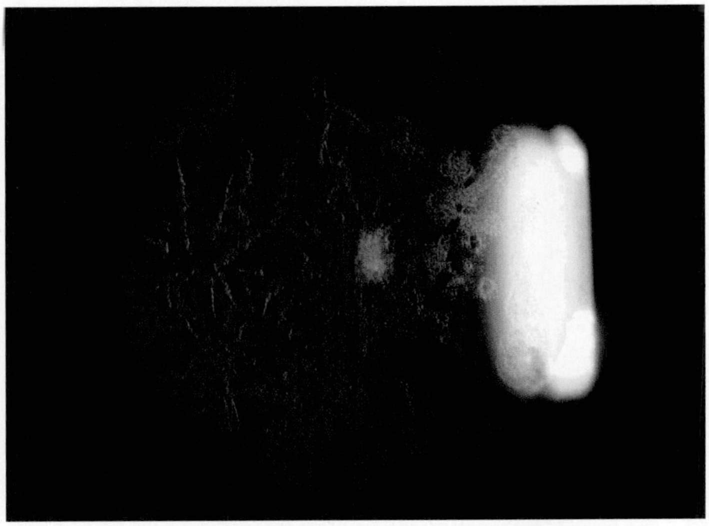

■ **Fig. 6.145** Same eye seen on retroillumination. (Courtesy of W. Lisch.)

Macular dystrophy

Inheritance is AR with the gene locus on 16q21. Onset is towards the end of the first decade with gradual visual deterioration.

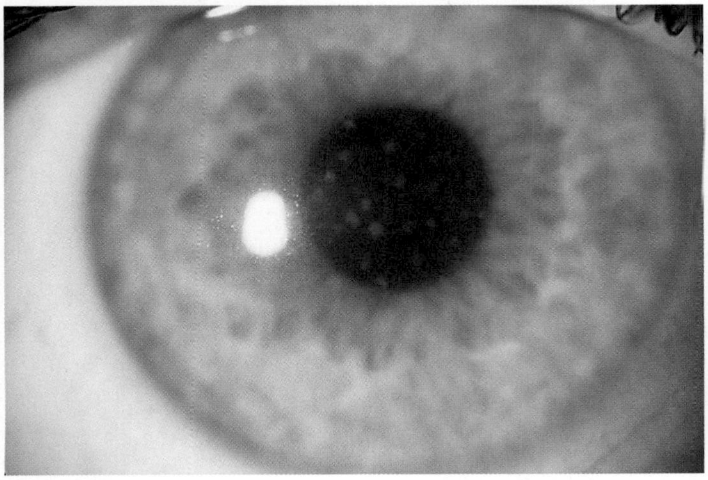

■ **Fig. 6.146** Greyish-white, dense, focal, poorly delineated spots in the superficial cornea with mild, diffuse stromal clouding. (Courtesy of A. Ridgway.)

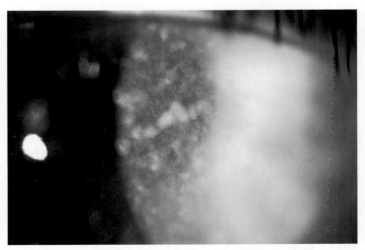

■ **Fig. 6.147** Increasing opacification and stromal haze. (Courtesy of A. Ridgway.)

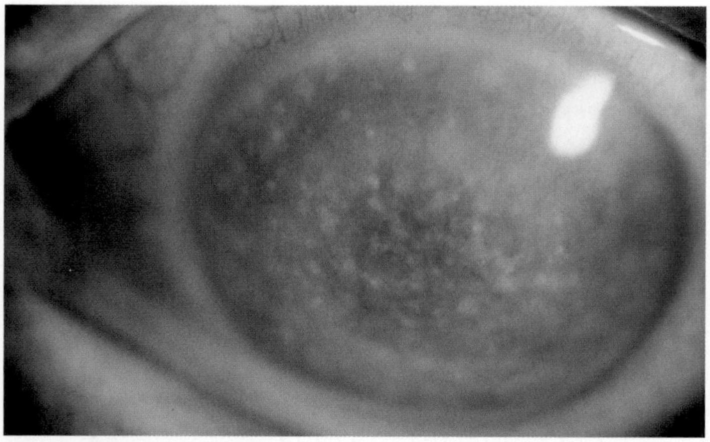

■ **Fig. 6.148** Involvement of full-thickness stroma up to the limbus. (Courtesy of A. Ridgway.)

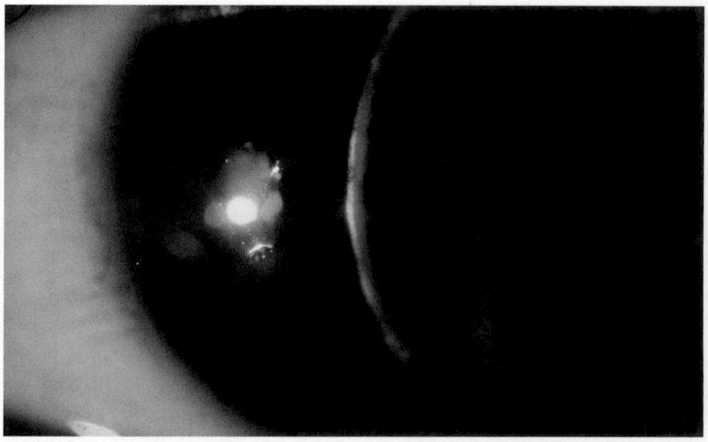

■ **Fig. 6.149** Mild corneal stromal thinning. (Courtesy of A. Ridgway.)

Gelatinous drop-like dystrophy

Inheritance is AR. Onset is in the first decade with severe photophobia, watering and visual impairment.

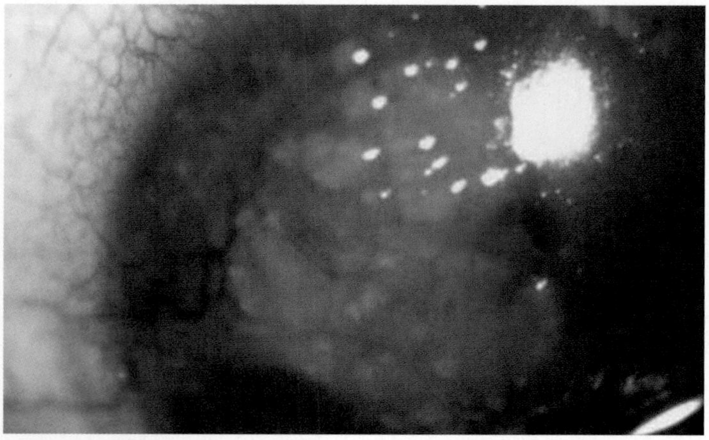

■ **Fig. 6.150** Multiple, grey, opaque, semi-spherical, gelatinous prominences. (Courtesy of Xin Tian.)

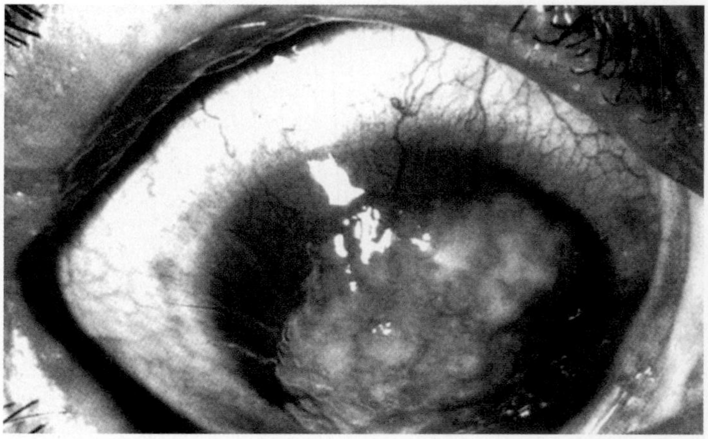

■ **Fig. 6.151** Gradual confluence and increase in size to form mulberry-like nodules. (Courtesy of T. A. Casey and K. W. Sharif.)

Central cloudy dystrophy of François

Inheritance is AD. Onset is early in the first decade.

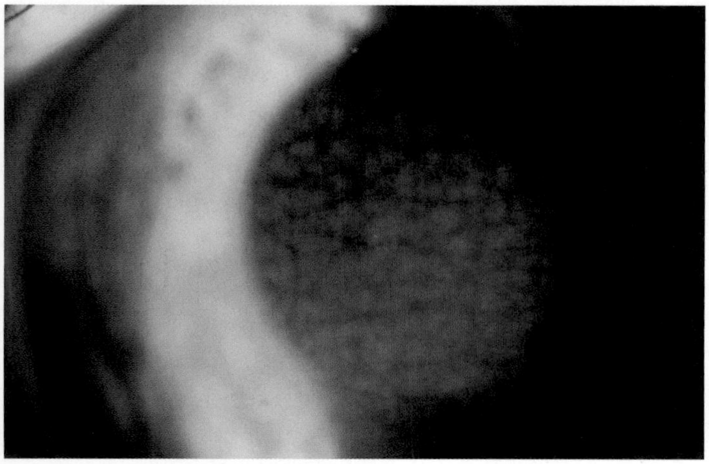

■ **Fig. 6.152** Multiple, central, greyish areas with polygonal stromal opacities and crack-like zones primarily involving the posterior half of the stroma, reminiscent of crocodile skin. (Courtesy of W. Lisch.)

Endothelial dystrophies

Fuchs endothelial dystrophy

Inheritance may occasionally be AD although the majority are sporadic.

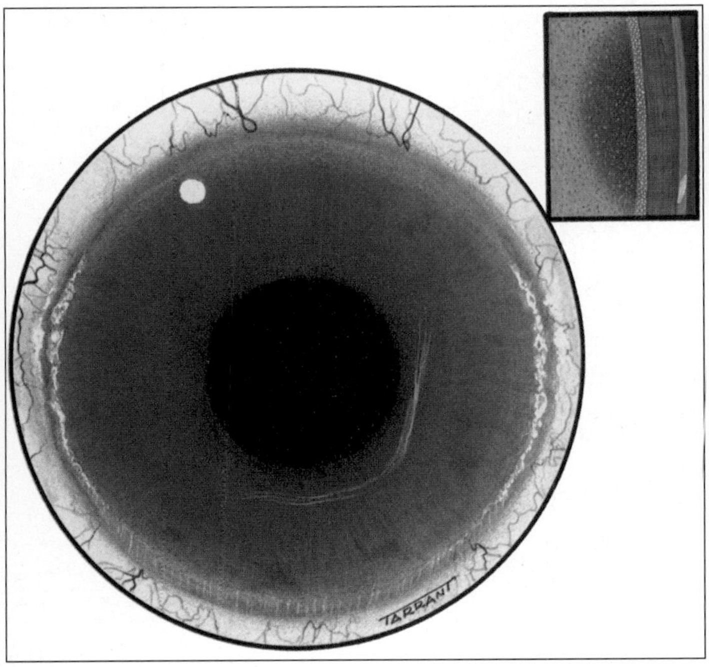

Fig. 6.153 Onset of this slowly progressive disease is in old age with the appearance of endothelial pigment dusting and guttata. (Courtesy of T. A. Casey and K. W. Sharif.)

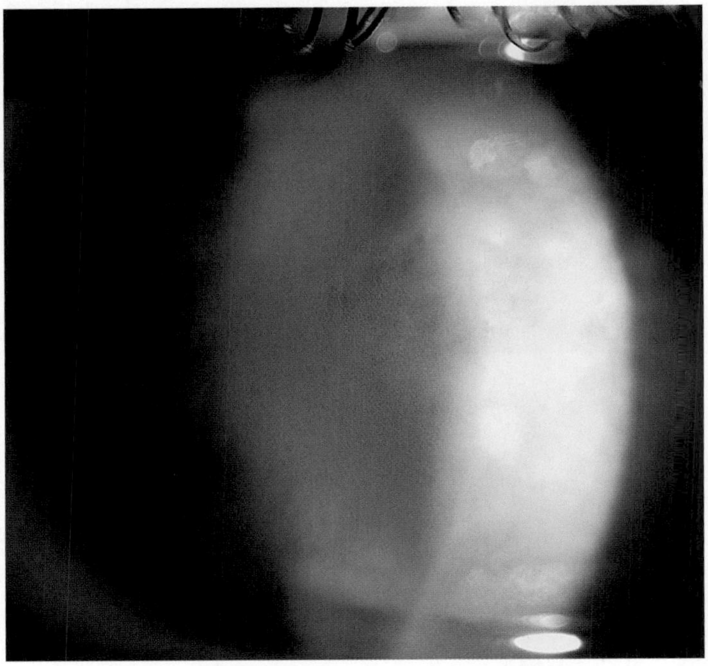

Fig. 6.154 Central epithelial oedema due to endothelial decompensation.

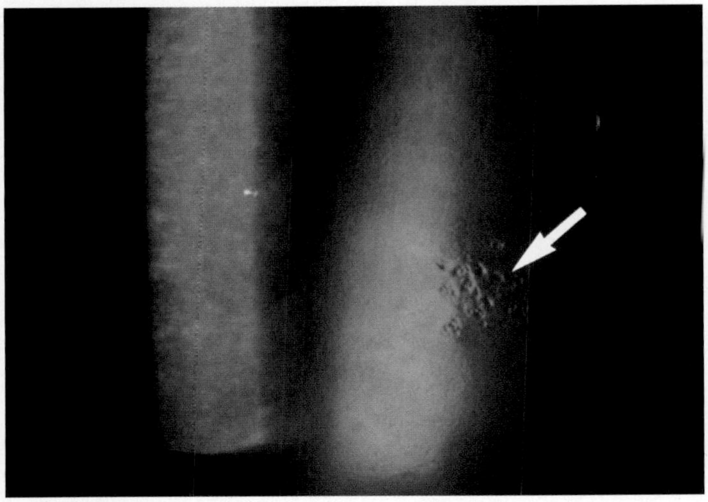

Fig. 6.155 Epithelial microcysts. (Courtesy of T. A. Casey and K. W. Sharif.)

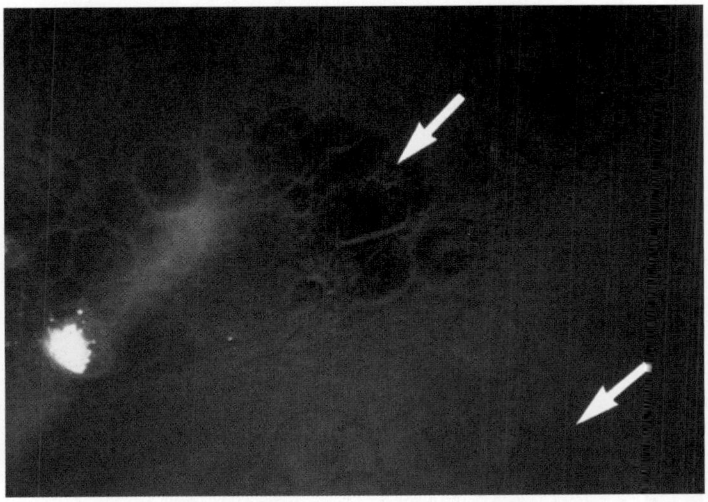

Fig. 6.156 Persistent epithelial oedema resulting in epithelial bullae (bullous keratopathy). (Courtesy of T. A. Casey and K. W. Sharif.)

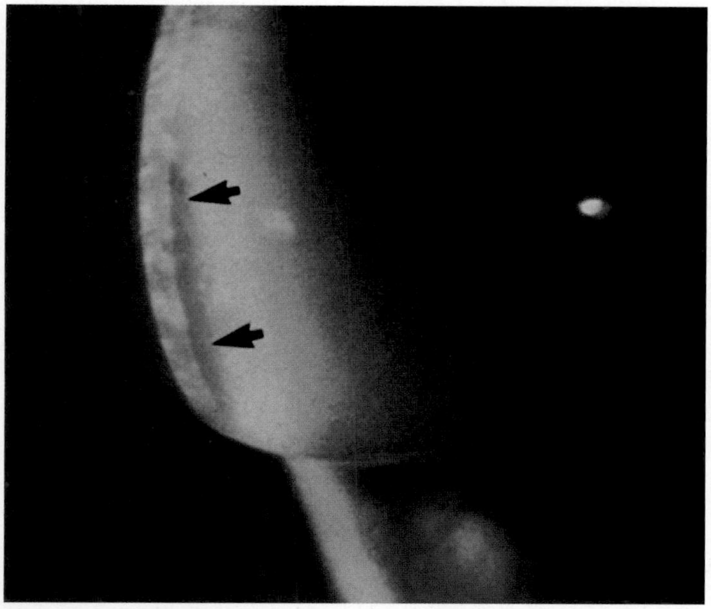

■ **Fig. 6.157** Coalescence of small bullae to form larger bullae. (Courtesy of T. A. Casey and K. W. Sharif.)

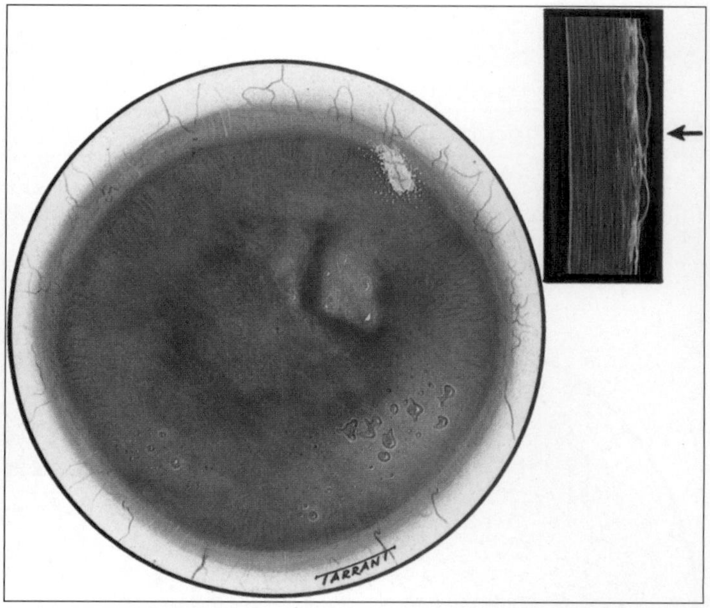

■ **Fig. 6.158** Subepithelial scarring, which may be followed by diminished corneal sensation, ulceration and vascularisation. (Courtesy of T. A. Casey and K. W. Sharif.)

Posterior polymorphous dystrophy

Inheritance is usually AD with the gene locus on chromosome 20. Onset is at birth or soon thereafter, although most cases are identified by chance in later life.

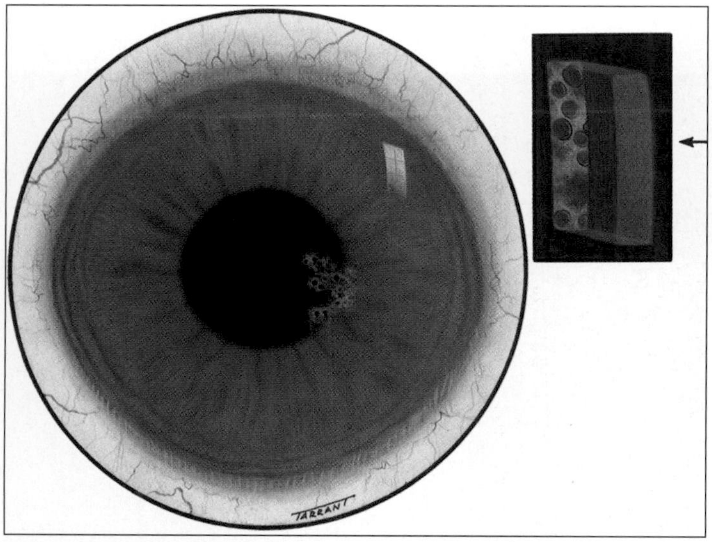

■ **Fig. 6.159** Endothelial vesicles. (Courtesy of T. A. Casey and K. W. Sharif.)

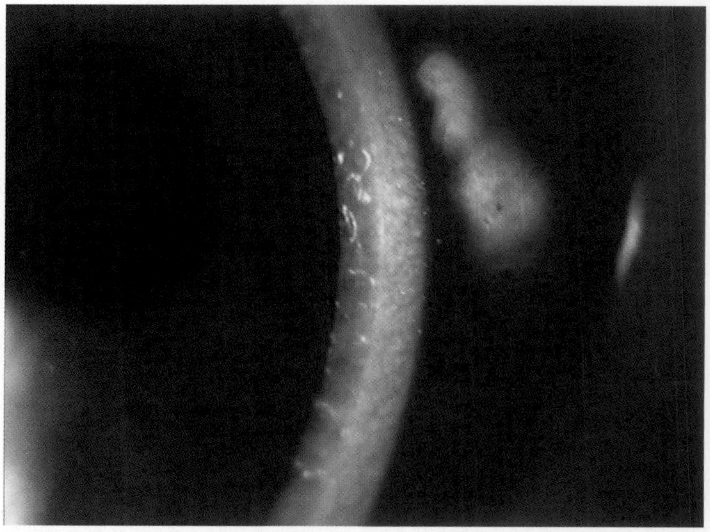

■ **Fig. 6.160** Coalescence of vesicles and grey opacification. (Courtesy of W. Lisch.)

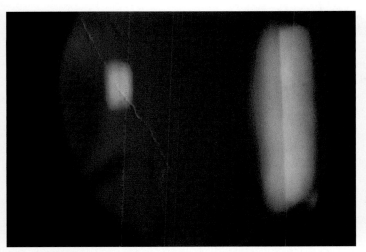

■ **Fig. 6.161** Subtle band-like lesions best seen on retroillumination. (Courtesy of W. Lisch.)

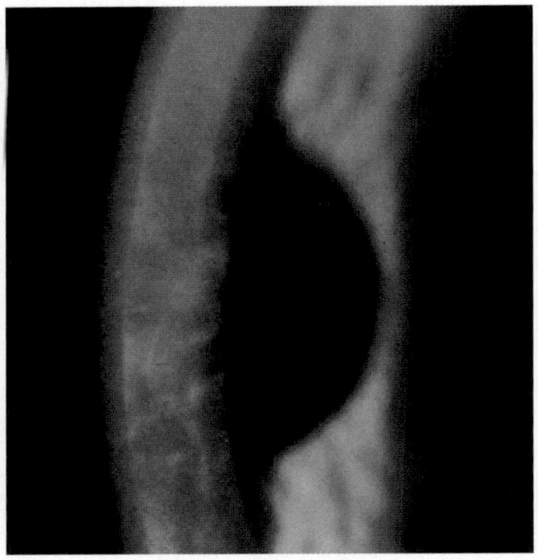

■ **Fig. 6.162** Stromal thickening and folds in Descemet membrane due to endothelial decompensation is uncommon. (Courtesy of T. A. Casey and K. W. Sharif.)

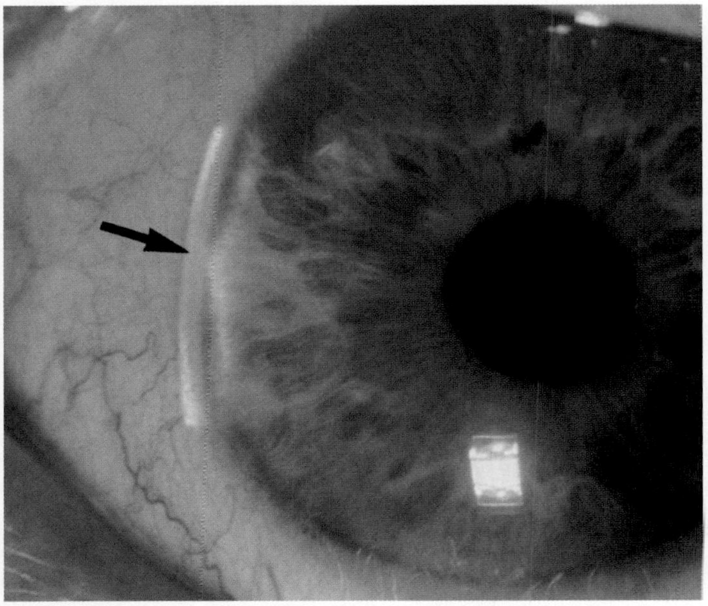

■ **Fig. 6.163** Small peripheral anterior synechiae are common. (Courtesy of T. A. Casey and K. W. Sharif.)

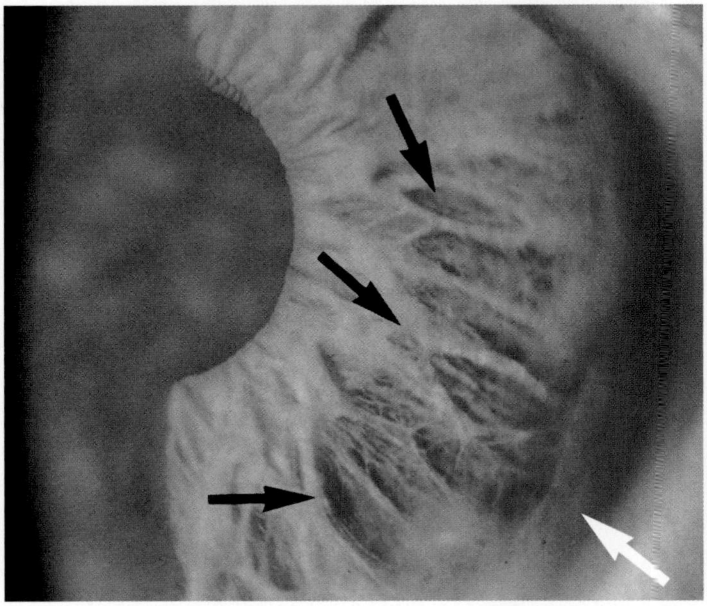

■ **Fig. 6.164** Broad-based iridocorneal adhesions (white arrow) and focal stromal iris atrophy (black arrows) are uncommon. (Courtesy of T. A. Casey and K. W. Sharif.)

Congenital hereditary endothelial dystrophy (CHED)

CHED is a rare dystrophy in which there is focal or generalised absence of corneal endothelium. There are two main forms CHED1 and CHED2, the latter being more severe. CHED1 is AD with the gene locus on 20p11.2–q11.2. CHED2 is AR with the gene locus on 20p13.

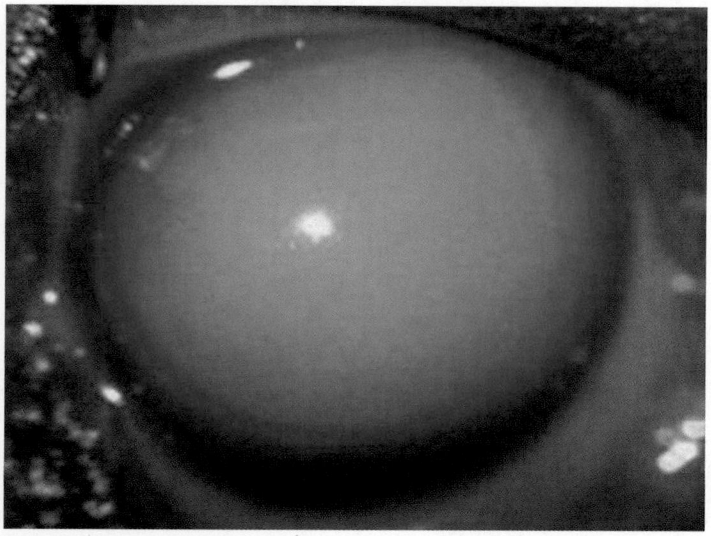

Fig. 6.165 Onset is at or shortly after birth with bilateral diffuse corneal oedema, which may have a ground-glass appearance. (Courtesy of K. Nischal.)

CORNEAL ECTASIA

Keratoconus

Keratoconus is a progressive disorder in which the cornea assumes an irregular conical shape. Onset occurs around puberty with slow progression thereafter, although the ectasia can become stationary at any time. Both eyes are affected, if only topographically, in almost all cases.

Classification

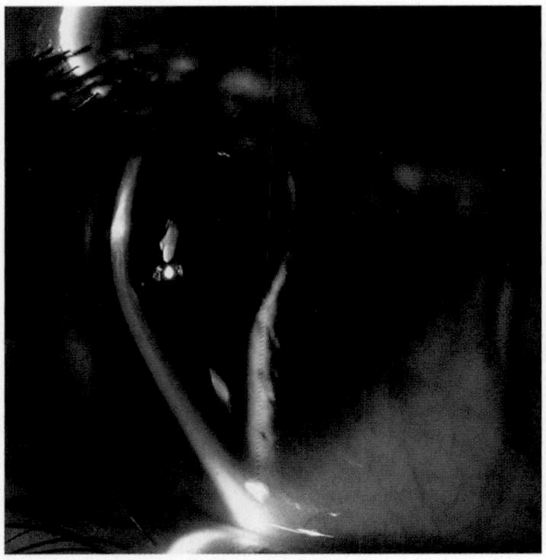

Fig. 6.166 Nipple cones are characterised by small size (5 mm) and steep curvature. The apex is central or paracentral and displaced inferonasally.

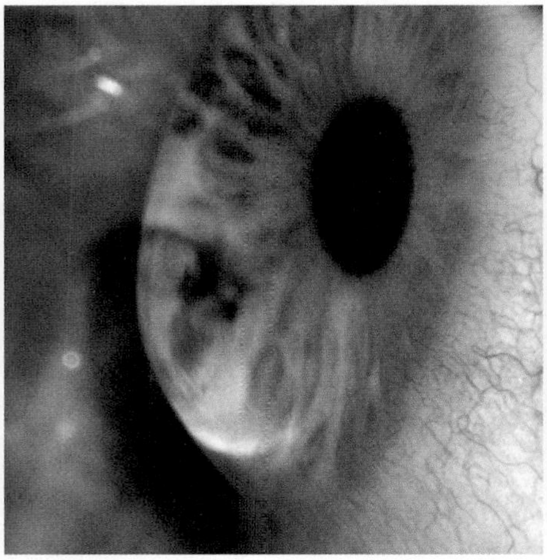

Fig. 6.167 Oval cones are larger (5–6 mm), ellipsoid and commonly decentred inferotemporally.

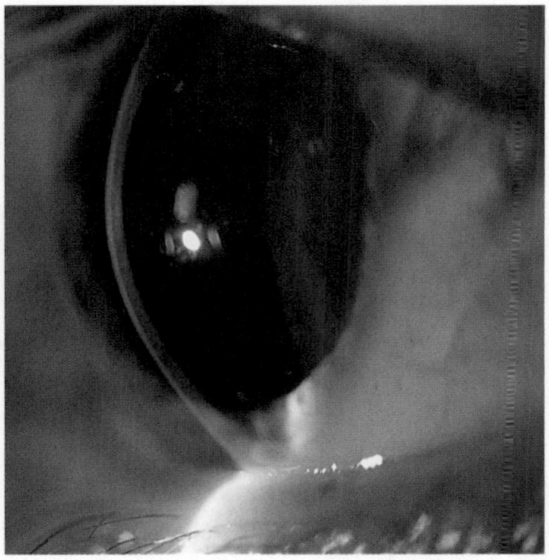

Fig. 6.168 Globus cones are the largest (>6 mm) and may involve over 75% of the cornea.

Signs

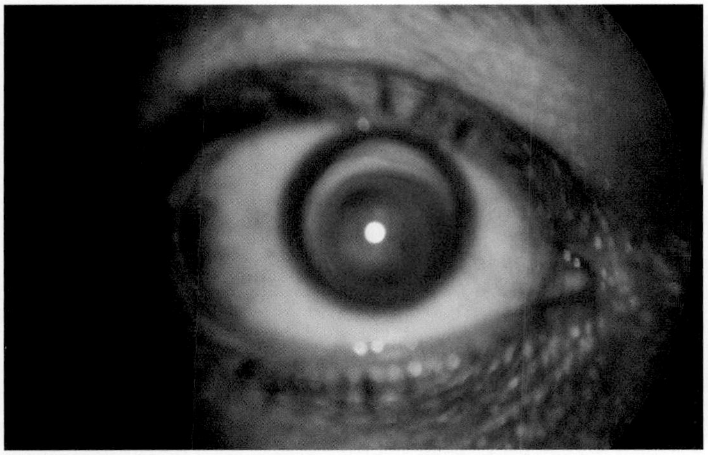

Fig. 6.169 Direct ophthalmoscopy from a distance of 30 cm shows an 'oil droplet' reflex; retinoscopy shows an irregular 'scissor' reflex.

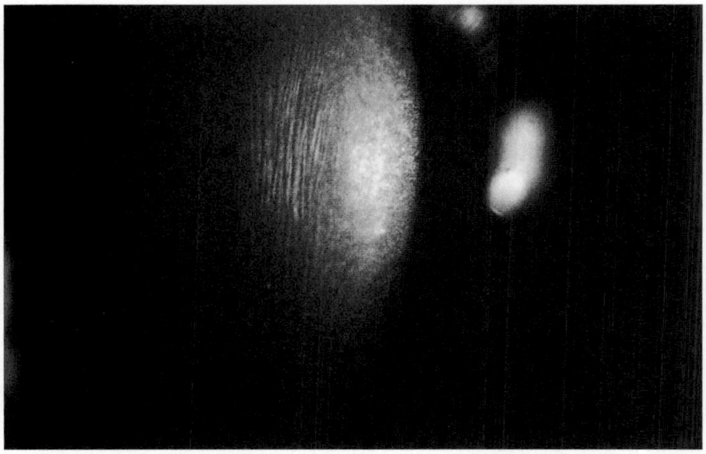

Fig. 6.170 Vogt striae are very fine, vertical, deep stromal lines that temporarily disappear with external pressure on the globe.

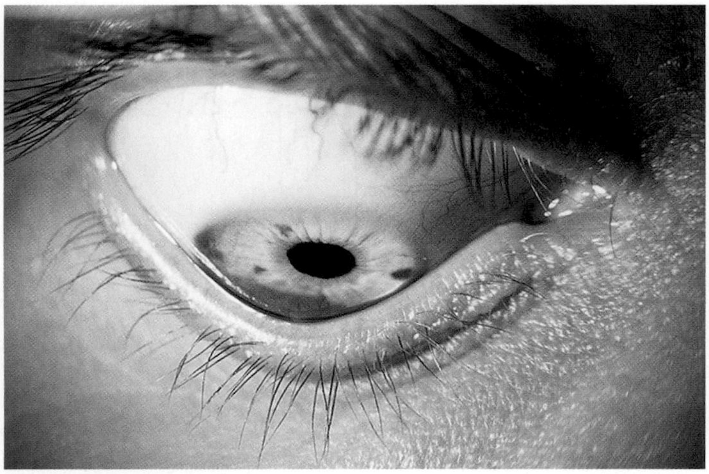

Fig. 6.171 Munson sign – bulging of the lower lid on downgaze.

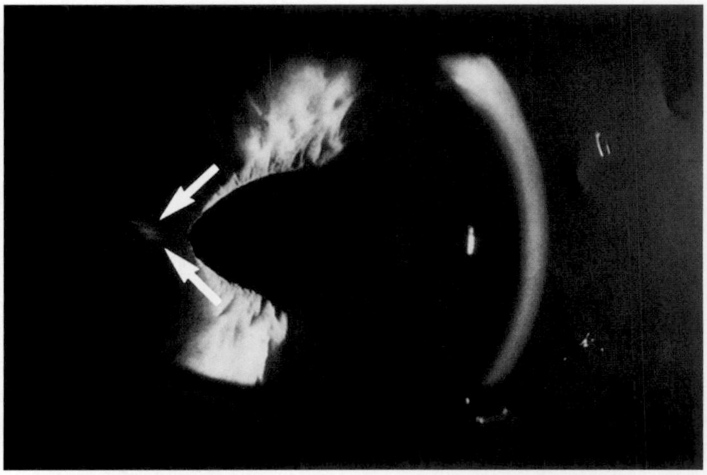

Fig. 6.172 Rezutti sign – arrowhead-shaped focus of light near the nasal limbus (arrows), produced by lateral illumination of the cornea. (Courtesy of T. A. Casey and K. W. Sharif.)

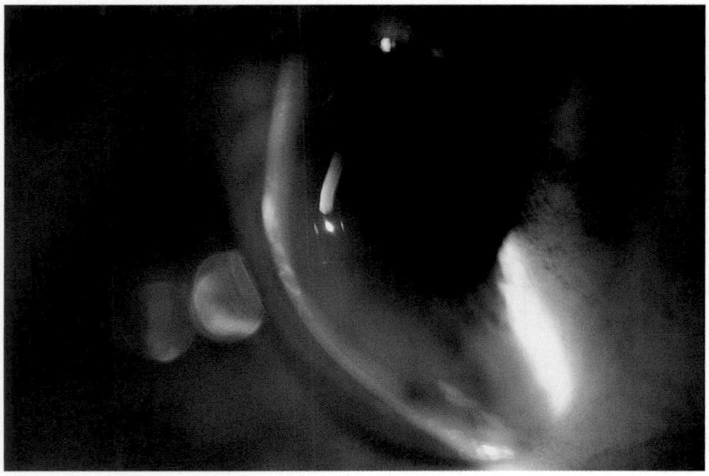

Fig. 6.173 Early apical stromal scarring.

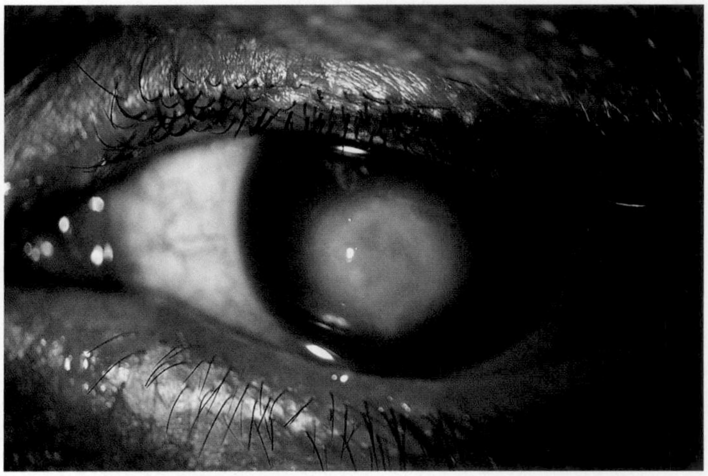

Fig. 6.174 Acute hydrops due to influx of aqueous into the cornea as a result of a rupture in Descemet membrane.

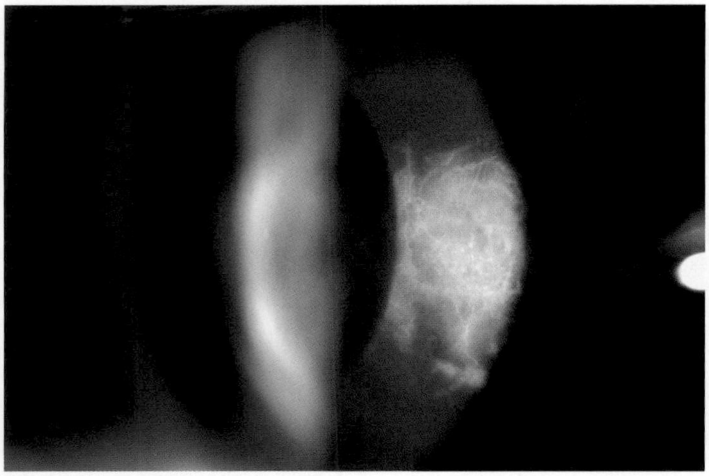

Fig. 6.175 Severe apical scarring following recurrent episodes of hydrops.

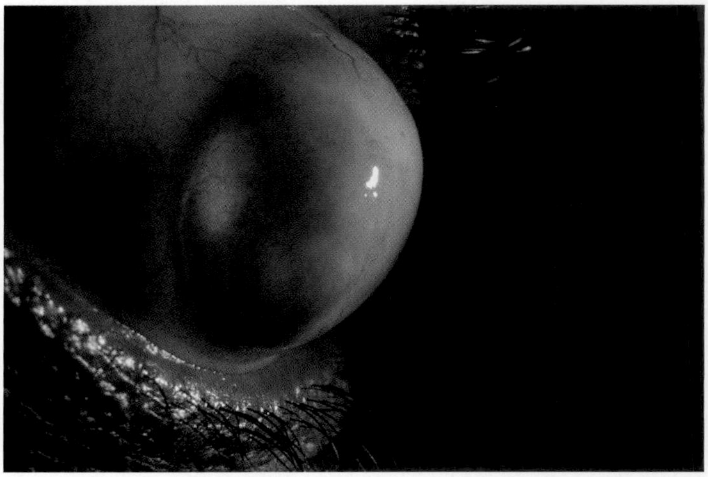

Fig. 6.176 Extensive ectasia, scarring and vascularisation in end-stage disease. (Courtesy of L. Merin.)

Ocular associations

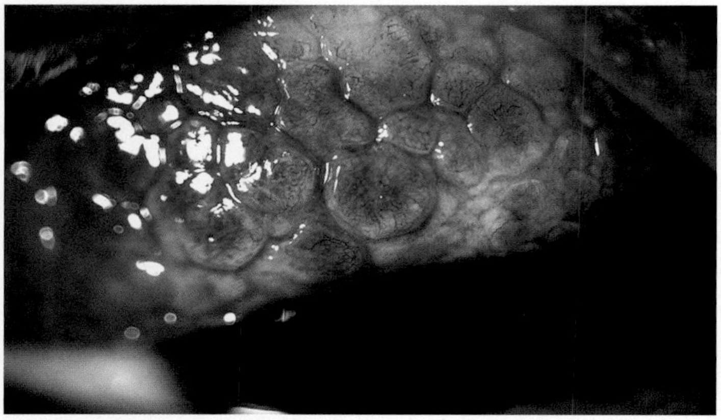

Fig. 6.177 Vernal keratoconjunctivitis.

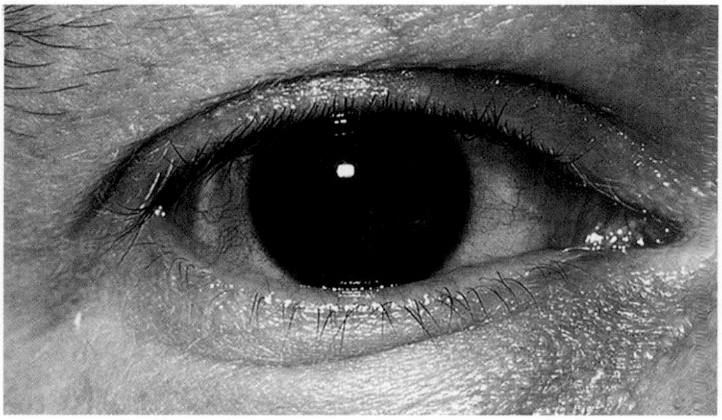

Fig. 6.178 Blue sclera.

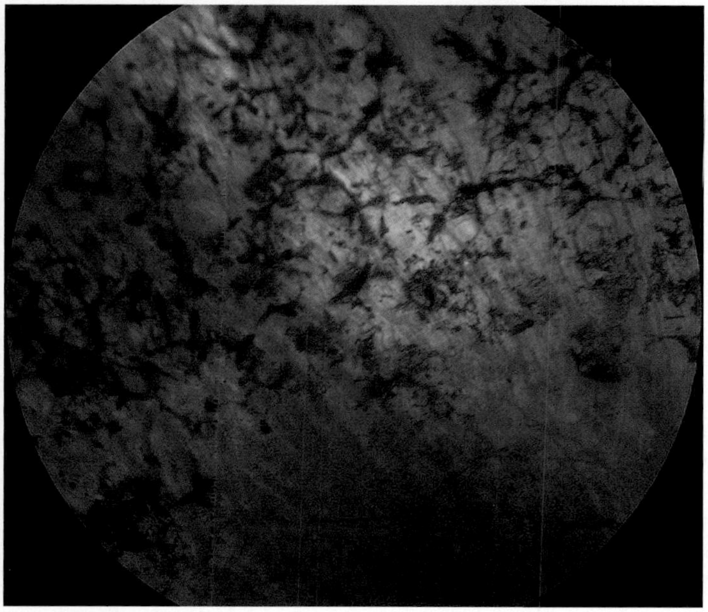

Fig. 6.179 Retinitis pigmentosa.

Important systemic associations

Down syndrome

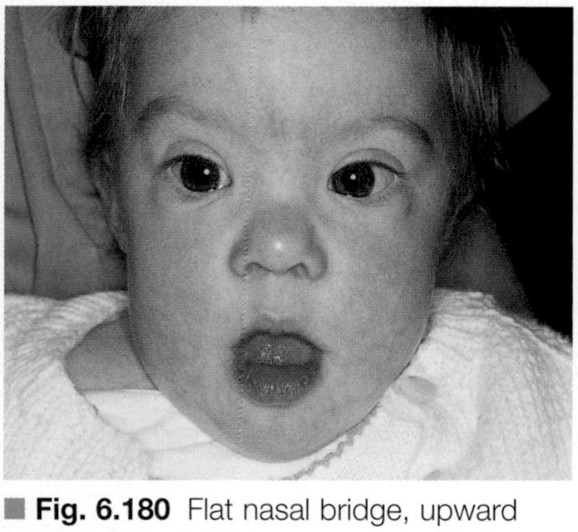

Fig. 6.180 Flat nasal bridge, upward sloping palpebral fissures, epicanthic folds, small mouth and protruding tongue, and small ears.

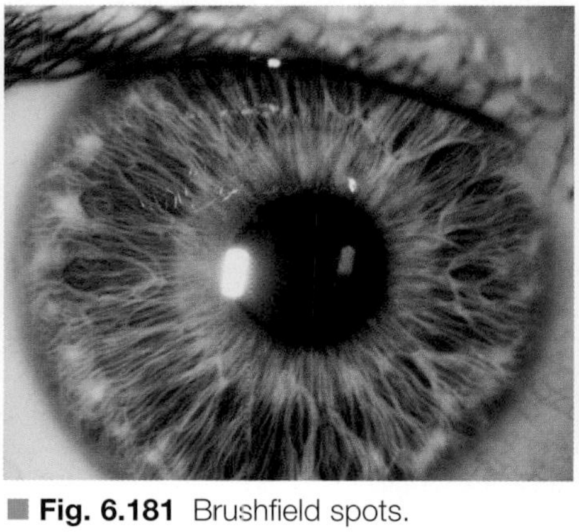

Fig. 6.181 Brushfield spots.

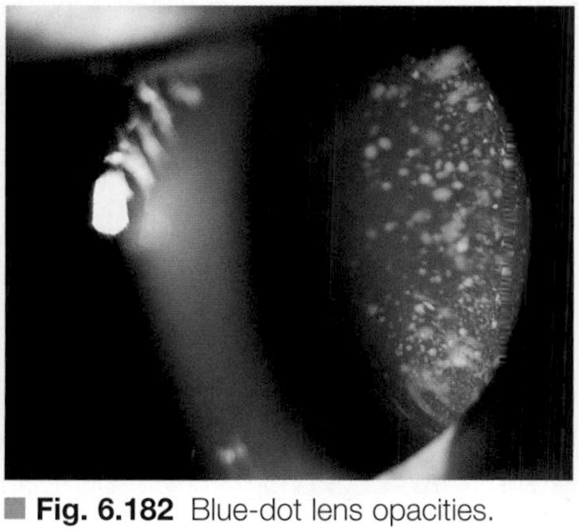

Fig. 6.182 Blue-dot lens opacities.

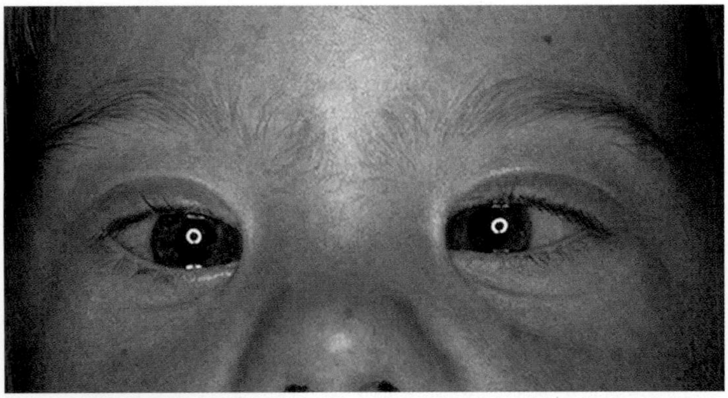

■ **Fig. 6.183** Predisposition to strabismus. (Courtesy of S. Ford and R. Marsh.)

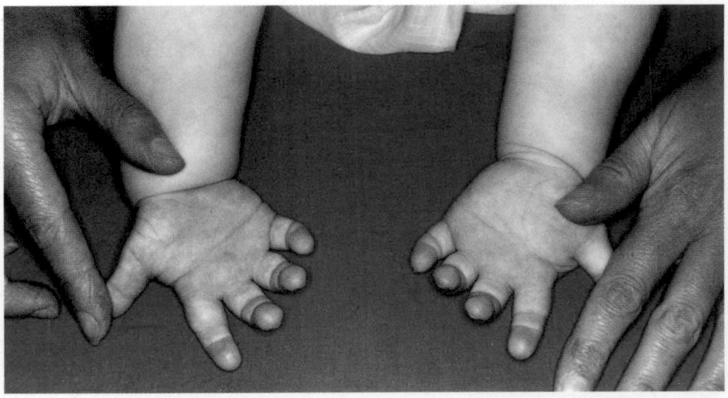

■ **Fig. 6.184** Single transverse palmar (simian) crease and a short incurved little finger (clinodactyly).

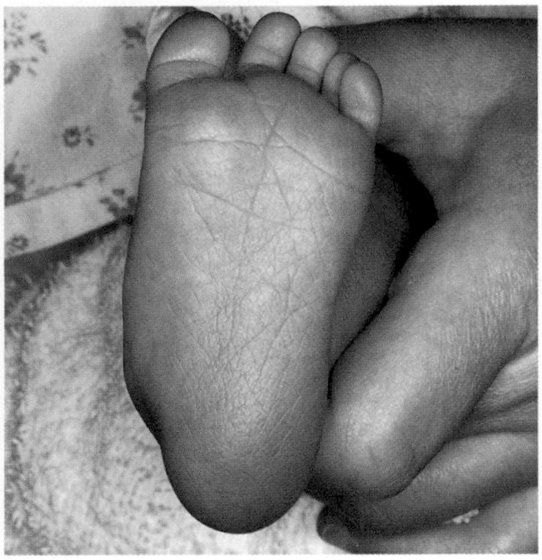

■ **Fig. 6.185** Wide separation between the first and second toes.

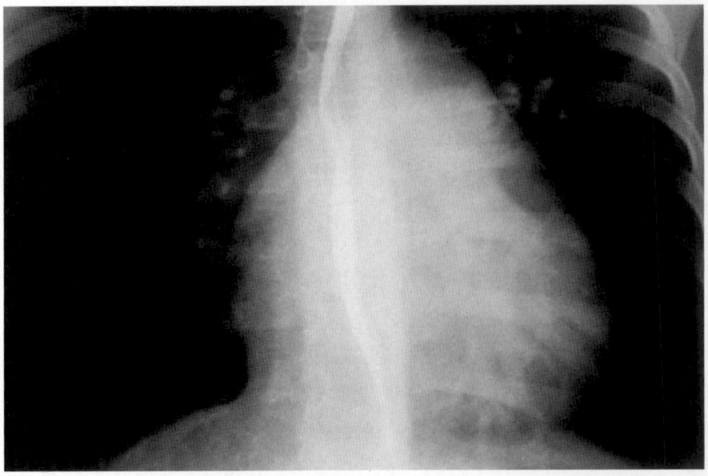

■ **Fig. 6.186** Congenital heart disease such as atrioseptal defect. (Courtesy of B. J. Zitelli and H. W. Davis.)

Ehlers–Danlos syndrome type 6 (ocular sclerotic)

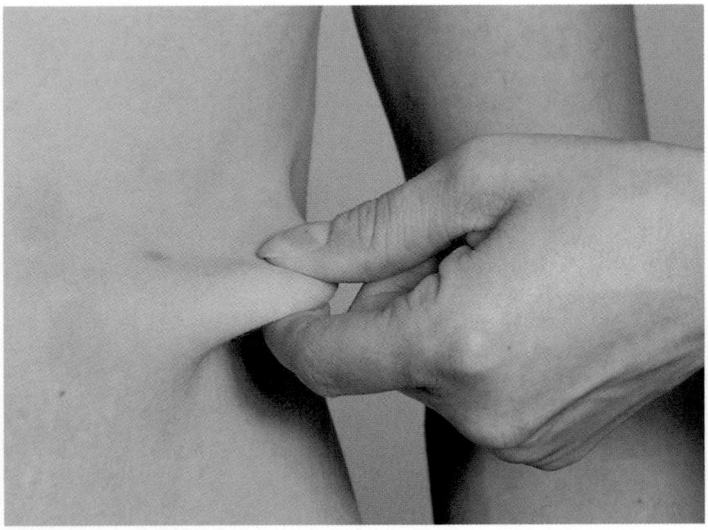

■ **Fig. 6.187** Cutaneous thinning and hyperelasticity. (Courtesy of M. A. Mir.)

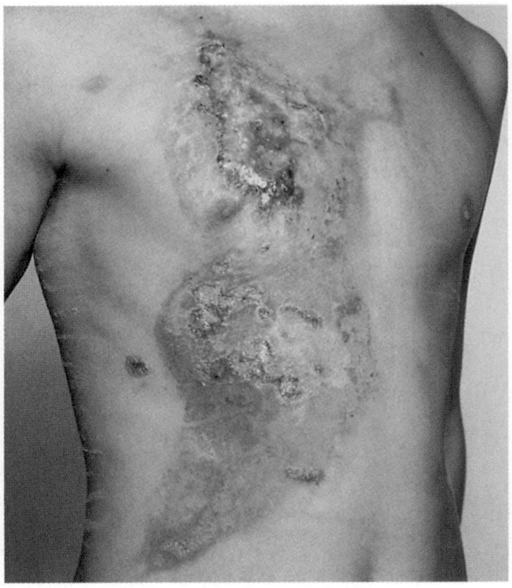

■ **Fig. 6.188** Slow cutaneous healing and easy (papyraceous) scarring. (Courtesy of M. A. Mir.)

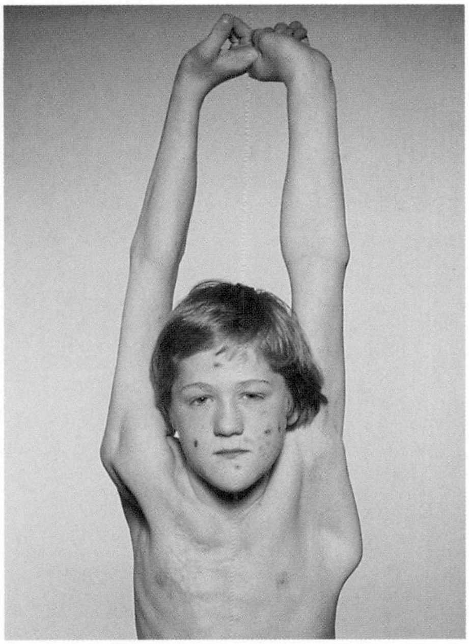

■ **Fig. 6.189** Joint hypermobility and easy dislocation. (Courtesy of M. A. Mir.)

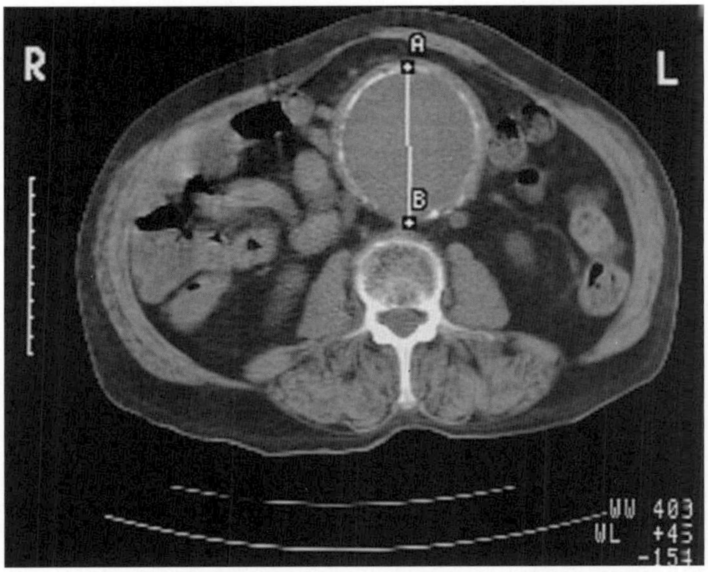

■ **Fig. 6.190** Dissecting aortic aneurysm. (Courtesy of L. Goldman and D. Ausiello.)

Posterior keratoconus

Posterior keratoconus is a very rare, unilateral, non-progressive condition.

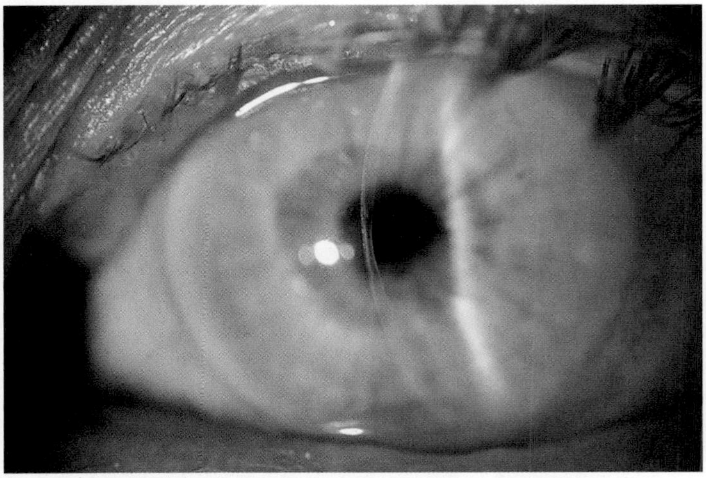

■ **Fig. 6.191** Increased curvature of the posterior corneal surface, which can be generalised or central. (Courtesy of S. Johns.)

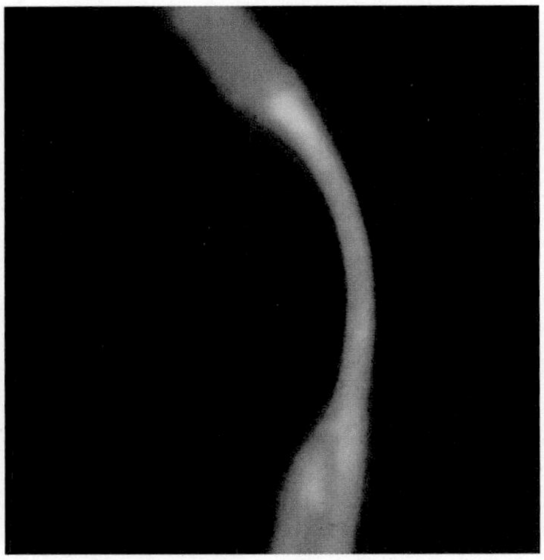

■ **Fig. 6.192** Magnified view of posterior keratoconus. (Courtesy of S. Boruchoff.)

Pellucid marginal degeneration

Pellucid marginal degeneration is a rare condition that may be initially misdiagnosed as keratoconus. Presentation is in the third to fifth decade with increasing astigmatism.

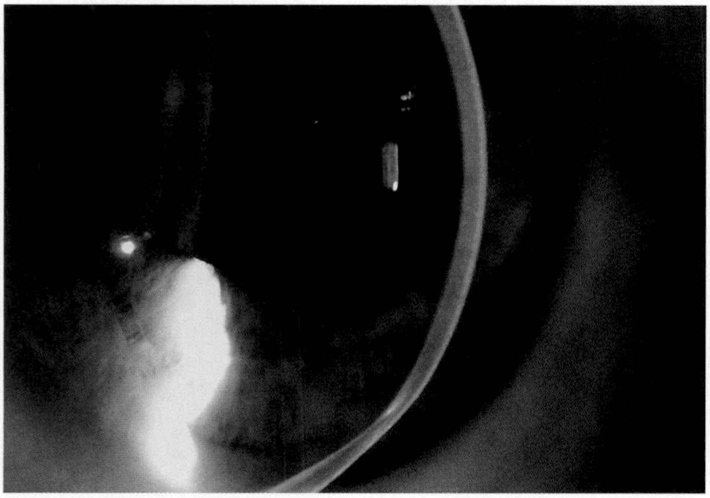

Fig. 6.193 Bilateral, slowly progressive, crescent-shaped band of inferior corneal thinning extending from 4 to 8 o'clock with slight protrusion of the cornea above the area of thinning. (Courtesy of R. Visser.)

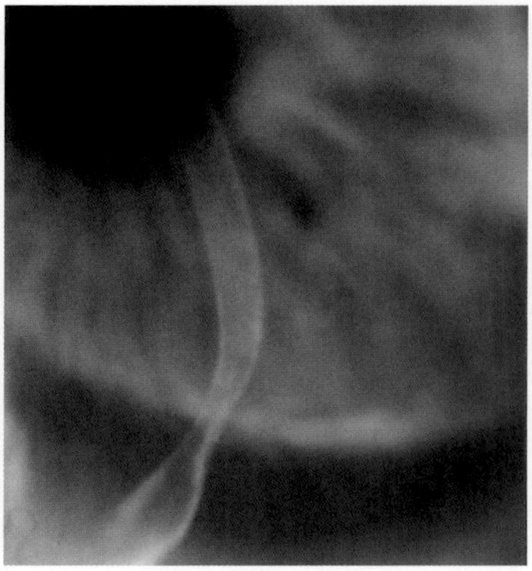

Fig. 6.194 A 2 mm interval of normal cornea separates the limbus from the protrusion. (Courtesy of S. Boruchoff.)

Keratoglobus

Keratoglobus is an extremely rare congenital condition in which the entire cornea is abnormally thin.

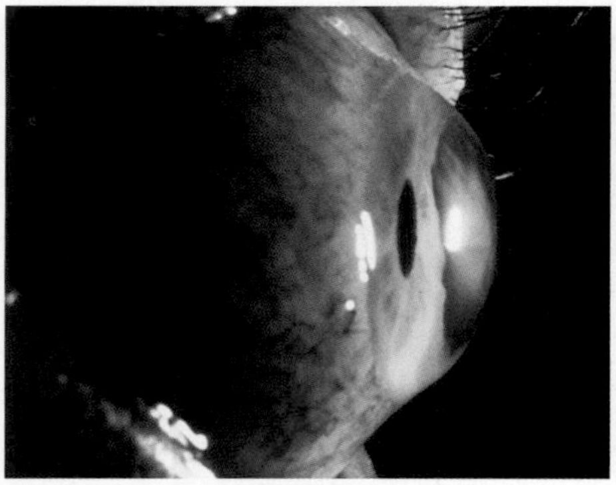

Fig. 6.195 In contrast to keratoconus, the cornea develops globular rather than conical ectasia. (Courtesy of L. Merin.)

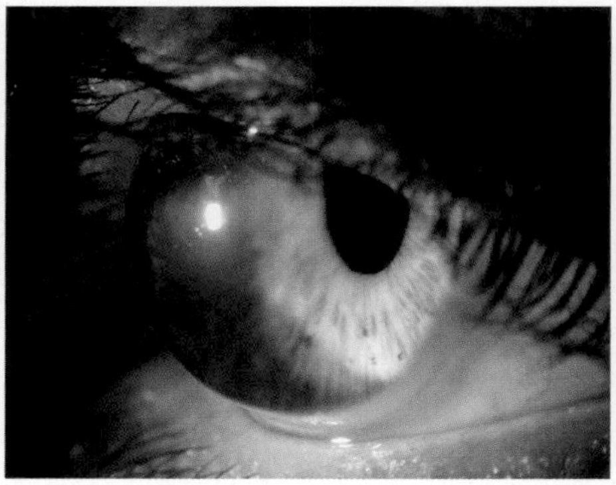

Fig. 6.196 More advanced keratoglobus.

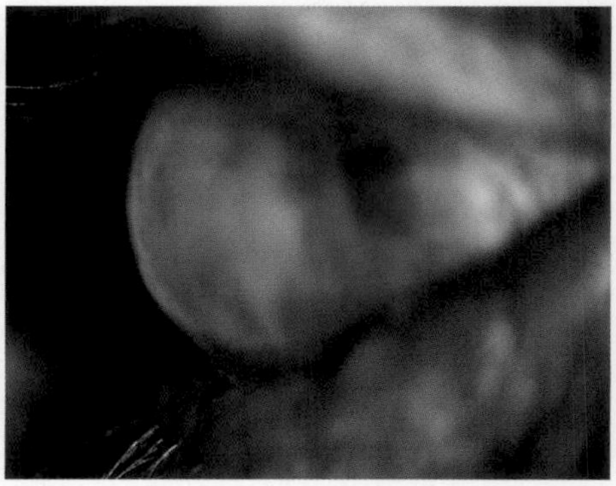

Fig. 6.197 Advanced keratoglobus with acute hydrops.

NEUROKERATOPATHIES

Neuroparalytic (exposure) keratopathy

Exposure keratopathy is the result of improper wetting of the ocular surface by the tear film because of inability to close the eyes on blinking (lagophthalmos).

Causes

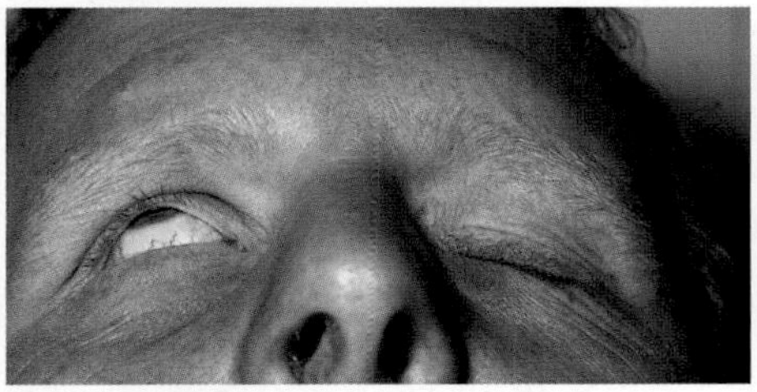

Fig. 6.198 Facial nerve palsy, particularly with a weak Bell phenomenon.

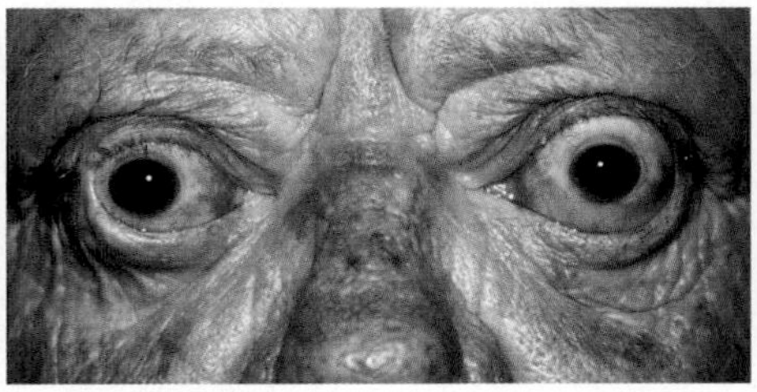

Fig. 6.199 Severe proptosis: note right lateral tarsorrhaphy.

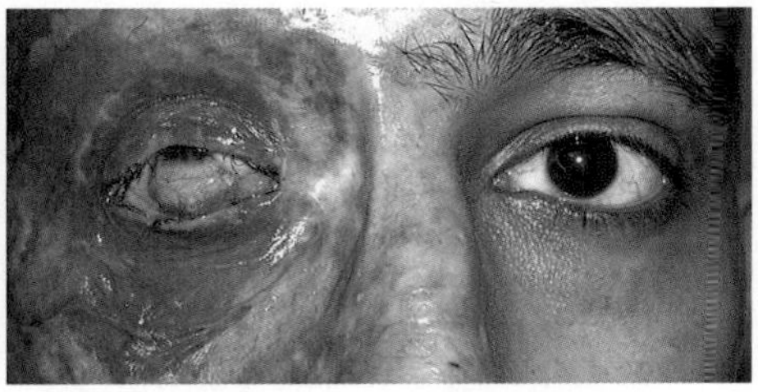

Fig. 6.200 Severe scarring of the eyelids.

Signs

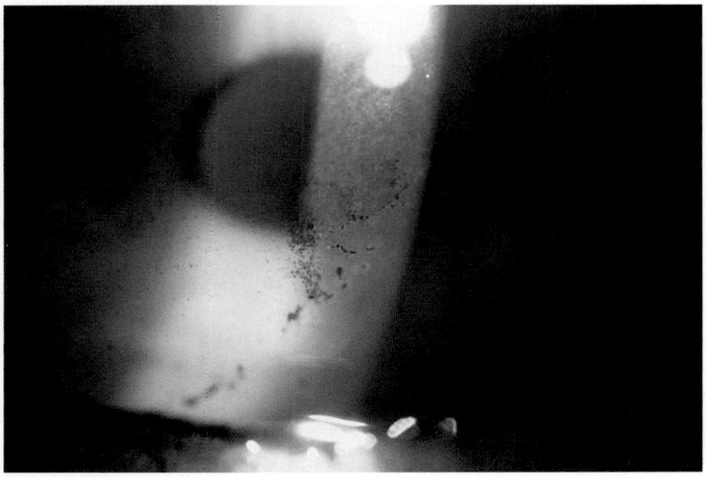

Fig. 6.201 Mild nferior punctate keratopathy.

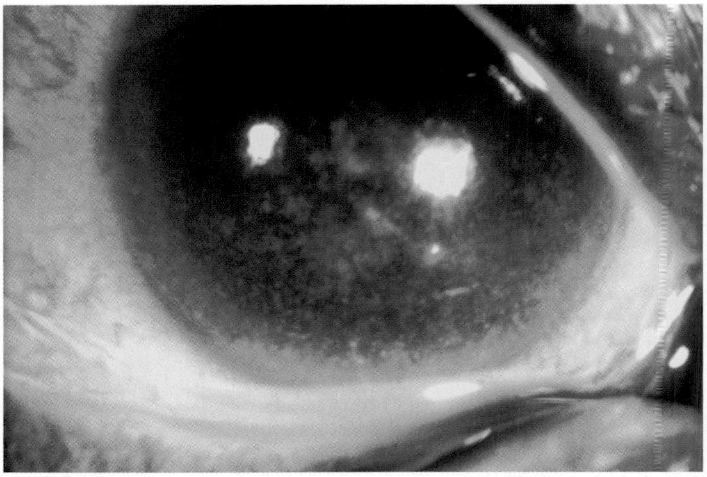

Fig. 6.202 More severe punctate keratopathy and early epithelial loss. (Courtesy of S. Ford and R. Marsh.)

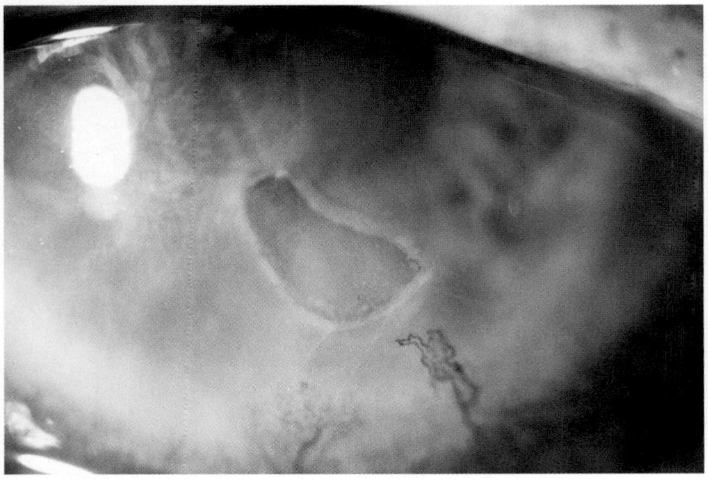

Fig. 6.203 Progressive epithelial loss.

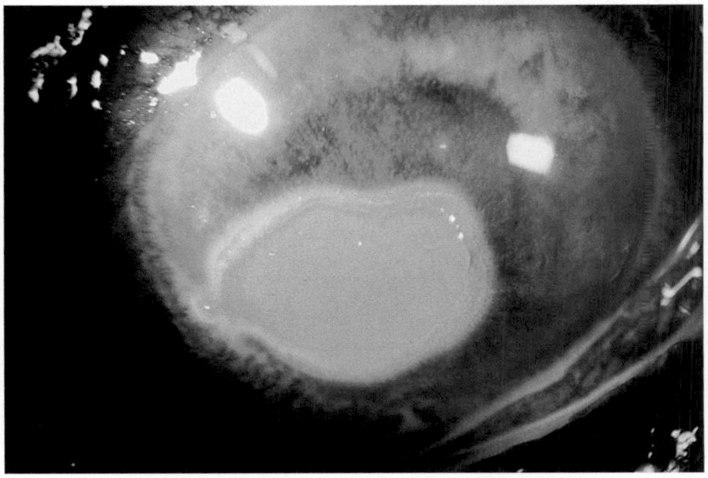

Fig. 6.204 Large ulcer stained with fluorescein.

Neurotrophic keratopathy

Neurotrophic keratopathy is caused by impairment of corneal sensory innervation.

Causes

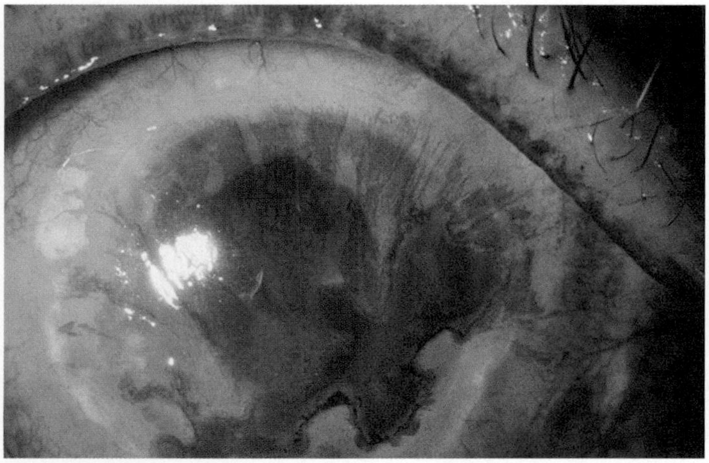

Fig. 6.205 Herpes simplex and herpes zoster keratitis. (Courtesy of R. Curtis.)

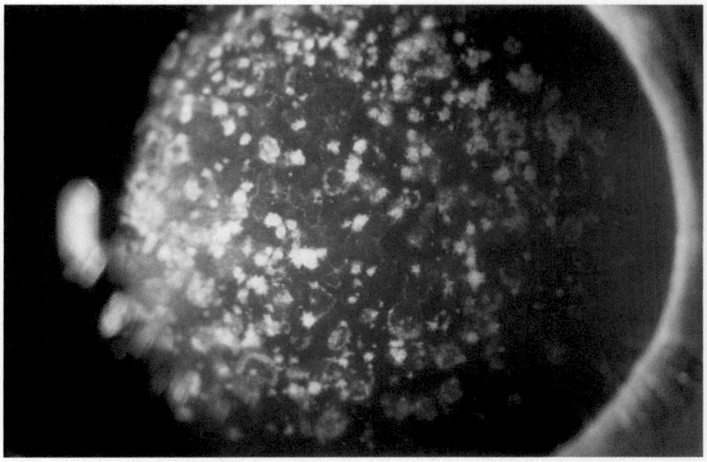

Fig. 6.206 Corneal dystrophies such as granular (shown here) and lattice. (Courtesy of L. Merin.)

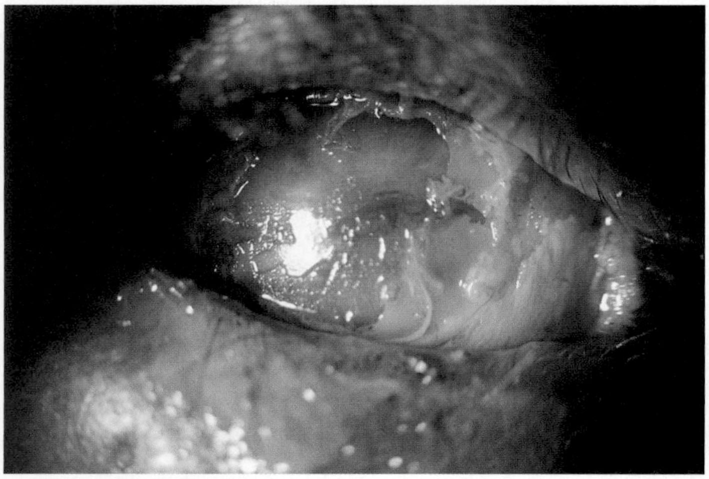

Fig. 6.207 Chemical burns.

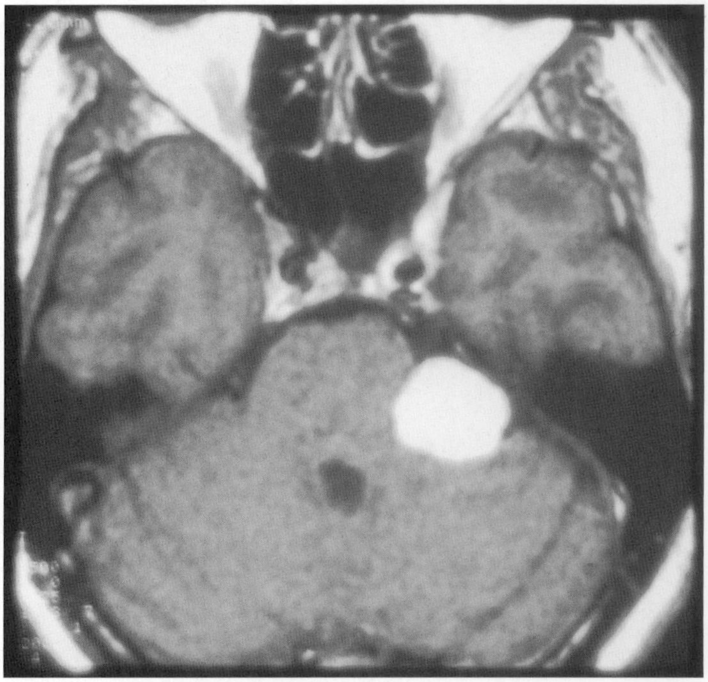

Fig. 6.208 Following surgical procedures for acoustic neuroma (shown here) and trigeminal neuralgia.

Signs

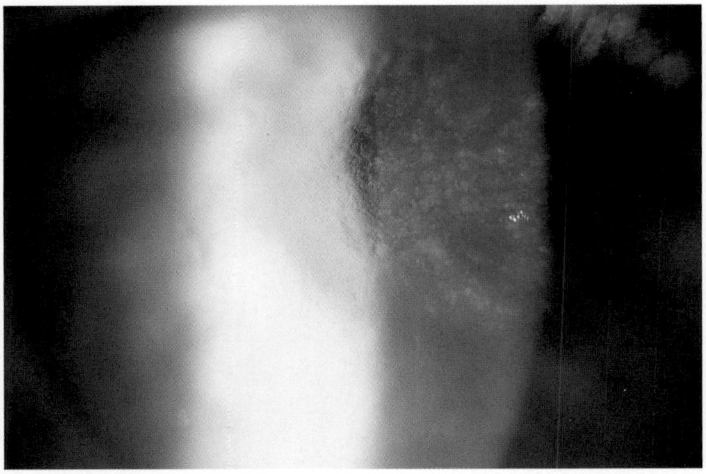

Fig. 6.209 Grey, slightly opaque and oedematous interpalpebral epithelium.

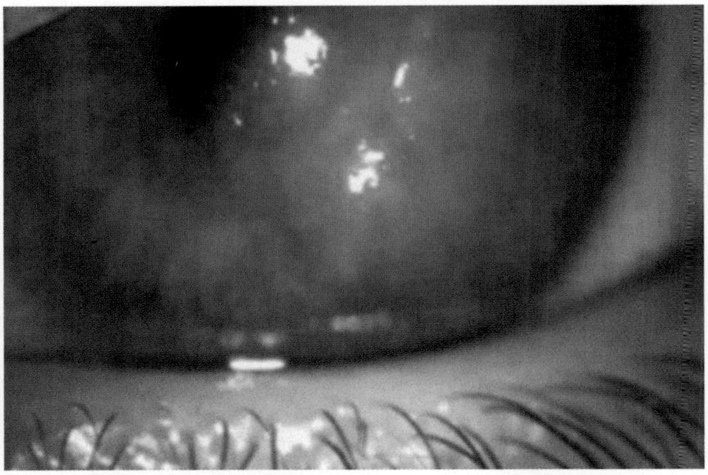

Fig. 6.210 Increasing epithelial haze and increased tear film break-up time. (Courtesy of S. Bonini.)

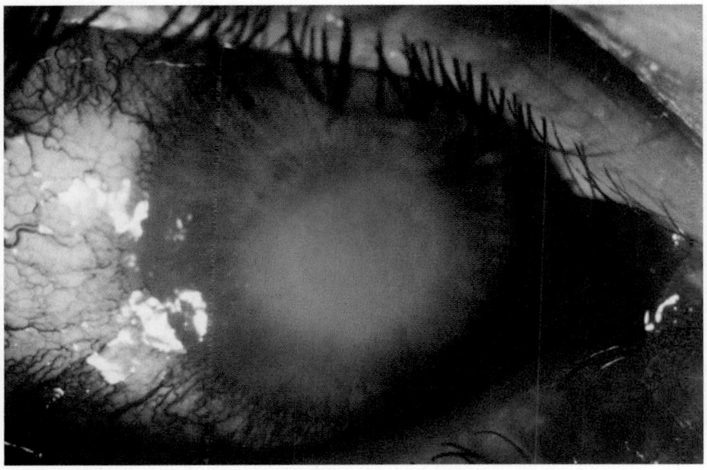

Fig. 6.211 Slow-healing epithelial defects surrounded by a rim of loose epithelium. (Courtesy of S. Bonini.)

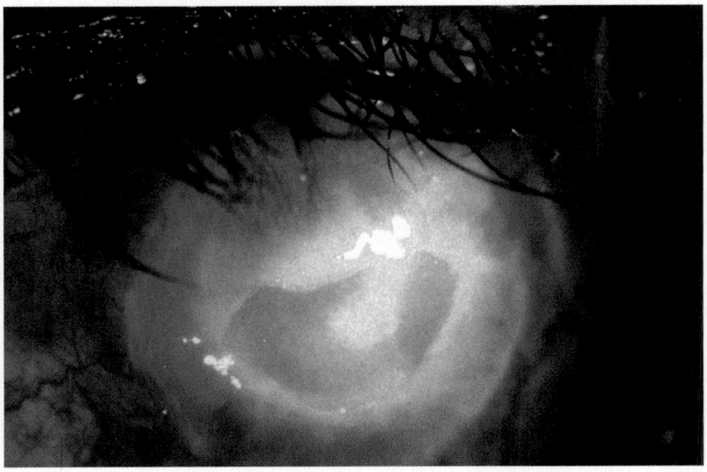

Fig. 6.212 Severe ulceration with clear-cut borders. (Courtesy of S. Bonini.)

DRUG-INDUCED KERATOPATHIES

Chrysiasis

Chrysiasis is the deposition of gold in living tissue, occurring after prolonged administration of gold, usually in the treatment of rheumatoid arthritis.

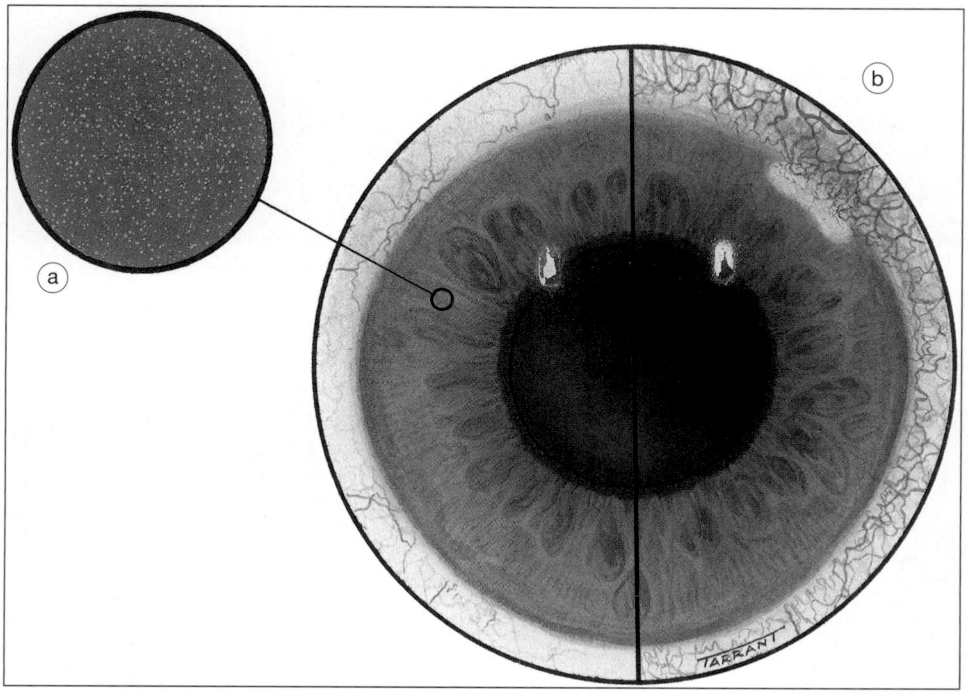

■ **Fig. 6.213** **(a)** Dust-like or glittering purple granules throughout the corneal stroma, more concentrated in the deep layers and the periphery. **(b)** Marginal keratitis may also occur.

Argyrosis

Argyrosis is a discoloration of ocular tissues secondary to silver deposits which may be iatrogenic or occupational.

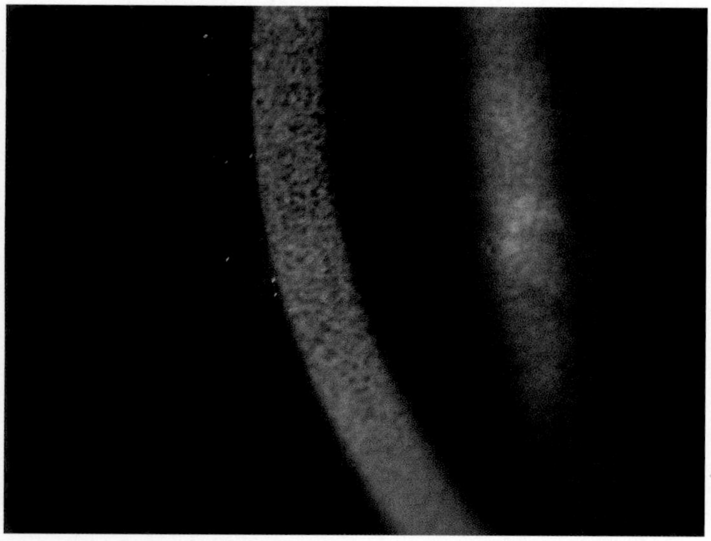

■ **Fig. 6.214** Greyish-brown, granular deposits with a metallic appearance in Descemet membrane. (Courtesy of L. Zografos.)

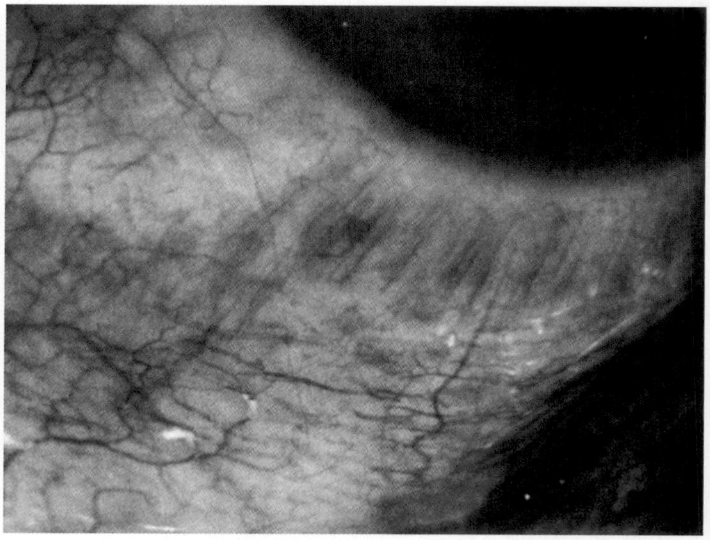

■ **Fig. 6.215** Dark greyish-brown conjunctival argyrosis. (Courtesy of L. Zografos.)

Vortex keratopathy (cornea verticillata)

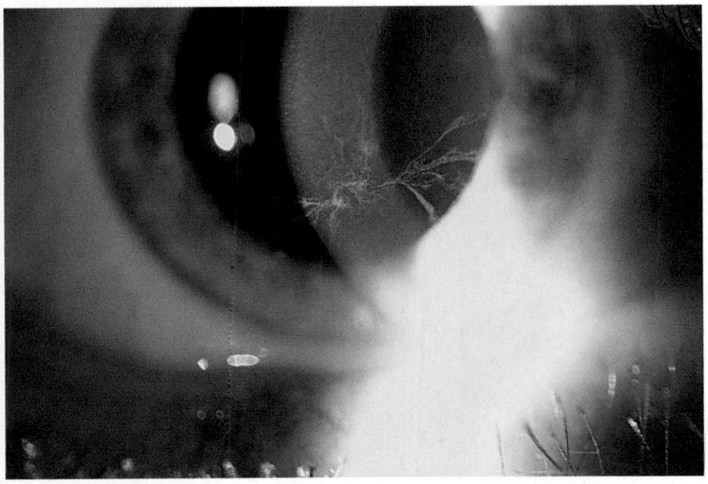

■ **Fig. 6.216** A whorl-like pattern of bilateral, fine, greyish or golden-brown, epithelial, arborising lines originating from a point below the pupil and swirling outwards, sparing the limbus.

Causes

Antimalarials (chloroquine and hydroxychloroquine)

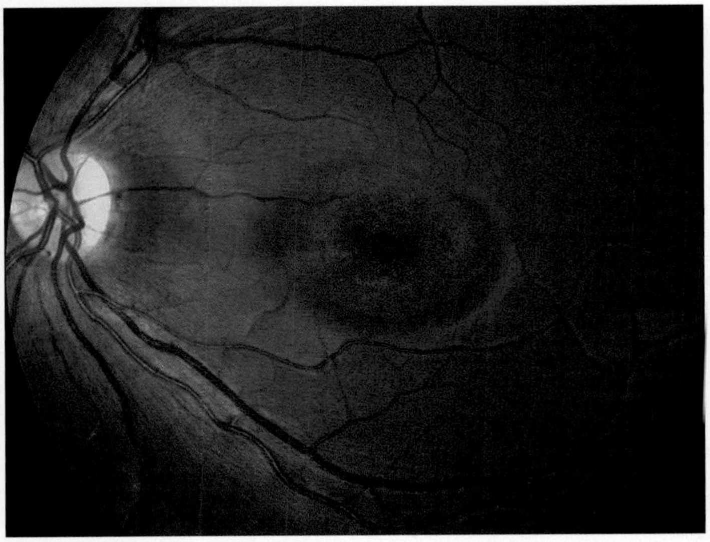

■ **Fig. 6.217** Unlike retinopathy, which may have a bull's eye configuration (shown here), keratopathy bears no relationship to dosage or duration of treatment. (Courtesy of Moorfields Eye Hospital.)

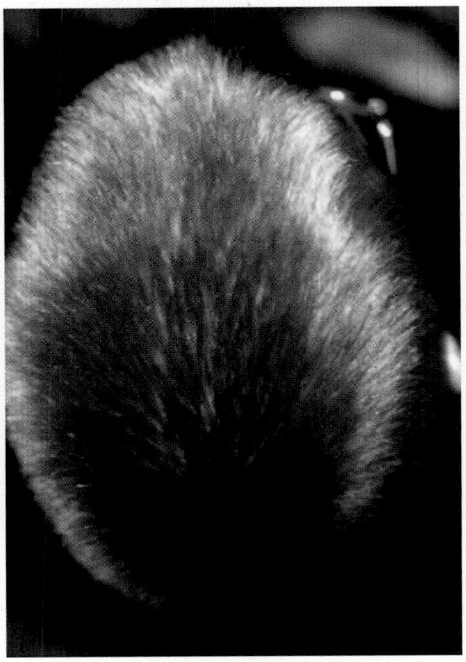

■ **Fig. 6.218** Depigmentation of hair is a rare side effect.

Amiodarone

Virtually all patients on amiodarone develop vortex keratopathy, which is reversible on discontinuation of medication.

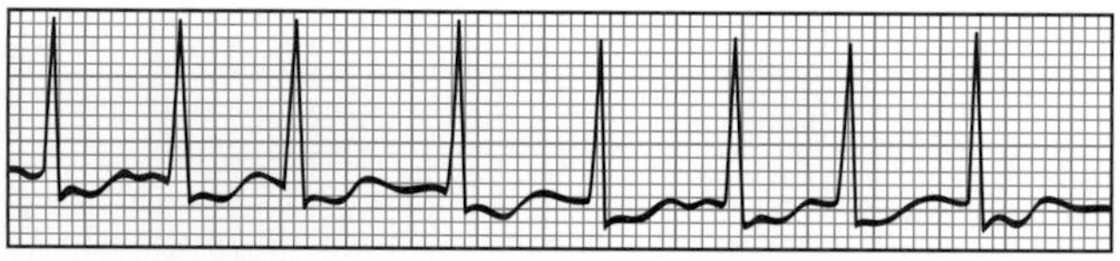

Fig. 6.219 Amiodarone is used to treat cardiac arrhythmias such as atrial fibrillation in which the pulse is irregularly irregular.

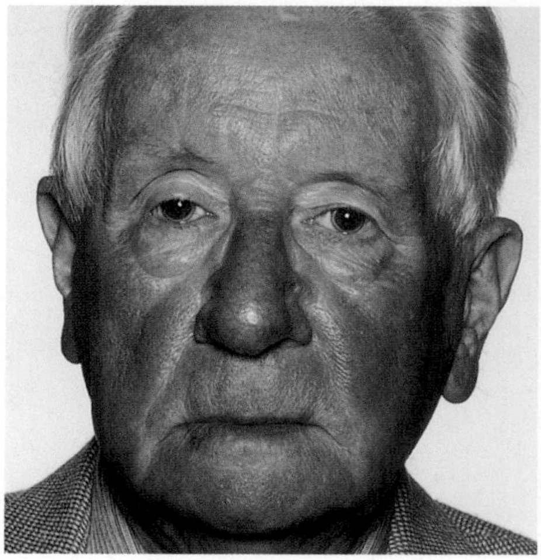

Fig. 6.220 Some patients on long-term therapy develop a bluish or slate-grey cutaneous hyperpigmentation. (Courtesy of A. F. Mir.)

Chlorpromazine

Chlorpromazine is used in the treatment of psychoses.

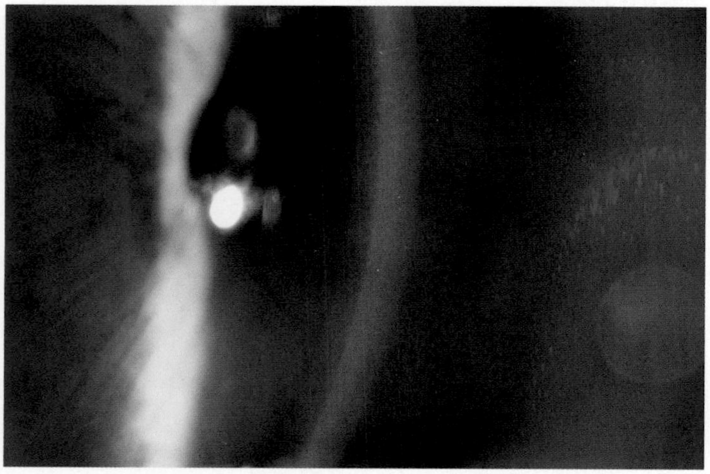

Fig. 6.221 Innocuous, diffuse, yellowish-brown granular deposits in the endothelium and deep stroma may develop with long-term therapy.

METABOLIC KERATOPATHIES

Cystinosis

Cystinosis is a rare, AR, metabolic disorder characterised by widespread tissue deposition of non-protein cystine crystals as a result of a defect in lysosomal transport.

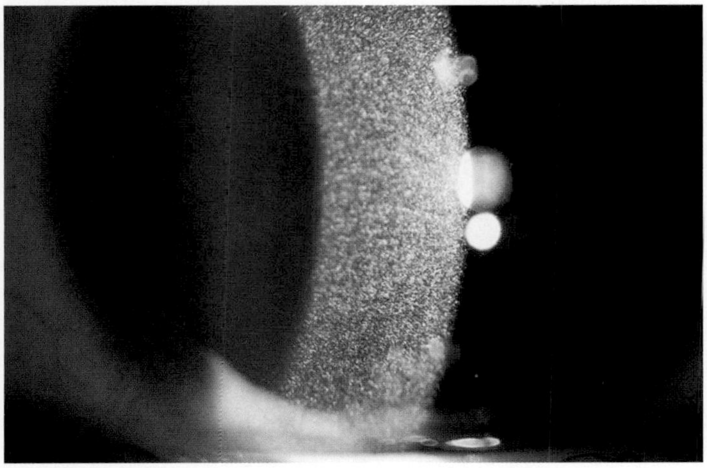

■ **Fig. 6.222** The diagnosis of cystinosis is made by finding cystine crystals in the cornea, which cause intense photophobia, blepharospasm, epithelial erosions and visual disability.

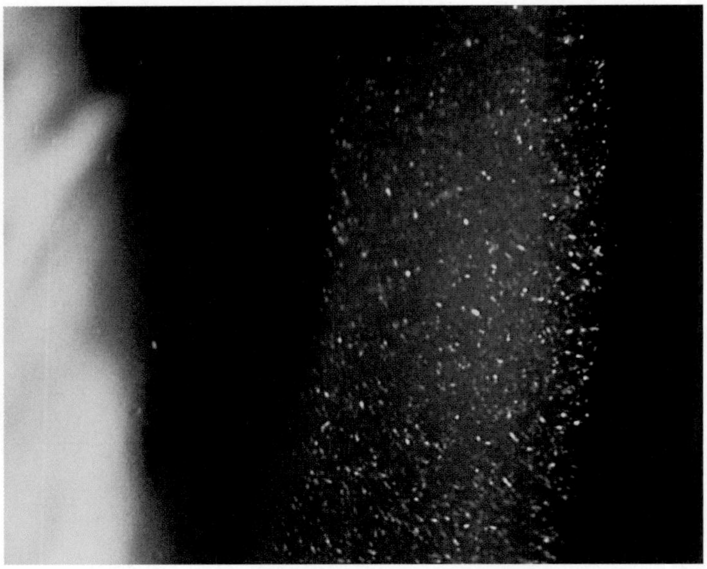

■ **Fig. 6.223** Magnified view. (Courtesy of L. Merin.)

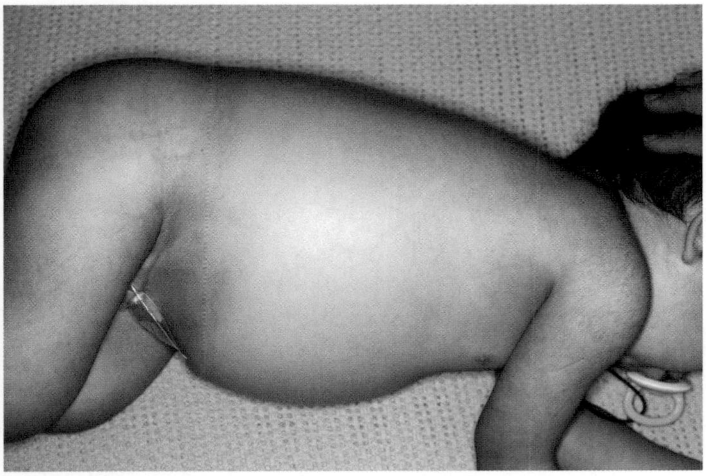

■ **Fig. 6.224** Children with the nephropathic form (Fanconi syndrome), which may cause ascites, often succumb before the second decade.

Wilson disease (hepatolenticular degeneration)

Wilson disease is a rare condition caused by a deficiency of caeruloplasmin resulting in the widespread deposition of copper in tissues. Presentation is between the ages of 5 and 30 with a combination of the following:

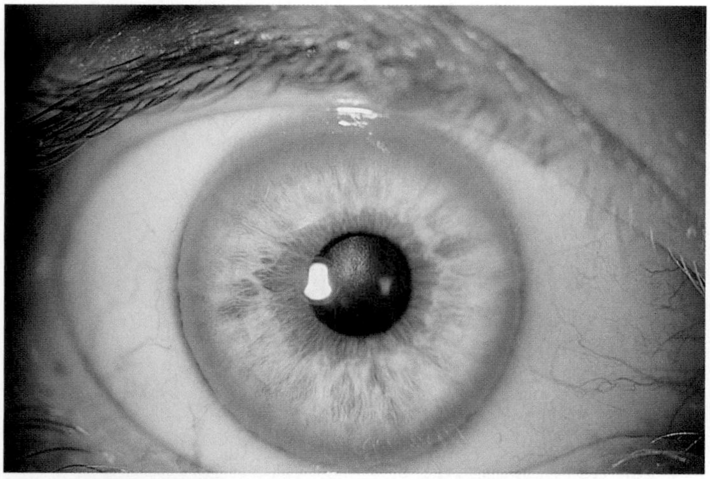

Fig. 6.225 Copper deposits in the peripheral part of Descemet membrane (Kayser–Fleischer ring) appear as a zone of granules that change colour under different types of illumination. (Courtesy of R. Chopdar.)

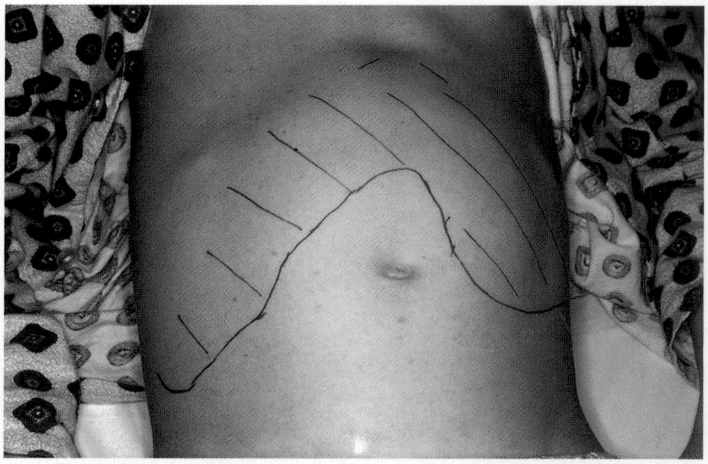

Fig. 6.227 Liver disease, which may give rise to hepatosplenomegaly.

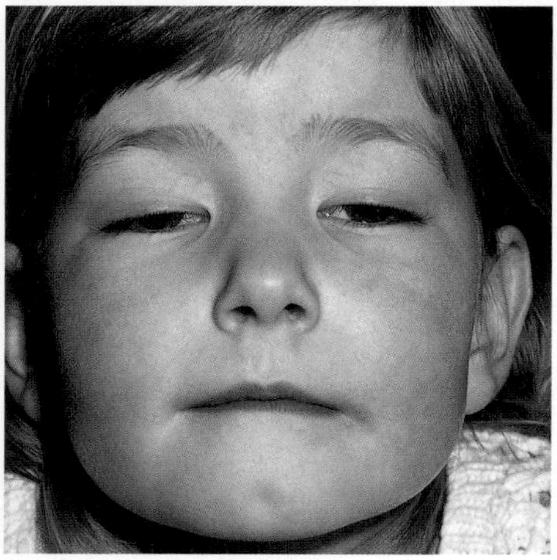

Fig. 6.226 Basal ganglion disease, which may cause an expressionless facies, parkinsonian tremor or athetoid movements.

Mucopolysaccharidoses

The mucopolysaccharidoses (MPS) are a group of inherited deficiencies of catabolic glycosidase necessary for the hydrolysis of mucopolysaccharides characterised by a wide spectrum of clinical severity.

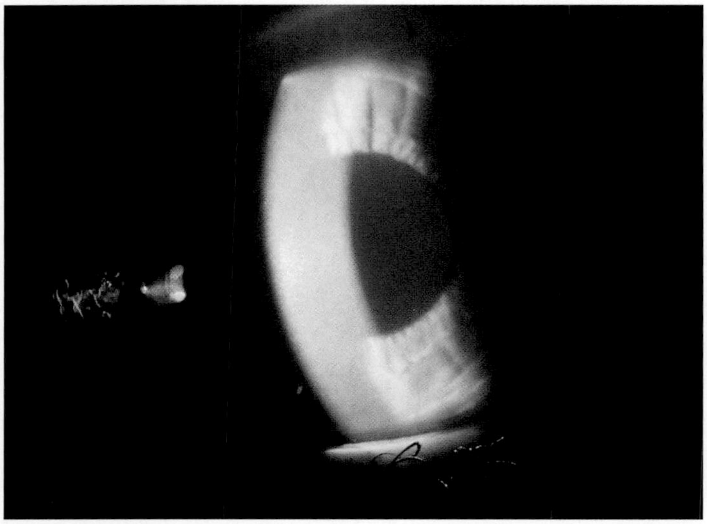

Fig. 6.228 Diffuse corneal clouding is most severe in Hurler and Scheie syndromes. (Courtesy of S. Ford and R. Marsh.)

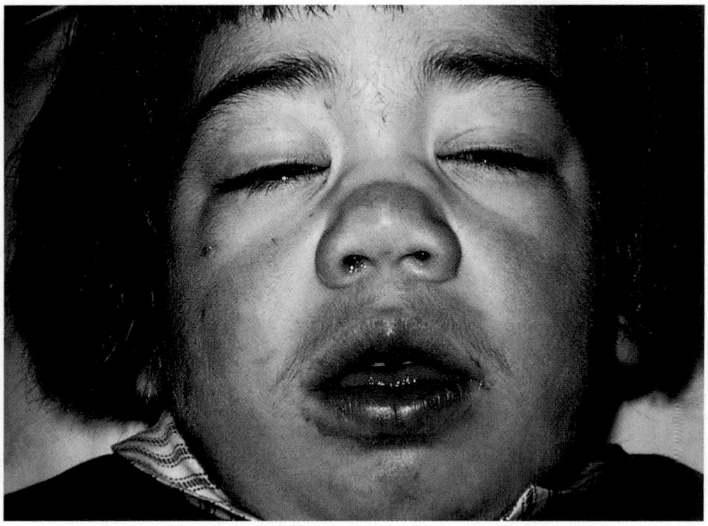

Fig. 6.229 Facial coarseness in Hurler syndrome.

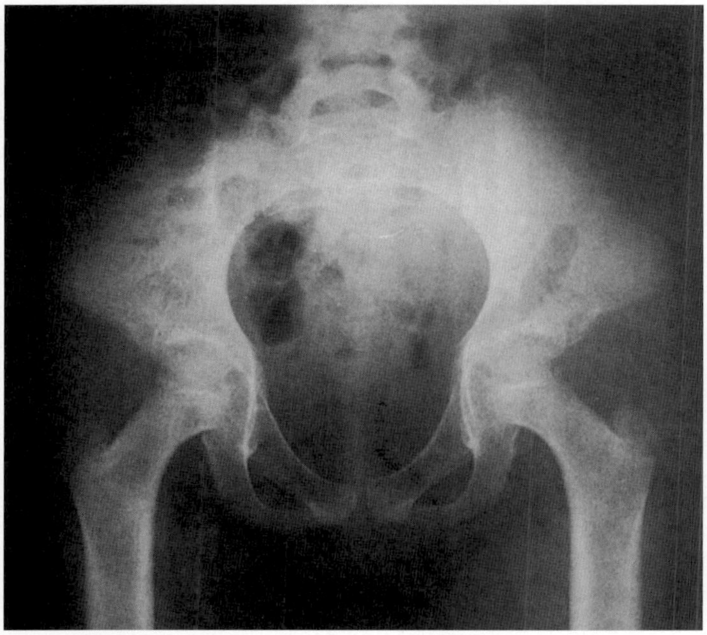

Fig. 6.230 Skeletal dysostosis in Hurler syndrome, showing abnormality of hip bone texture and development. (Courtesy of B. M. Ansell, S. Rudge and J. G. Schaller.)

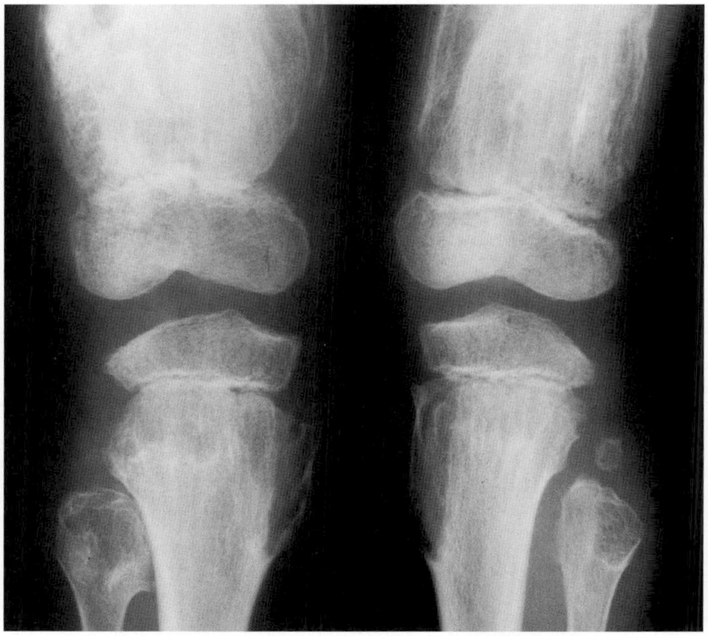

Fig. 6. 231 Distinct skeletal dysplasia in Morquio syndrome. (Courtesy of S. Ghiacy.)

Fabry disease (angiokeratoma corporis diffusum)

Fabry disease is an X-linked lysosomal storage disorder caused by deficiency of alpha-galactosidase.

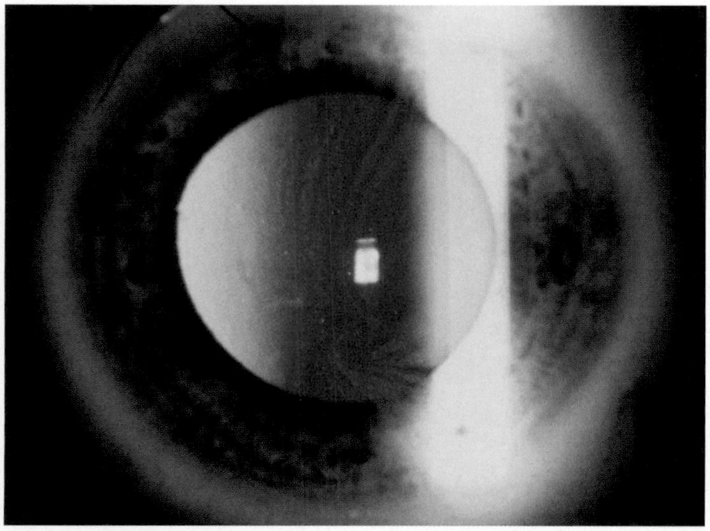

Fig. 6.232 Faint but extensive vortex keratopathy seen on retroillumination. (Courtesy of W. Lisch.)

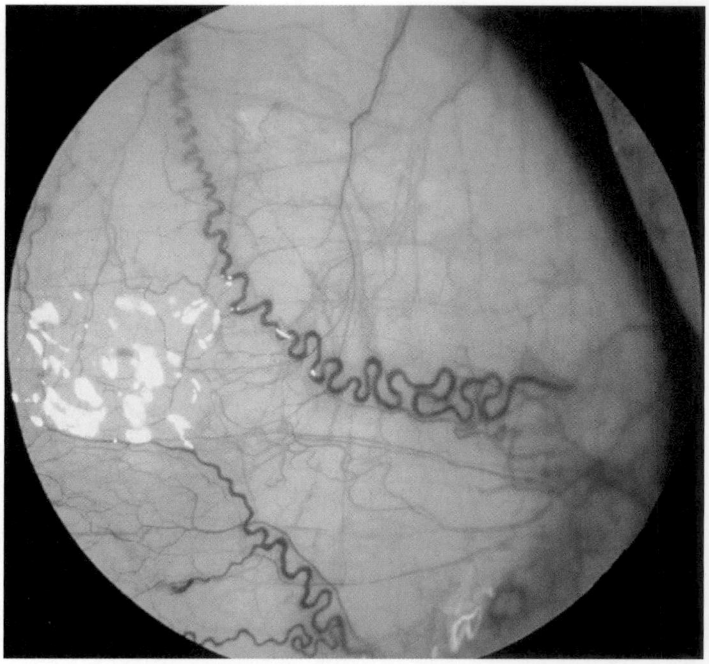

Fig. 6.233 Conjunctival vascular tortuosity. (Courtesy of W. Lisch.)

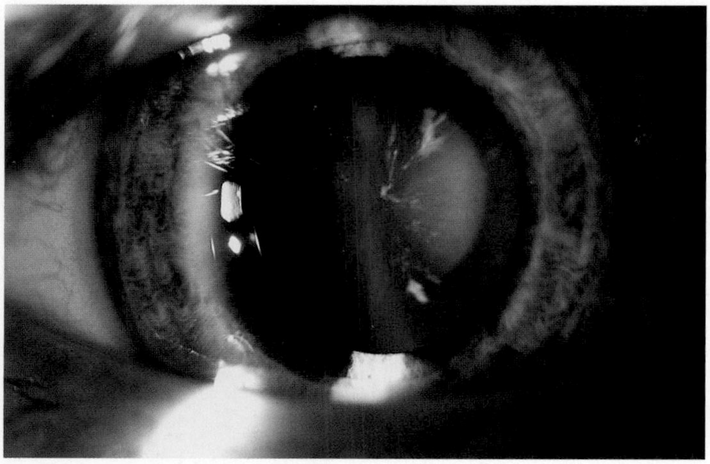

Fig. 6.234 Wedge-shaped lens opacities.

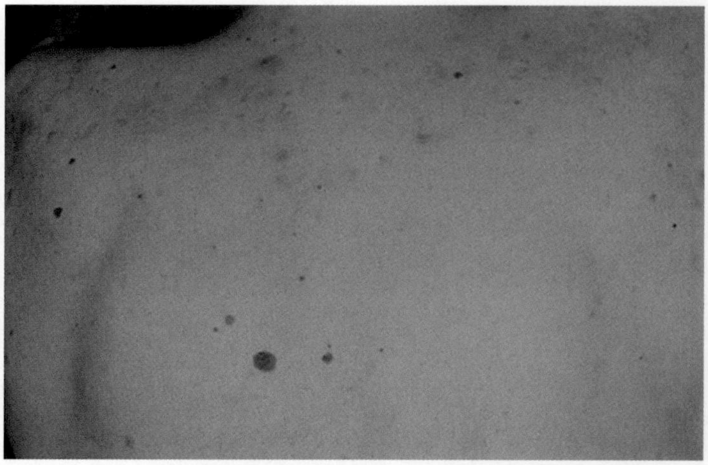

Fig. 6.235 Small, reddish skin papules (angiokeratomas), especially over the trunk. (Courtesy of B. J. Zitelli and H. W. Davis.)

Lecithin–cholesterol–acyltransferase deficiency (Norum disease)

This is an AR disease characterised by hyperlipidaemia, early atheroma, anaemia and renal failure.

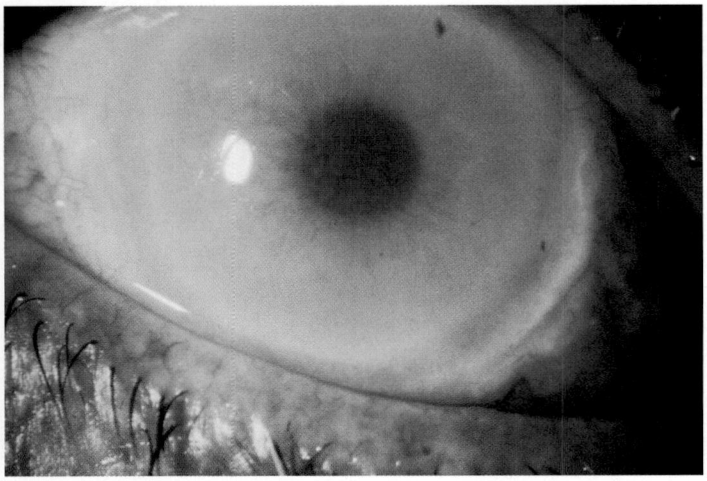

Fig. 6.236 Progressive corneal opacification due to lipid crystal deposition with arcus-like changes extending on to the sclera.

Immunoprotein deposits

Diffuse or focal immunoprotein deposition is a relatively uncommon manifestation of several systemic diseases, including multiple myeloma, Waldenström macroglobulinaemia, monoclonal gammopathy of unknown cause, certain lymphoproliferative disorders and leukaemia.

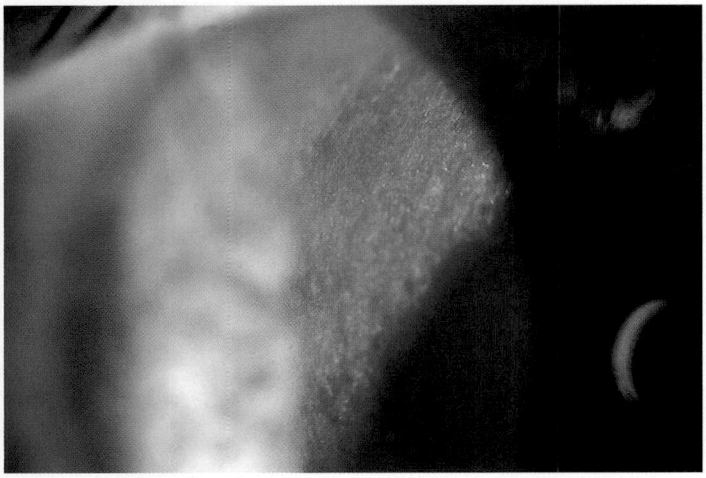

Fig. 6.237 Bilateral band of punctate, flake-like opacities in the posterior stroma.

CONGENITAL ANOMALIES

Microcornea

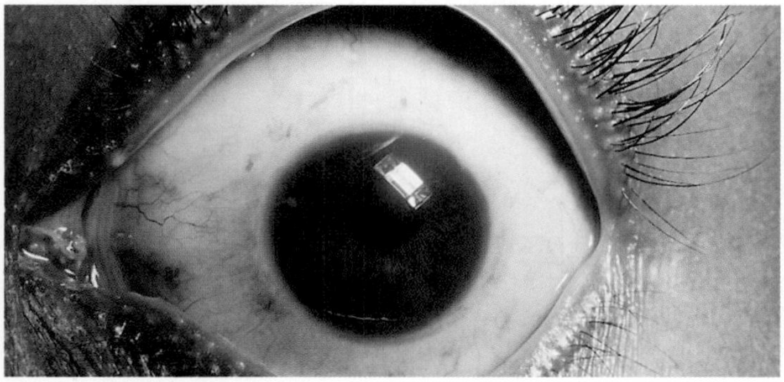

Fig. 6.238 The adult corneal diameter is 10 mm or less, the anterior chamber is shallow but other dimensions are normal. (Courtesy of J. Salmon.)

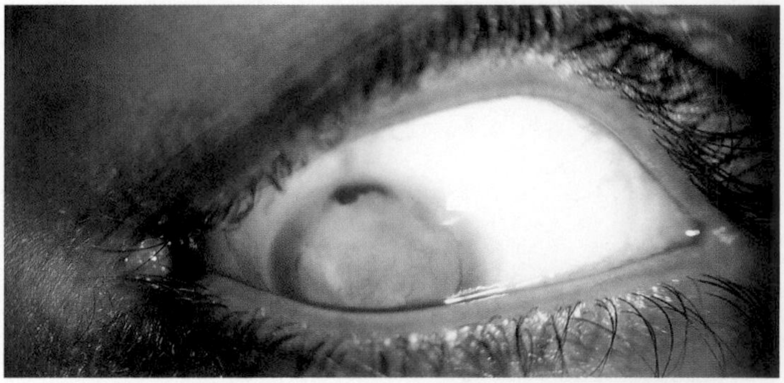

Fig. 6.239 Vision-threatening associations include glaucoma, cataract and leukoma.

Microphthalmos

A microphthalmic eye is one with a severely reduced axial length. It may be simple or colobomatous.

Simple

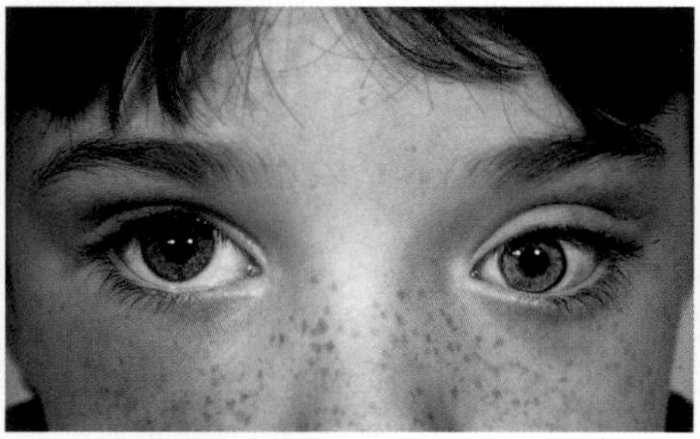

Fig. 6.240 Mild unilateral microphthalmos.

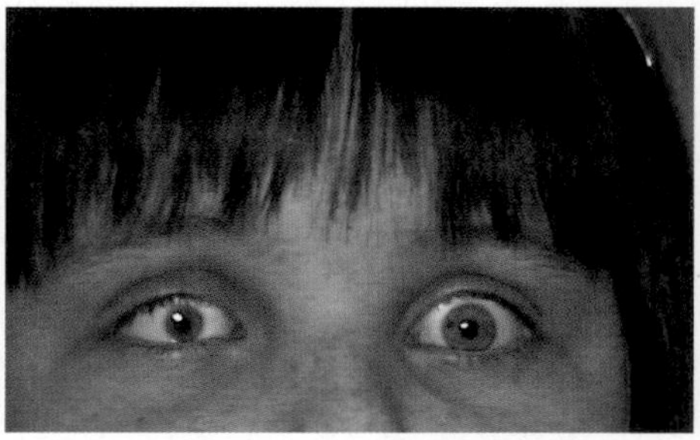

Fig. 6.241 Severe unilateral microphthalmos. (Courtesy of M. Parulekar.)

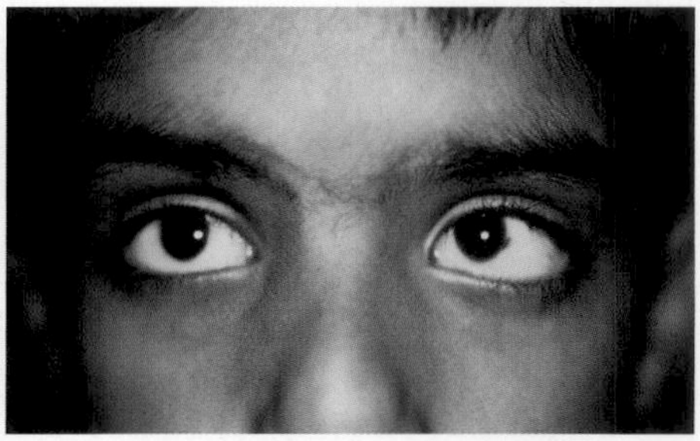

Fig. 6.242 Bilateral moderate microphthalmos.

Colobomatous

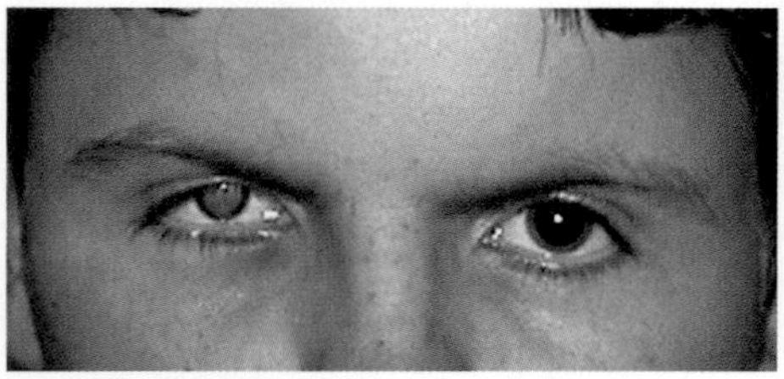

Fig. 6.243 Unilateral colobomatous microphthalmos. (Courtesy of M. Parulekar.)

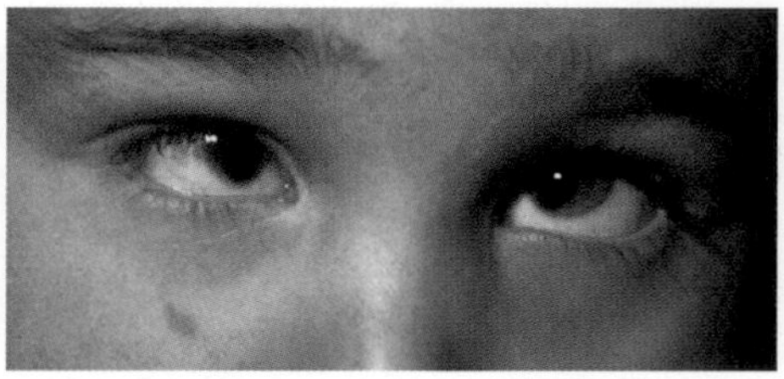

Fig. 6.244 Unilateral microphthalmos and bilateral iris colobomas. (Courtesy of S. Ford and R. Marsh.)

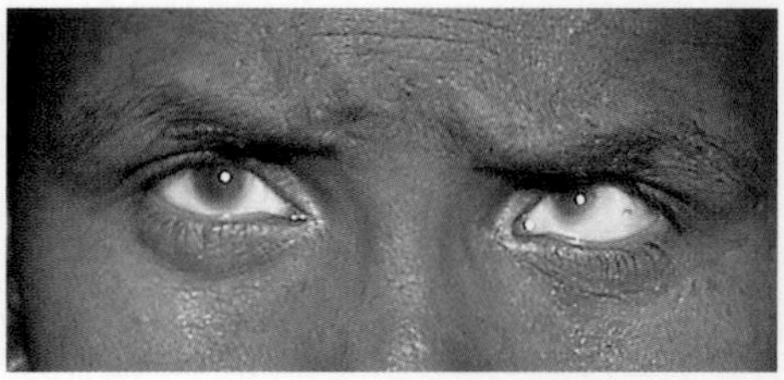

Fig. 6.245 Severe bilateral colobomatous microphthalmos. (Courtesy of M. Parulekar.)

Megalocornea

Megalocornea is a non-progressive bilateral X-linked recessive disorder.

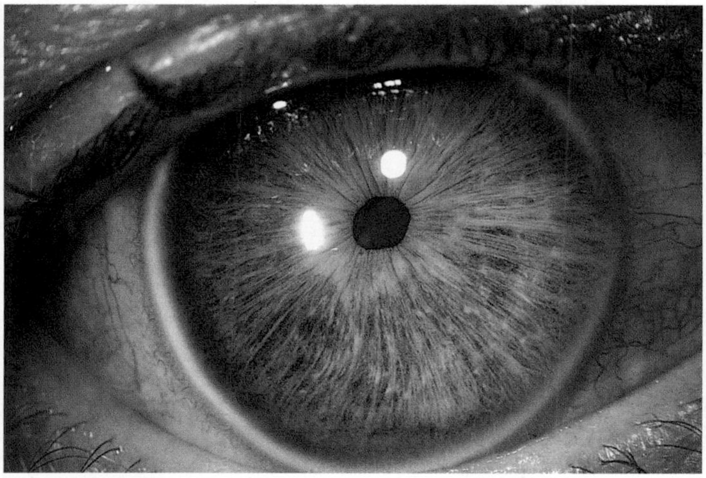

■ **Fig. 6.246** Corneal diameter is over 13 mm in the absence of raised intraocular pressure.

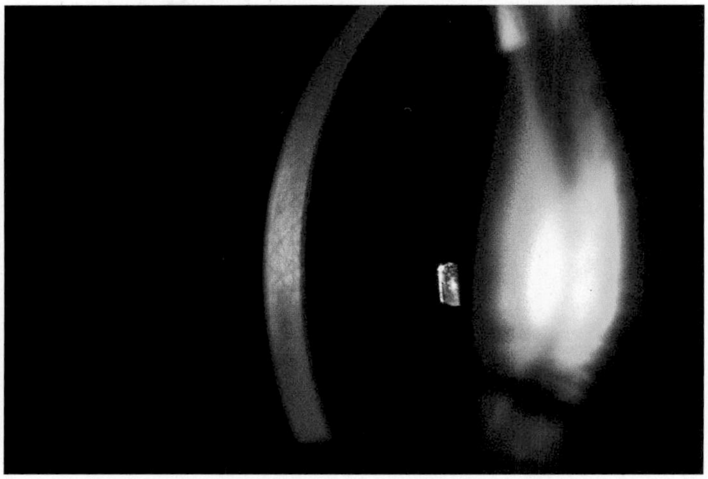

■ **Fig. 6.247** Slit view of very deep anterior chamber.

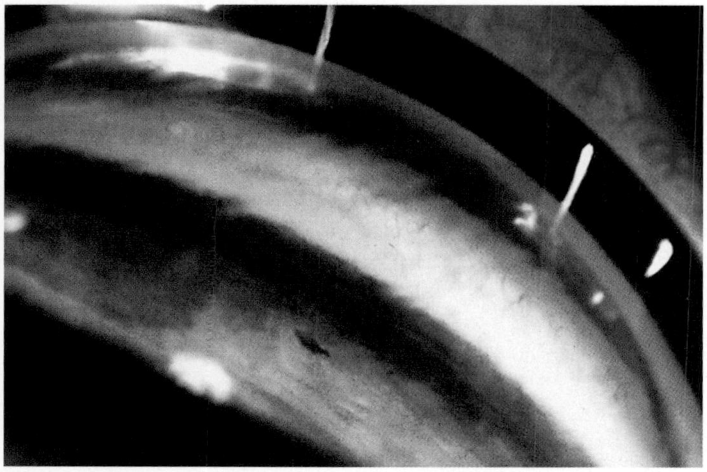

■ **Fig. 6.248** Gonioscopy shows a very wide angle and trabecular hyperpigmentation due to pigment dispersion.

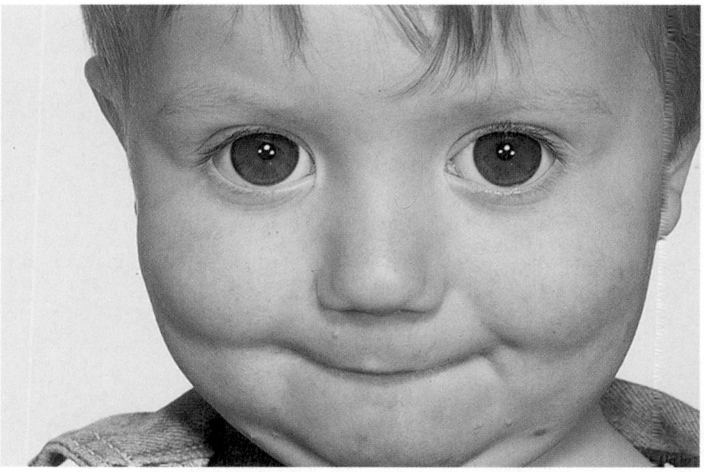

■ **Fig. 6.249** A child with megalocornea.

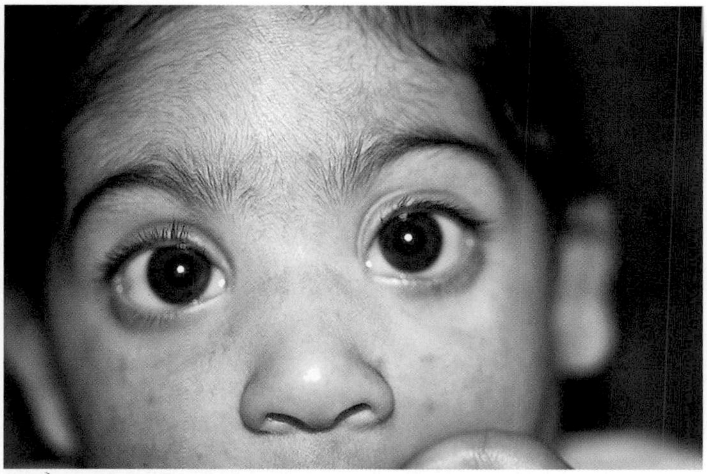

■ **Fig. 6.250** Pseudomegalocornea in a child with microcephaly (small head).

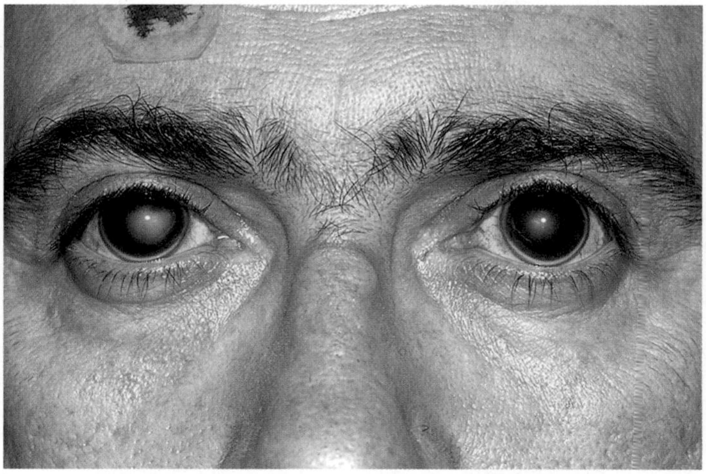

■ **Fig. 6.251** Megalocornea and bilateral cataracts.

Cornea plana

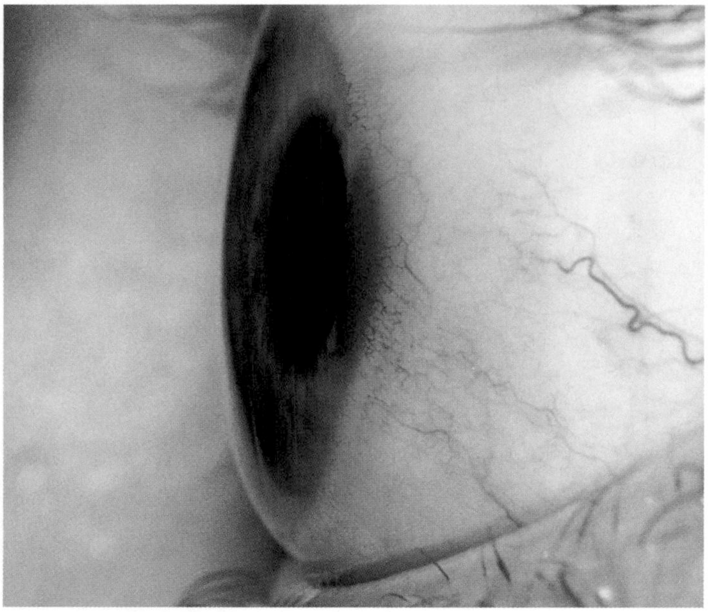

Fig. 6.252 Severe decrease in corneal curvature (K reading 20–30 D), hypermetropia, shallow anterior chamber and predisposition to angle-closure glaucoma. (Courtesy of R. Visser.)

Sclerocornea

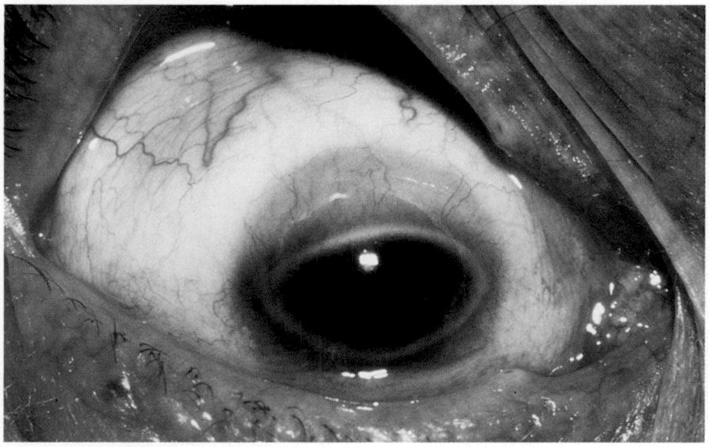

Fig. 6.253 Opacification and vascularisation of the cornea; if this is restricted to the periphery the resulting 'scleralisation' makes the cornea look small. (Courtesy of A. Shun-Shin.)

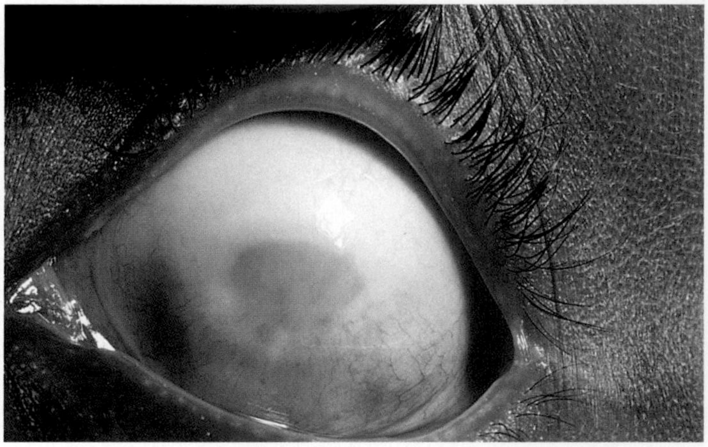

Fig. 6.254 Severe sclerocornea. (Courtesy of J. Salmon.)

Keratectasia

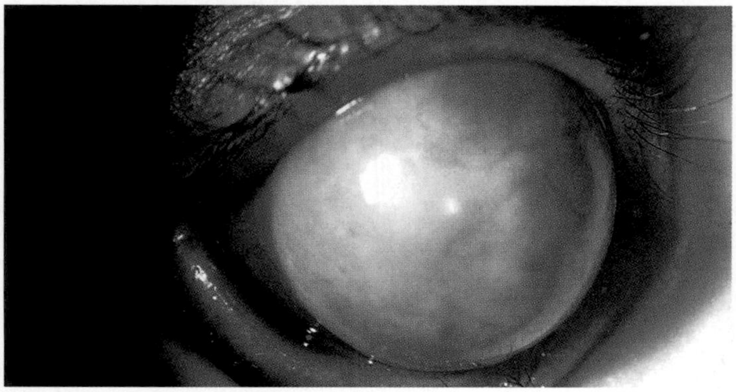

Fig. 6.255 Protuberance, usually unilateral, between the eyelids of an opaque cornea. (Courtesy of U. Raina.)

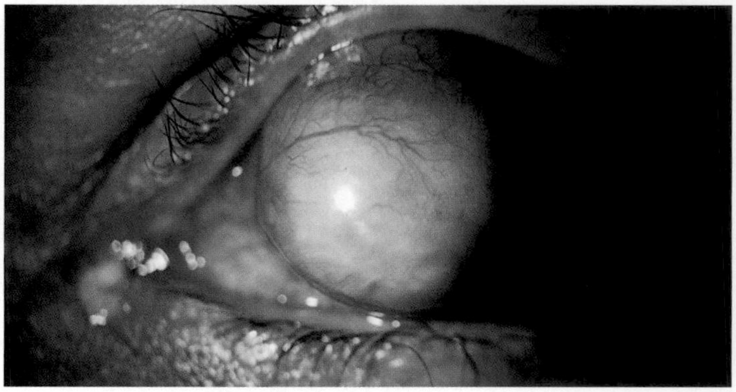

Fig. 6.256 Vascularised keratectasia.

CHAPTER 7

LENS

ACQUIRED CATARACT

Age-related cataract

Anterior subcapsular

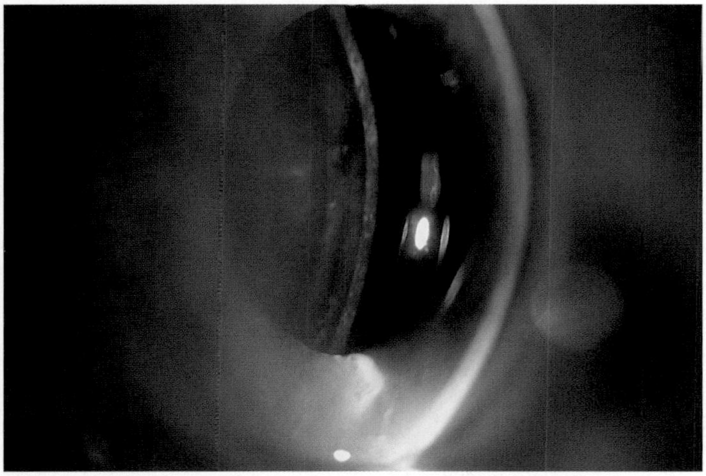

Fig. 7.1 The opacity lies under the lens capsule and is associated with fibrous metaplasia of the lens epithelium.

Posterior subcapsular

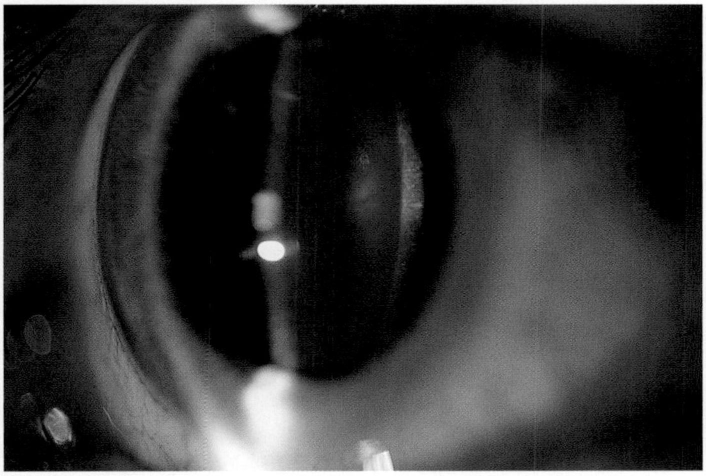

Fig. 7.2 The opacity lies in front of the posterior capsule and manifests a vacuolated, granular or plaque-like appearance.

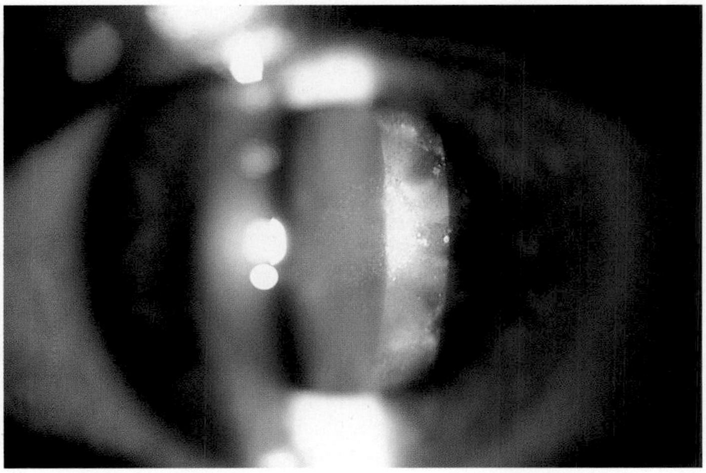

Fig. 7.3 More advanced posterior subcapsular cataract.

Nuclear

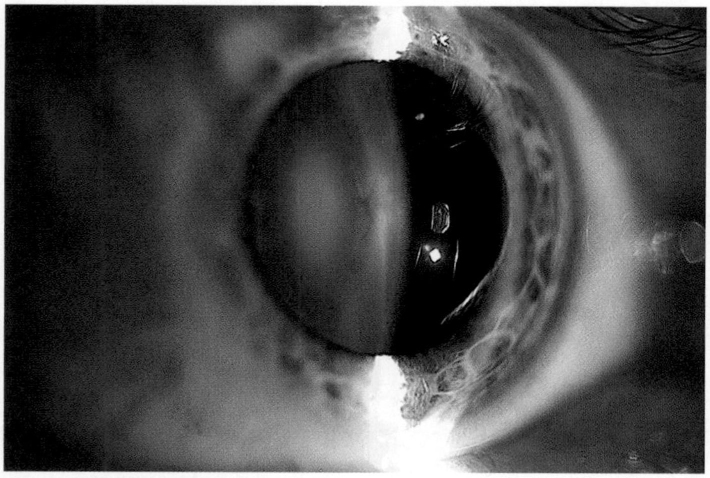

■ **Fig. 7.4** The nucleus is yellowish-brown due to the deposition of urochrome pigment.

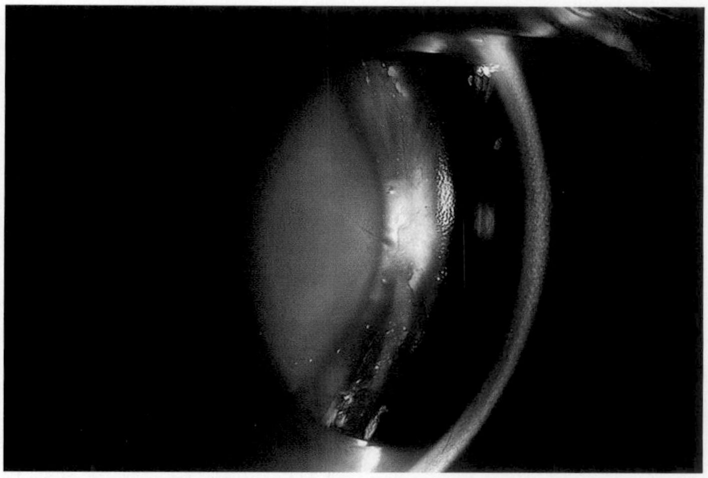

■ **Fig. 7.5** More advanced nuclear cataract.

Cortical

The opacity may involve the anterior, posterior or equatorial cortex.

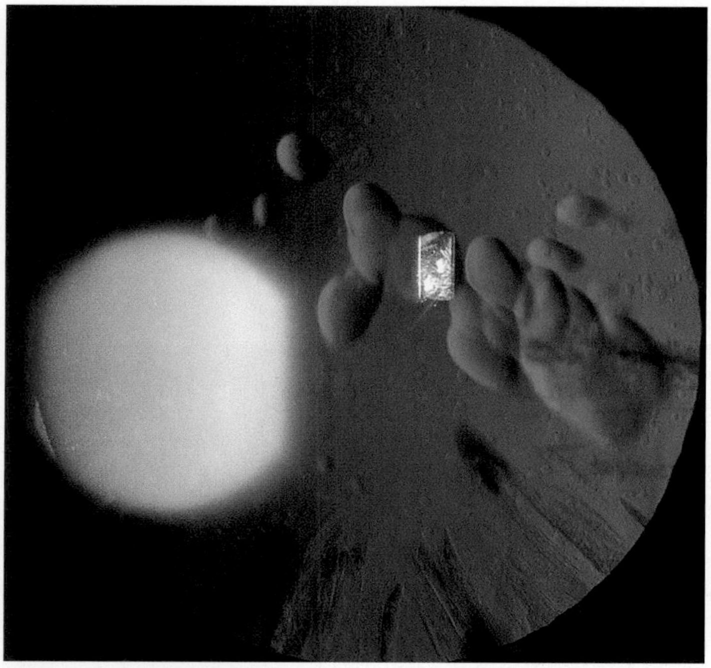

■ **Fig. 7.6** Early cortical opacities associated with vacuoles and water clefts.

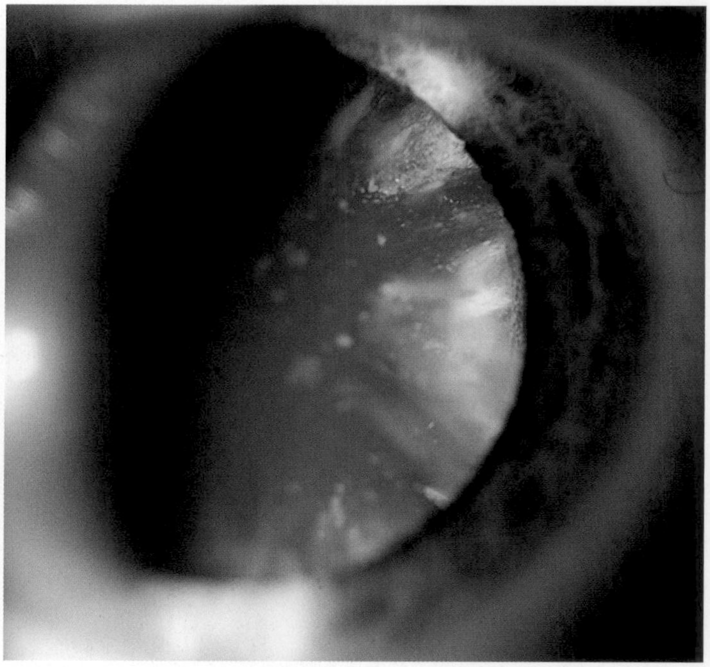

■ **Fig. 7.7** Cuneiform (wedge-shaped) cortical cataract.

Christmas tree

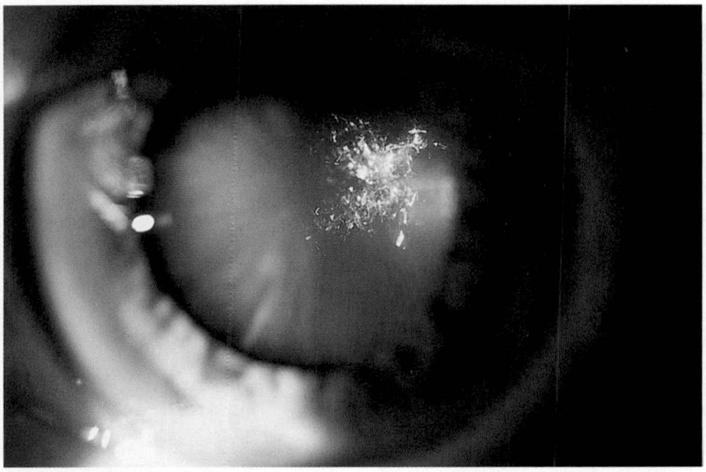

■ **Fig. 7.8** Polychromatic, needle-like deposits in the deep cortex and nucleus.

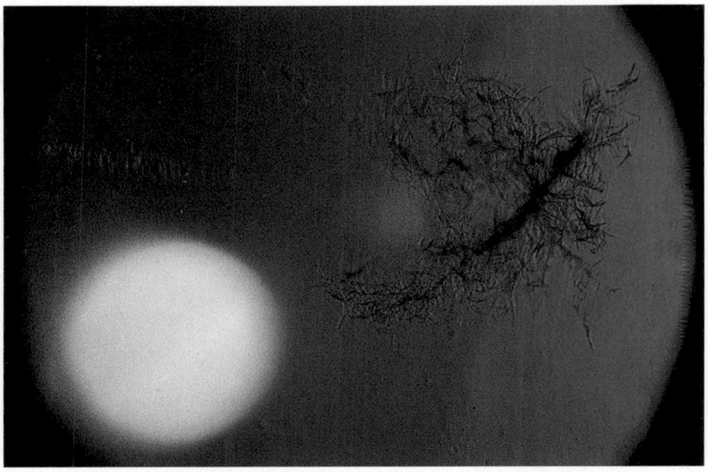

■ **Fig. 7.9** Same eye seen on retroillumination.

Mature and hypermature

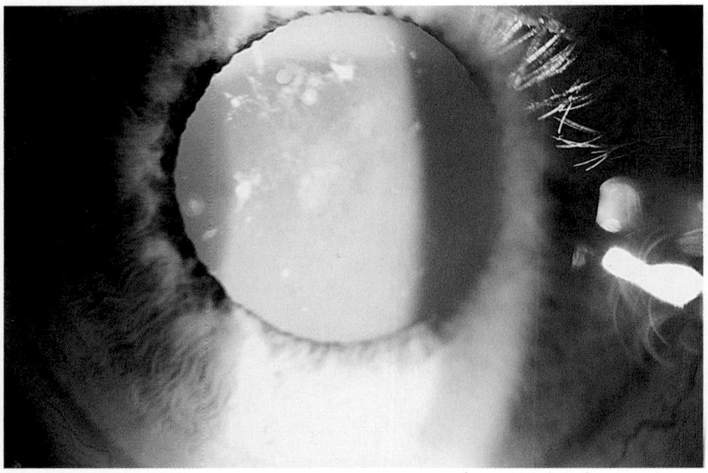

■ **Fig. 7.10** Mature cataract in which the lens is completely opaque.

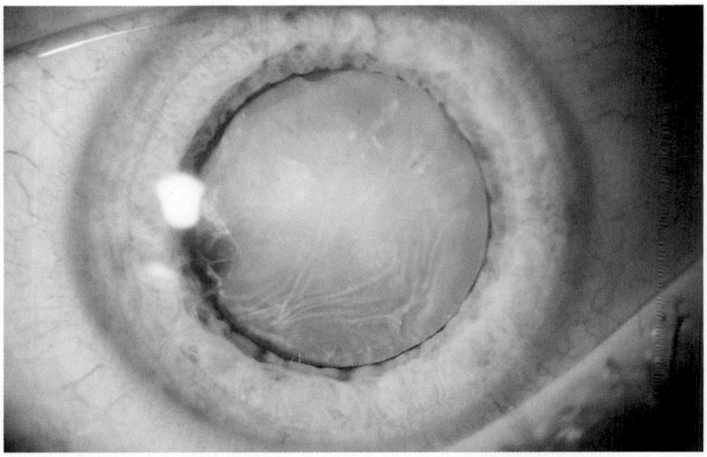

■ **Fig. 7.11** A hypermature cataract in which the lens has a shrunken appearance and the anterior lens capsule is wrinkled as a result of leakage of water out of the lens.

Morgagnian

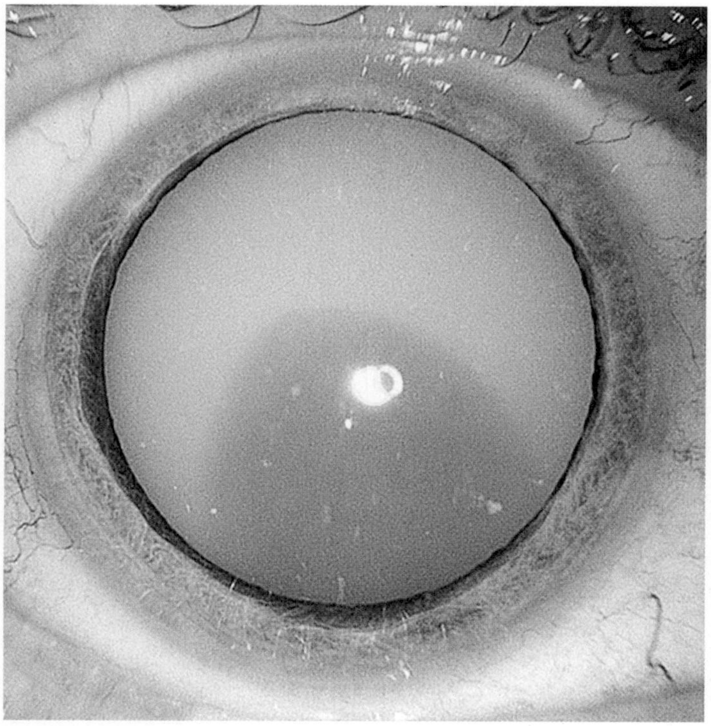

■ **Fig. 7.12** Cortical liquefaction with inferior sinking of the nucleus.

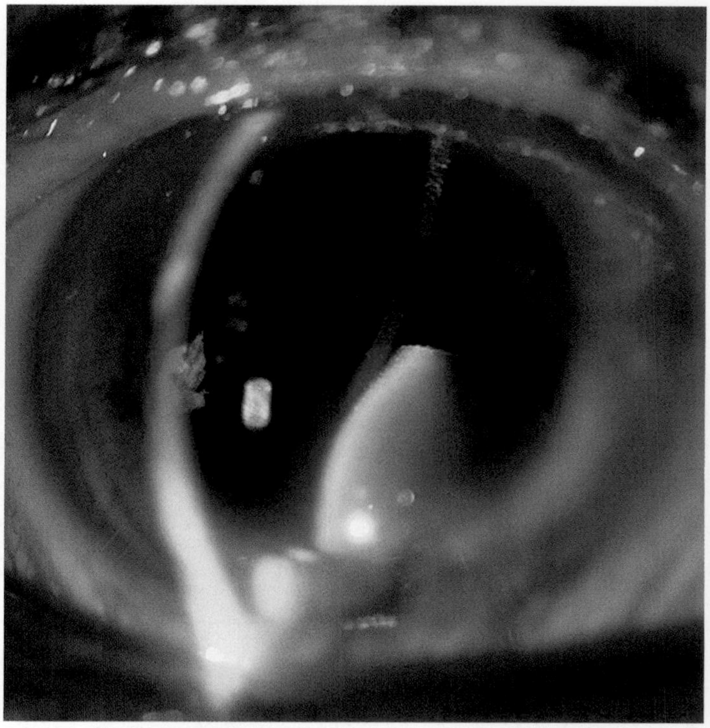

■ **Fig. 7.13** Total liquefaction of the lens with inferior dislocation of the nucleus. (Courtesy of P. Gili.)

Presenile cataract

Diabetic

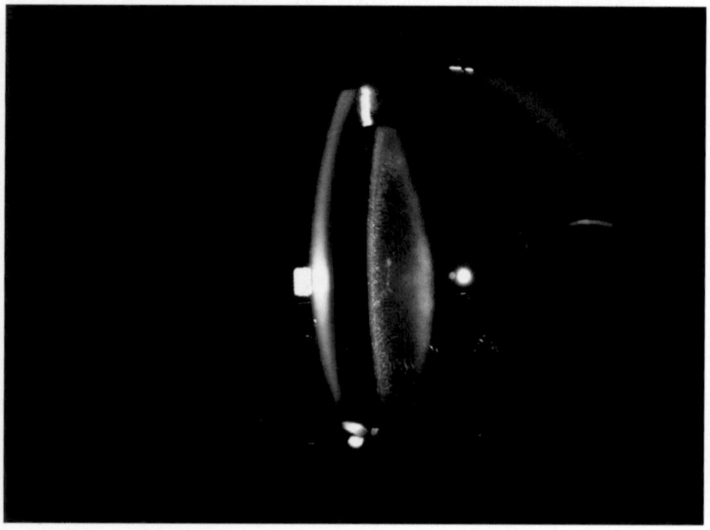

■ **Fig. 7.14** Classic acute diabetic cataract is characterised by snowflake cortical opacities occurring in the young diabetic. Such a cataract may resolve spontaneously or become mature within a few days. (Courtesy of A. Fielder.)

Myotonic

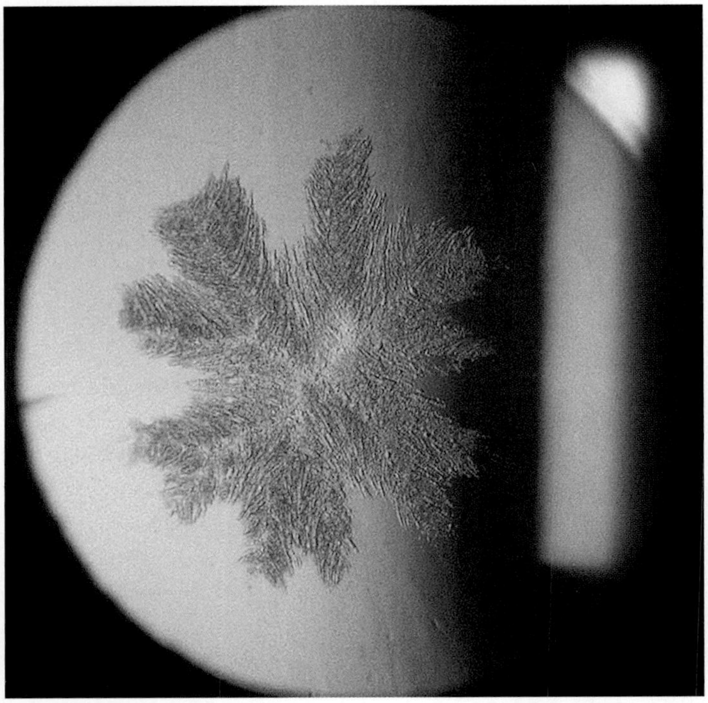

■ **Fig. 7.15** Stellate posterior subcapsular cataract. (Courtesy of L. Merin.)

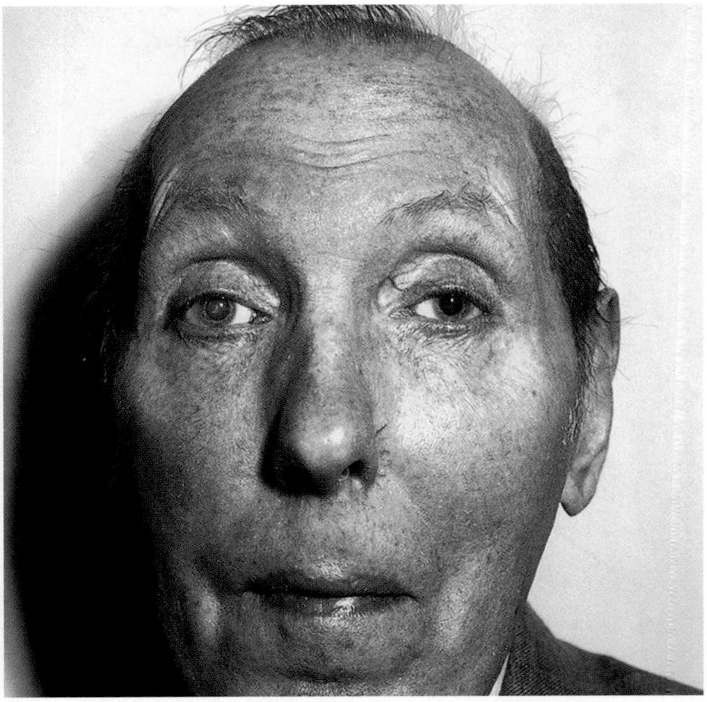

■ **Fig. 7.16** Mournful facial expression, frontal baldness and right cataract.

Atopic

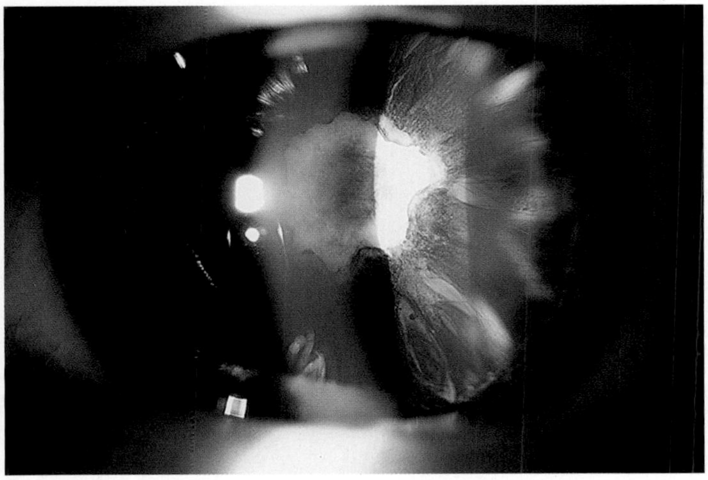

■ **Fig. 7.17** Dense, shield-like anterior subcapsular plaque that wrinkles the anterior capsule is characteristic.

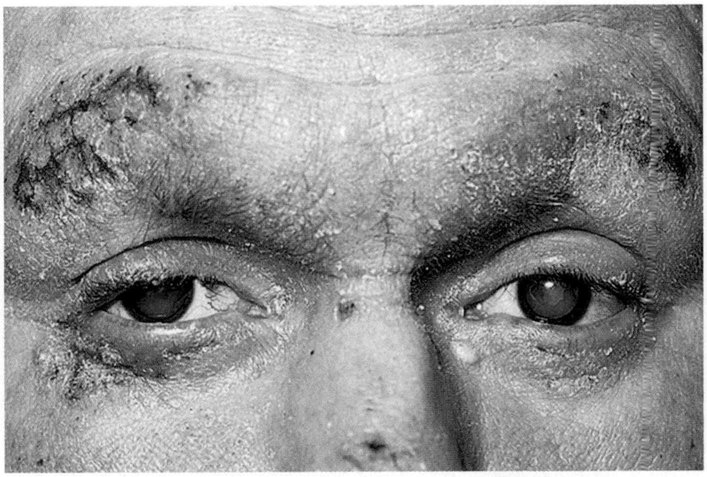

■ **Fig. 7.18** The opacities are often bilateral and may become mature quickly.

Drug-induced cataract

Steroids

Steroids, both systemic and topical, are cataractogenic.

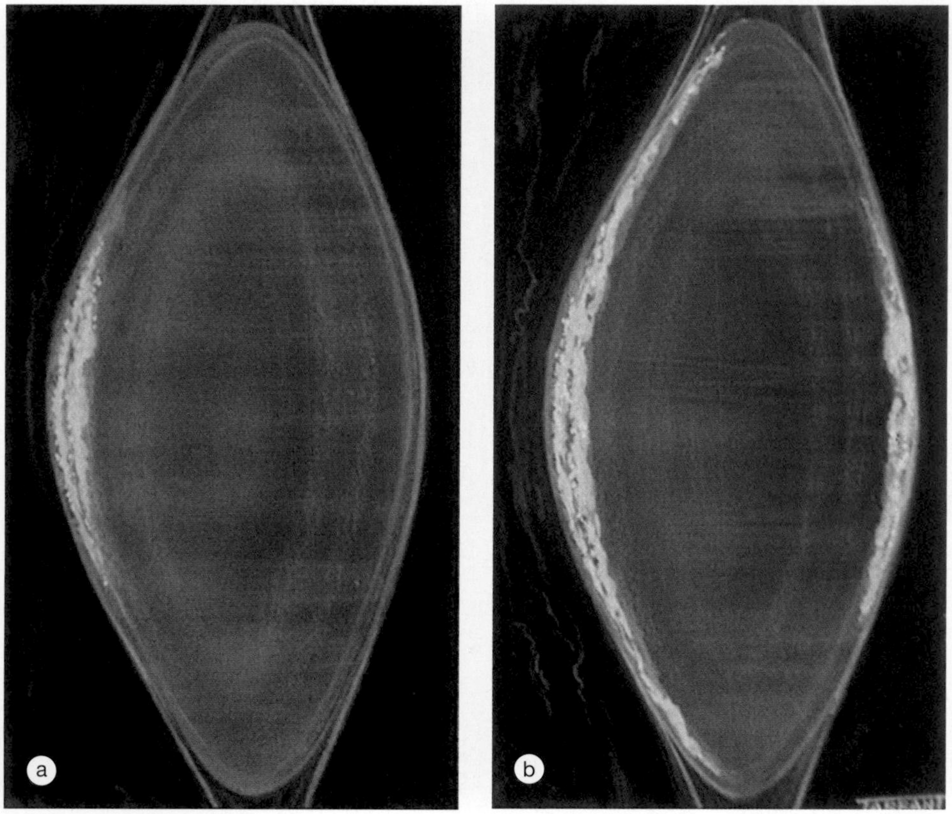

Fig. 7.19 **(a)** The lens opacities are initially posterior subcapsular **(b)**; later the anterior subcapsular region becomes affected.

Chlorpromazine

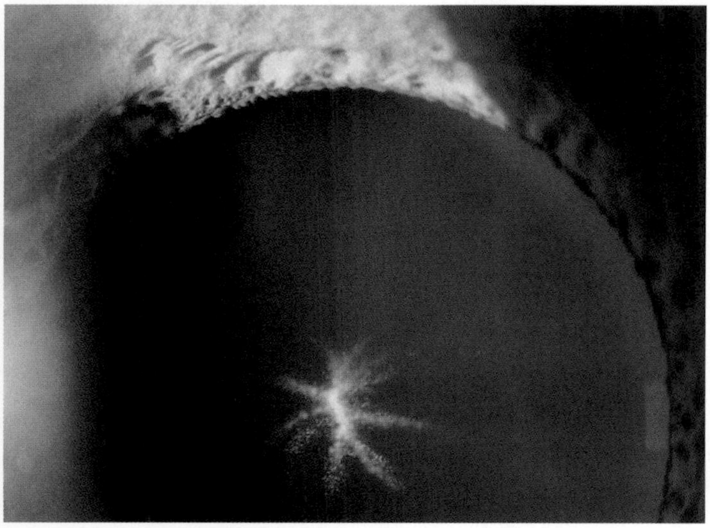

Fig. 7.20 Innocuous, fine, stellate, yellowish-brown granules on the anterior lens capsule within the pupillary area. (Courtesy of R. Curtis.)

Secondary cataract

Secondary (complicated) cataract develops as a result of some other ocular disease such as:

Chronic anterior uveitis

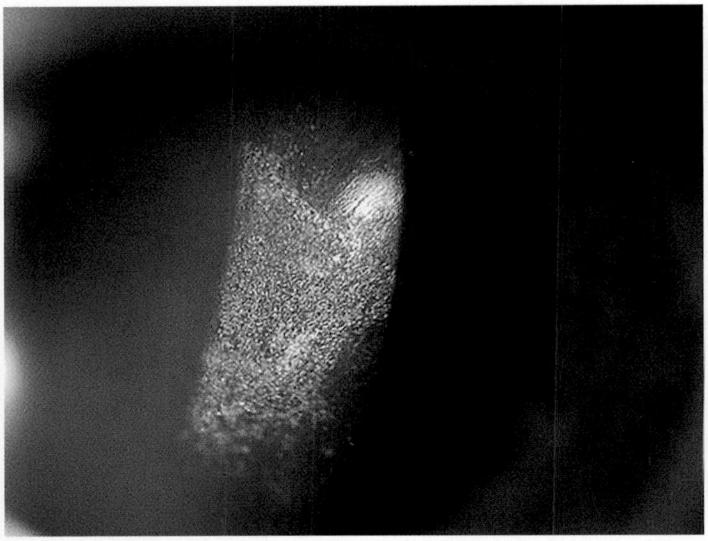

Fig. 7.21 Polychromatic posterior subcapsular granules.

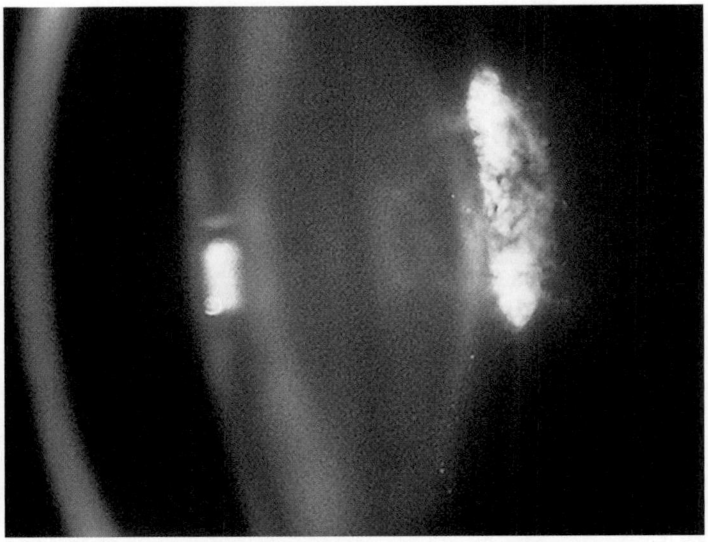

Fig. 7.22 Posterior subcapsular cataract.

Acute congestive angle closure glaucoma

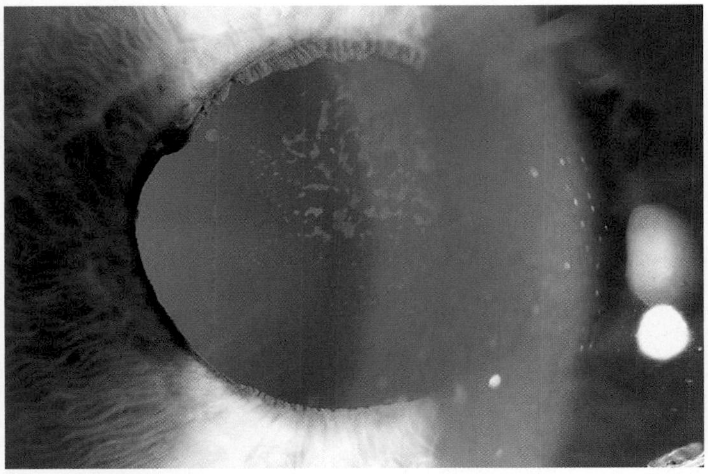

Fig. 7.23 Small, grey-white, anterior, subcapsular or capsular opacities within the pupillary area (*glaukomflecken*).

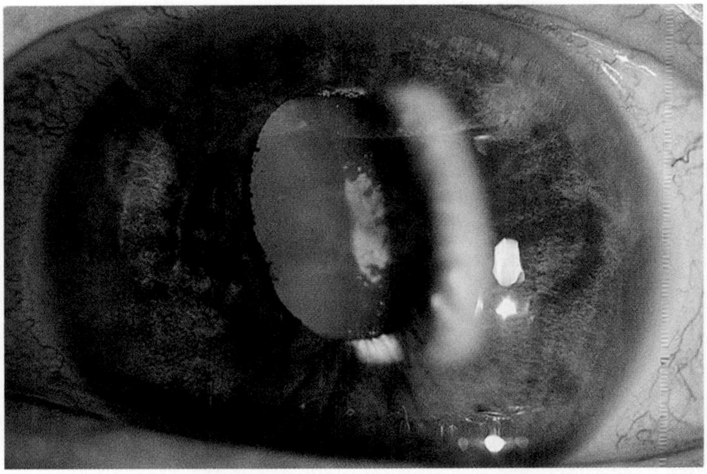

Fig. 7.24 More severe *glaukomflecken*.

CONGENITAL CATARACT

Isolated hereditary cataracts

Isolated hereditary cataract is most frequently autosomal dominant (AD) but may be autosomal recessive (AR) or X-linked (XL).

Nuclear

The opacity is confined the embryonic nucleus of the lens.

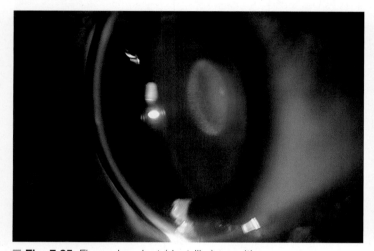

Fig. 7.25 Fine pulverulent (dust-like) opacities.

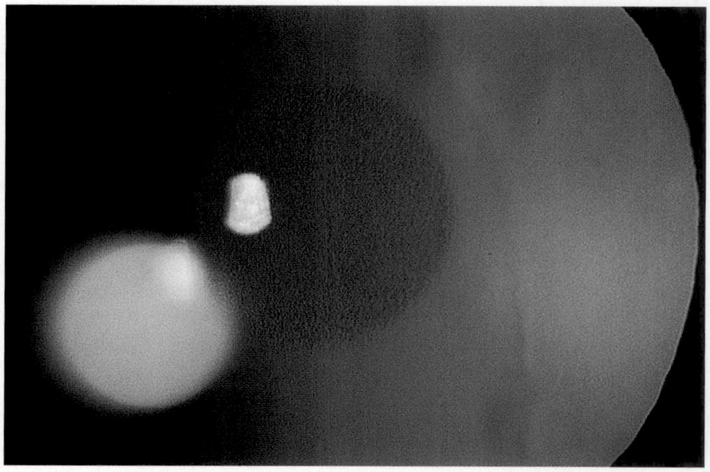

Fig. 7.26 Same eye seen on retroillumination.

Lamellar

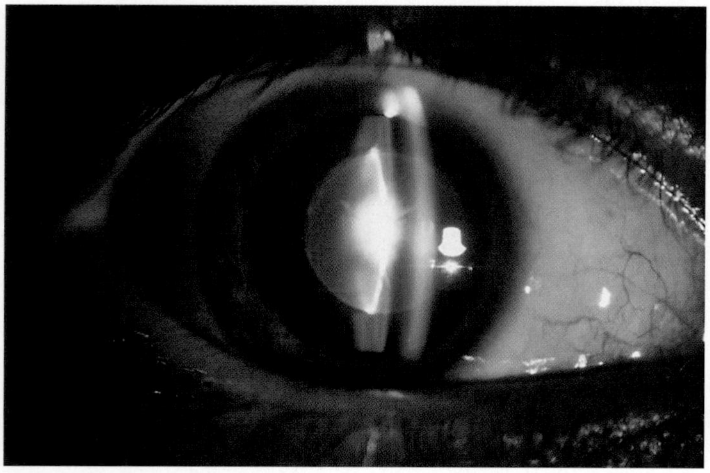

Fig. 7.27 The opacity is sandwiched between clear nucleus and cortex.

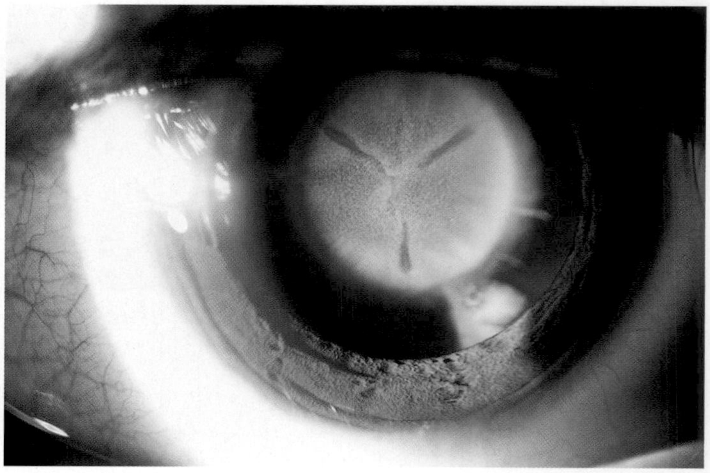

Fig. 7.28 The cataract may be associated with radial extensions (riders).

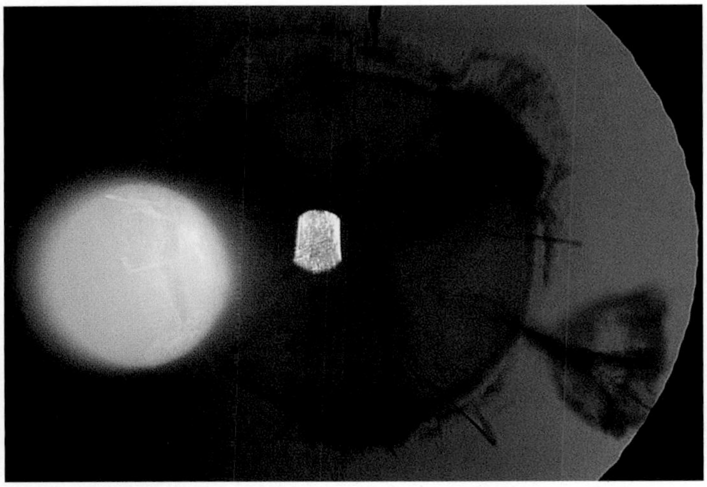

■ **Fig. 7.29** Same eye seen on retroillumination.

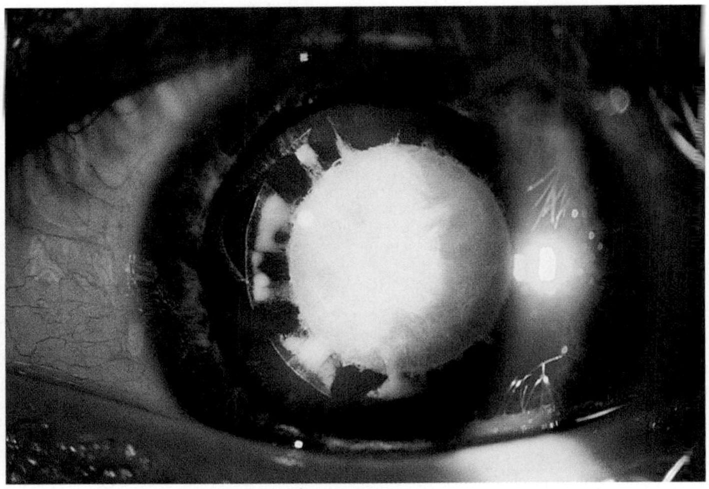

■ **Fig. 7.30** Dense lamellar cataract with riders.

Sutural

The opacity follows the anterior or posterior Y suture.

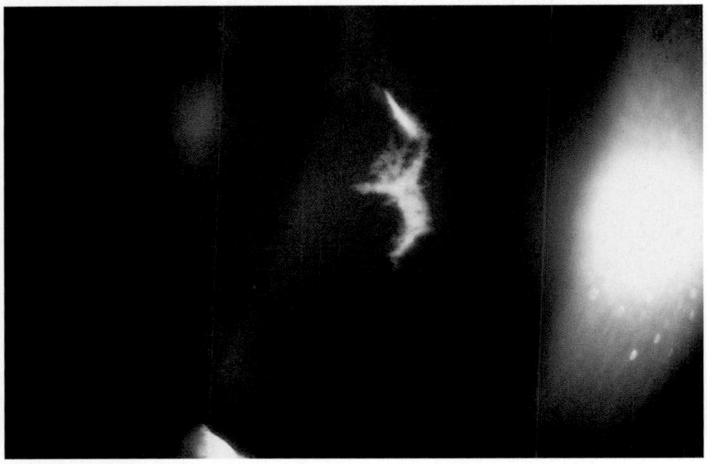

■ **Fig. 7.31** Sutural cataract.

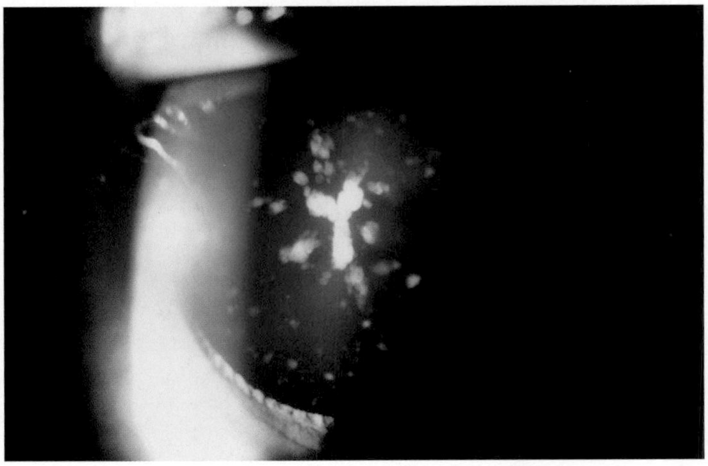

■ **Fig. 7.32** Sutural and blue dot opacities.

Anterior polar

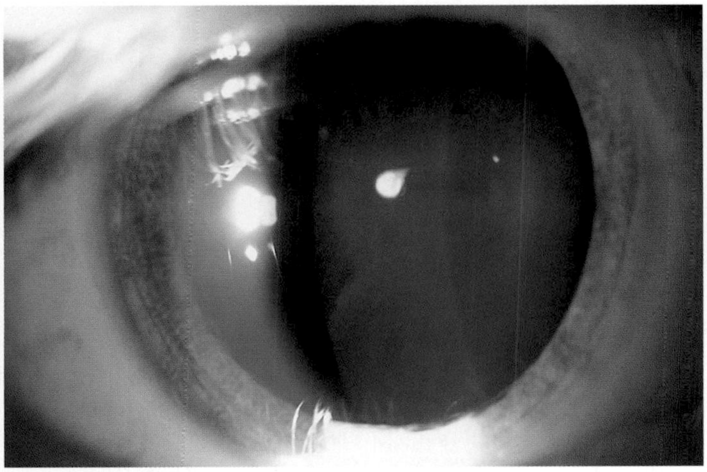

■ **Fig. 7.33** Flat anterior polar cataract.

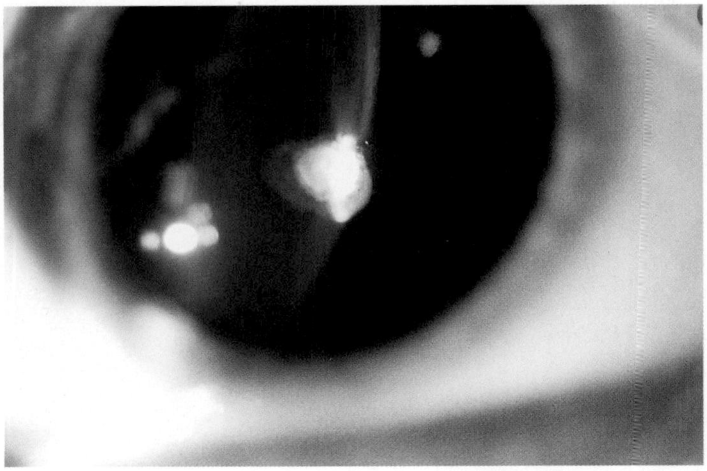

■ **Fig. 7.34** Anterior polar cataract projecting as a conical opacity into the anterior chamber (pyramidal cataract).

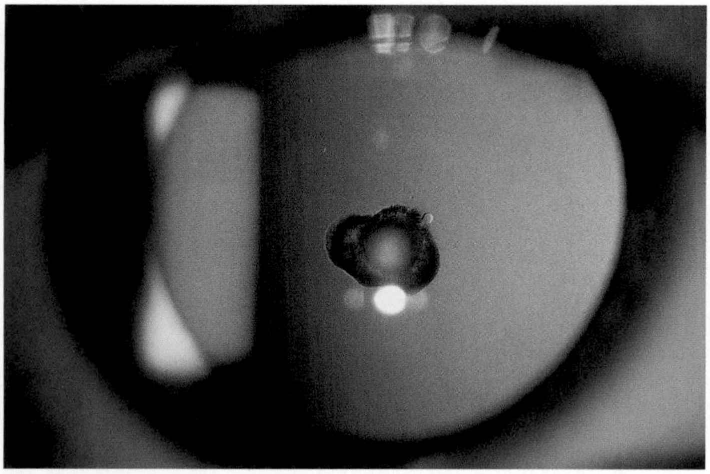

Fig. 7.35 Same eye seen on retroillumination.

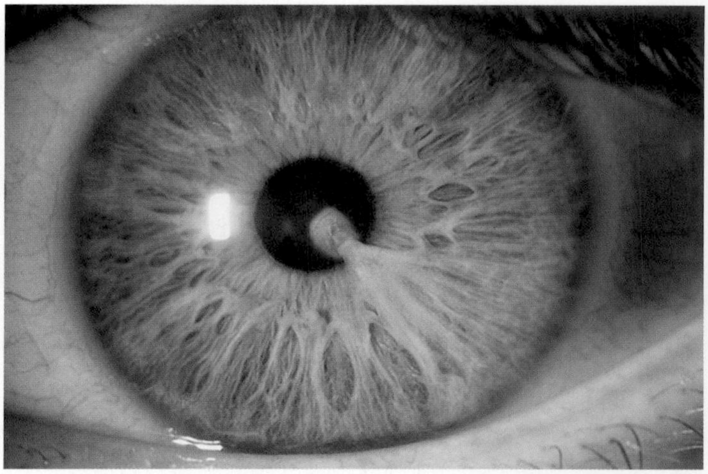

Fig. 7.36 Anterior polar opacity associated with a persistent pupillary membrane.

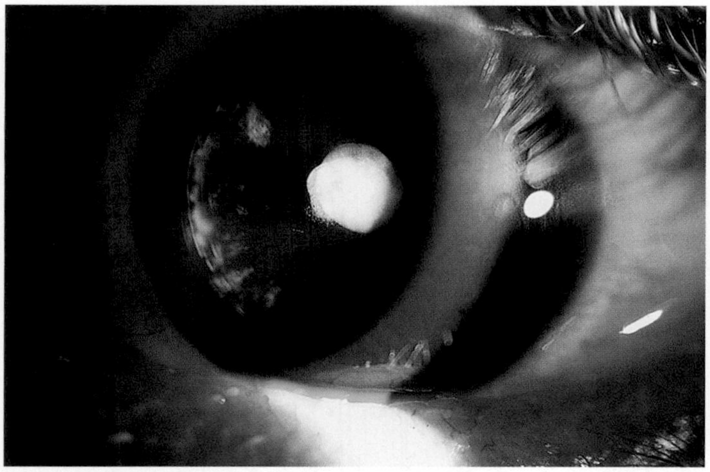

Fig. 7.37 Anterior polar cataract in aniridia.

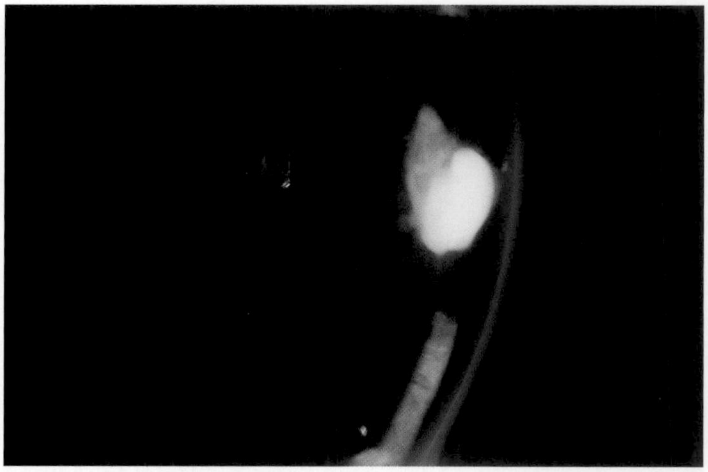

Fig. 7.38 Anterior polar cataract in Peters anomaly.

Posterior polar

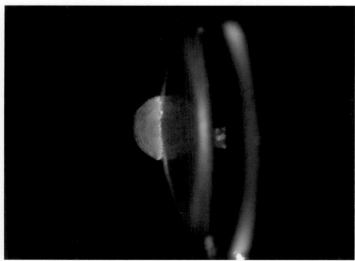

Fig. 7.39 A posterior polar opacity may be occasionally associated with persistent hyaloid remnants (Mittendorf dots), posterior lenticonus or persistent hyperplastic primary vitreous. (Courtesy of L. Merin.)

Other congenital cataracts

Coronary (supranuclear)

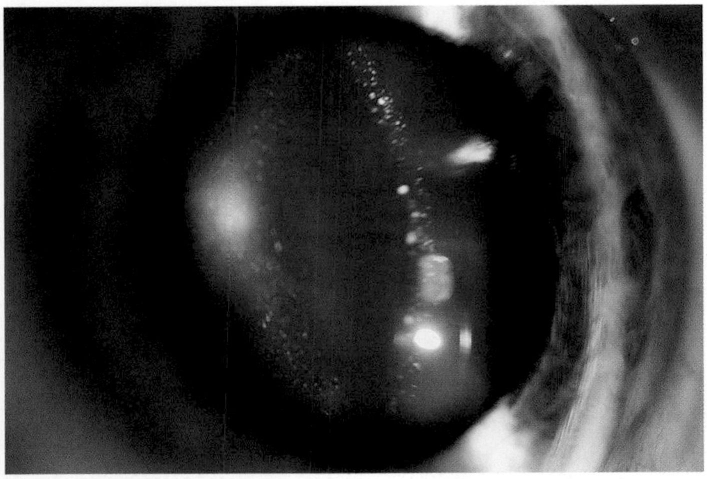

■ **Fig. 7.40** Round opacities in the deep cortex that surround the nucleus like a crown, which are usually sporadic and only occasionally hereditary.

Blue dot (cataracta punctata caerulea)

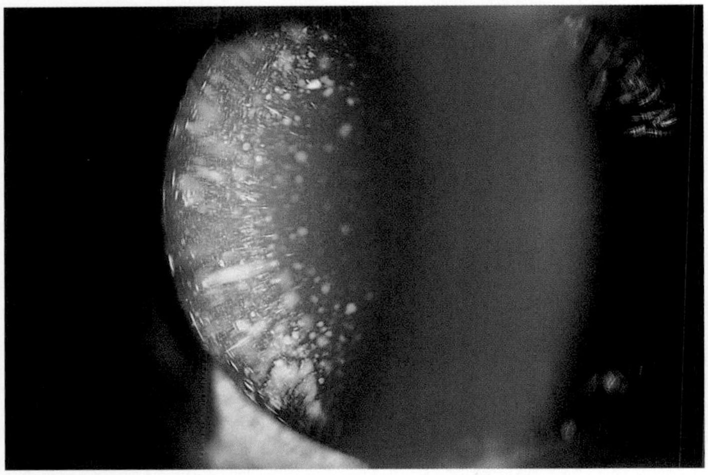

■ **Fig. 7.41** Blue dots are innocuous and typically occur in patients with Down syndrome.

■ **Fig. 7.42** Same eye seen on retroillumination.

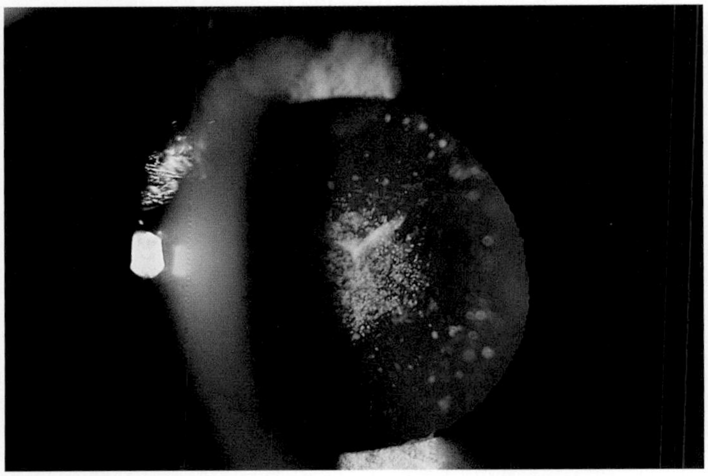

■ **Fig. 7.43** Blue dots may coexist with other opacities, such as sutural in this case.

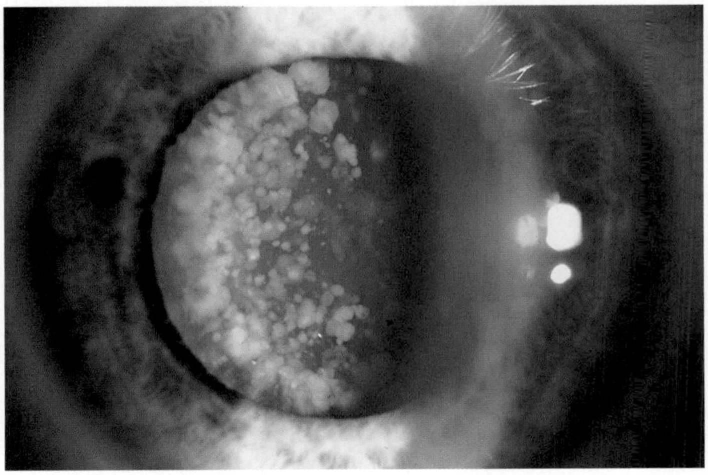

■ **Fig. 7.44** Dense blue dot cataract.

Systemic associations of congenital cataract

Galastosaemia

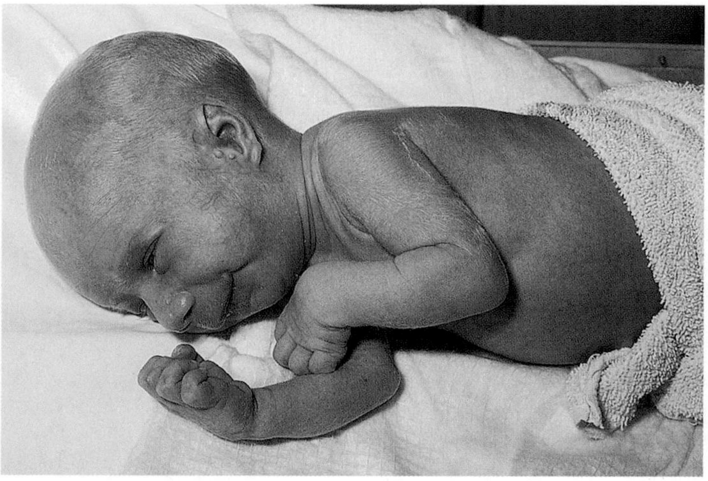

■ **Fig. 7.45** Systemic features of this AR condition include failure to thrive, lethargy, vomiting and diarrhoea.

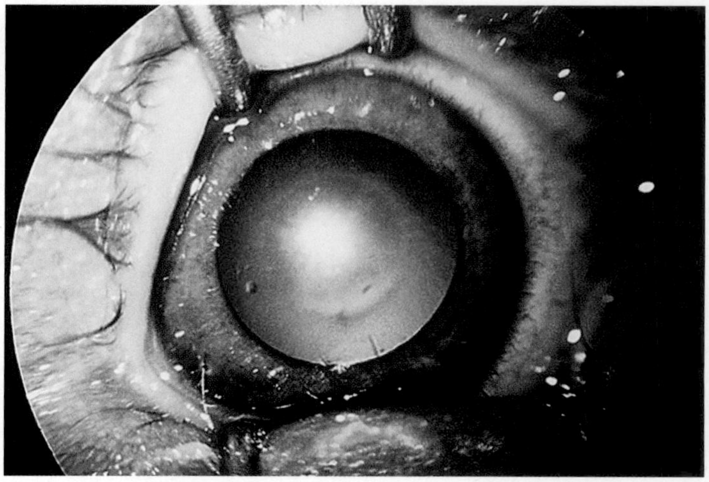

■ **Fig. 7.46** Central 'oil droplet' opacity develops within the first few days or weeks of life in a large percentage of babies. (Courtesy of K. Nischal.)

Lowe (oculocerebrorenal) syndrome

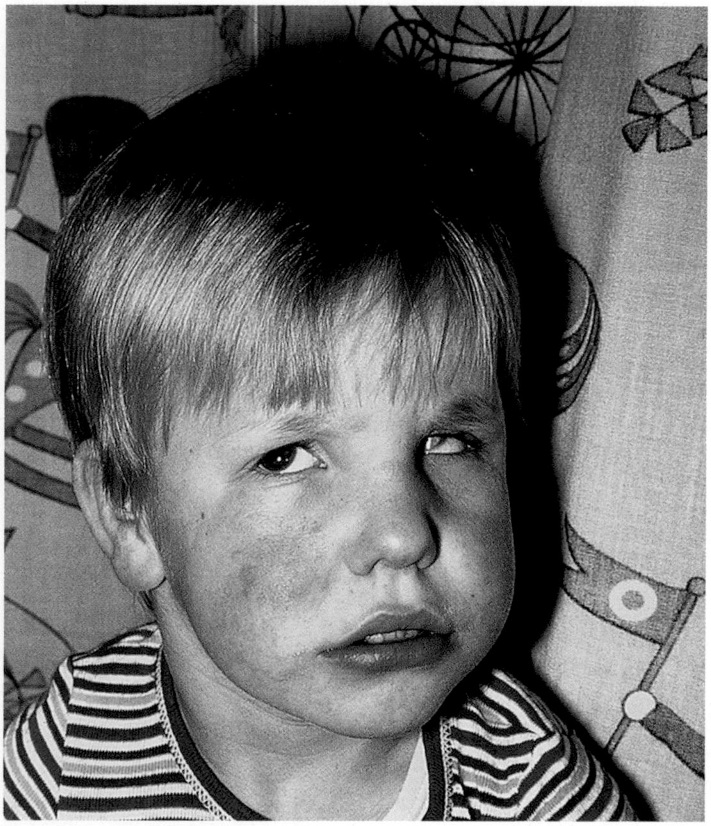

■ **Fig. 7.47** Systemic features include mental handicap, renal disease, muscular hypotonia, frontal prominence and sunken eyes. Cataract is universal and is associated with glaucoma in 50% of cases.

Hallermann–Streiff–Francois syndrome

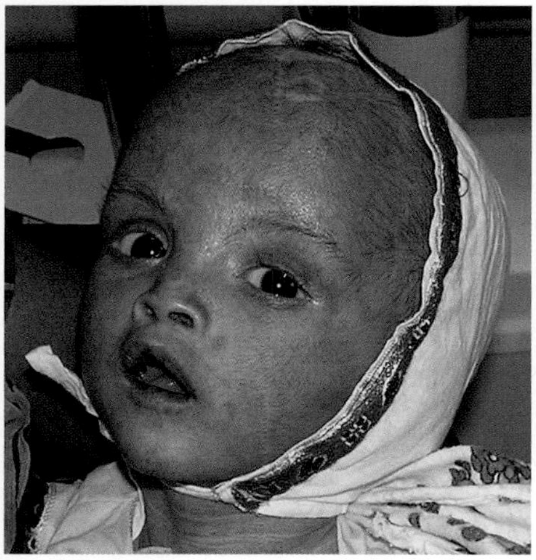

■ **Fig. 7.48** Systemic features include frontal prominence, small beaked nose, baldness, progeria, micrognathia and pointed chin, short stature and hypodontia. (Courtesy of M. Parulekar.)

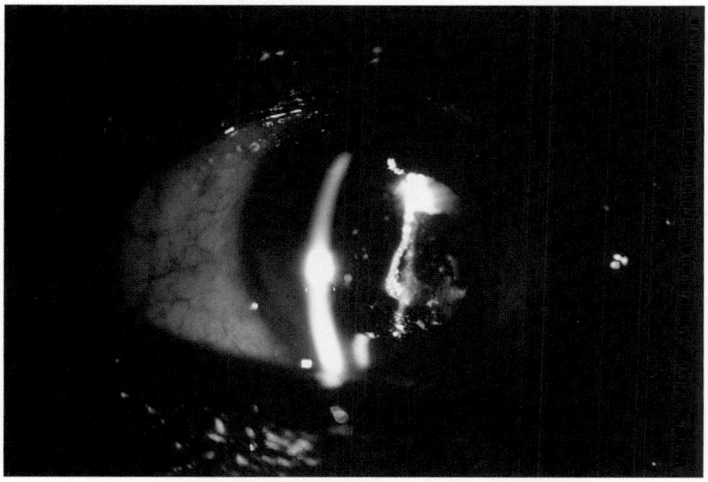

■ **Fig. 7.49** A membranous cataract is typical. It is due to reabsorption of lens material leaving behind residual chalky-white matter sandwiched between the anterior and posterior capsules.

Congenital rubella

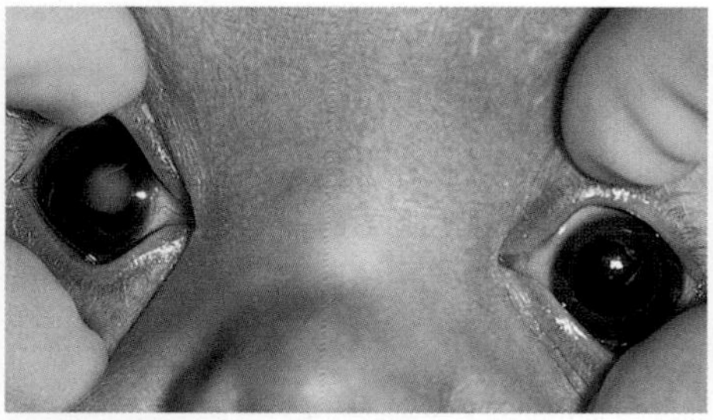

■ **Fig. 7.50** Unilateral or bilateral pearly nuclear cataracts. (Courtesy of W. Aclimandos.)

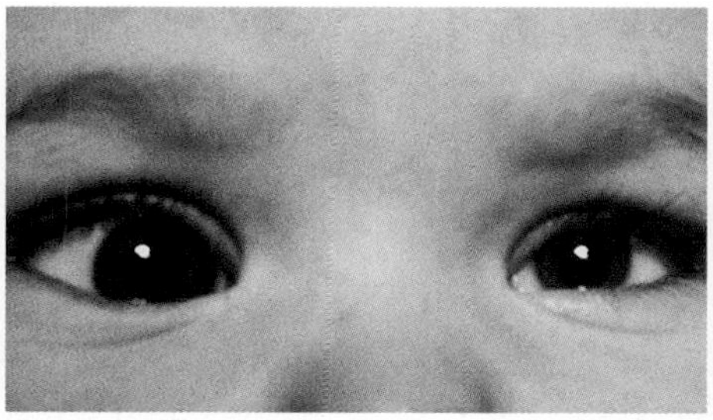

■ **Fig. 7.51** Microphthalmos. (Courtesy of S. Ford and R. Marsh.)

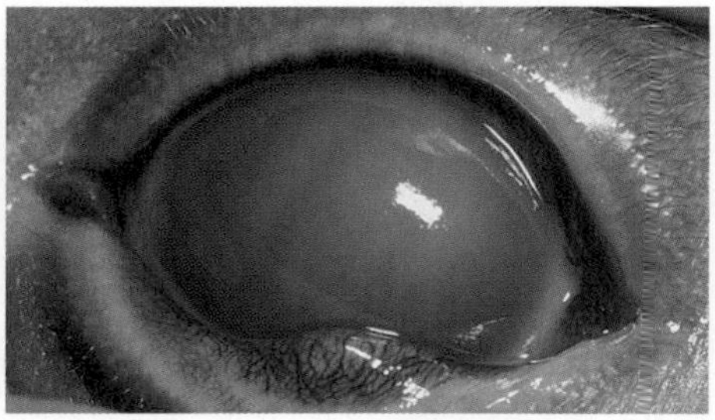

■ **Fig. 7.52** Corneal haze may be caused by keratitis or less commonly elevation of intraocular pressure. (Courtesy of L. Merin.)

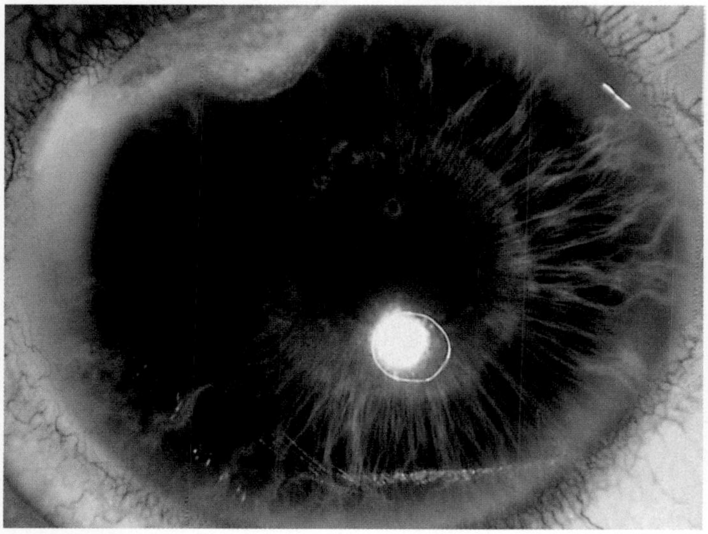

■ **Fig. 7.53** Iris hypoplasia.

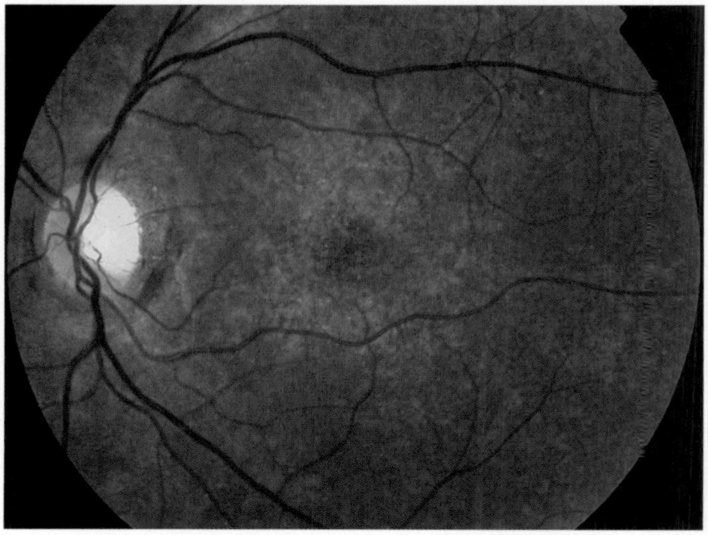

■ **Fig. 7.54** Pigmentary retinopathy. (Courtesy of Moorfields Eye Hospital.)

ANOMALIES OF LENS SHAPE

Coloboma

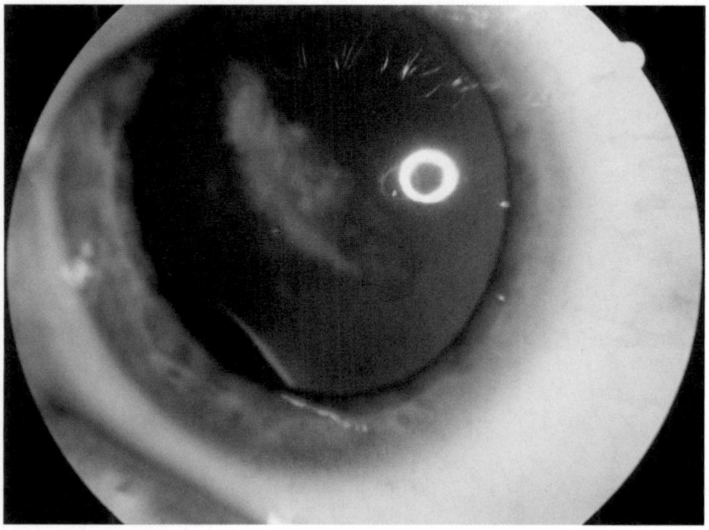

■ **Fig. 7.55** Notching (segmental agenesis) at the inferior equator with corresponding absence of zonules.

Posterior lenticonus

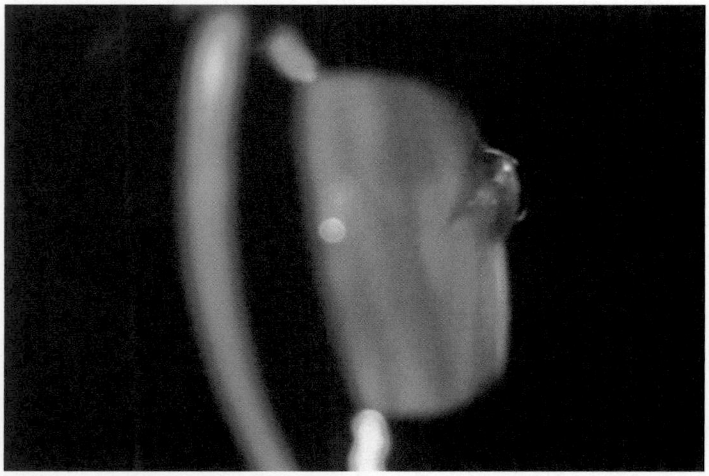

■ **Fig. 7.56** A bulge of the posterior axial zone of the lens into the vitreous associated with local thinning or absence of the capsule.

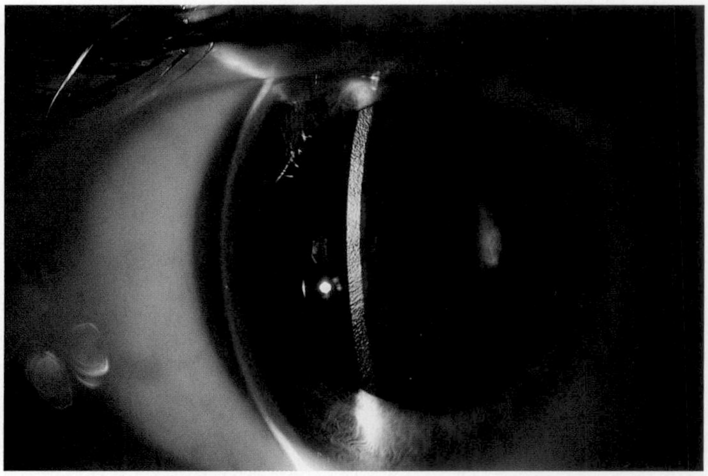

■ **Fig. 7.57** Posterior lenticonus associated with a mild posterior polar opacity.

Anterior lenticonus

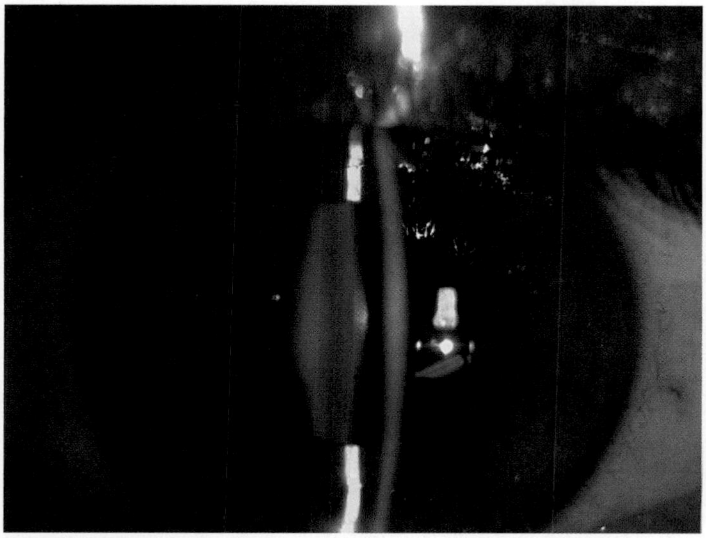

■ **Fig. 7.58** Bilateral axial projection of the anterior surface of the lens found in about 90% of patients with Alport syndrome. (Courtesy of M. Khairallah.)

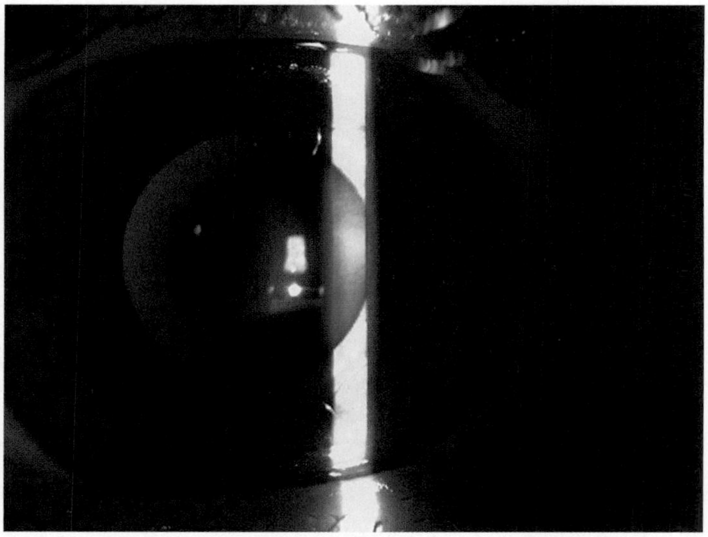

■ **Fig. 7.59** Same eye seen on retroillumination. (Courtesy of M. Khairallah.)

Microspherophakia

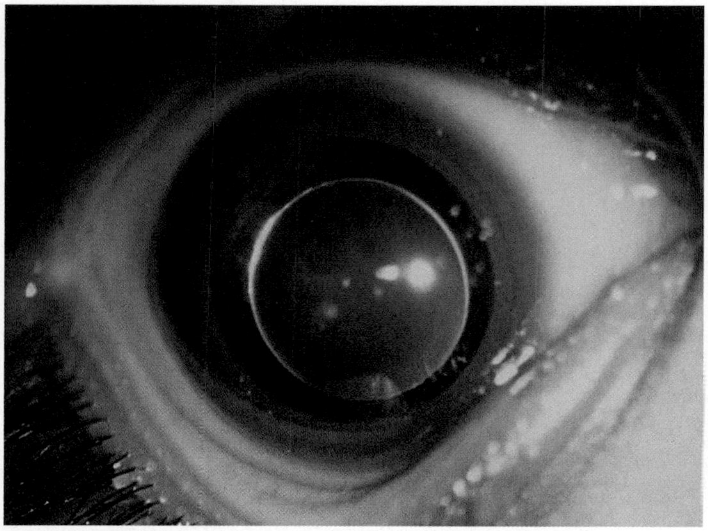

■ **Fig. 7.60** A lens with a small diameter and spherical shape. (Courtesy of U. Raina.)

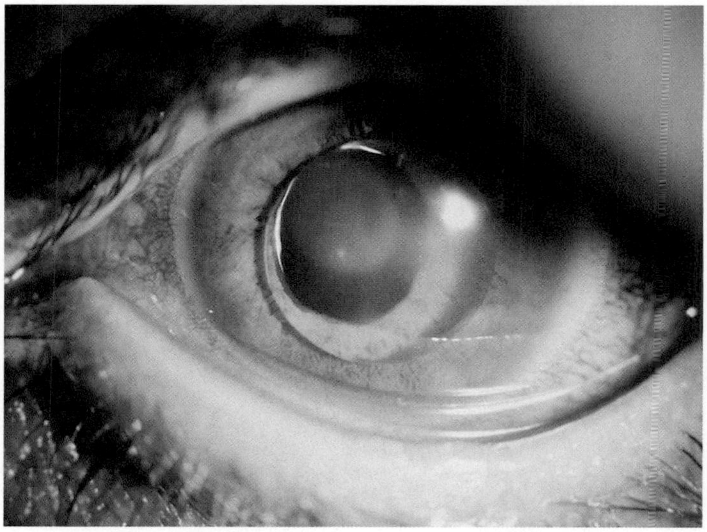

■ **Fig. 7.61** Dislocation into the anterior chamber is a serious complication.

HEREDITARY ECTOPIA LENTIS

Ectopia lentis refers to a displacement of the lens from its normal position. Acquired causes include trauma, a large eye (i.e. high myopia, buphthalmos), anterior uveal tumours and hypermature cataract. Hereditary causes include the following:

Without systemic associations

Familial ectopia lentis

Inheritance is AD.

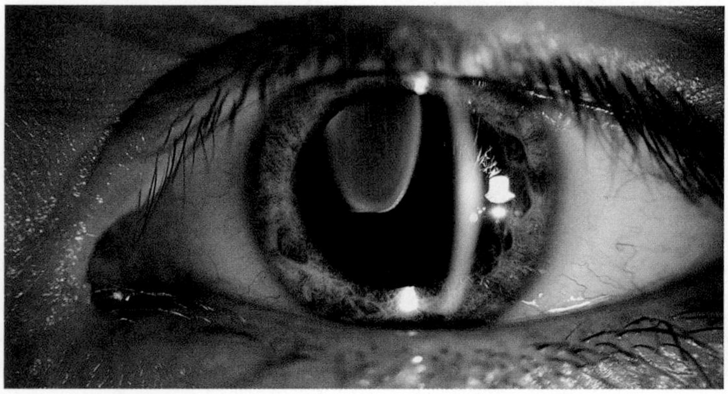

Fig. 7.62 Bilateral, symmetrical, superior subluxation.

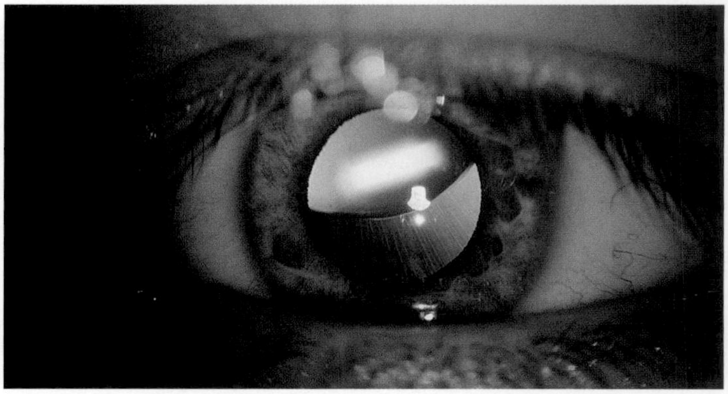

Fig. 7.63 Same eye seen on retroillumination.

Ectopia lentis et pupillae

Inheritance is AR.

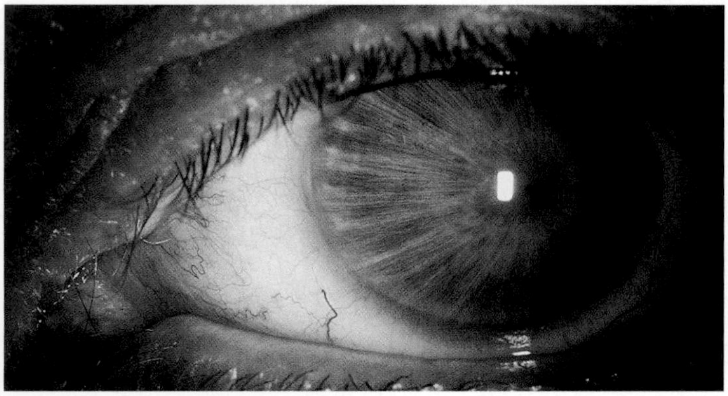

Fig. 7.64 The pupils are displaced, small and slit-like.

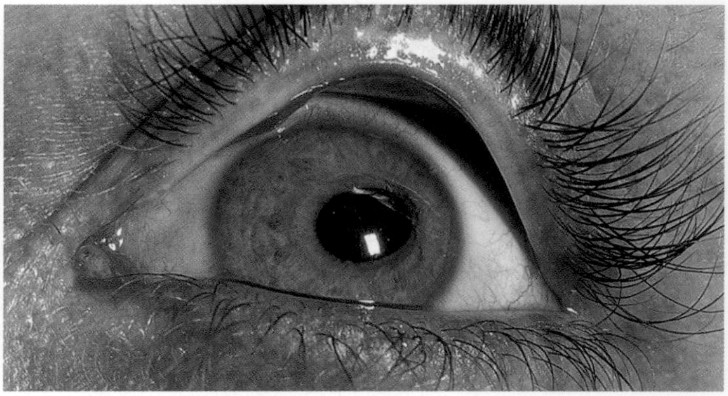

Fig. 7.65 Although dilatation is poor it can be seen that the lens and pupil are displaced in opposite directions.

Aniridia

Aniridia is occasionally associated with ectopia lentis.

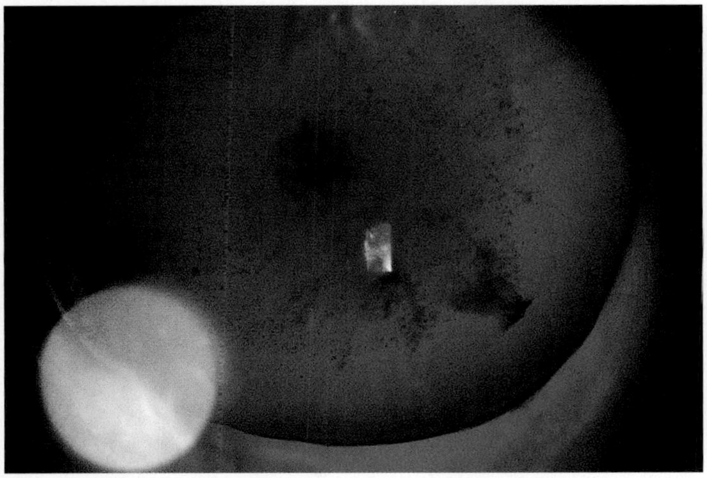

Fig. 7.66 Superior subluxation of a clear lens in aniridia.

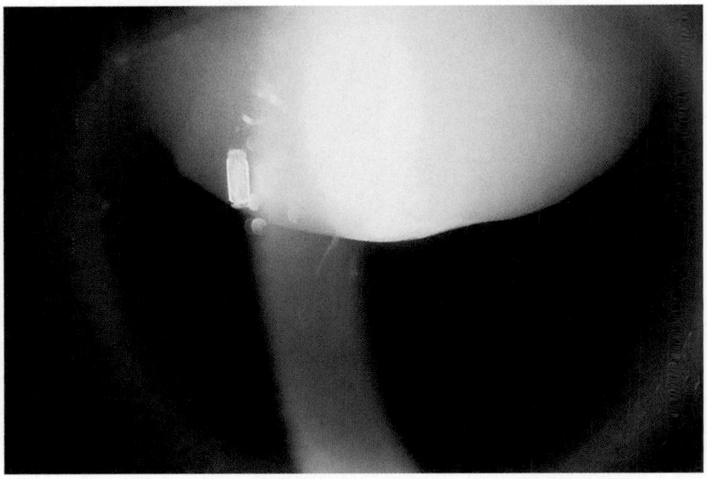

Fig. 7.67 Superior subluxation of a cataractous lens in aniridia.

With systemic associations

Marfan syndrome

Marfan syndrome is an AD disorder of connective tissue.

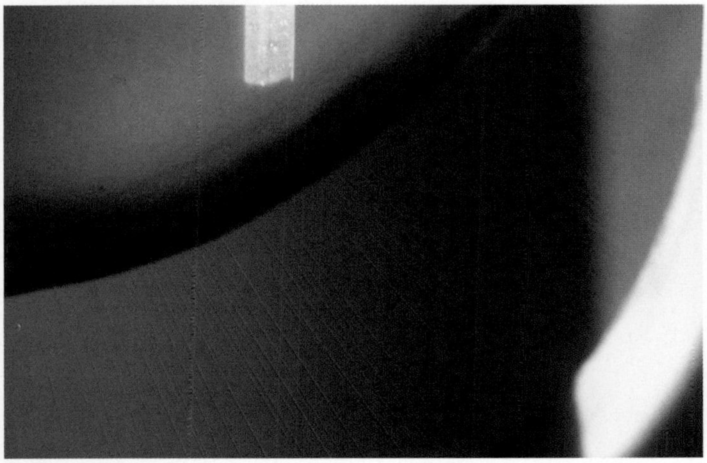

Fig. 7.68 Ectopia lentis is bilateral, most frequently superotemporal but may be in any meridian. Because the zonules are frequently intact, accommodation is retained. (Courtesy of L. Merin.)

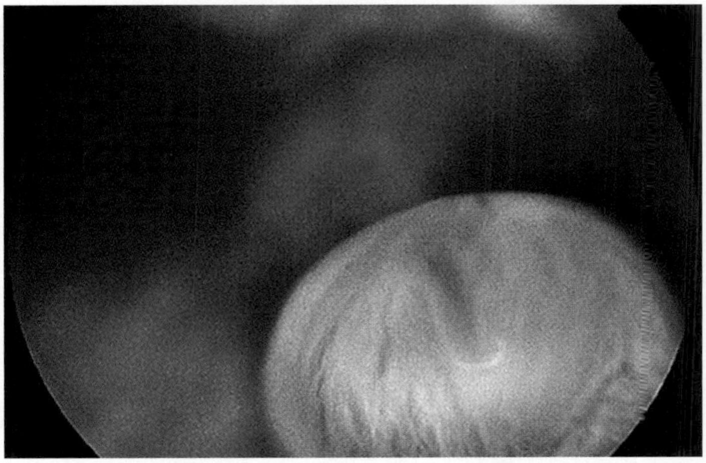

Fig. 7.69 Dislocation into the vitreous is uncommon. (Courtesy of S. Milewski.)

Systemic signs

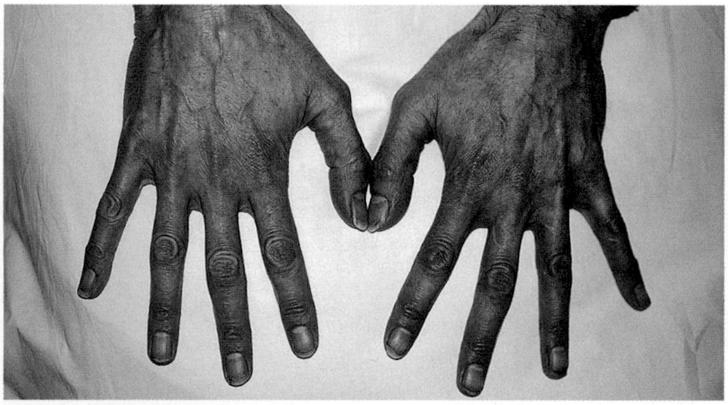

■ **Fig. 7.70** Arachnodactyly of the fingers.

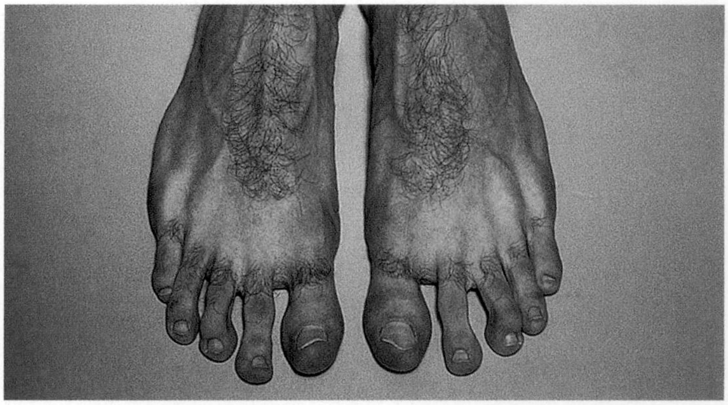

■ **Fig. 7.71** Arachnodactyly of the toes. (Courtesy of M. A. Mir.)

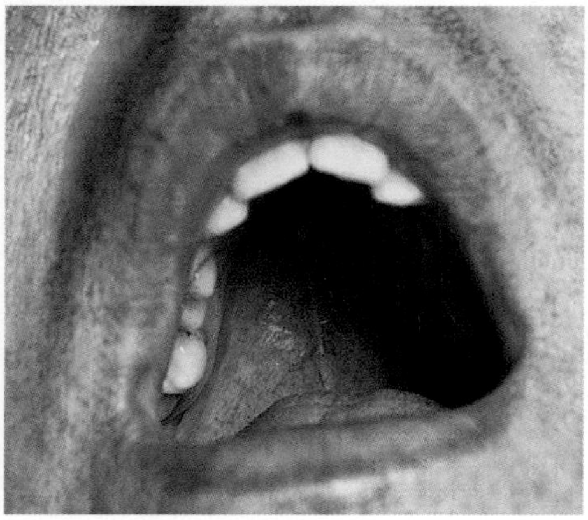

■ **Fig. 7.72** A narrow and high-arched (gothic) palate. (Courtesy of M. A. Mir.)

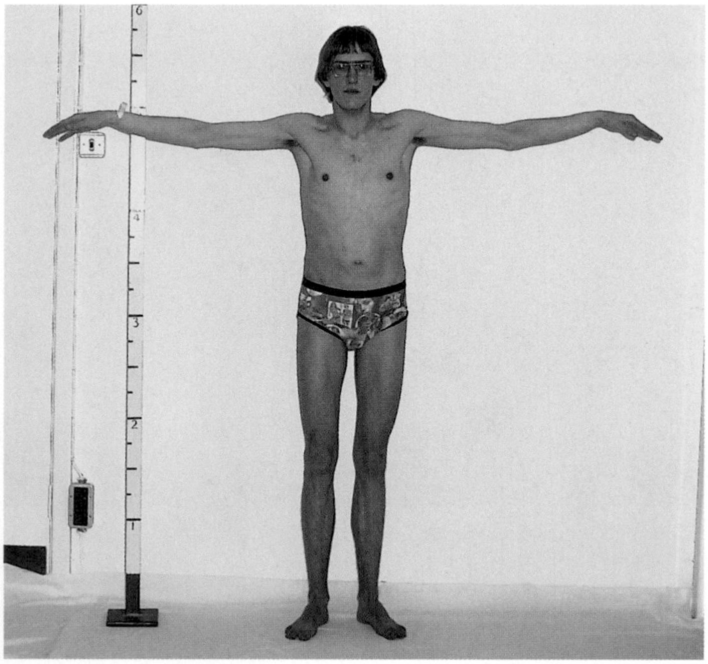

■ **Fig. 7.73** Tall thin stature with disproportionately long limbs compared with the trunk (arm span > height.)

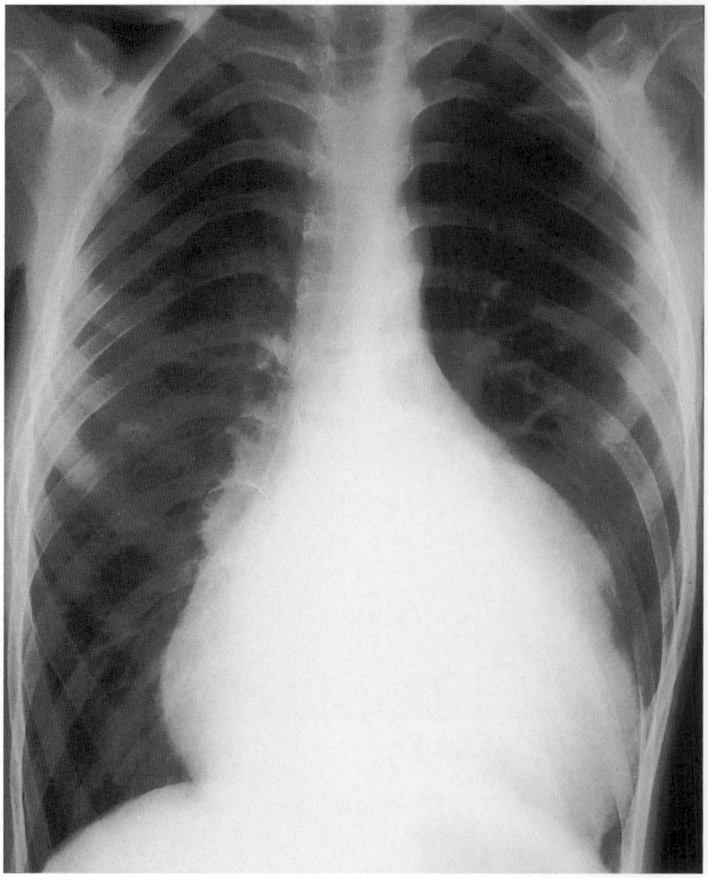

■ **Fig. 7.74** Cardiovascular disease such as dilatation of the ascending aorta leading to aortic incompetence and heart failure; also note the elongated chest. (Courtesy of S. Ghiacy.)

Weill–Marchesani syndrome

Weill–Marchesani syndrome is an AD or AR, connective tissue disease, conceptually the converse of Marfan syndrome.

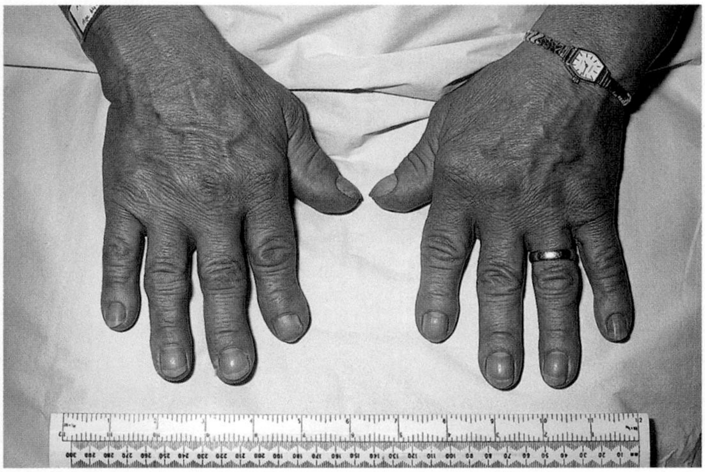

Fig. 7.75 Short, stubby hands (brachydactyly) with stiff fingers. Other features include short stature and mental handicap.

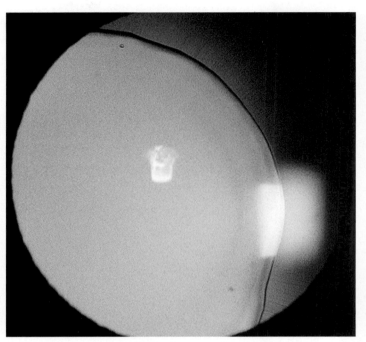

Fig. 7.76 Inferior ectopia lentis occurs in about 50% of cases during the teens or early twenties.

Homocystinuria

Homocystinuria is an AR inborn error of metabolism that results in systemic accumulation of homocysteine and methionine.

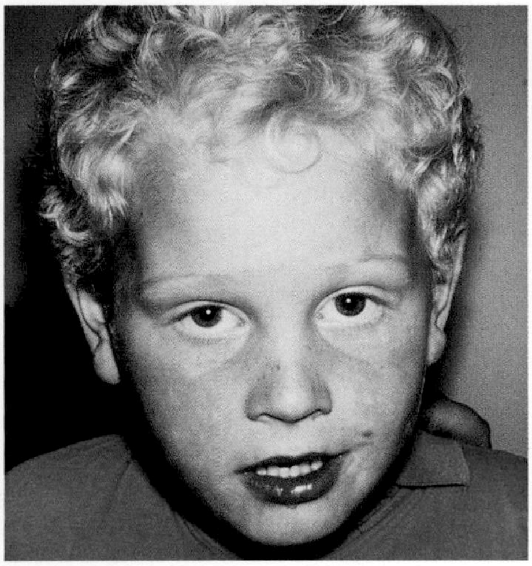

Fig. 7.77 Fair complexion, marfanoid habitus and a tendency to thrombotic episodes.

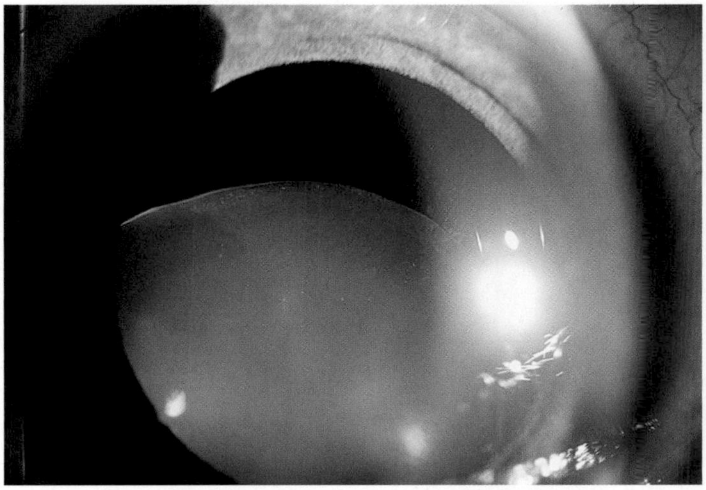

Fig. 7.78 Inferonasal ectopia lentis with disintegration of the zonules usually occurs by the age of 10 years.

COMPLICATIONS OF CATARACT SURGERY

Operative complications

Damage to the iris

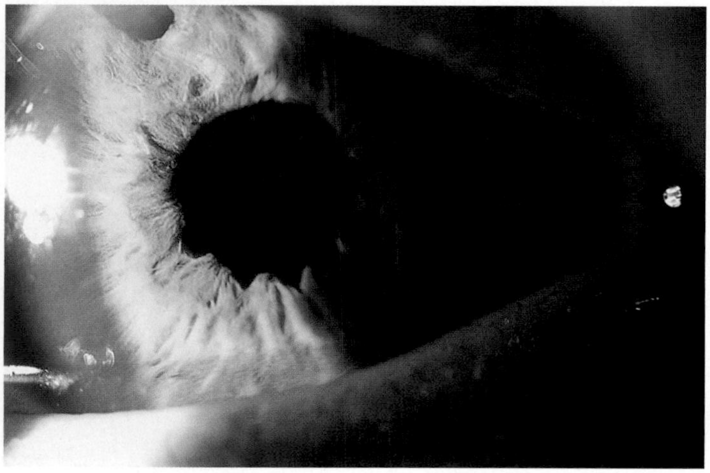

Fig. 7.79 The iris sphincter may be inadvertently damaged during phacoemulsification particularly if mydriasis is poor.

Posterior capsular rupture

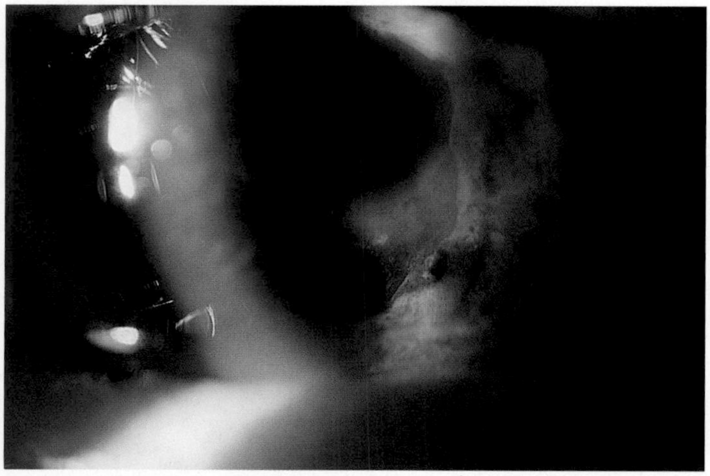

Fig. 7.80 Postoperative appearance.

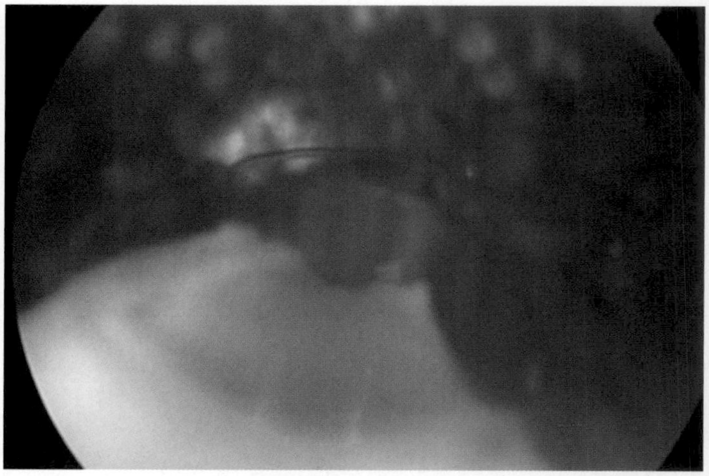

Fig. 7.81 Dislocation of fragments of lens material into the vitreous cavity, and occasionally also the intraocular lens (IOL), is rare.

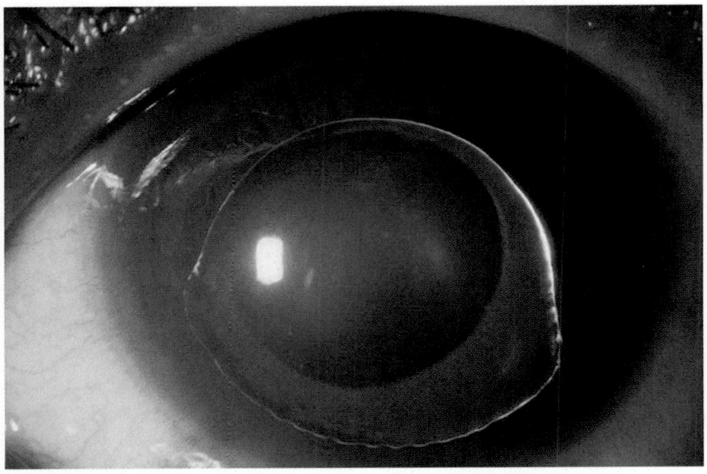

■ **Fig. 7.82** The lens material may subsequently migrate into the anterior chamber. (Courtesy of R. Curtis.)

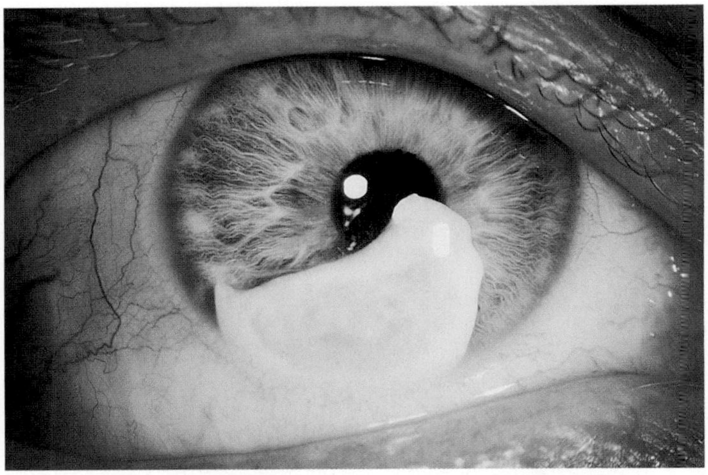

■ **Fig. 7.83** Large pieces of dense lens material may cause endothelial damage.

Vitreous loss

Vitreous loss may give rise to the following problems:

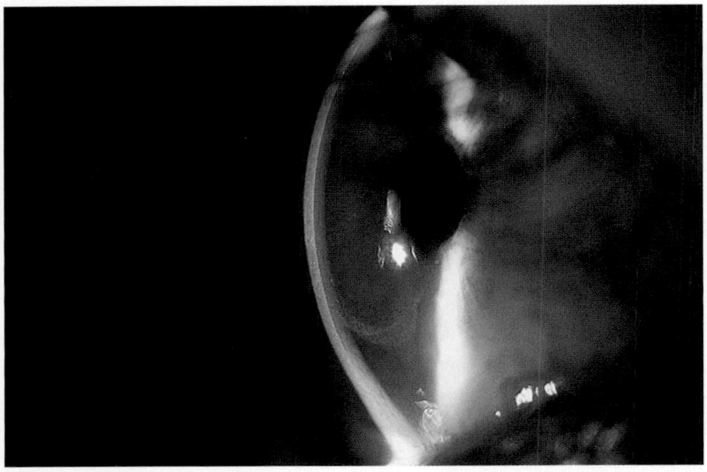

■ **Fig. 7.84** Postoperative vitreous touch which may result in endothelial decompensation.

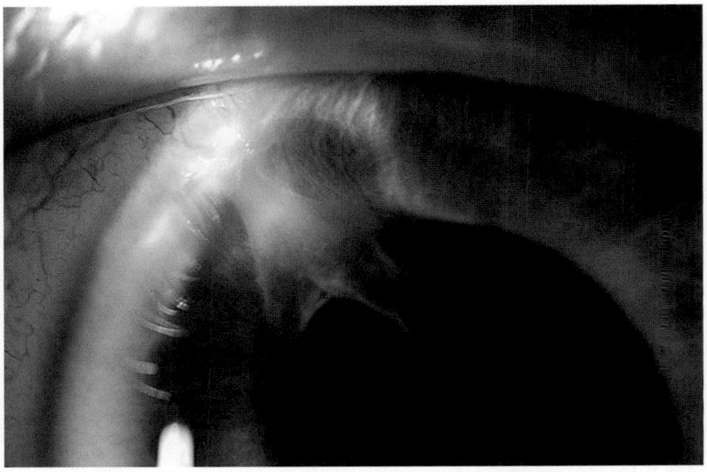

■ **Fig. 7.85** Vitreous incarceration in the incision site.

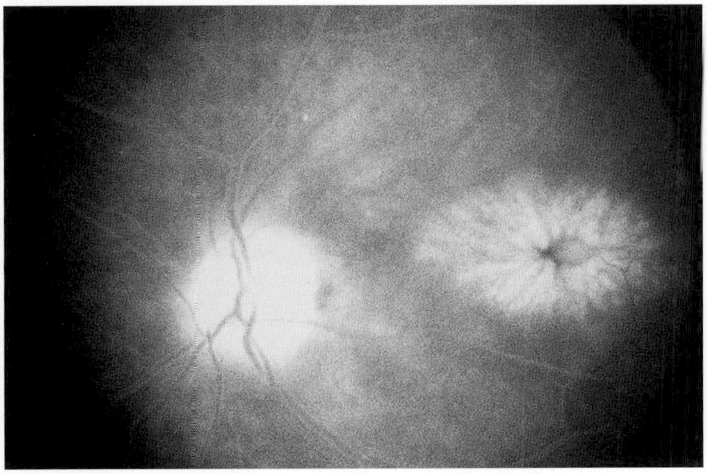

■ **Fig. 7.86** FA shows the characteristic flower-petal pattern of hyperfluorescence of cystoid macular oedema, which may occur as a result of vitreous loss and incarceration. (Courtesy of A. Frohlichstein.)

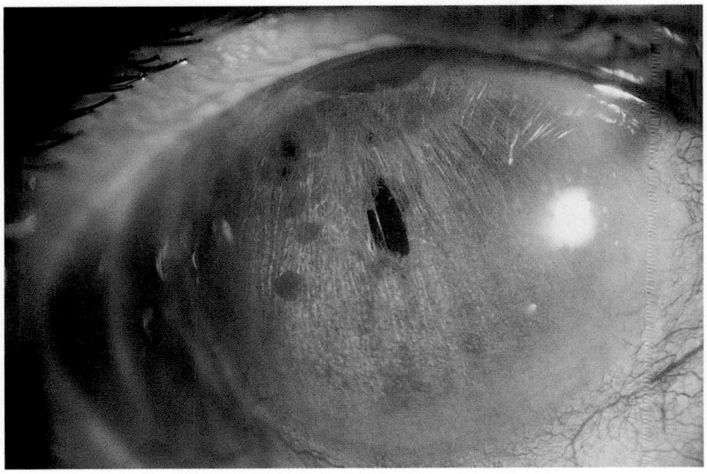

■ **Fig. 7.87** Updrawn pupil may also be associated with vitreous loss. In this case a second pupil has been made with a YAG laser.

Expulsive haemorrhage

A bleed into the suprachoroidal space is rare but very serious because it may result in extrusion of intraocular contents or apposition of retinal surfaces.

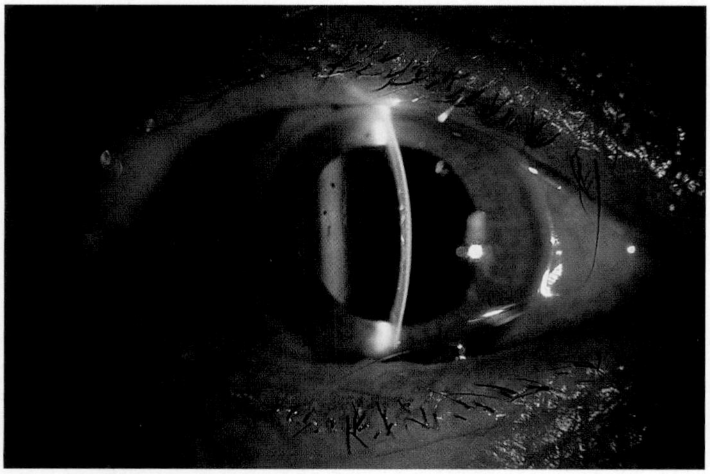

Fig. 7.88 Postoperative appearance.

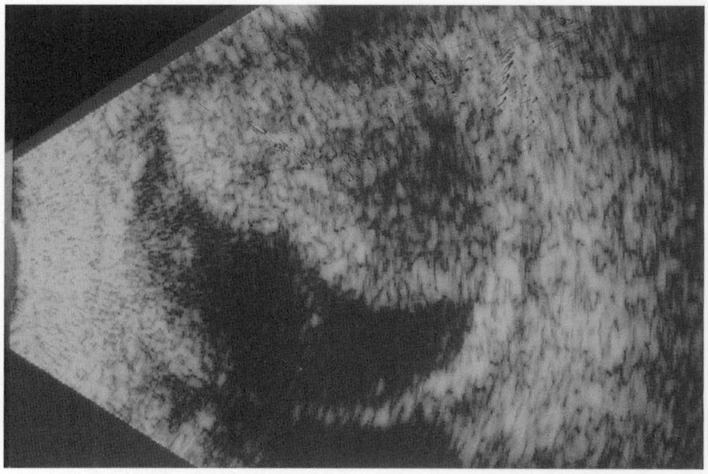

Fig. 7.89 Ultrasonogram shows a large suprachoroidal haemorrhage.

Postoperative complications

Corneal oedema

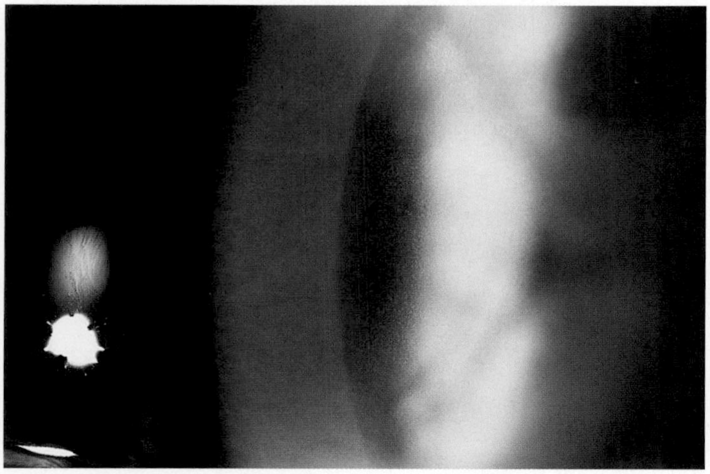

Fig. 7.90 Mild transient corneal oedema may occur as a result of endothelial damage during surgery.

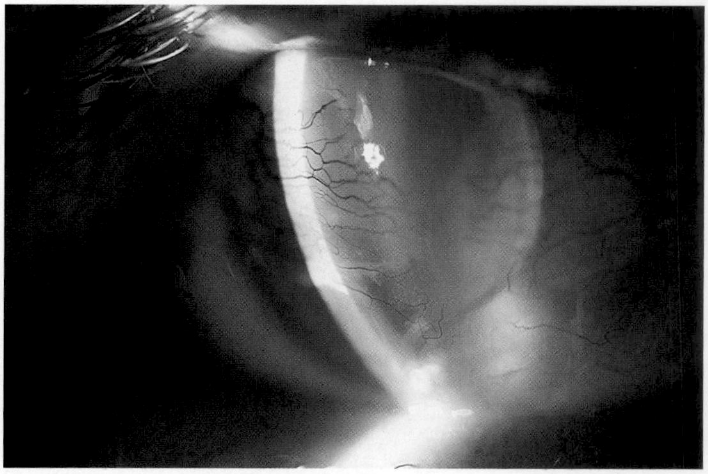

Fig. 7.91 Severe persistent corneal oedema, which may be associated with neovascularisation, is uncommon and may be caused by progressive endothelial decompensation by an anterior chamber IOL.

Iris prolapse

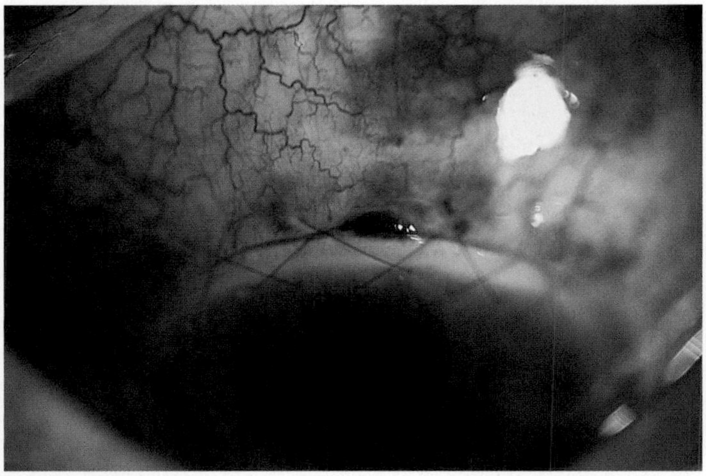

■ **Fig. 7.92** Iris prolapse may occur after large-incision surgery.

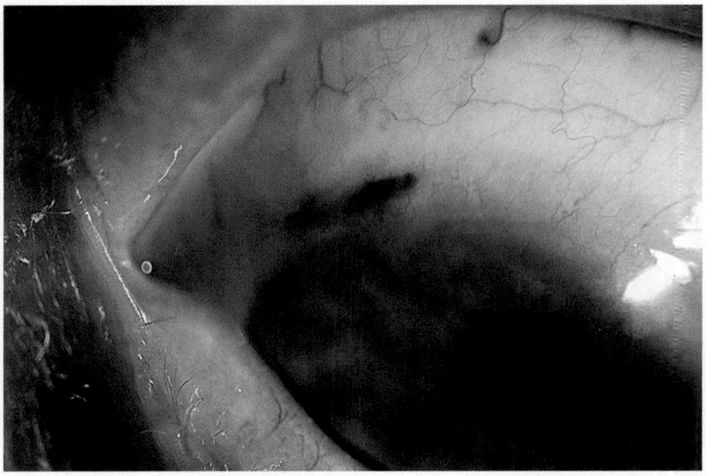

■ **Fig. 7.93** If untreated, a small iris prolapse may atrophy.

Malposition of IOL

Although uncommon, malposition may be associated with both optical and structural problems.

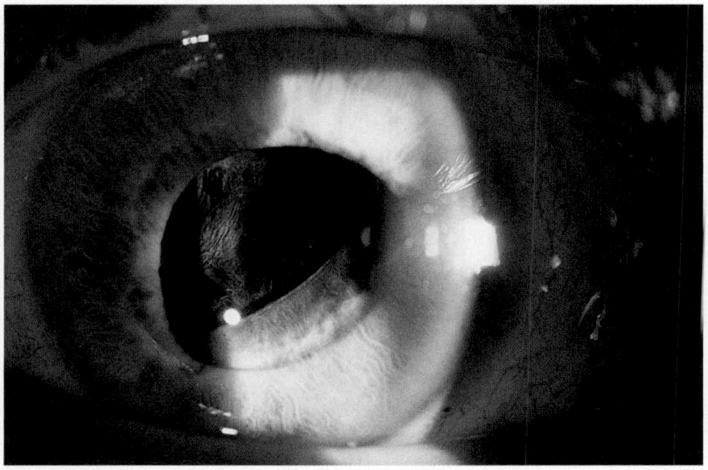

■ **Fig. 7.94** Entrapment of the IOL in the pupil.

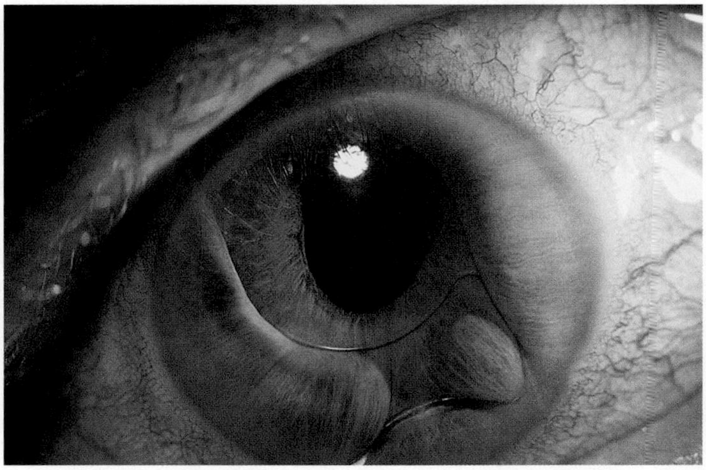

■ **Fig. 7.95** Iris bombé due to pupil block may occur with an anterior chamber IOL in the absence of an adequate peripheral iridectomy.

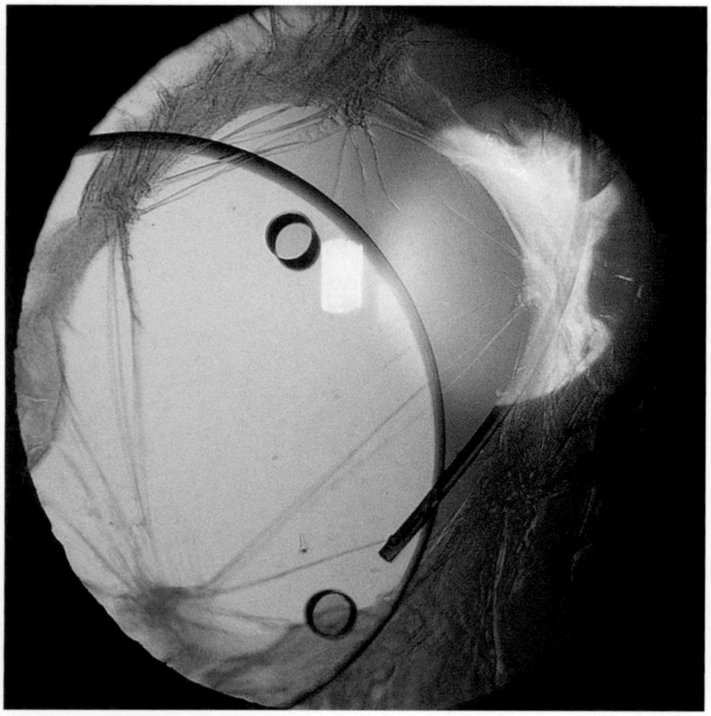

■ **Fig. 7.96** Decentration of the IOL may be caused by postoperative capsular contraction and result in annoying visual symptoms such as glare and monocular diplopia.

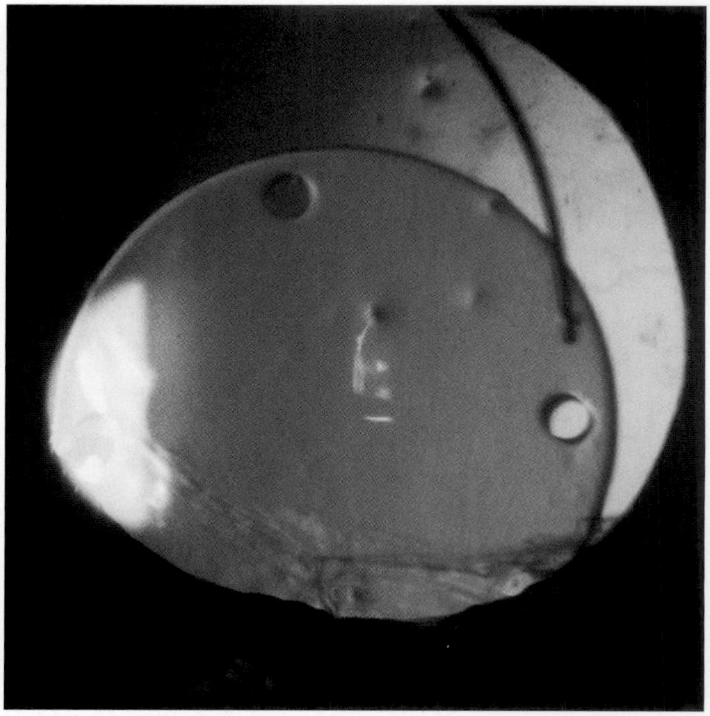

■ **Fig. 7.97** Decentration may also be caused by poor technique when one haptic has been inserted into the capsular bag and the other into the ciliary sulcus.

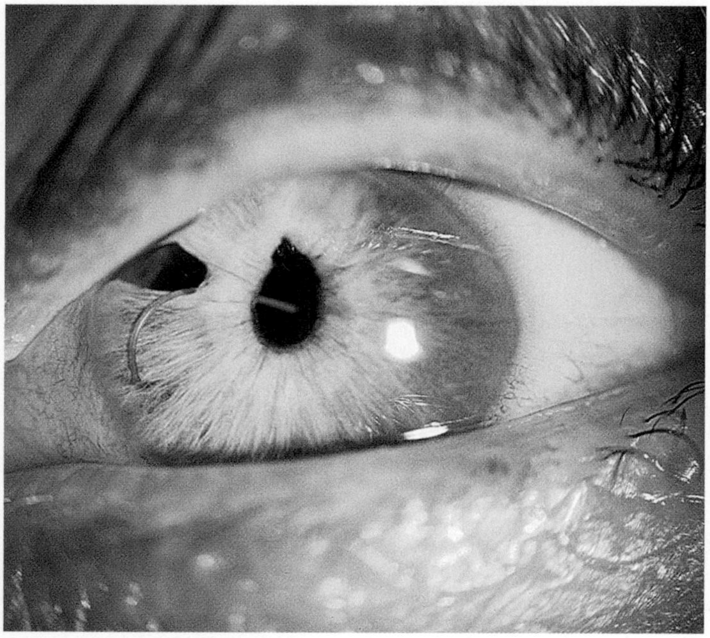

■ **Fig. 7.98** Posterior dislocation ('sunset' syndrome) is very rare and may be associated with zonular rupture during implantation or follow YAG laser capsulotomy.

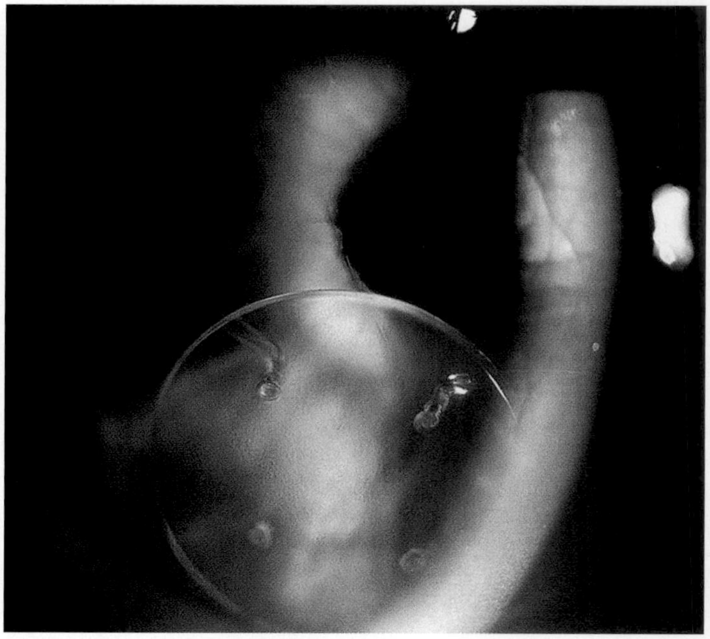

■ **Fig. 7.99** Dislocation into the anterior chamber of an old-type pupil-fixation IOL.

Acute postoperative endophthalmitis

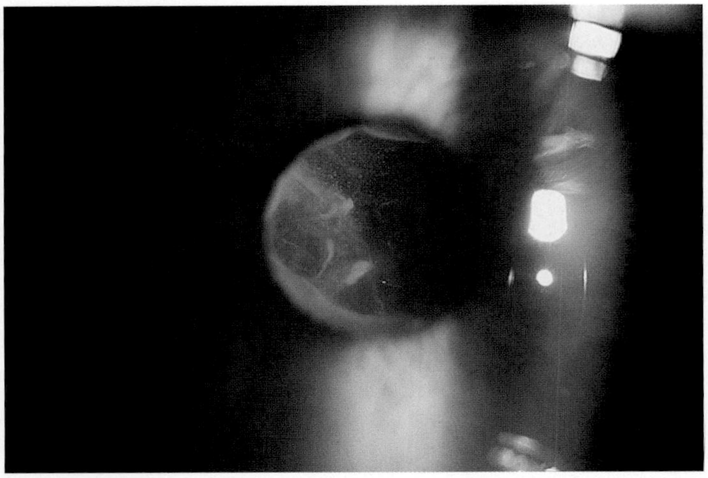

■ **Fig. 7.100** Fibrinous exudate in the pupil.

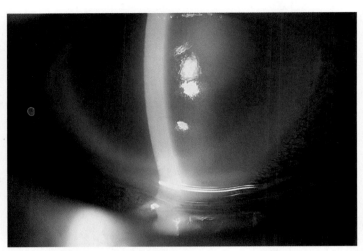

■ **Fig. 7.101** Extensive fibrinous exudate.

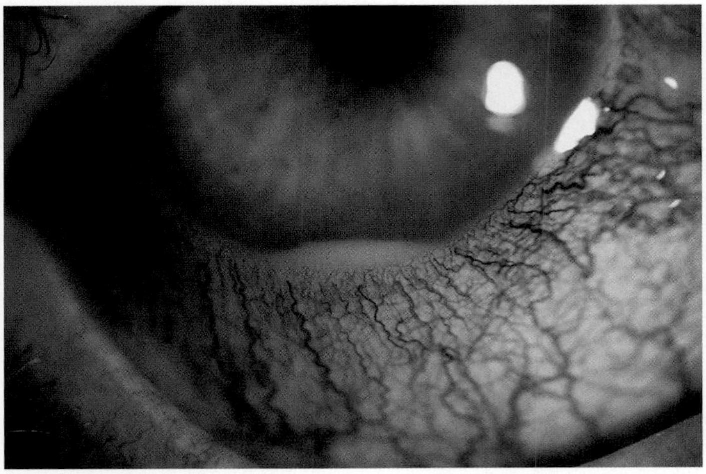

■ **Fig. 7.102** Small hypopyon.

■ **Fig. 7.103** Increasing vitreous haze.

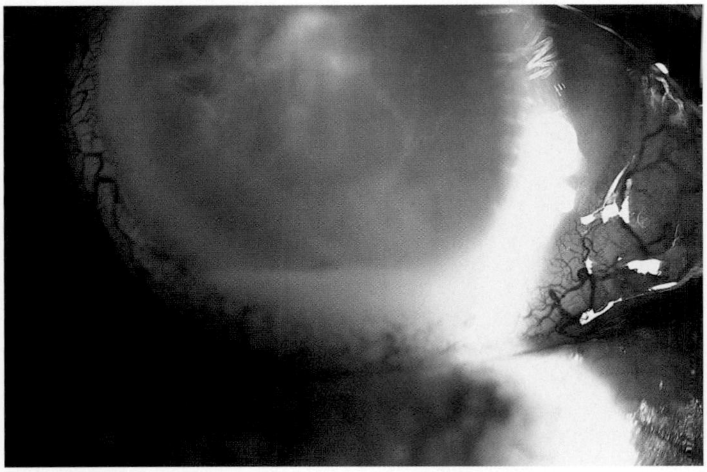

■ **Fig. 7.104** Fibrinous exudate with larger hypopyon.

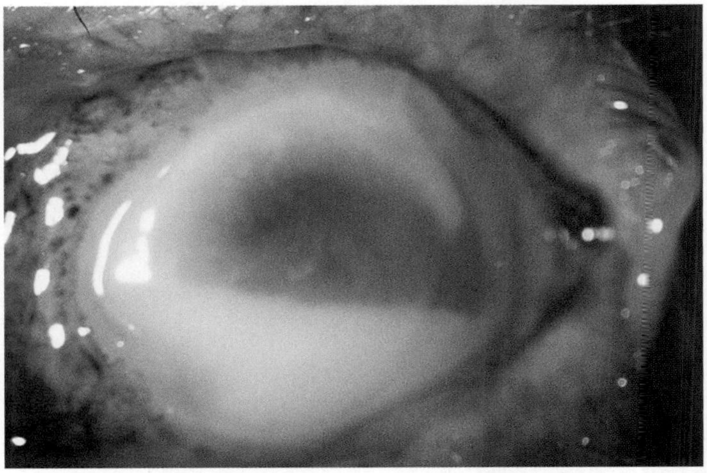

■ **Fig. 7.105** Very large hypopyon.

Delayed-onset chronic indolent endophthalmitis

Chronic endophthalmitis occurs when an organism of low virulence becomes trapped within the capsular bag.

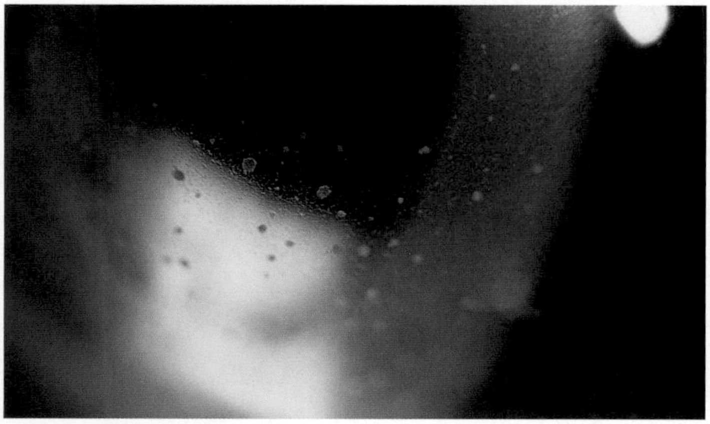

■ **Fig. 7.106** Low-grade anterior uveitis, sometimes with granulomatous features such as mutton-fat keratic precipitates.

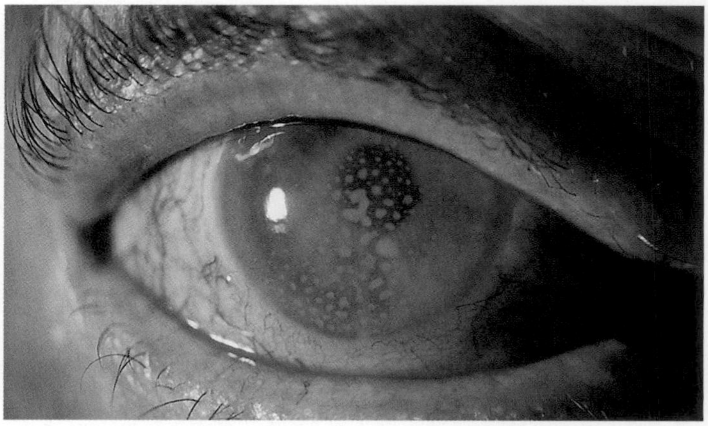

■ **Fig. 7.107** Gradual worsening of anterior uveitis with increase in mutton-fat keratic precipitates.

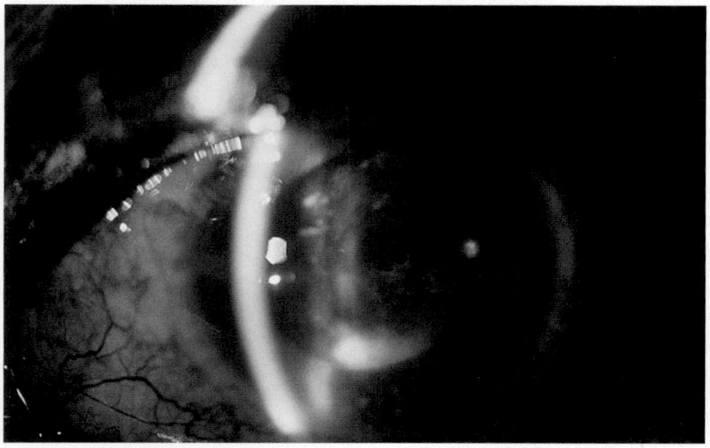

■ **Fig. 7.108** An enlarging white capsular plaque is highly suggestive of infection by *Propionibacterium acnes*.

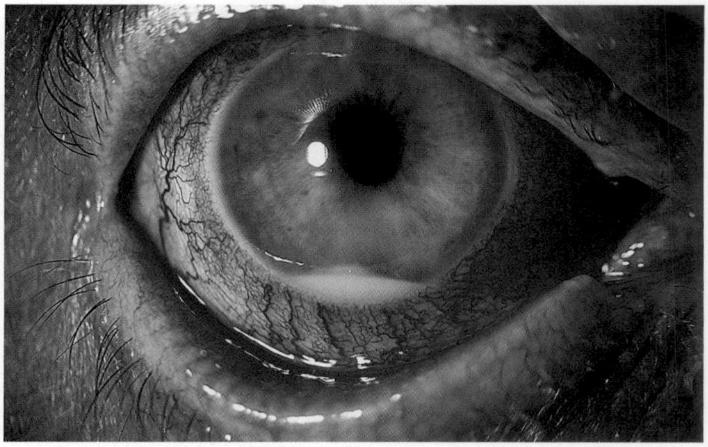

■ **Fig. 7.109** Further gradual worsening of uveitis with a small hypopyon.

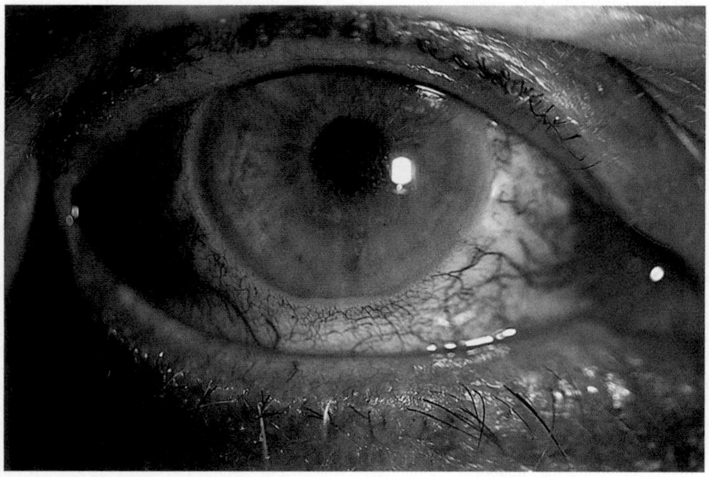

■ **Fig. 7.110** Good initial response to topical steroids.

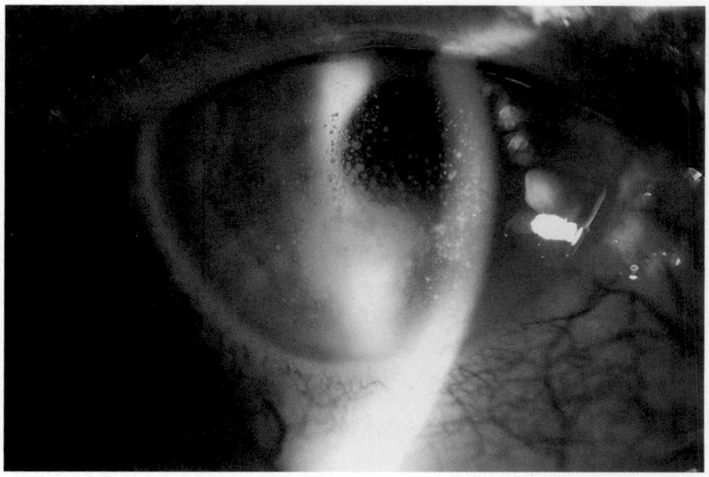

■ **Fig. 7.111** Recurrence and often worsening of uveitis soon after cessation of treatment.

Capsular opacification

Elschnig pearls

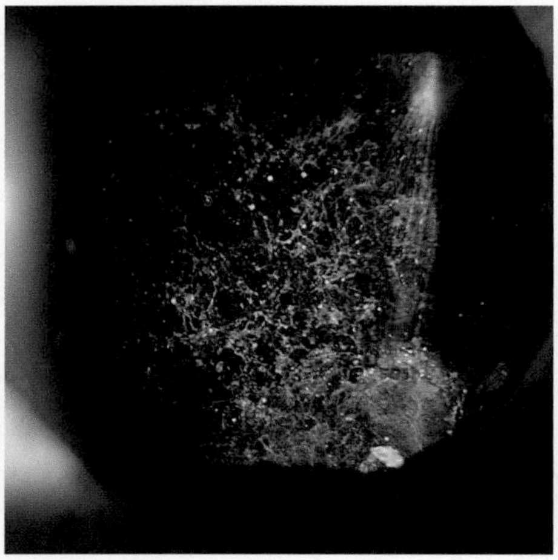

Fig. 7.112 Small elschnig pearls.

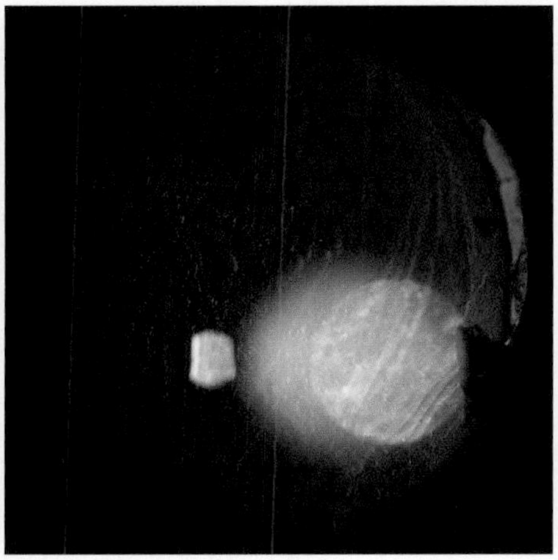

Fig. 7.113 Same eye on retroillumination.

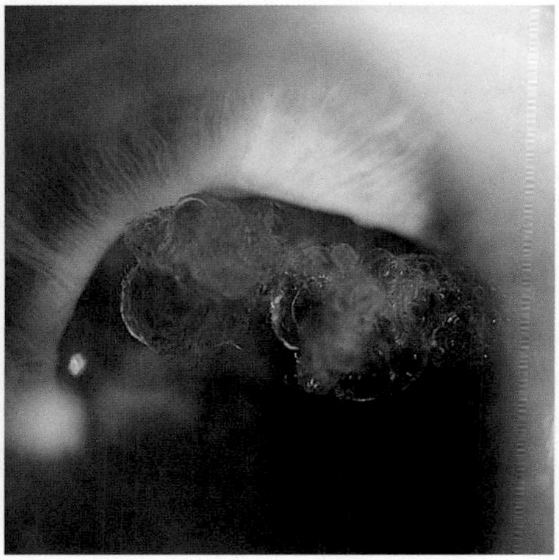

Fig. 7.114 Large Elschnig pearls.

Posterior capsular fibrosis

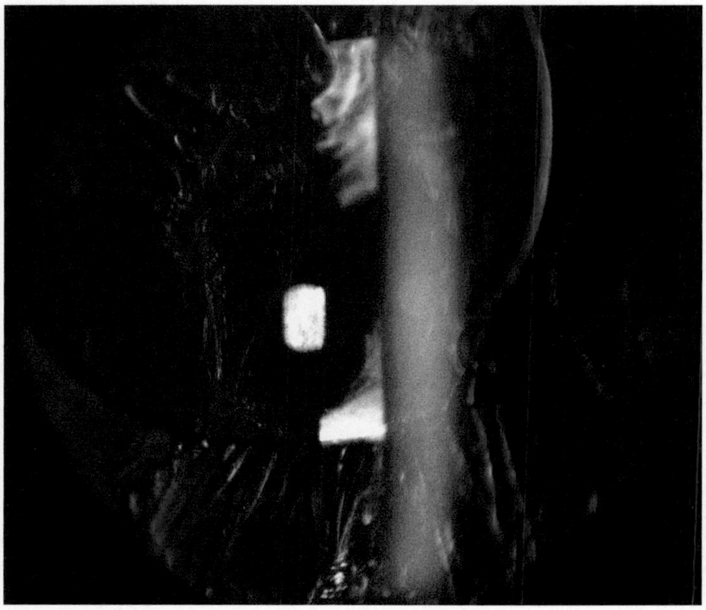

Fig. 7.115 Fibrosis is less common than Elschnig pearl formation and usually appears earlier. (Courtesy of P. Gili.)

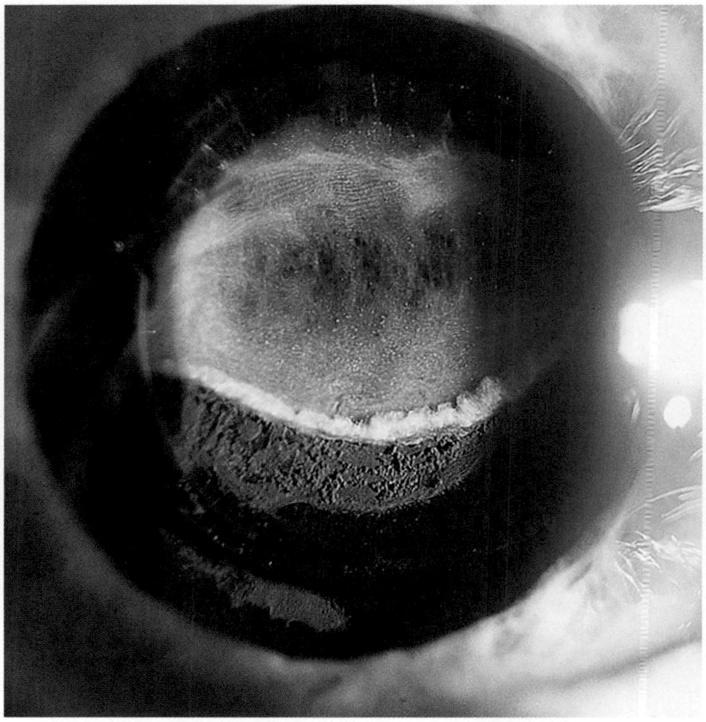

Fig. 7.116 Very severe capsular fibrosis and pigment depcsition on the IOL.

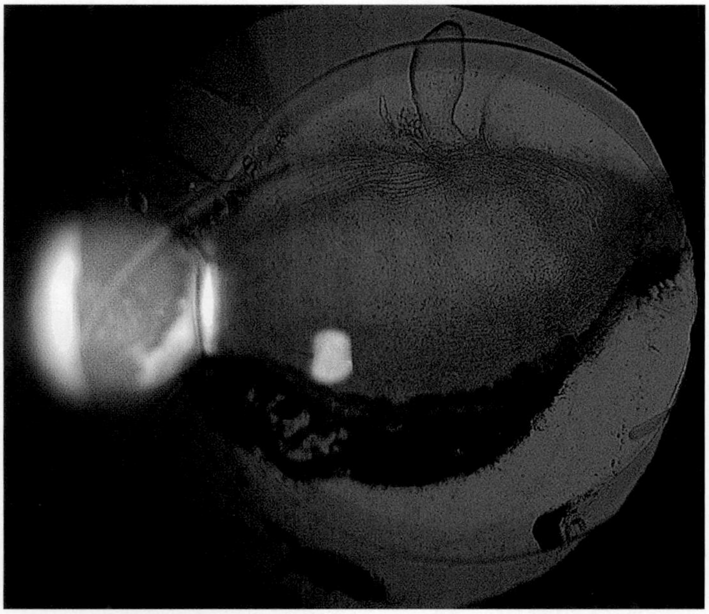

Fig. 7.117 View of the same eye on retroillumination.

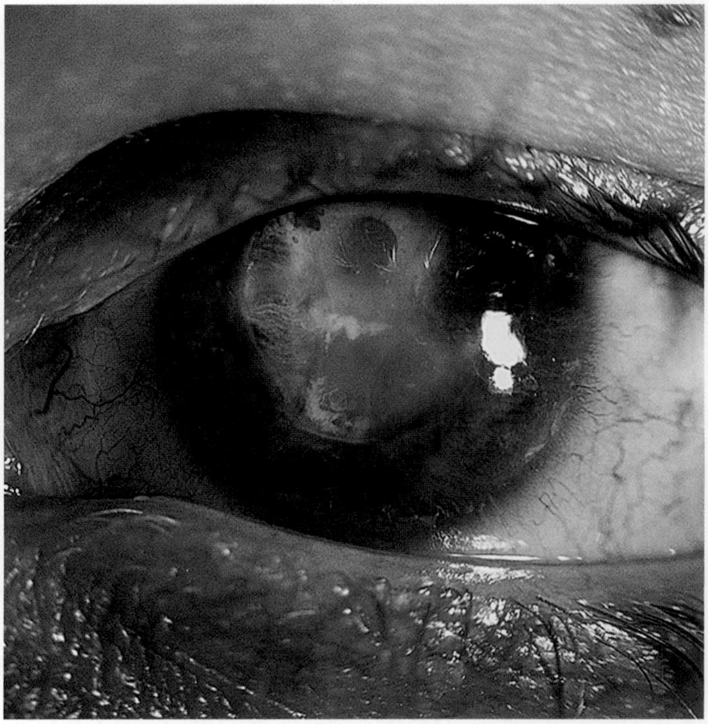

Fig. 7.118 Very severe capsular fibrosis and synechiae to the IOL following cataract surgery in a child with chronic uveitis associated with juvenile idiopathic arthritis.

Anterior capsular fibrosis

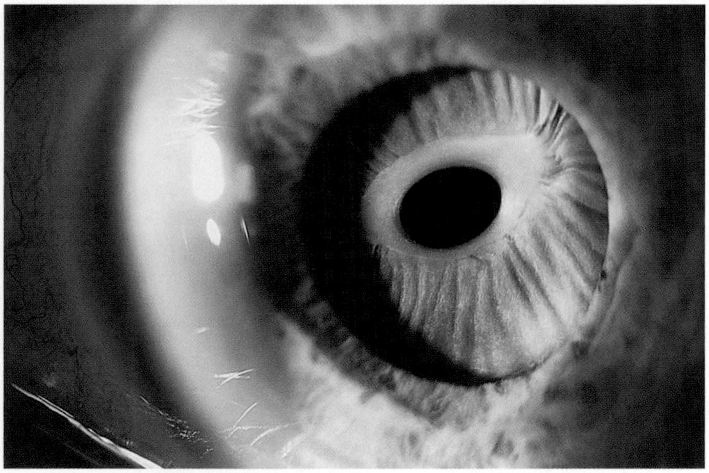

Fig. 7.119 Severe fibrosis resulting in shrinkage and constriction of the capsulorrhexis (capsulophimosis).

Soemmerring ring

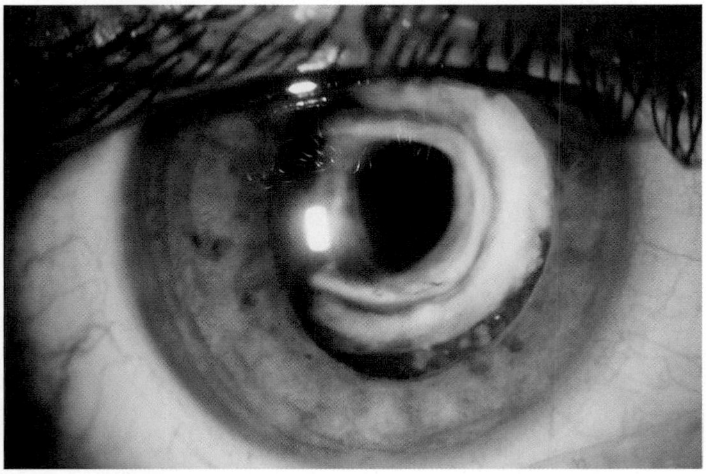

■ **Fig. 7.120** Encapsulation of proliferated epithelium within the remnants of the anterior and posterior capsule, which may develop following inadequate surgery for congenital cataract.

Miscellaneous complications

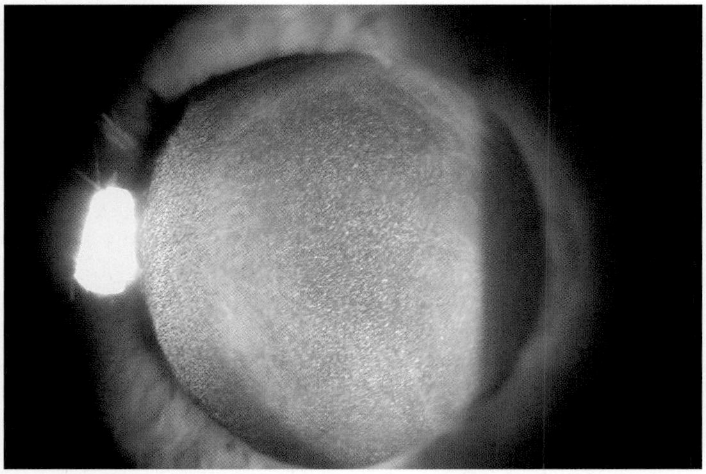

■ **Fig. 7.121** Opacification of the IOL is very rare. (Courtesy of R. Curtis.)

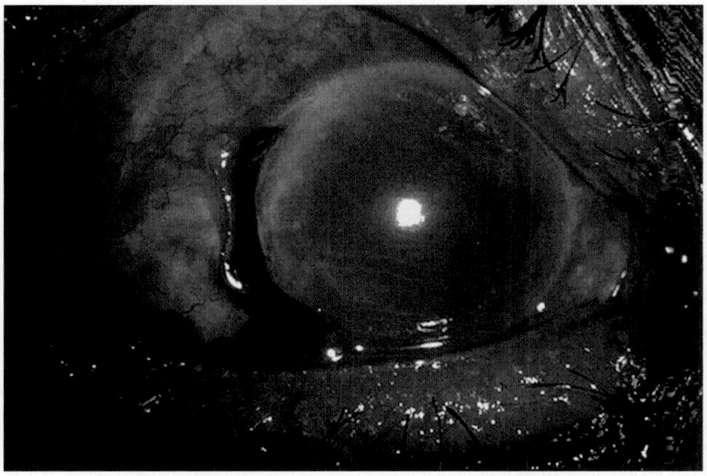

■ **Fig. 7.122** Extrusion of the IOL through a large incision is also very rare. (Courtesy of S. Ford and R. Marsh.)

CHAPTER 8

GLAUCOMA

NORMAL OPTIC NERVE HEAD

Neuroretinal rim

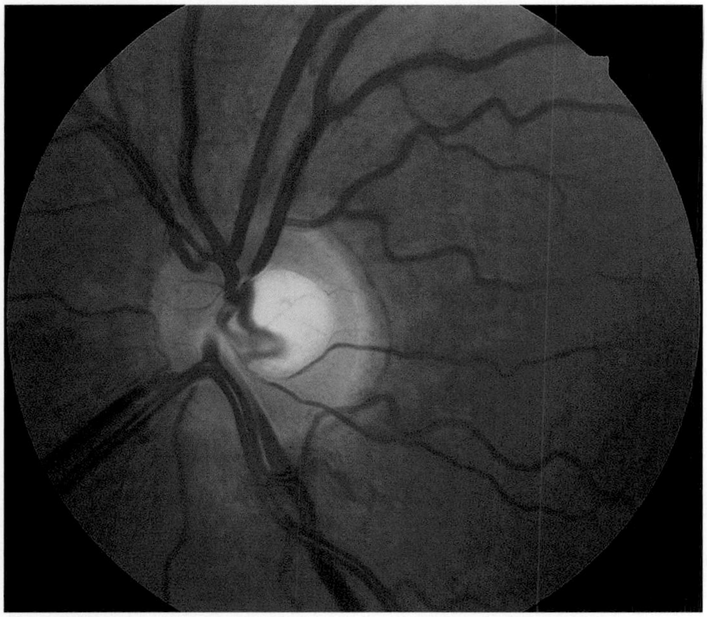

■ **Fig. 8.1** The neuroretinal rim consists of neural tissue between the outer edge of the cup and the disc margin. The normal healthy rim has an orange or pink colour and shows a characteristic configuration. The inferior rim is the broadest, followed by superior nasal and temporal ('ISNT').

Optic cup

The cup may have one of three main appearances:

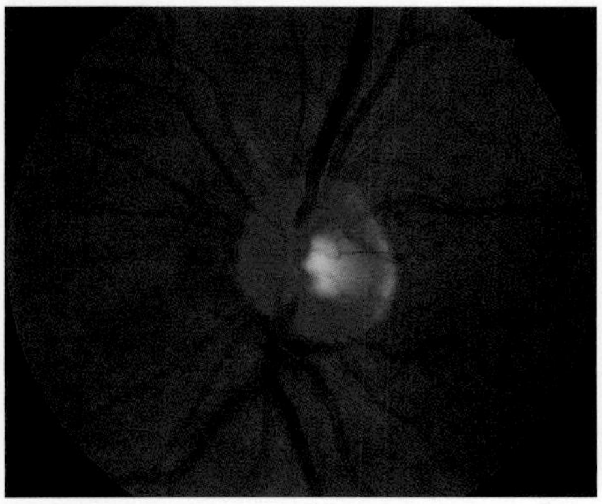

■ **Fig. 8.2** A small, dimple-like central cup.

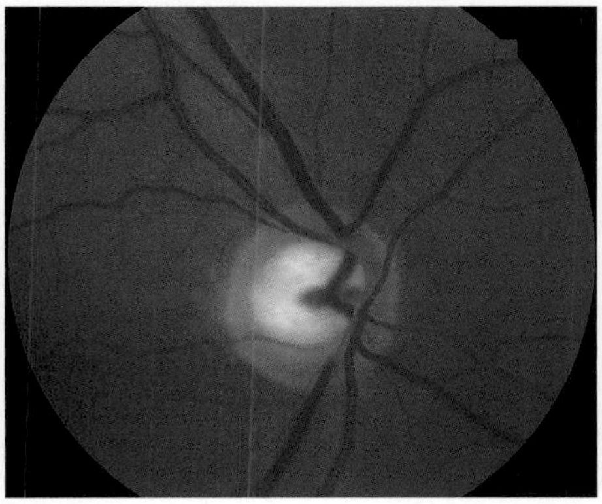

■ **Fig. 8.3** A punched-out, deep central cup.

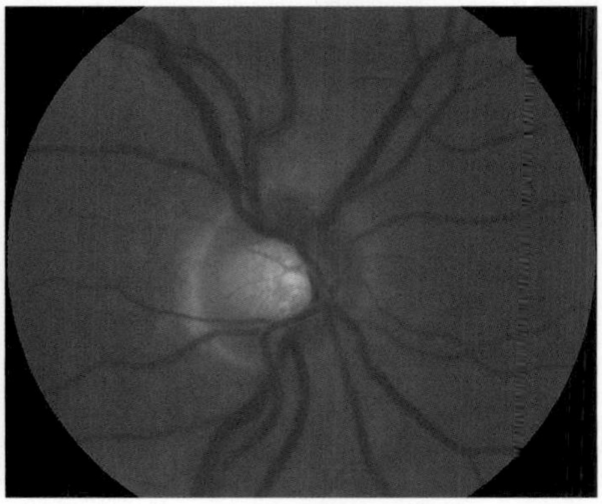

■ **Fig. 8.4** A cup with a sloping temporal wall.

Cup–disc ratio

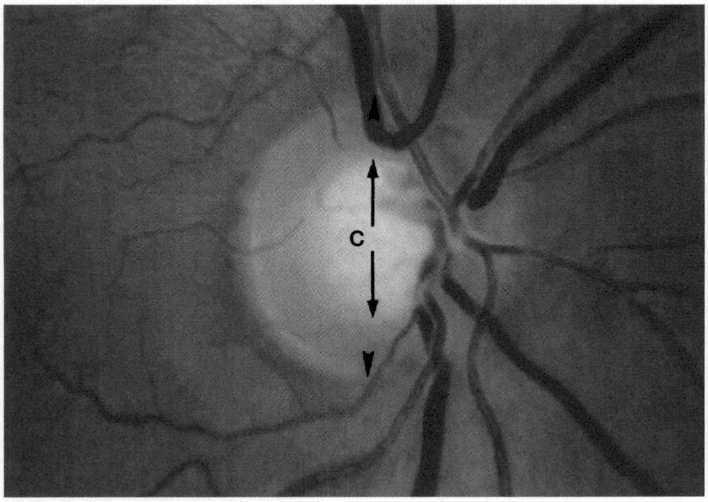

■ **Fig. 8.5** The cup–disc ratio indicates the diameter of the cup expressed as a fraction of the diameter of the disc. Most normal eyes have a vertical cup–disc ratio of 0.3 or less. (Courtesy of J. Salmon.)

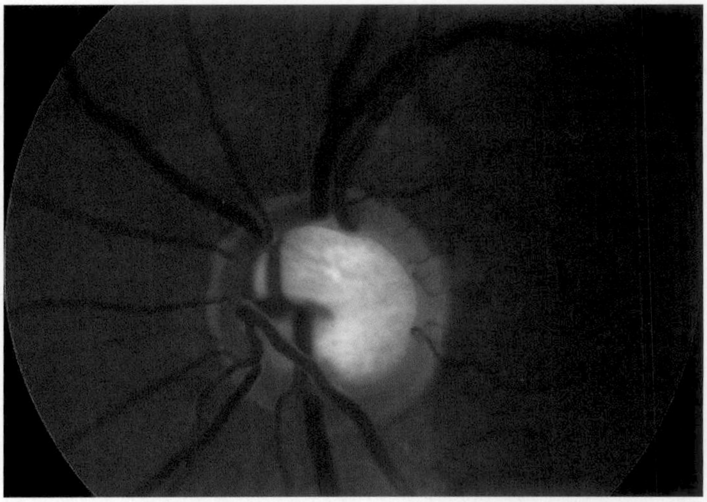

■ **Fig. 8.6** Only 2% of normal eyes have a ratio greater than 0.7.

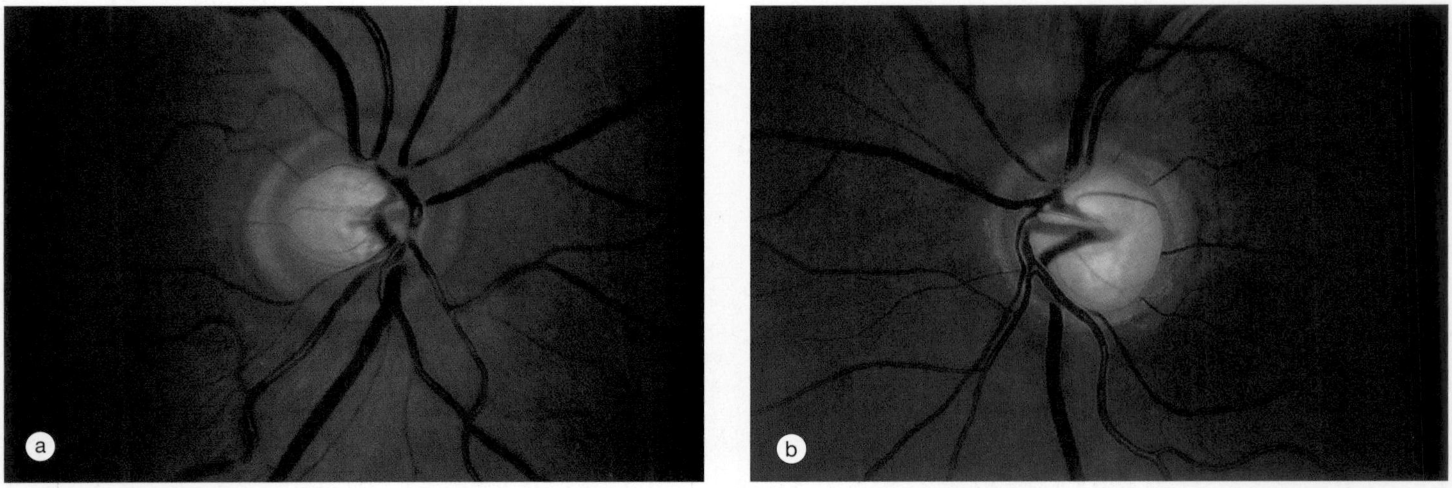

■ **Fig. 8.7** In any individual, asymmetry of 0.2 or more between the eyes should be regarded with suspicion until glaucoma has been excluded.

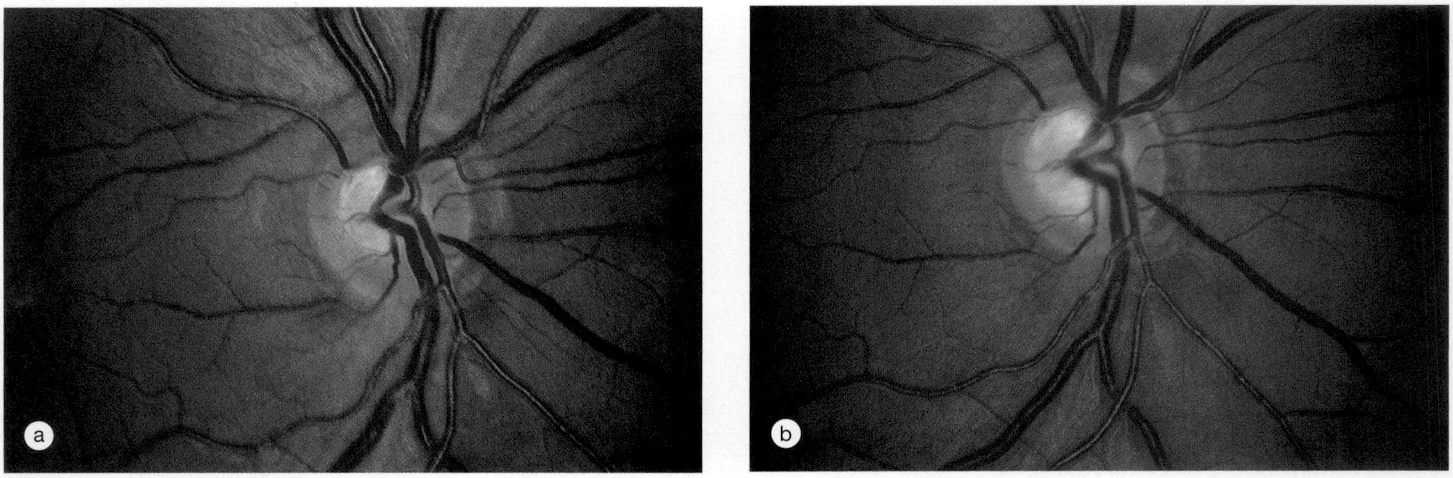

■ **Fig. 8.8** Optic disc damage is superimposed upon physiological cupping present prior to the onset of raised intraocular pressure (IOP). **(a)** If an eye with a small cup develops glaucoma; **(b)** the cup will increase in size but, during the early stages, its dimensions may still be smaller than that of a large physiological cup. An estimation of cup size alone is therefore of limited value in the diagnosis of early glaucoma, unless it is found to be increasing.

SIGNS OF GLAUCOMATOUS DAMAGE

Retinal nerve fibre layer defects

In glaucoma subtle retinal nerve fibre layer defects precede the development of detectable optic disc and visual field changes.

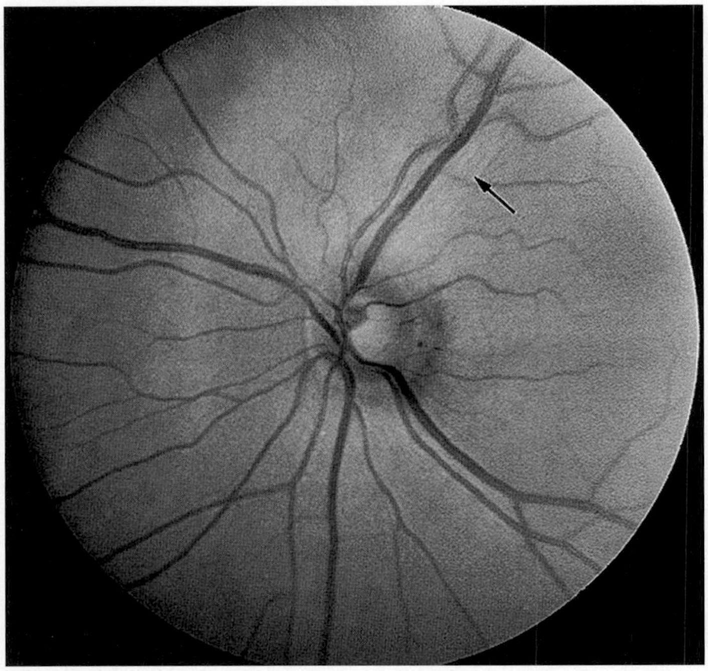

Fig. 8.9 Early localised damage is characterised by slit defects in the retinal nerve fibre layer.

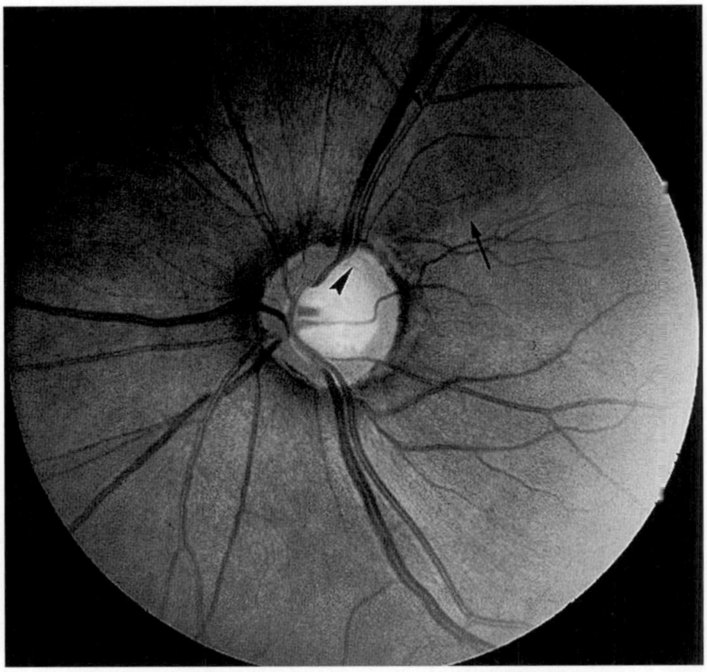

Fig. 8.10 The atrophic area becomes darker as a result of enhanced visualisation of the retinal pigment epithelium, and there is baring of larger retinal blood vessels.

Parapapillary changes

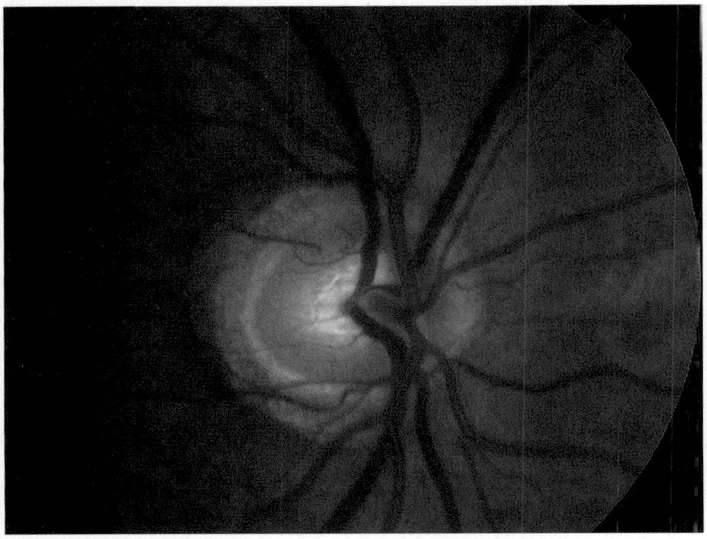

Fig. 8.11 These consist of: an inner 'beta' zone of chorioretinal atrophy concentrically surrounded by an outer 'alpha' zone displaying variable irregular retinal pigment epithelial changes. The beta zone is larger and occurs more frequently in patients with primary open-angle glaucoma (POAG) than in normal individuals.

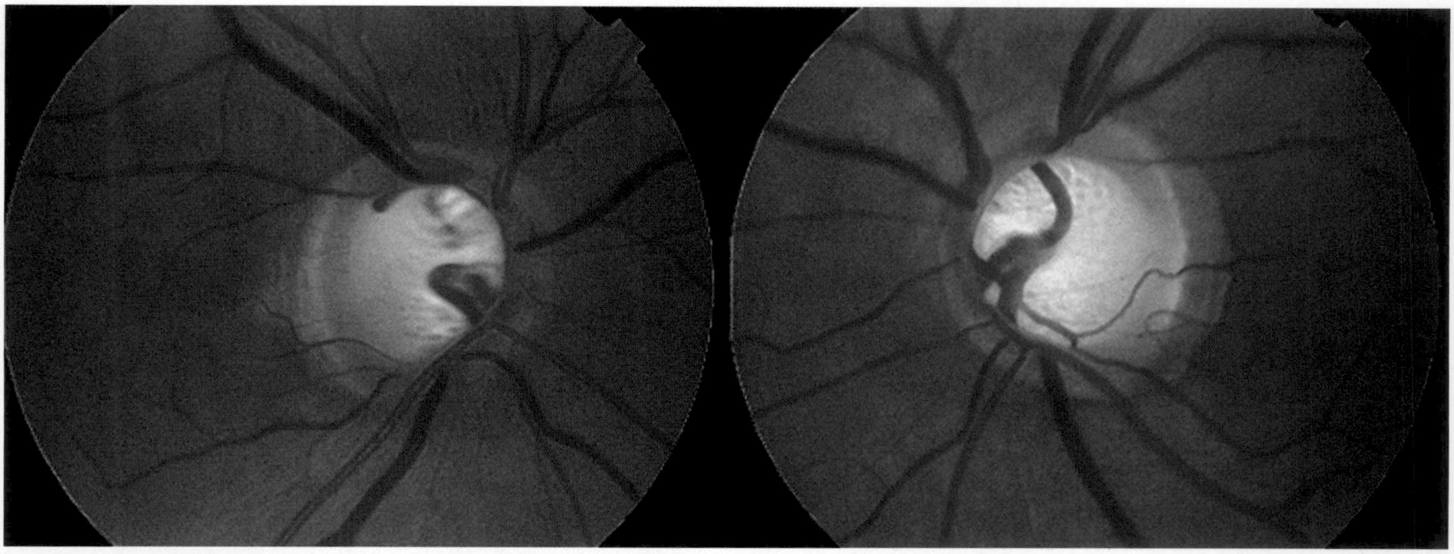

■ **Fig. 8.12** Mild asymmetrical parapapillary changes.

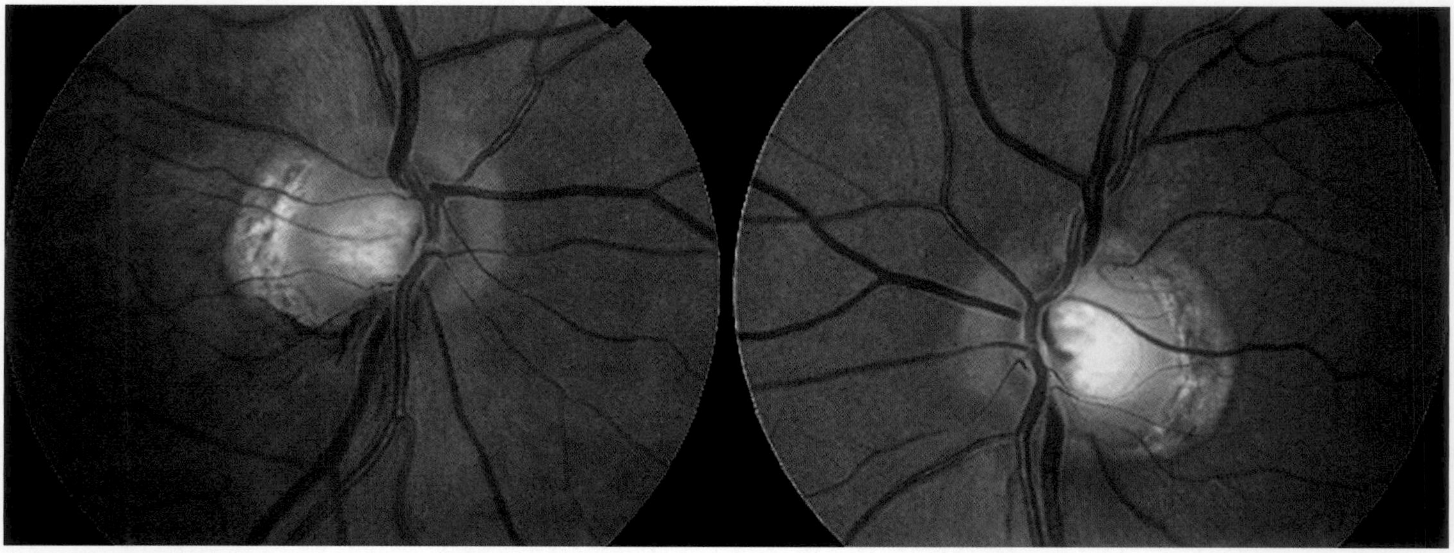

■ **Fig. 8.13** More severe symmetrical parapapillary changes.

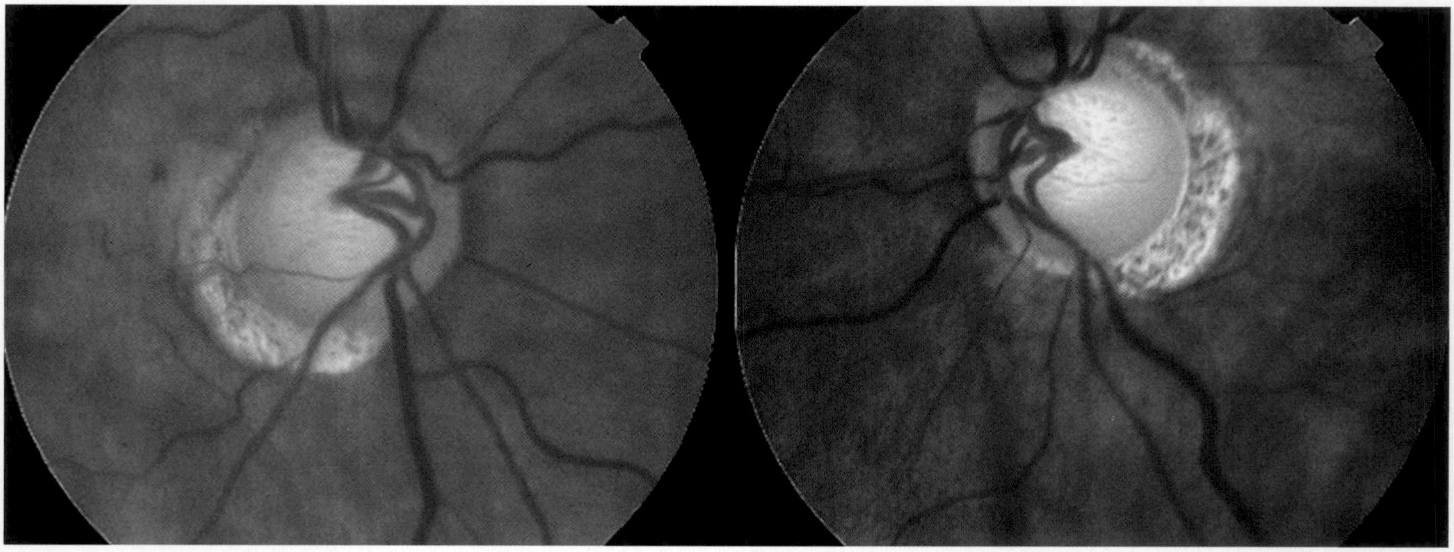

■ **Fig. 8.14** Very severe asymmetrical parapapillary changes in advanced POAG. The changes are more severe in the left eye, which also shows more advanced cupping.

Optic nerve head

Subtypes of glaucomatous damage

The appearance and pattern of disc damage may correlate with subtypes of glaucoma and provide clues as to the pathogenic mechanisms involved as follows:

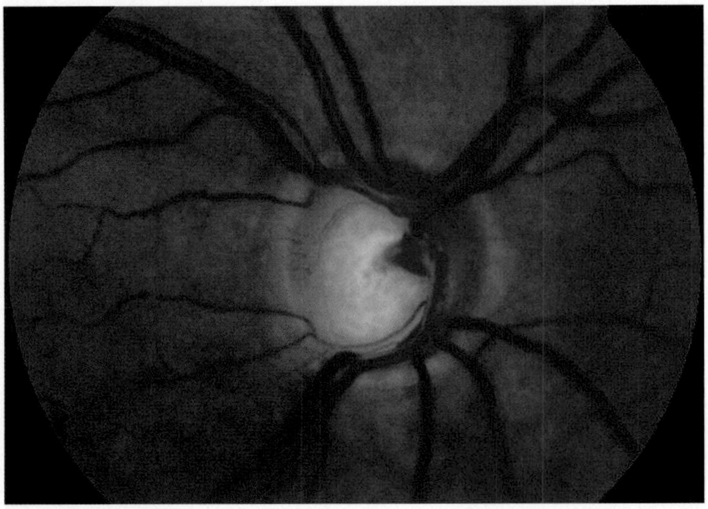

Fig. 8.15 Type 1 (focal ischaemic) disc is characterised by tissue loss at the superior and/or inferior poles (polar notching) and an otherwise relatively intact neuroretinal rim.

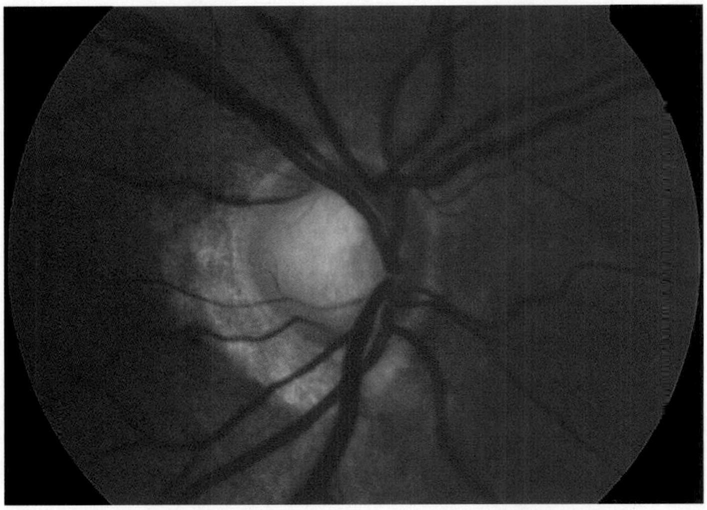

Fig. 8.16 Type 2 (myopic glaucomatous) disc is characterised by polar notching and a temporal crescent in the absence of degenerative myopia.

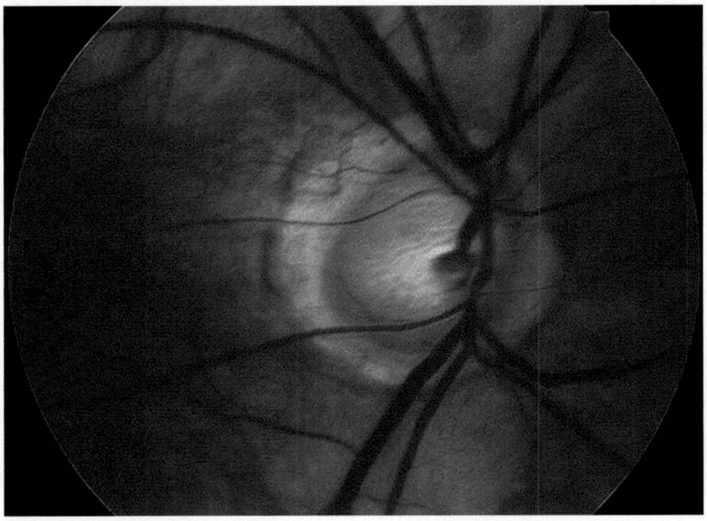

Fig. 8.17 Type 3 (senile sclerotic) disc is characterised by a shallow, saucerised cup and a gently sloping neuroretinal rim, a 'motheaten appearance' and parapapillary atrophy.

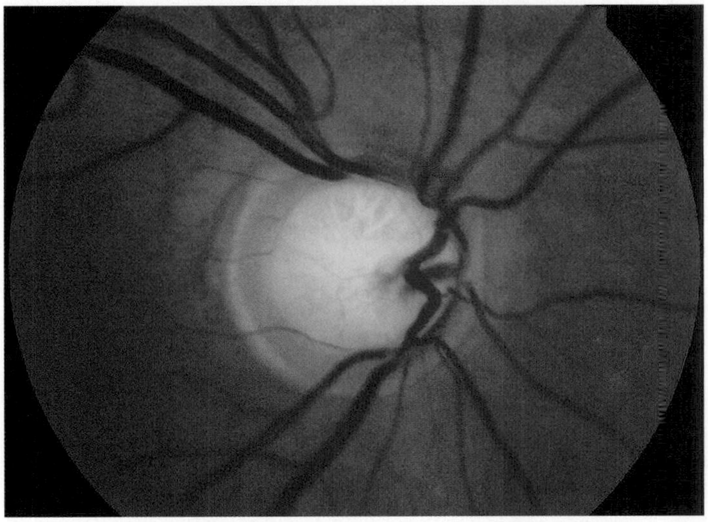

Fig. 8.18 Type 4 (concentrically enlarging) disc is characterised by thinning of the entire neuroretinal rim without notching.

Acute congestive angle-closure glaucoma

Acute congestive angle closure is a sight-threatening emergency, manifesting with painful loss of vision due to sudden and total closure of the angle.

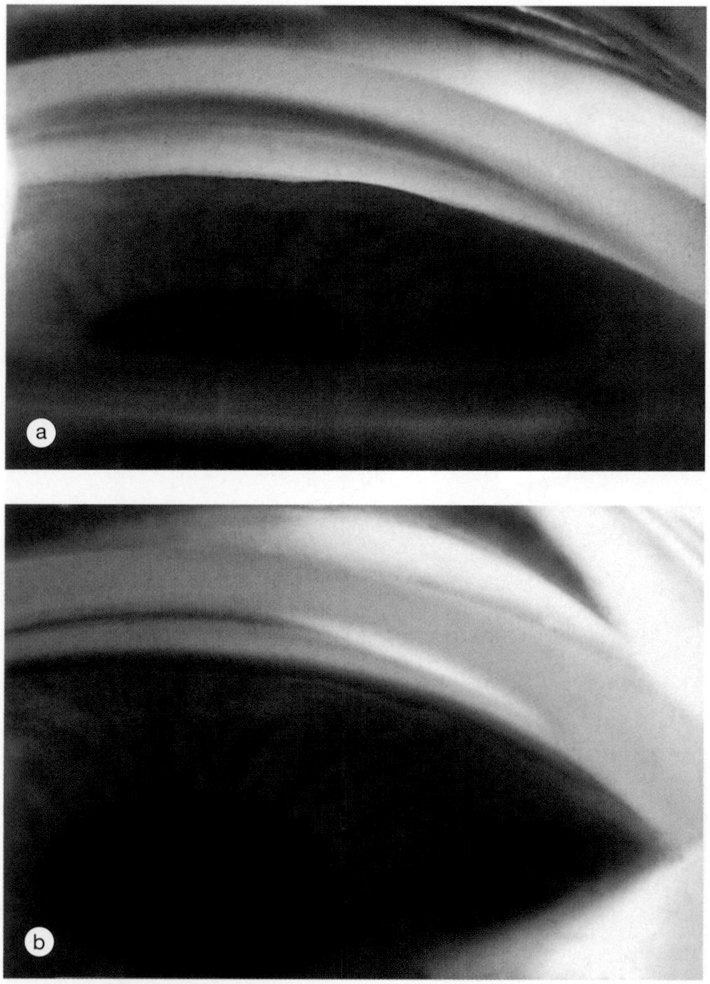

■ **Fig. 8.29** **(a)** Gonioscopy shows complete peripheral iridocorneal contact (Shaffer grade 0). **(b)** Open angle after YAG laser peripheral iridotomy.

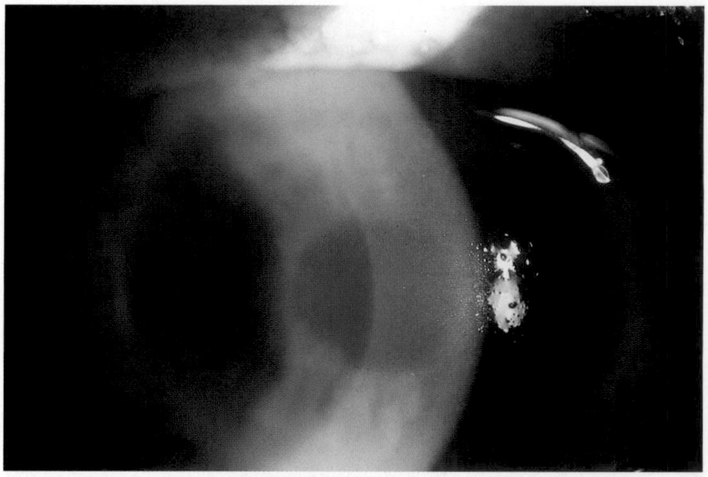

■ **Fig. 8.30** Corneal epithelial oedema and a fixed, semi-dilated pupil.

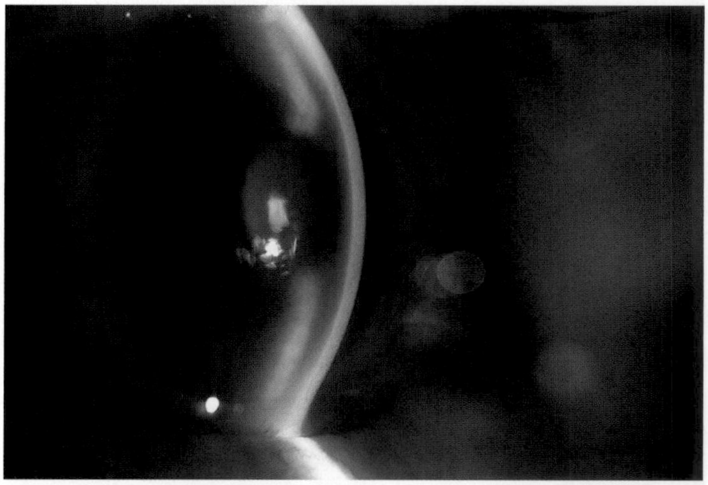

■ **Fig. 8.31** Shallow anterior chamber with peripheral iridocorneal contact.

Postcongestive angle-closure glaucoma

The postcongestive stage occurs after the IOP has been normalised.

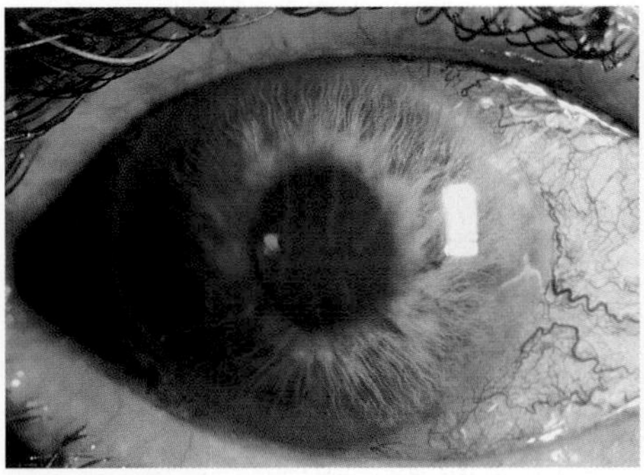

Fig. 8.32 Folds in Descemet membrane, if the IOP has been reduced rapidly. (Courtesy of S. Ford and R. Marsh.)

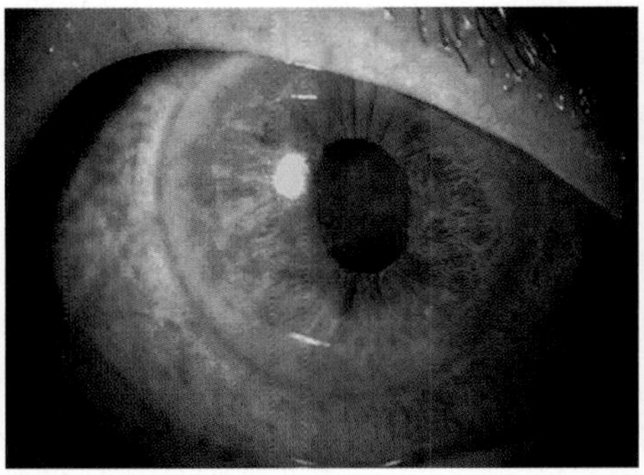

Fig. 8.33 Stromal iris atrophy and a fixed, semi-dilated, oval pupil. (Courtesy of S. Ford and R. Marsh.)

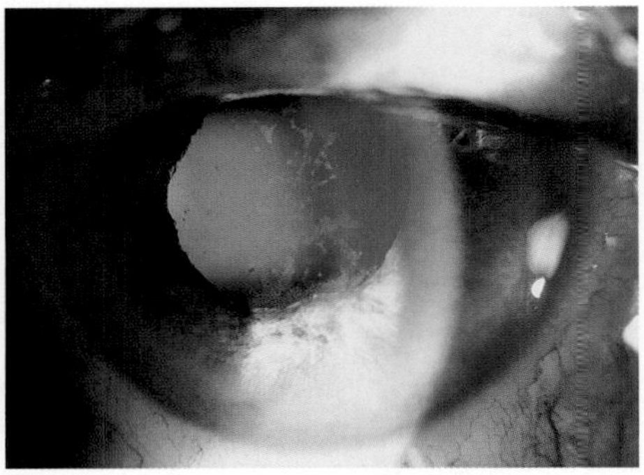

Fig. 8.34 Posterior synechiae.

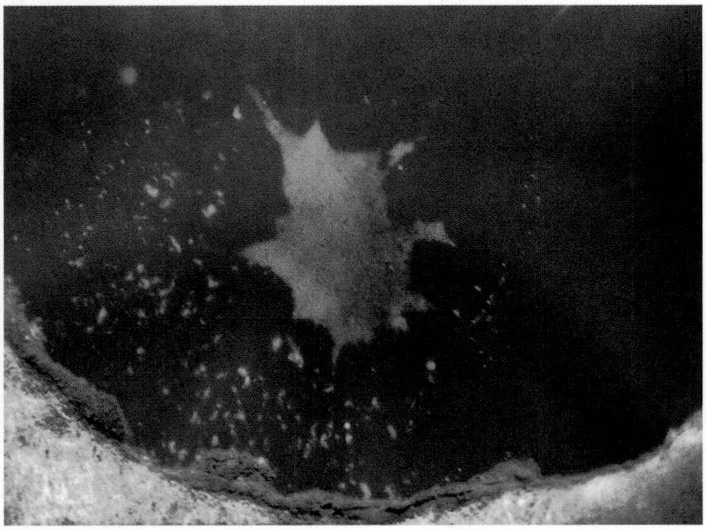

Fig. 8.35 Small, grey-white anterior subcapsular or capsular lens opacities in the pupillary zone (*glaukomflecken*) are diagnostic of a previous congestive attack. (Courtesy of L. Merin.)

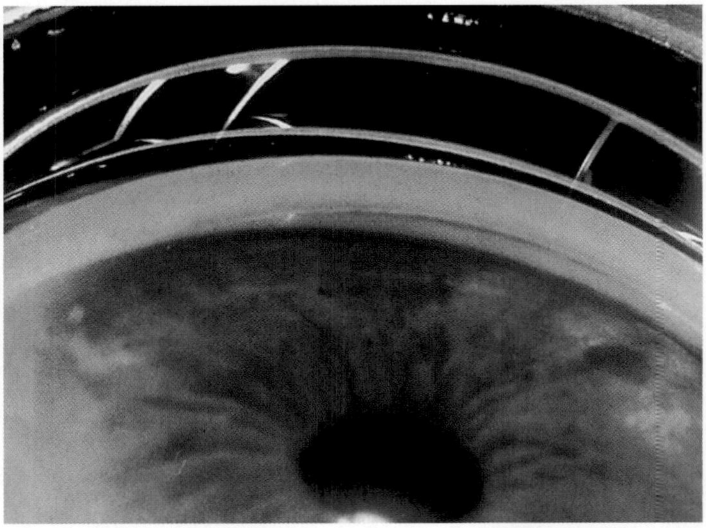

Fig. 8.36 Narrow angle with trabecular hyperpigmentation.

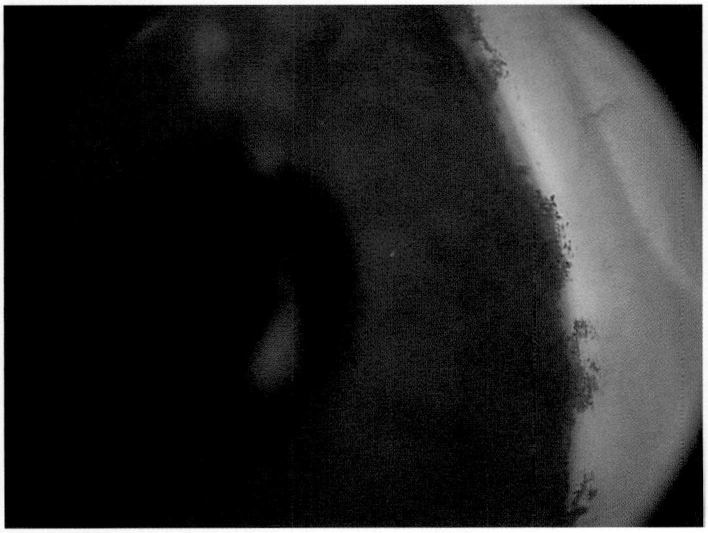

Fig. 8.37 Partial synechial angle closure.

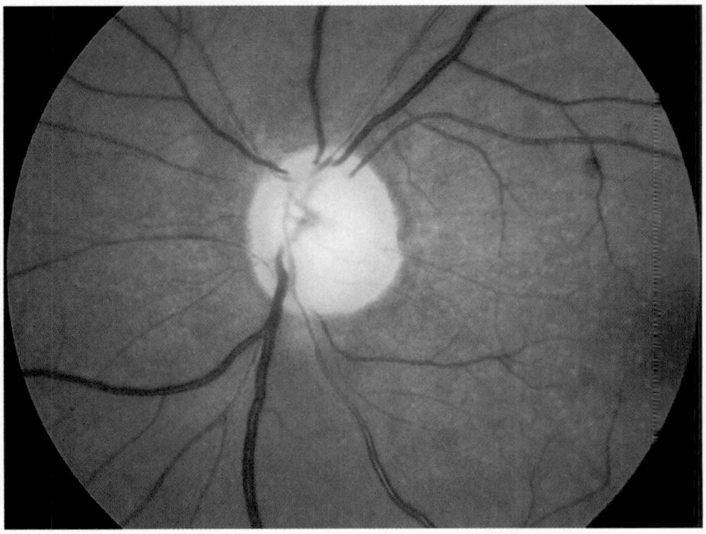

Fig. 8.38 Optic atrophy as a result of infarction. (Courtesy of J. Salmon.)

PSEUDOEXFOLIATION GLAUCOMA

The pseudoexfoliation (PEX) syndrome is a relatively common cause of chronic open-angle glaucoma.

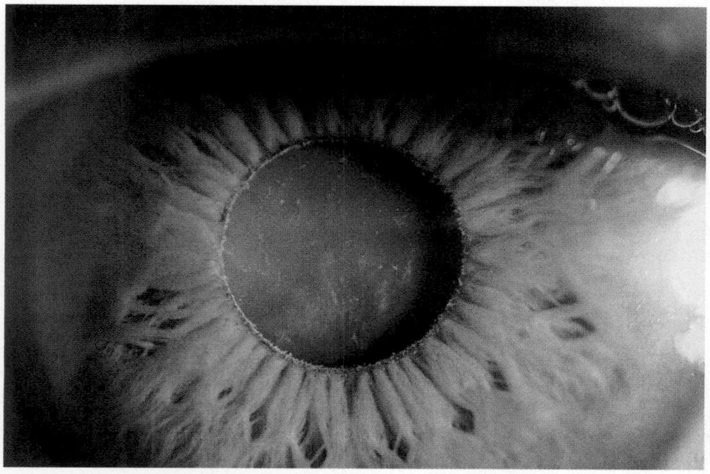

Fig. 8.39 PEX on the pupillary margin with defects of the pupillary ruff (frill).

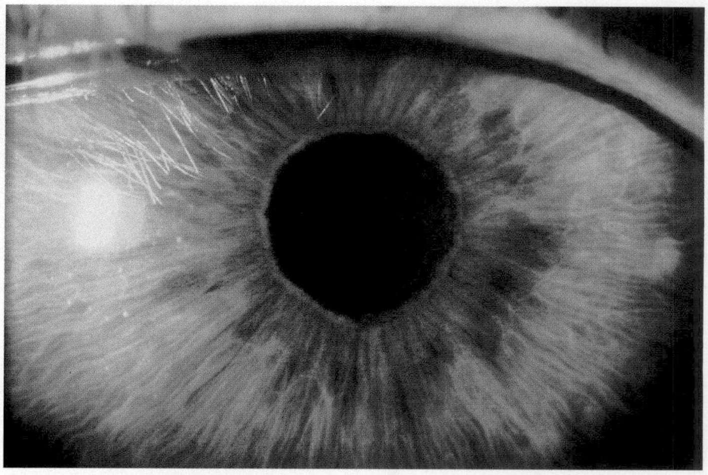

Fig. 8.40 Sphincter atrophy.

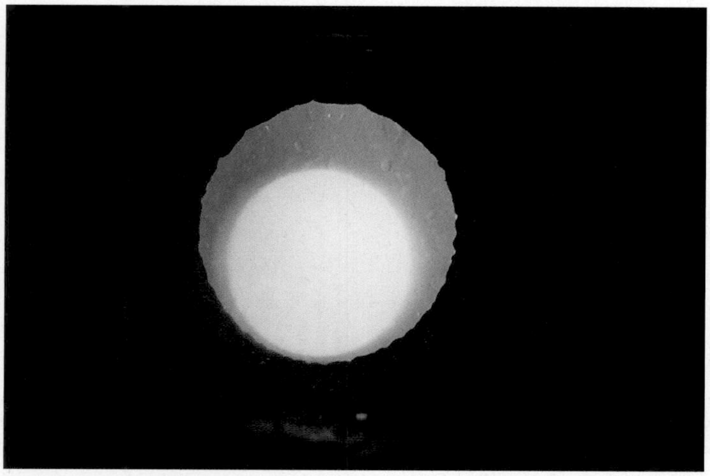

Fig. 8.41 'Motheaten' transillumination defects corresponding to the sphincter atrophy.

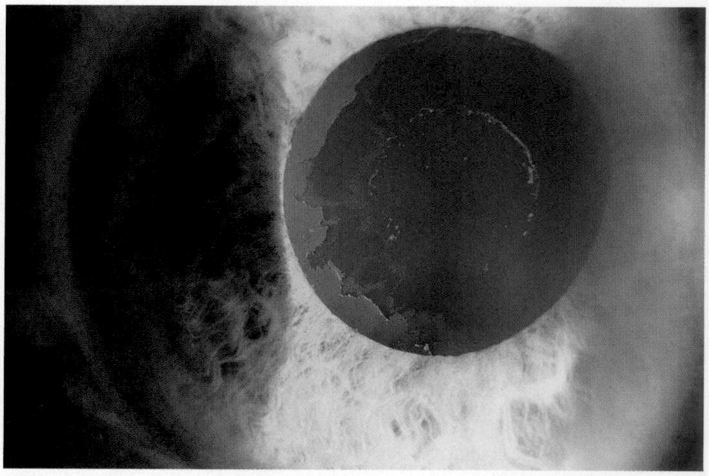

Fig. 8.42 A central disc of PEX on the anterior lens surface and a peripheral band separated by a clear zone.

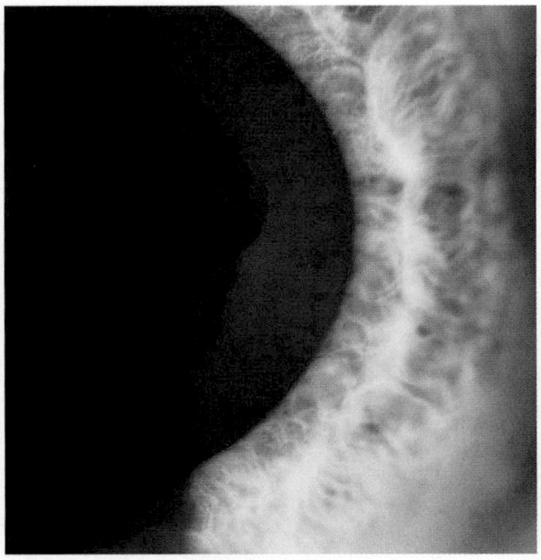

■ **Fig. 8.43** The peripheral band of PEX is granular and has a well-demarcated inner border.

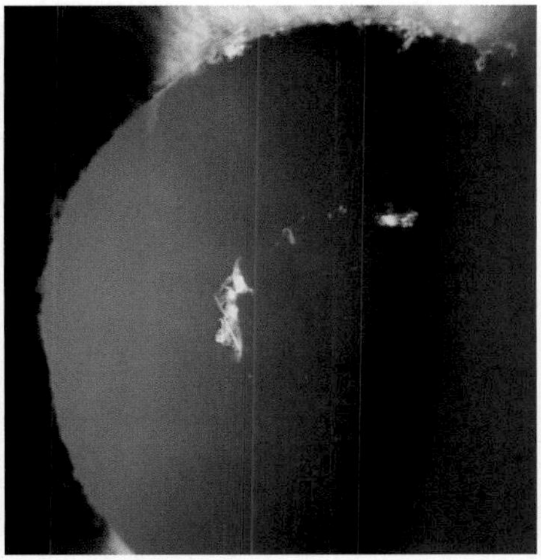

■ **Fig. 8.44** The margin of the central disc may be ill-defined or absent.

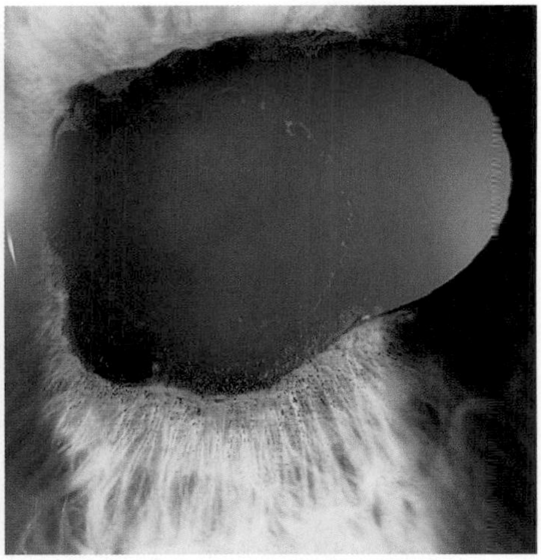

■ **Fig. 8.45** Posterior synechiae may contribute to poor pupillary dilatation.

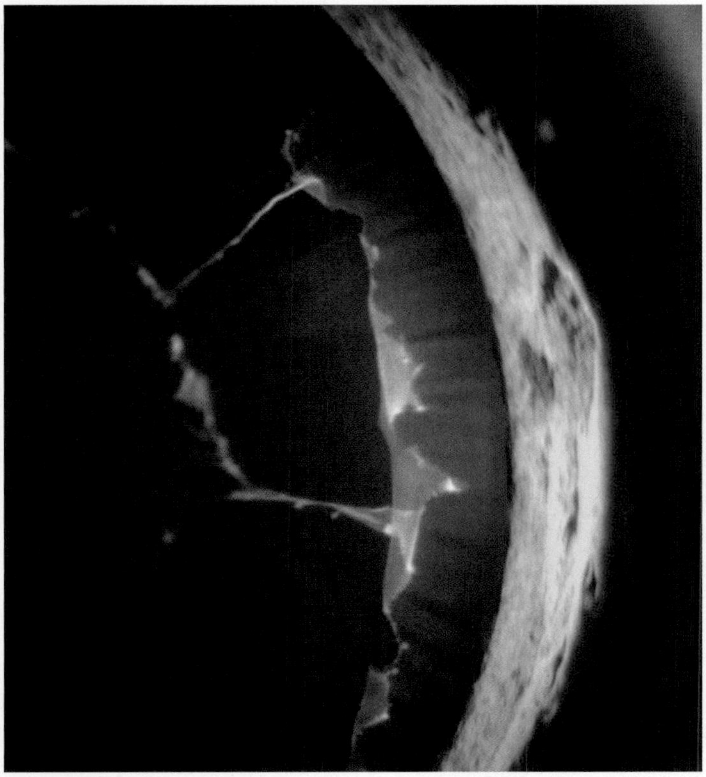

■ **Fig. 8.46** The edge of the peripheral band may contain rolled-up fragments. (Courtesy of R. Curtis.)

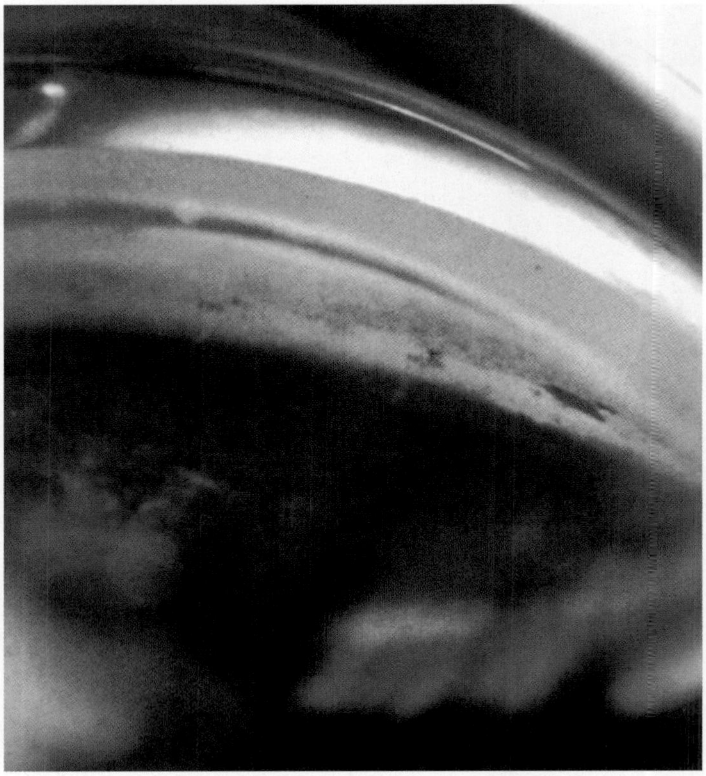

■ **Fig. 8.47** Narrow angle, trabecular hyperpigmentation, a scalloped band of pigment running on to Schwalbe line (Sampaolesi line) and 'dandruff-like' deposits of PEX in the angle.

PIGMENTARY GLAUCOMA

The pigment dispersion syndrome characterised by the liberation of pigment granules from the iris pigment epithelium and their deposition throughout the anterior segment. About 15% of patients develop glaucoma.

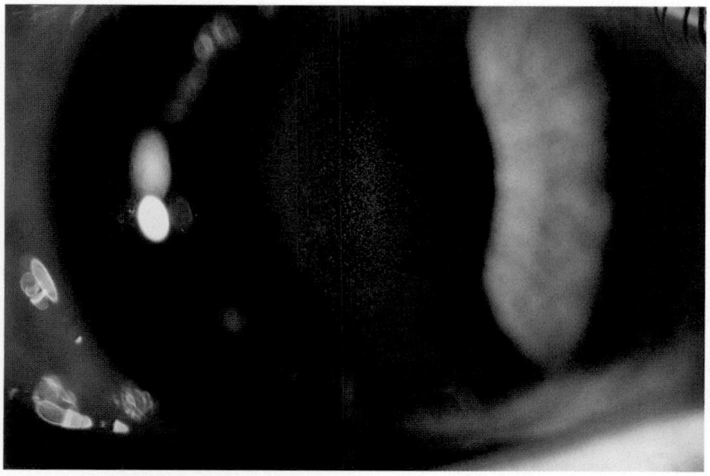

■ **Fig. 8.48** Pigment deposition on the endothelium, in a vertical spindle-shaped distribution (Krukenberg spindle).

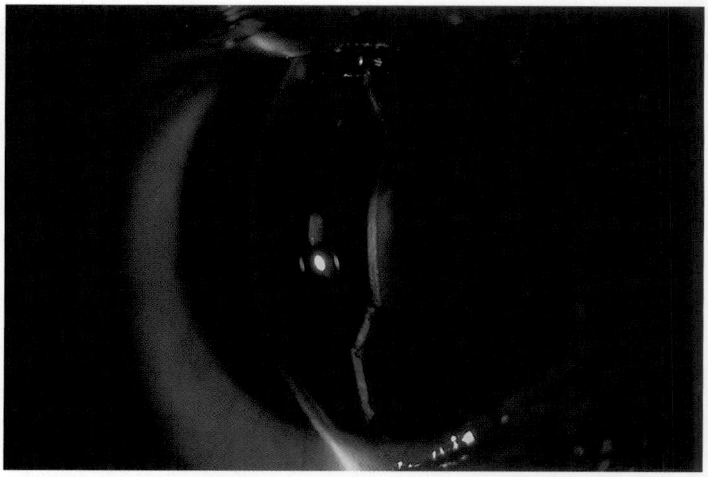

■ **Fig. 8.49** Very deep anterior chamber and a concave shape of the mid-peripheral iris.

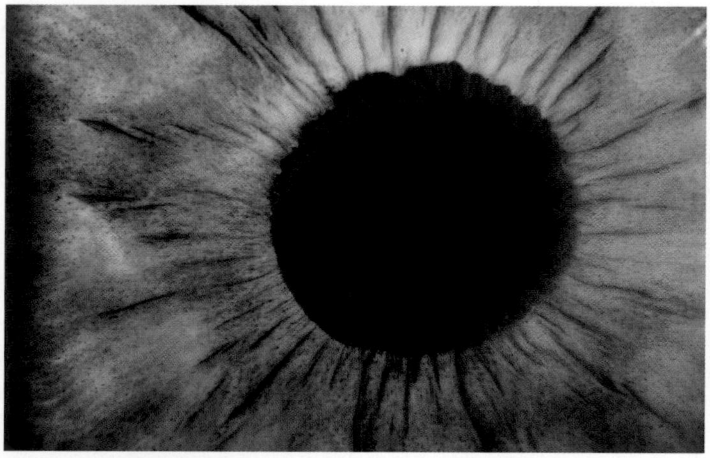

■ **Fig. 8.50** Partial loss of the pupillary ruff and fine pigment granules on the iris surface.

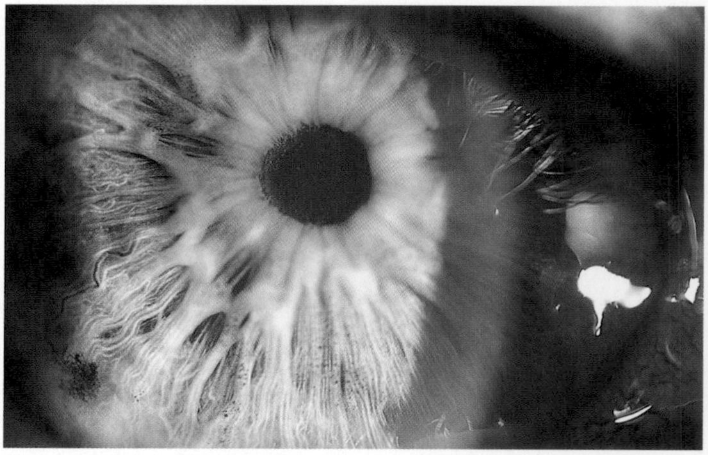

■ **Fig. 8.51** The pigment granules extending on to the lens.

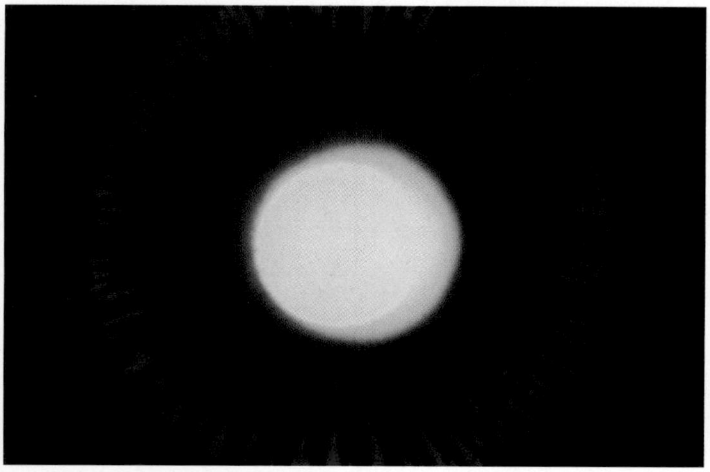

■ **Fig. 8.52** Iris pigment epithelial atrophy gives rise to radial slit-like transillumination defects. (Courtesy of L. Merin.)

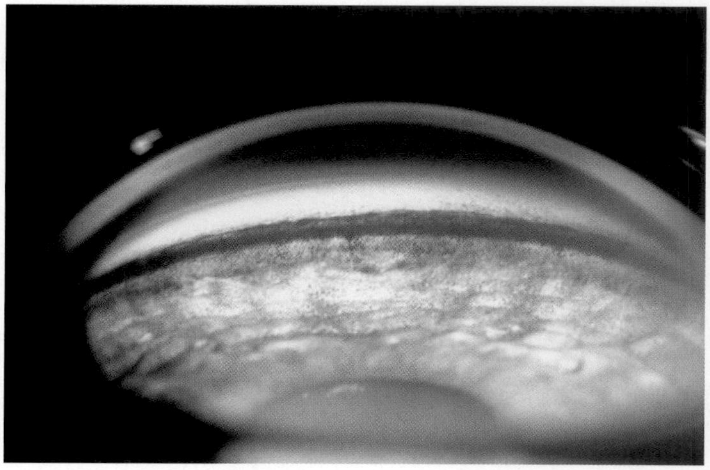

■ **Fig. 8.53** Homogeneous trabecular hyperpigmentation is most marked over the posterior trabeculum and may also be seen on or anterior to Schwalbe line. (Courtesy of L. Merin.)

NEOVASCULAR GLAUCOMA

Neovascular glaucoma is a serious condition that occurs as a result of iris neovascularisation (rubeosis iridis) secondary to diffuse chronic retinal ischaemia.

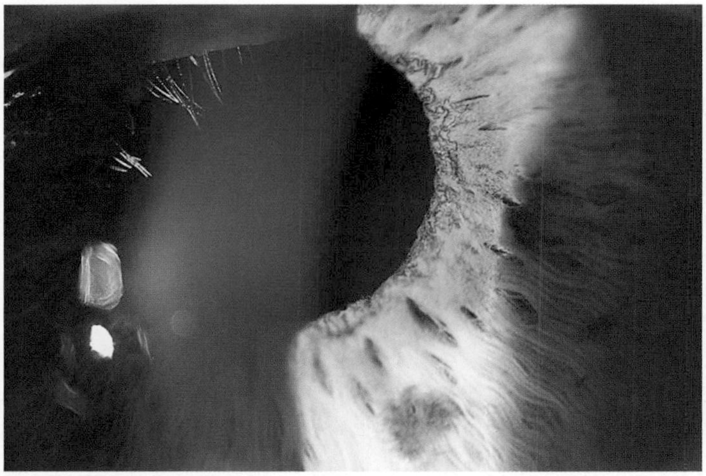

Fig. 8.54 Tiny, dilated capillary tufts or red spots develop at the pupillary margin and may be missed unless the iris is examined carefully under high magnification.

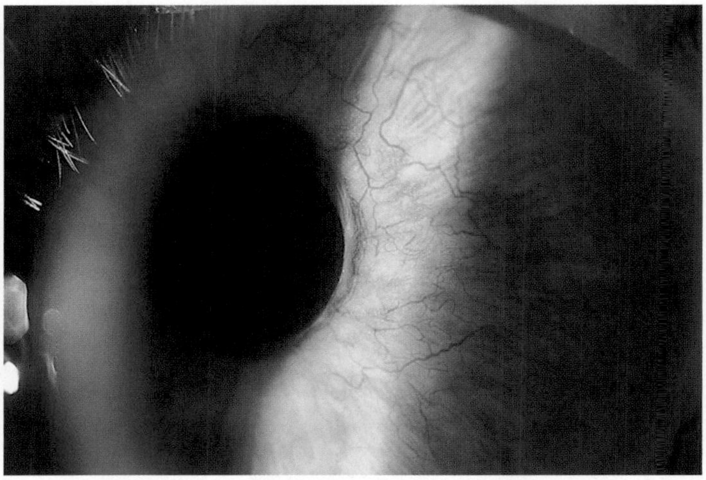

Fig. 8.55 The new vessels grow radially over the surface of the iris towards the angle, sometimes joining dilated blood vessels at the collarette.

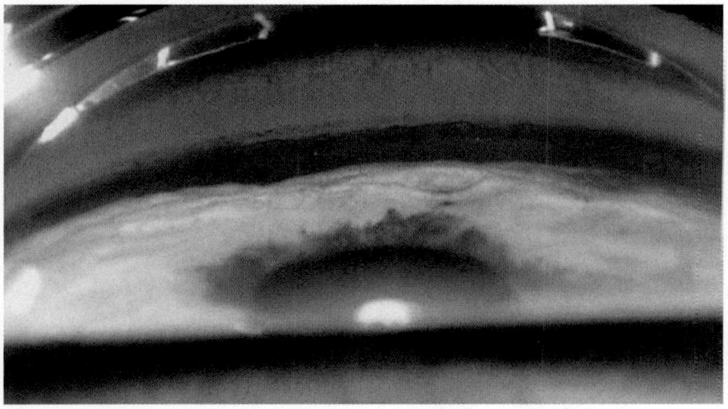

Fig. 8.56 The new blood vessels invade the angle and form a fibrovascular membrane that blocks the trabeculum.

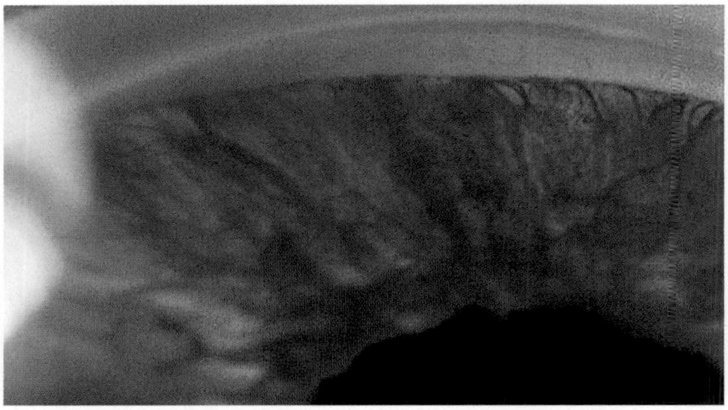

Fig. 8.57 The angle becomes progressively closed by contraction of fibrovascular tissue in a zipper-like fashion.

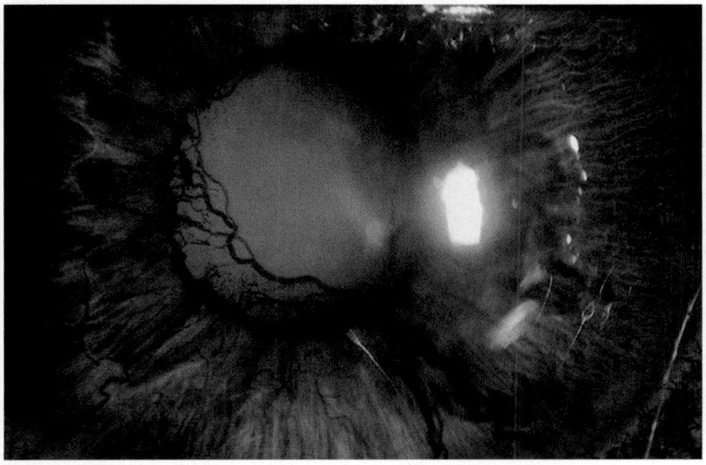

Fig. 8.58 The rubeosis may extend on to the anterior lens surface.

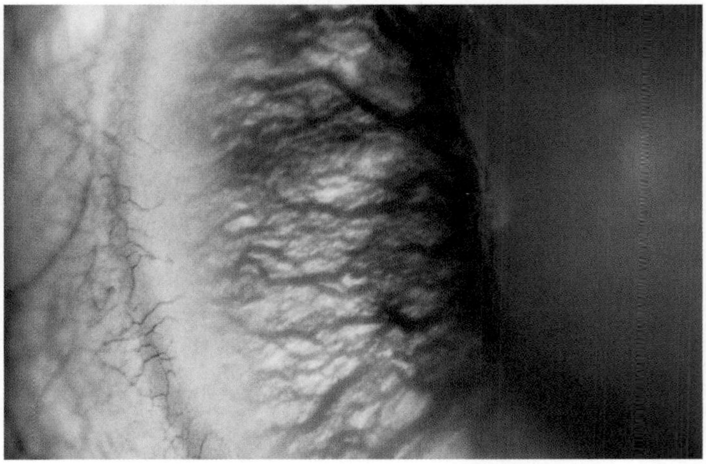

Fig. 8.59 Extremely severe rubeosis in end-stage disease.

INFLAMMATORY GLAUCOMA

Secondary glaucoma is the most common cause of visual loss in young individuals with chronic anterior uveitis.

Angle-closure glaucoma with pupil block

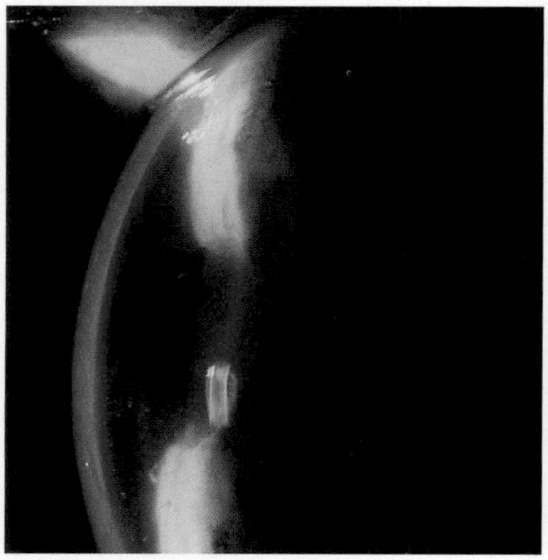

Fig. 8.60 Posterior synechiae extending for 360° (seclusio pupillae), which obstruct aqueous flow from the posterior to the anterior chamber.

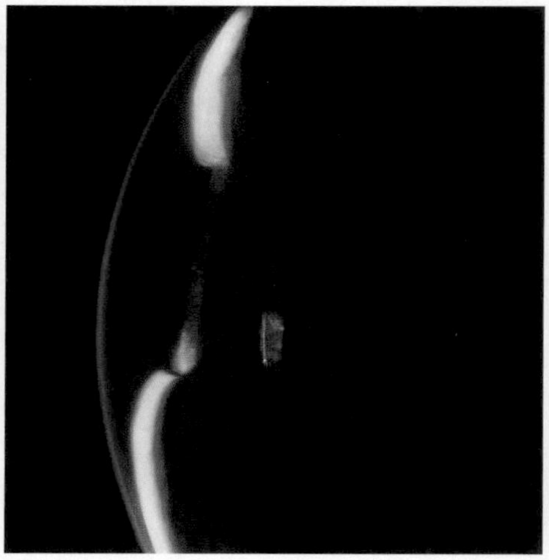

Fig. 8.61 The resultant increased pressure in the posterior chamber produces anterior bowing of the peripheral iris (iris bombé).

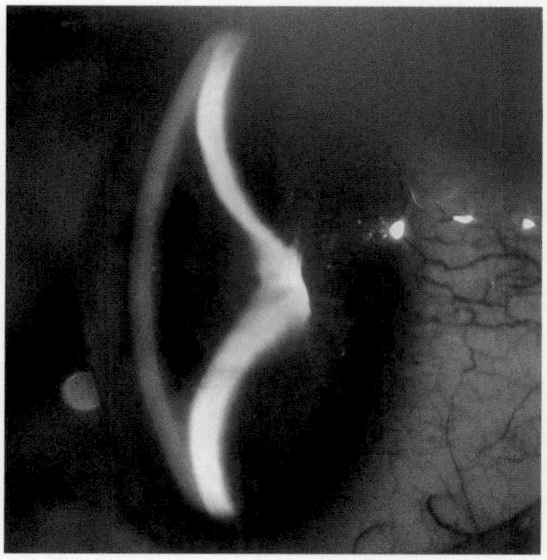

Fig. 8.62 Angle closure due to apposition of the peripheral iris to the trabeculum and peripheral cornea.

Angle-closure glaucoma without pupil block

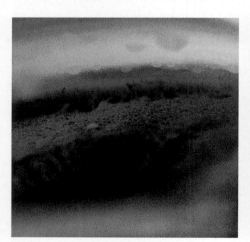

Fig. 8.63 Deposition of inflammatory debris in the angle.

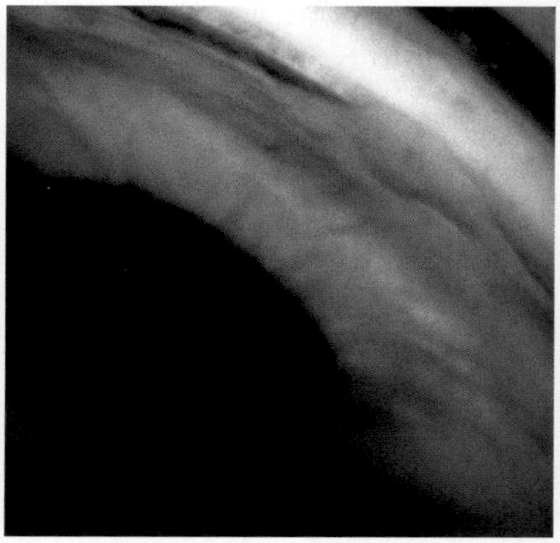

Fig.8.64 Subsequent organisation and contraction of debris pulls the peripheral iris over the trabeculum. (Courtesy of R. Curtis.)

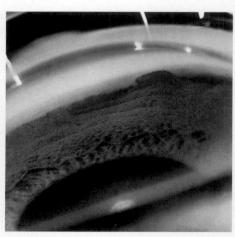

Fig. 8.65 Progressive synechial angle closure.

LENS-RELATED GLAUCOMA

Phacolytic (lens protein) glaucoma

Phacolytic glaucoma is an open-angle glaucoma occurring in association with a hypermature cataract.

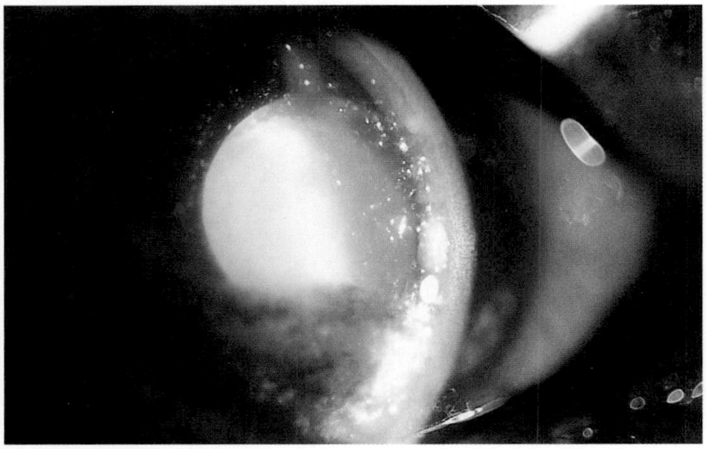

Fig. 8.66 The anterior chamber is deep and the aqueous manifests floating white particles consisting of lens-protein-laden macrophages.

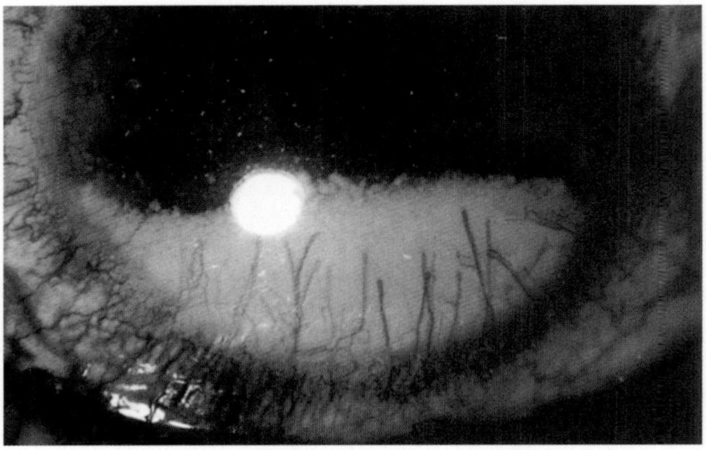

Fig. 8.67 A pseudohypopyon may form if many particles settle inferiorly.

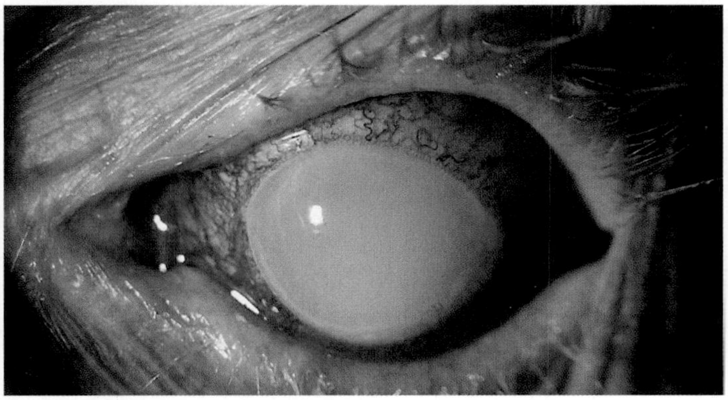

Fig. 8.68 Total pseudohypopyon.

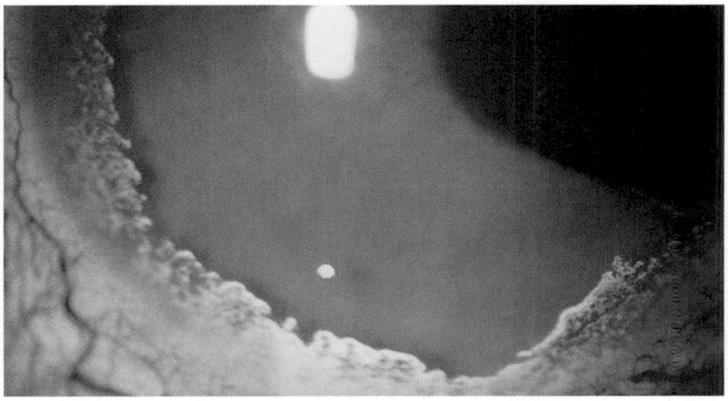

Fig. 8.69 Residual particles in the anterior chamber following incomplete irrigation.

Phacomorphic glaucoma

Phacomorphic glaucoma is an acute angle-closure glaucoma precipitated by an intumescent cataract.

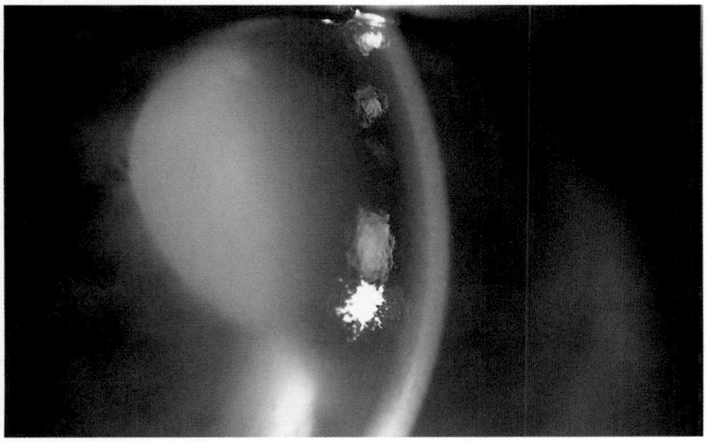

Fig. 8.70 Corneal epithelial oedema due to acute elevation of IOP, a shallow anterior chamber, dilated pupil and cataract.

Lens dislocation into the anterior chamber

Causes include blunt ocular trauma, eyes with weak zonules and microspherophakia.

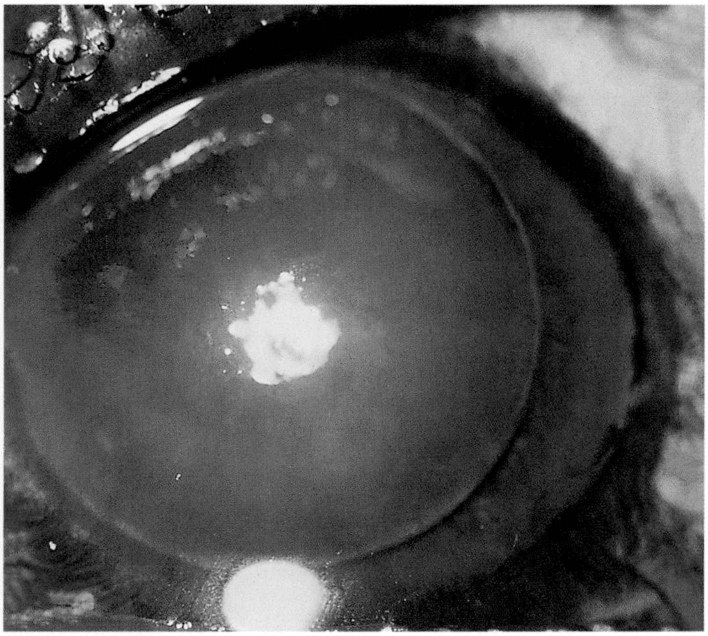

■ **Fig. 8.71** Acute pupil block and sudden severe elevation of IOP.

Lens incarceration in the pupil

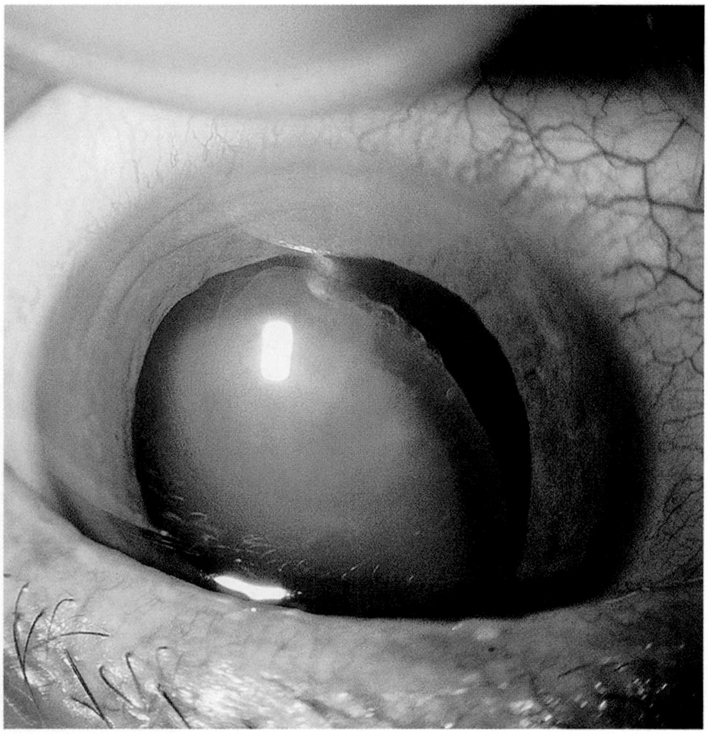

■ **Fig. 8.72** The rise in IOP is caused by pupil block in which only part of the zonules have been disrupted so that the intact zonules act as a hinge.

IRIDOCORNEAL ENDOTHELIAL SYNDROME

Iridocorneal endothelial syndrome typically affects one eye of a middle-aged woman. It consists of the following three very rare and frequently overlapping disorders: (a) progressive iris atrophy, (b) iris naevus (Cogan–Reese) syndrome and (c) Chandler syndrome.

Progressive iris atrophy

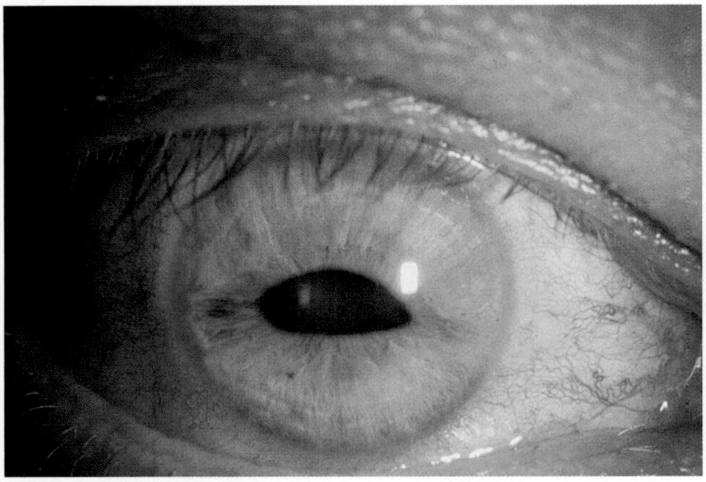

■ **Fig. 8.73** Displacement of the pupil (corectopia) and mild stromal iris atrophy. (Courtesy or R. Curtis.)

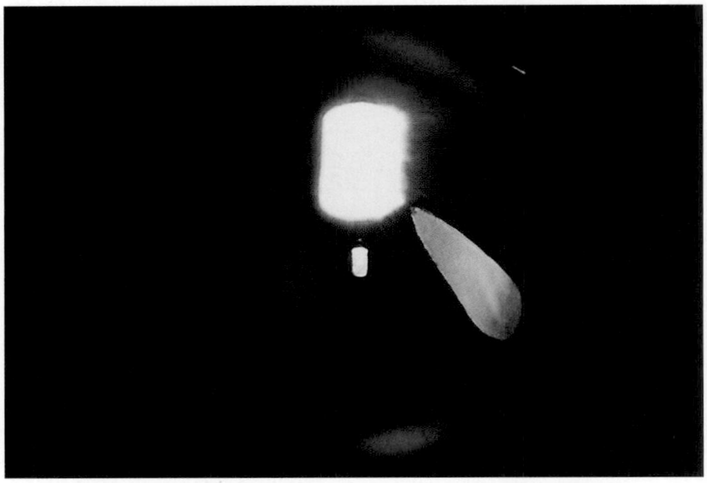

■ **Fig. 8.74** Iris atrophy resulting in a supernumerary pupil (pseudopolycoria). (Courtesy of R. Curtis.)

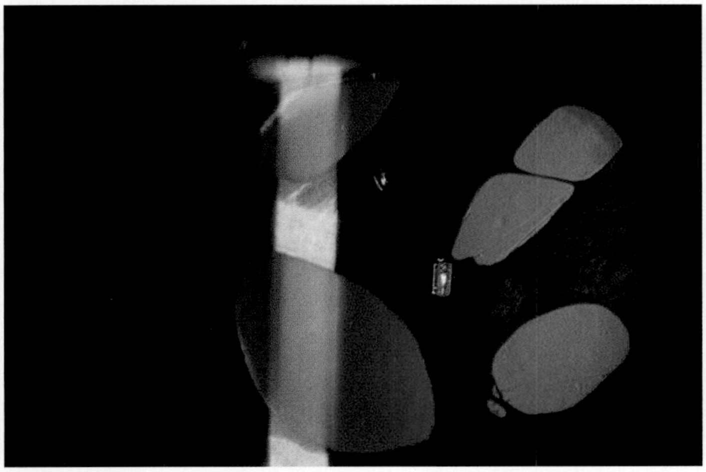

■ **Fig. 8.75** Multifocal pseudopolycoria. (Courtesy of R. Curtis.)

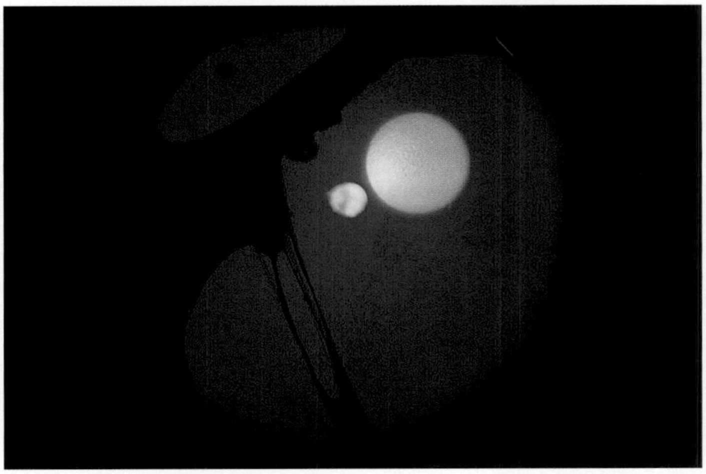

■ **Fig. 8.76** Extreme iris atrophy.

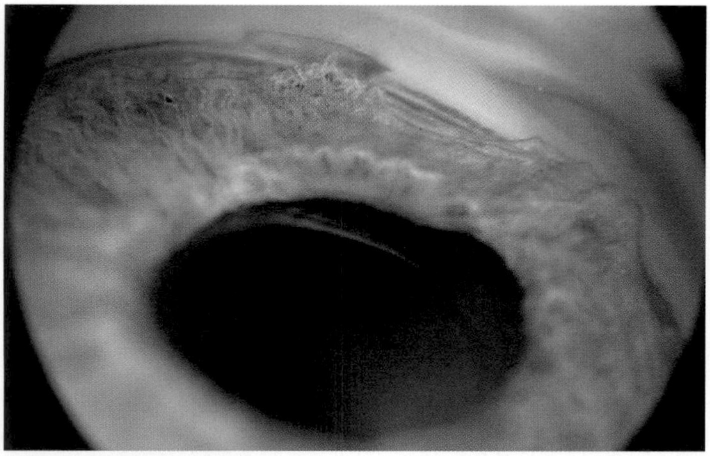

■ **Fig. 8.77** Broad-based peripheral anterior synechiae extending anterior to Schwalbe line. (Courtesy of L. MacKeen.)

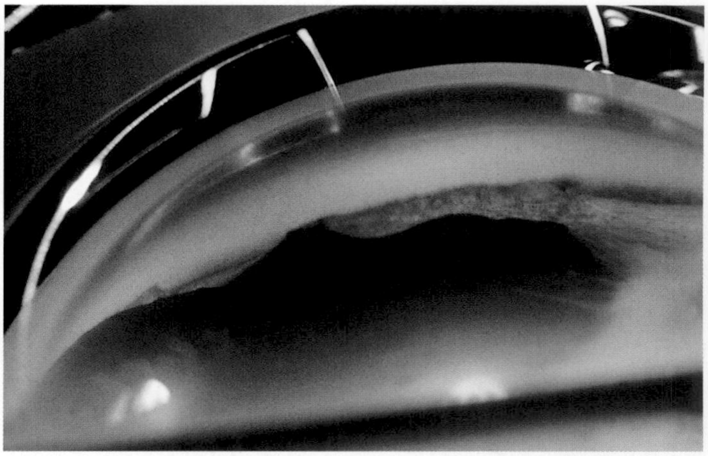

■ **Fig. 8.78** Extensive angle closure.

Cogan–Reese syndrome

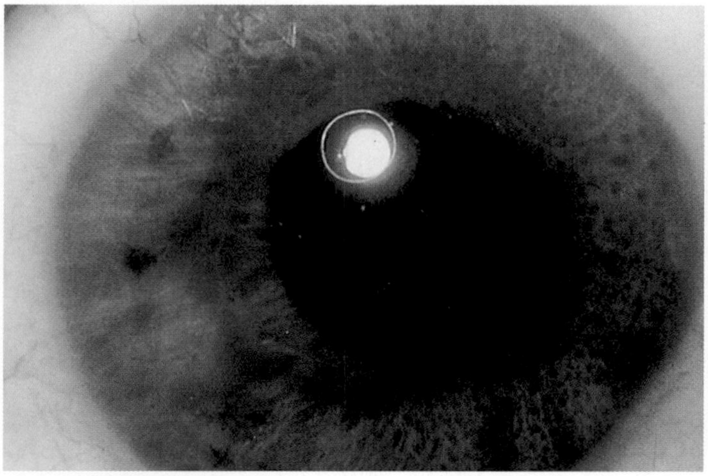

■ **Fig. 8.79** Multiple iris nodules with either absent or mild–moderate iris atrophy.

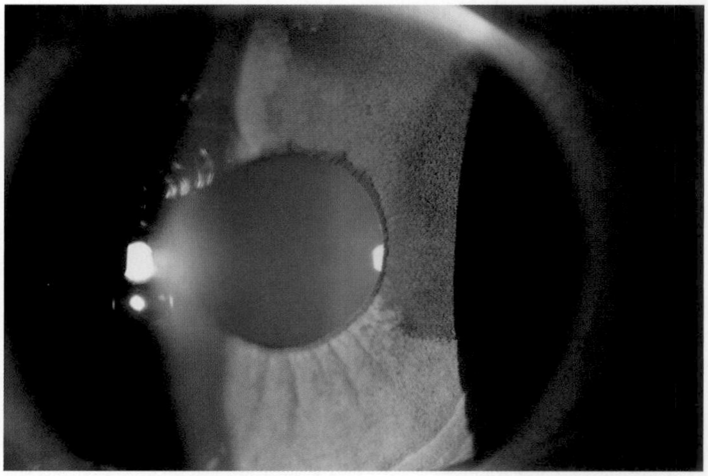

■ **Fig. 8.80** A diffuse iris naevus may be present in some cases.

Chandler syndrome

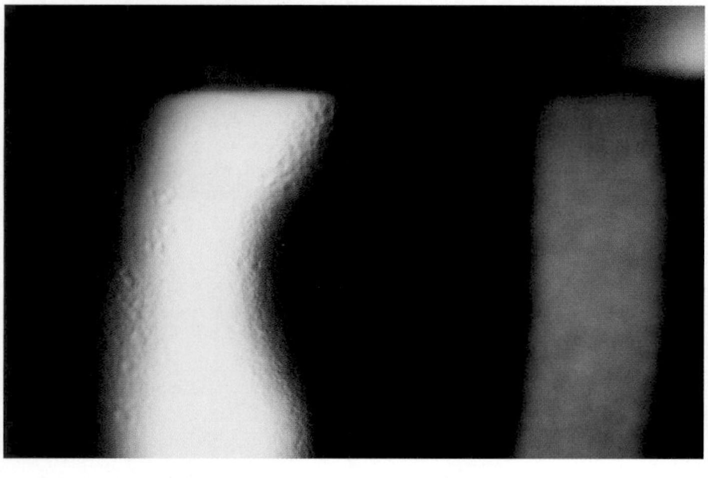

■ **Fig. 8.81** 'Hammered-silver' corneal endothelial abnormalities with absent or mild iris changes.

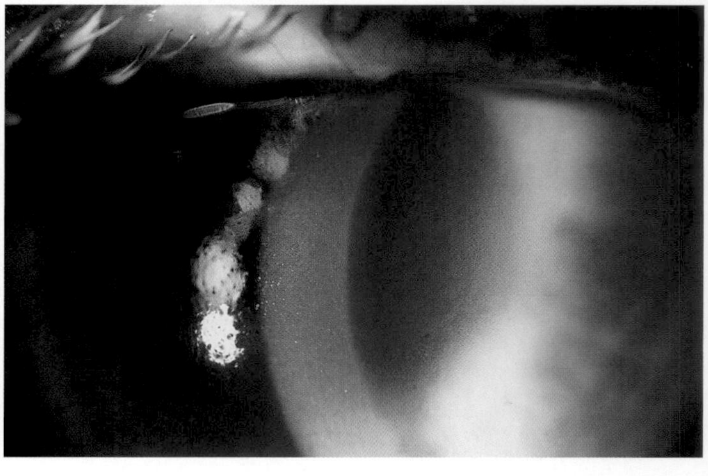

■ **Fig. 8.82** Endothelial decompensation and corneal oedema may occur in advanced cases.

MISCELLANEOUS SECONDARY GLAUCOMAS

Ghost cell glaucoma

Ghost cell glaucoma is due to trabecular obstruction by degenerate erythrocytes ('ghost cells').

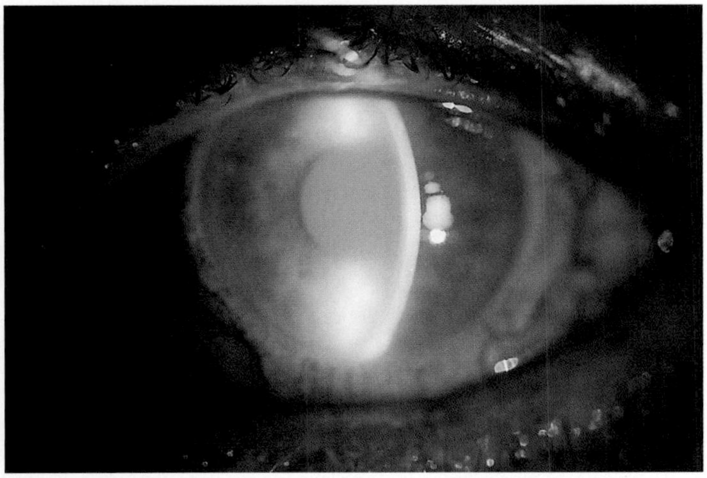

Fig. 8.83 The aqueous exhibits reddish-brown or khaki particles

Glaucoma in epithelial ingrowth

Epithelial ingrowth is a rare and serious complication of anterior segment surgery or trauma. It is characterised by the proliferation of sheets of epithelial cells over the posterior cornea, trabeculum, iris and ciliary body.

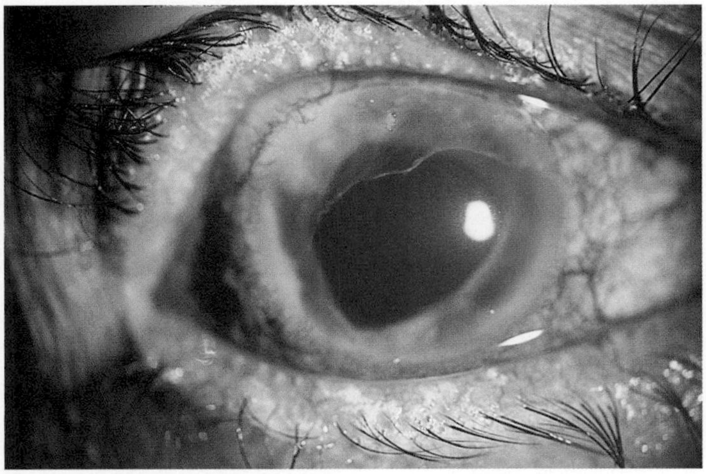

Fig. 8.84 A translucent posterior corneal membrane with a scalloped border and pupillary distortion.

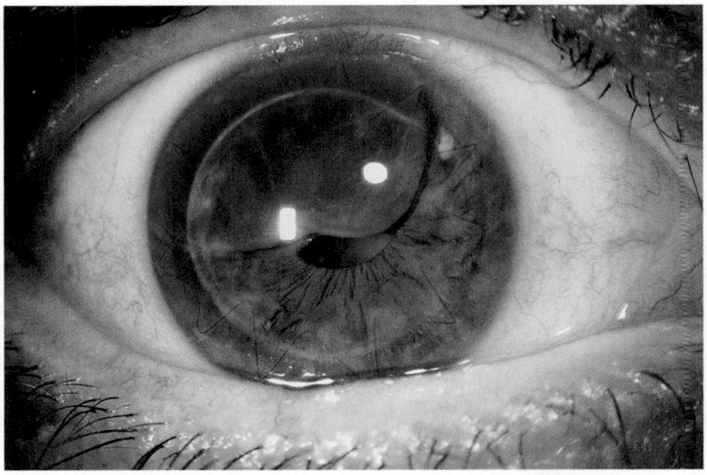

Fig. 8.85 Cystic anterior chamber ingrowth is less frequently associated with glaucoma. This case occurred following corneal grafting.

Glaucoma in iridoschisis

Iridoschisis is characterised by splitting of the iris stroma and is often associated with underlying angle-closure glaucoma.

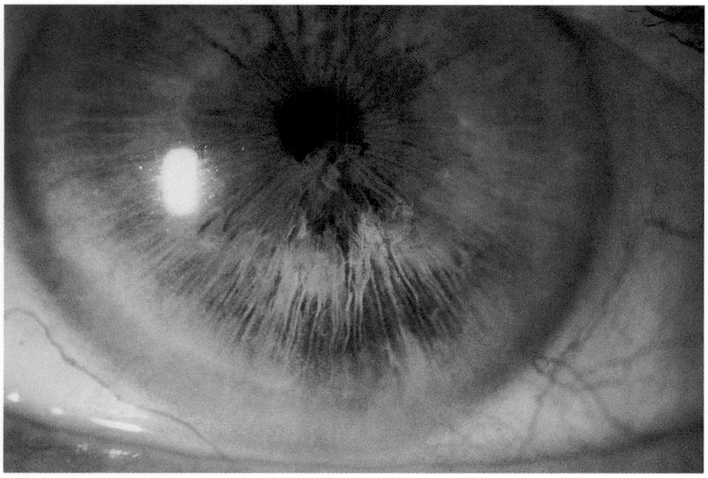

■ **Fig. 8.86** Mild iridoschisis.

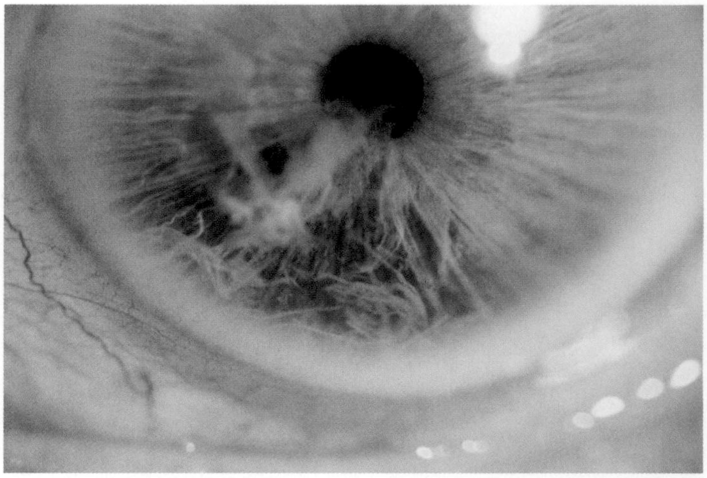

■ **Fig. 8.87** Moderately severe iridoschisis.

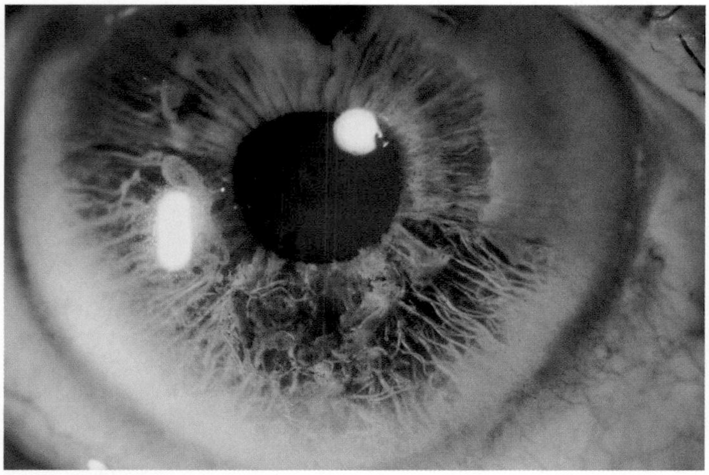

■ **Fig. 8.88** More extensive iridoschisis.

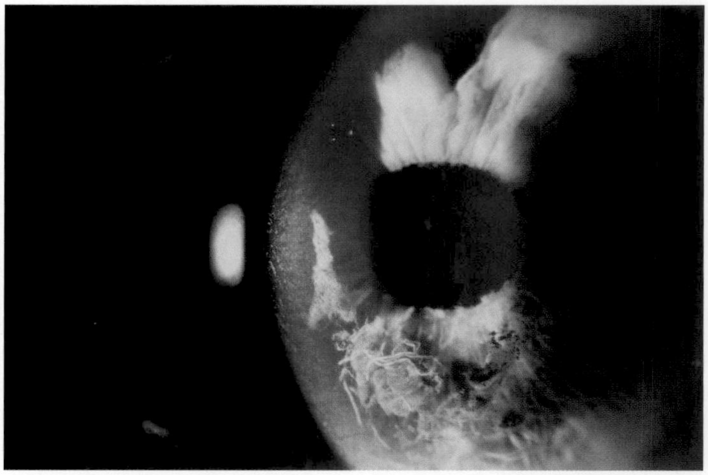

■ **Fig. 8.89** Very severe iridoschisis with disintegration of iris fibrils; note the peripheral iridectomy.

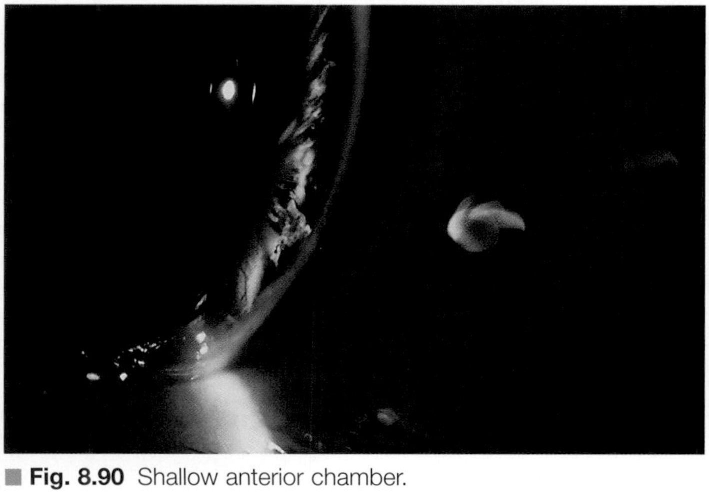

■ **Fig. 8.90** Shallow anterior chamber.

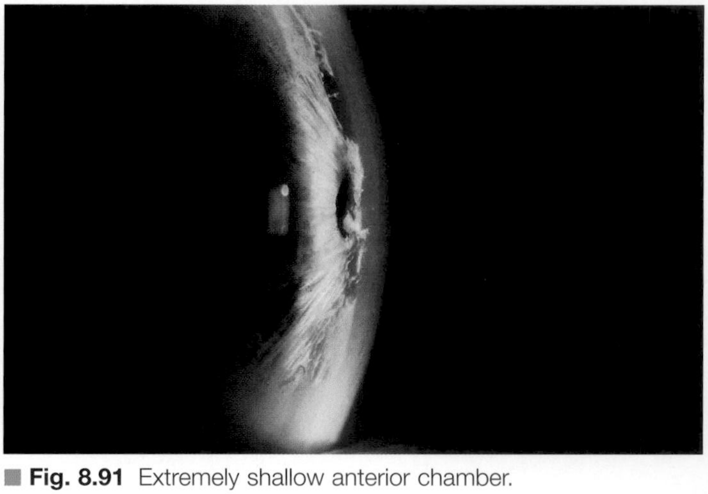

■ **Fig. 8.91** Extremely shallow anterior chamber.

Glaucoma associated with raised episcleral venous pressure

Causes

Carotid–cavernous fistula

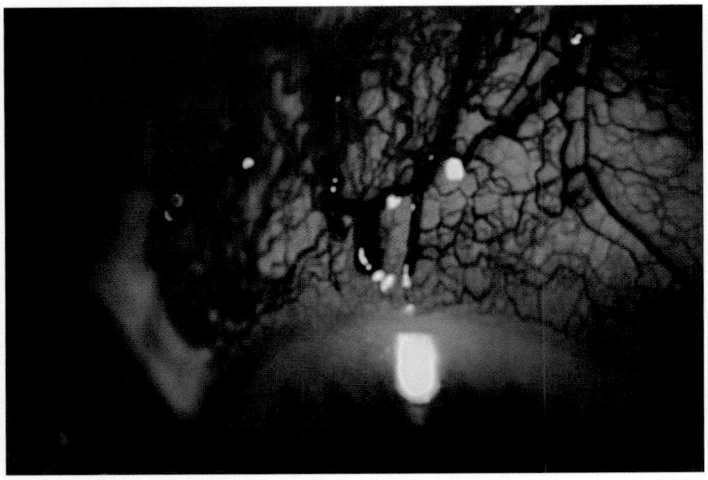

Fig. 8.92 Dilated episcleral vessels.

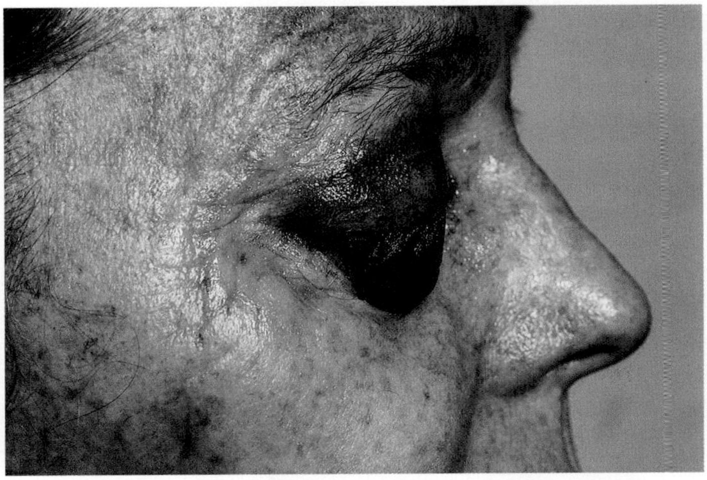

Fig. 8.93 Pulsetile proptosis and haemorrhagic chemosis.

Sturge–Weber syndrome

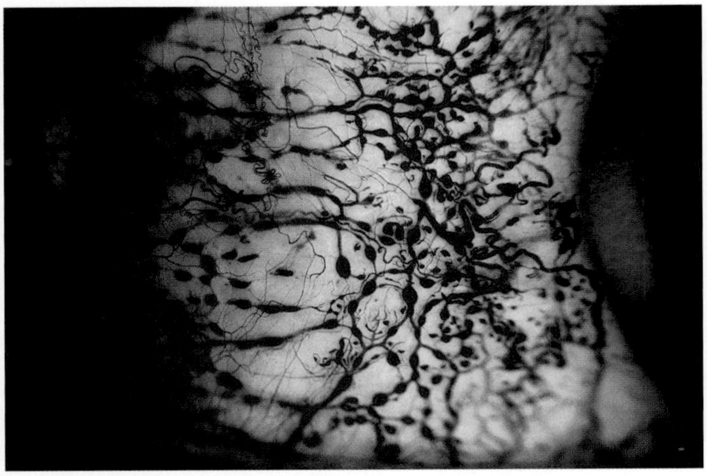

Fig. 8.94 Episcleral haemangioma.

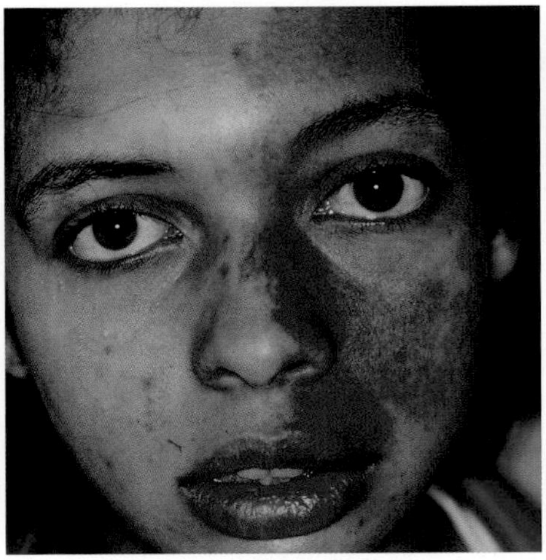

Fig. 8.95 Naevus flammeus and mild left buphthalmos. (Courtesy of J. Salmon.)

Superior vena caval obstruction

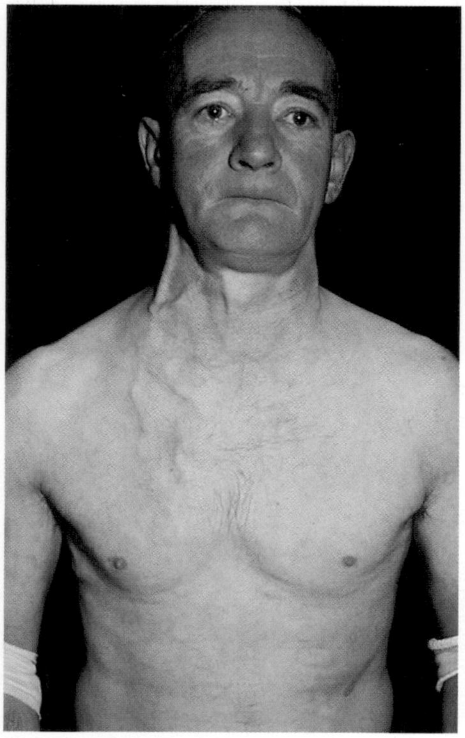

Fig. 8.96 Facial suffusion associated with dilated blood vessels of the neck and chest. (Courtesy of M. A. Mir.)

Gonioscopy

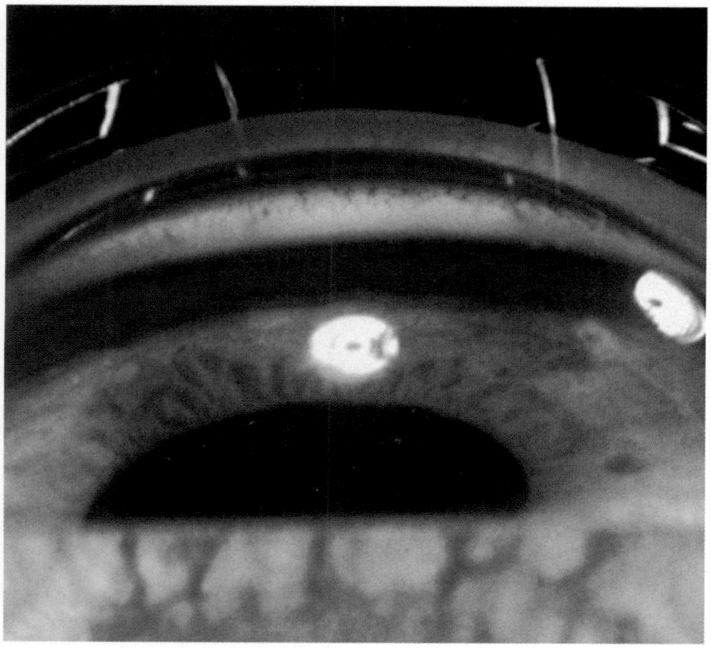

Fig. 8.97 Open angle with blood in Schlemm canal.

Glaucoma in intraocular tumours

Approximately 5% of eyes with intraocular tumours develop a secondary elevation of IOP. Depending on the location of the tumour one or more of the following mechanisms may be responsible:

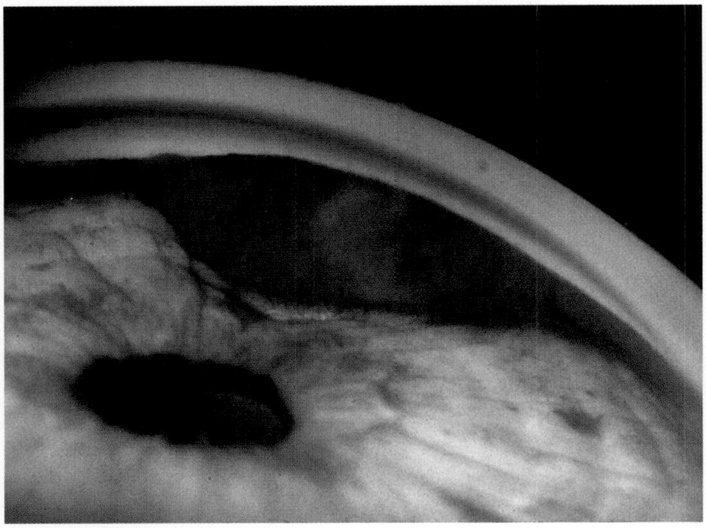

Fig. 8.98 Direct trabecular invasion by a solid iris melanoma. (Courtesy of R. Curtis.)

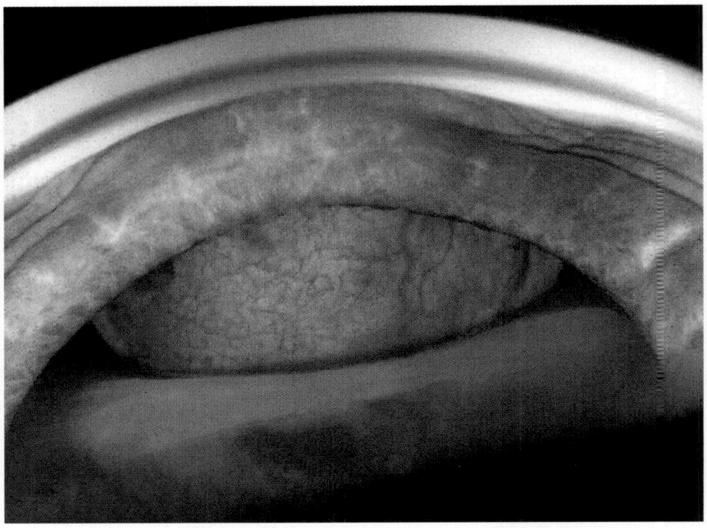

Fig. 8.99 Secondary angle closure due to anterior displacement of the iris–lens diaphragm by a large ciliary body melanoma.

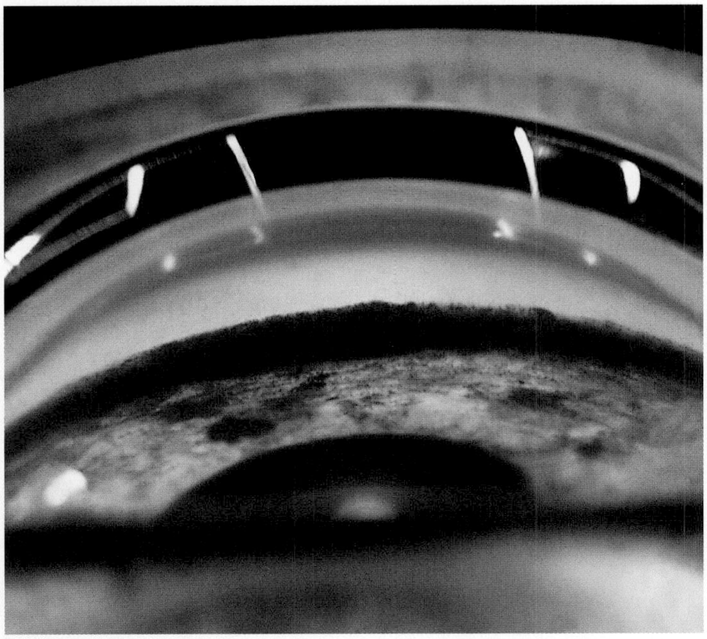

Fig. 8.100 Direct trabecular invasion by a diffuse iris melanoma.

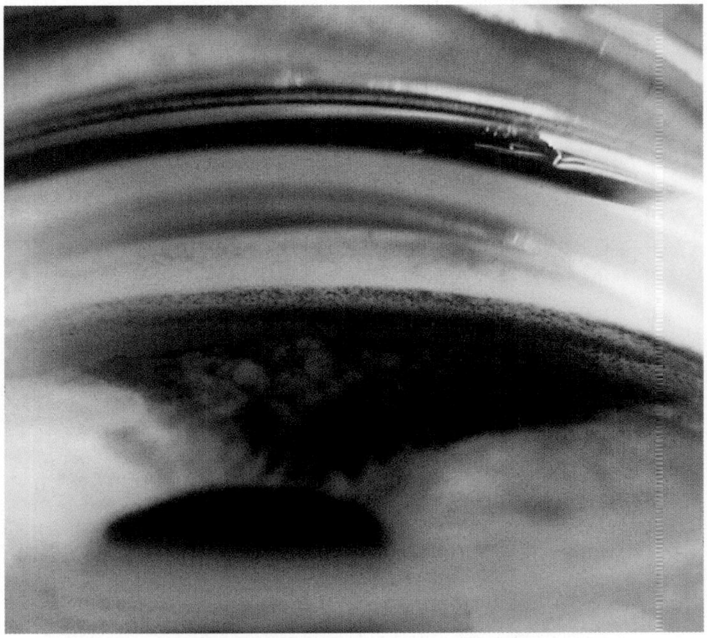

Fig. 8.101 Melanomalytic glaucoma due to trabecular blockage by macrophages that have ingested pigment and tumour cells. The resulting trabecular hyperpigmentation may mimic pigment dispersion syndrome.

PRIMARY CONGENITAL GLAUCOMA

Impaired aqueous outflow in primary congenital glaucoma is caused by maldevelopment of the angle of the anterior chamber, unassociated with any other major ocular anomalies (isolated trabeculodysgenesis).

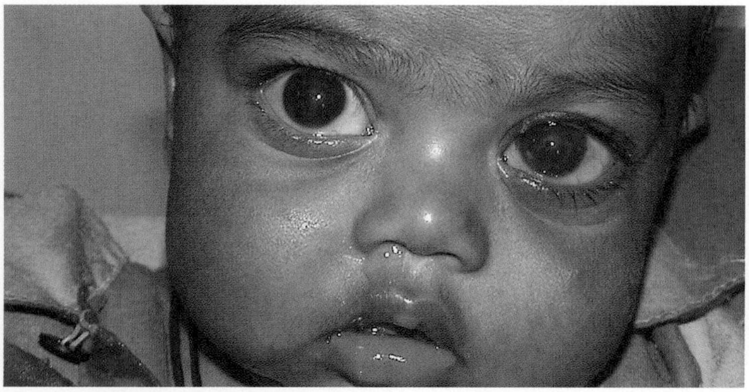

Fig. 8.102 Corneal haze due to corneal oedema is often the first sign noticed by the parents. (Courtesy of M. Parulekar.)

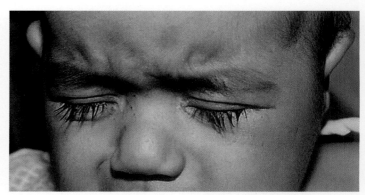

Fig. 8.103 Corneal irritation may cause lacrimation, photophobia and blepharospasm. (Courtesy of U. Raina.)

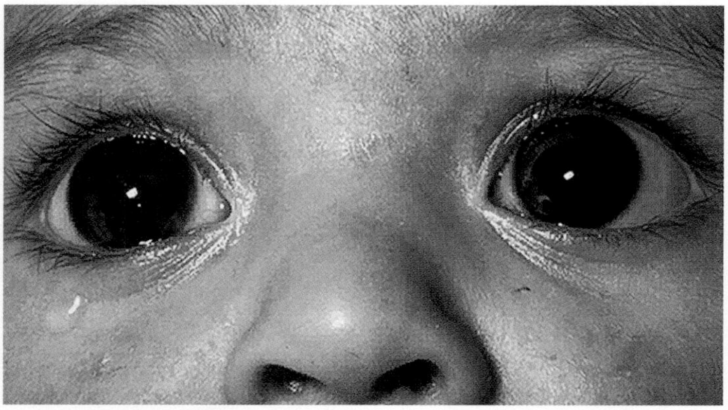

Fig. 8.104 Mild bilateral symmetrical buphthalmos. (Courtesy of S. Ford and R. Marsh.)

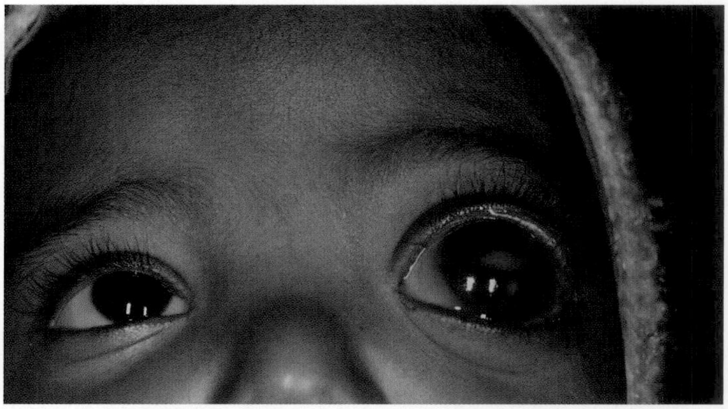

Fig. 8.105 Buphthalmos is not usually reported by the parents unless it is unilateral and advanced. (Courtesy of U. Raina.)

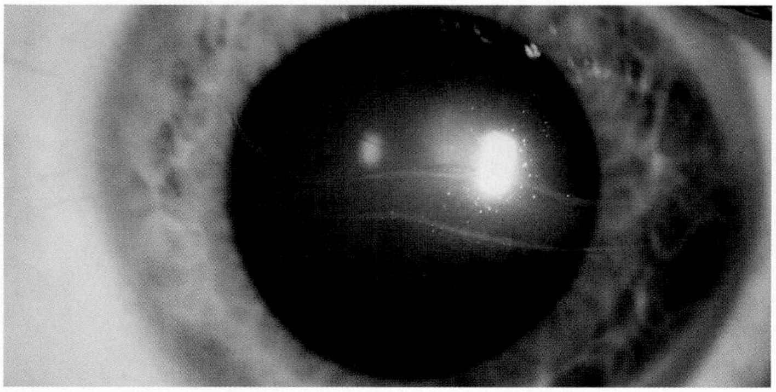

Fig. 8.106 Haab striae represent healed breaks in Descemet membrane and appear as horizontal curvilinear lines.

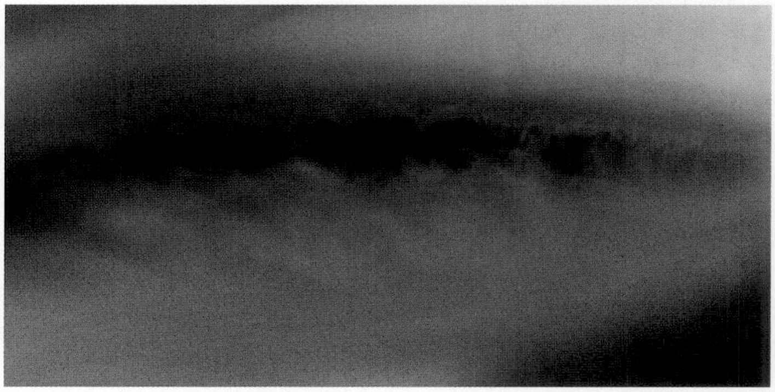

Fig. 8.107 Absence of the angle recess, with the iris inserted directly into the surface of the trabeculum and obscuration of angle structures by bridging iris tissue.

IRIDOCORNEAL DYSGENESIS

Iridocorneal dysgenesis consists of the following rare, bilateral overlapping congenital disorders involving the cornea and iris, some of which may be associated with glaucoma.

Axenfeld–Rieger syndrome

Axenfeld anomaly

Axenfeld anomaly is rarely associated with glaucoma.

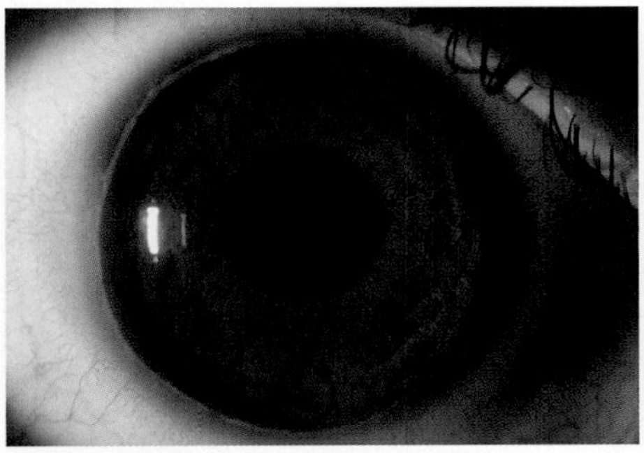

Fig. 8.108 Prominent anteriorly displaced Schwalbe line (posterior embryotoxon). (Courtesy of P. Gili.)

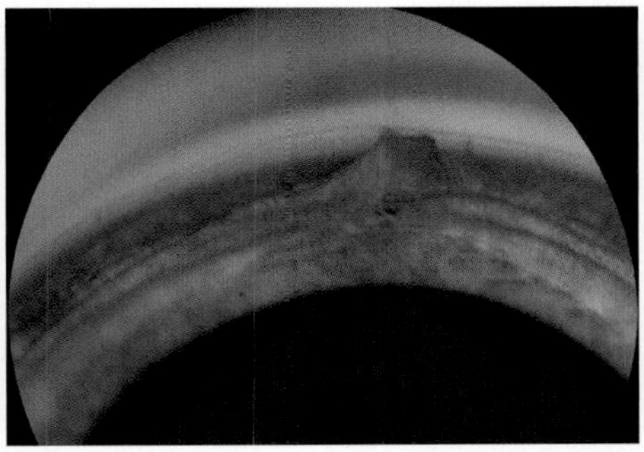

Fig. 8.109 Strands of peripheral iris attached to posterior embryotoxon. (Courtesy of L. MacKeen.)

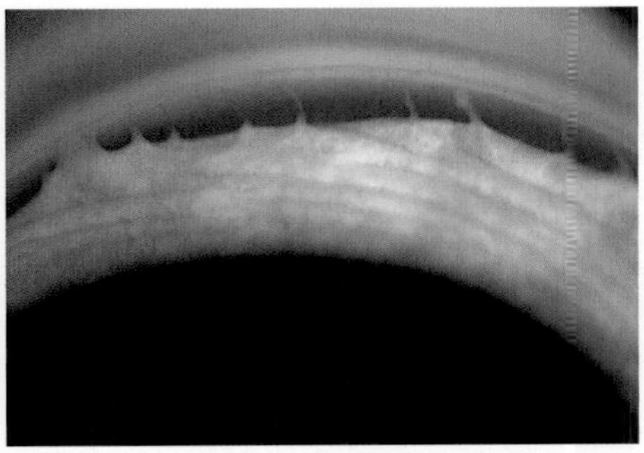

Fig. 8.110 More extensive involvement. (Courtesy of L. MacKeen.)

Rieger anomaly

Rieger anomaly is associated with glaucoma in 50% of cases.

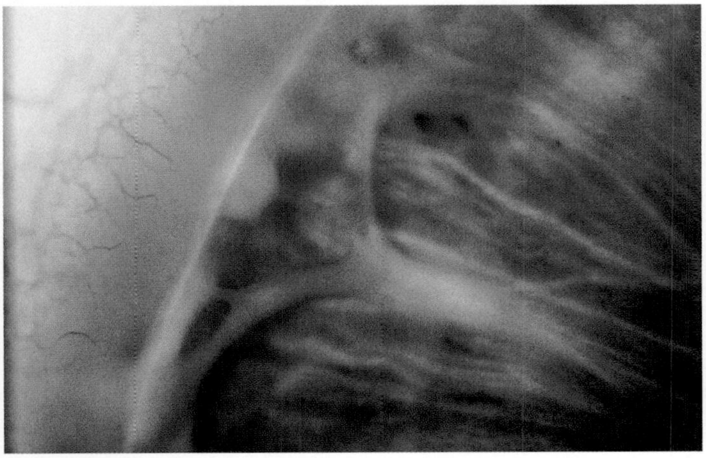

Fig. 8.111 Posterior embryotoxon.

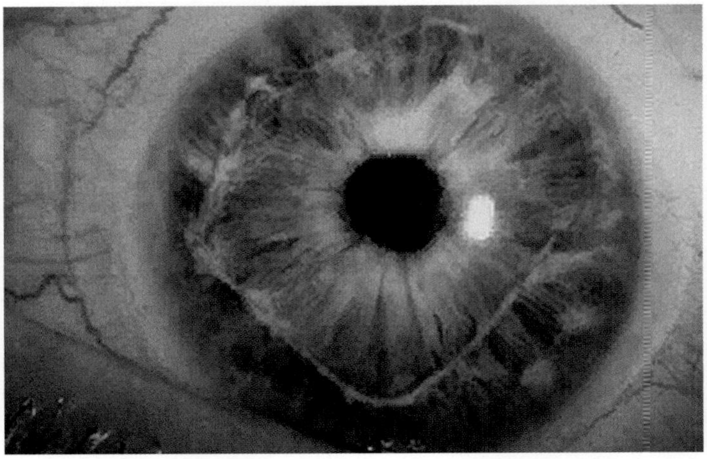

Fig. 8.112 Schwalbe line may become detached. (Courtesy of S. Ford and R. Marsh.)

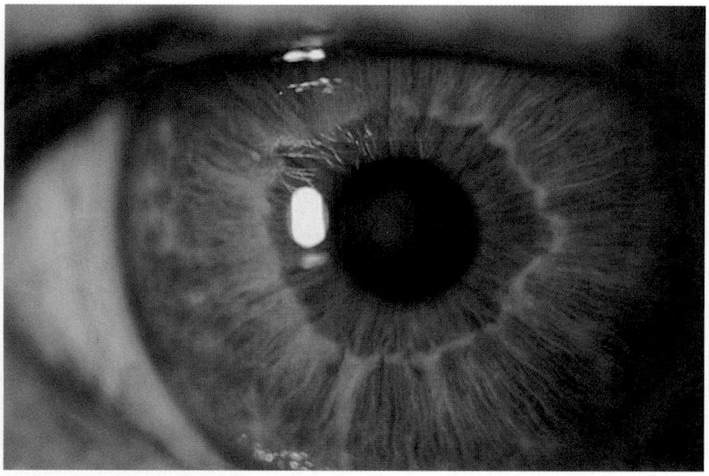

Fig. 8.113 Early iris stromal hypoplasia.

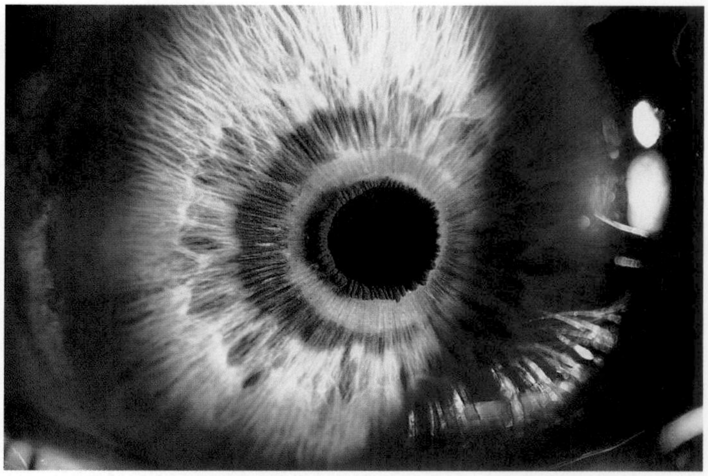

Fig. 8.114 Iris stromal hypoplasia resulting in prominence of the sphincter pupillae.

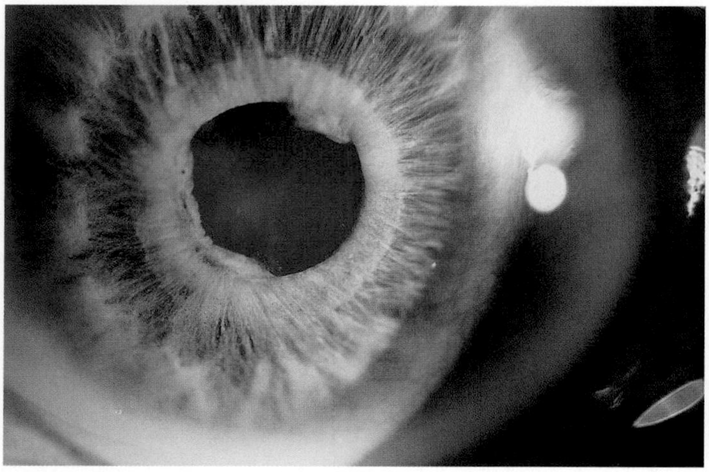

Fig. 8.115 More severe stromal hypoplasia.

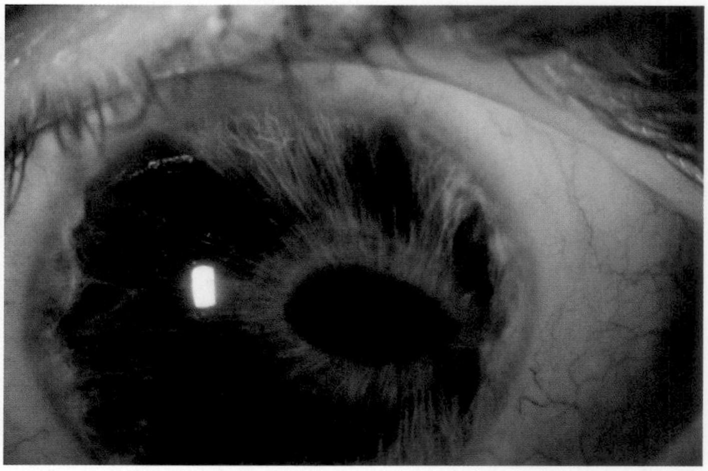

Fig. 8.116 Corectopia and stromal hypoplasia.

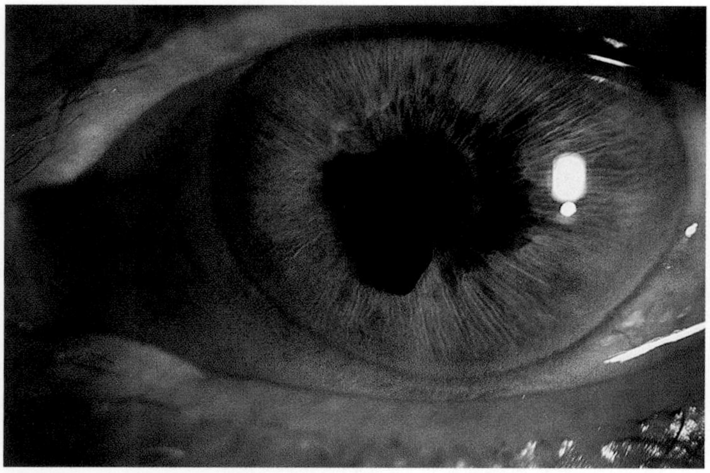

Fig. 8.117 Ectropion uveae and stromal hypoplasia.

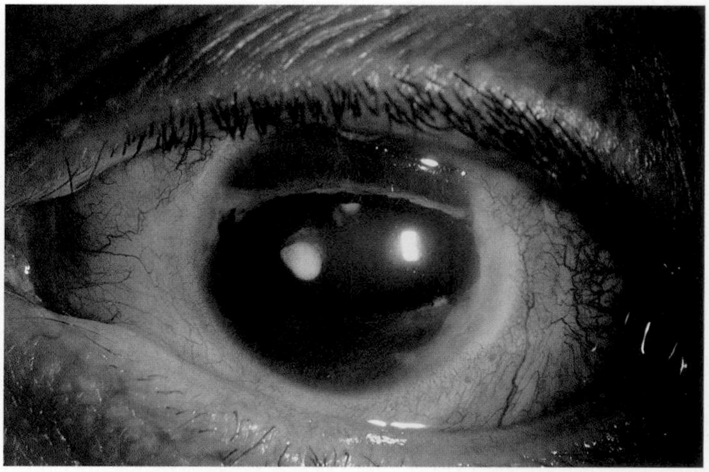

Fig. 8.118 Corectopia, ectropion uveae and stromal hypoplasia.

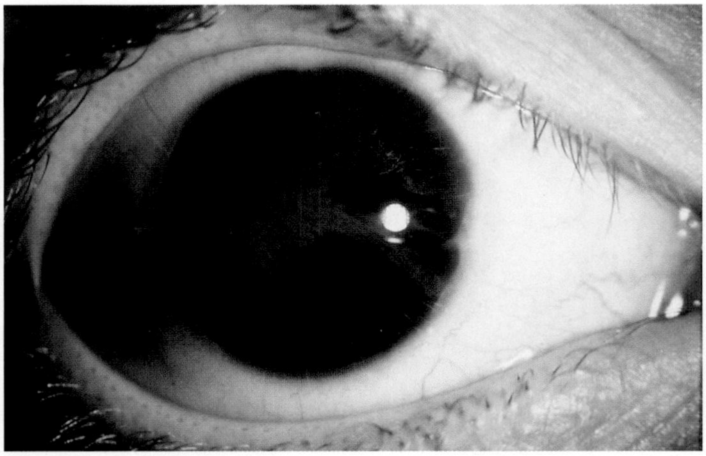

Fig. 8.119 Corectopia and full-thickness iris defects.

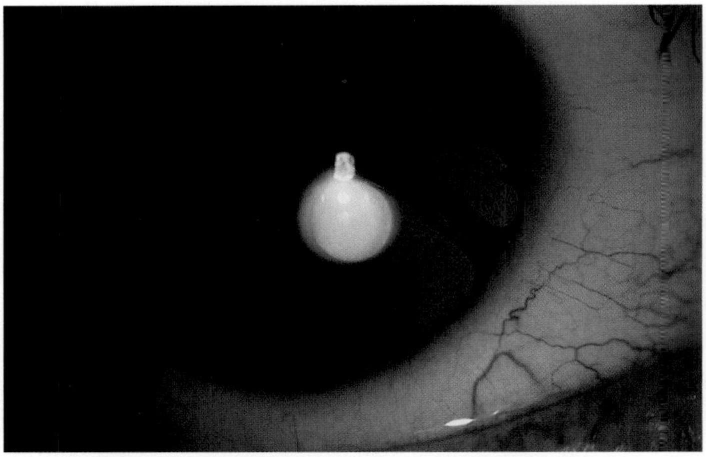

Fig. 8.120 Retroillumination of full-thickness iris defects.

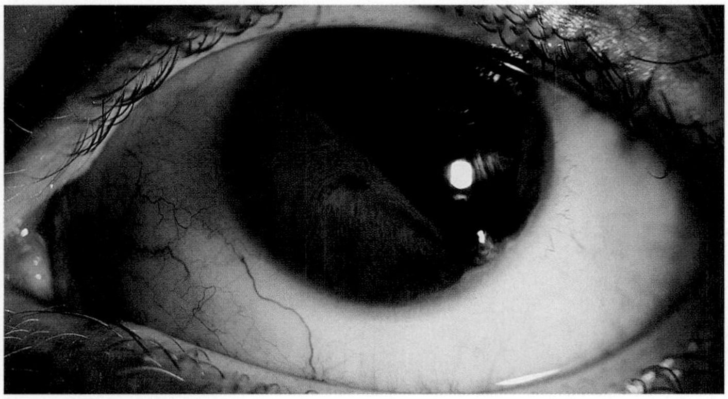

Fig. 8.121 Very severe iris atrophy.

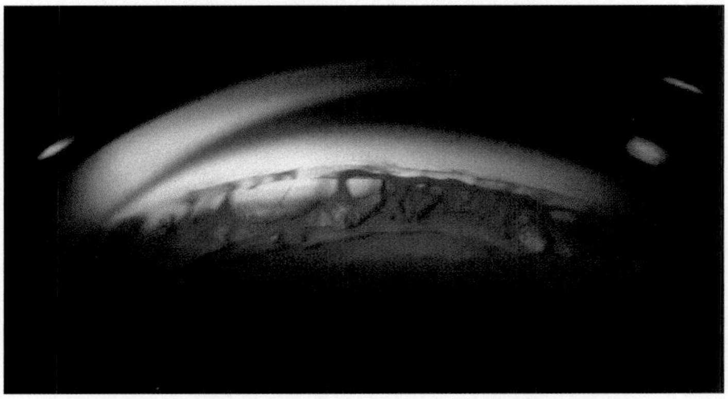

Fig. 8.122 Extensive peripheral anterior synechiae extending anterior to Schwalbe line. (Courtesy of P. Gili.)

Rieger syndrome

Rieger syndrome consists of Rieger anomaly in association with the following extraocular malformations:

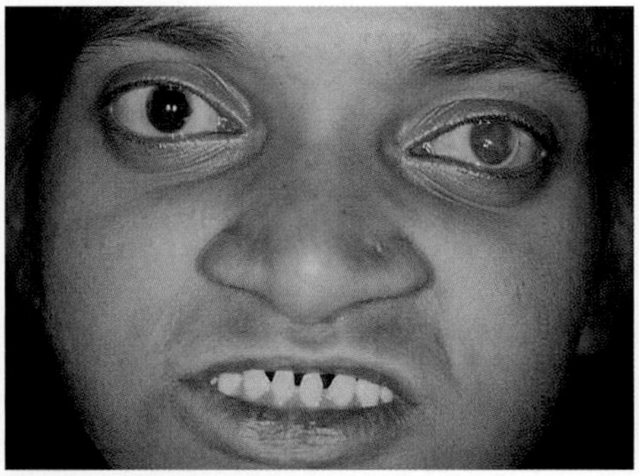

Fig. 8.123 Facial anomalies include maxillary hypoplasia, broad nasal bridge, telecanthus and hypertelorism. (Courtesy of U. Raina.)

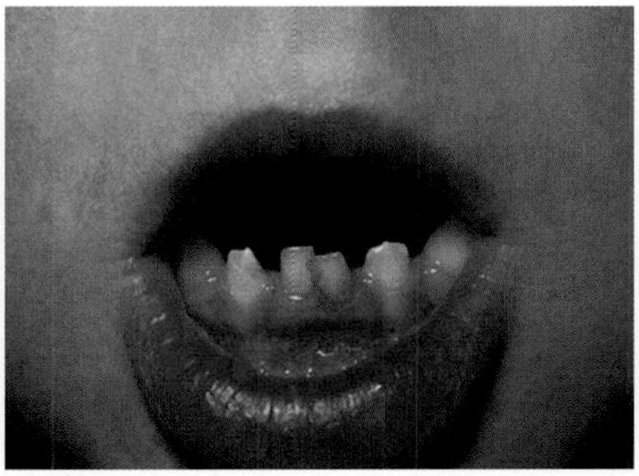

Fig. 8.124 Dental anomalies consist of hypodontia (few teeth) and microdontia (small teeth). (Courtesy of S. Ford and R. Marsh.)

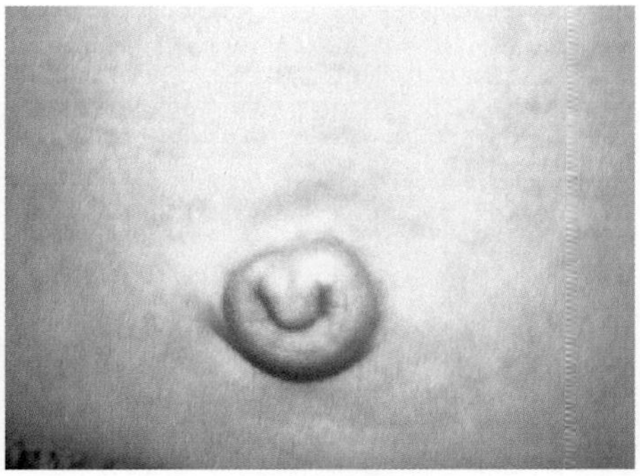

Fig. 8.125 Redundant paraumbilical skin. (Courtesy of K. Nischal.)

Peters anomaly

Peters anomaly is an extremely rare but serious condition which is associated with glaucoma in about 50% of cases due to an angle anomaly.

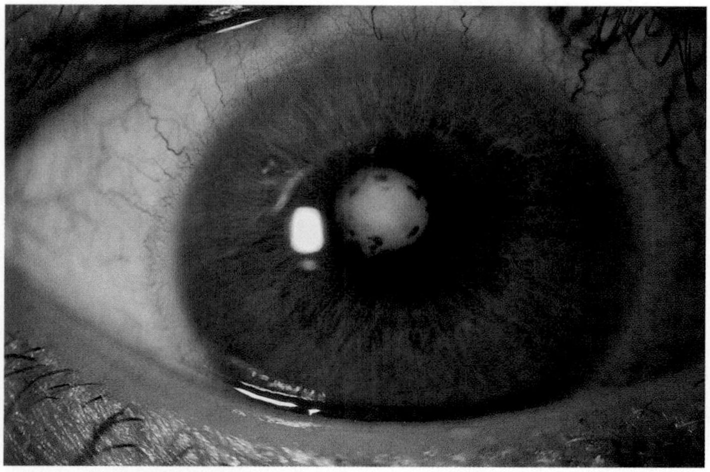

Fig. 8.126 Corneal opacity of variable density, with an underlying posterior corneal defect.

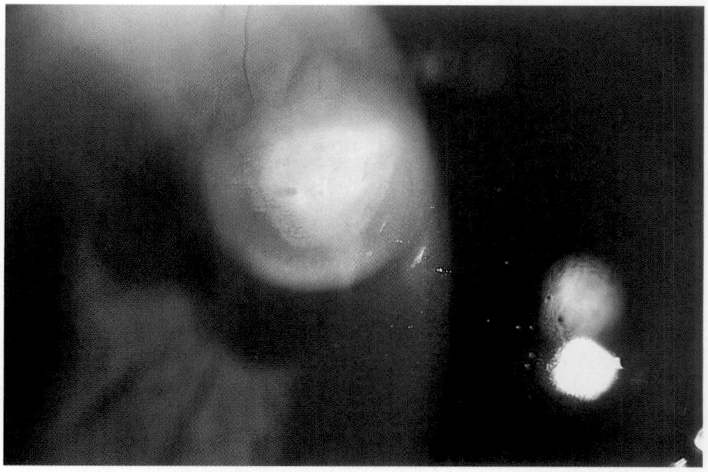

Fig. 8.127 Larger corneal opacity.

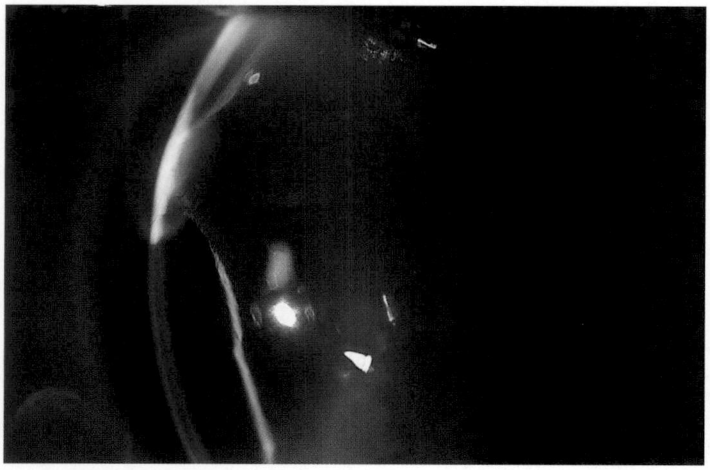

Fig. 8.128 Strands of iris tissue adhere to the margin of the opacity.

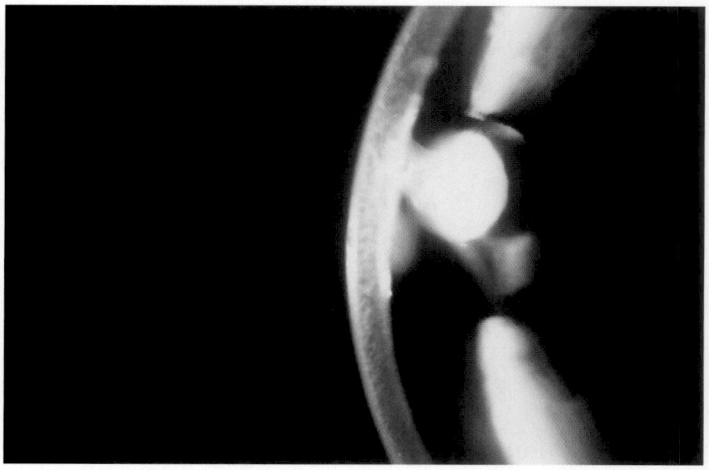

Fig. 8.129 Keratolenticular adhesion.

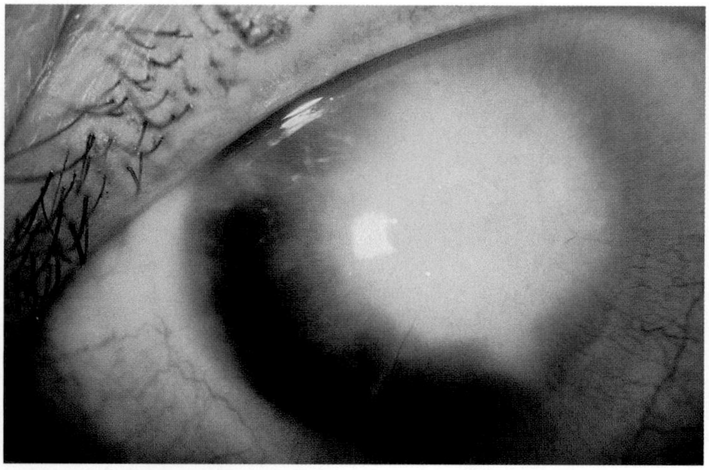

Fig. 8.130 Very severe Peters anomaly. (Courtesy of S. Ford and R. Marsh.)

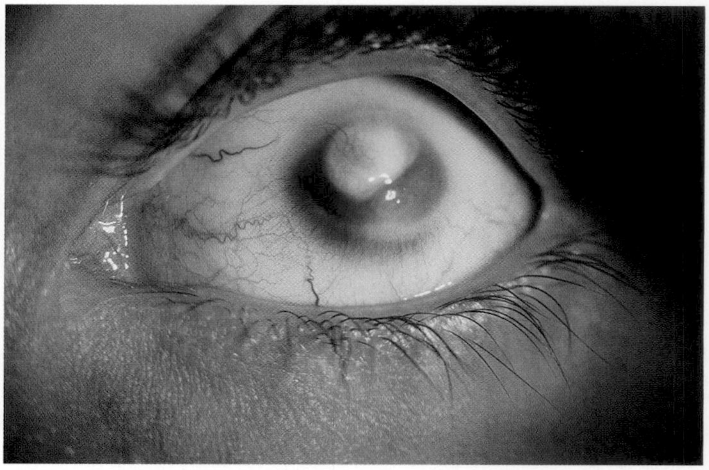

Fig. 8.131 Peters anomaly in a microphthalmic eye is uncommon.

Aniridia

Aniridia is associated with glaucoma in 75% of cases.

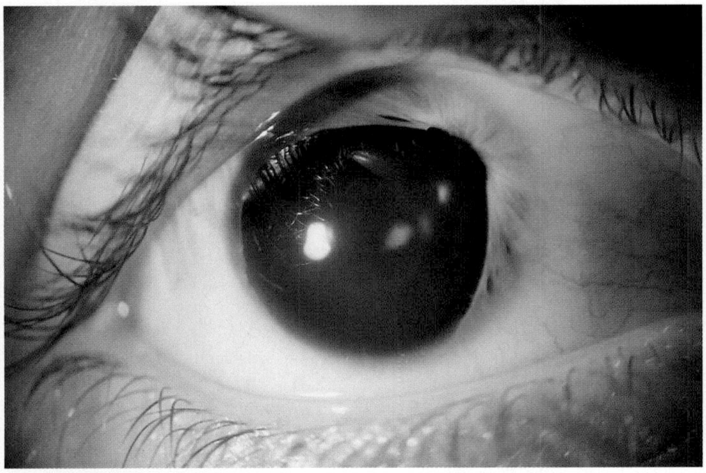

Fig. 8.132 Partial aniridia.

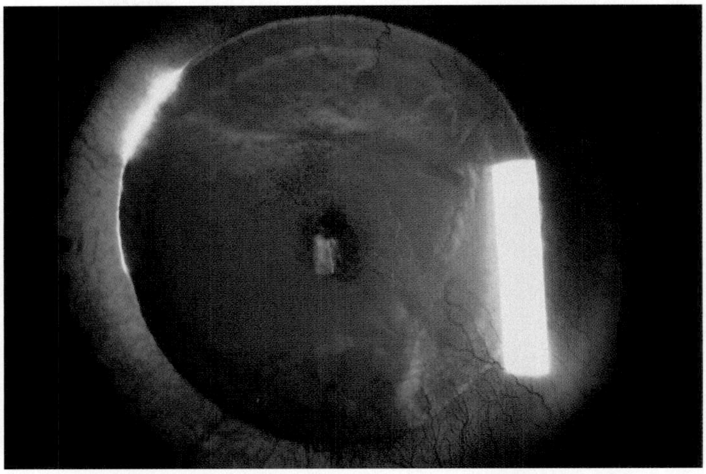

Fig. 8.133 Total aniridia seen on retroillumination with peripheral corneal vascularisation secondary to limbal stem cell deficiency. (Courtesy of L. Merin.)

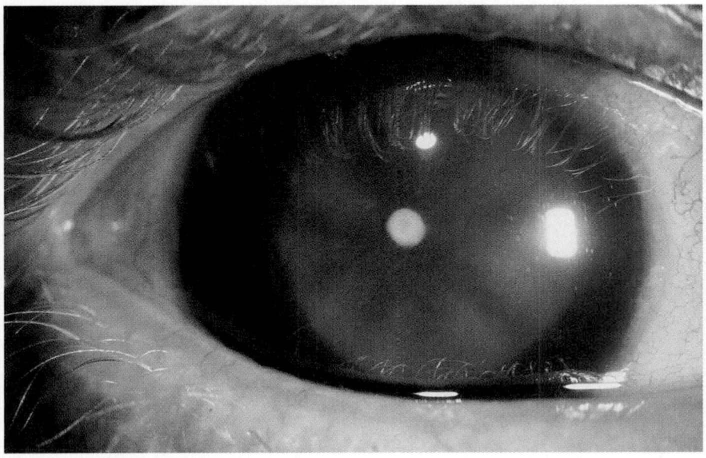

Fig. 8.134 Total aniridia with a small anterior polar and a large nuclear cataract.

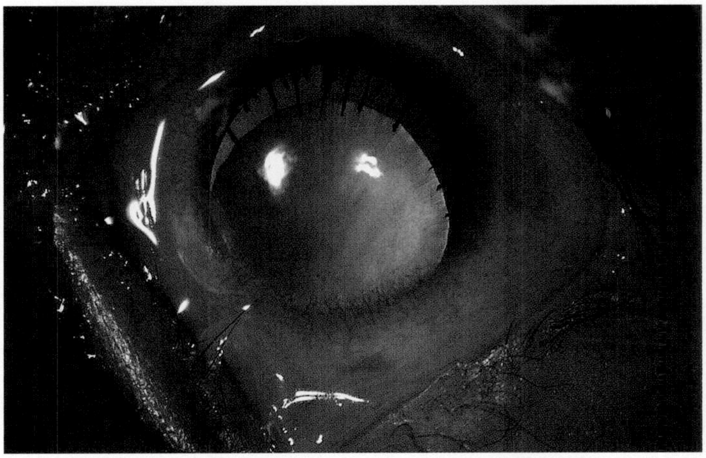

Fig. 8.135 Aniridia and inferior lens subluxation (Courtesy of U. Raina.)

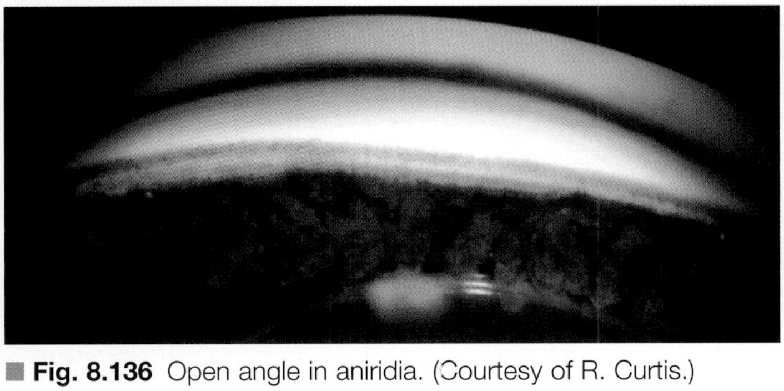

Fig. 8.136 Open angle in aniridia. (Courtesy of R. Curtis.)

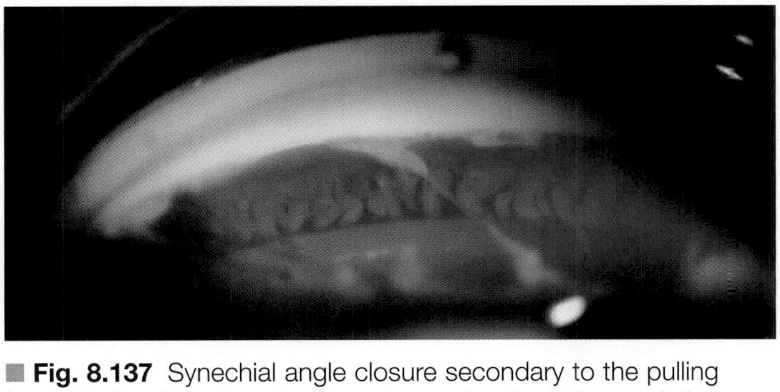

Fig. 8.137 Synechial angle closure secondary to the pulling forward of rudimentary iris tissue by contraction of pre-existing fibres that bridge the angle.

COMPLICATIONS OF GLAUCOMA SURGERY

Trabeculectomy

Shallow anterior chamber

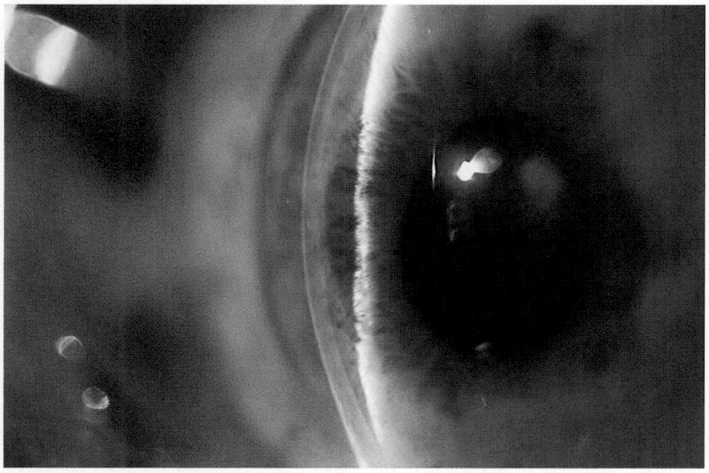

Fig. 8.138 Grade 1: peripheral iris–corneal apposition.

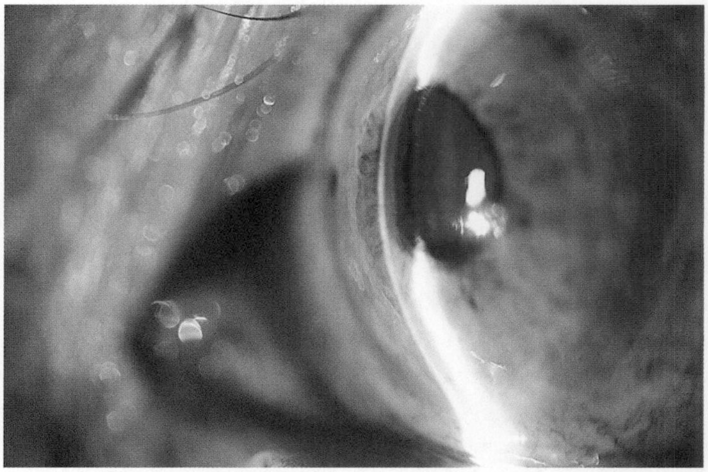

Fig. 8.139 Grade 2: pupillary border–corneal apposition.

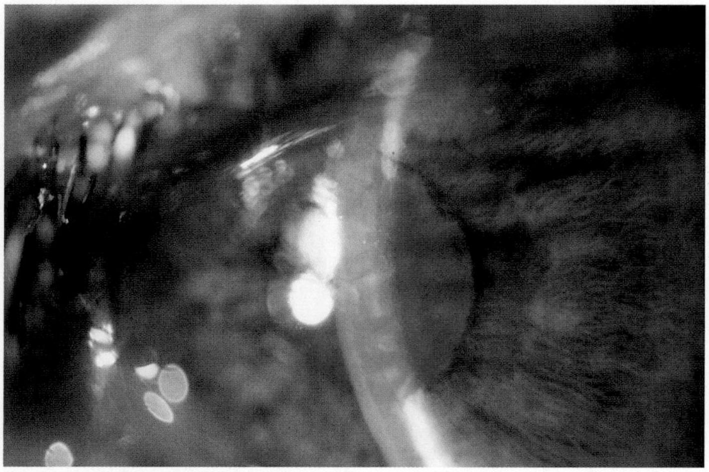

Fig. 8.140 Grade 3: lenticulo-corneal apposition resulting in corneal oedema.

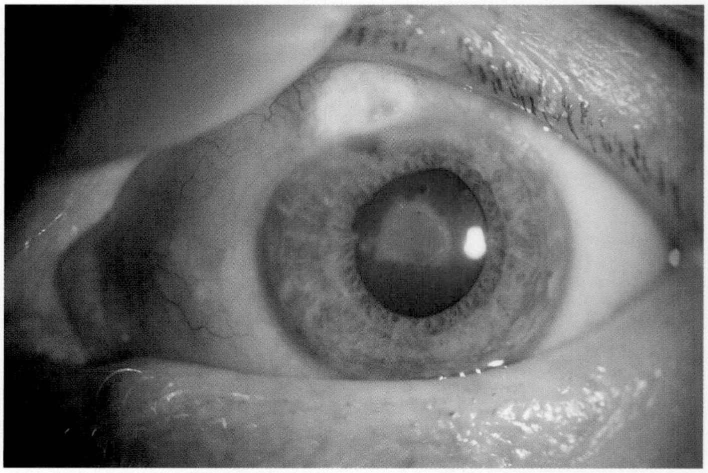

Fig. 8.141 Anterior cataract resulting from prolonged lenticulo-corneal apposition.

Overfiltration

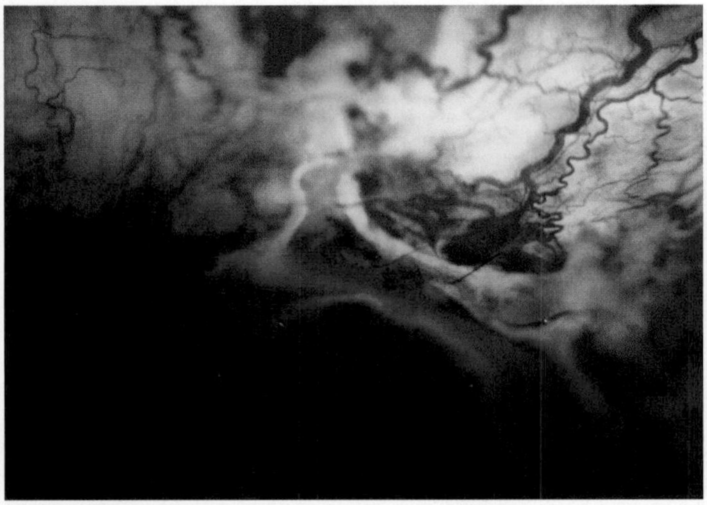

■ **Fig. 8.142** Positive Seidel test characterised by dilution of fluorescein by escaping aqueous.

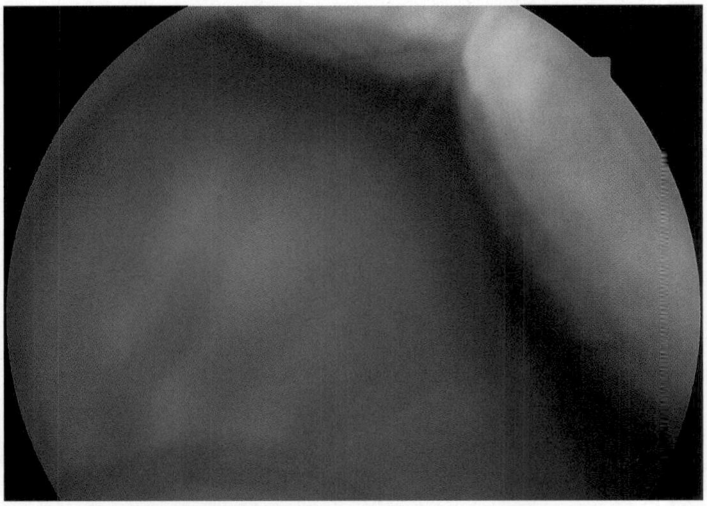

■ **Fig. 8.143** Choroidal detachment.

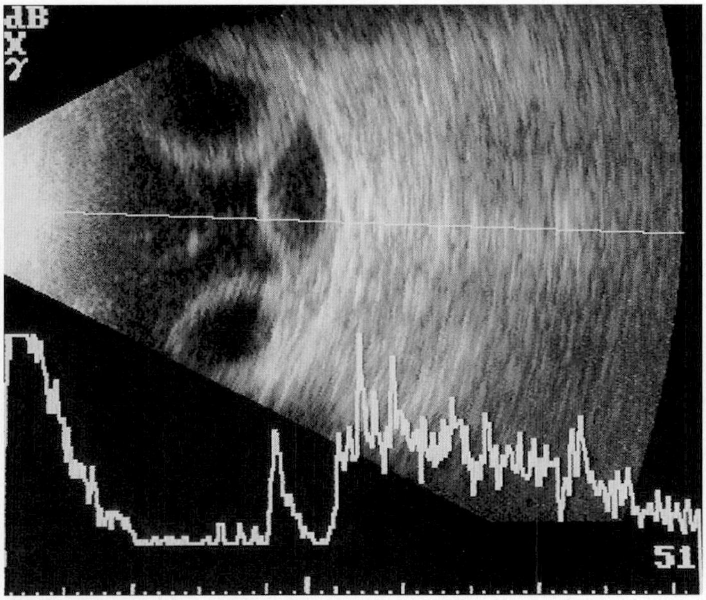

■ **Fig. 8.144** Ultrasound of choroidal detachments.

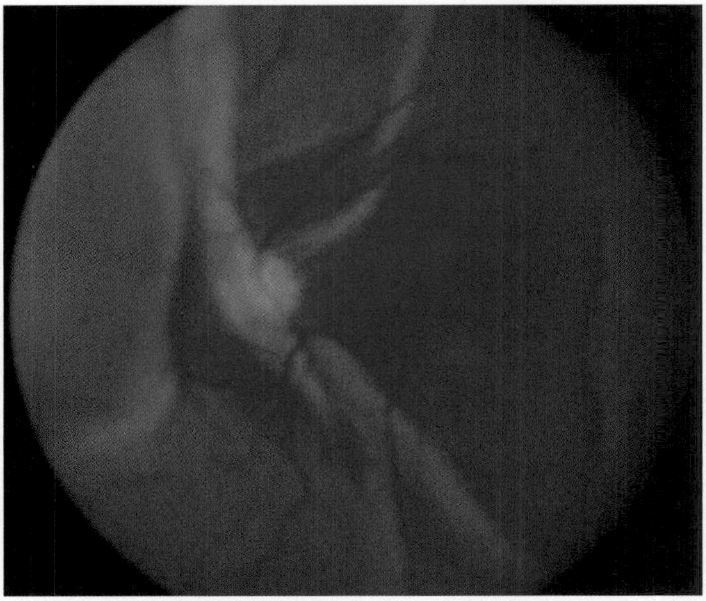

■ **Fig. 8.145** Chorioretinal folds in a hypotonous eye, which may be associated with maculopathy.

Poor filtration

Signs of good filtration

Good filtration is characterised by a low IOP and a bleb with one of the following appearances:

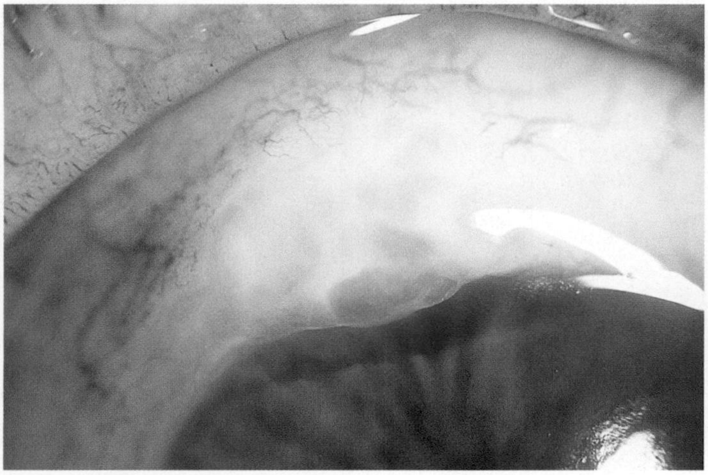

Fig. 8.146 Type 1 has a thin and polycystic appearance.

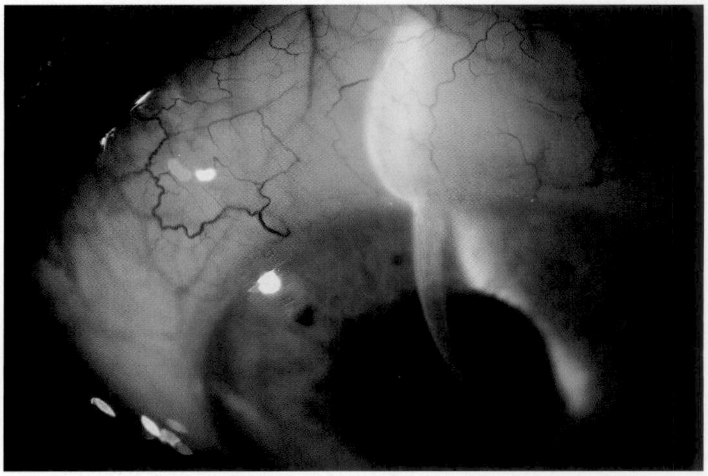

Fig. 8.147 Type 2 is shallow, thin-walled and diffuse with a relatively avascular appearance in comparison with the surrounding conjunctiva.

Signs of poor filtration

Poor filtration is characterised by increasing IOP and a bleb with one of the following appearances:

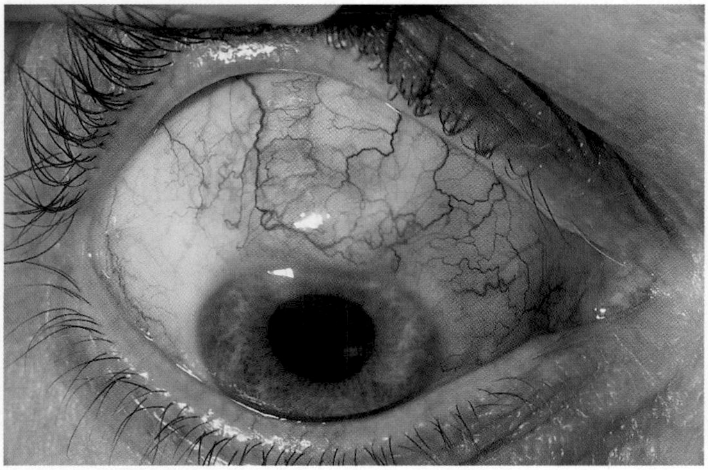

Fig. 8.148 Type 3, due to episcleral fibrosis, is flat, unassociated with microcystic spaces and manifests engorged surface blood vessels. (Courtesy of J. Salmon.)

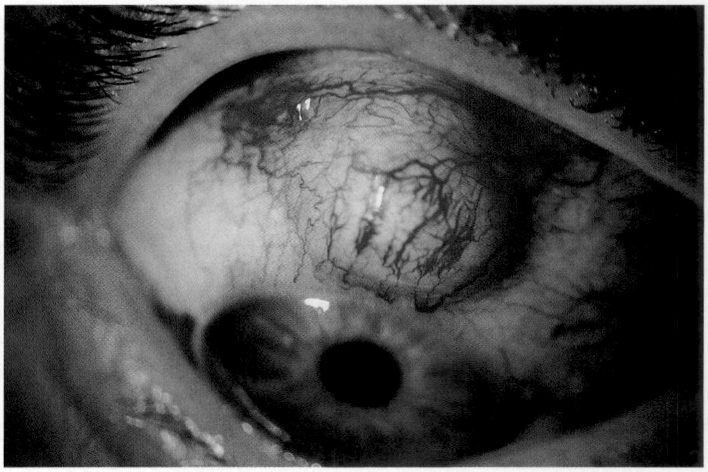

Fig. 8.149 Type 4 is an encapsulated bleb (Tenon cyst), which is characterised by a localised, highly elevated, dome-shaped cavity with engorged surface blood vessels. (Courtesy of S. Ford and R. Marsh.)

Infection

Blebitis

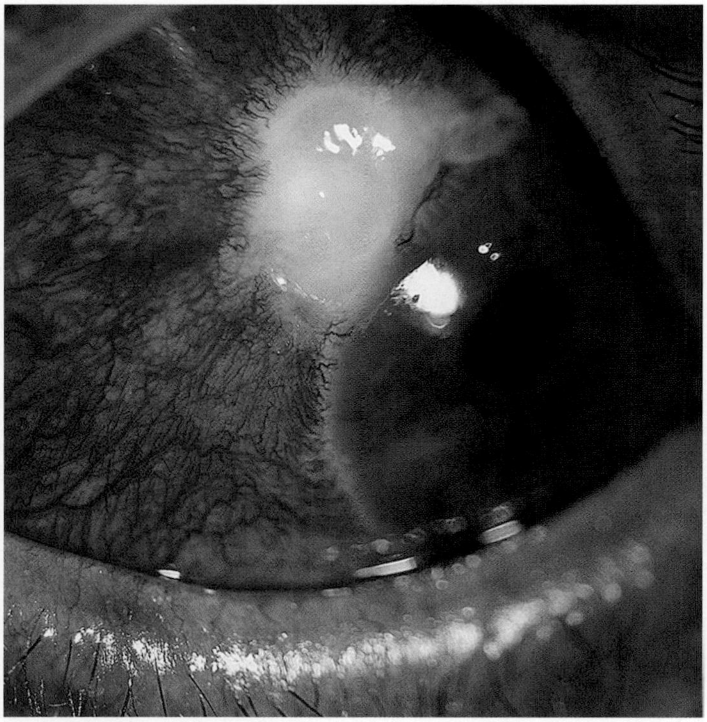

■ **Fig. 8.150** A white drainage bleb with surrounding conjunctival inflammation that may be associated with anterior uveitis but not vitritis.

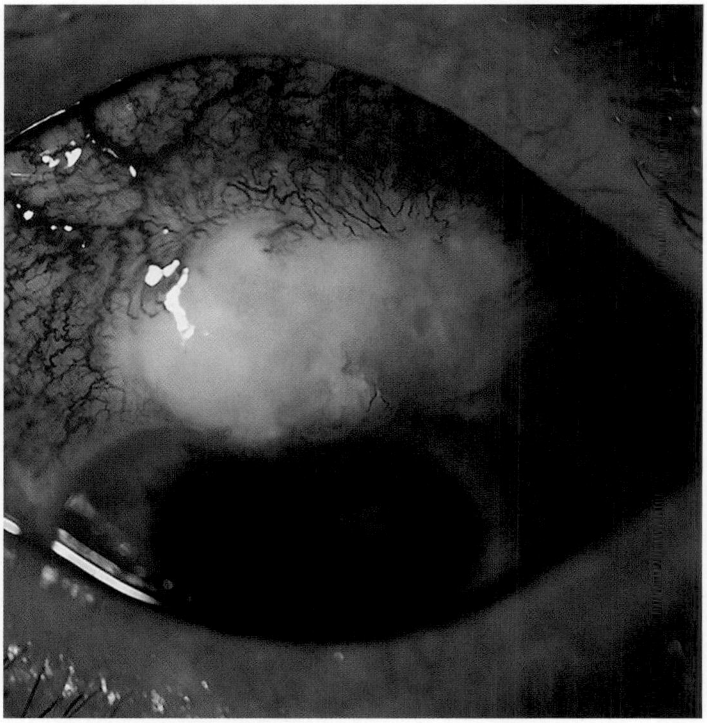

■ **Fig. 8.151** More severe blebitis.

Bleb-associated endophthalmitis

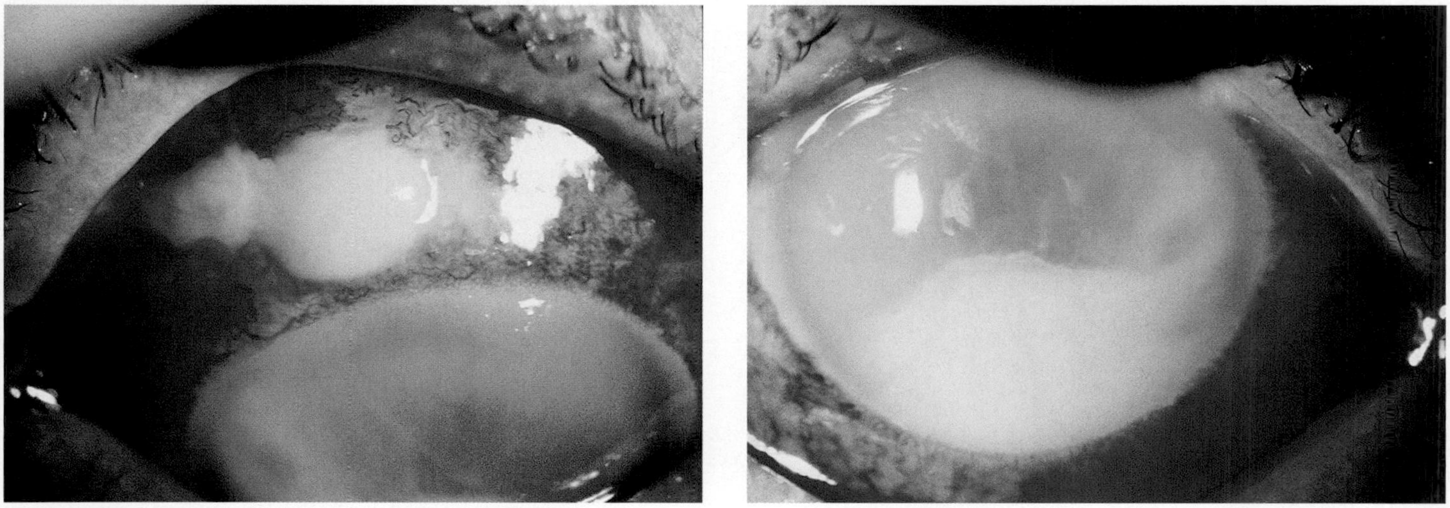

■ **Fig. 8.152** Very severe bleb-associated endophthalmitis.

Drainage implants

Because shunts are used in severely compromised eyes, the complication rate tends to be greater than following trabeculectomy.

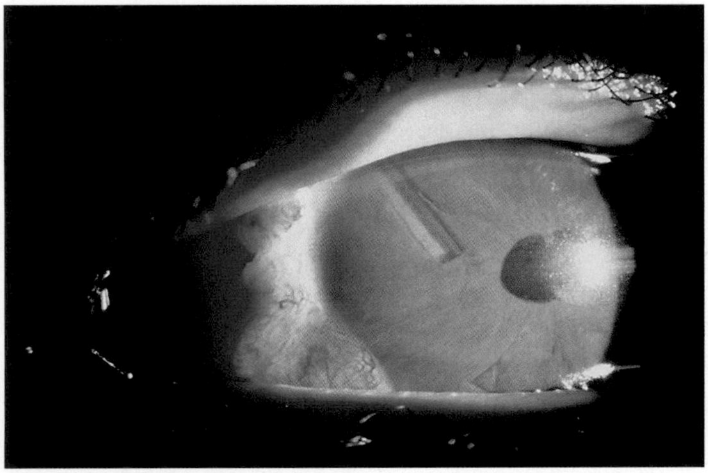

Fig. 8.153 If the occluding suture is loose, excessive drainage may occur as a result of leakage around or down the tube and result in hypotony and a shallow anterior chamber. (Courtesy of J. Salmon.)

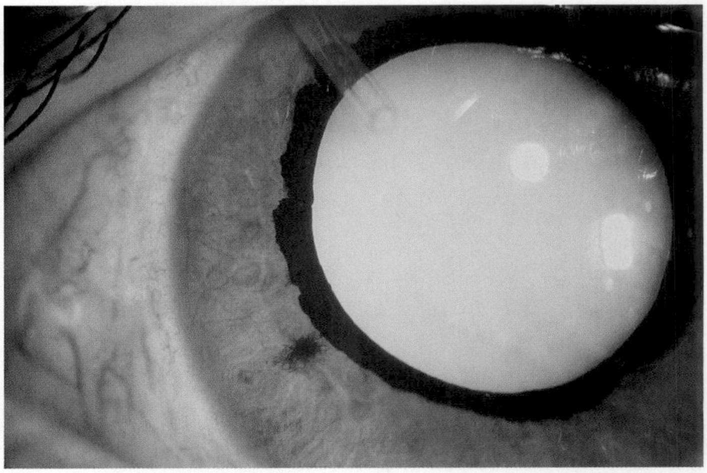

Fig. 8.154 Cataract may develop if the end of the tube touches the lens.

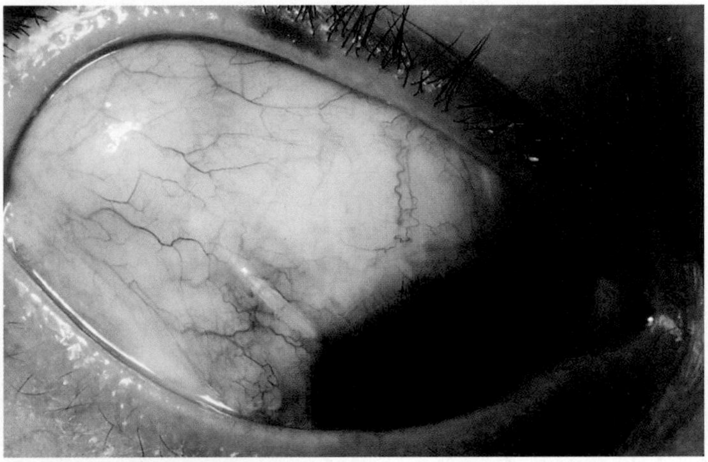

Fig. 8.155 Tube erosion through the sclera and conjunctiva. (Courtesy of J. Salmon.)

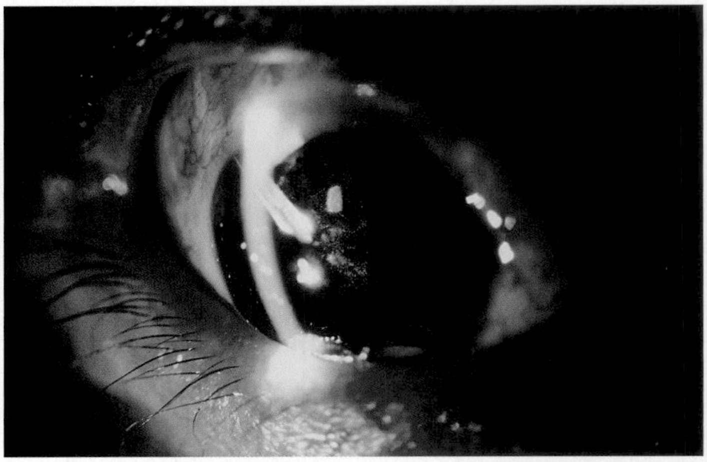

Fig. 8.156 Drainage failure may occur as a result of blockage of the end of the tube by vitreous, blood or iris tissue. (Courtesy of J. Salmon.)

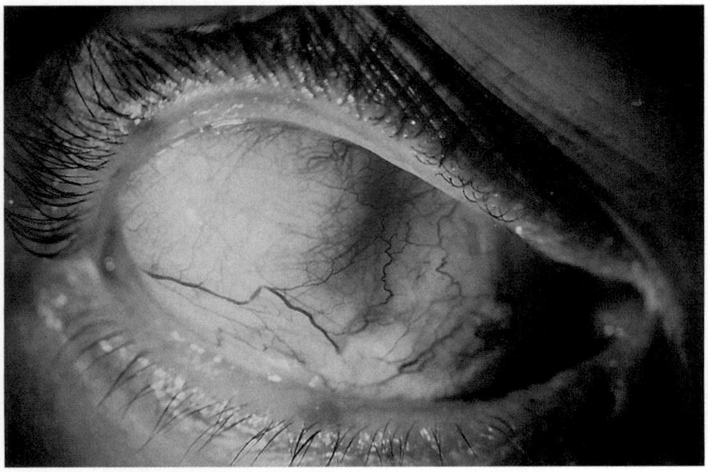

Fig. 8.157 Bleb encapsulation over the footplate, which may result in poor drainage. (Courtesy of J. Salmon.)

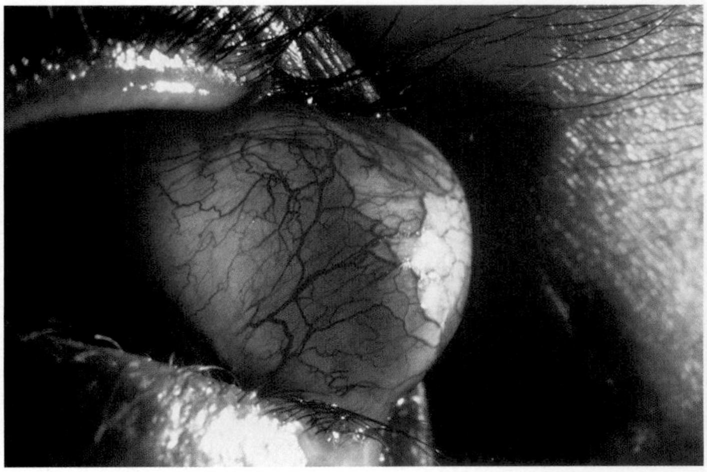

Fig. 8.158 Tenon cyst formation resulting in poor drainage. (Courtesy of L. Merin.)

CHAPTER 9

INTRAOCULAR TUMOURS

IRIS TUMOURS

Freckle

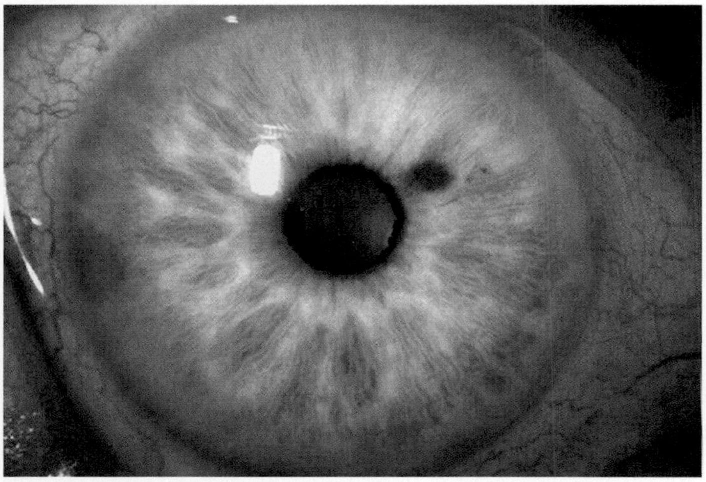

■ **Fig. 9.1** A freckle is an extremely common, tiny, pigmented lesion. (Courtesy of S. Ford and R. Marsh.)

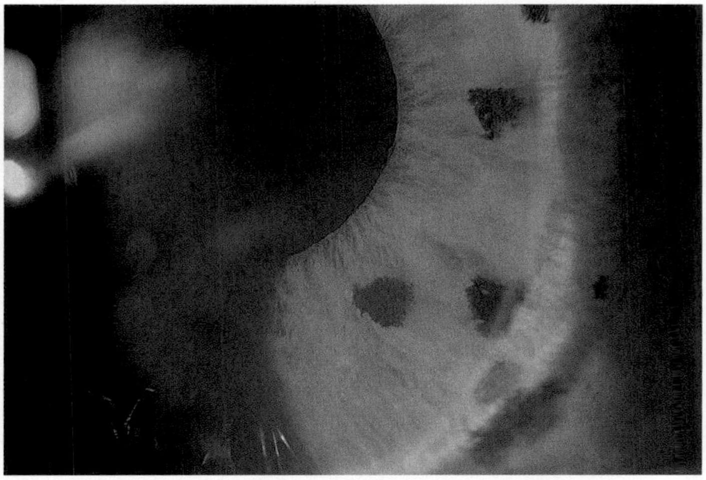

■ **Fig. 9.2** Freckles are often multiple and bilateral.

Naevus

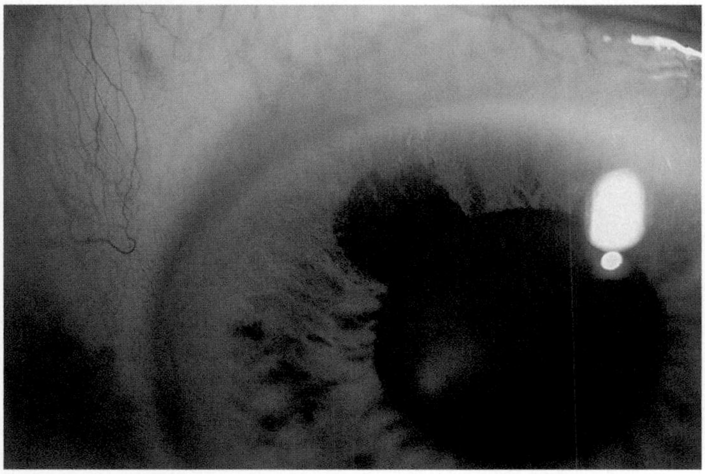

■ **Fig. 9.3** A typical naevus is a superficial, pigmented, flat or slightly elevated lesion.

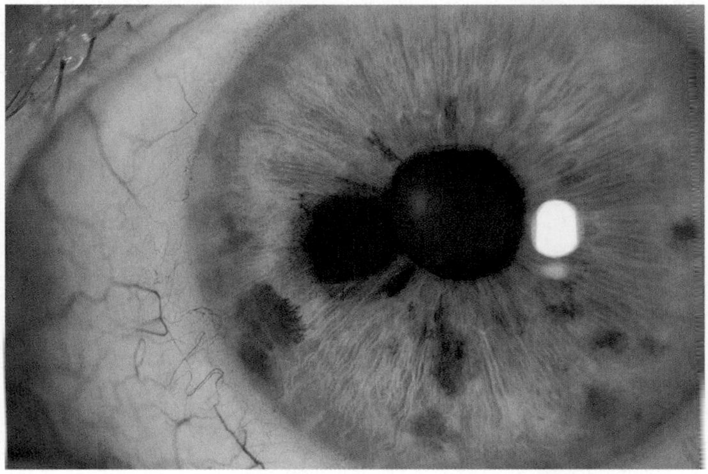

■ **Fig. 9.4** A small naevus with coexisting freckles.

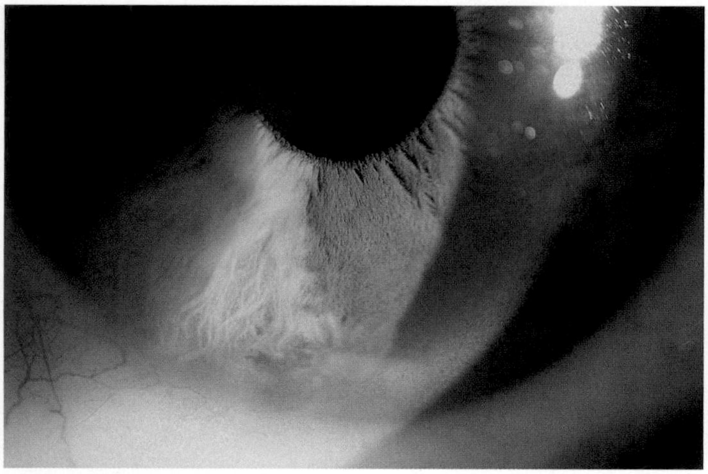

Fig. 9.5 A large flat naevus.

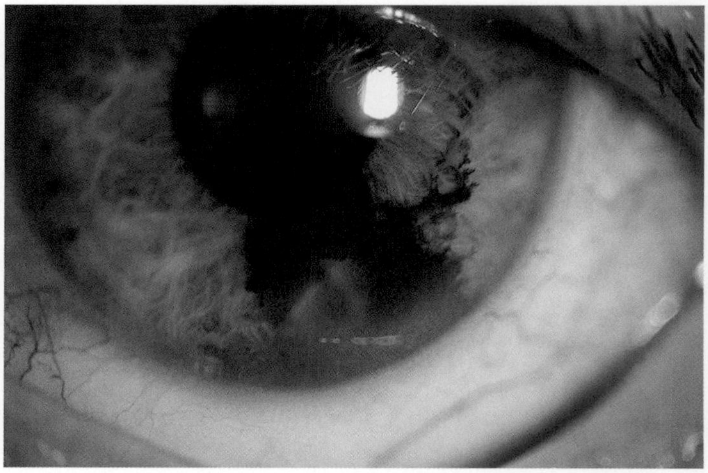

Fig. 9.6 A large, slightly elevated naevus.

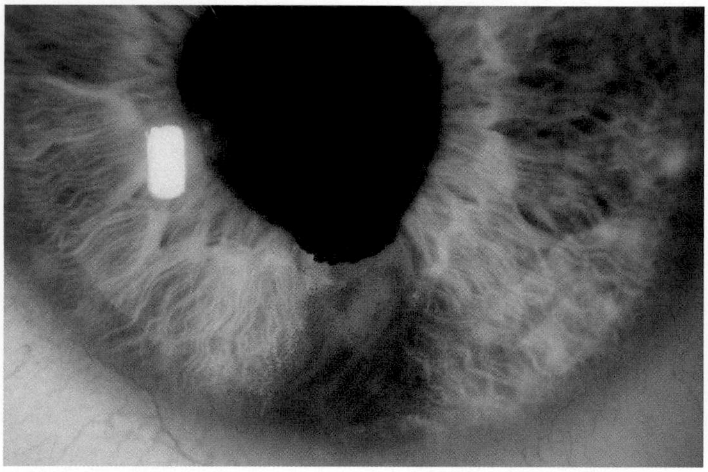

Fig. 9.7 A large naevus may occasionally cause mild distortion of the pupil and ectropion uveae.

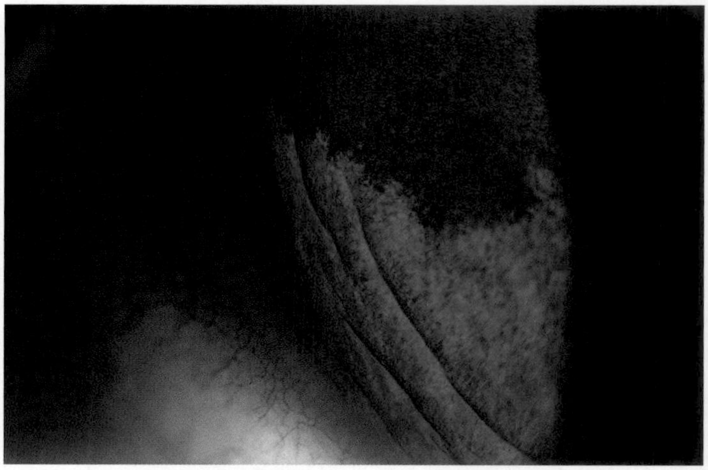

Fig. 9.8 A diffuse naevus obscuring normal iris crypts.

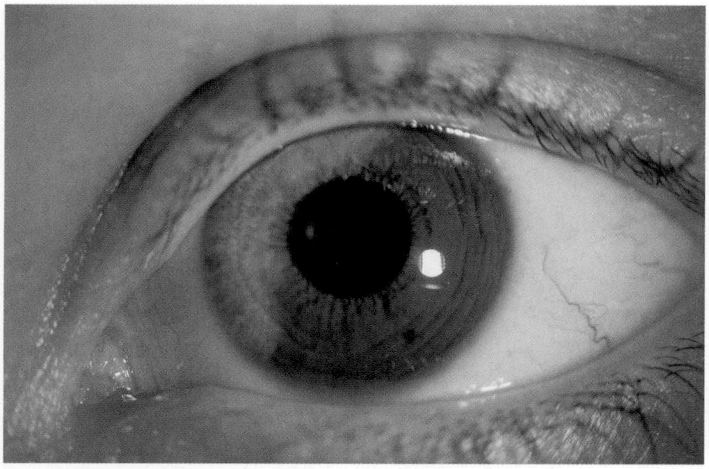

Fig. 9.9 A very large diffuse naevus may give rise to hyperchromic heterochromia and is occasionally associated with the Cogan–Reese syndrome.

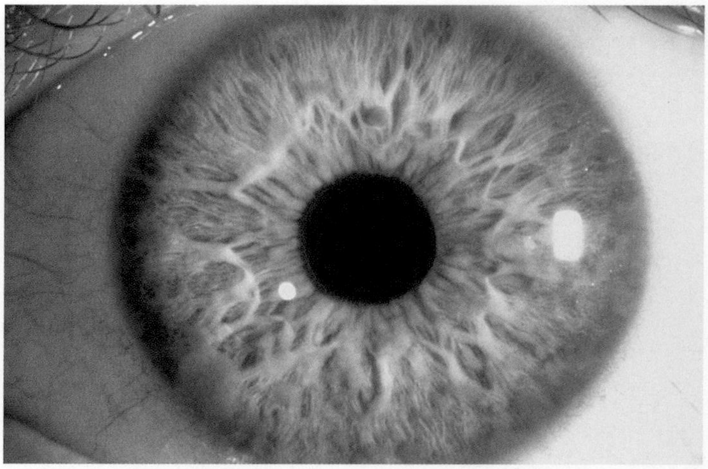

Fig. 9.10 Lisch nodules are multiple, small, bilateral, melanocytic hamartomas found after the age of 16 years in virtually all patients with neurofibromatosis-1 (Courtesy of L. Merin.)

Melanoma

Iris melanomas may be circumscribed or diffuse and may show varying degrees of pigmentation and vascularity. They account for 5% of uveal melanomas and invariably arise from the inferior half of the iris.

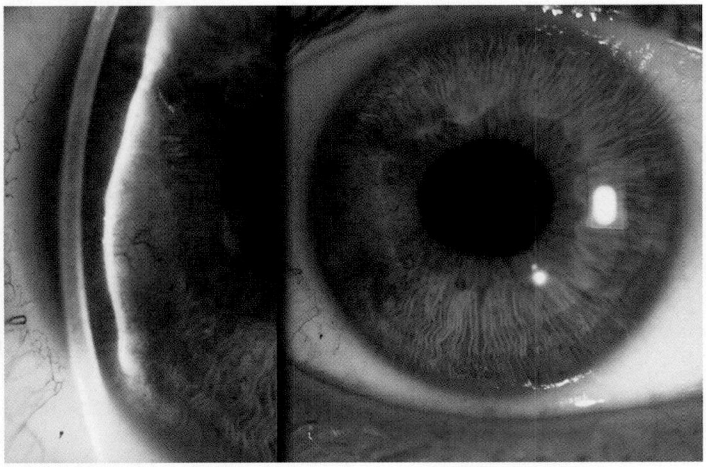

Fig. 9.11 Large, lightly pigmented melanoma with surface vessels. (Courtesy of P. Gili.)

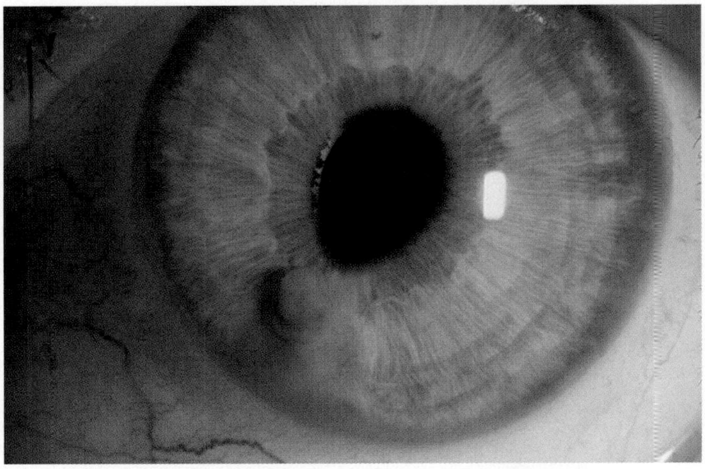

Fig. 9.12 Small, lightly pigmented melanoma with slight distortion of the pupil. (Courtesy of R. Curtis.)

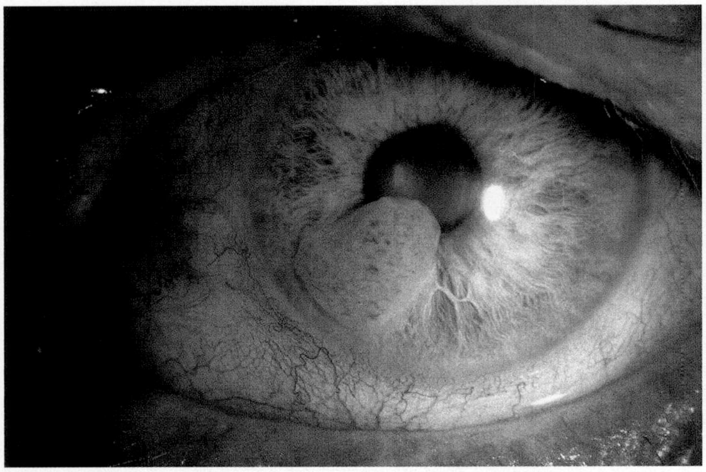

Fig. 9.13 Lightly pigmented melanoma with prominent surface vasculature.

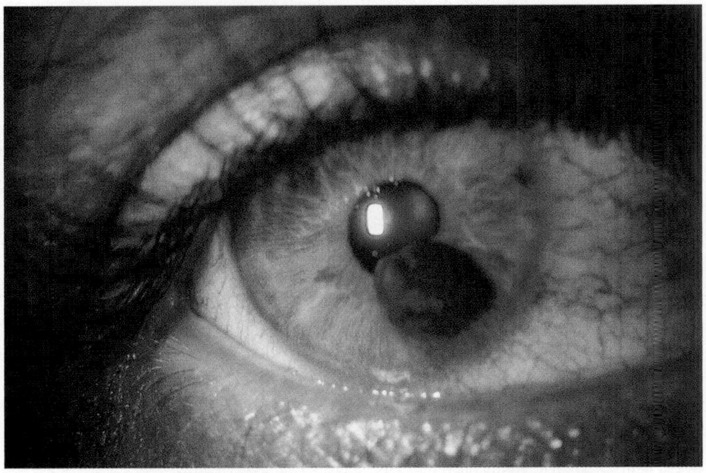

Fig. 9.14 Highly pigmented melanoma in which vessels are difficult to detect.

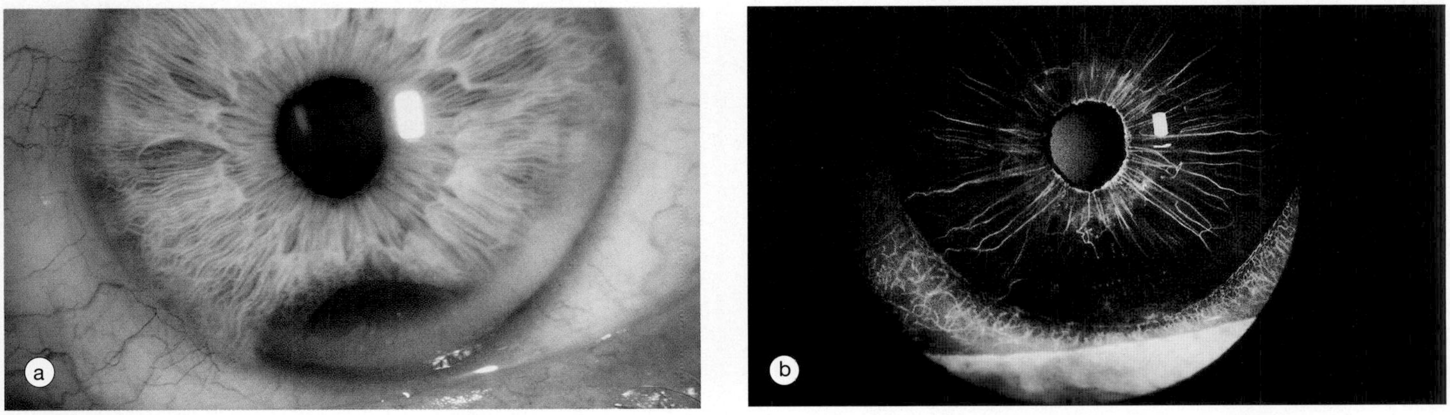

Fig. 9.15 **(a)** Small pigmented melanoma. (**b**) FA shows corresponding blockage of iris vascular fluorescence.

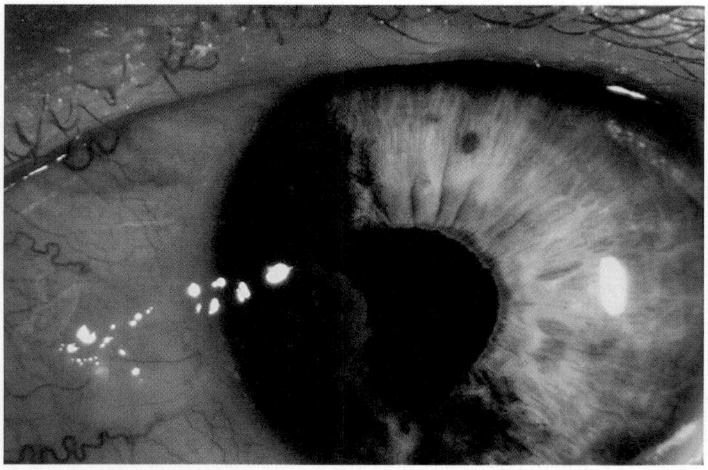

Fig. 9.16 Very large nodular melanoma.

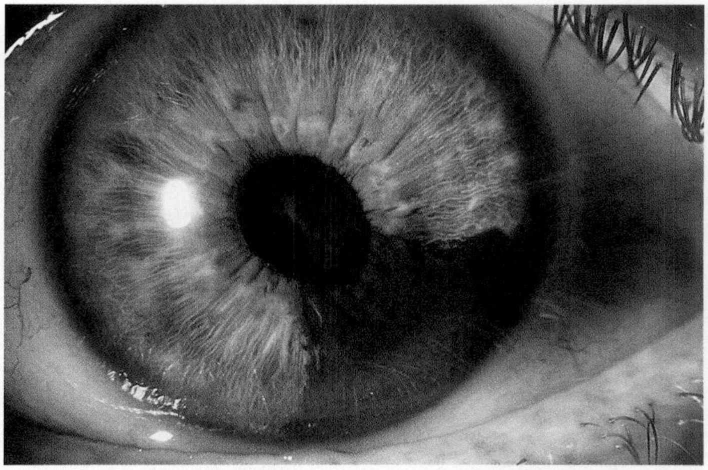

Fig. 9.17 Diffuse melanoma causing pupillary distortion, ectropion uveae and localised cataract.

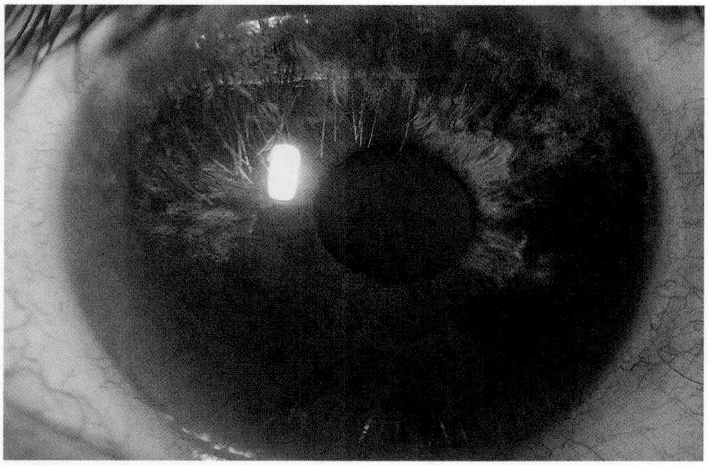

Fig. 9.18 Extensive diffusely growing melanoma is rare and may give rise to ipsilateral hyperchromic heterochromia. (Courtesy of S. Ford and R. Marsh.)

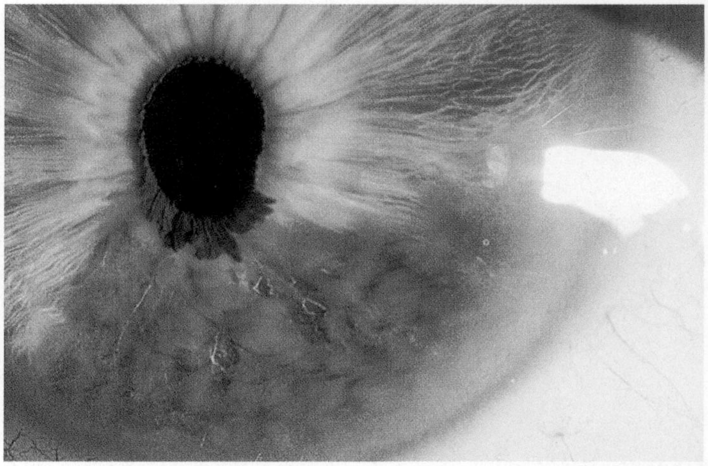

Fig. 9.19 'Tapioca melanoma' characterised by multiple surface nodules is very rare. (Courtesy or B. Damato.)

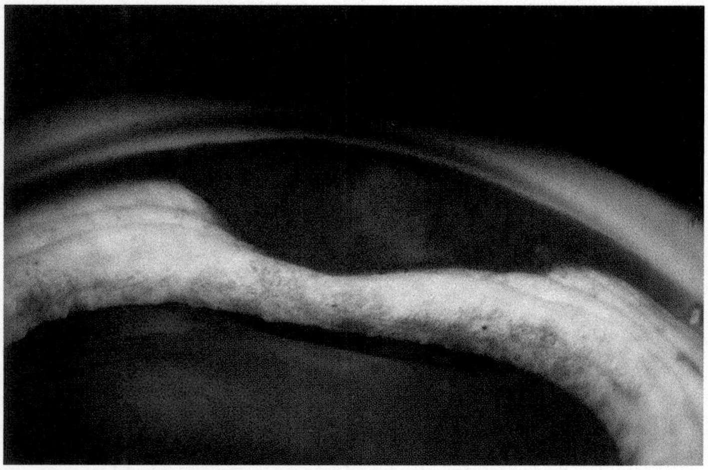

Fig. 9.20 Localised angle involvement by melanoma. (Courtesy or R. Curtis.)

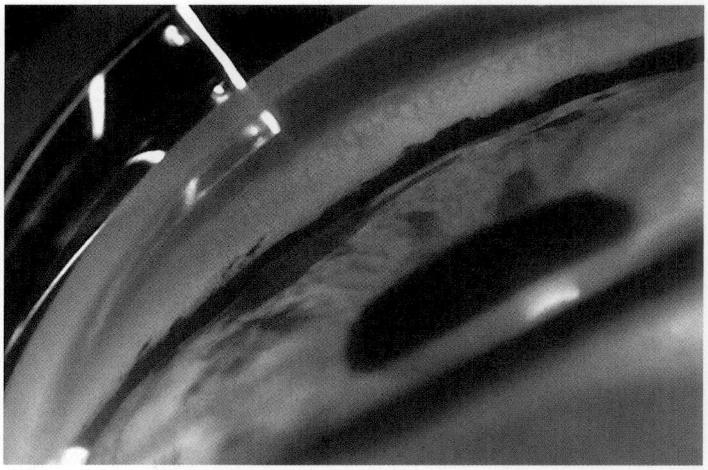

Fig. 9.21 Diffuse angle involvement by melanoma may result in elevation of intraocular pressure.

Adenoma of the iris pigment epithelium

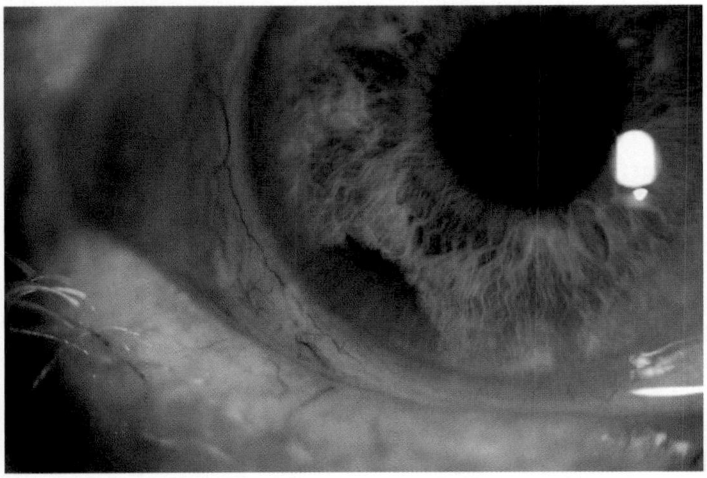

■ **Fig. 9.22** Dark grey-black nodule with a smooth surface, most frequently in the peripheral iris.

Leiomyoma

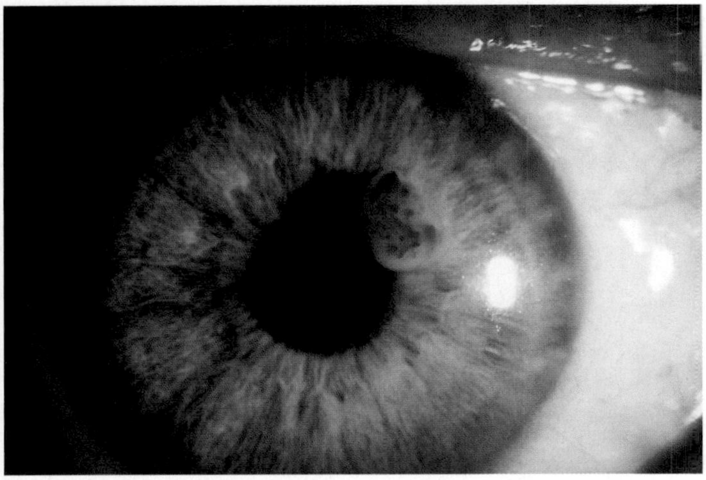

■ **Fig. 9.23** The appearance is similar to that of an amelanotic melanoma except that it is not necessarily confined to the inferior half of the iris. (Courtesy of S. Ford and R. Marsh.)

Juvenile xanthogranuloma

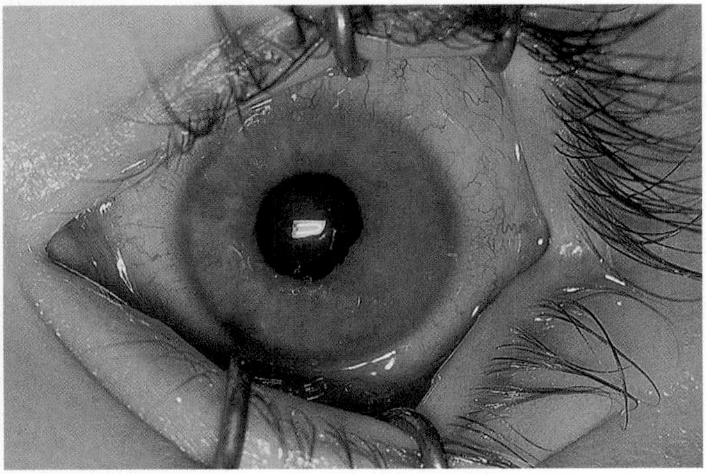

■ **Fig. 9.24** A yellow, vascularised lesion which may give rise to spontaneous hyphaema.

Racemose haemangioma

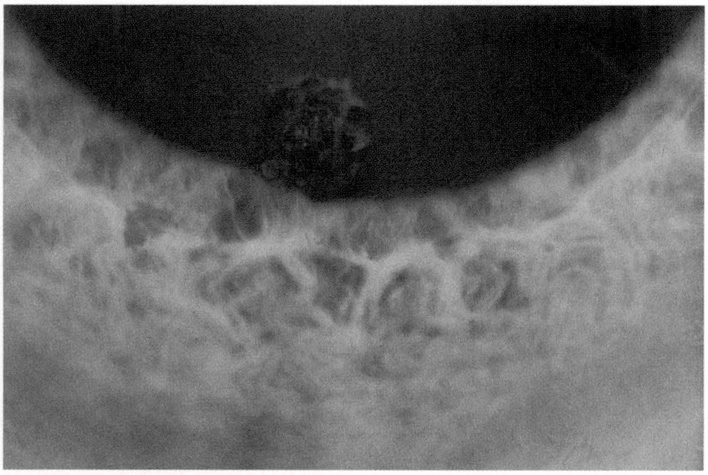

Fig. 9.25 An extremely rare tumour that resembles a cluster of grapes. (Courtesy of M. Prost.)

Metastasis

Iris metastases are much less common than choroidal deposits.

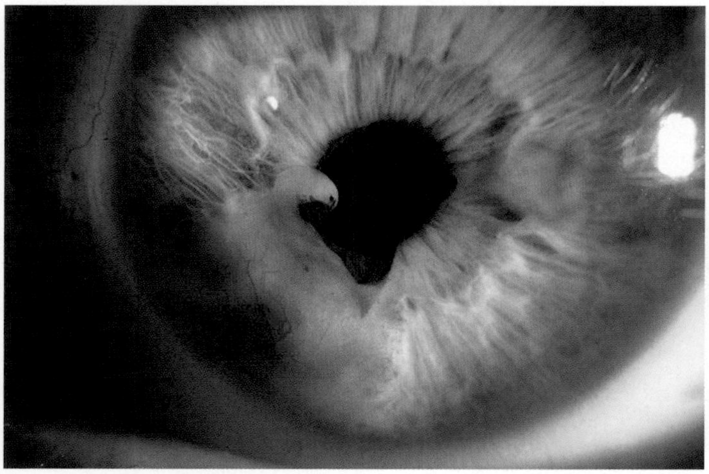

Fig. 9.26 A solitary, pink or yellow, fast-growing mass (Courtesy of R. Curtis.)

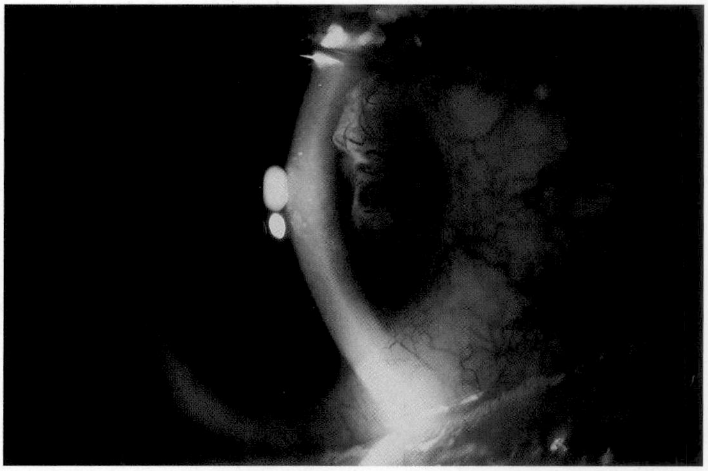

Fig. 9.27 Very vascular metastasis from cutaneous melanoma with spontaneous hyphaema.

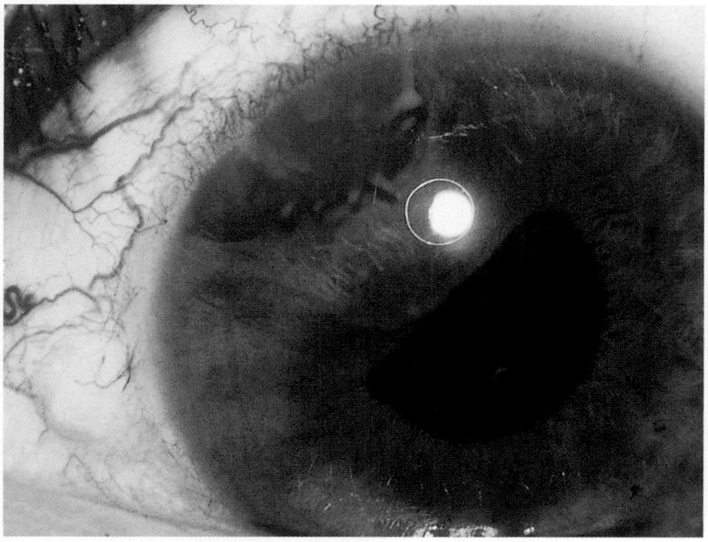

Fig. 9.28 Haemorrhagic metastatic breast carcinoma.

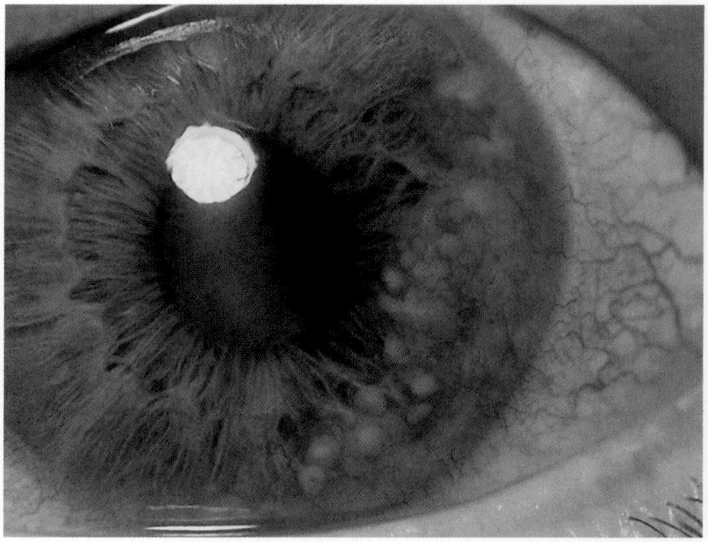

Fig. 9.29 Multiple small, pale deposits are uncommon.

IRIS CYSTS

Primary cysts

Primary iris cysts are rare curiosities that arise from the pigment epithelium or, rarely, the stroma.

Epithelial

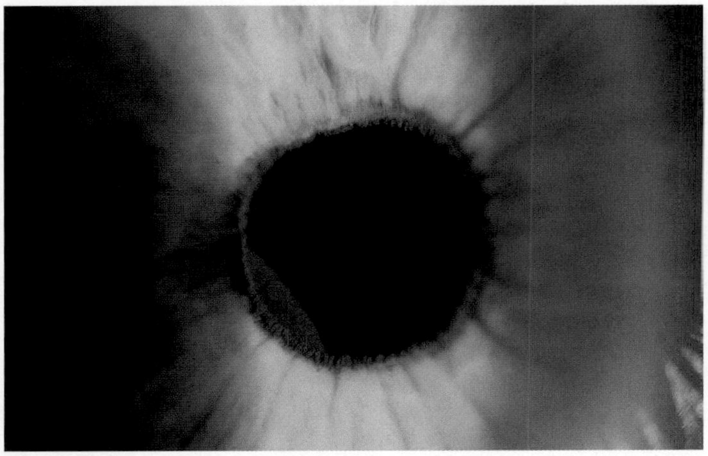

Fig. 9.30 Unilateral, solitary, dark brown, globular structure that transilluminates.

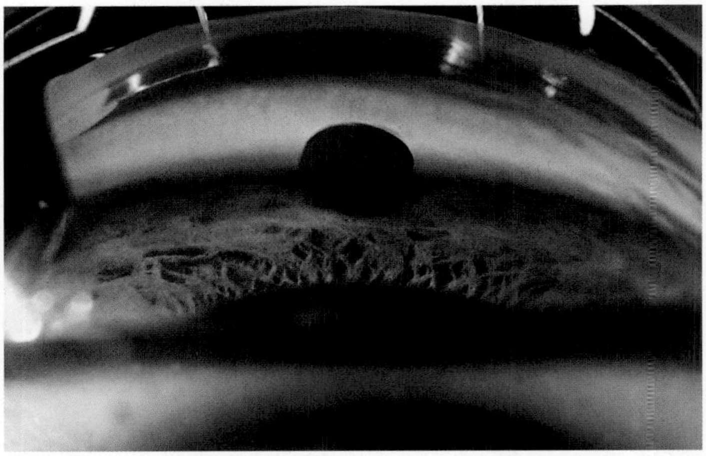

Fig. 9.31 A dislodged cyst in the angle.

Stromal

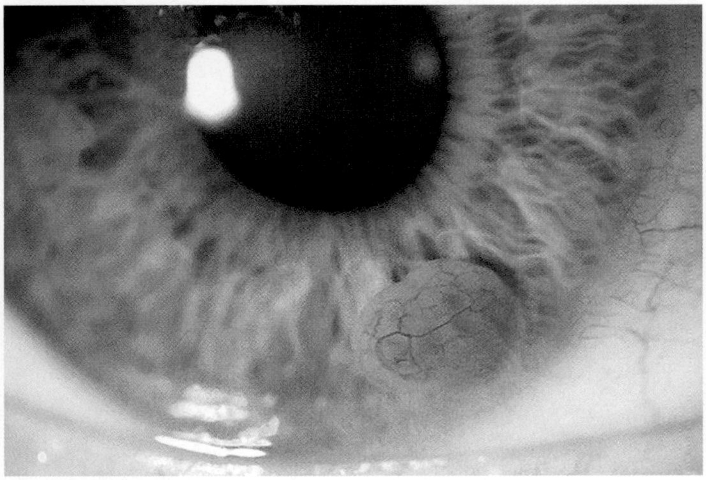

Fig. 9.32 A solitary, unilateral, smooth structure containing fluic with a translucent anterior wall.

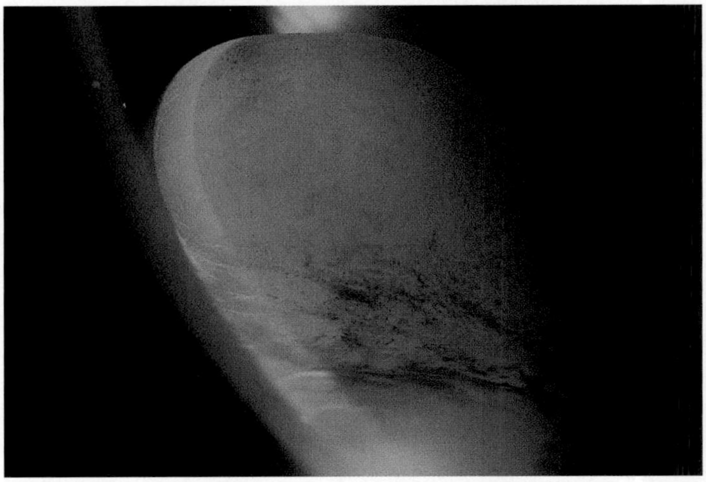

Fig. 9.33 A large cyst touching the corneal endothelium.

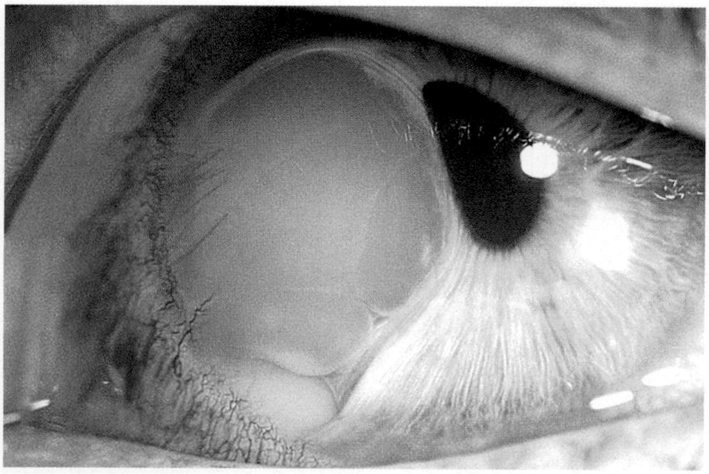

Fig. 9.34 A cyst with a fluid–debris level reminiscent of a pseudohypopyon.

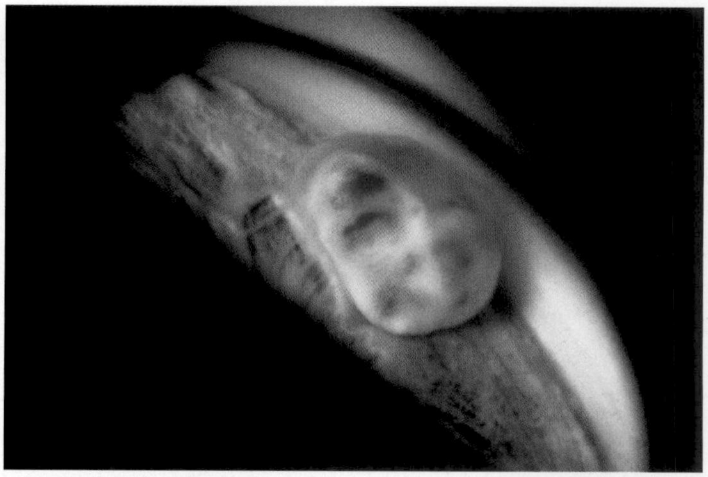

Fig. 9.35 Occasionally the cyst may break free from the iris. (Courtesy of R. Curtis.)

Secondary cysts

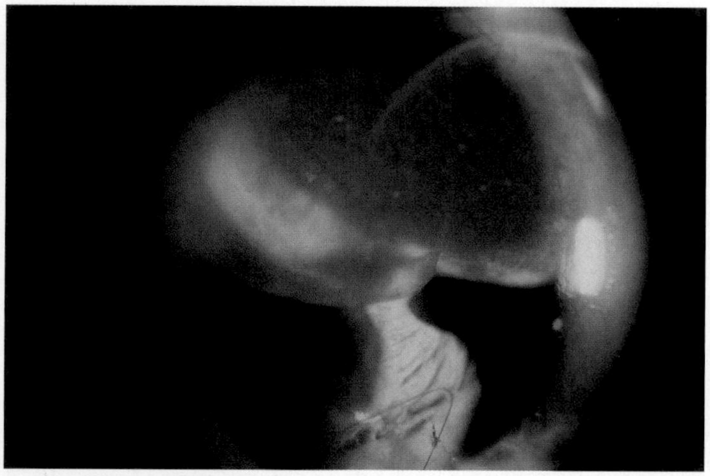

Fig. 9.36 Implantation cysts develop following penetrating or surgical trauma. They are usually translucent, filled with fluid and may be connected to the wound.

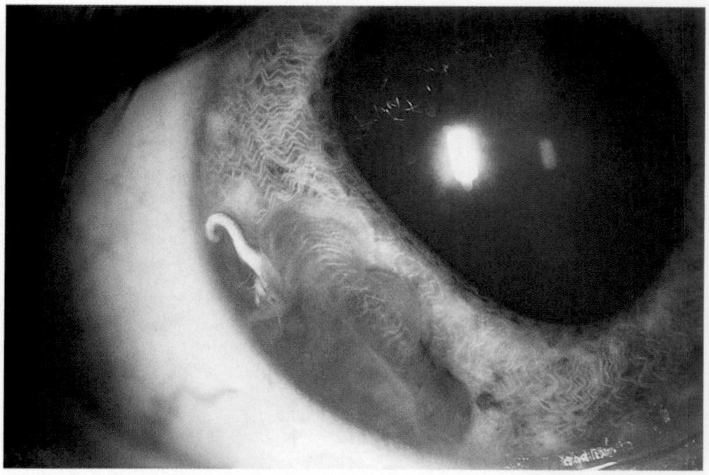

Fig. 9.37 Parasitic cysts are very rare.

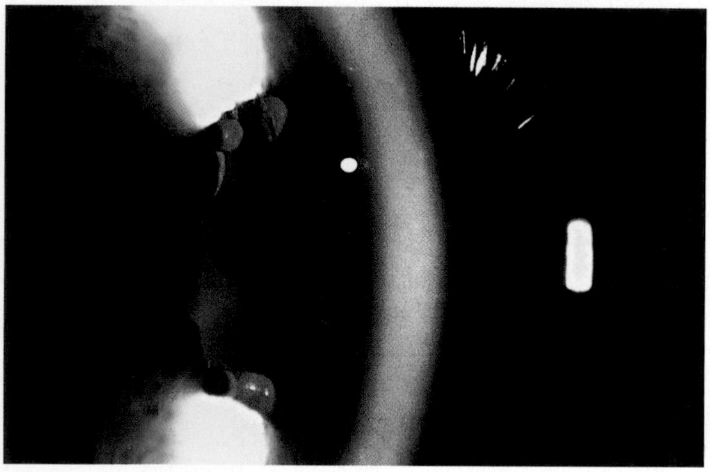

Fig. 9.38 Cysts caused by the prolonged use of long-acting miotics are small, multiple and located at the pupillary border.

CILIARY BODY TUMOURS AND CYSTS

Melanoma

Ciliary body melanomas account for about 10% of uveal melanomas.

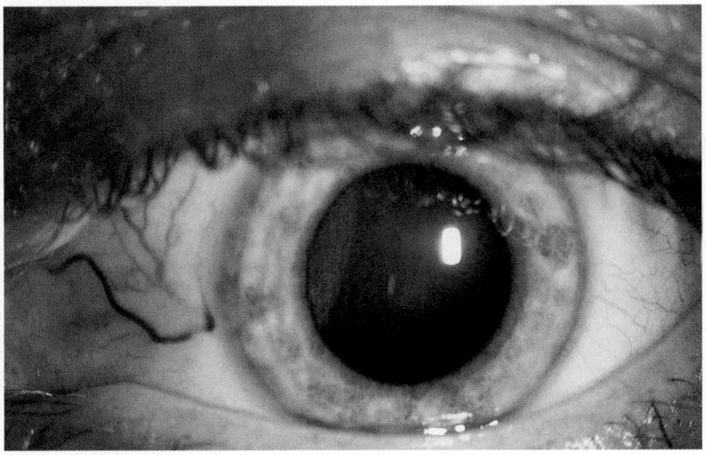

Fig. 9.39 Dilated episcleral blood vessel in the same quadrant as the tumour (sentinel vessels).

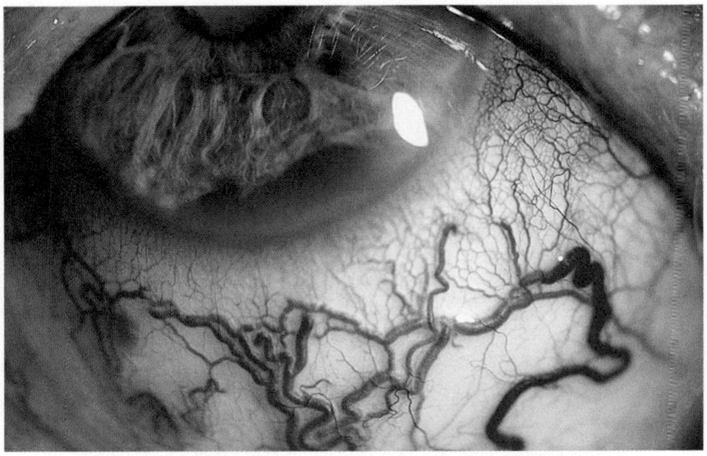

Fig. 9.40 More extensive sentinel vessels and extension of tumour through the iris root. (Courtesy of B. Damato.)

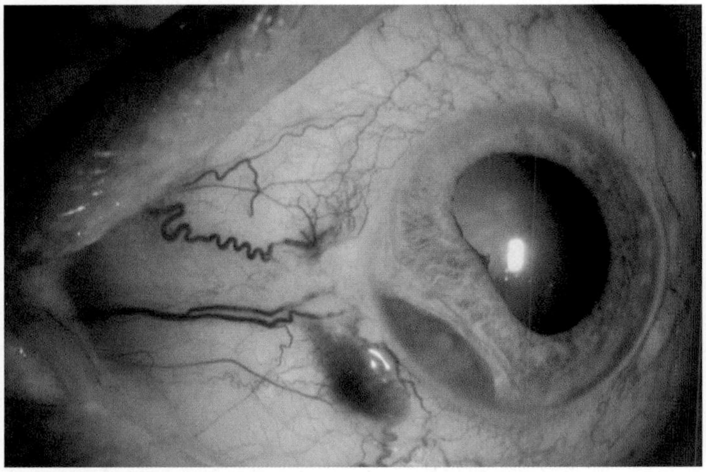

Fig. 9.41 Sentinel vessels and early extraocular extension through the scleral emissary vessels as well as extension through the iris root. (Courtesy of R. Curtis.)

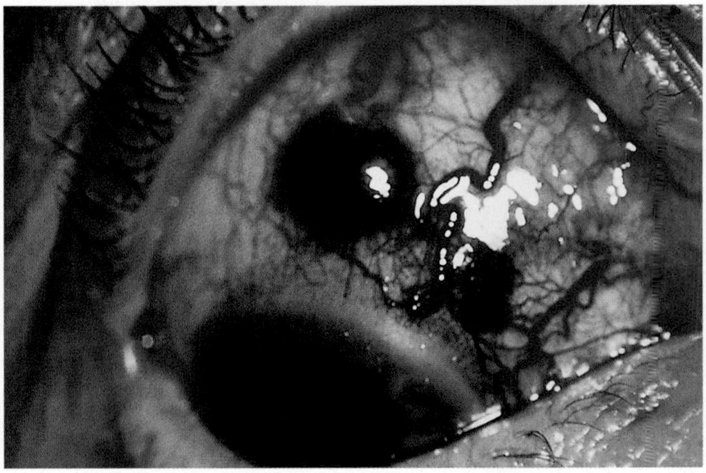

Fig. 9.42 Extensive extraocular extension, which may mimic a conjunctival melanoma.

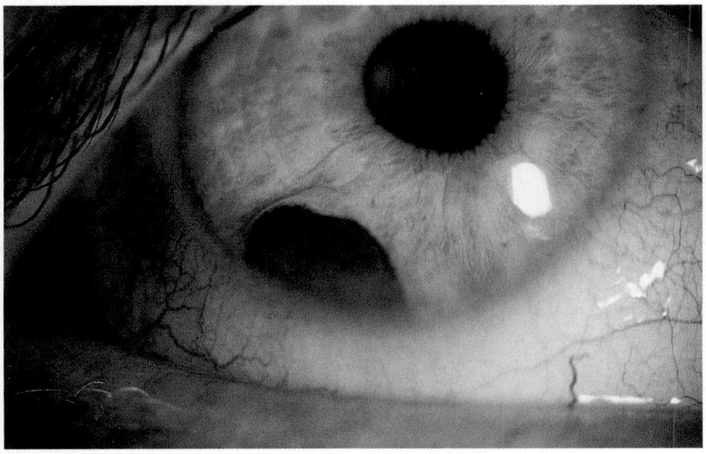

Fig. 9.43 More advanced extension through the iris root.

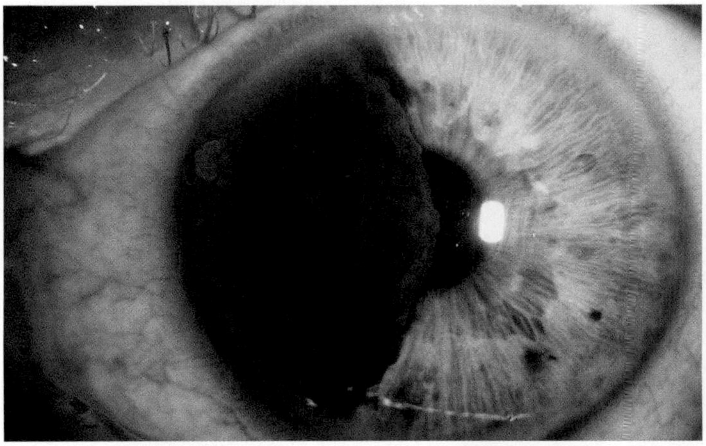

Fig. 9.44 Very extensive anterior segment extension, which may mimic an iris melanoma.

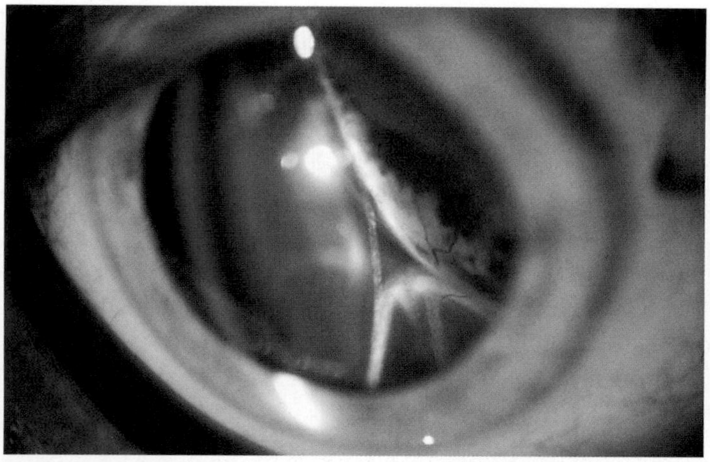

Fig. 9.45 Ciliary body melanoma causing lens subluxation and inferior retinal detachment. (Courtesy of C. Barry.)

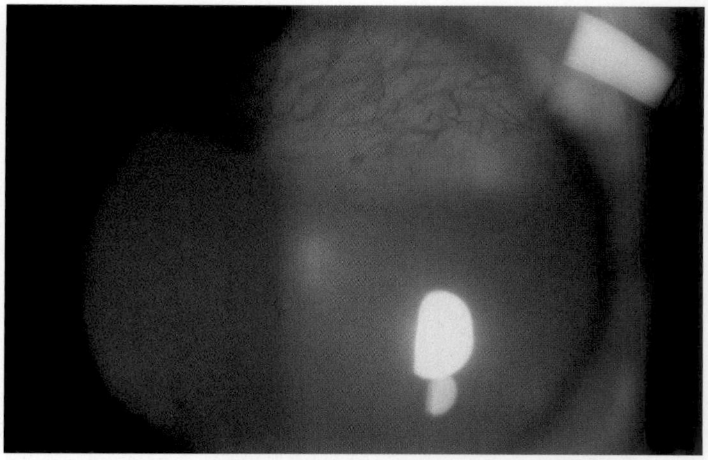

Fig. 9.46 Ciliary body melanoma seen against the red reflex.

Medulloepithelioma (diktyoma)

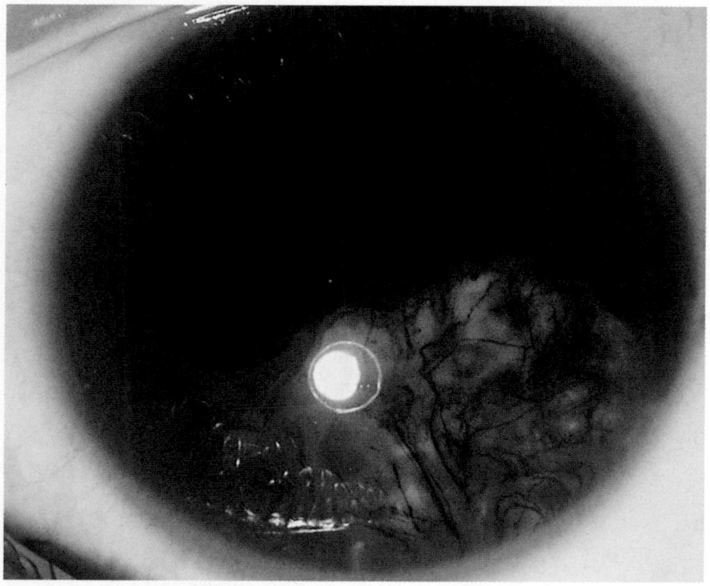

Fig. 9.47 Medulloepithelioma is a very rare malignant tumour that typically presents in childhood as a solid or cystic ciliary body or anterior chamber mass containing grey-white opacities consisting of cartilage.

Cyst

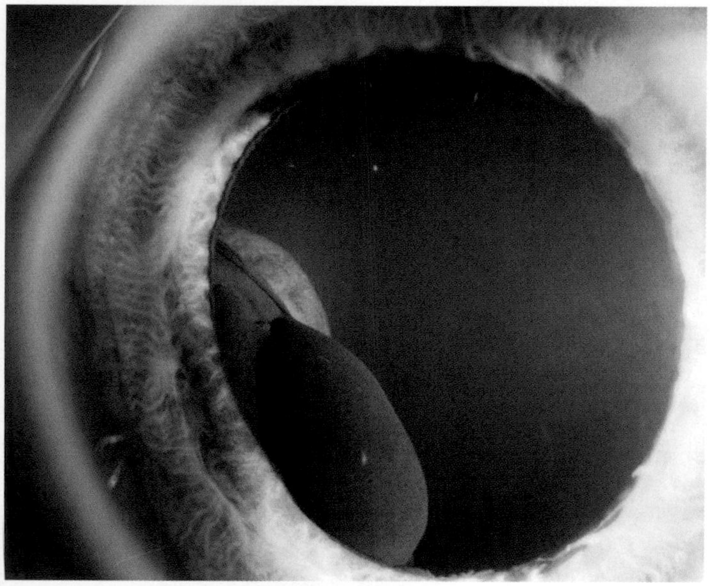

Fig. 9.48 Epithelial ciliary body cysts are congenital and similar in appearance to their iris counterparts. (Courtesy of R. Curtis.)

TUMOURS OF THE CHOROID

Naevus

Choroidal naevi are present in 5–10% of the population. The vast majority are innocous and asymptomatic.

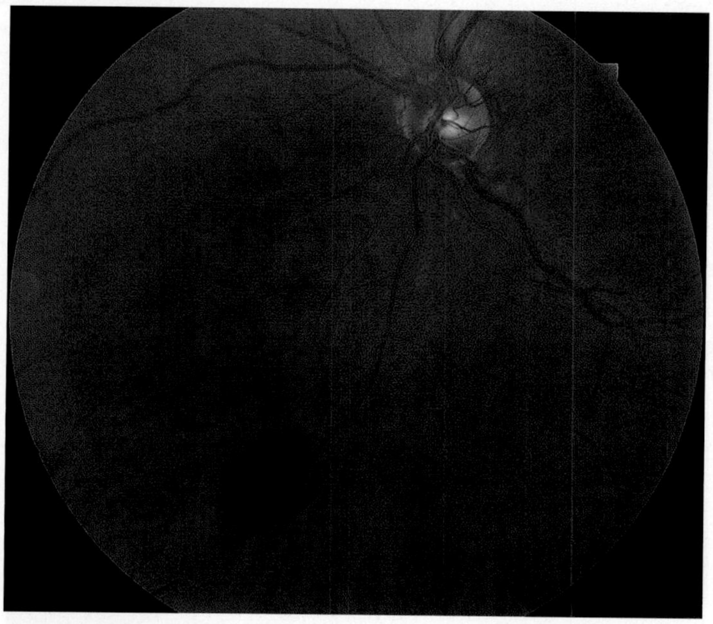

■ **Fig. 9.49** A small, postequatorial, oval or circular, slate-blue or grey lesion with detectable but not sharp borders which is 1 mm or less in thickness and less than 5 mm in diameter.

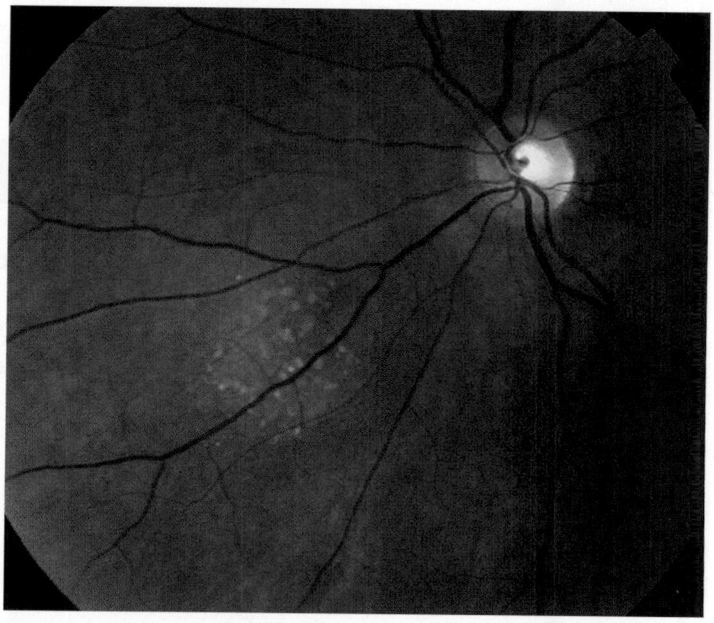

■ **Fig. 9.50** Surface drusen may be present, particularly in the central area of a larger lesion.

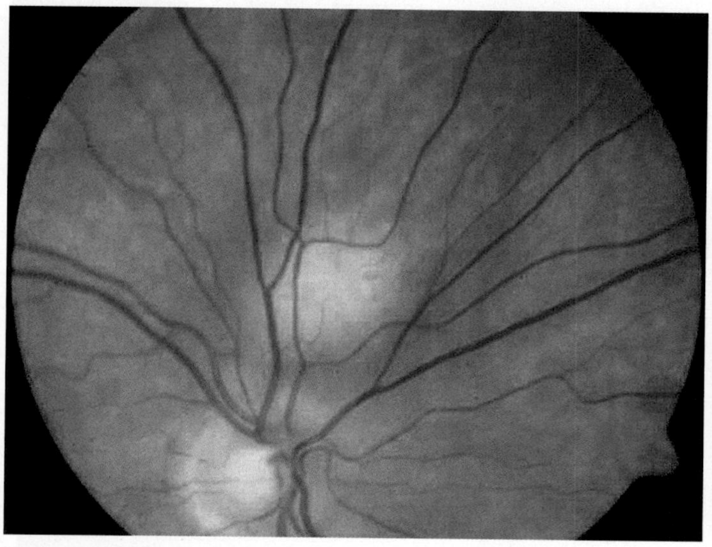

■ **Fig. 9.51** An amelanotic naevus is rare. (Courtesy of B. Damato.)

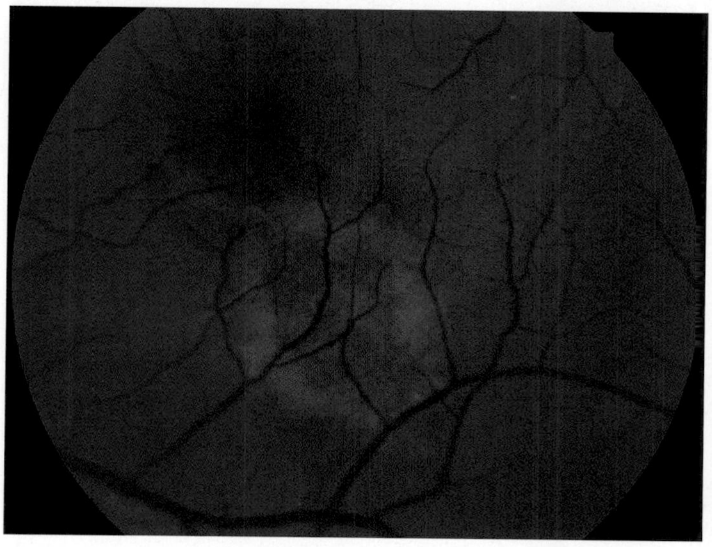

■ **Fig. 9.52** A 'halo' naevus surrounded by a pale zone resembling choroidal atrophy is uncommon.

thickness, particularly if touching the disc margin.

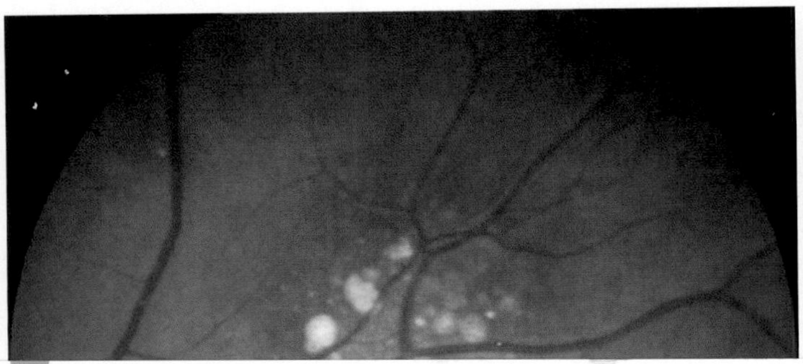

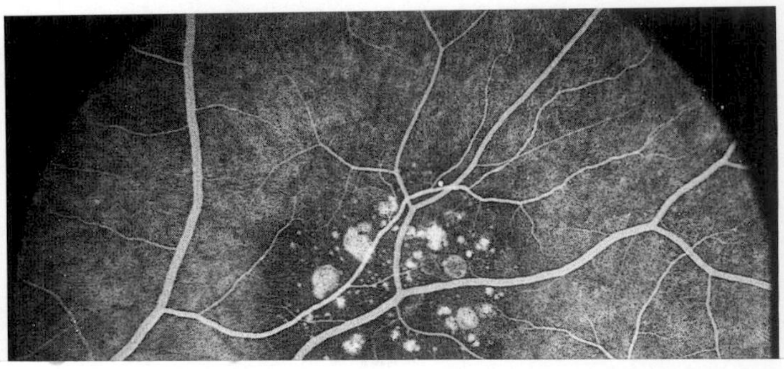

Melanoma

Choroidal melanoma is the most common primary intraocular malignancy in adults.

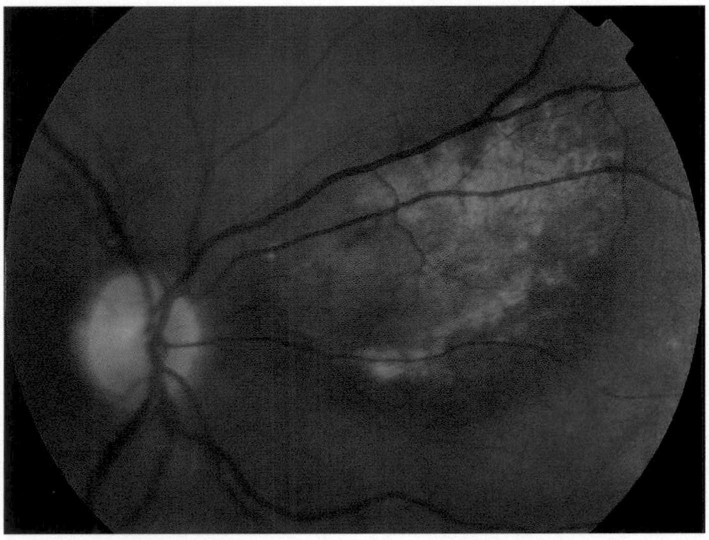

Fig. 9.60 A subretinal, dome-shaped, grey mass with surface orange lipofuscin pigment.

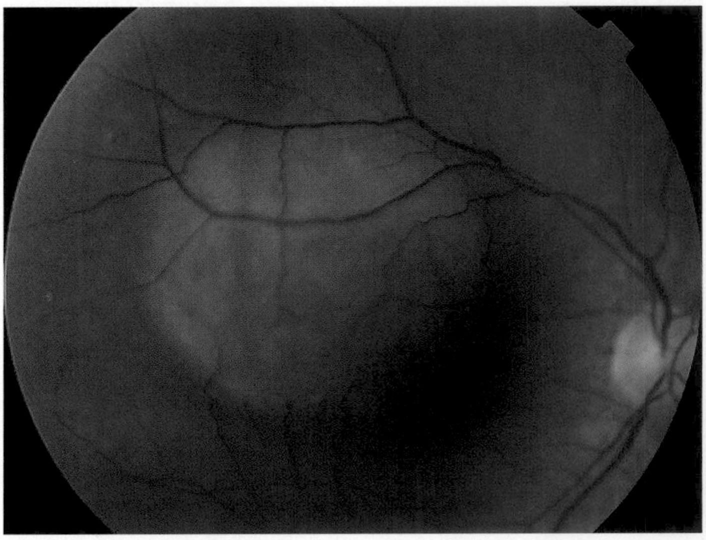

Fig. 9.61 A grey mass without surface lipofuscin pigment.

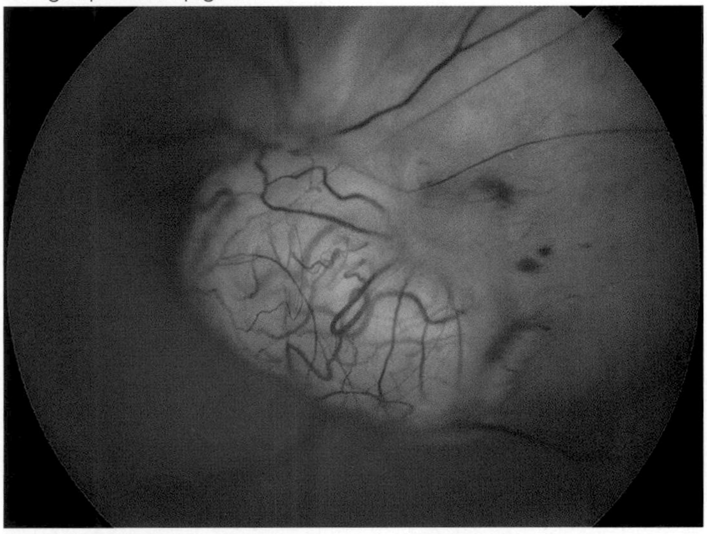

Fig. 9.62 If the tumour breaks through Bruch membrane it acquires a mushroom-shaped appearance, with visible blood vessels if the tumour is amelanotic.

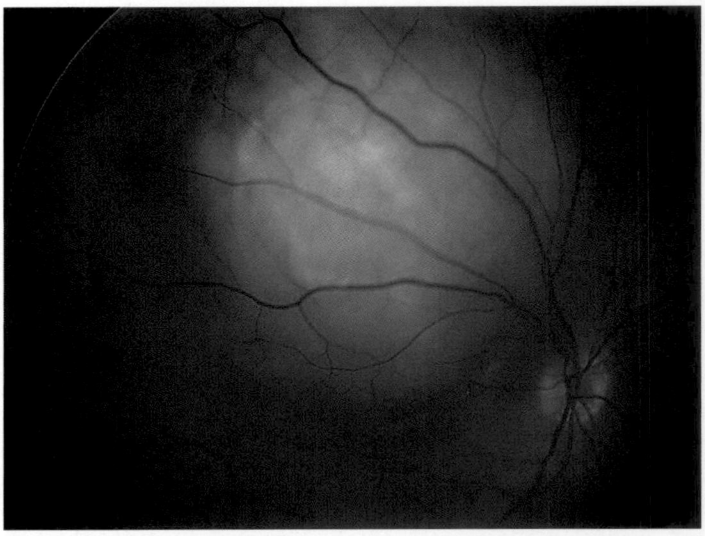

Fig. 9.63 An amelanotic mass with a thin layer of overlying subretinal fluid initially confined to the surface of the tumour. (Courtesy of C. Barry.)

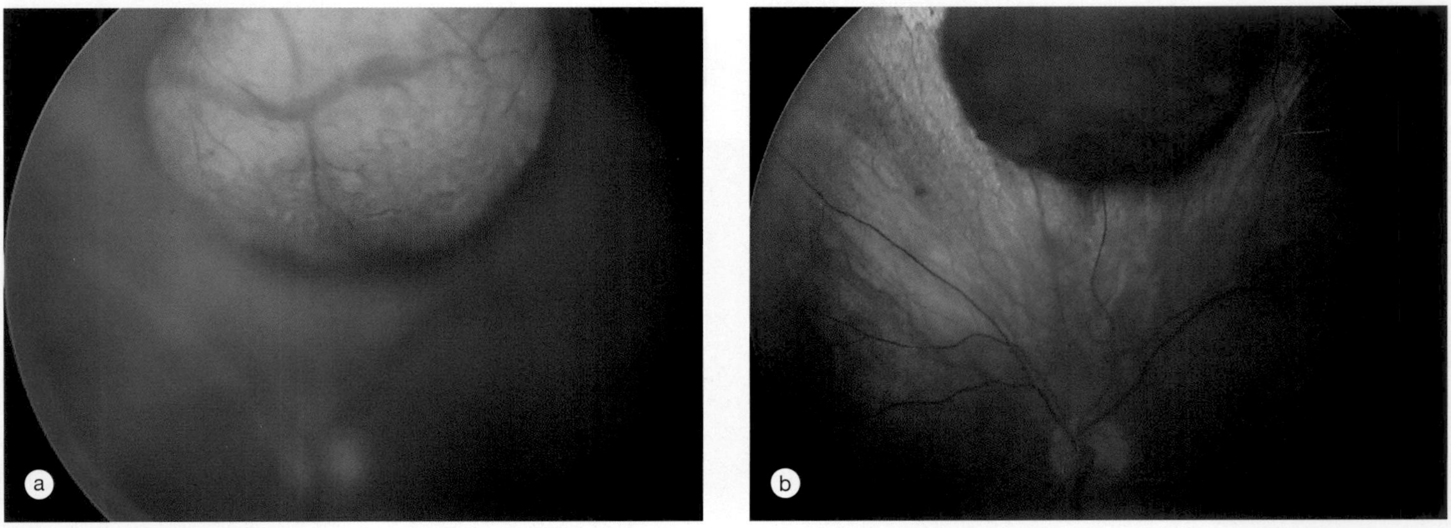

Fig. 9.64 Choroidal melanoma. **(a)** Before radiotherapy. **(b)** Increase in pigmentation following treatment. (Courtesy of C. Barry.)

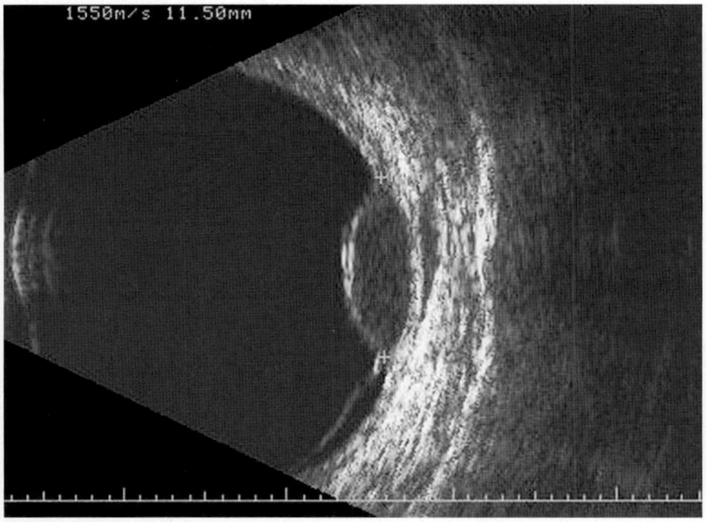

■ **Fig. 9.65** US shows the characteristic acoustic hollowness, choroidal excavation and orbital shadowing. (Courtesy of B. Damato.)

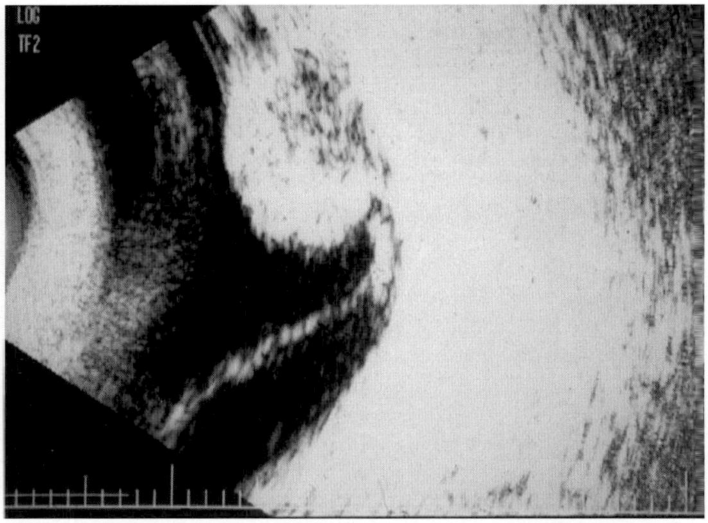

■ **Fig. 9.66** US shows a collar-stud configuration with inferior retinal detachment. (Courtesy of M. Hamza.)

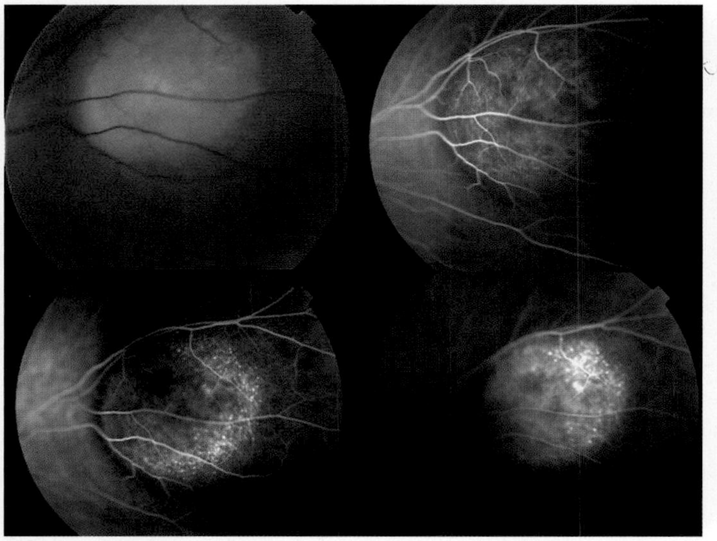

■ **Fig. 9.67** FA typically shows mottled fluorescence during the arteriovenous phase and then progressive leakage and staining.

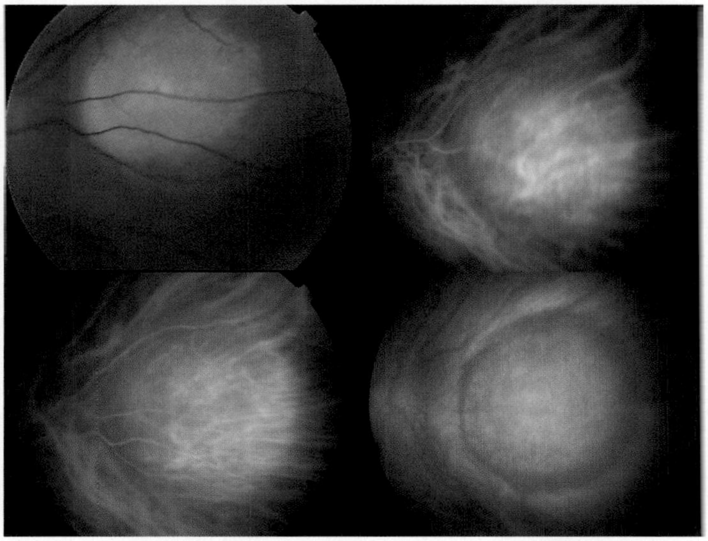

■ **Fig. 9.68** ICG provides more information about the extent of the tumour, because there is less interference caused by RPE changes.

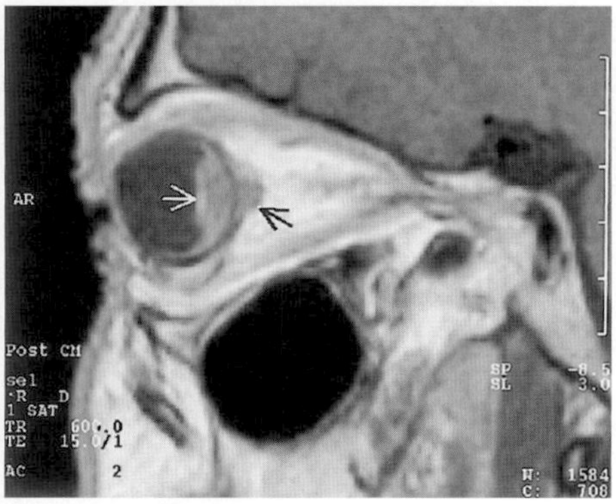

■ **Fig. 9.69** MRI shows that choroidal melanomas are hyperintense in T1-weighted images; the black arrow shows extraocular extension. (Courtesy of M. Karolczak-Kulesza.)

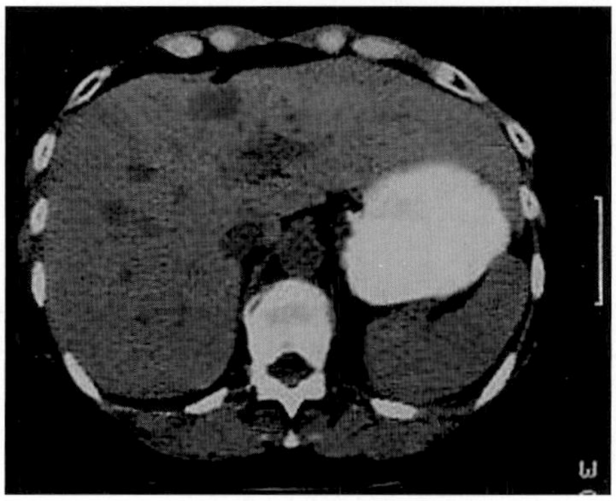

■ **Fig. 9.70** CT shows multiple hypointense liver metastases from choroidal melanoma.

Circumscribed haemangioma

Circumscribed haemangioma is a rare slow-growing hamartoma.

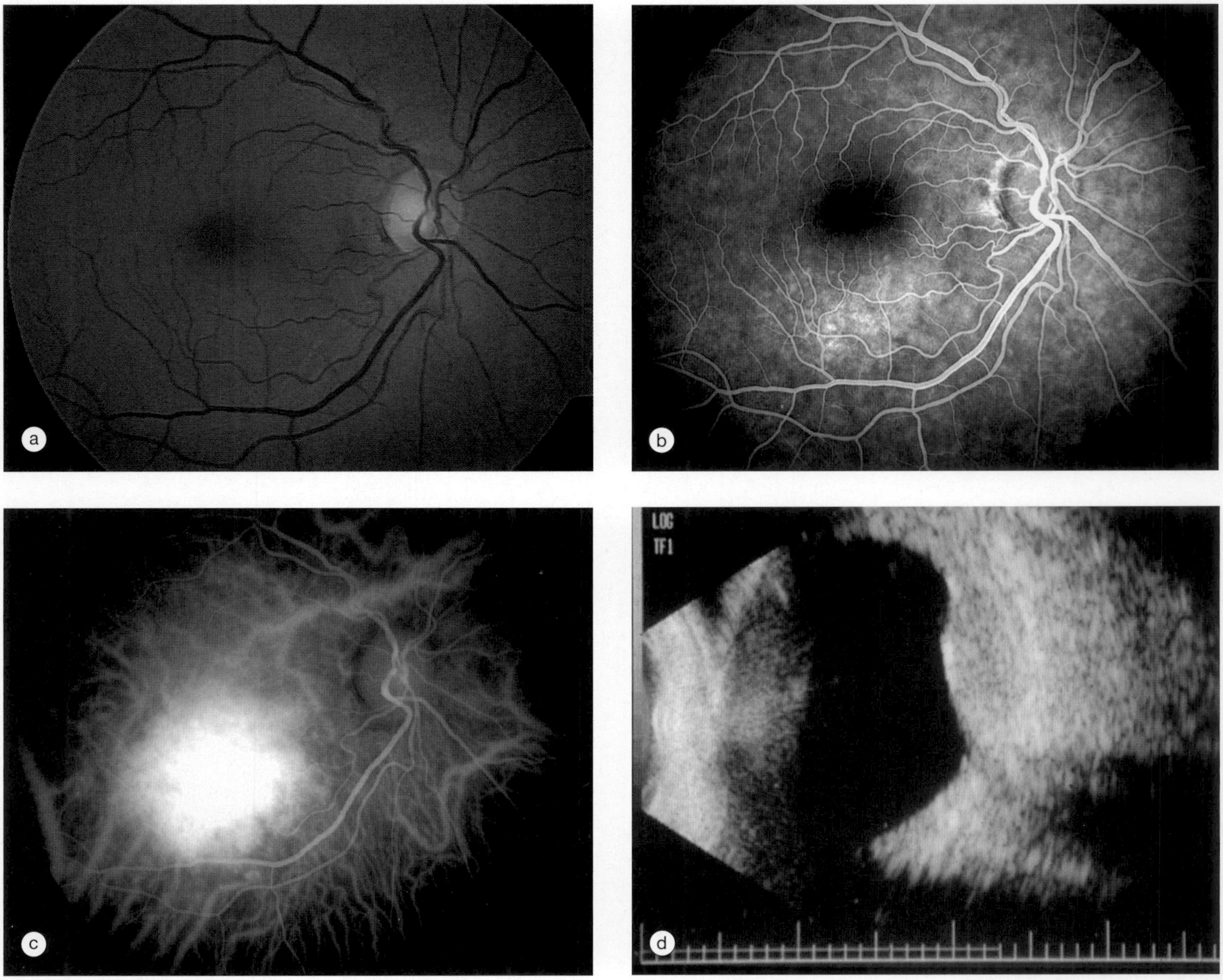

Fig. 9.71 **(a)** Circumscribed choroidal haemangioma. **(b)** FA shows early rapid hyperfluorescence. **(c)** ICG shows lacy hyperfluorescence in the early frames (shown here) and hypofluorescence ('washout') at 20 minutes. **(d)** US shows a low convex dome with a sharp anterior surface and high internal reflectivity without choroidal excavation or orbital shadowing. (Courtesy of M. Hamza and P. Gili.)

Diffuse choroidal haemangioma

Diffuse choroidal haemangioma usually affects over half of the choroid and enlarges very slowly. It occurs almost exclusively in patients with Sturge–Weber syndrome.

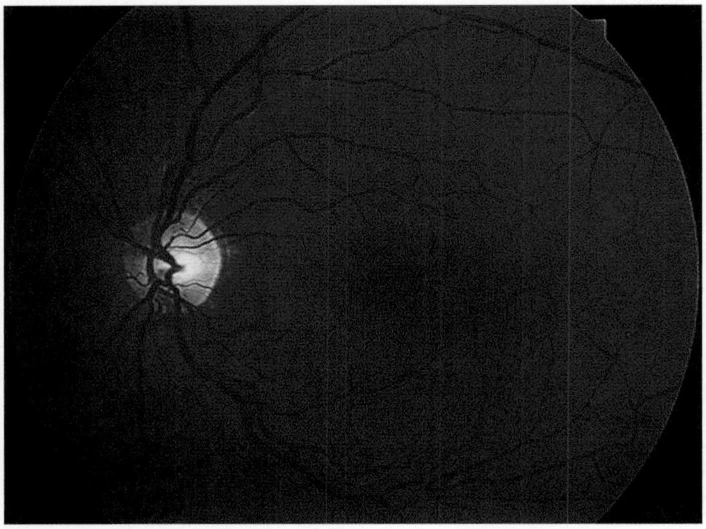

Fig. 9.72 The tumor has a deep red, 'tomato ketchup' colour.

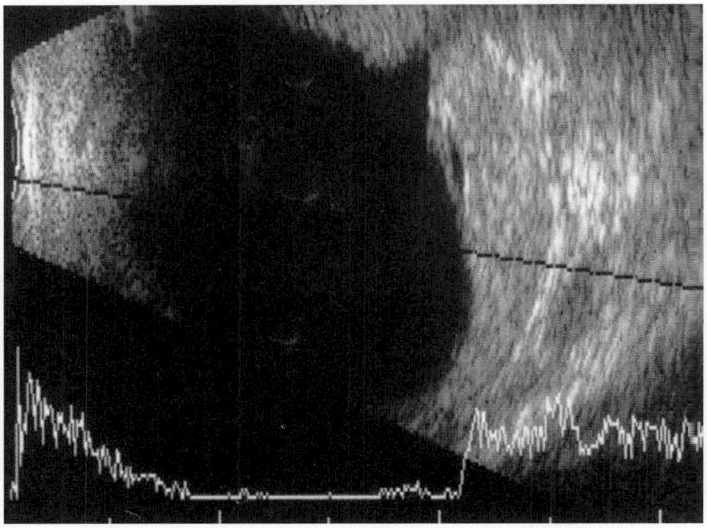

Fig. 9.73 US shows diffuse choroidal thickening.

Melanocytoma

Melanocytoma is a rare, distinctive, heavily pigmented lesion that is seen most frequently in the optic nerve head in dark-skinned individuals.

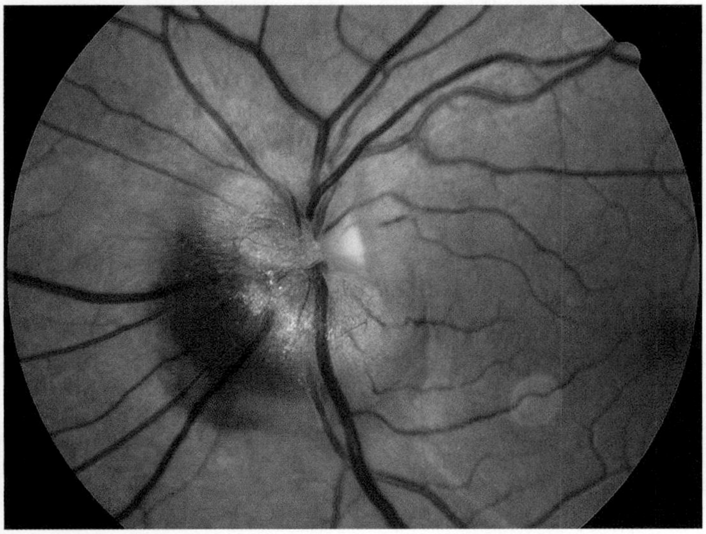

Fig. 9.74 A dark brown or black lesion with feathery edges within the retinal nerve fibre layer that typically extends over the inferior edge of the disc.

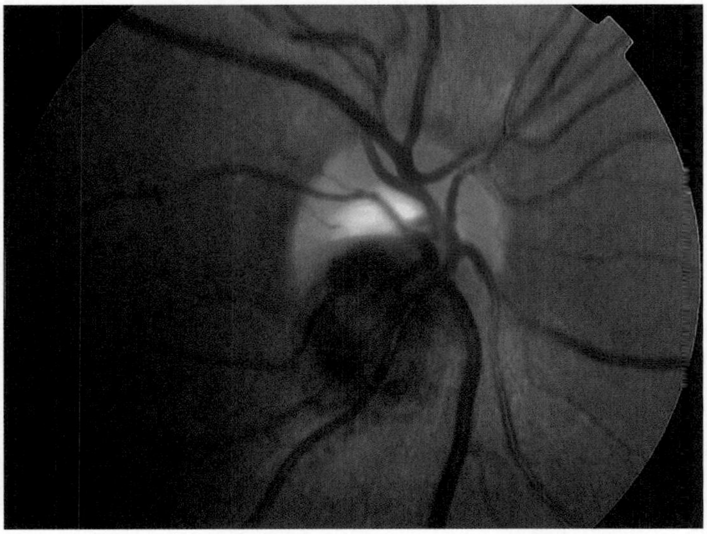

Fig. 9.75 A highly pigmented melanocytoma.

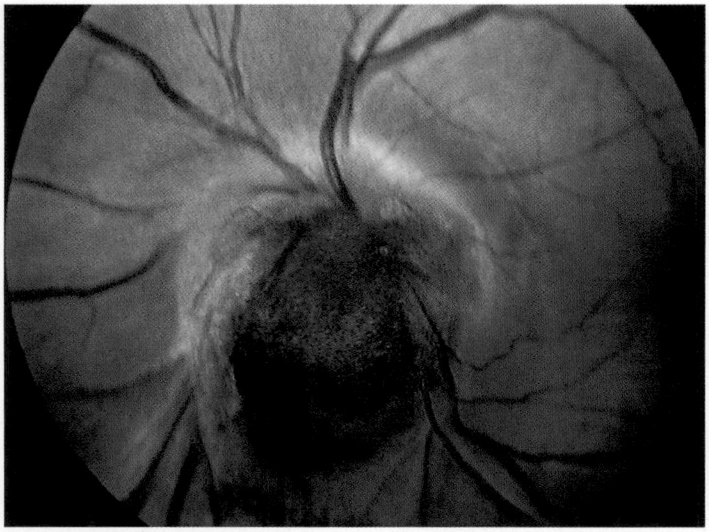

■ **Fig. 9.76** Occasionally the tumour occupies the entire disc surface.

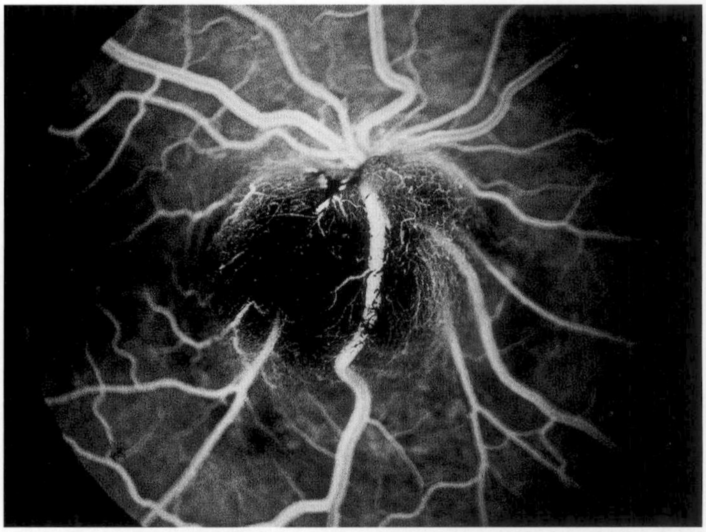

■ **Fig. 9.77** FA shows hypofluorescence of deeper vessels due to blockage.

Osteoma

Choroidal osteoma (osseous choristoma) is a very rare, benign, slow-growing tumour that typically affects females. Both eyes are affected in about 25% of cases but not usually simultaneously.

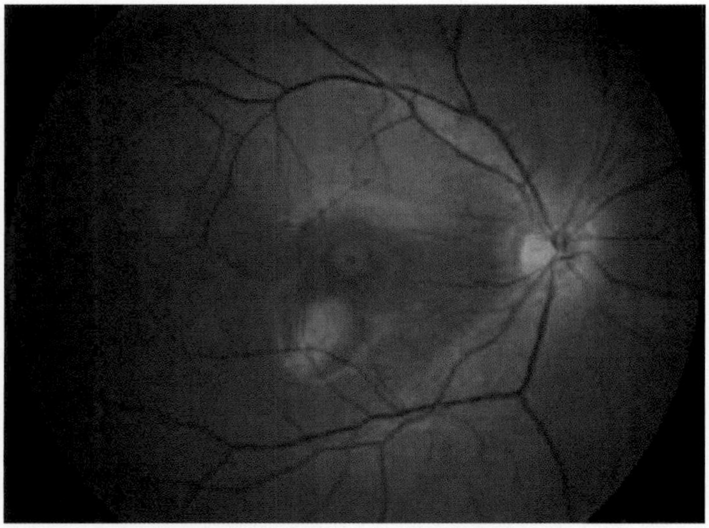

■ **Fig. 9.78** A placoid, orange-yellow, well-defined lesion at the posterior pole. (Courtesy of B. Damato.)

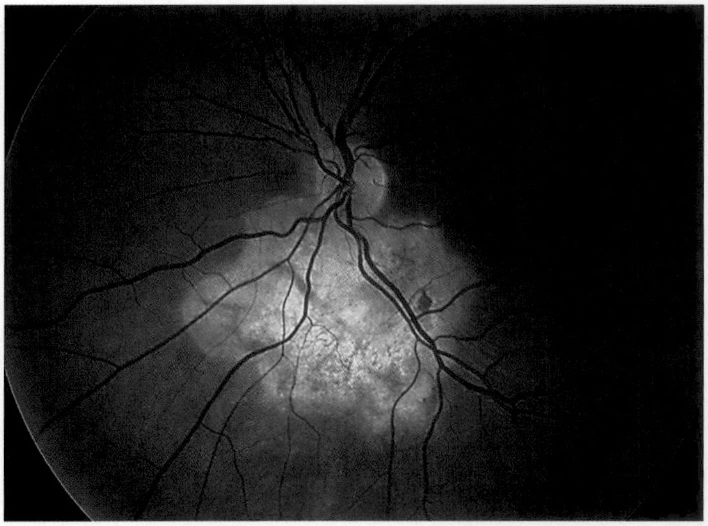

■ **Fig. 9.79** Larger lesions have scalloped borders and are frequently juxtapapillary. (Courtesy of C. Barry.)

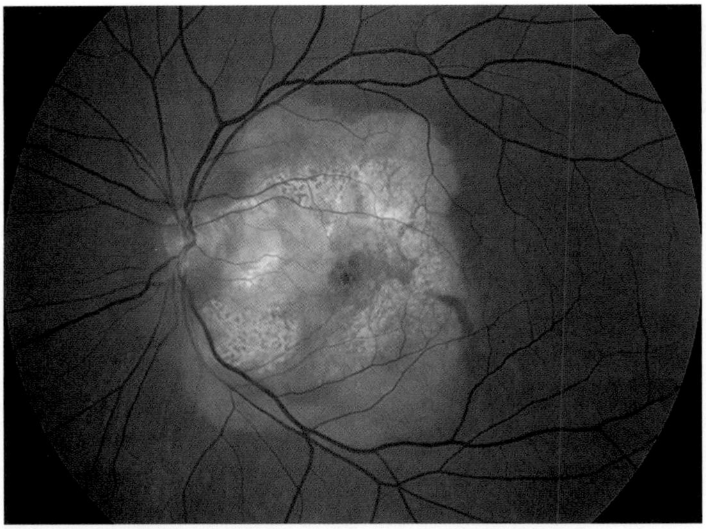

■ **Fig. 9.80** Visual loss may occur as a result of macular involvement or secondary choroidal neovascularisation. (Courtesy of C. Barry.)

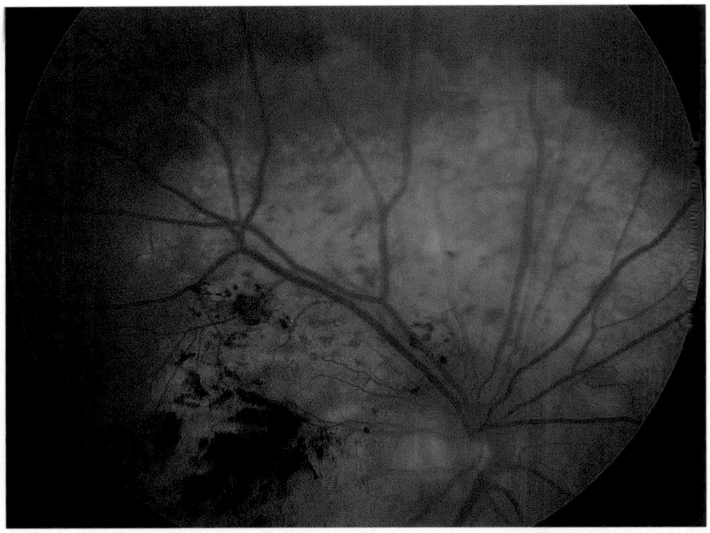

■ **Fig. 9.81** Long-standing lesion showing overlying RPE hyperplasia.

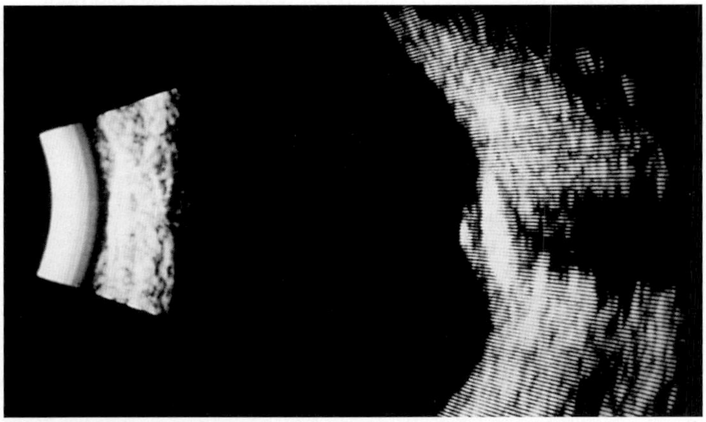

■ **Fig. 9.82** US shows a very dense highly reflective lesion (bone), which causes linear orbital shadowing.

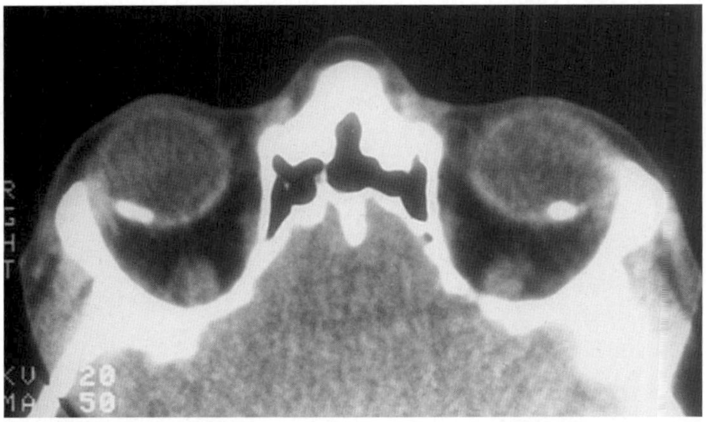

■ **Fig. 9.83** CT demonstrates the same features as bone; note bilateral involvement. (Courtesy of C. Barry.)

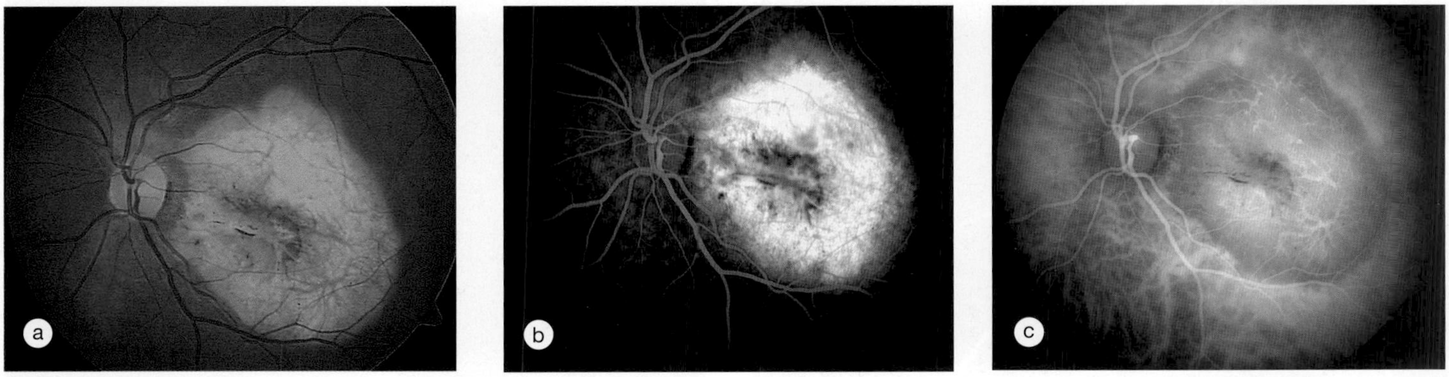

■ **Fig. 9.84** **(a)** Choroidal osteoma. **(b)** FA shows irregular, diffuse mottled hyperfluorescence during the early and late phases. **(c)** ICG shows early hypofluorescence and late staining. (Courtesy of P. Gili.)

TUMOURS OF THE RETINA

Retinoblastoma

Retinoblastoma is the most common primary intraocular malignancy of childhood.

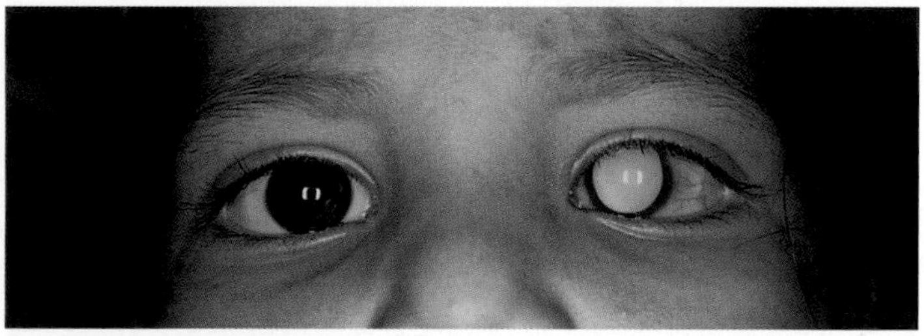

■ **Fig. 9.94** Leukocoria (white pupillary reflex) is the commonest presenting feature and may be first noticed in family photographs. (Courtesy of U. Raina.)

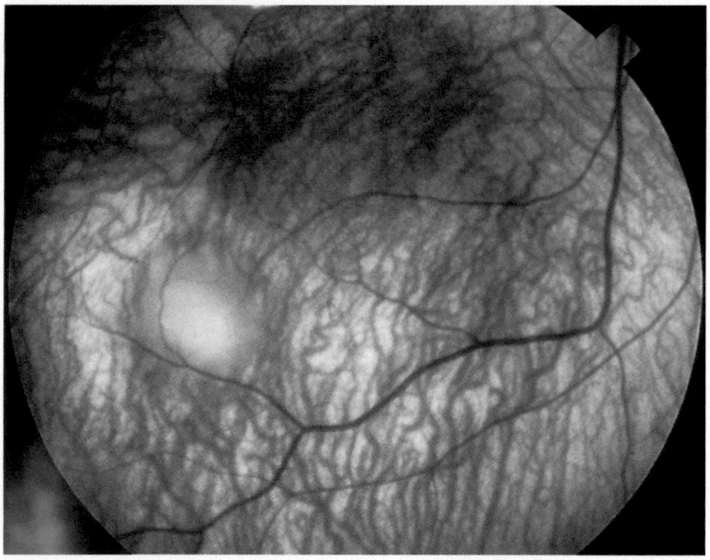

■ **Fig. 9.95** An early tumour is a placoid white lesion that may be associated with white flecks of calcification.

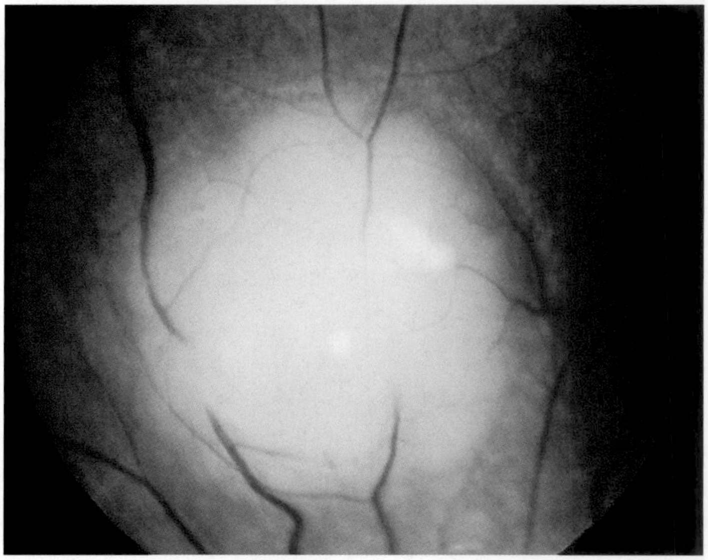

■ **Fig. 9.96** A larger placoid tumour.

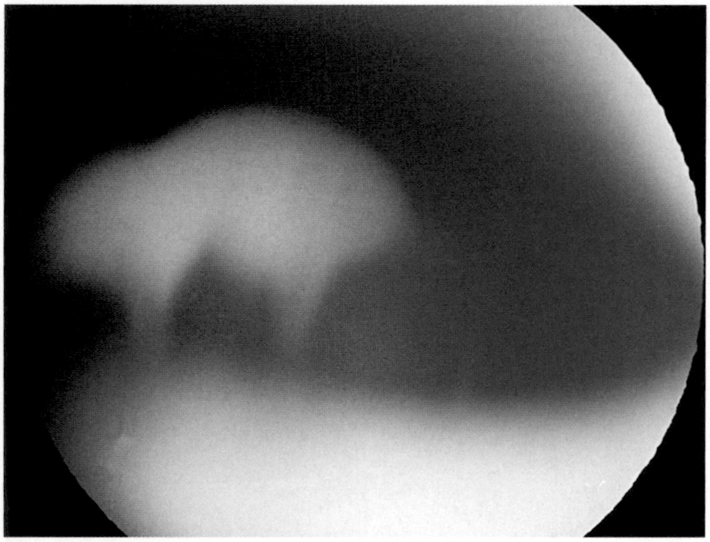

■ **Fig. 9.97** A small peripheral tumour may be overlooked unless scleral indentation is performed.

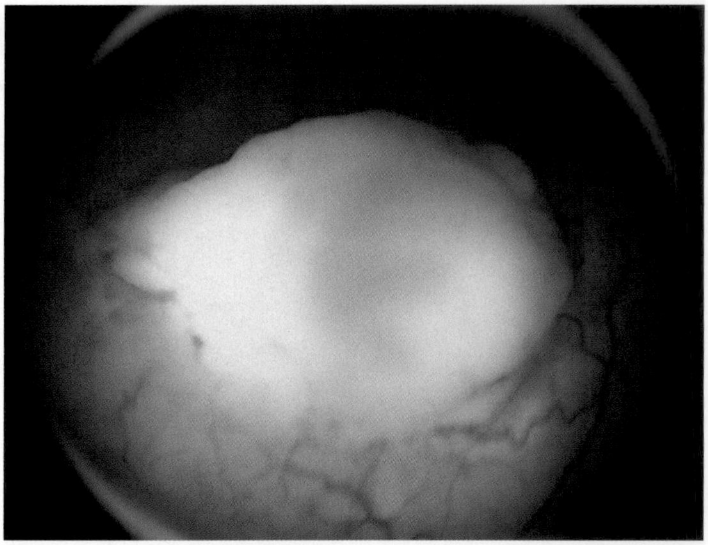

■ **Fig. 9.98** An endophytic tumour projects into the vitreous as a white mass. (Courtesy of L. Merin.)

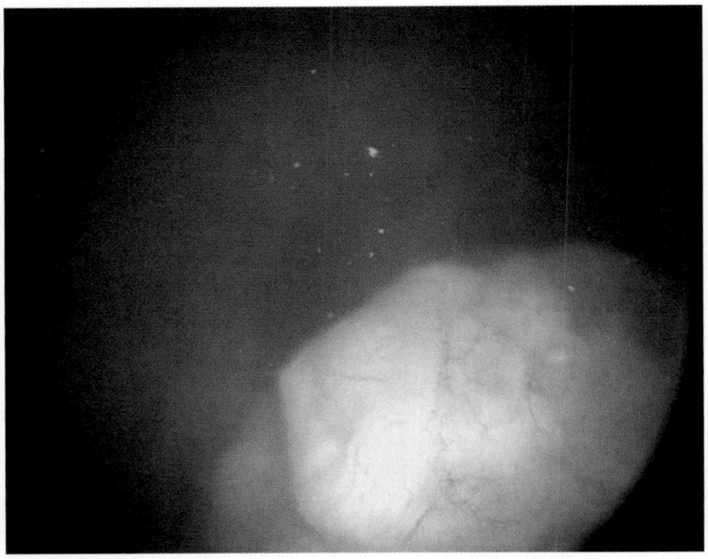

■ **Fig. 9.99** Endophytic tumour with vitreous seeding. (Courtesy of B. Gallie.)

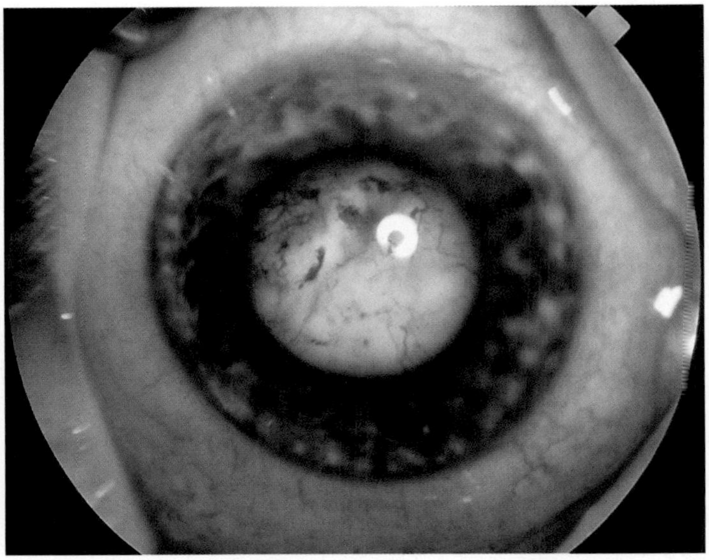

■ **Fig. 9.100** Retinoblastoma with surface vessels filling the vitreous cavity.

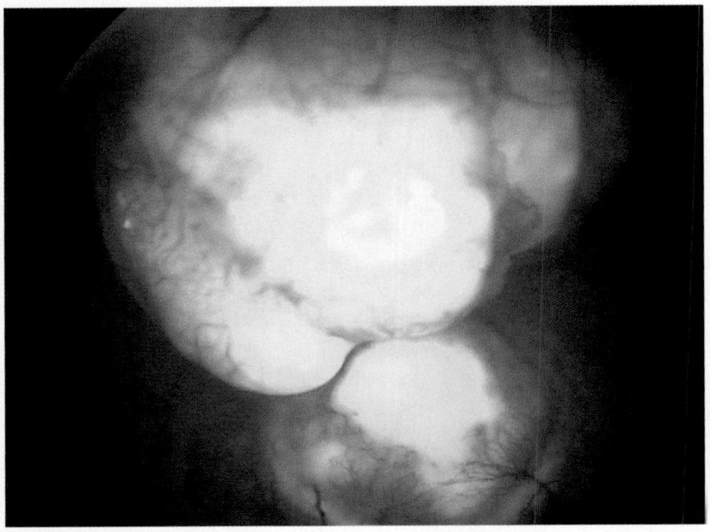

■ **Fig. 9.101** An exophytic tumour grows outwards as a subretinal multilobulated mass and detaches the retina. (Courtesy of L. MacKeen.)

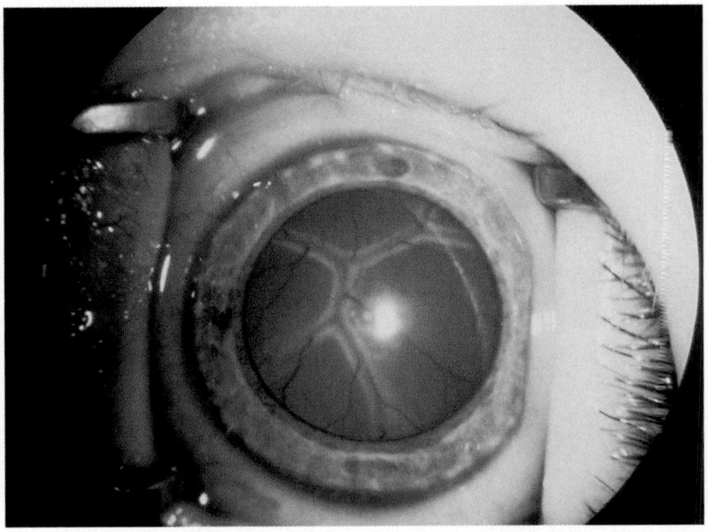

■ **Fig. 9.102** An exophytic tumour may be difficult to visualise if the subretinal fluid is deep.

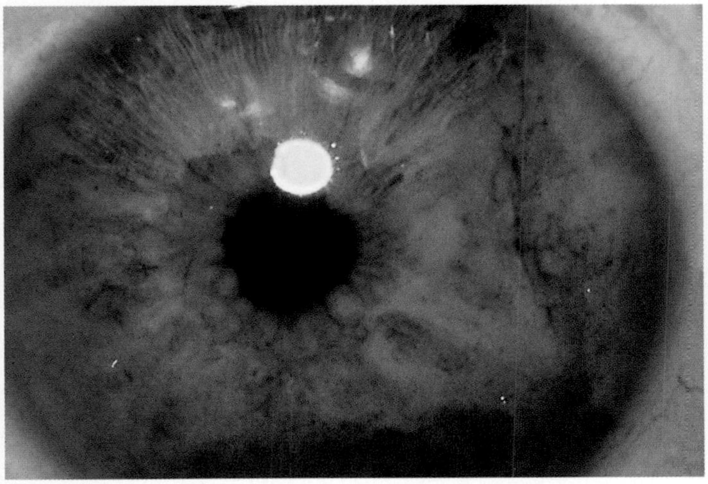

■ **Fig. 9.103** Iris involvement by multiple nodules and hyphaema may occur in older children with diffuse tumours.

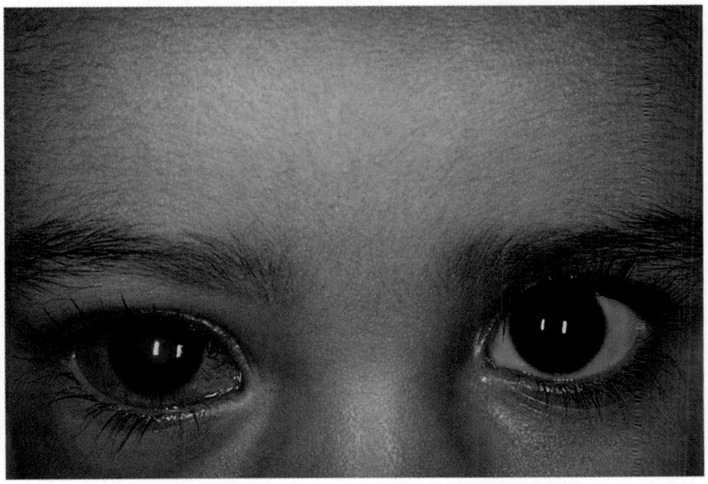

■ **Fig. 9.104** A red eye may be caused by tumour-induced inflammation or secondary glaucoma. (Courtesy of U. Raina.)

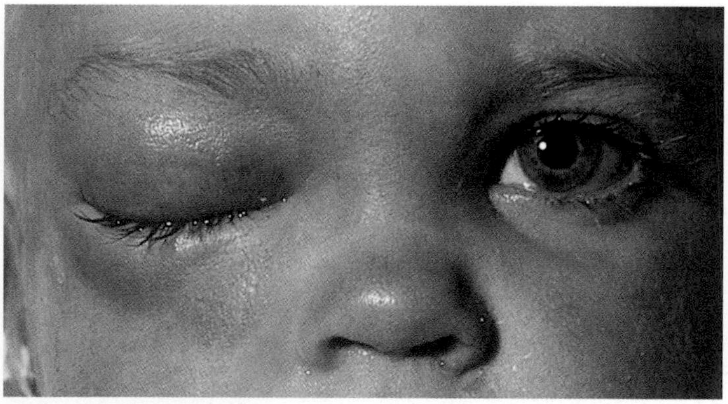

Fig. 9.105 Orbital inflammation mimicking orbital or preseptal cellulitis may occur with necrotic tumours and does not necessarily imply extraocular extension.

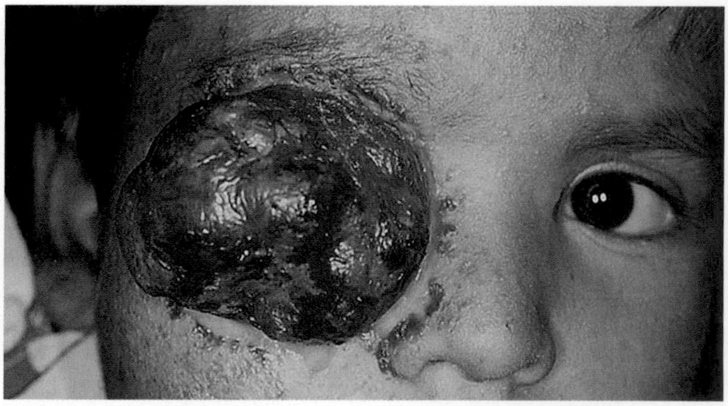

Fig. 9.106 Orbital invasion with proptosis and bone invasion may occur in neglected cases. (Courtesy of U. Raina.)

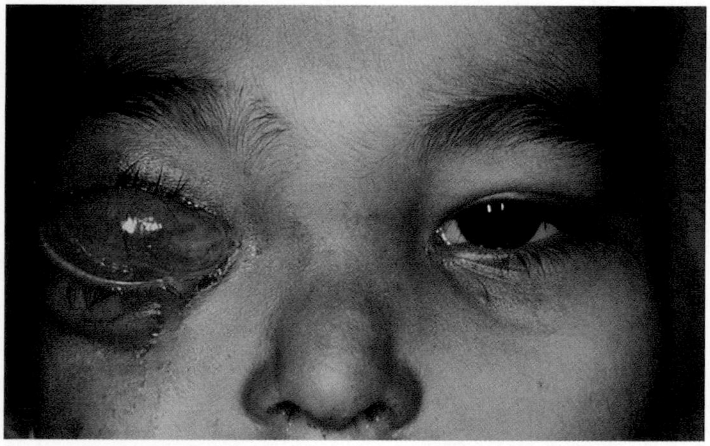

Fig. 9.107 Orbital recurrence of retinoblastoma following enucleation. (Courtesy of U. Raina.)

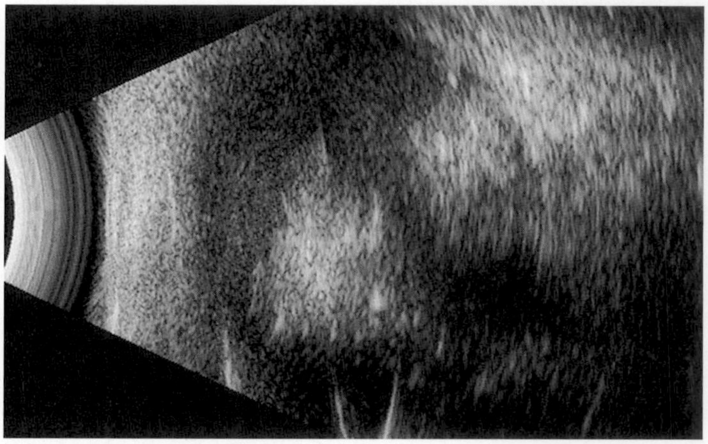

Fig. 9.108 US is used mainly to assess tumour size. It also detects calcification within the tumour and is helpful in the diagnosis of simulating lesions such as Coats disease. (Courtesy of A. Singh.)

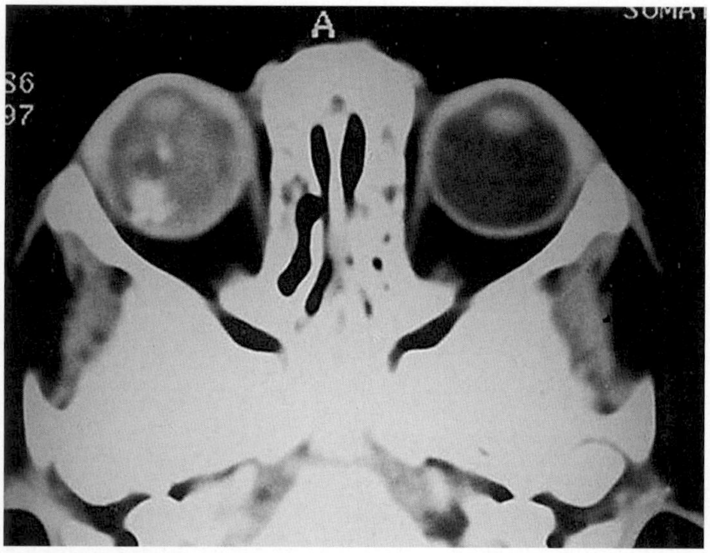

Fig. 9.109 CT may show gross involvement of the optic nerve, tumour calcification and extraocular extension. (Courtesy of U. Raina.)

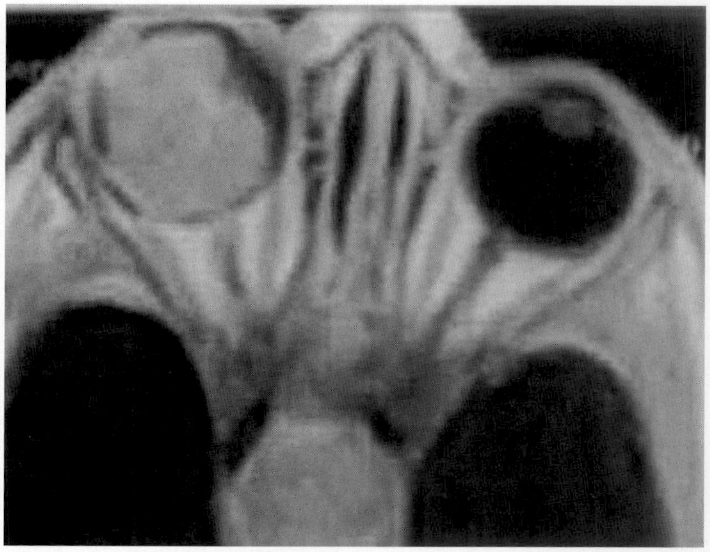

Fig. 9.110 MRI cannot detect calcification but is superior to CT for optic nerve evaluation and for detection of a pinealoblastoma. This figure shows a large retinoblastoma in the right eye and a pinealoblastoma. (Courtesy of J. Pe'er.)

Astrocytoma

Astrocytoma is a rare, benign tumour that does not usually threaten vision. About 50% of patients with tuberous sclerosis have fundus astrocytomas, which may be multiple and bilateral.

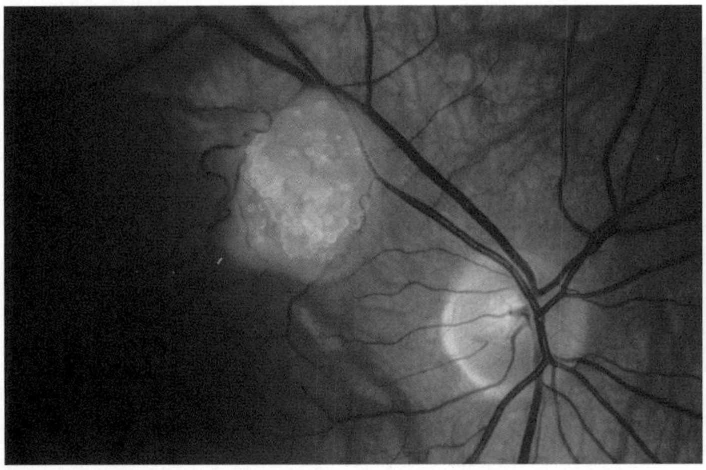

Fig. 9.111 A semi-translucent, mulberry-like nodule. (Courtesy of L. Merin.)

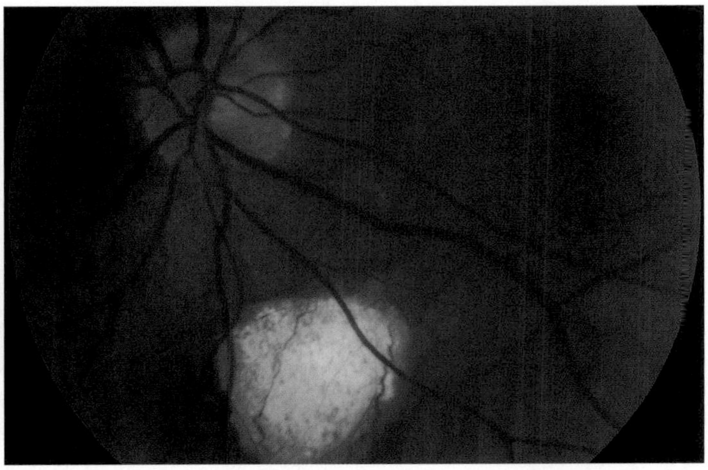

Fig. 9.112 A white, well-circumscribed plaque. (Courtesy of C. Barry.)

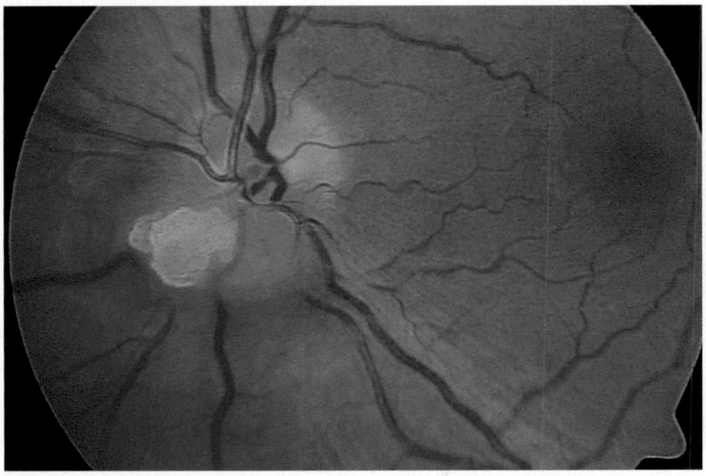

Fig. 9.113 A peripapillary lesion. (Courtesy of P. Gili.)

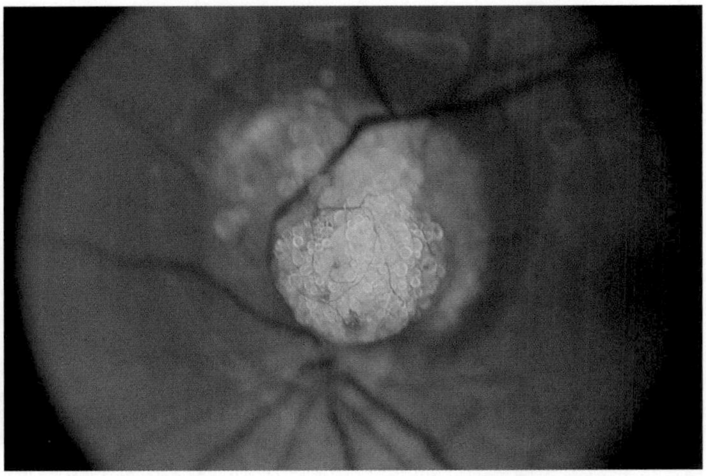

Fig. 9.114 A very large peripapillary lesion. (Courtesy of T. Link.)

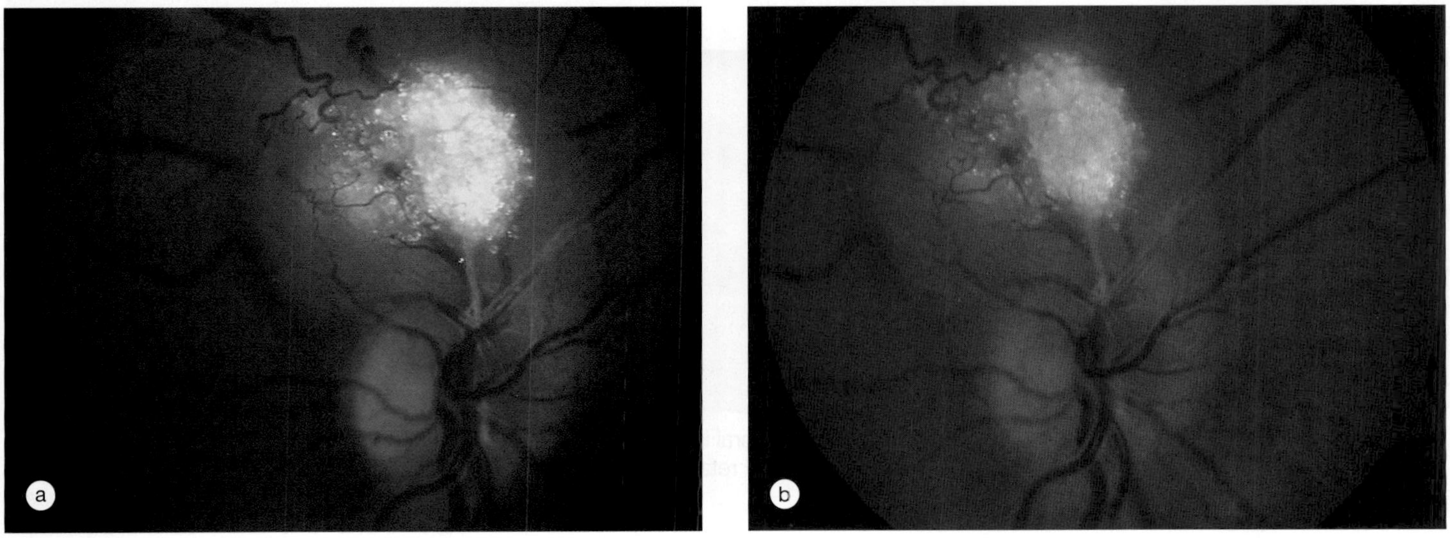

Fig. 9.115 **(a)** Astrocytoma. **(b)** Red-free image showing autofluorescence. (Courtesy of P. Gili.)

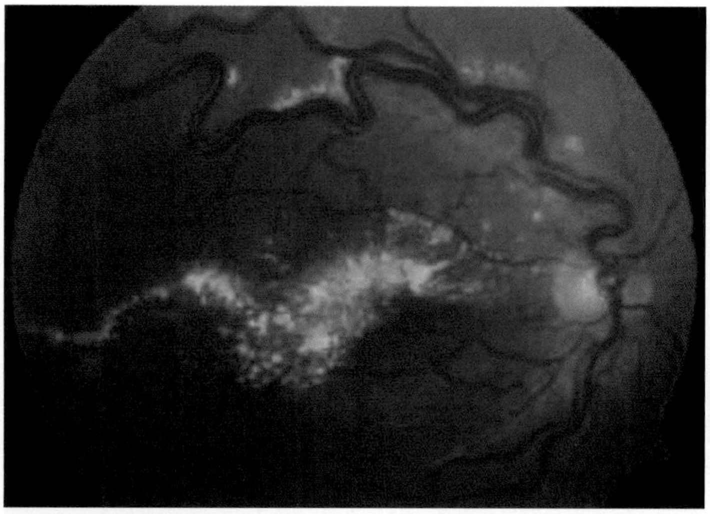

Fig. 9.128 Hard exudate formation in the macula is a major cause of visual morbidity. (Courtesy of B. Damato.)

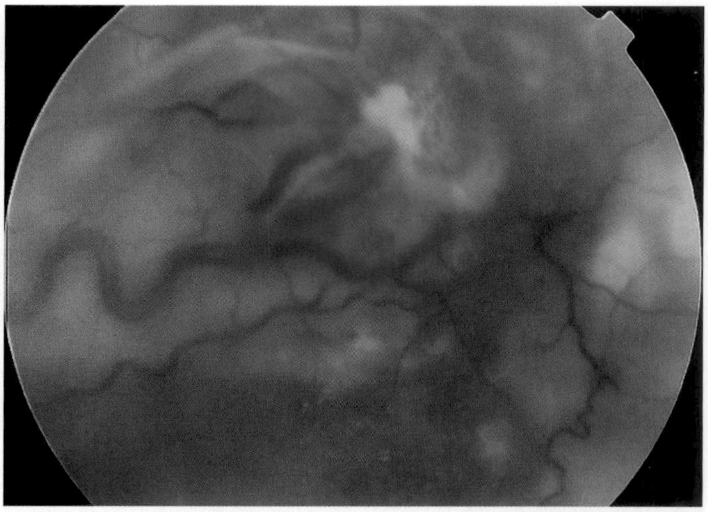

Fig. 9.129 Hard exudate formation around the tumour and exudative retinal detachment are caused by leakage.

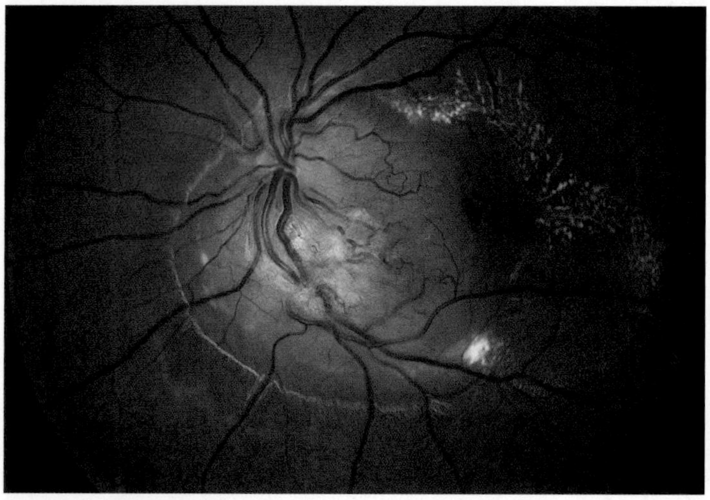

Fig. 9.130 An exophytic optic disc haemangioma is a diffuse placoid lesion with dilated blood vessels. (Courtesy of P. Saine.)

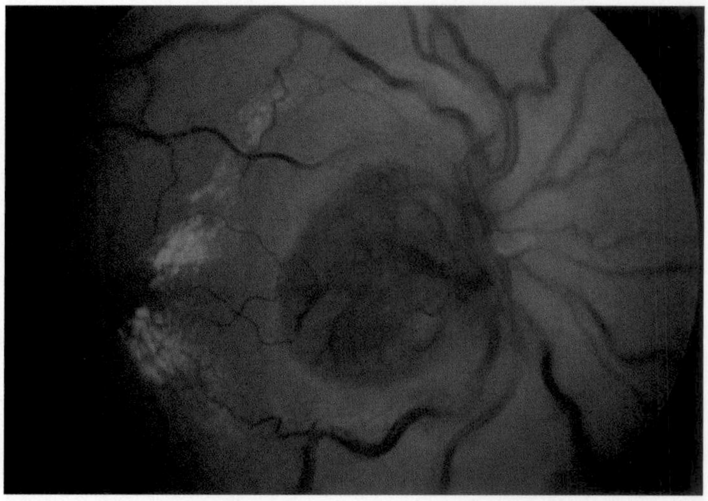

Fig. 9.131 An endophytic optic disc haemangioma protrudes into the vitreous and typically causes visual loss due to hard exudate formation at the macula. (Courtesy of K. Nischal.)

Von Hippel–Lindau disease

About 50% of patients with solitary capillary haemangiomas and virtually all patients with multiple lesions have von Hippel–Lindau disease, which is an autosomal dominant condition.

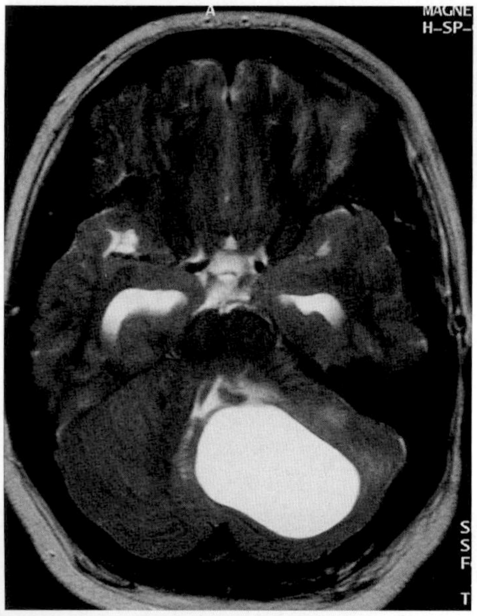

Fig. 9.132 Axial MRI scan showing a cystic cerebellar haemangioblastoma. (Courtesy of A. Singh.)

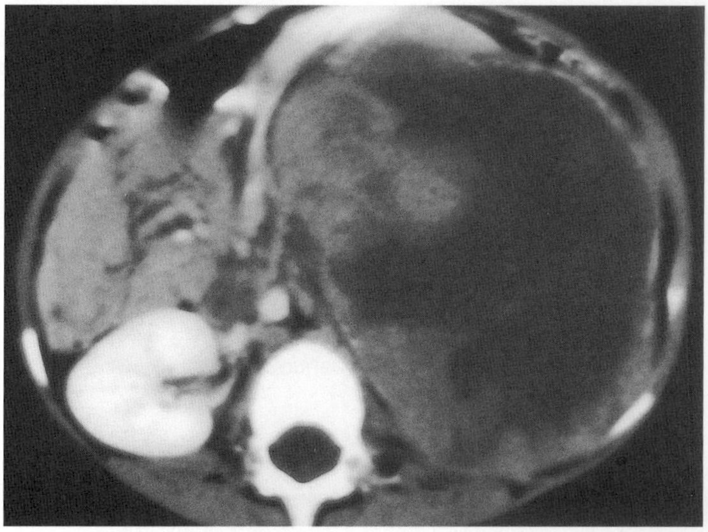

Fig. 9.133 Axial CT of the abdomen showing a large renal carcinoma right of midline. (Courtesy of G. Wilkinson.)

Cavernous haemangioma

Cavernous haemangioma of the retina or optic nerve head is a rare, congenital, unilateral, vascular hamartoma.

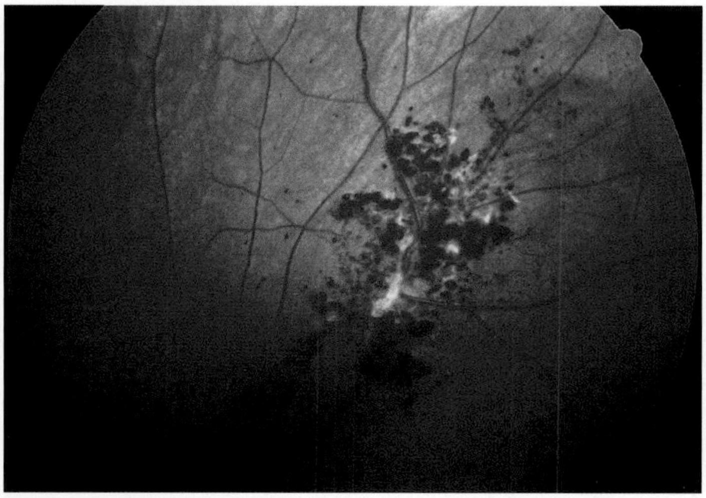

■ **Fig. 9.134** Sessile clusters of saccular aneurysms resembling a 'bunch of grapes' on the retina. (Courtesy of C. Barry.)

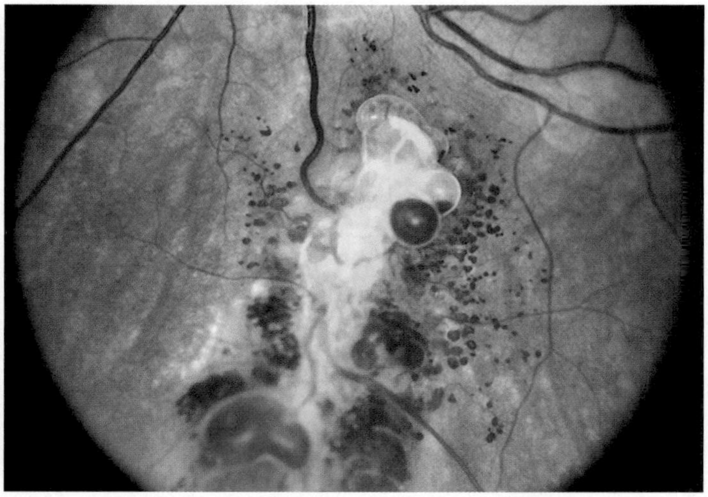

■ **Fig. 9.135** Larger cavernous haemangioma. (Courtesy of C. Barry.)

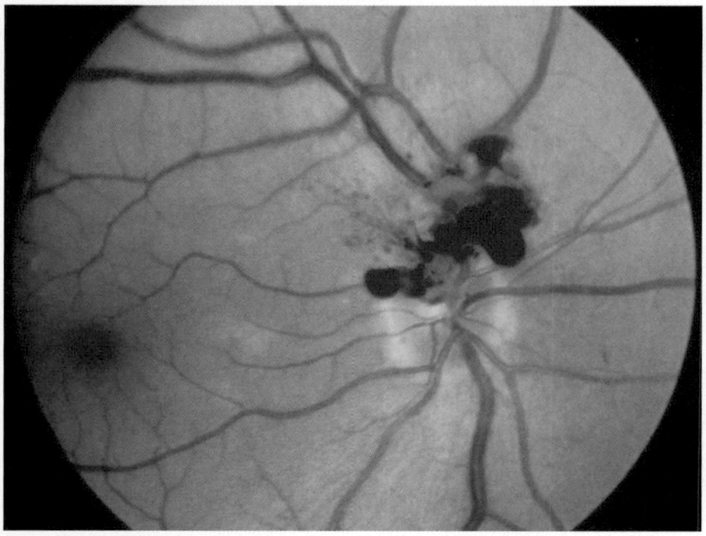

■ **Fig. 9.136** Cavernous haemangioma of the optic nerve head (Courtesy of P. Morse.)

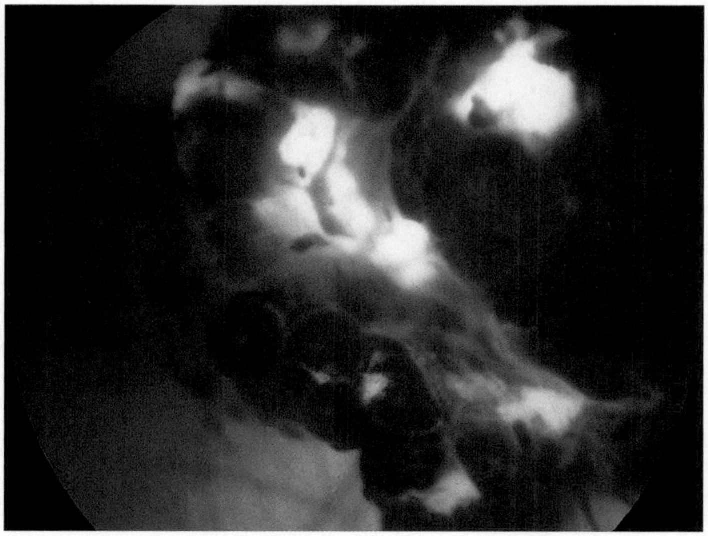

■ **Fig. 9.137** Very large cavernous haemangioma. (Courtesy of T. Link.)

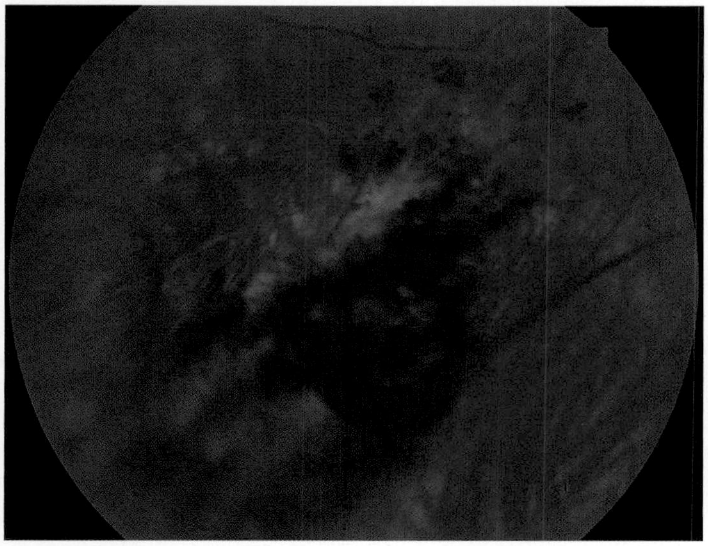

■ **Fig. 9.138** Vitreous haemorrhage is uncommon and usually innocuous.

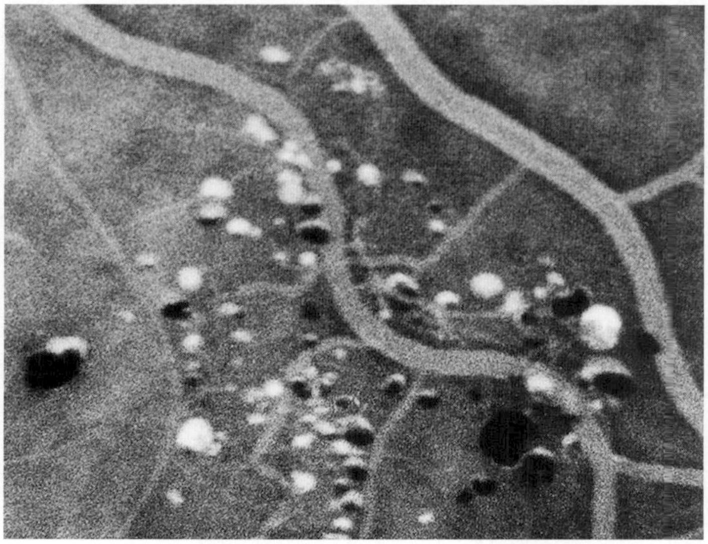

■ **Fig. 9.139** FA showing fluid levels due to the separation of red cells from plasma.

Racemose haemangioma

Racemose haemangioma is a rare, usually unilateral, congenital malformation. Some patients have similar ipsilateral lesions involving the midbrain, basofrontal region and posterior fossa (Wyburn–Mason syndrome).

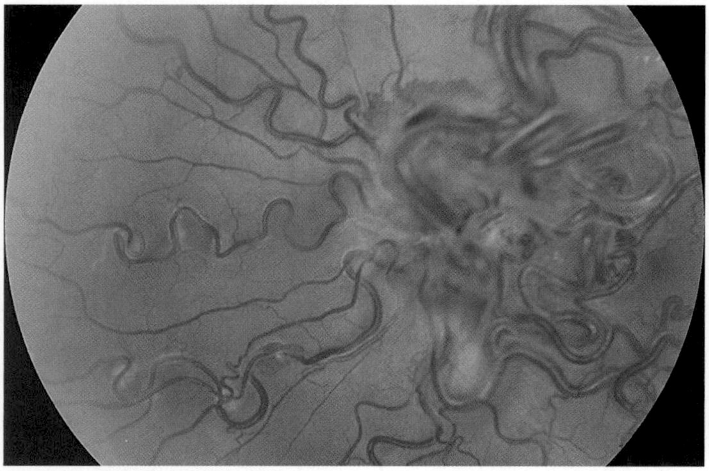

Fig. 9.140 Enlarged, tortuous blood vessels, which are often more numerous than in a normal fundus, with the vein and artery appearing similar. (Courtesy of S. Milewski.)

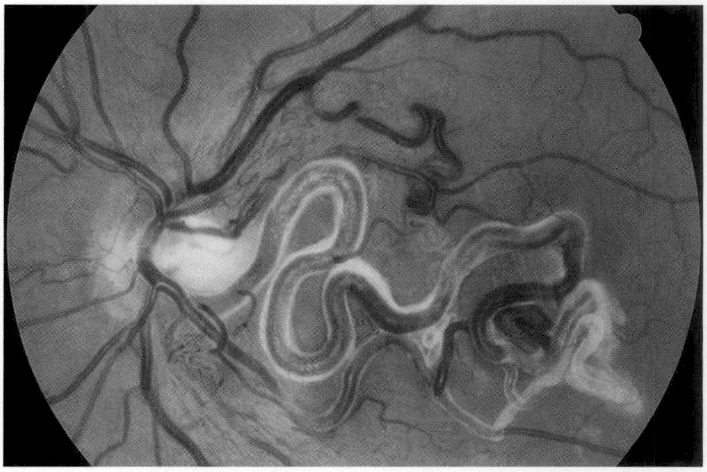

Fig. 9.141 Vascular sclerosis may occur in long-standing cases.

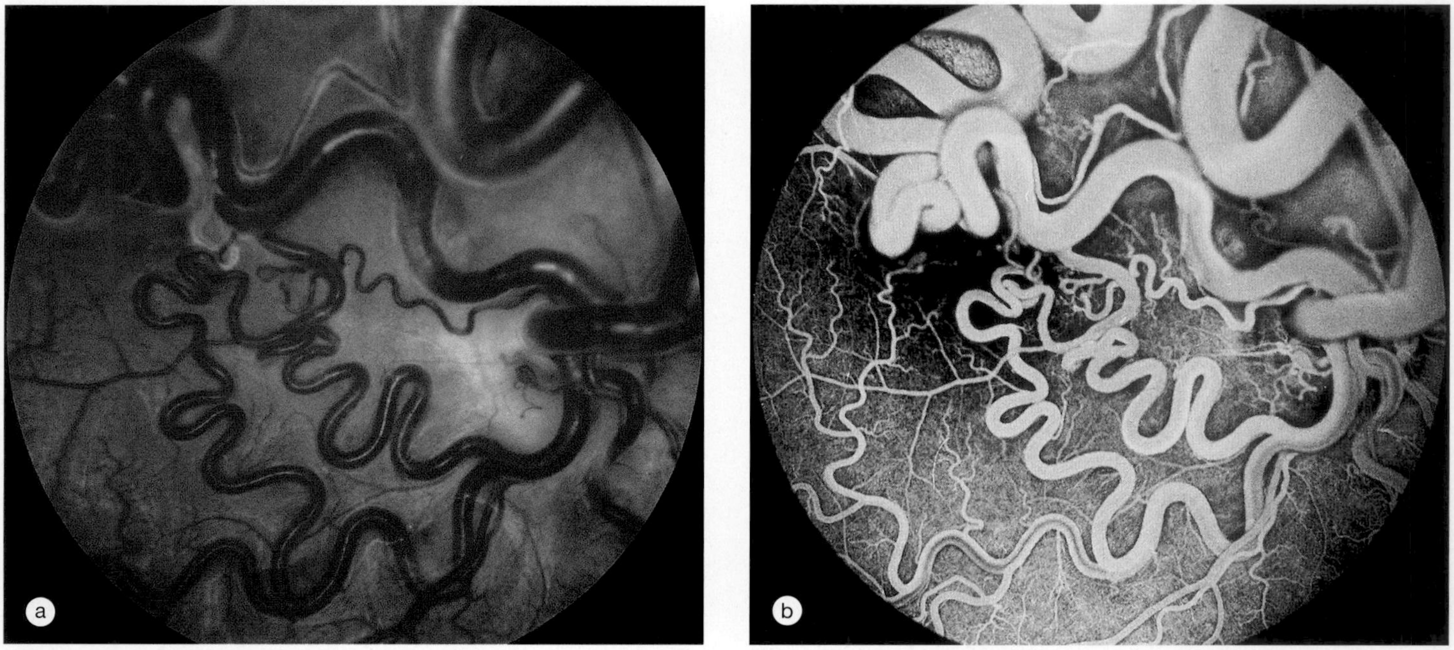

Fig. 9.142 **(a)** Racemose haemangioma. **(b)** FA shows marked vascular hyperfluorescence but absence of leakage.

Primary intraocular-central nervous system lymphoma

This is an uncommon, highly malignant, large B-cell (non-Hodgkin) lymphoma.

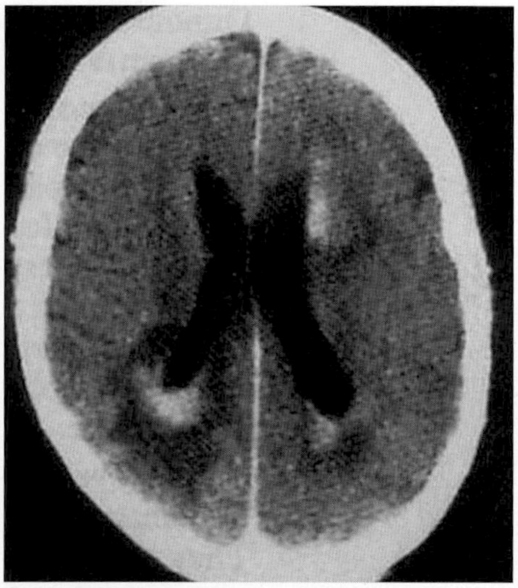

Fig. 9.143 Axial CT showing periventricular lymphomatous lesions. (Courtesy of P. Trend, M. Swash and C. Kennard.)

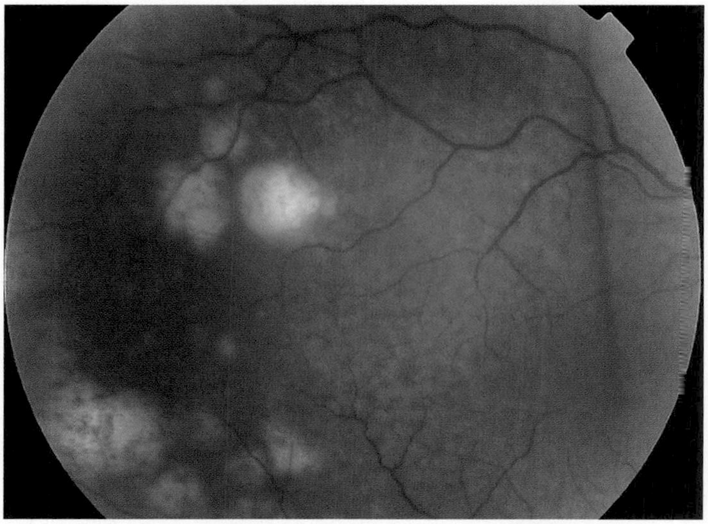

Fig. 9.144 Multifocal, yellowish, oval subretinal infiltrates.

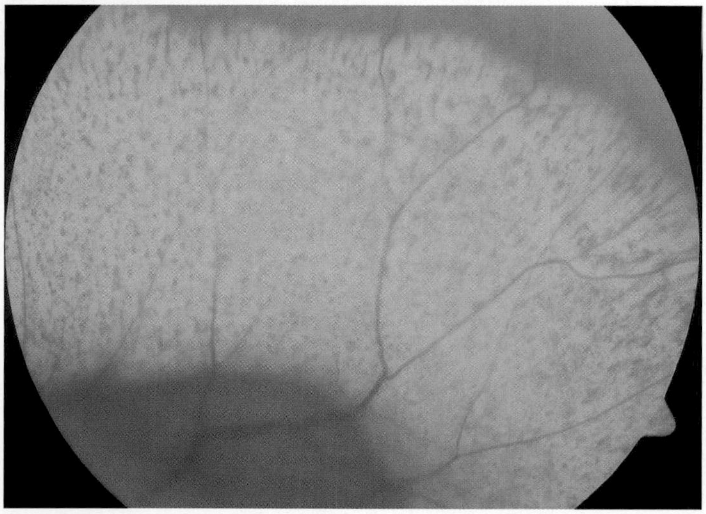

Fig. 9.145 Occasionally coalescence of the subretinal infiltrates may form a ring encircling the equator, which is pathognomonic for lymphoma. (Courtesy of B. Damato.)

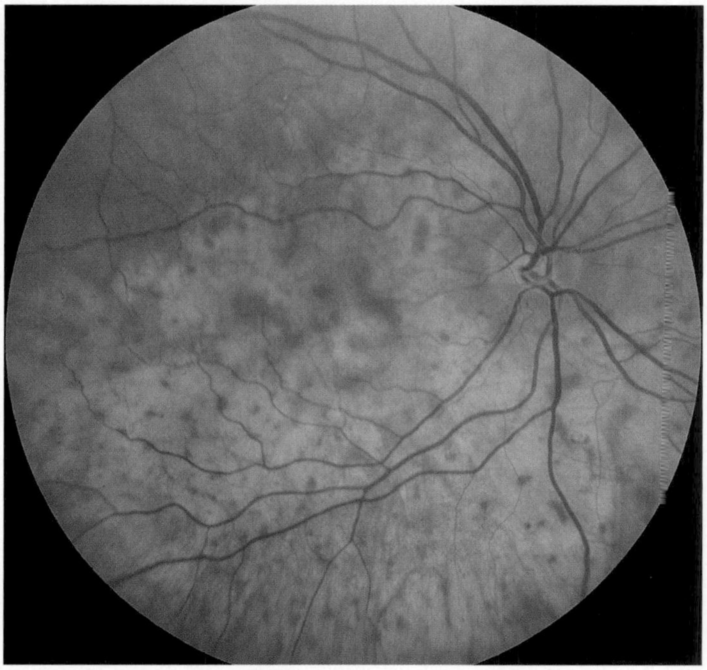

Fig. 9.146 Diffuse retinal or subretinal infiltration.

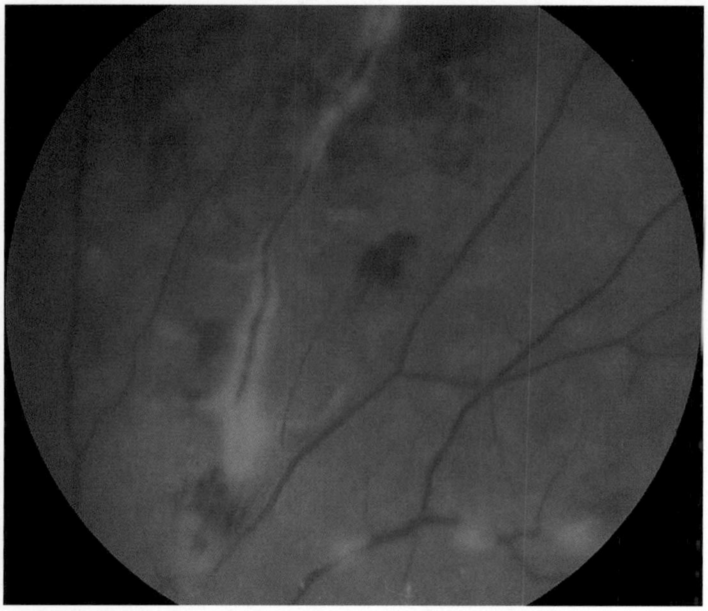

Fig. 9.147 Haemorrhagic retinal vasculitis. (Courtesy of C. Barry.)

TUMOURS OF THE RETINAL PIGMENT EPITHELIUM

Congenital hypertrophy of the retinal pigment epithelium (CHRPE)

Typical

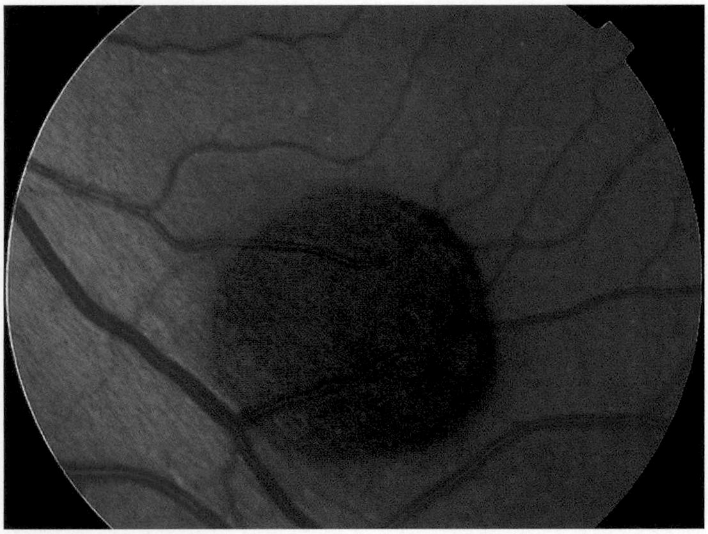

Fig. 9.148 A unilateral, flat, dark-grey or black, well-demarcated, round or oval lesion 1–3 disc diameters in size.

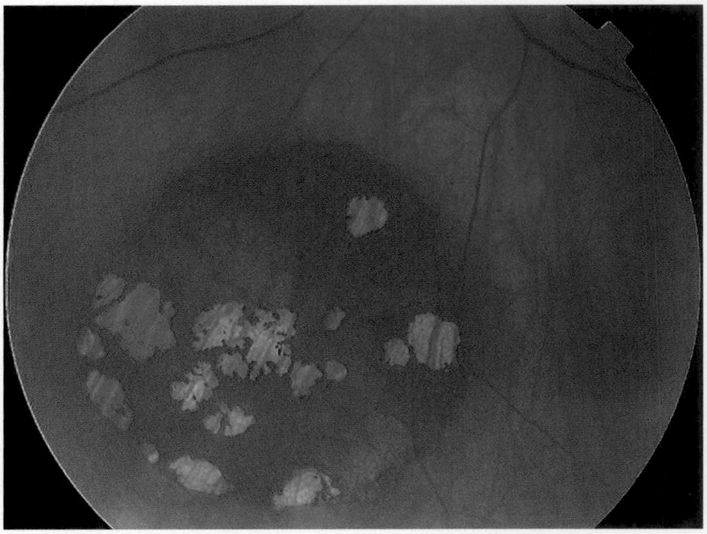

Fig. 9.149 Depigmented lacunae, which often enlarge or coalesce, may be present, particularly in older patients.

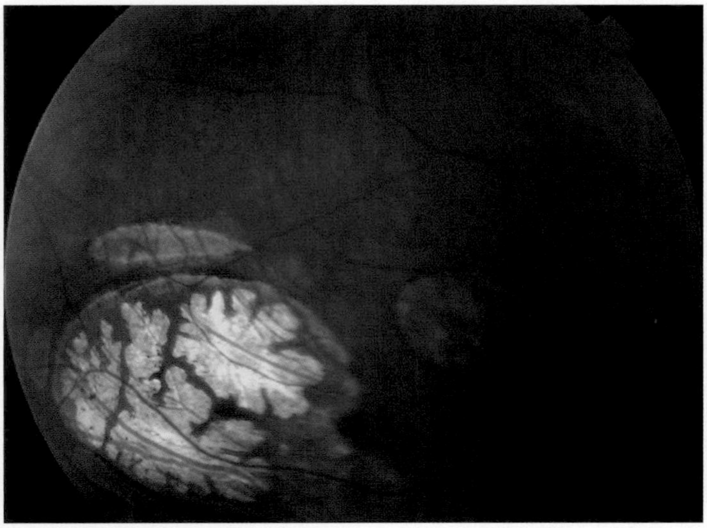

Fig. 9.150 Some lesions may become depigmented with only a thin residual rim of pigment.

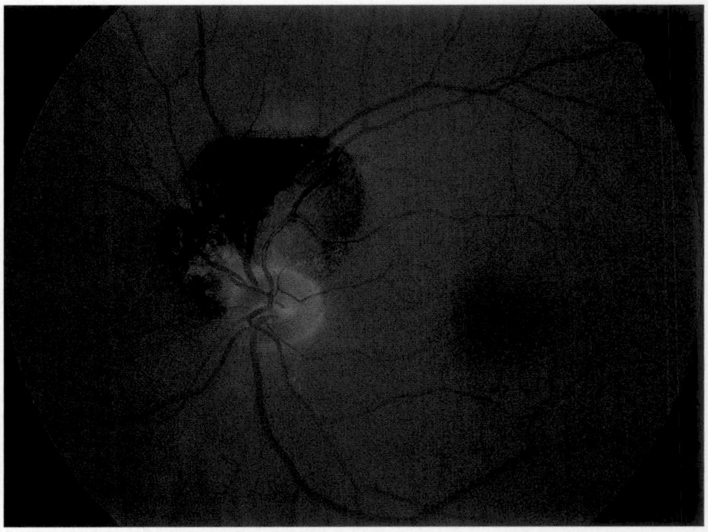

Fig. 9.151 Juxtapapillary CHRPE is uncommon.

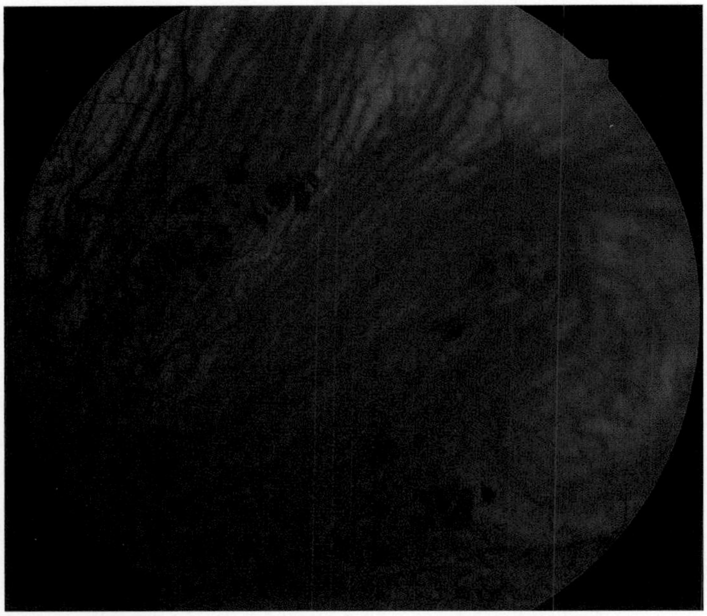

■ **Fig. 9.152** Grouped CRPE is characterised by multiple lesions, often organised in a pattern simulating animal footprints (bear-track pigmentation) with the smaller spots located more centrally.

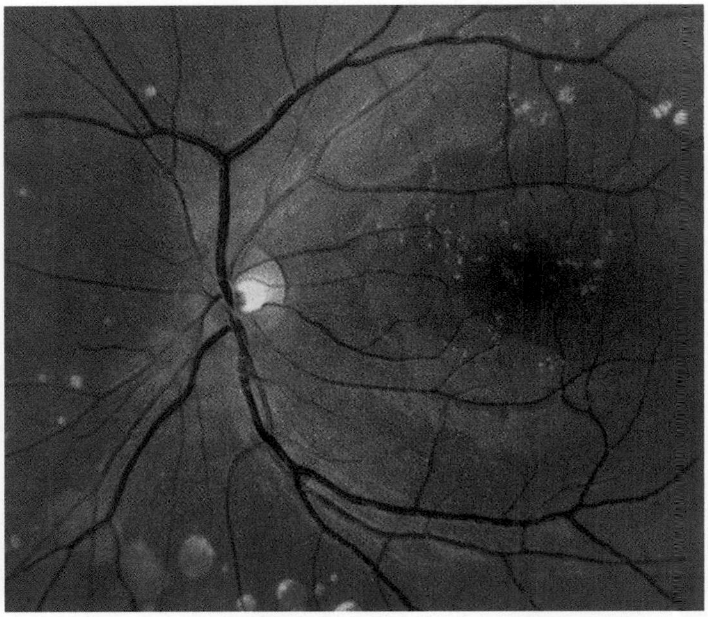

■ **Fig. 9.153** Occasionally the lesions may be depigmented (polar bear tracks).

Atypical

Atypical CHRPE is less common but may have important systemic implications.

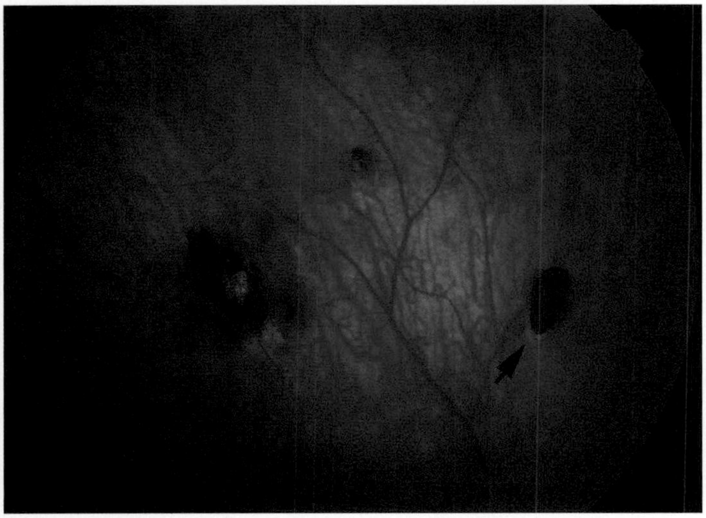

■ **Fig. 9.154** Oral or spindle-shaped lesions with hypopigmentation at one end (arrow), which are multiple, widely separated and bilateral. (Courtesy of C. Barry.)

Familial adenomatous polyposis (FAP)

FAP is a dominantly inherited condition characterised by adenomatous polyps throughout the rectum and colon, which usually start to develop in adolescence. Over 80% of patients with FAP manifest atypical CHRPE.

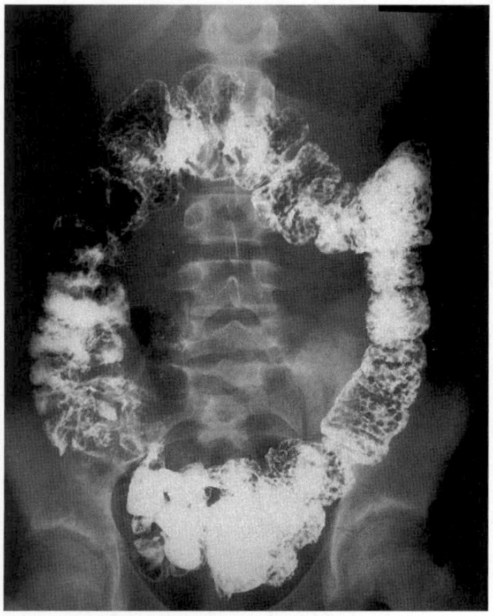

Fig. 9.155 Barium enema showing adenomatous polyposis.

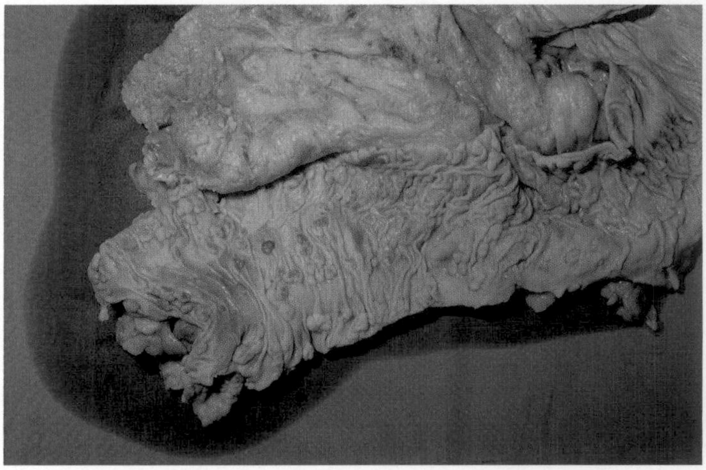

Fig. 9.156 If untreated, virtually all patients with FAP develop carcinoma of the colorectal region by the age of 50 years.

Gardner syndrome

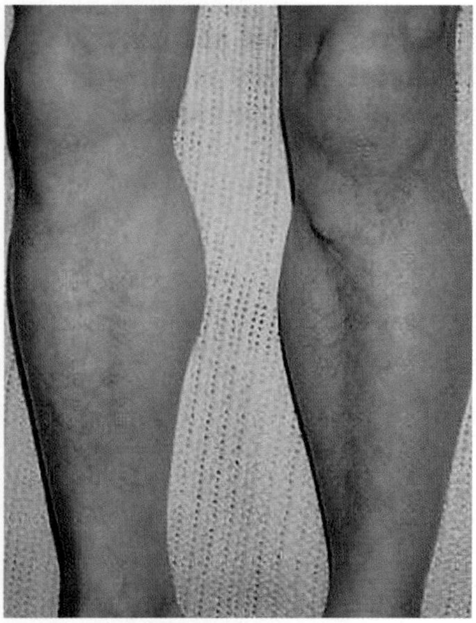

Fig. 9.157 This is characterised by atypical CHRPE, FAP, osteomas (shown here) and epidermoid cysts.

Turcot syndrome

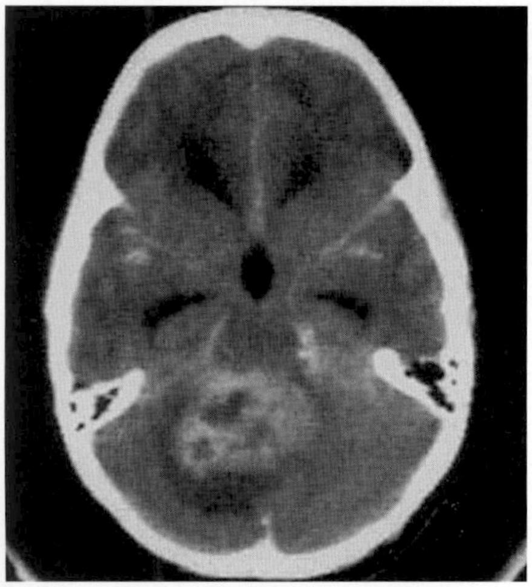

Fig. 9.158 This is characterised by atypical CHRPE, FAP and brain tumours, particularly medulloblastoma (shown here) and astrocytoma. (Courtesy of P. Trend, M. Swash and C. Kennard.)

Combined hamartoma of the retina and retinal pigment epithelium

Combined hamartoma of the retina and RPE is a rare, usually unilateral malformation, which predominantly affects males.

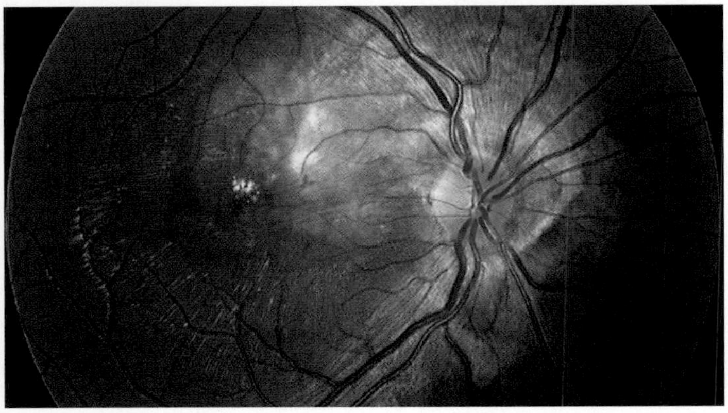

Fig. 9.159 An early flat juxtapapillary hamartoma showing intra- and epiretinal gliosis without distortion.

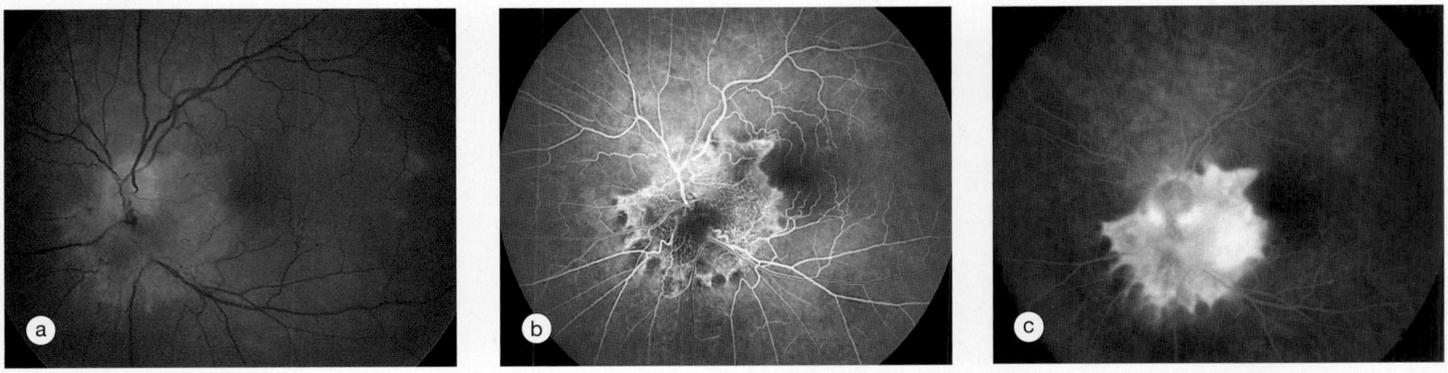

Fig. 9.160 **(a)** A slightly elevated juxtapapillary lesion with mild distortion. **(b)** FA early venous phase highlights a fine network of dilated capillaries and vascular tortuosity. **(c)** Late phase shows marked hyperfluorescence due to leakage. (Courtesy of C. Barry.)

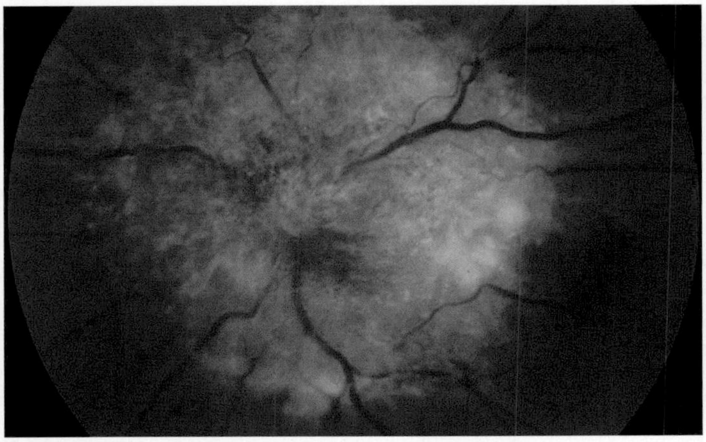

Fig. 9.161 An advanced peripapillary hamartoma showing marked gliosis and partial obscuration of disc vasculature.

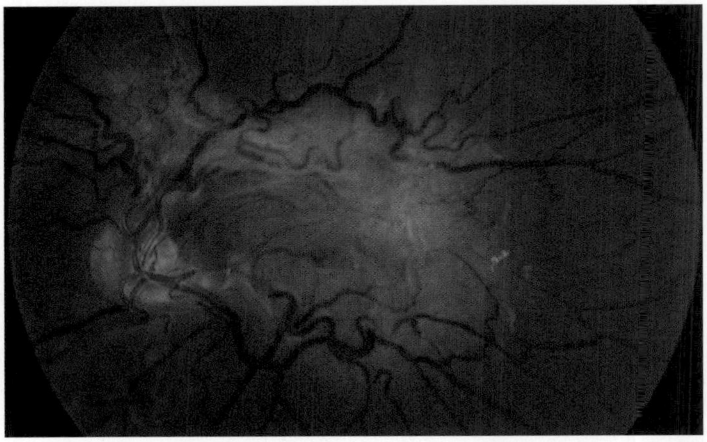

Fig. 9.162 Large hamartoma involving the posterior pole causing severe distortion of the vascular arcades. (Courtesy of P. Gili.)

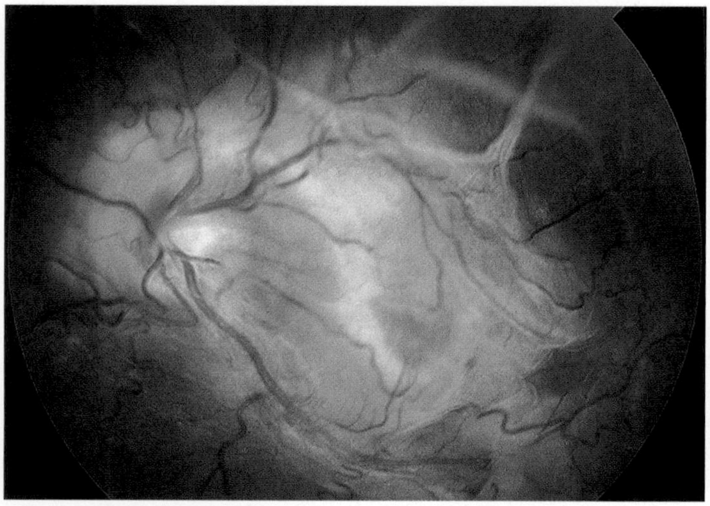

Fig. 9.163 Large hamartoma involving the posterior pole with extensive epiretinal gliosis and distortion. (Courtesy of S. Milewski.)

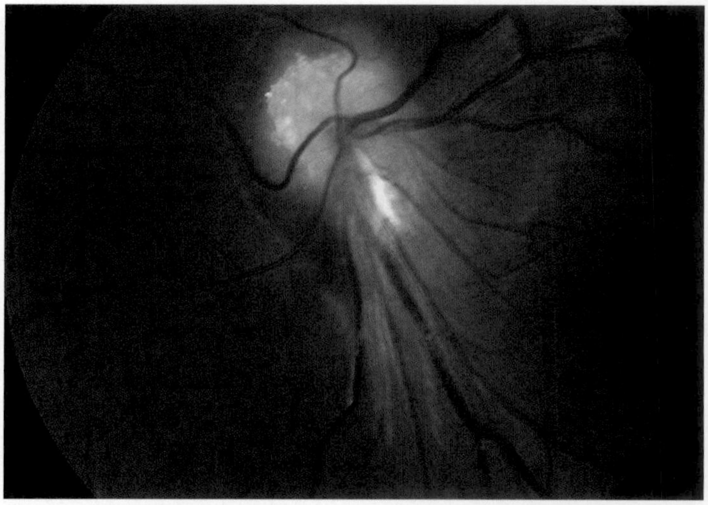

Fig. 9.164 A peripheral lesion is characterised by a linear ridge associated with retinal distortion and vascular stretching; also note optic disc drusen.

Congenital hamartoma of the retinal pigment epithelium

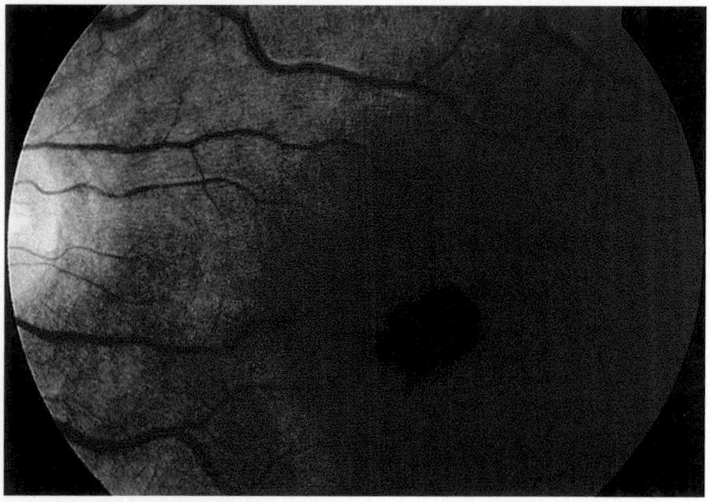

Fig. 9.165 This is a rare, small, jet-black lesion typically located adjacent to the fovea.

Solitary albinotic naevus of the retinal pigment epithelium

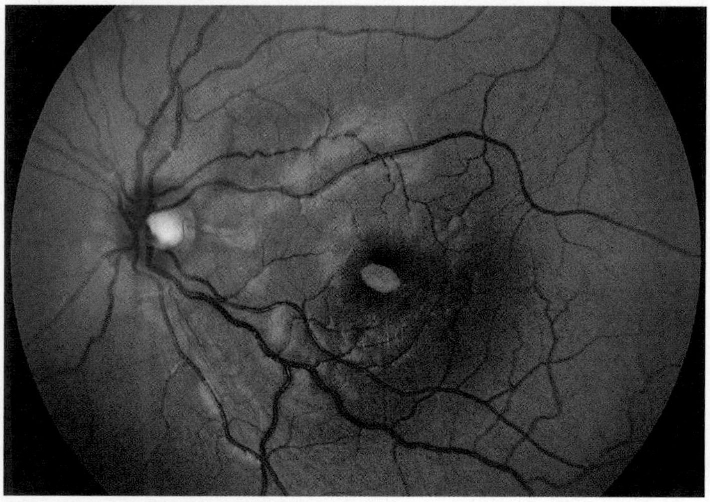

Fig. 9.166 Hypopigmented, reddish-orange, oval or fish-shaped lesion, similar in shape to atypical CHRPE, at the posterior pole or peripheral fundus.

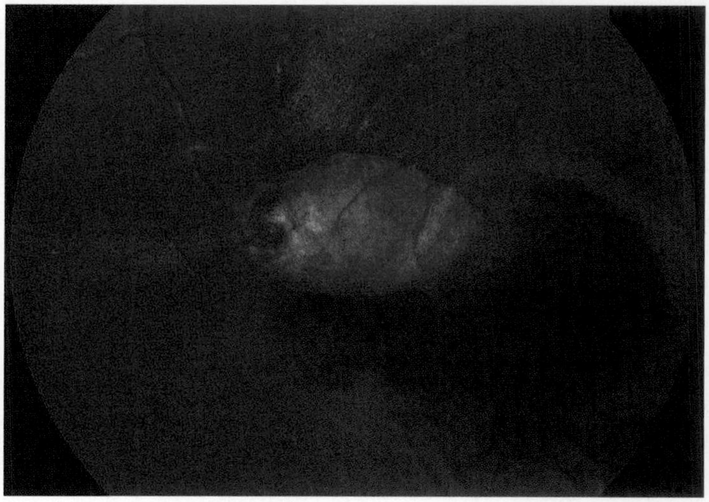

Fig. 9.167 Magnified view of a similar lesion in another patient.

CHAPTER 10

UVEITIS

ANTERIOR UVEITIS

Signs

Circumcorneal (ciliary) injection

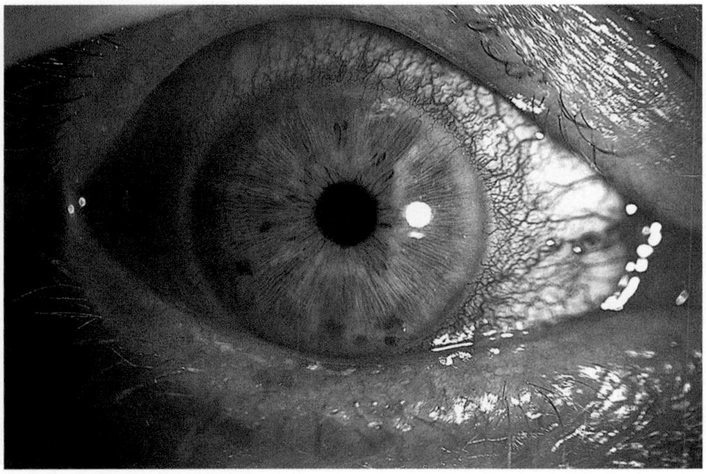

■ **Fig. 10.1** Ciliary injection occurs in acute anterior uveitis and has a violaceous hue; also note miosis.

Keratic precipitates (KP)

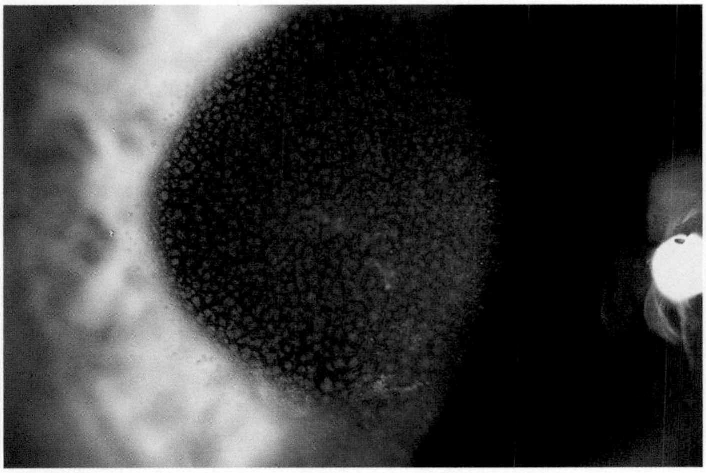

■ **Fig. 10.2** Endothelial dusting by myriads of cells occurs in acute anterior uveitis and during subacute exacerbations of chronic uveitis.

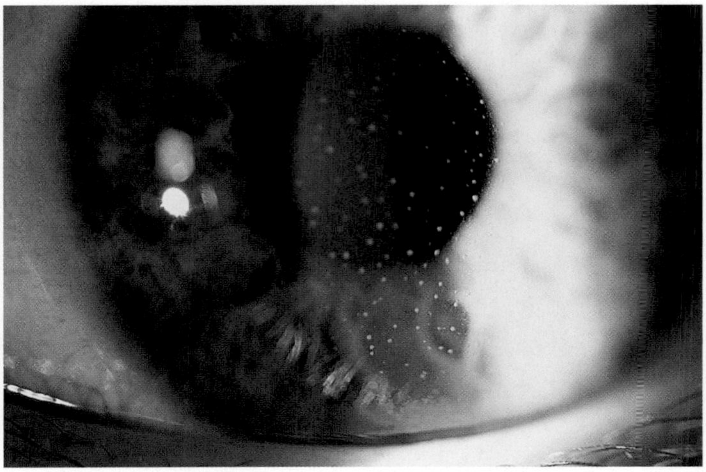

■ **Fig. 10.3** Medium-sized KP occur in most types of acute and chronic anterior uveitis.

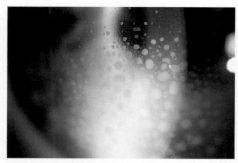

■ **Fig. 10.4** Large 'mutton fat' KP typically occur in granulomatous uveitis.

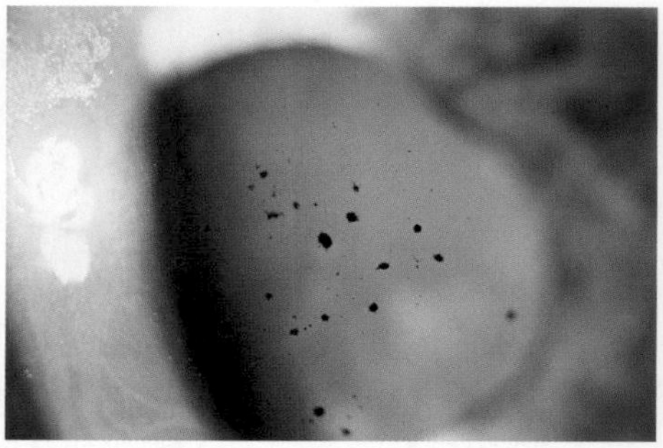

■ **Fig. 10.5** Old KP are pigmented.

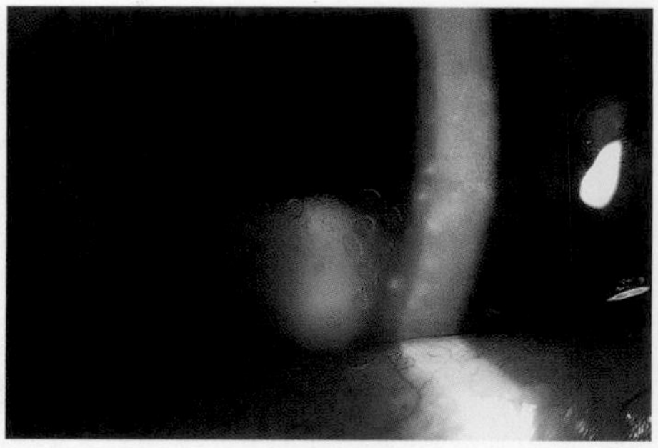

■ **Fig. 10.6** Old, large KP may leave a 'ground-glass' endothelial imprint.

Aqueous

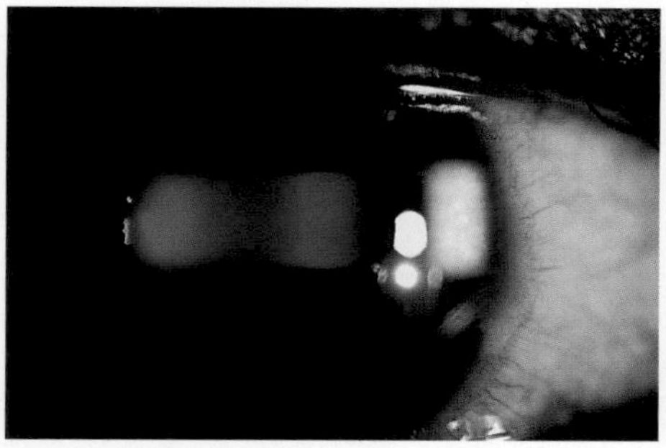

■ **Fig. 10.7** Flare and cells, the extent of which is proportional to the severity of inflammation.

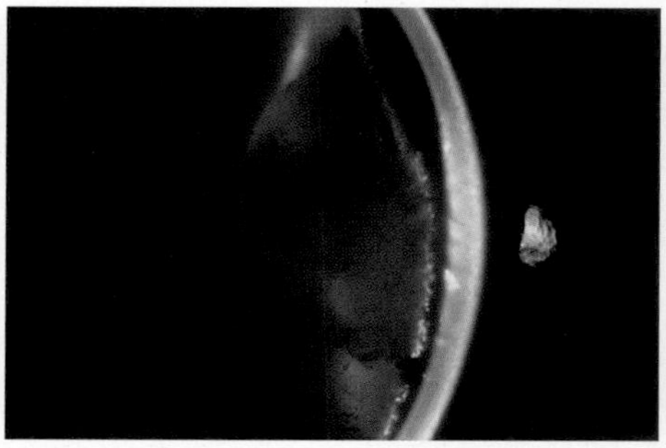

■ **Fig. 10.8** A fibrinous exudate is indicative of severe acute anterior uveitis, especially in patients positive for HLA-B27.

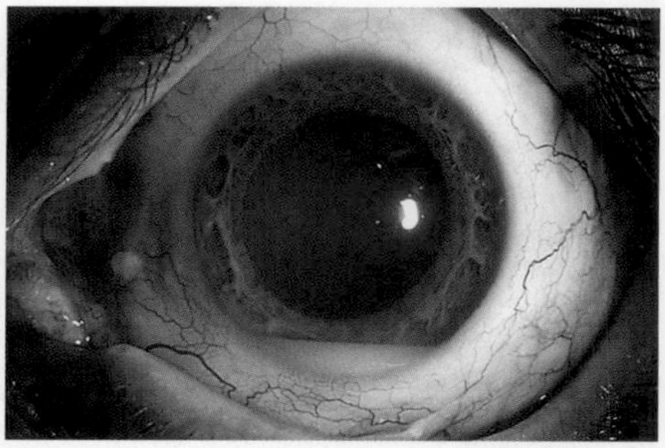

■ **Fig. 10.9** Hypopyon occurs in very severe acute anterior uveitis.

Iris nodules

Nodules are a feature of granulomatous inflammation.

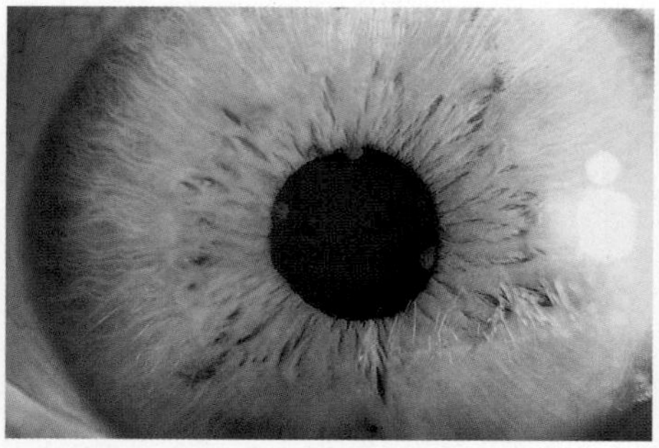

■ **Fig. 10.10** Koeppe nodules are small and situated at the pupillary border.

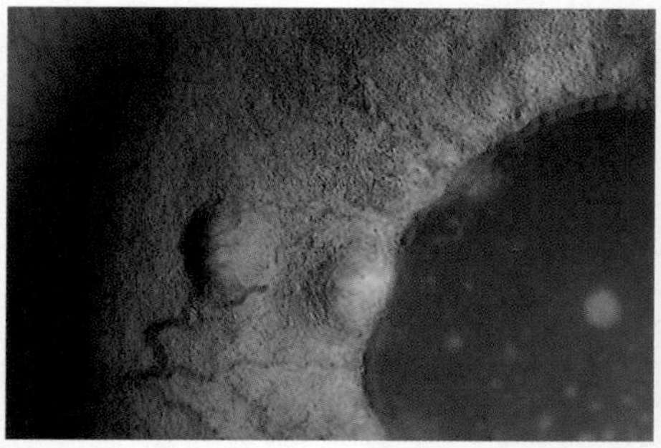

■ **Fig. 10.11** Busacca nodules are less common and located on the surface of the iris. (Courtesy of C. Pavesio.)

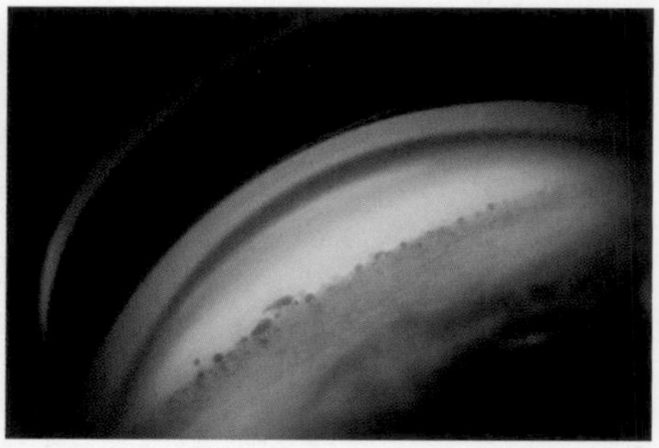

■ **Fig. 10.12** Nodules in the chamber angle. (Courtesy of R. Curtis.)

Complications

Synechiae

Posterior synechiae

Posterior synechiae are adhesions between the iris and anterior lens capsule.

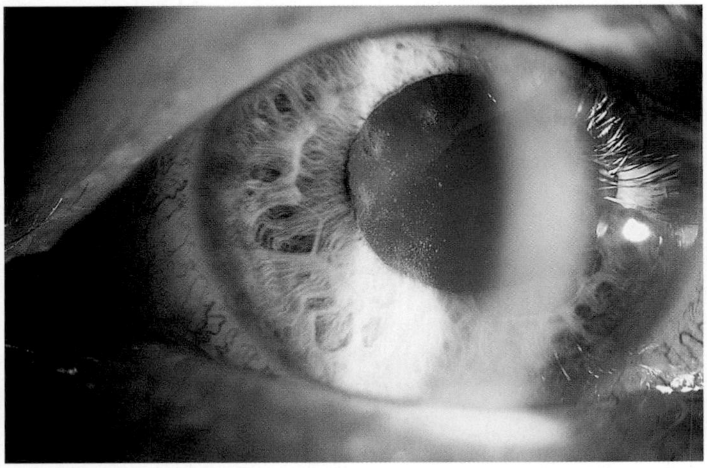

■ **Fig.10.13** Two small posterior synechiae in acute anterior uveitis.

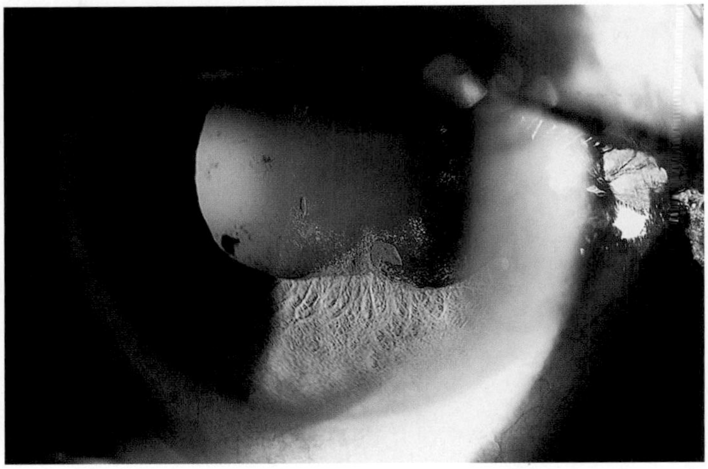

■ **Fig. 10.14** More extensive posterior synechiae.

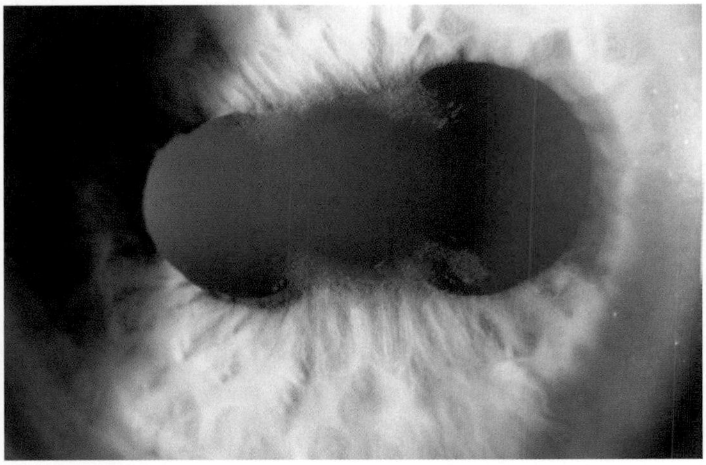

■ **Fig. 10.15** Strong posterior synechiae that cannot be broken by dilating the pupil. (Courtesy of L. Merin.)

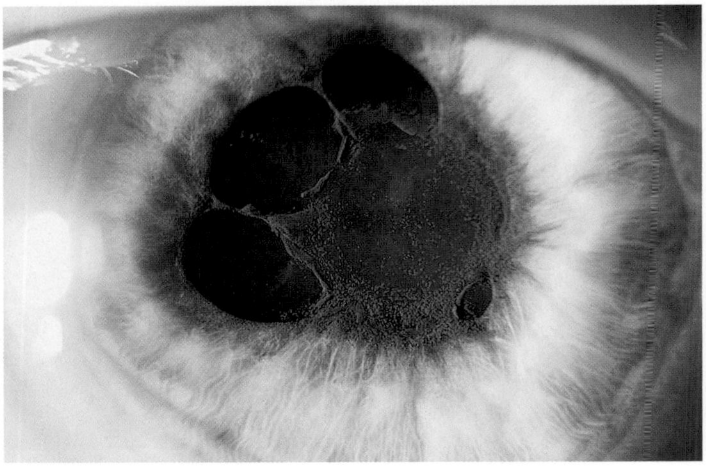

■ **Fig. 10.16** Extensive posterior synechiae with a sheet of pigment on the anterior lens capsule.

Peripheral anterior synechiae

Peripheral anterior synechiae (PAS) extend from the peripheral iris to the trabecular meshwork and peripheral cornea.

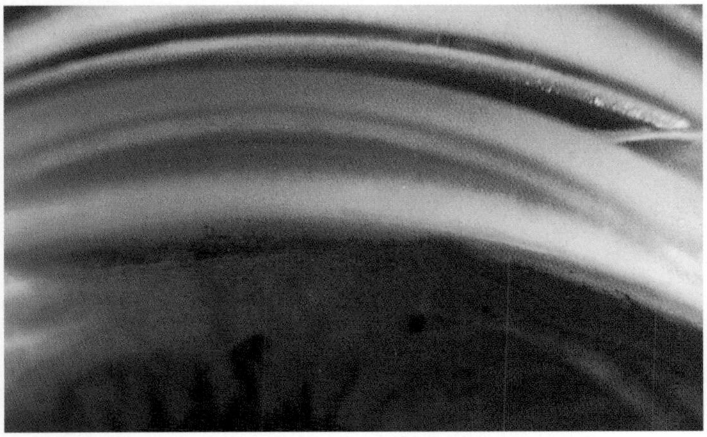

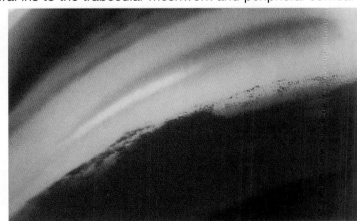

■ **Fig. 10.17** Early PAS involving the trabecular meshwork.

■ **Fig. 10.18** Extensive broad PAS.

Band keratopathy

Band keratopathy may occur in chronic anterior uveitis, especially in children.

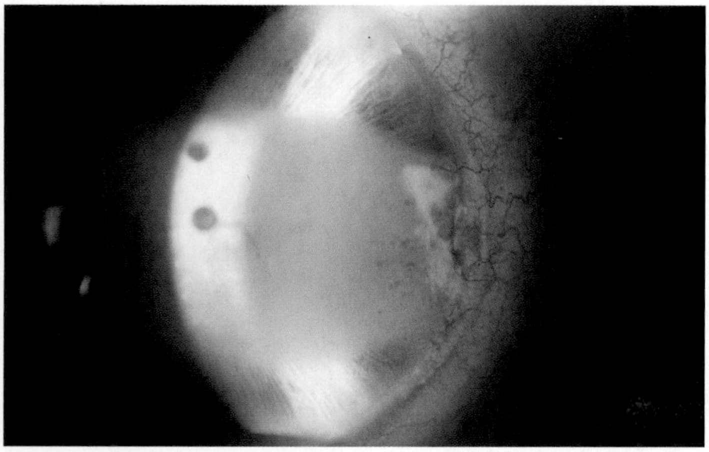

Fig. 10.19 Interpalpebral corneal deposition of calcium.

Cataract

Secondary lens opacities may occur in chronic anterior uveitis.

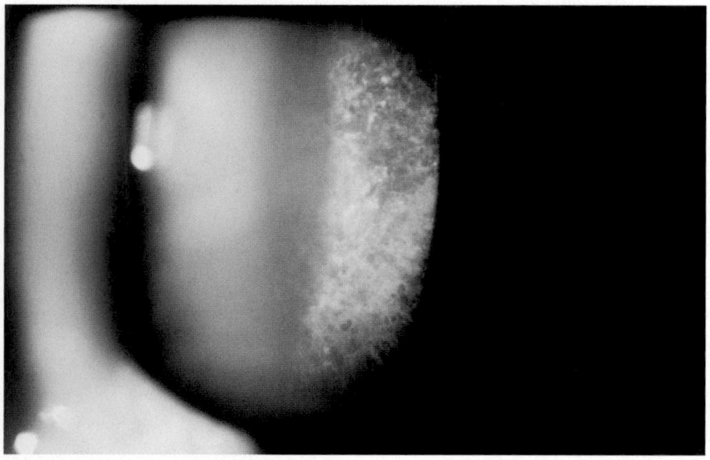

Fig. 10.20 The opacity is typically posterior subcapsular.

Phthisis bulbi

Phthisis bulbi may be the end result of severe uncontrolled chronic anterior uveitis.

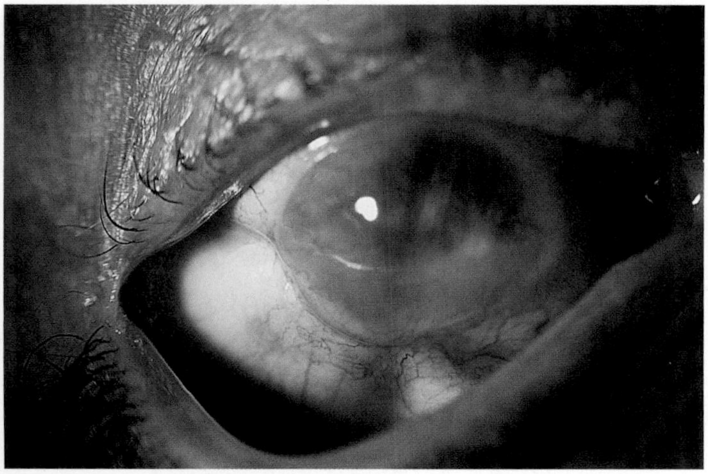

Fig. 10.21 A soft, shrunken globe.

COMMON SPECIFIC UVEITIS ENTITIES

Fuchs heterochromic cyclitis

Fuchs heterochromic cyclitis is a chronic, non-granulomatous, unilateral anterior uveitis of insidious onset.

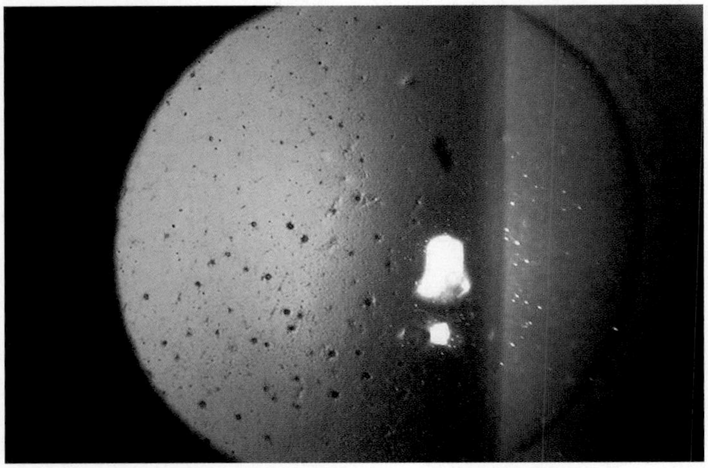

■ **Fig. 10.22** KPs are small, round or stellate, grey-white in colour and scattered throughout the corneal endothelium. Feathery fibrin filaments may be seen in between the KP. (Courtesy of C. Pavesio.)

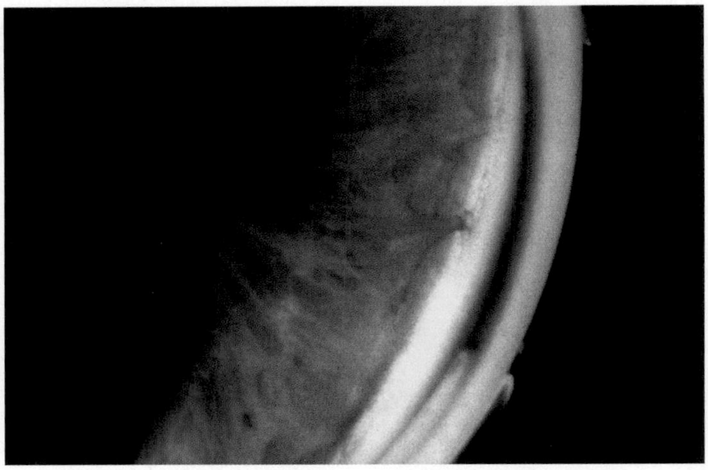

■ **Fig. 10.23** Small, irregular PAS and twig-like angle vessels. (Courtesy of R. Curtis.)

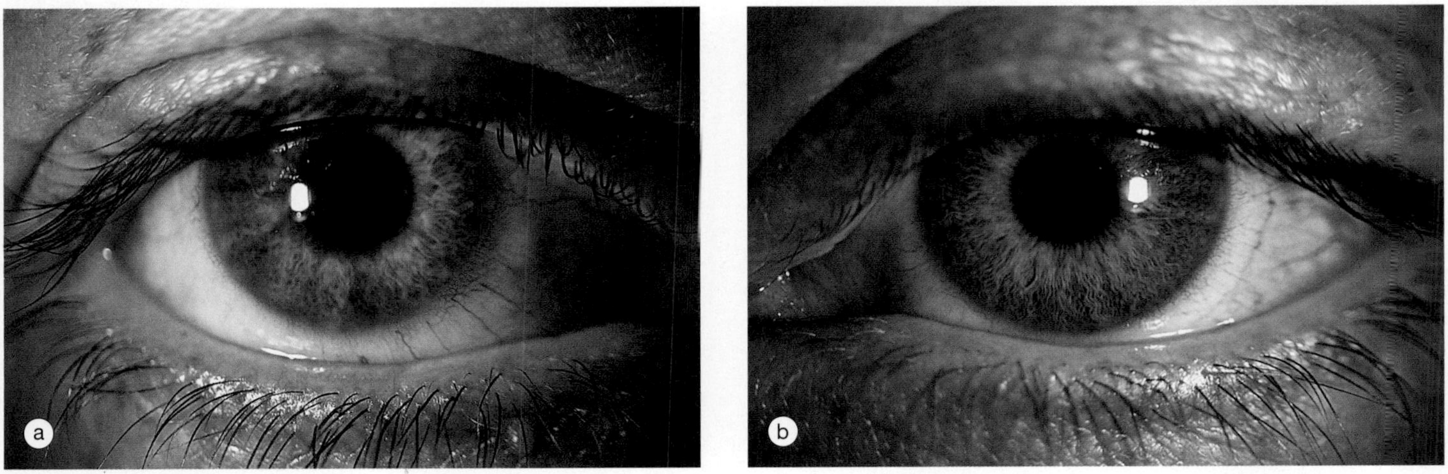

■ **Fig. 10.24** **(a)** Loss of iris crypts and early stromal atrophy. **(b)** Normal fellow eye for comparison.

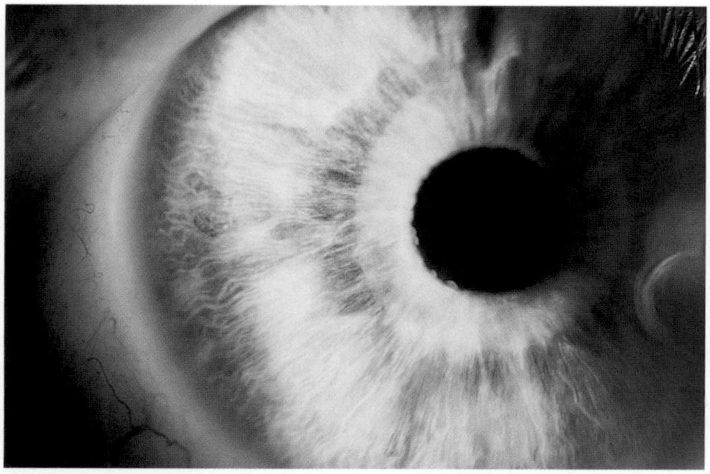

■ **Fig. 10.25** Advanced stromal atrophy makes the affected iris appear dull, with loss of detail, giving rise to a washed-out appearance, particularly in the pupillary zone; also note a few Koeppe nodules.

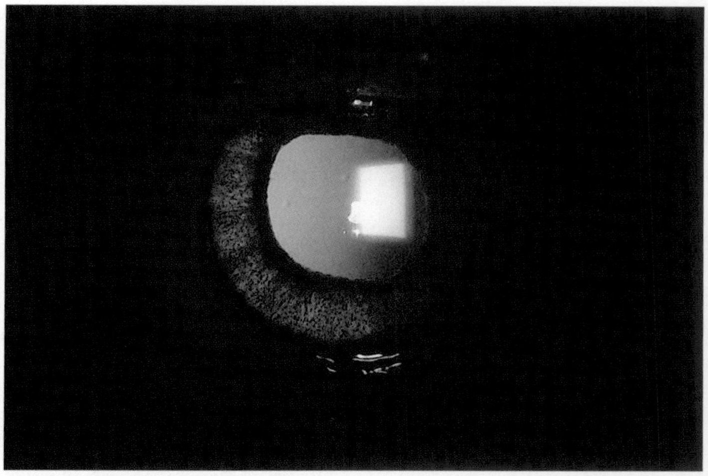

■ **Fig. 10.26** Severe posterior pigment layer iris atrophy seen on retroillumination.

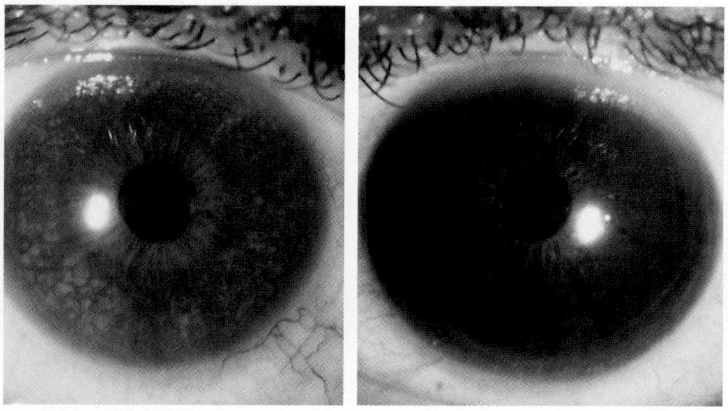

■ **Fig. 10.27** Heterochromia iridis, in which the affected eye (right) is usually hypochromic.

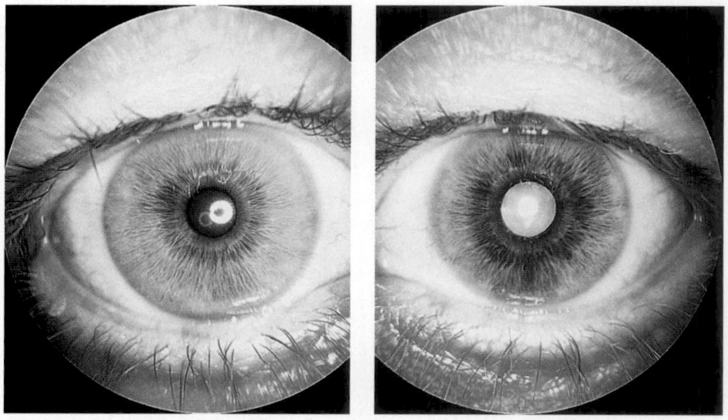

■ **Fig. 10.28** Occasionally the affected eye (left) is slightly hyperchromic because stromal atrophy allows the pigment layer to show through; note the mature cataract.

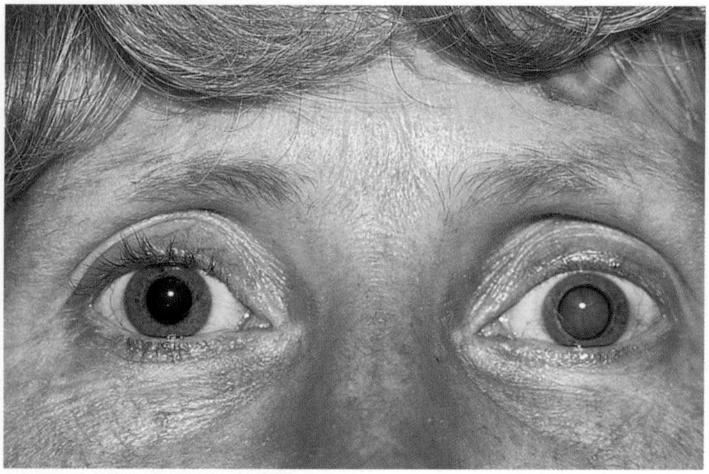

■ **Fig. 10.29** Cataract (left eye) is extremely common and does not differ from that associated with other types of anterior uveitis.

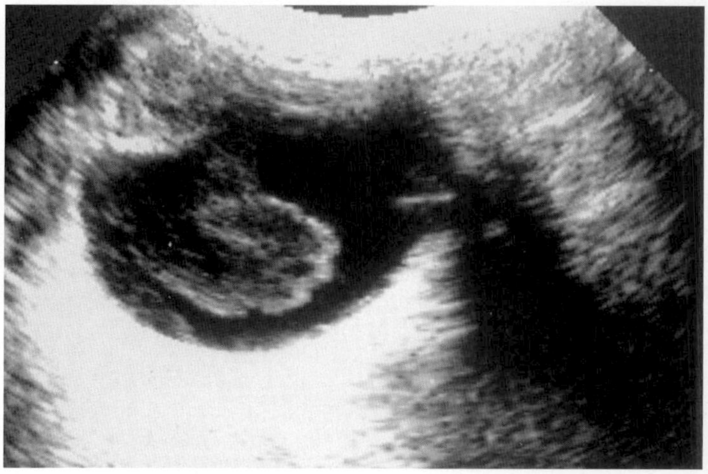

■ **Fig. 10.30** US showing vitreous opacities. (Courtesy of C. Pavesio.)

Intermediate uveitis

Intermediate uveitis is an idiopathic, insidious, inflammatory disease affecting the pars plana, peripheral retina and underlying choroid. Systemic diseases that may be associated with 'secondary intermediate uveitis' include sarcoidosis, Lyme disease, non-Hodgkin B-cell lymphoma, cat-scratch fever, multiple sclerosis and Whipple disease.

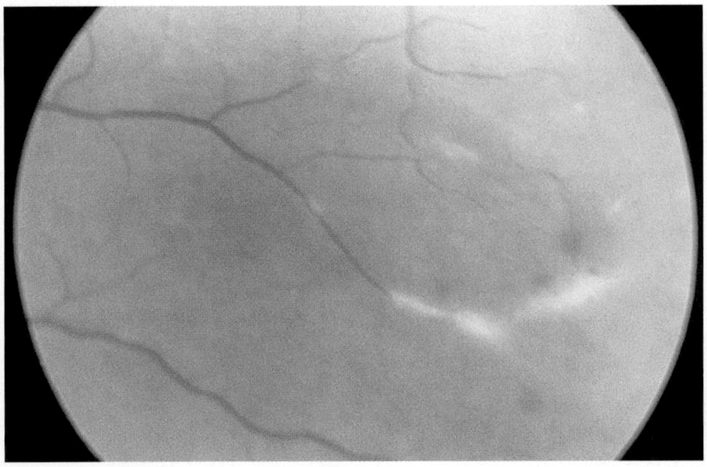

Fig. 10.31 Mild peripheral periphlebitis.

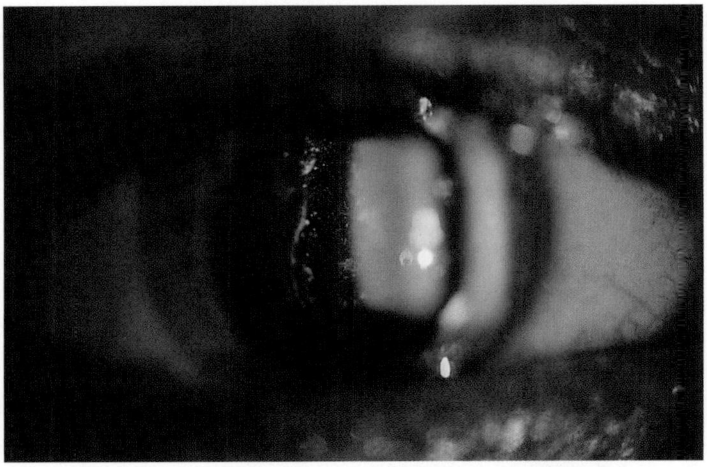

Fig. 10.32 Vitritis with cells in the anterior vitreous.

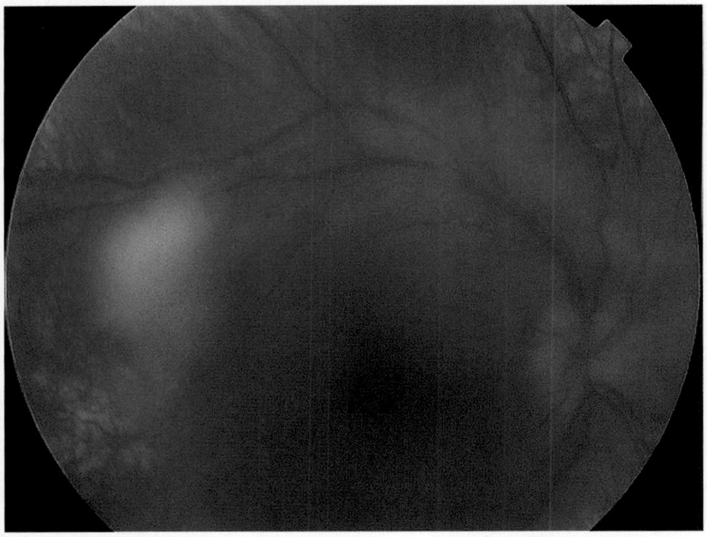

Fig. 10.33 Vitreous haze and a gelatinous vitreous exudate ('snowball' or 'cotton ball').

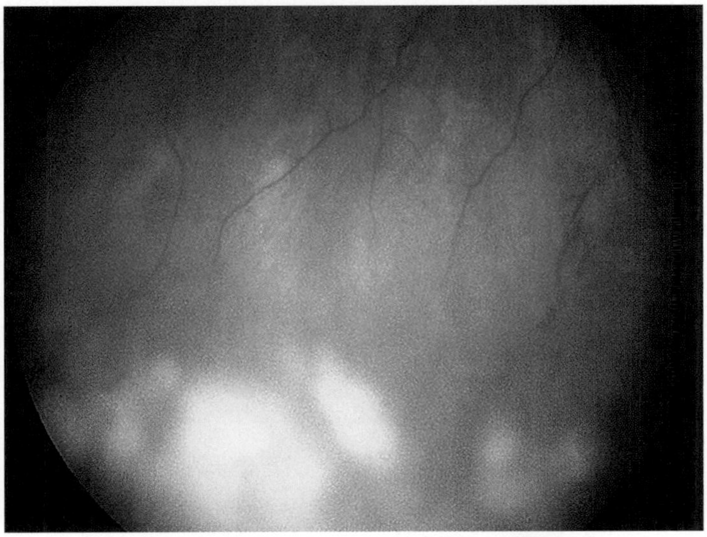

Fig. 10.34 Increase in number and size of 'cotton balls'.

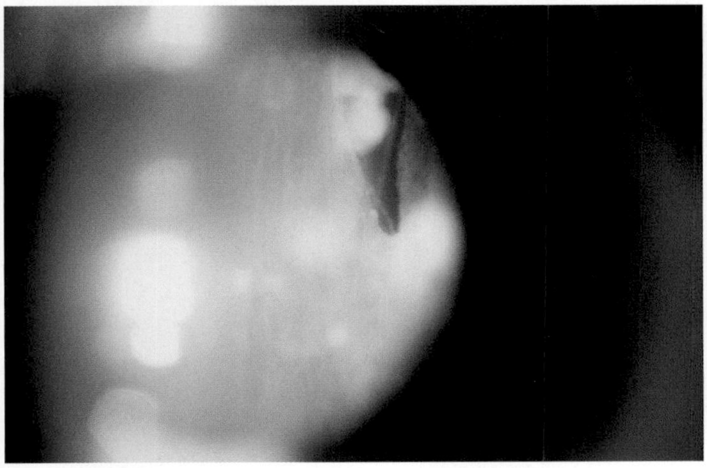

Fig. 10.35 Condensation of cotton balls and severe vitreous opacification.

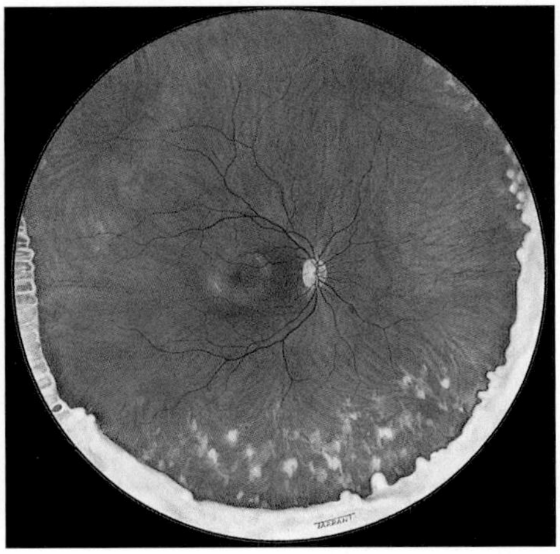

Fig. 10.36 Snowbanking is the hallmark of pars planitis.

UVEITIS IN ARTHROPATHIES

Spondyloarthropathies

Ankylosing spondylitis

Ankylosing spondylitis (AS) primarily involves the sacroiliac joints and axial skeleton. Some patients also have ulcerative colitis. Acute anterior uveitis occurs in about 30% of cases.

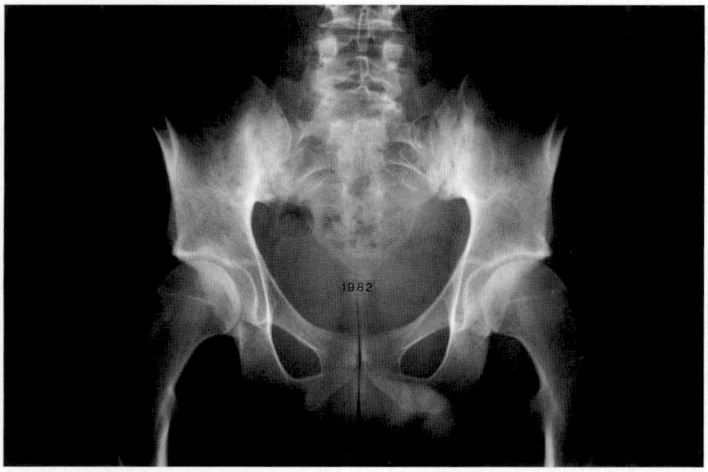

Fig. 10.37 Bilateral, symmetrical sclerosis and bony obliteration of the sacroiliac joints.

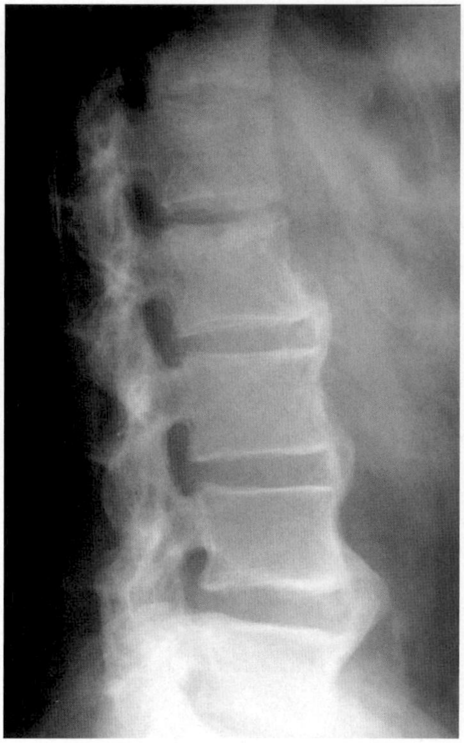

Fig. 10.38 Severe spinal involvement with bony bridging by syndesmophytes (bamboo spine). (Courtesy of S. Ghiacy.)

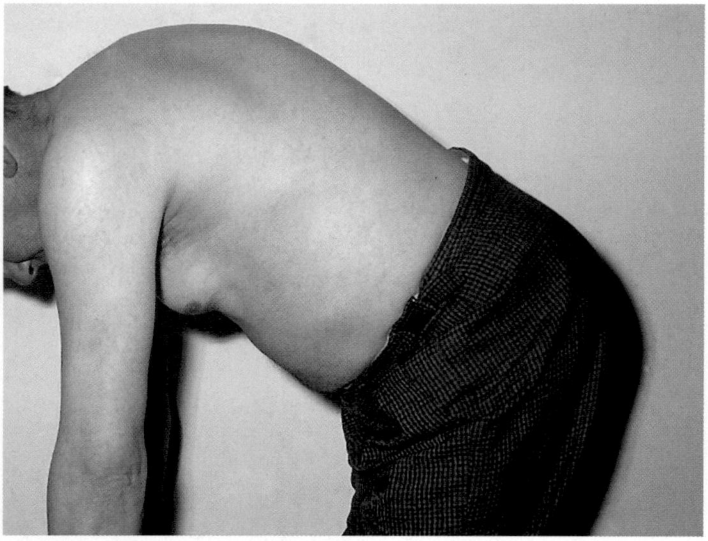

Fig. 10.39 Limitation of spinal flexion.

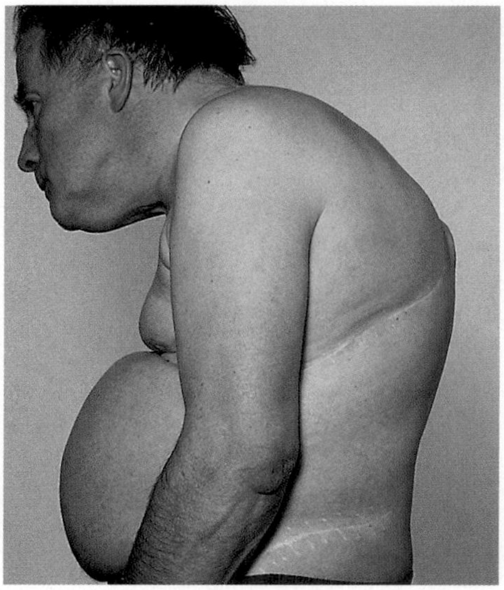

Fig. 10.40 Severe fixed thoracic kyphosis producing a question-mark appearance. (Courtesy of M. A. Mir.)

Reiter syndrome

Reiter syndrome is characterised by the triad of urethritis, conjunctivitis and arthritis. Acute anterior uveitis occurs in about 20% of cases.

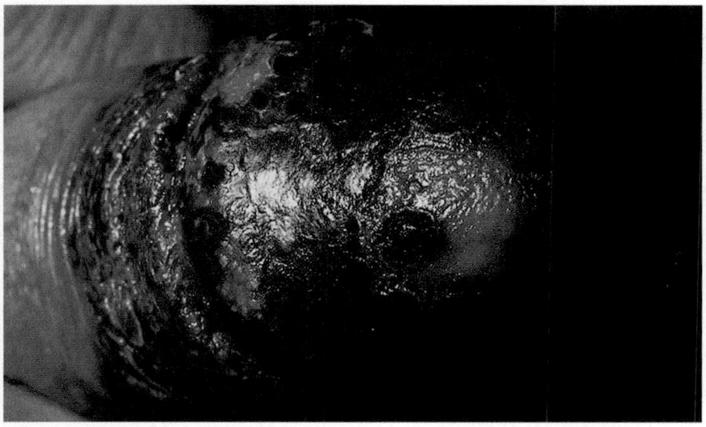

Fig. 10.41 Severe circinate balanitis. (Courtesy of R. T. D. Emond, P. D. Welsby and H. A. K. Rowland.)

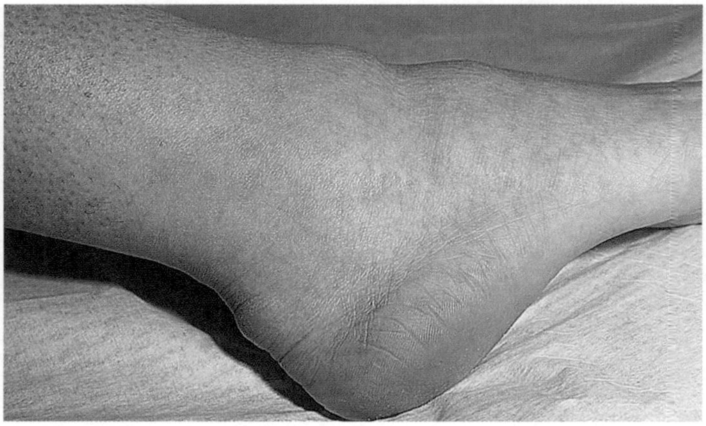

Fig. 10.42 Achilles tendinitis and arthritis.

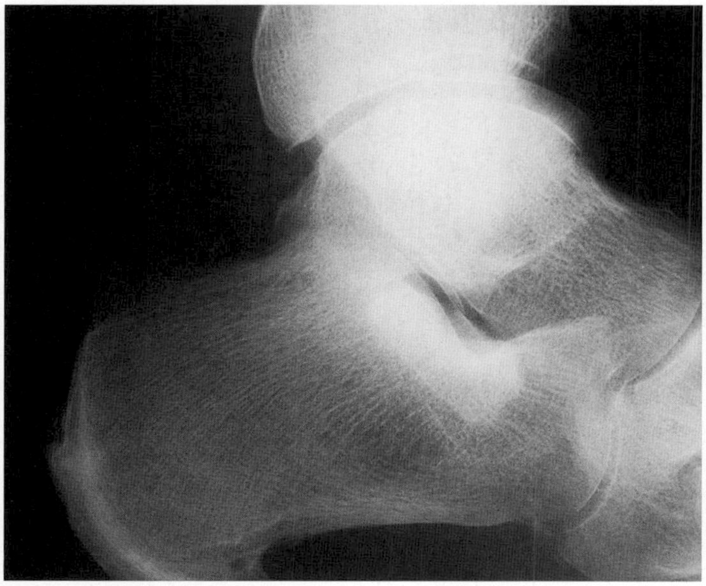

Fig. 10.43 Periostitis resulting in calcaneal spur formation is typical.

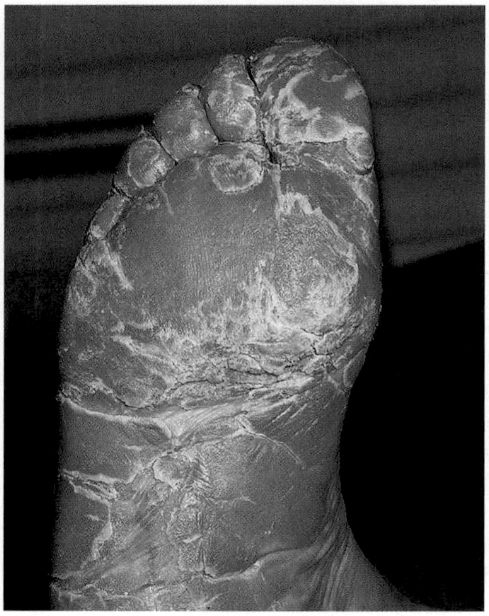

Fig. 10.44 Keratoderma blenorrhagica is characterised by painless crusty plaques on the soles or palms.

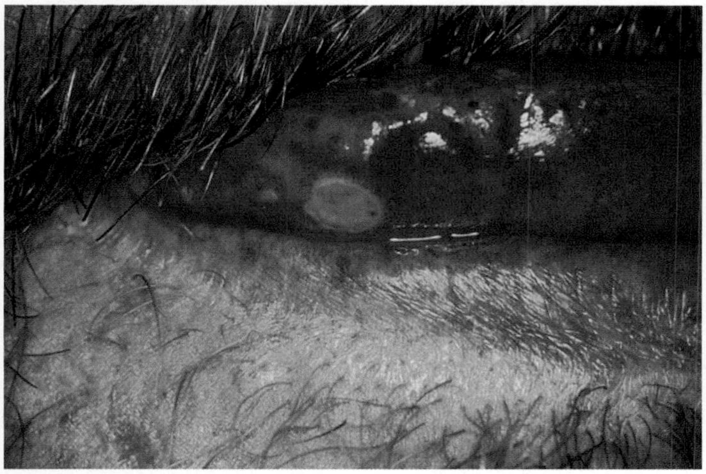

Fig. 10.45 Transient painless mouth ulcers.

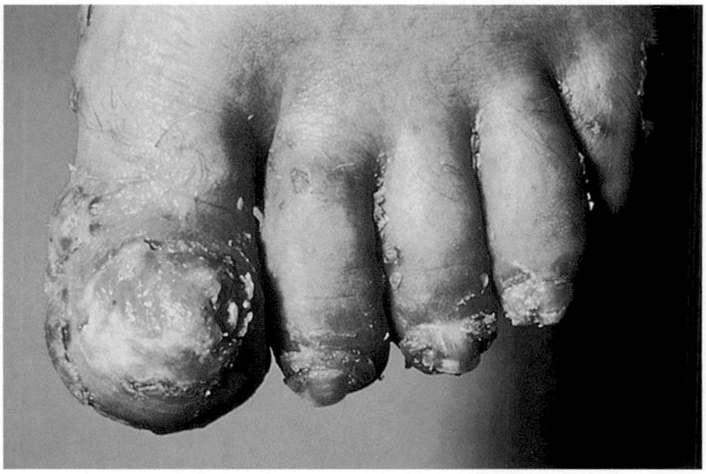

Fig. 10.46 Nail dystrophy with subungual keratosis. (Courtesy of M. A. Mir.)

Psoriatic arthritis

Psoriatic arthritis affects about 7% of patients with psoriasis. Anterior uveitis is uncommon.

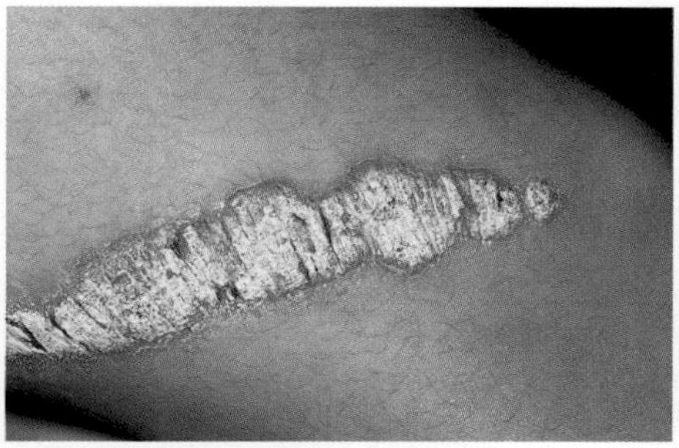

Fig. 10.47 Plaque psoriasis is characterised by well-demarcated silvery plaques, often on extensor surfaces and the scalp.

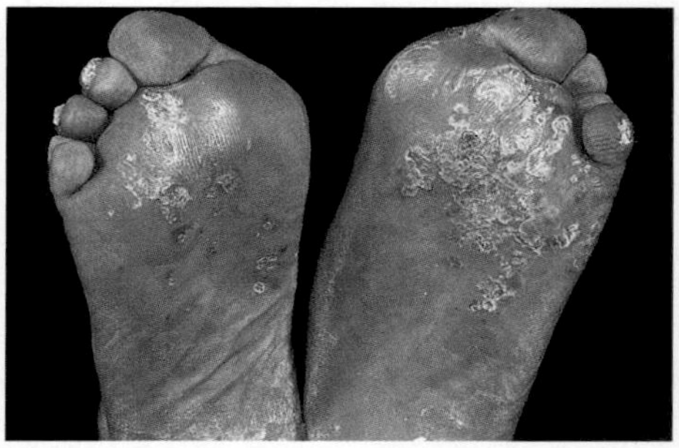

Fig. 10.48 Pustular psoriasis typically involves the soles and palms.

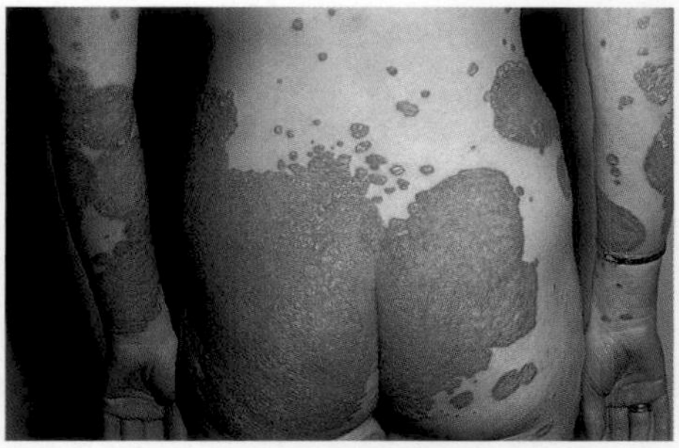

Fig. 10.49 Erythrodermic psoriasis is characterised by severe erythema and scaling involving the trunk and limbs.

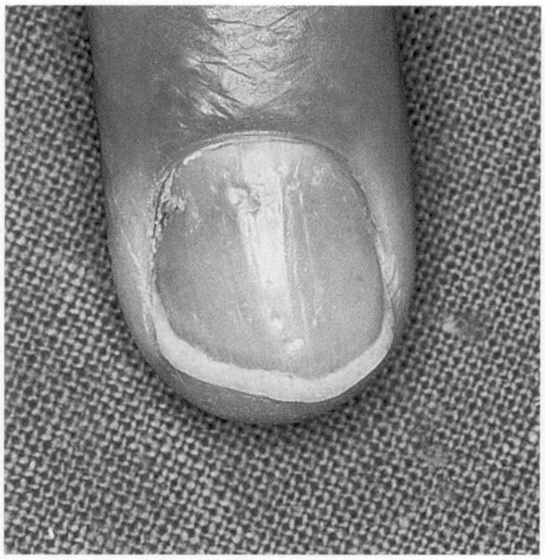

Fig. 10.50 Mild nail pitting is very common.

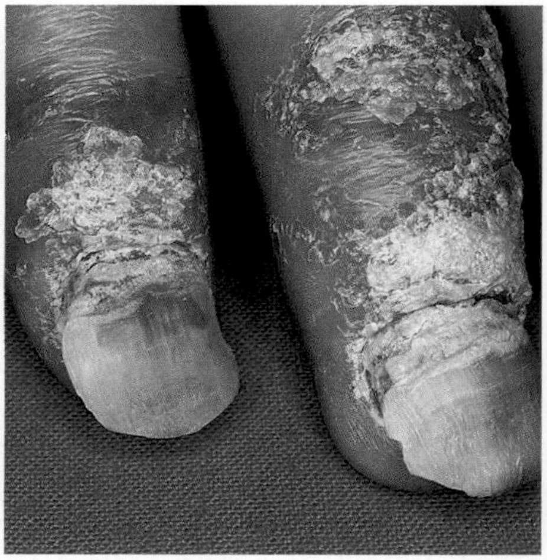

Fig. 10.51 Severe psoriasis and early onycholysis.

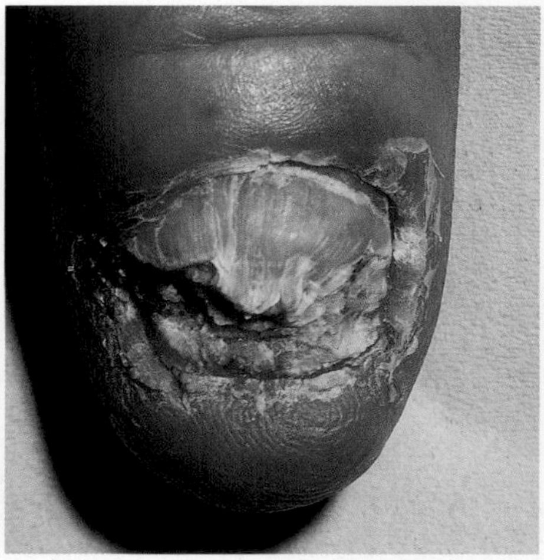

Fig. 10.52 Severe onycholysis and subungual keratosis.

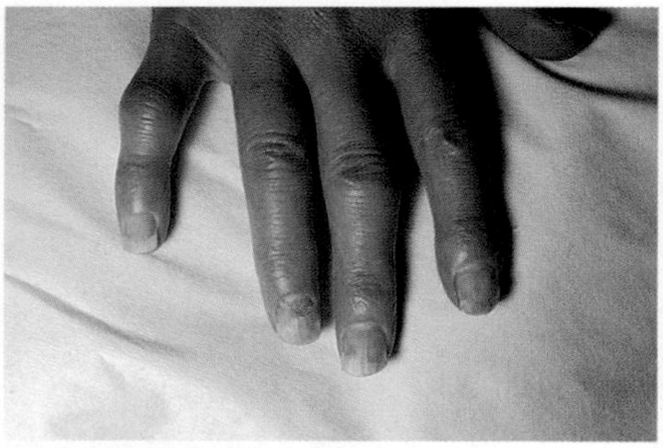

Fig. 10.53 Mild nail dystrophy associated with arthritis involving distal interphalangeal joints, resulting in sausage-shaped fingers.

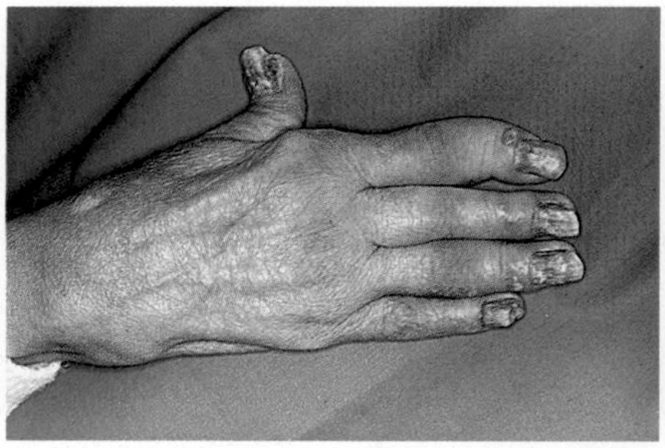

Fig. 10.54 More severe arthritis and nail dystrophy.

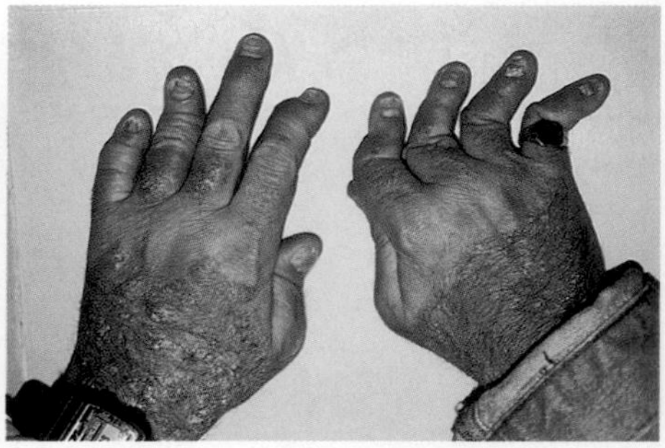

Fig. 10.55 Arthritis mutilans.

Juvenile arthritis

Juvenile idiopathic arthritis

Juvenile idiopathic arthritis (JIA) develops in children before the age of 16 years.

Pauciarticular-onset JIA

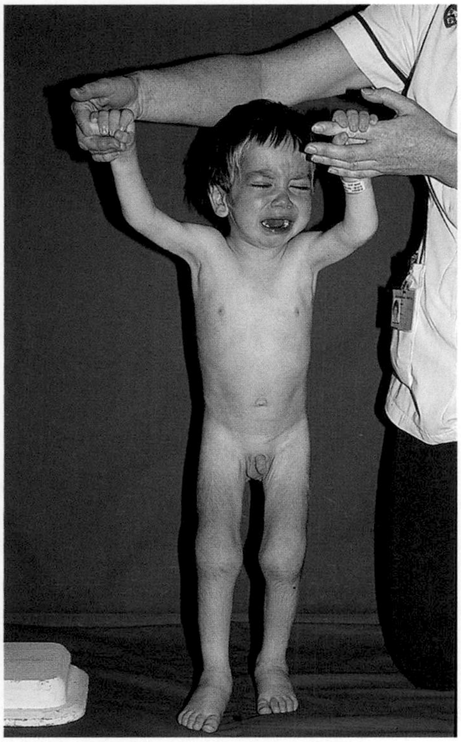

Fig. 10.56 Children at highest risk are those with early pauciarticular-onset JIA in whom four or fewer joints are involved and who are positive for antinuclear antibodies.

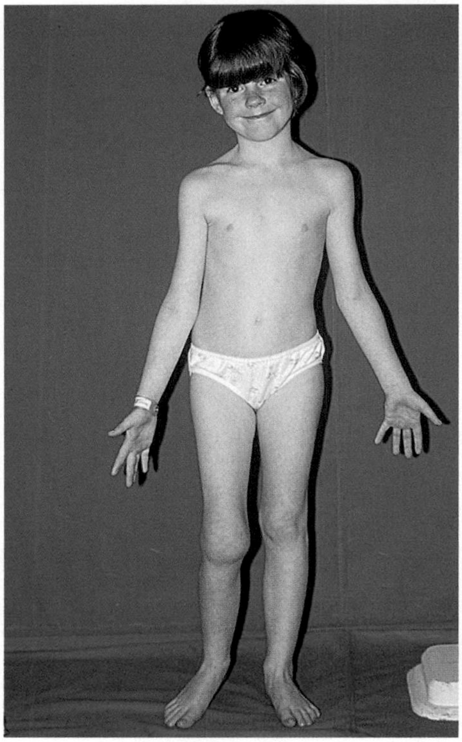

Fig. 10.57 In some cases only one joint is involved, typically the knee, but the risk of uveitis may still be significant.

Polyarticular-onset JIA

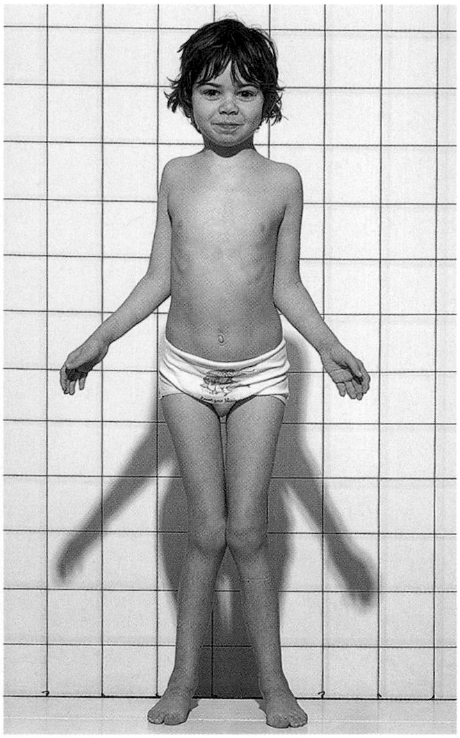

Fig. 10.58 The risk of uveitis is less in older children with polyarticular-onset JIA in whom more than four joints are involved.

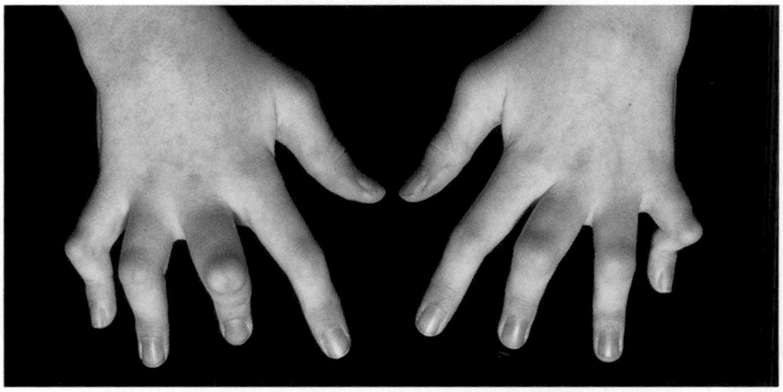

Fig. 10.59 Severe involvement of the hands is uncommon.

Systemic-onset JIA

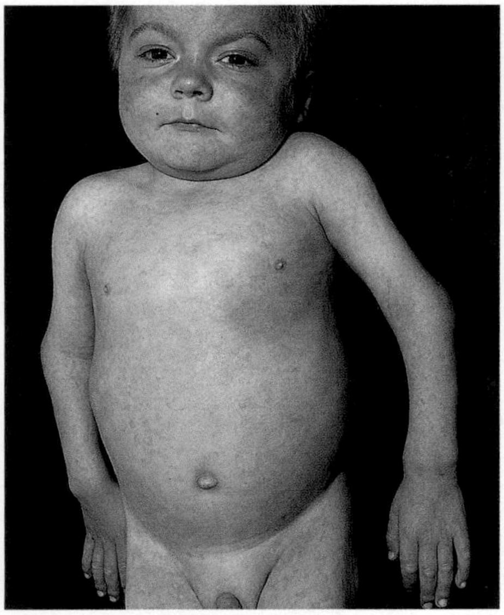

Fig. 10.60 There is no risk of uveitis in children with systemic-onset JIA, which is characterised by fever, rash and hepatosplenomegaly.

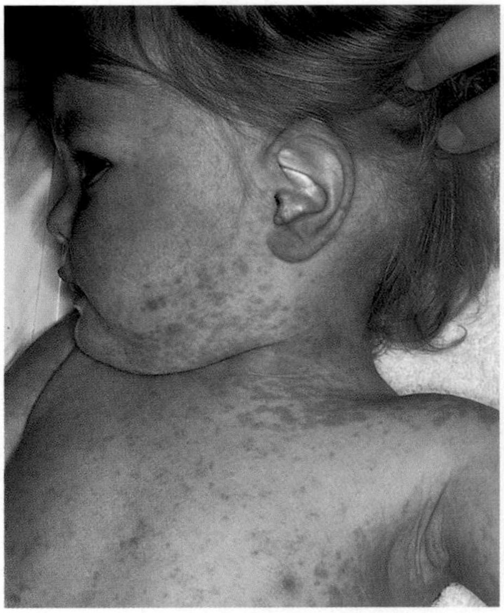

Fig. 10.61 Transient non-itchy maculopapular rash in systemic-onset JIA.

Juvenile ankylosing spondylitis

Juvenile AS is uncommon and typically affects boys around the age of 10 years.

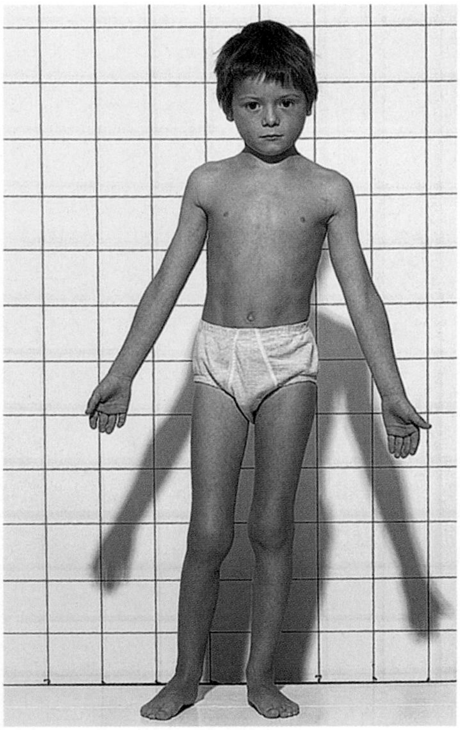

Fig. 10.62 In contrast to adult AS, children tend to present with peripheral joint involvement but, like adults, may develop acute anterior uveitis.

UVEITIS IN INFLAMMATORY BOWEL DISEASE

Ulcerative colitis

Ulcerative colitis is an idiopathic, chronic, relapsing disease involving the rectum and colon. Acute anterior uveitis occurs in about 5% of cases, although the risk is much higher in patients with associated AS.

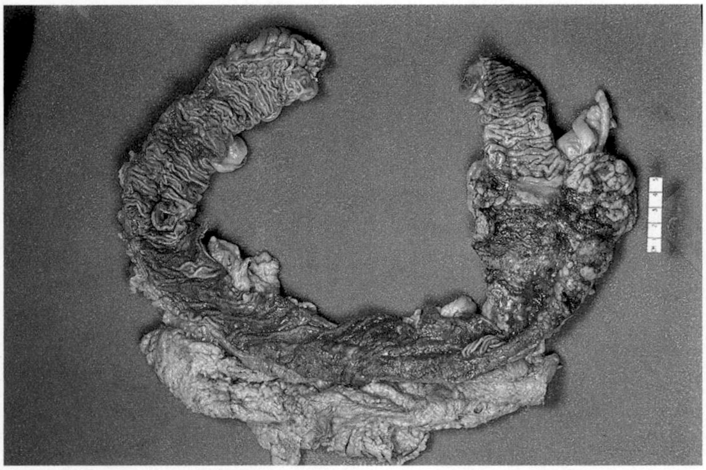

Fig. 10.63 Diffuse surface ulceration of the mucosa with the development of crypt abscesses and pseudopolyposis. Patients with long-standing disease carry an increased risk of developing carcinoma.

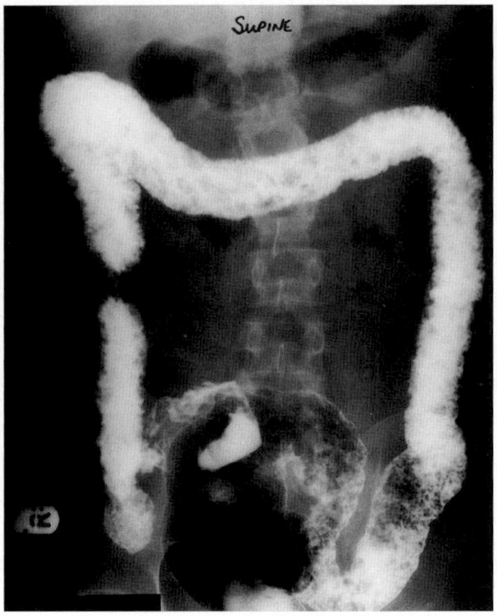

Fig. 10.64 Barium enema showing pseudopolyps, loss of haustral markings and straightening of the colon.

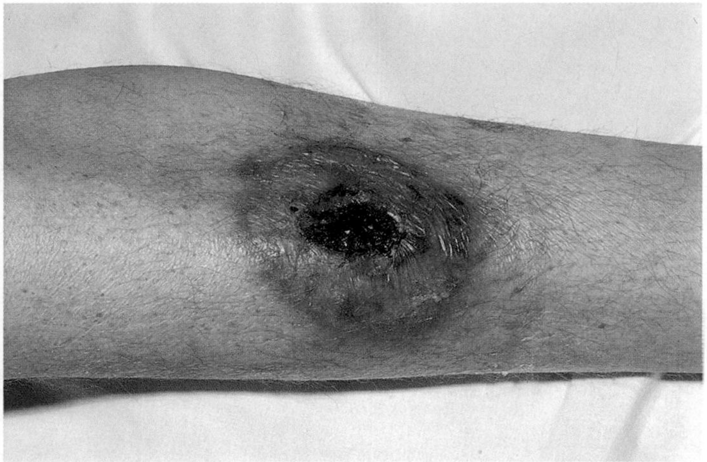

Fig. 10.65 Pyoderma gangrenosum, which is characterised by necrosis and irregular ulceration, typically appears during the acute phase and resolves when the colitis is controlled.

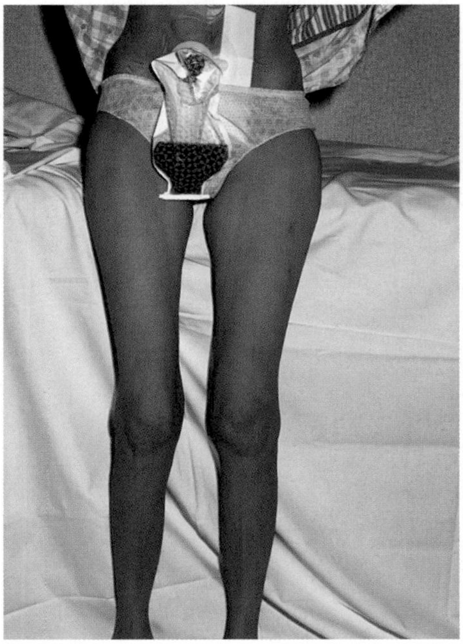

Fig. 10.66 Colectomy and ileostomy is required in about 50% of patients with extensive disease

Crohn disease

Crohn disease is an idiopathic, chronic, relapsing disease that most frequently involves the ileocaecal region, but any part of the gastrointestinal tract may be affected from mouth to anus. Acute anterior uveitis occurs in about 3% of patients.

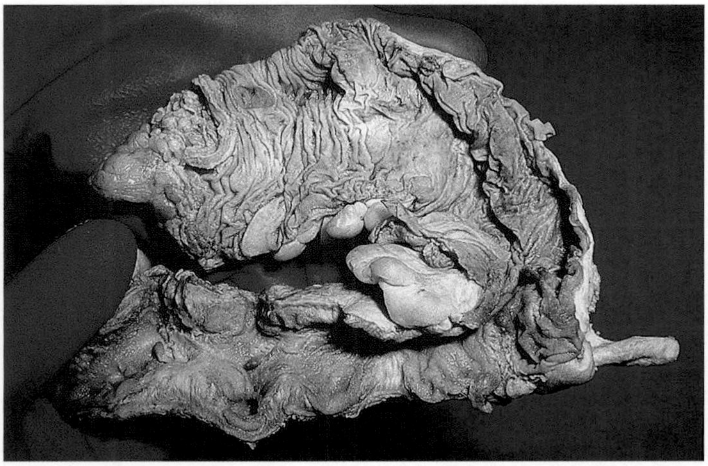

Fig. 10.67 Crohn disease affecting the ileocaecal region.

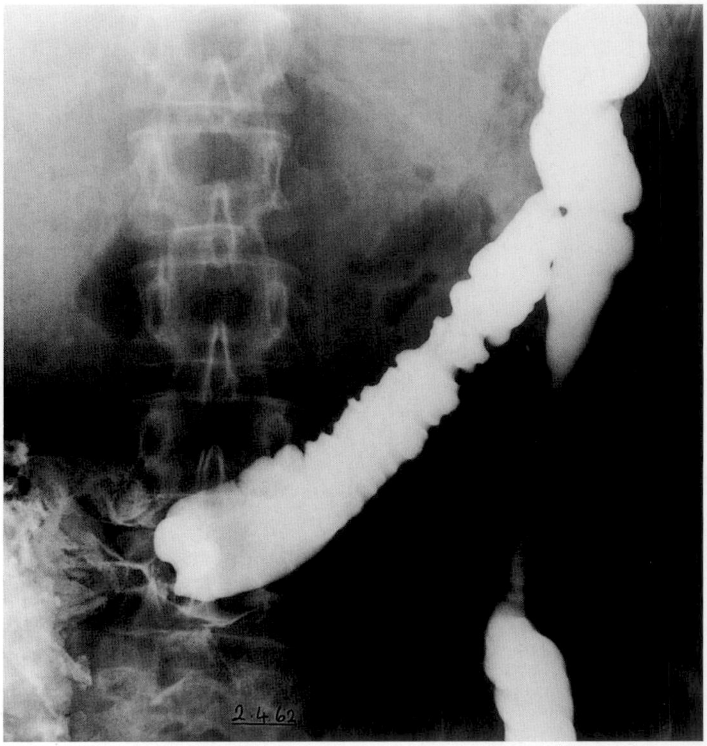

Fig. 10.68 Barium enema shows a stricture.

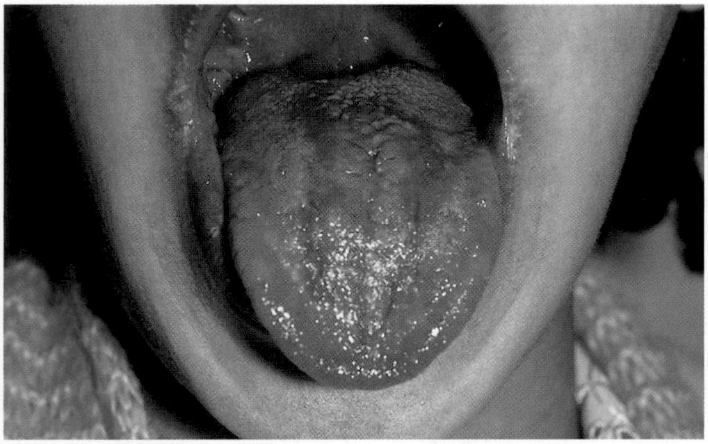

Fig. 10.69 Glossitis, which may be associated with aphthous ulceration.

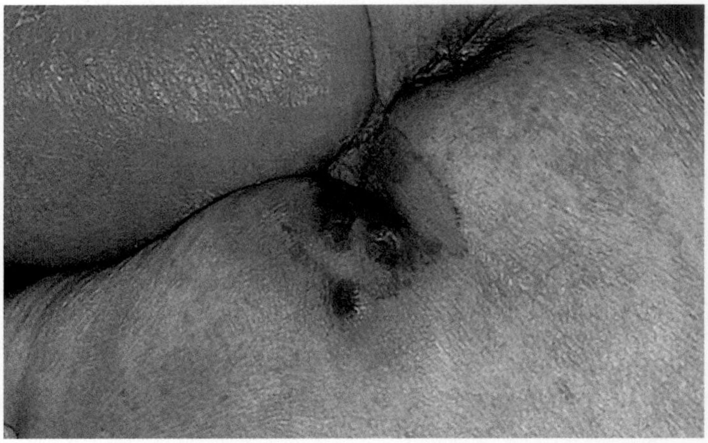

Fig. 10.70 Perianal abscess and fistula formation. (Courtesy of P. C. Hayes and N. D. C. Finlayson.)

UVEITIS IN NON-INFECTIOUS SYSTEMIC DISEASES

Sarcoidosis

Sarcoidosis is an idiopathic, multisystem, granulomatous disorder, more common in patients of African descent than in Caucasians.

General systemic signs

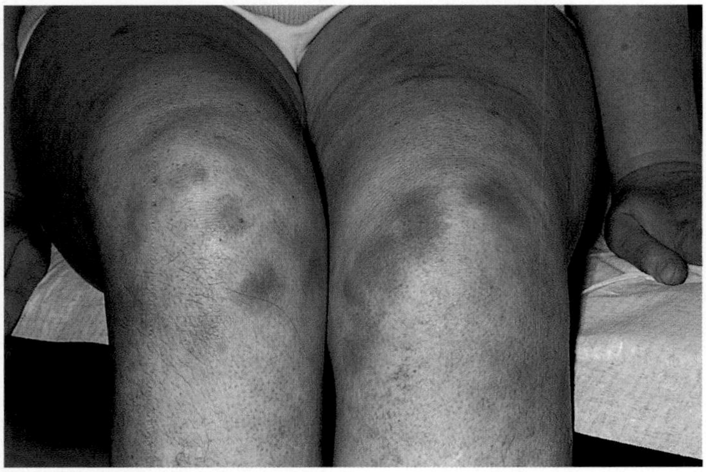

Fig. 10.71 Erythema nodosum occurs in acute sarcoidosis and, in combination with bilateral hilar adenopathy and arthralgia, forms part of Lofgren syndrome.

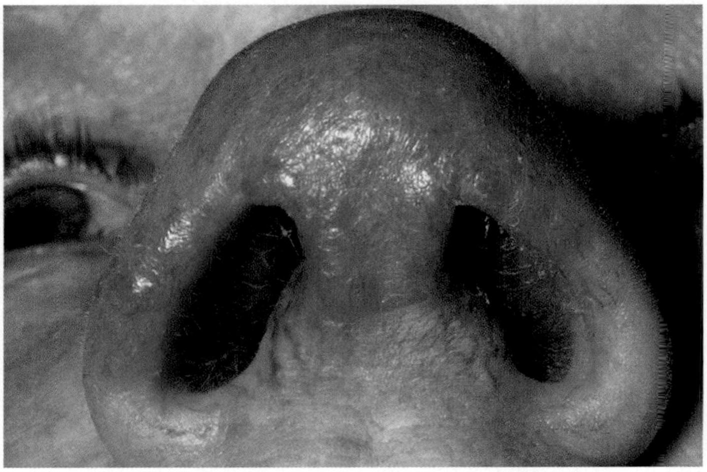

Fig. 10.72 Lupus pernio is characterised by indurated purple-blue skin lesions typically involving the nose, cheeks and ears. (Courtesy of M. A. Mir.)

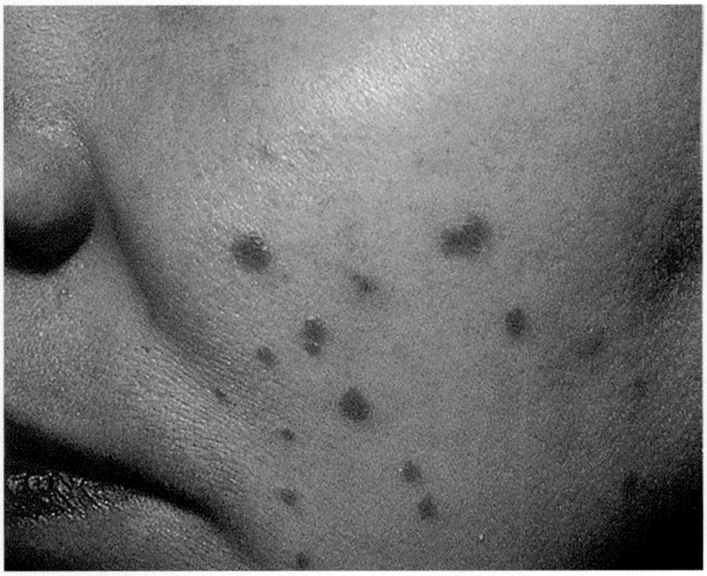

Fig. 10.73 Mild, reddish maculopapular lesions on the cheek. (Courtesy of M. A. Mir.)

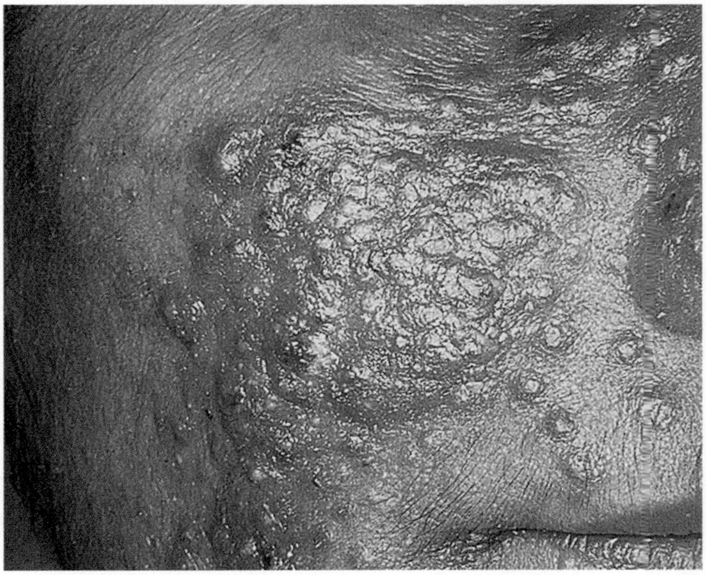

Fig. 10.74 Nodular granulomatous infiltration of the cheek.

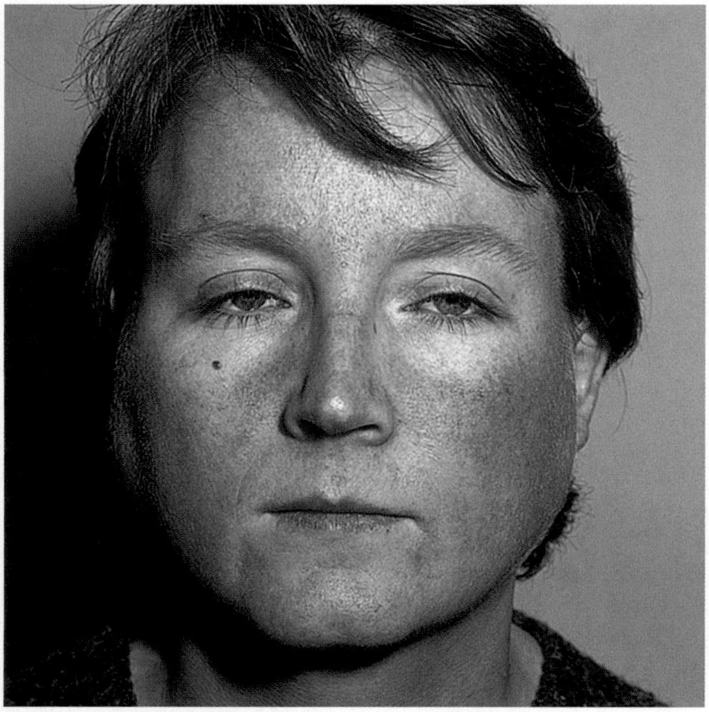

■ **Fig. 10.75** Parotid enlargement typically occurs in Heerfordt syndrome, which also manifests fever and acute anterior uveitis (uveoparotid fever).

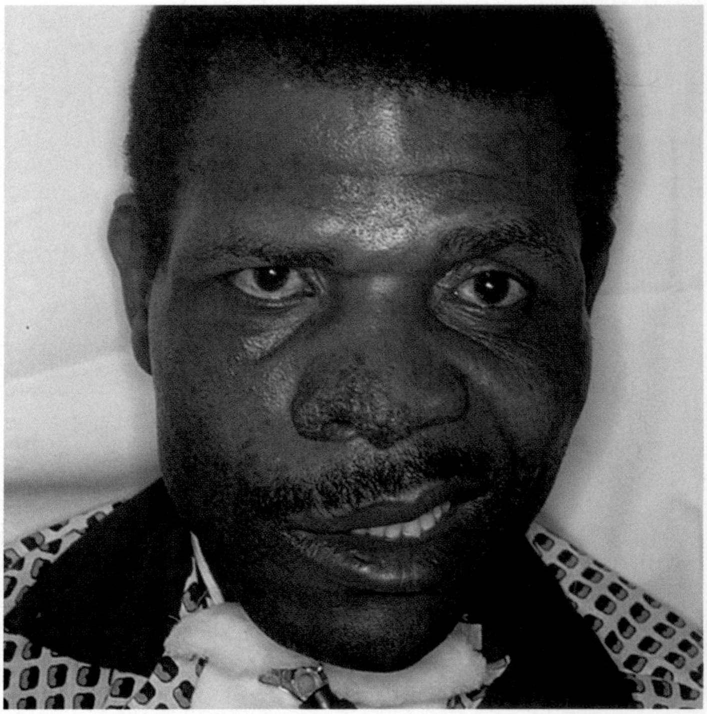

■ **Fig. 10.76** Seventh nerve palsy may also form part of Heerfordt syndrome. Also note granulomatous infiltration of the nose and tracheostomy.

Progression of pulmonary involvement

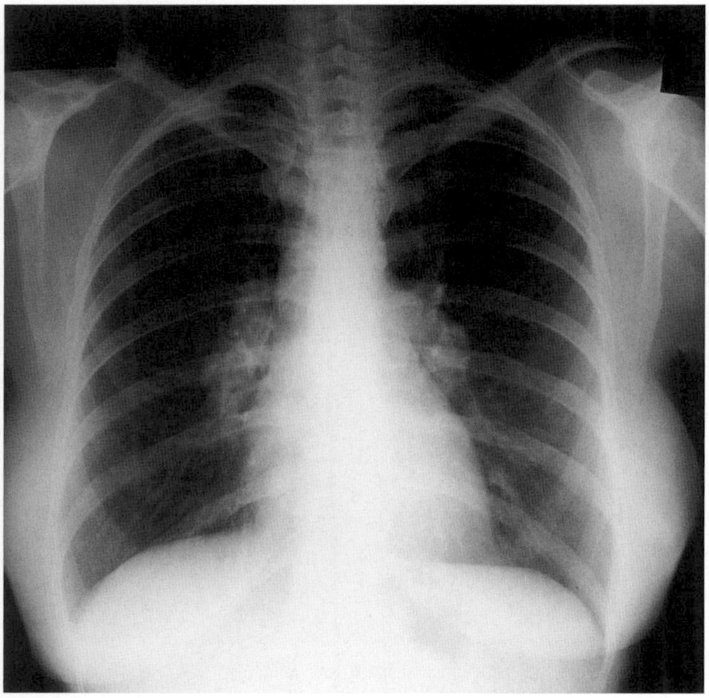

■ **Fig. 10.77** Stage 1 pulmonary involvement, characterised by bilateral symmetrical hilar glandular enlargement, forms part of Lofgren syndrome.

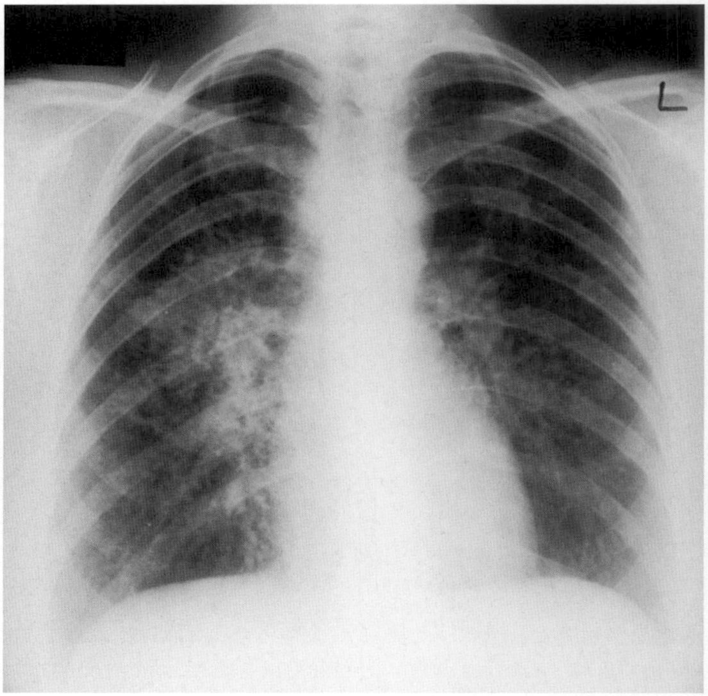

■ **Fig. 10.78** Stage 2: hilar enlargement and diffuse pulmonary infiltrates.

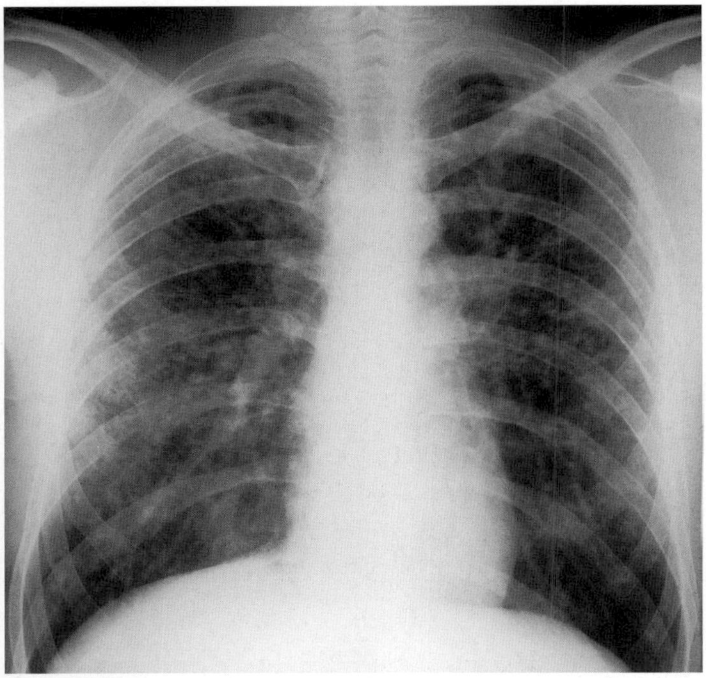

■ **Fig. 10.79** Stage 3: diffuse pulmonary shadowing without hilar enlargement.

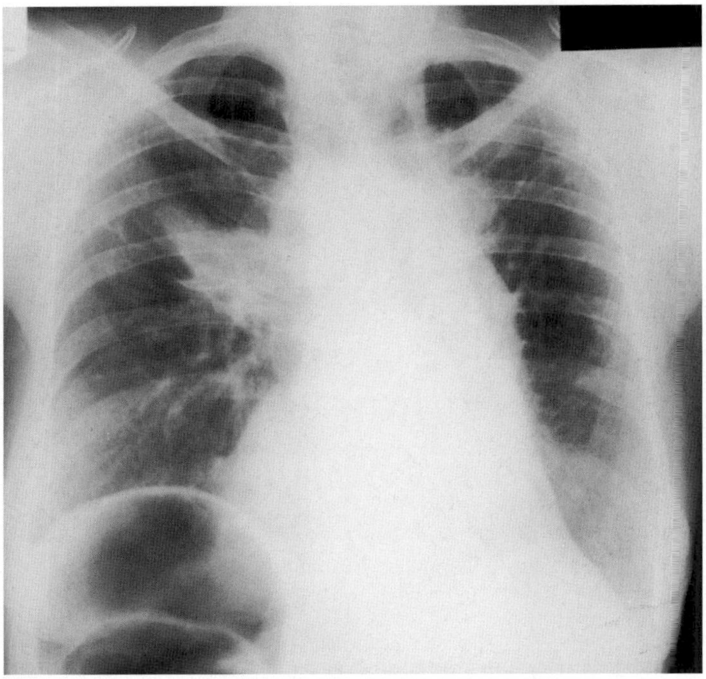

■ **Fig. 10.80** Stage 4: pulmonary fibrosis, which may progress to pulmonary hypertension and cor pulmonale.

Ocular signs

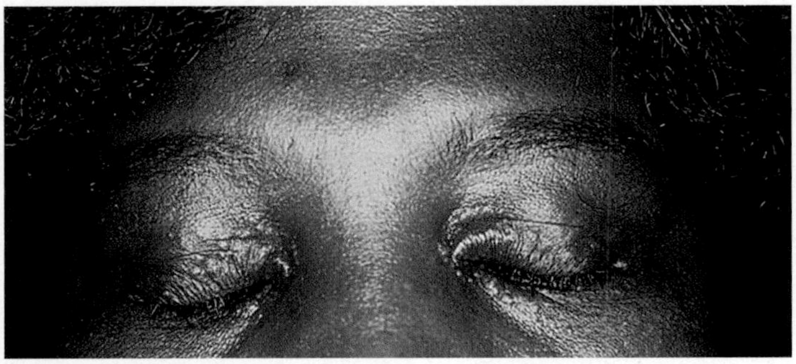

■ **Fig. 10.81** Mild nodular granulomatous involvement of the upper eyelids.

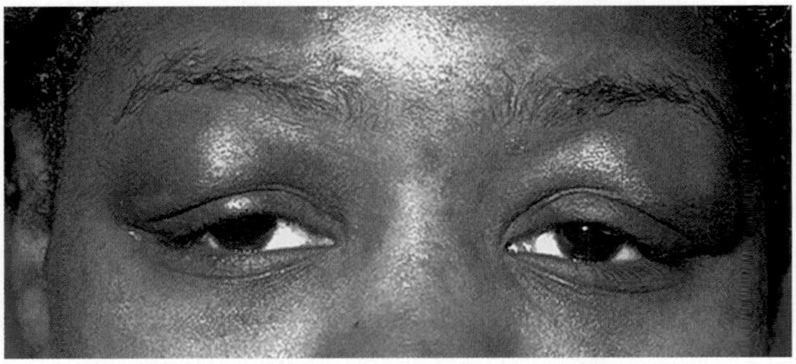

■ **Fig. 10.82** Lacrimal gland involvement may result in keratoconjunctivitis sicca. (Courtesy of S. Ford and R. Marsh.)

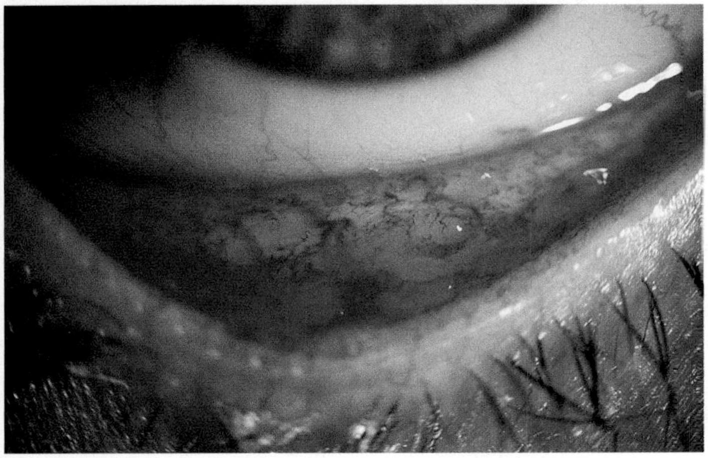

■ **Fig. 10.83** Small conjunctival granulomas that may be used for biopsy.

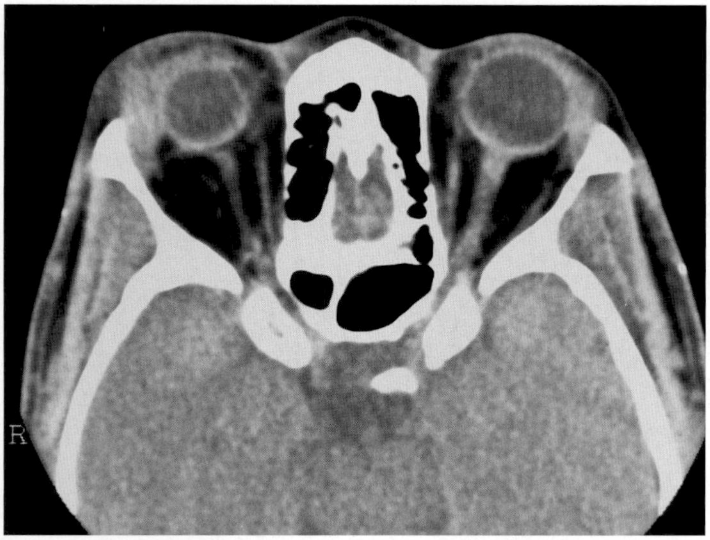

■ **Fig. 10.84** Axial CT showing bilateral lacrimal gland enlargement.

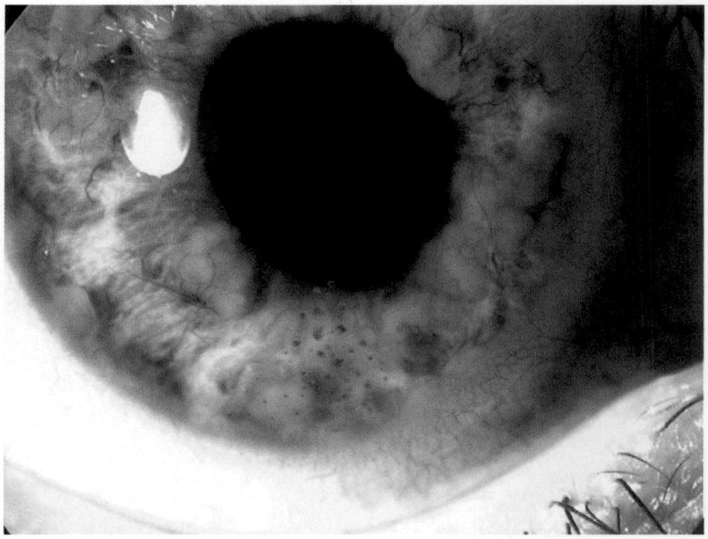

■ **Fig. 10.85** Large iris nodules in chronic granulomatous anterior uveitis which typically affects older patients with chronic lung disease. (Courtesy of C. Pavésio.)

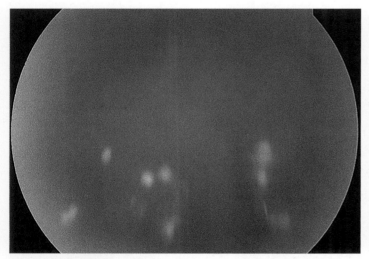

■ **Fig. 10.86** Vitreous 'cotton balls' in 'secondary' intermediate uveitis is common.

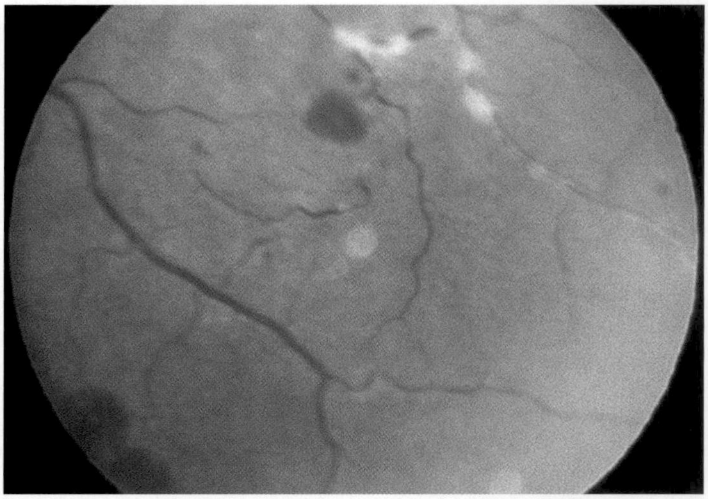

■ **Fig. 10.87** Mild periphlebitis characterised by perivenous infiltration.

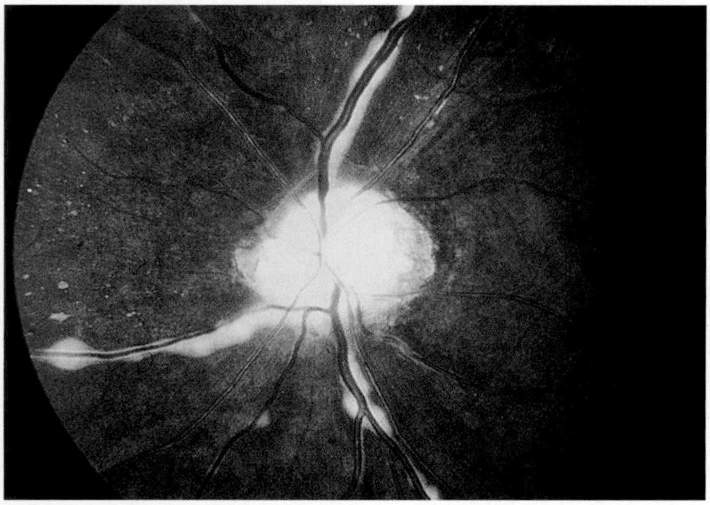

■ **Fig. 10.88** Severe periphlebitis with 'candle wax drippings'. (Courtesy of P. Morse.)

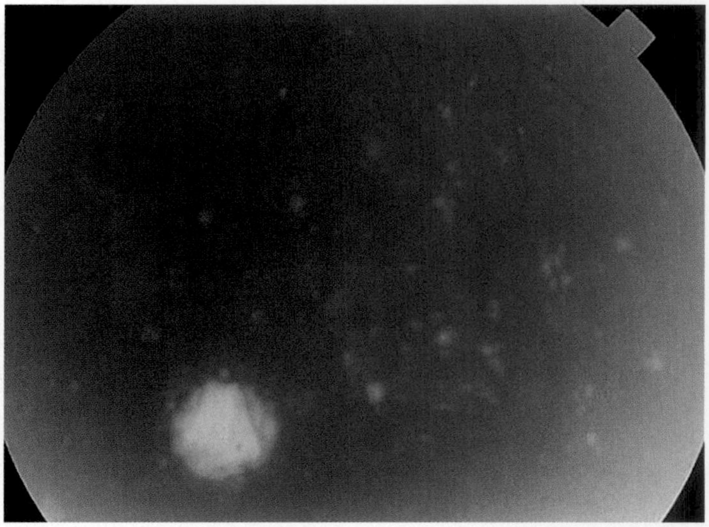

■ **Fig. 10.89** Multiple, small, pale-yellow choroidal infiltrates with a 'punched-out' are common. (Courtesy of C. Pavésio.)

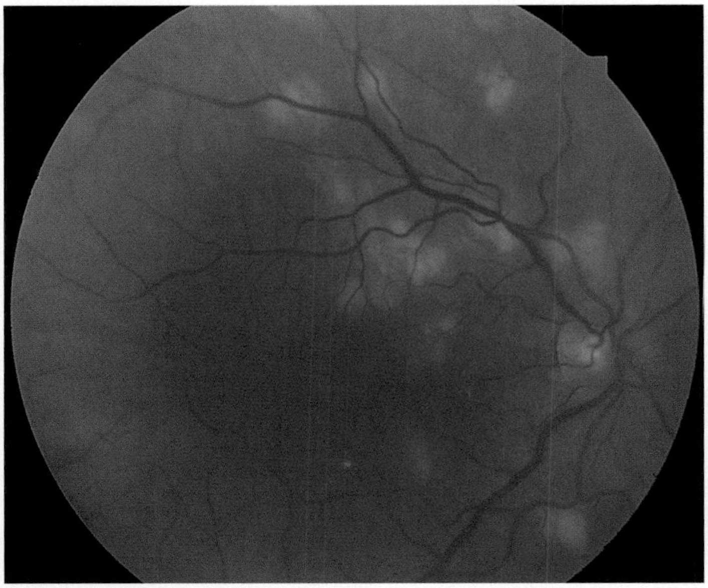

■ **Fig. 10.90** Larger, confluent infiltrates.

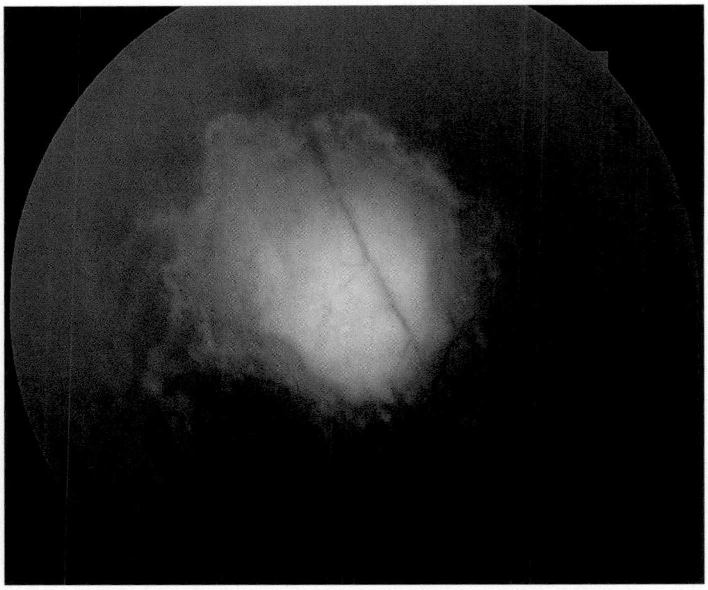

■ **Fig. 10.91** Large solitary granulomas are rare.

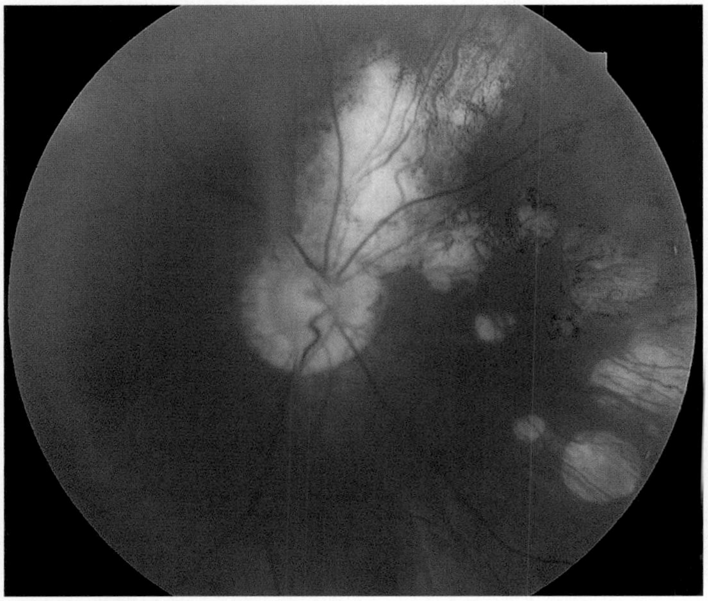

■ **Fig. 10.92** Multifocal choroiditis.

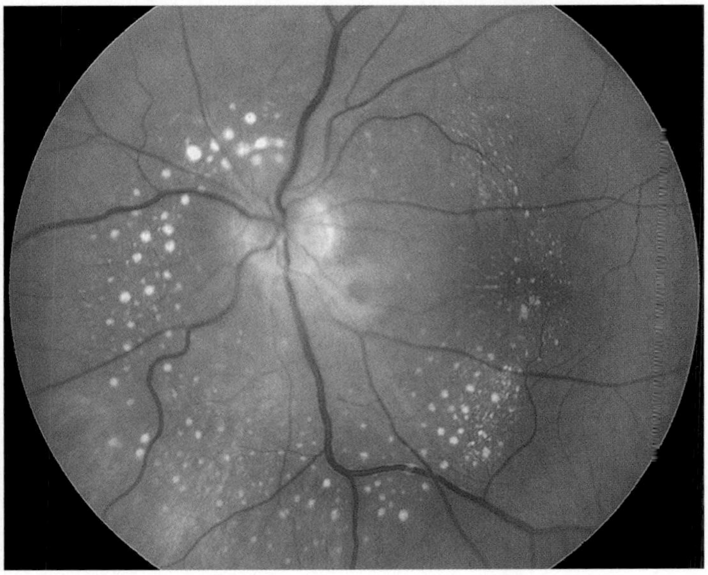

■ **Fig. 10.93** Small retinal granulomas.

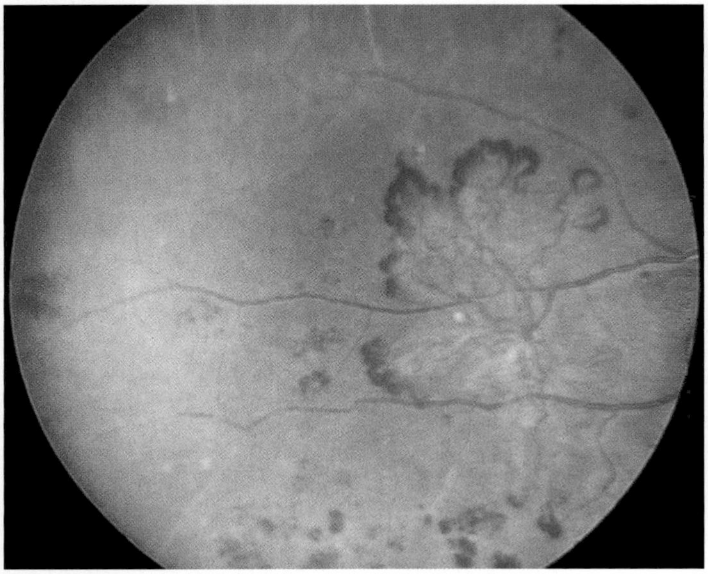

■ **Fig. 10.94** Peripheral retinal neovascularisation.

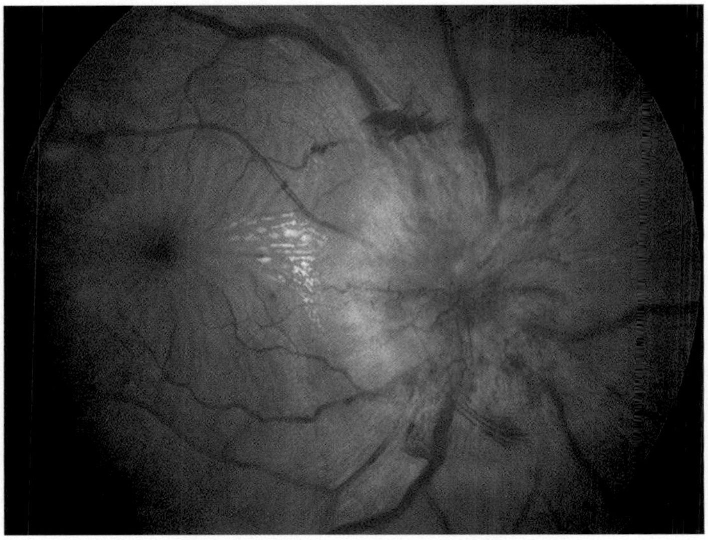

■ **Fig. 10.95** Optic disc swelling due to infiltration or raised intracranial pressure.

Behçet syndrome

Behçet syndrome is an idiopathic, recurrent, multisystem vasculitis that may involve both veins and arteries.

Systemic signs

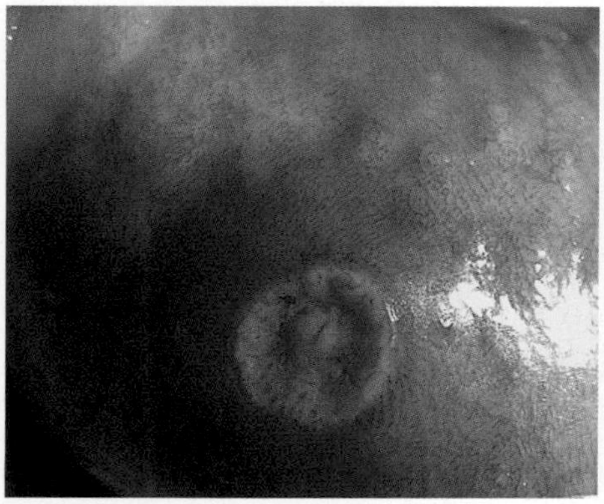

Fig. 10.96 Recurrent oral ulcers.

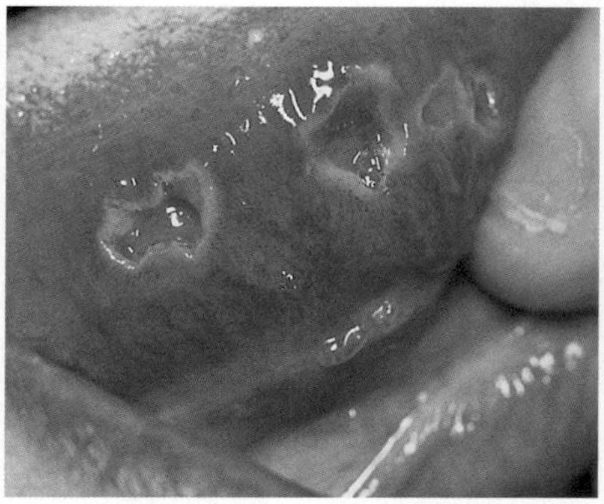

Fig. 10.97 The ulcers are often multiple and deep. (Courtesy of M. A. Mir.)

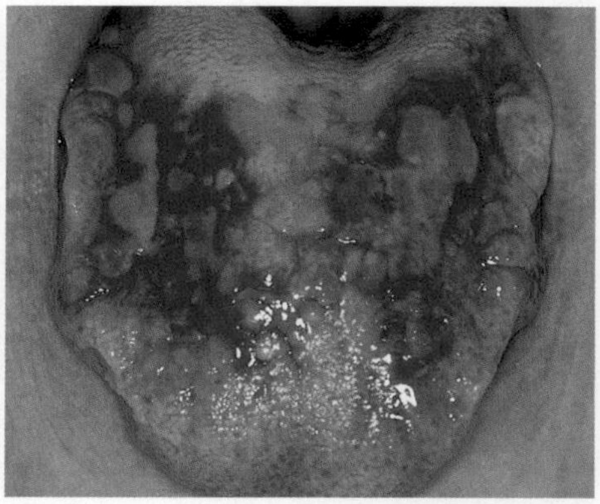

Fig. 10.98 Severe confluent ulceration is uncommon. (Courtesy of P. Saine.)

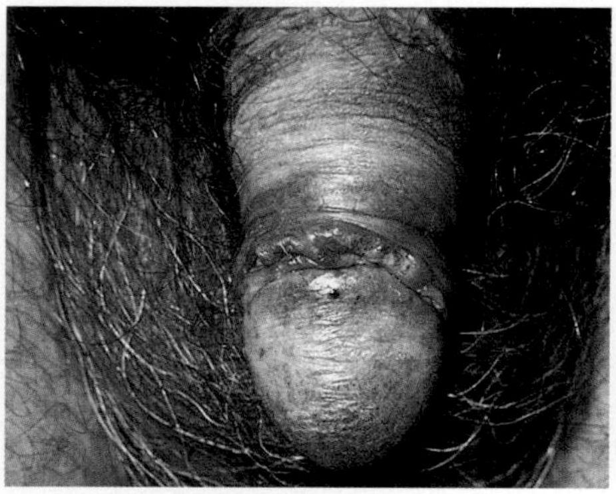

Fig. 10.99 Recurrent genital ulceration.

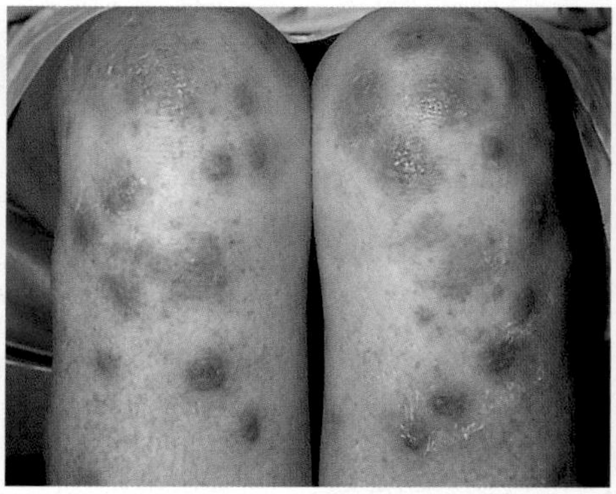

Fig. 10.100 Erythema-nodosum-like lesions. (Courtesy of B. Noble.)

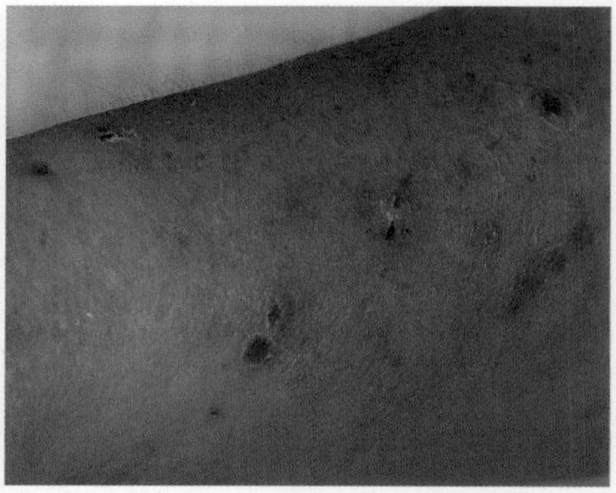

Fig. 10.101 Acneiform nodules. (Courtesy of P. Saine.)

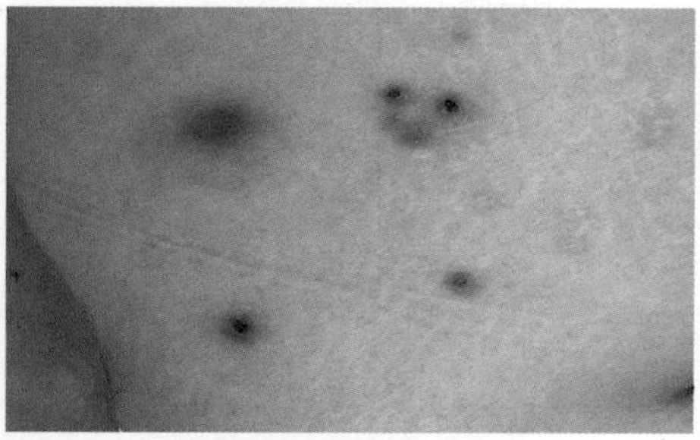

Fig. 10.102 Papulopustular lesions. (Courtesy of P. Saine.)

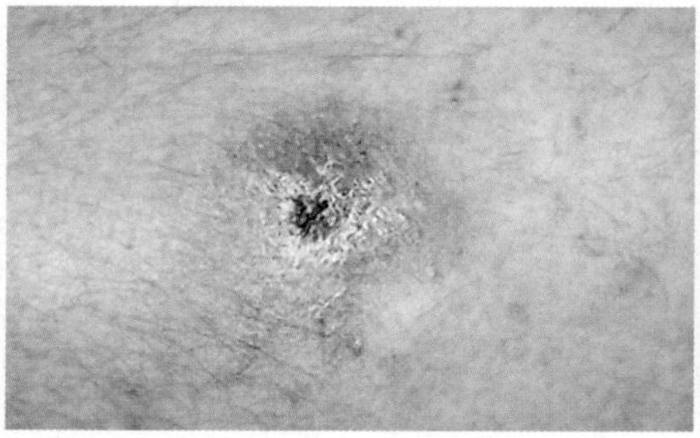

Fig. 10.103 Formation of a pustule 48 hours following an intradermal prick with a needle (positive pathergy test). (Courtesy of B. Noble.)

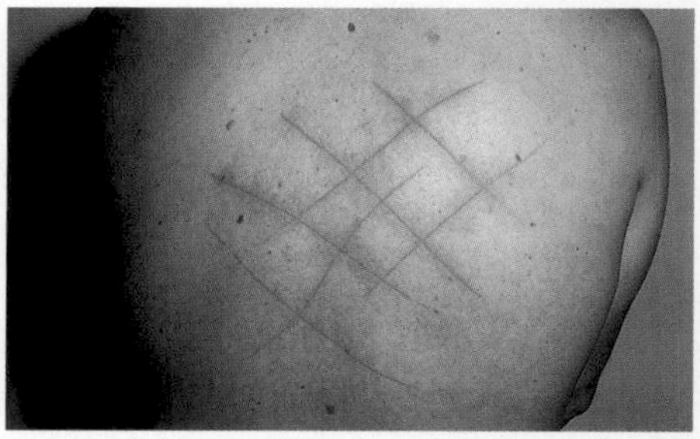

Fig. 10.104 Cutaneous hypersensitivity (dermatographism) demonstrated by the appearance of weals after firmly stroking the skin.

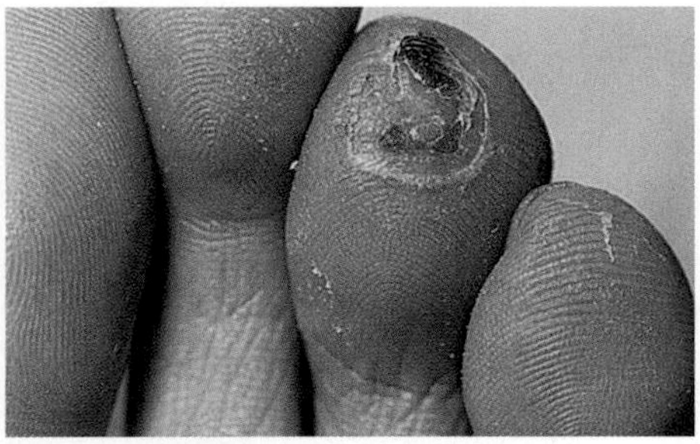

Fig. 10.105 Cutaneous vasculitis.

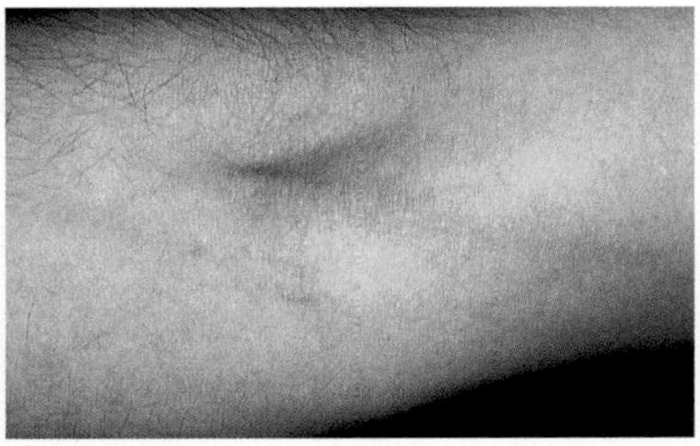

Fig. 10.106 Migratory superficial thrombophlebitis.

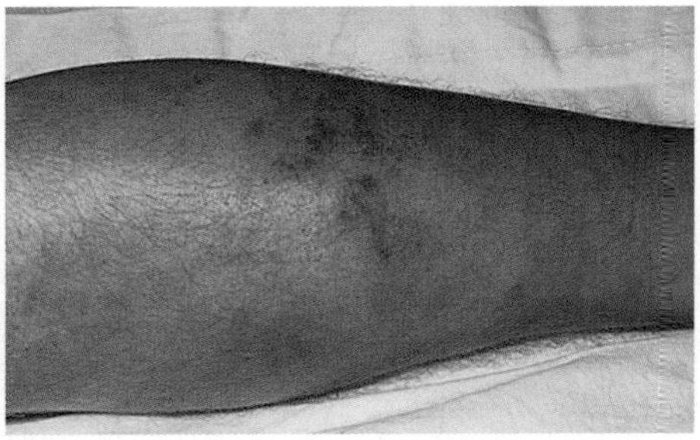

Fig. 10.107 Deep vein thrombosis.

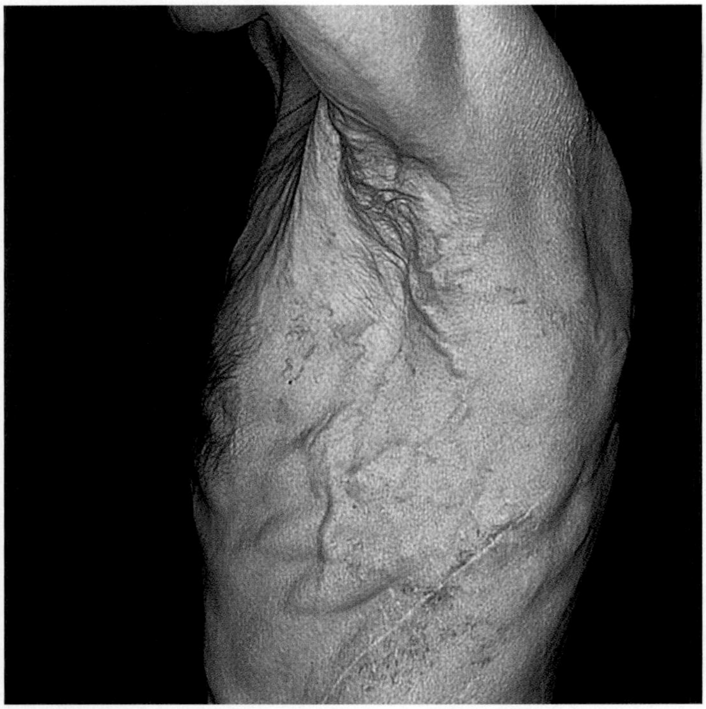

Fig. 10.108 Deep obliterative thrombophlebitis, which may give rise to compensatory dilatation of the superficial veins.

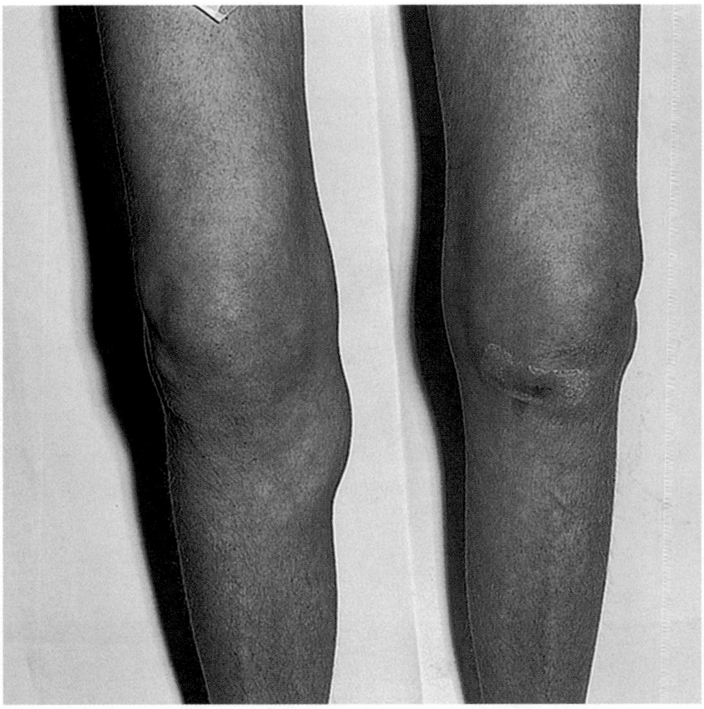

Fig. 10.109 Arthritis involving the knees and ankles, and occasionally sacroiliitis.

Ocular signs

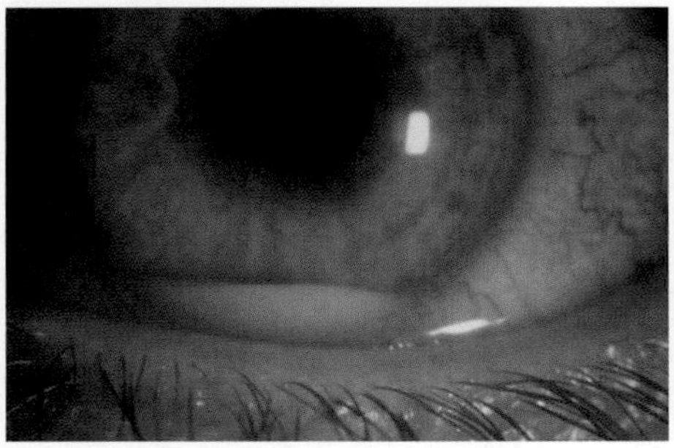

Fig. 10.110 Acute recurrent anterior uveitis, which may be simultaneously bilateral and frequently associated with a transient mobile hypopyon. (Courtesy of A. Curi.)

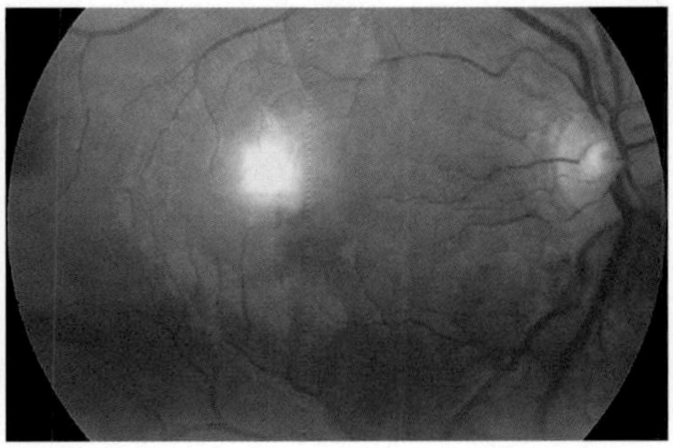

Fig. 10.111 Transient superficial retinal infiltrates. (Courtesy of B. Noble.)

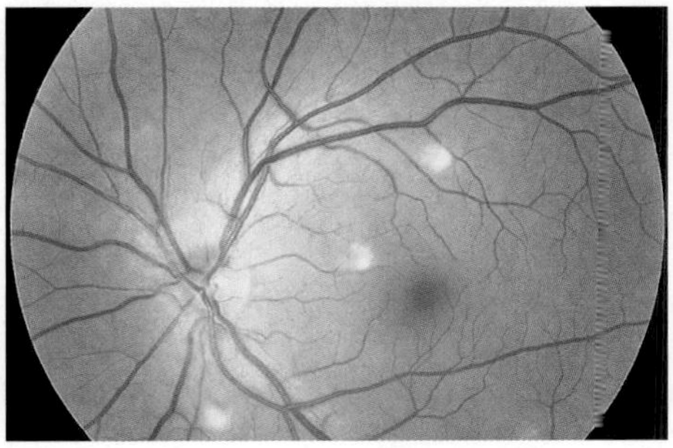

Fig. 10.112 Multiple retinal infiltrates. (Courtesy of S. Milewski.)

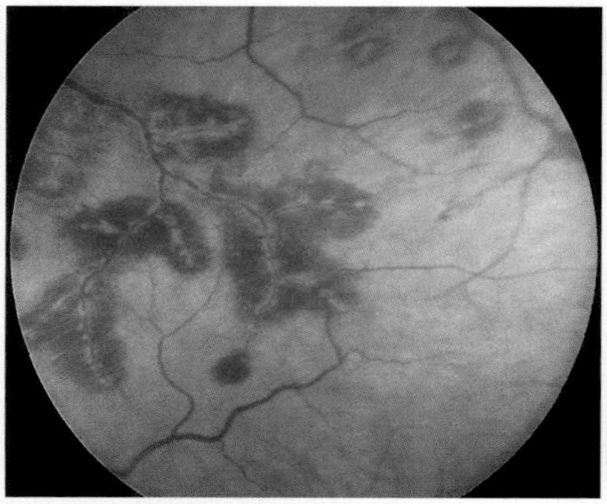

Fig. 10.113 Retinal periphlebitis. (Courtesy of P. Frith.)

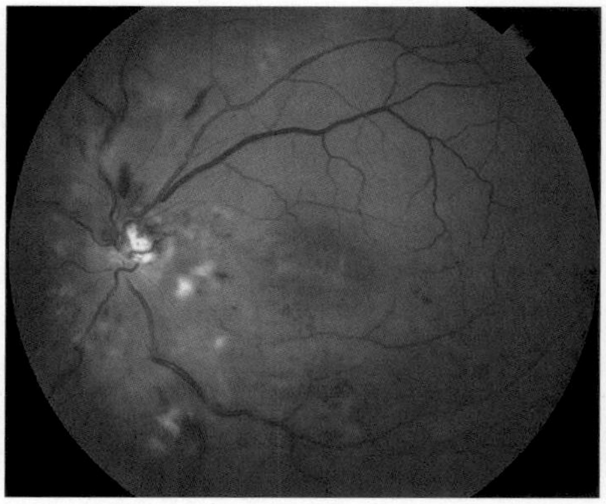

Fig. 10.114 Optic disc vasculitis.

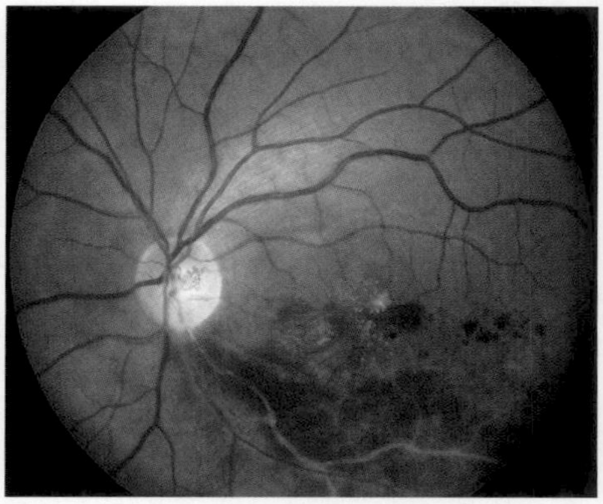

Fig. 10.115 Occlusive periphlebitis. (Courtesy of S. Ford and R. Marsh.)

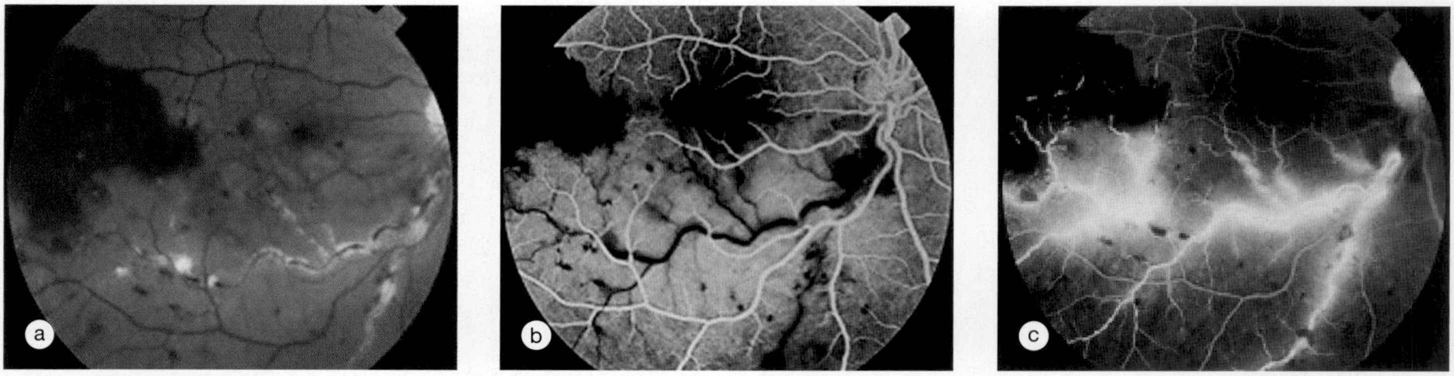

Fig. 10.116 **(a)** Severe occlusive retinal periphlebitis with a large intraretinal haemorrhage. **(b)** FA early phase shows delayed filling of the involved vein. **(c)** Late staining. (Courtesy of A. Abu El-Asrar.)

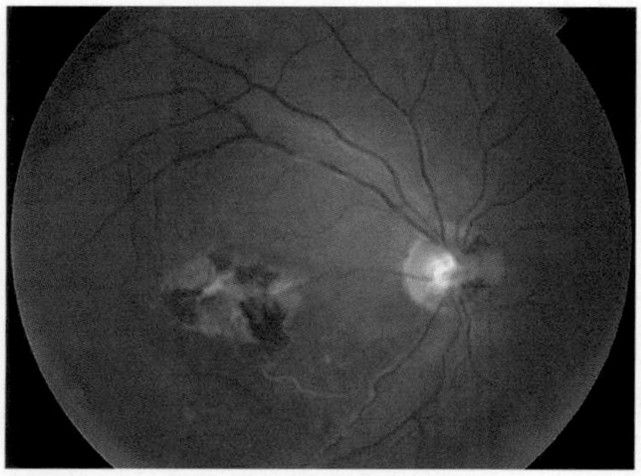

Fig. 10.117 Residual venous sheathing and chorioretinal scarring at the macula. (Courtesy of A. Dick.)

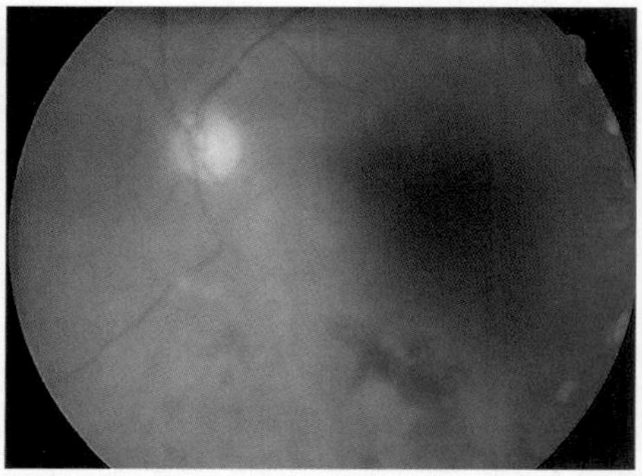

Fig. 10.118 Vitritis is universal and may be severe and persistent. (Courtesy of A. Curi.)

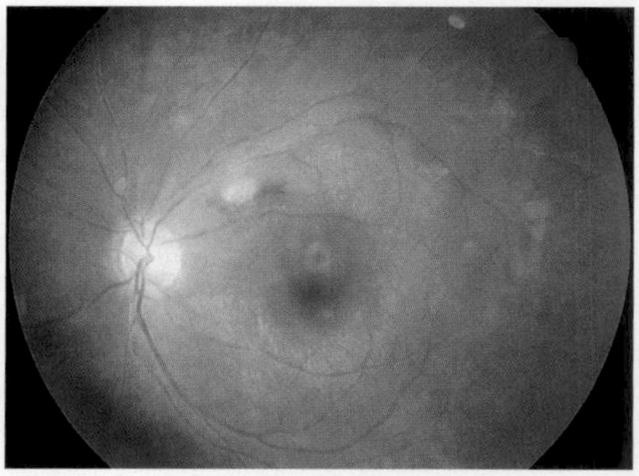

Fig. 10.119 End-stage disease characterised by optic atrophy and attenuation of veins and arteries. (Courtesy of B. Noble.)

Vogt–Koyanagi–Harada syndrome

Vogt–Koyanagi–Harada disease is an idiopathic, multisystem disorder that typically affects Hispanics, Japanese and pigmented individuals.

Systemic signs

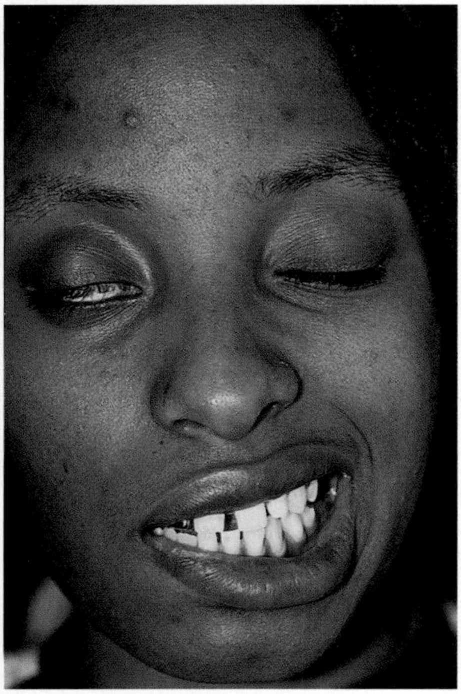

Fig. 10.120 The prodromal phase is characterised by neurological and auditory manifestations.

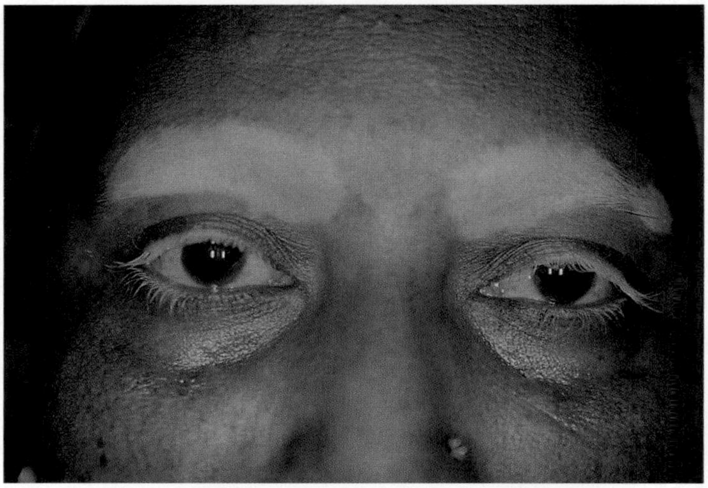

Fig. 10.121 The convalescent phase is characterised by localised alopecia, poliosis and vitiligo. (Courtesy of U. Raina.)

Ocular signs

Vogt–Koyanagi syndrome

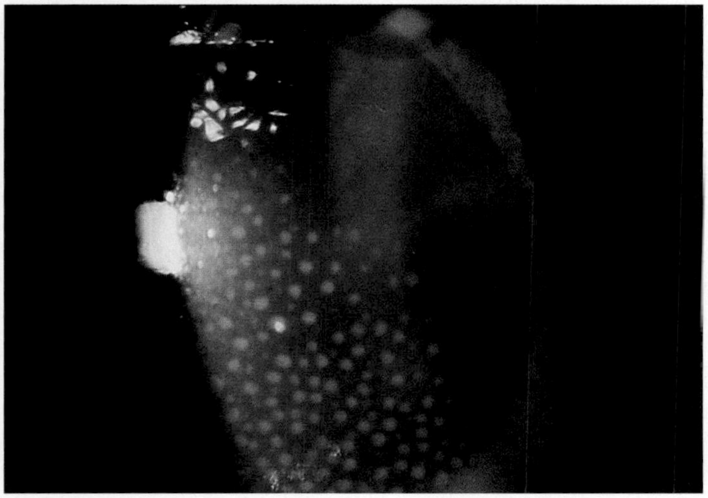

Fig. 10.122 The acute uveitic phase is characterised by bilateral granulomatous anterior uveitis.

Harada disease

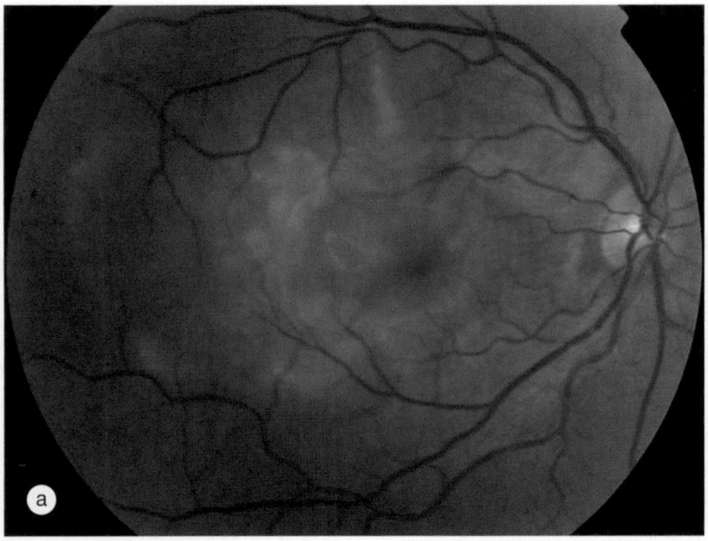

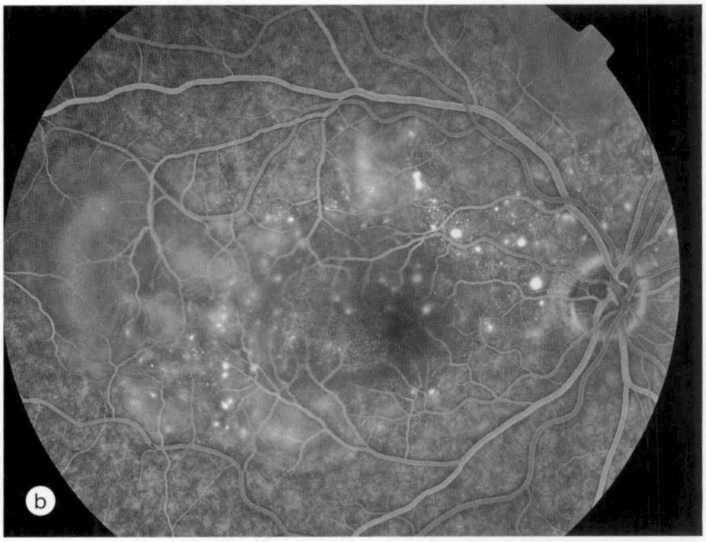

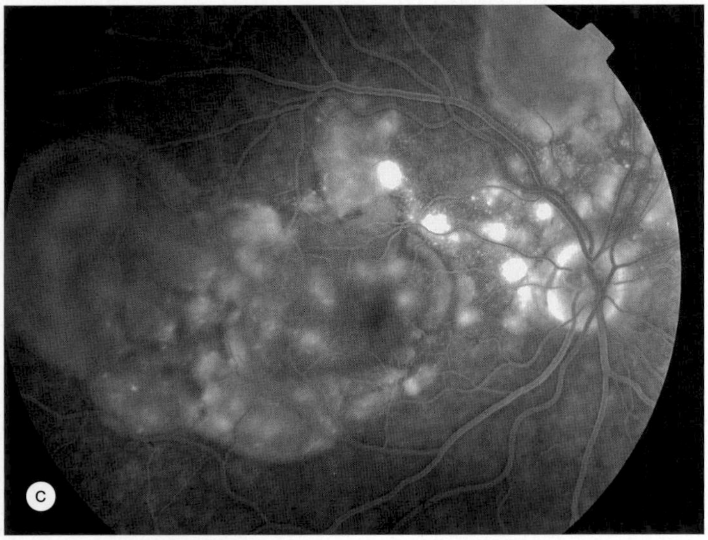

■ **Fig. 10.123** **(a)** Multifocal detachments of the sensory retina with small folds in the macula and around the disc. **(b)** FA venous phase shows pinpoint hyperfluorescent spots at the macula and more diffuse hyperfluorescence temporally. **(c)** Late phase shows a large area of hyperfluorescence due to pooling of dye under the sensory retina. (Courtesy of C. Pavésio.)

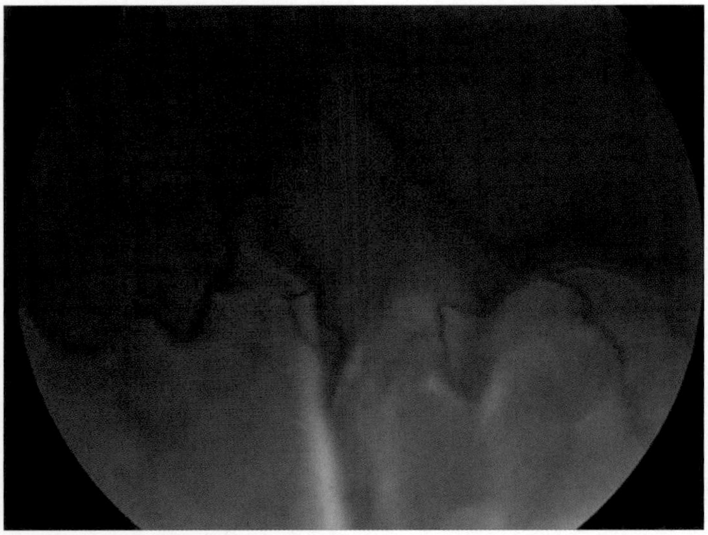

■ **Fig. 10.124** Bilateral bullous exudative retinal detachment may develop.

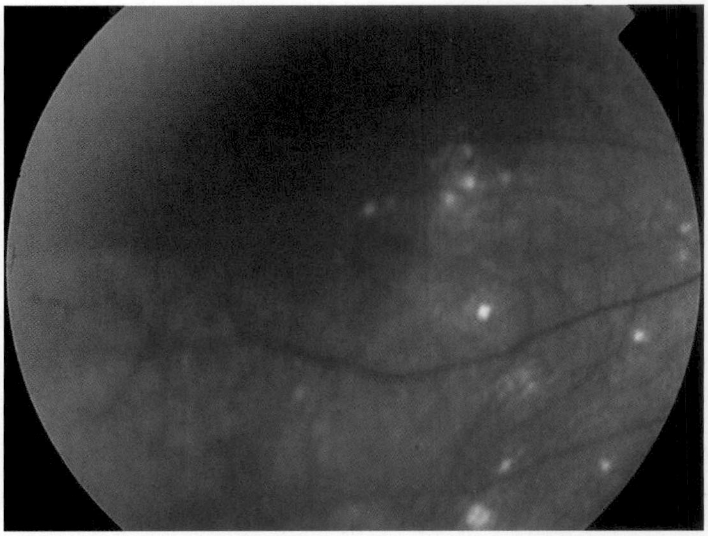

■ **Fig. 10.125** The convalescent phase is characterised by numerous, small, peripheral depigmented spots ('sunset glow' fundus). (Courtesy of C. Pavésio.)

PARASITIC UVEITIS

Toxoplasmosis

Toxoplasma gondii is an obligate intracellular protozoan. The cat is the definitive host of the parasite and other animals are intermediate hosts.

Congenital signs

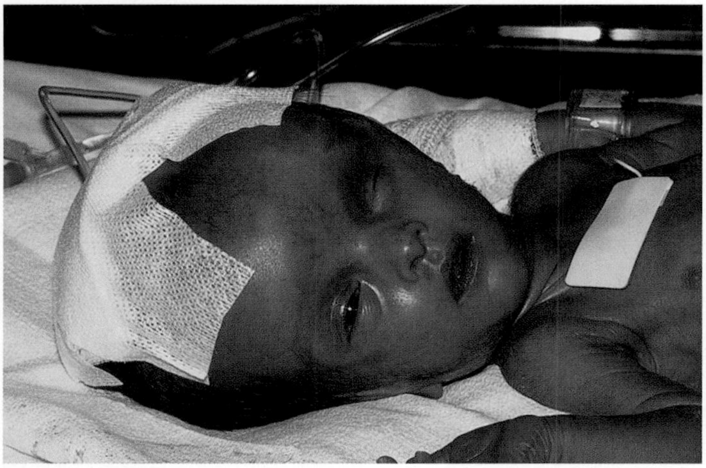

Fig. 10.126 Infection during late pregnancy may result in convulsions, paralysis, hydrocephalus and visceral involvement; also note left anophthalmos. (Courtesy of M. Szreter.)

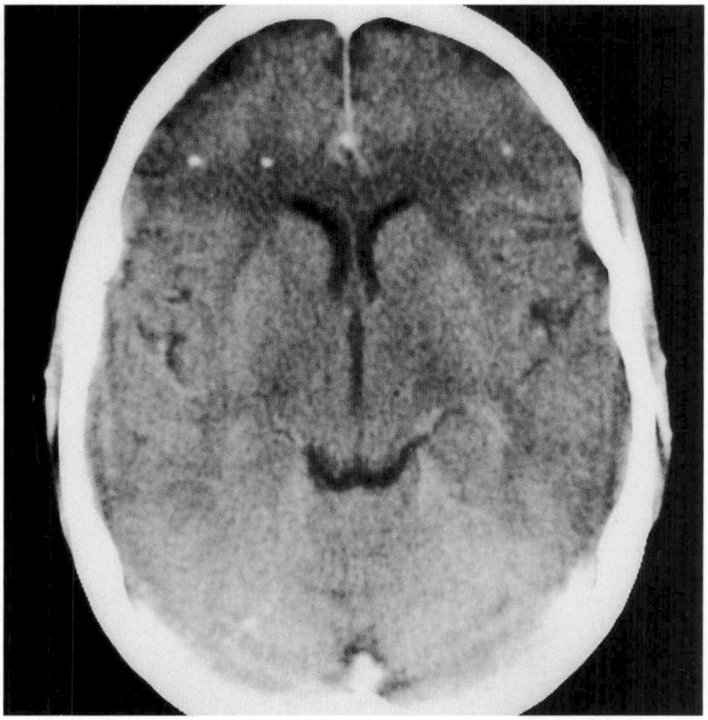

Fig. 10.127 Axial CT showing small foci of cerebral calcification.

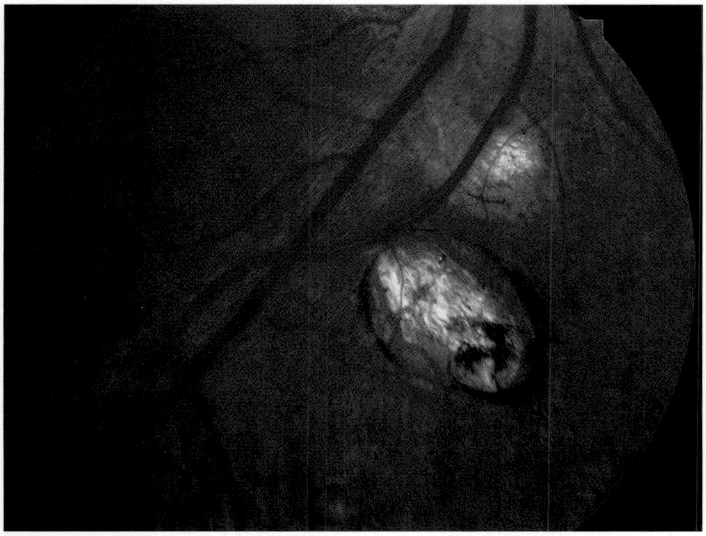

Fig. 10.128 Asymptomatic peripheral chorioretinal scars.

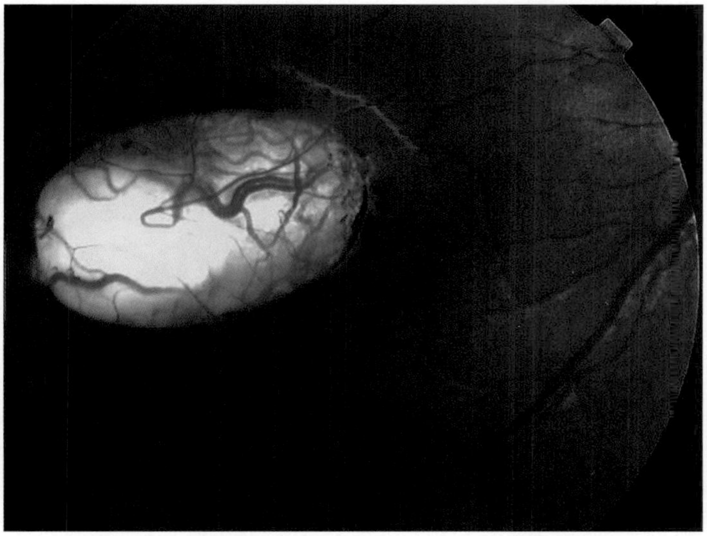

Fig. 10.129 Large macular scar.

Retinitis

Active

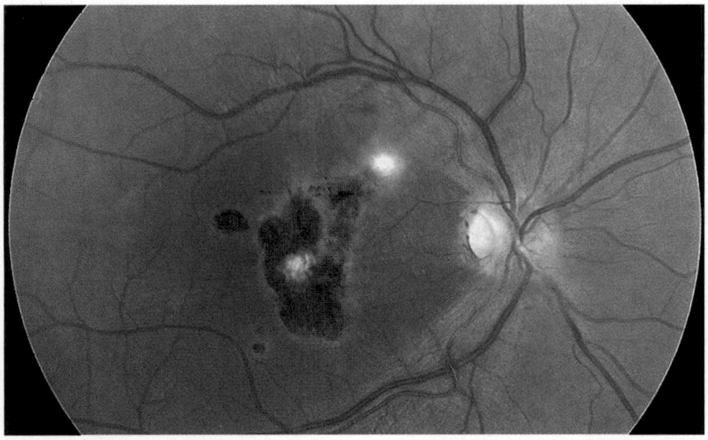

Fig. 10.130 Solitary inflammatory focus near an old pigmented scar ('satellite lesion'). In this case the scar is much larger than the active lesion.

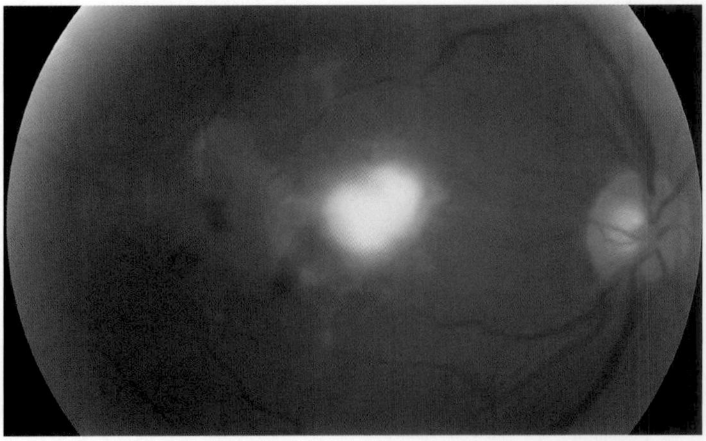

Fig. 10.131 Very large macular focus. (Courtesy of L. Merin.)

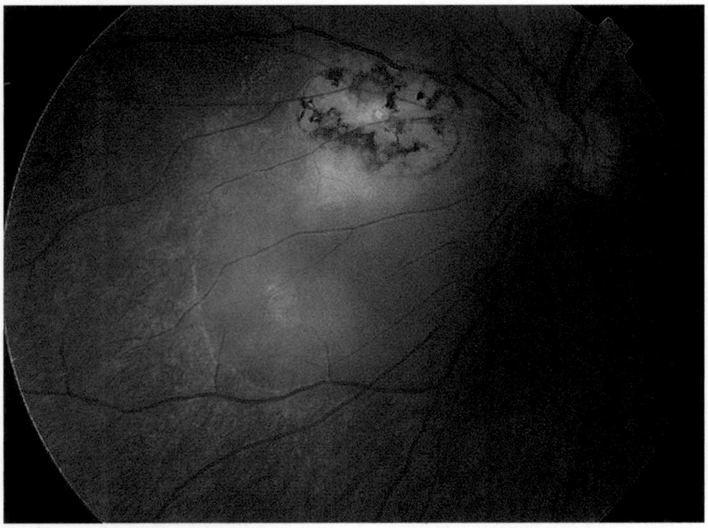

Fig. 10.132 Retinitis with adjacent shallow sensory retinal elevation.

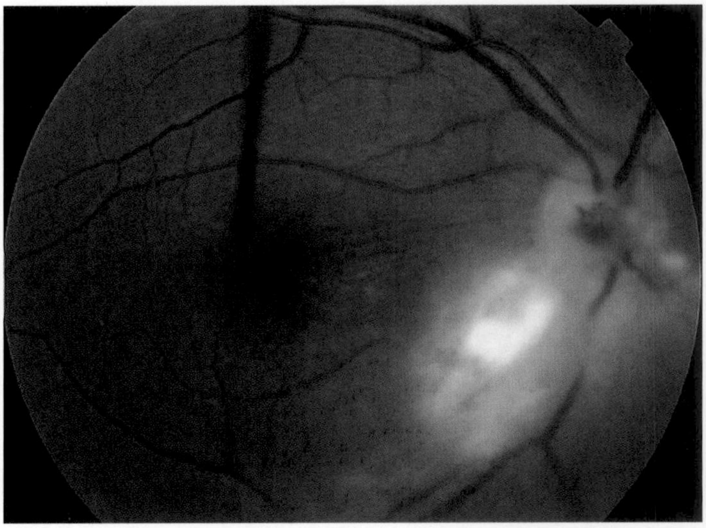

Fig. 10.133 Juxtapapillary retinitis with overlying vitreous haze.

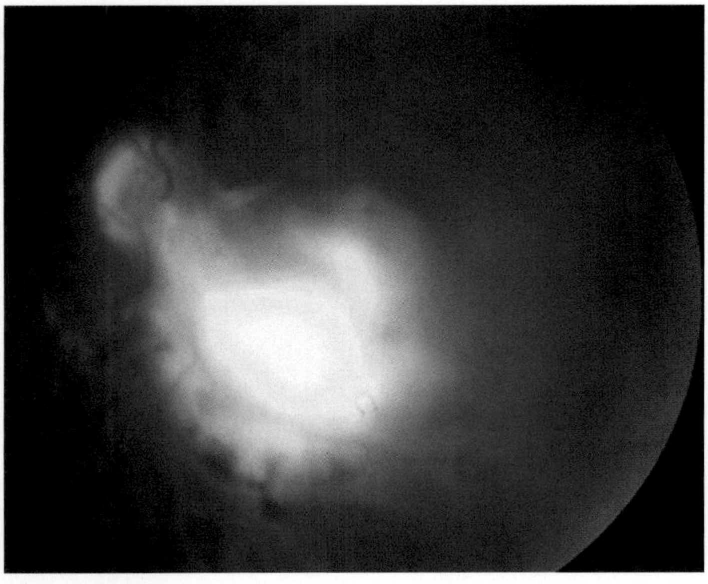

Fig. 10.134 Severe juxtapapillary retinitis with moderate vitreous haze. (Courtesy of C. de A. Garcia.)

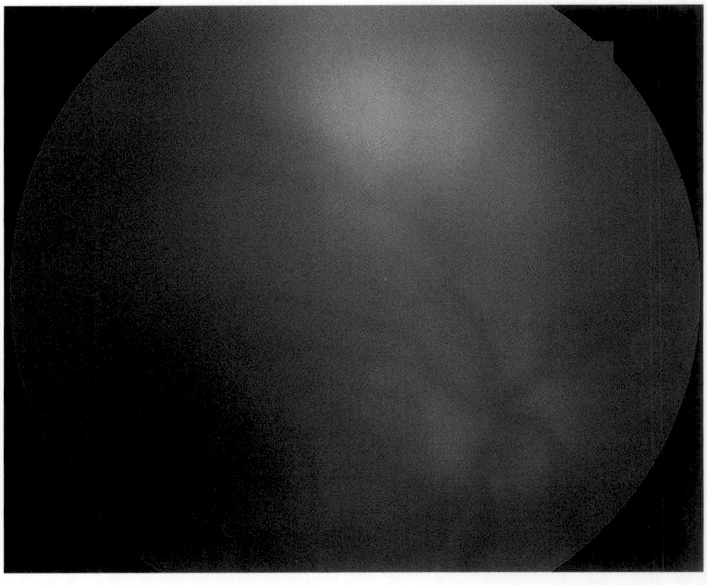

Fig. 10.135 Very severe vitritis in which the inflammatory focus is discernible ('headlight in the fog' appearance); 'spill-over' anterior uveitis may also be severe.

Inactive

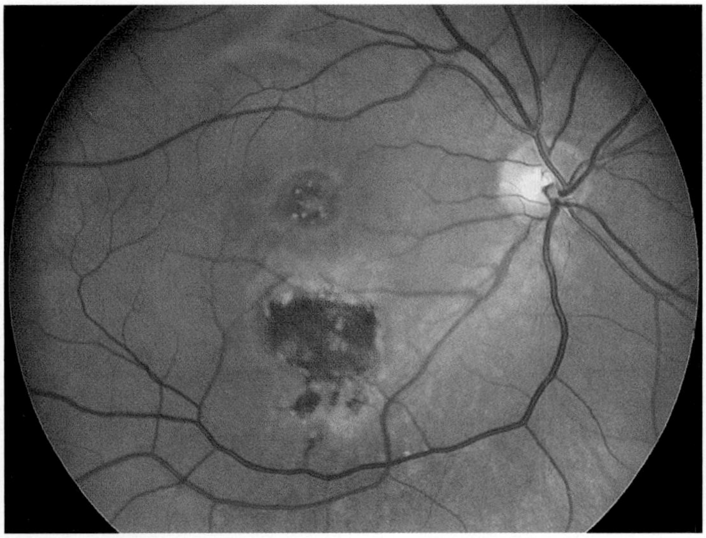

■ **Fig. 10.136** Macular pseudohole above a scar.

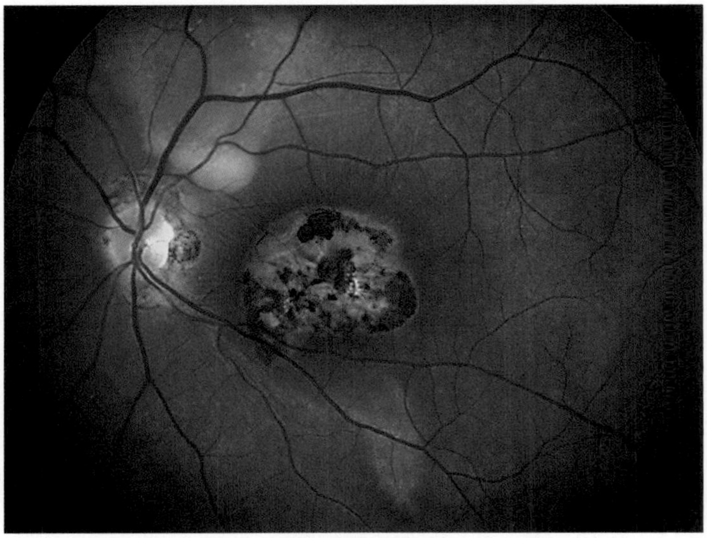

■ **Fig. 10.137** Macular scar and subretinal exudation above the disc. (Courtesy of C. Barry.)

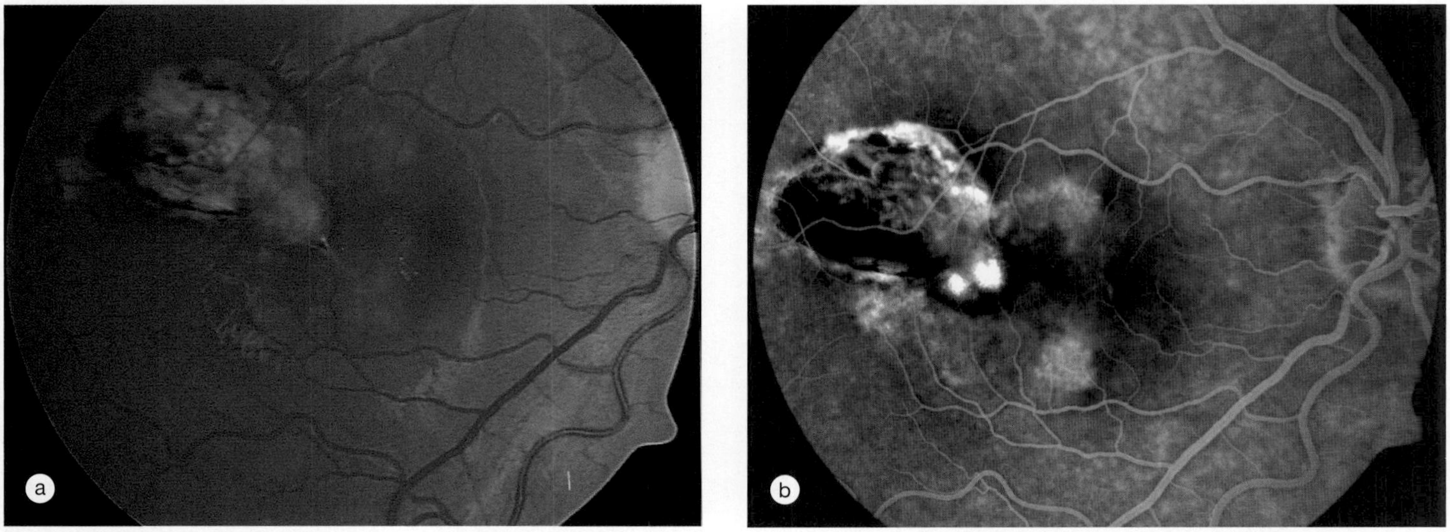

■ **Fig. 10.138** **(a)** Choroidal neovascularisation resulting in subretinal scarring is uncommon. **(b)** FA showing two areas of hyperfluorescence at the macula. (Courtesy of P. Gili.)

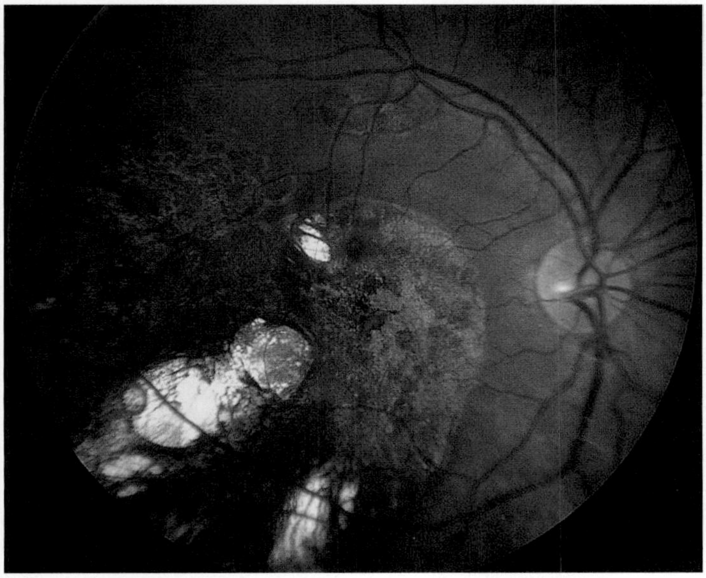

■ **Fig. 10.139** Very severe confluent macular scarring is rare.

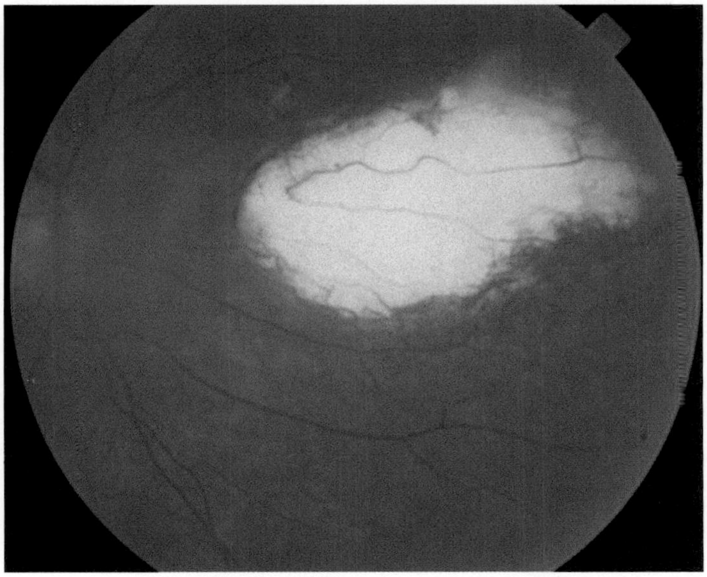

■ **Fig. 10.140** Confluent peripheral scarring is uncommon. (Courtesy of S. Milewski.)

Toxocariasis

Toxocariasis is caused by a common intestinal ascarid (roundworm) of dogs, *Toxocara canis*.

Chronic endophthalmitis

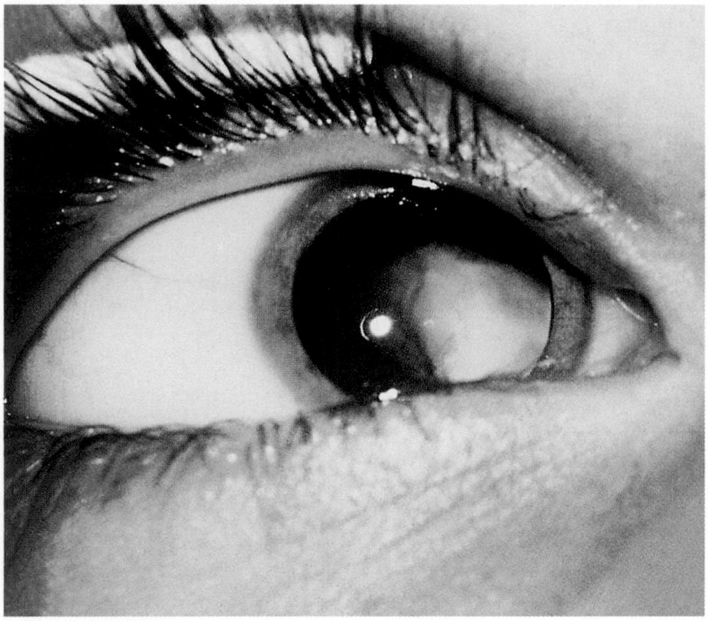

Fig. 10.141 Presentation is in childhood with leukocoria, strabismus or unilateral visual loss.

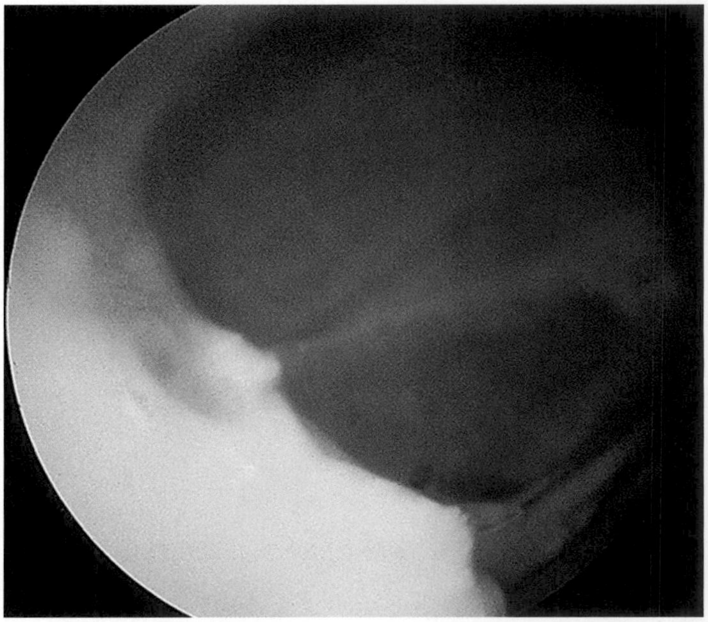

Fig. 10.142 The peripheral retina and pars plana may be covered by a dens, greyish-white exudate, similar to the 'snowbanking' seen in pars planitis. (Courtesy of S. Lightman.)

Posterior pole granuloma

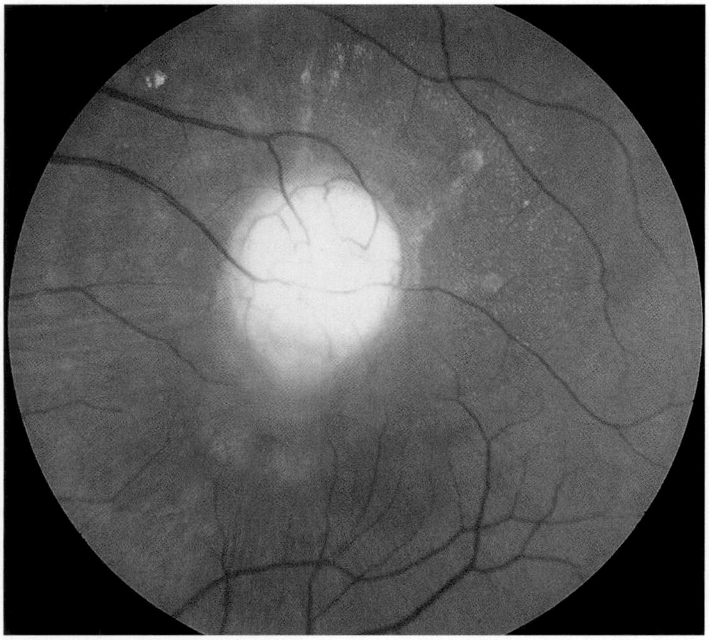

Fig. 10.143 Yellow-white granuloma at the posterior pole.

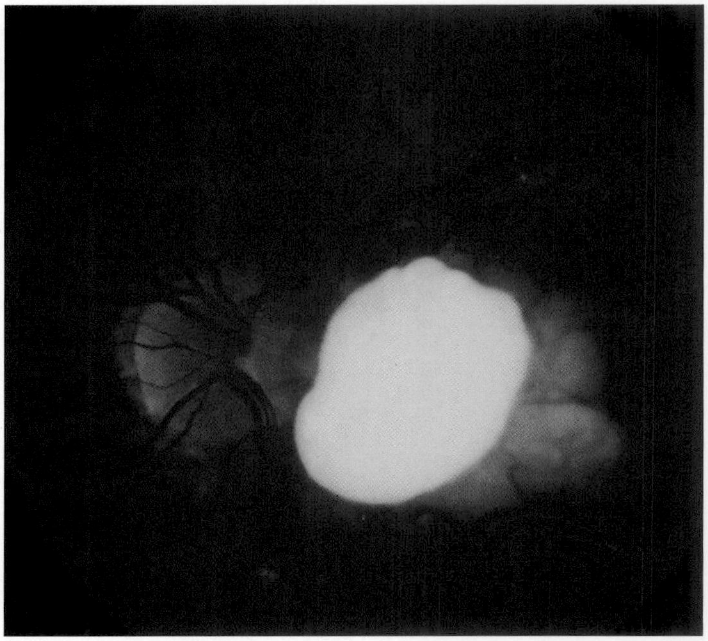

Fig. 10.144 Large granuloma associated with vascular distortion.

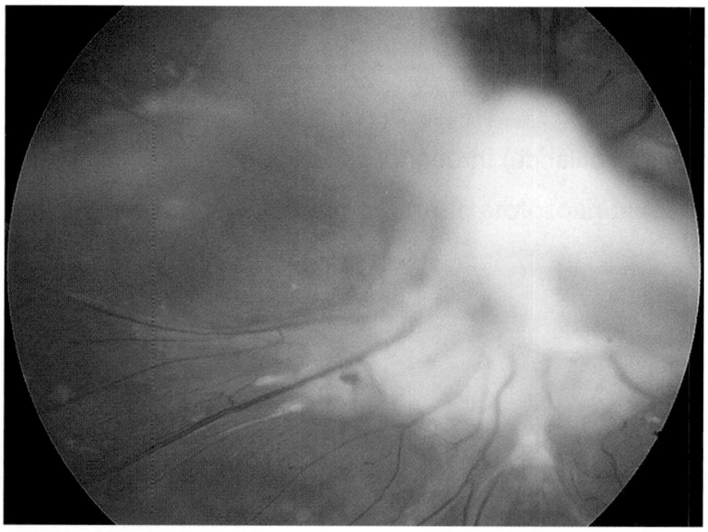

■ **Fig. 10.145** Optic disc granuloma with secondary tractional retinal detachment.

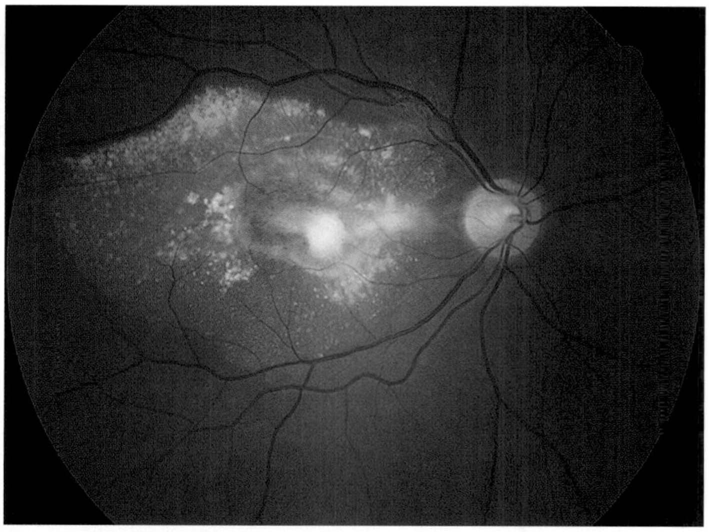

■ **Fig. 10.146** Small macular granuloma surrounded by hard exudates. (Courtesy of L. Merin.)

Peripheral granuloma

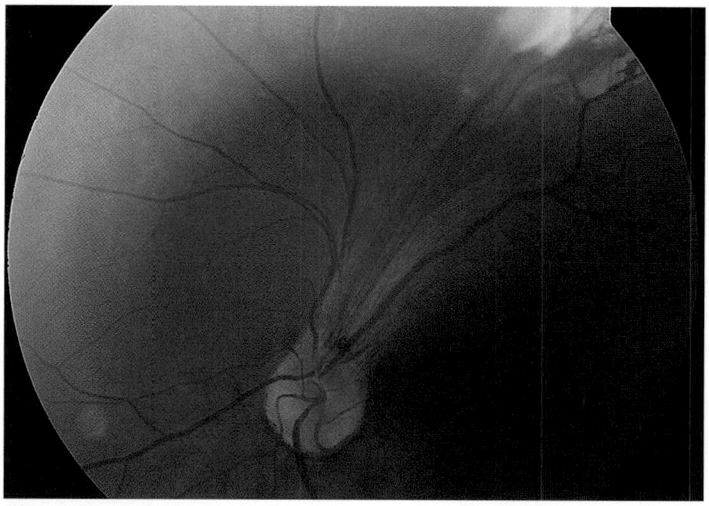

■ **Fig. 10.147** Small equatorial granuloma with traction band.

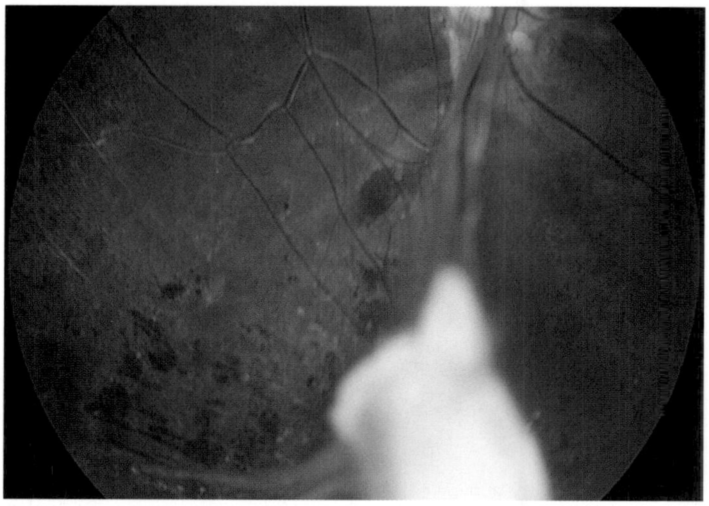

■ **Fig. 10.148** Large peripheral granuloma with traction band distorting the inferior part of the disc. (Courtesy of K. Rahman.)

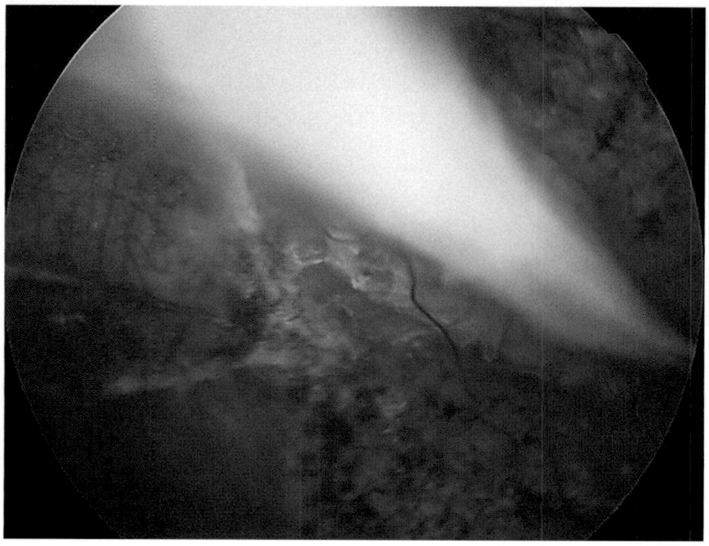

■ **Fig. 10.149** Very dense traction band. (Courtesy of C. Barry.)

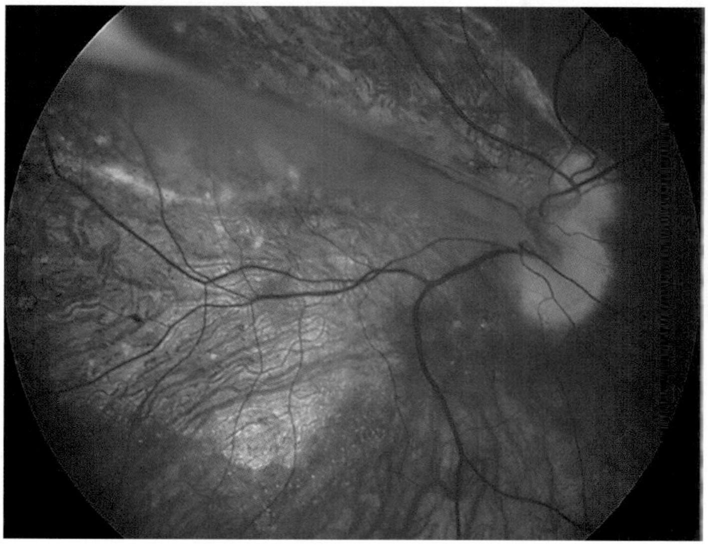

■ **Fig. 10.150** 'Dragging' of the disc and straightening of blood vessels by a traction band. (Courtesy of C. Barry.)

VIRAL RETINITIS

Cytomegalovirus (CMV) retinitis

CMV retinitis affects patients with AIDS, which is caused by the human immunodeficiency virus.

Systemic signs of AIDS

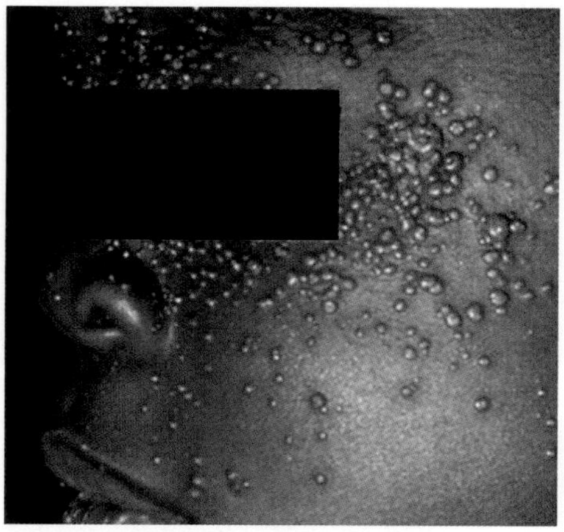

Fig. 10.167 Severe molluscum contagiosum. (Courtesy of B. J. Zitelli and H. W. Davis.)

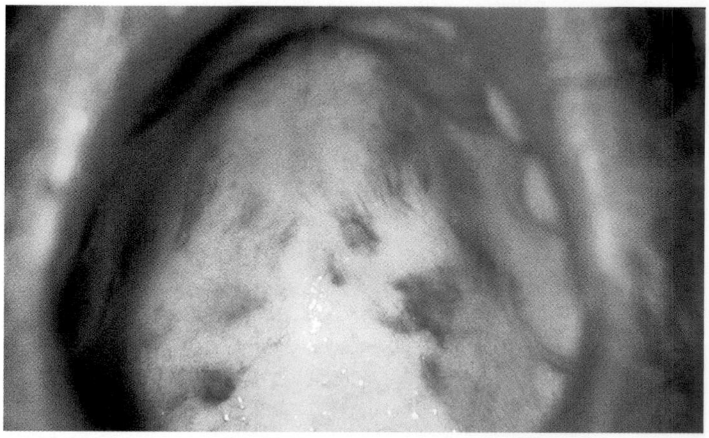

Fig. 10.168 Severe oral candidiasis, which may spread to the oesophagus.

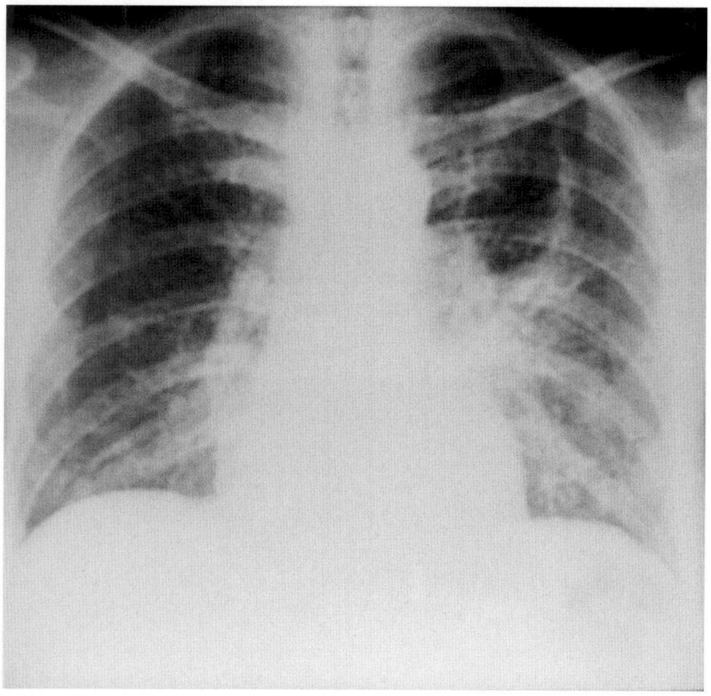

Fig. 10.169 *Pneumocystis carinii* pneumonia.

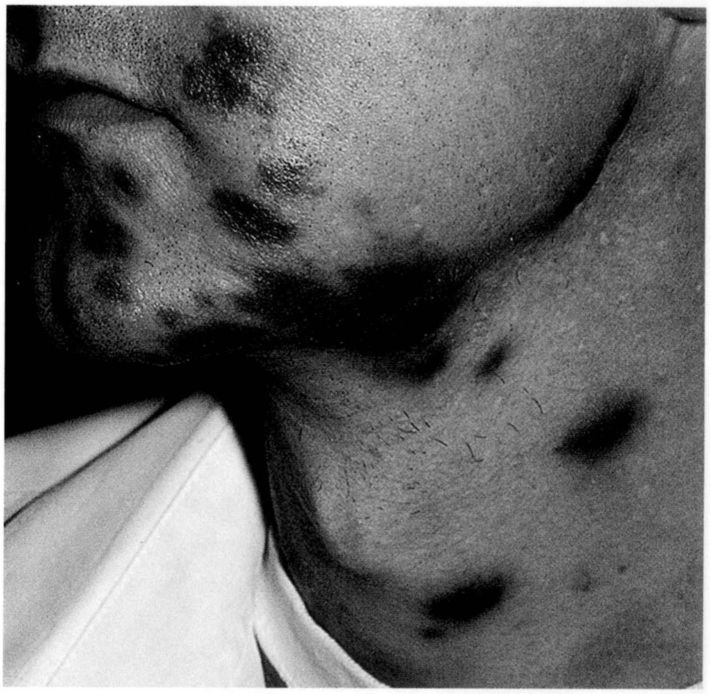

Fig. 10.170 Extensive cutaneous Kaposi sarcoma.

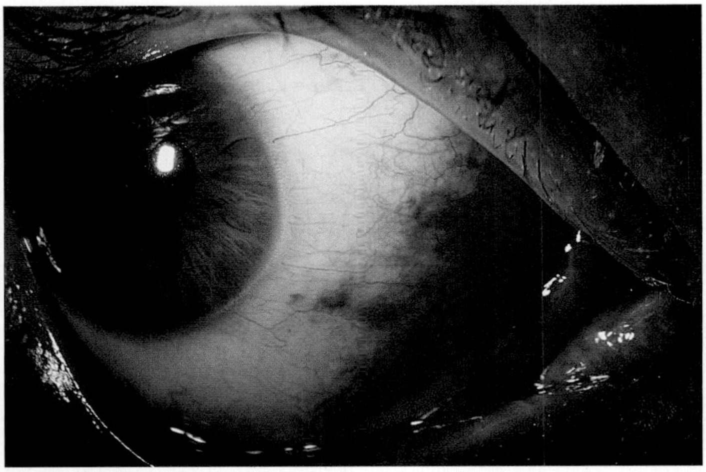

■ **Fig. 10.171** Conjunctival Kaposi sarcoma.

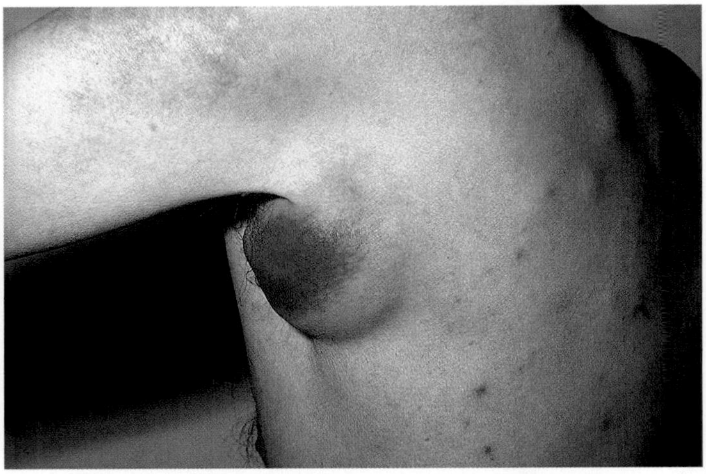

■ **Fig. 10.172** Non-Hodgkin B-cell lymphoma.

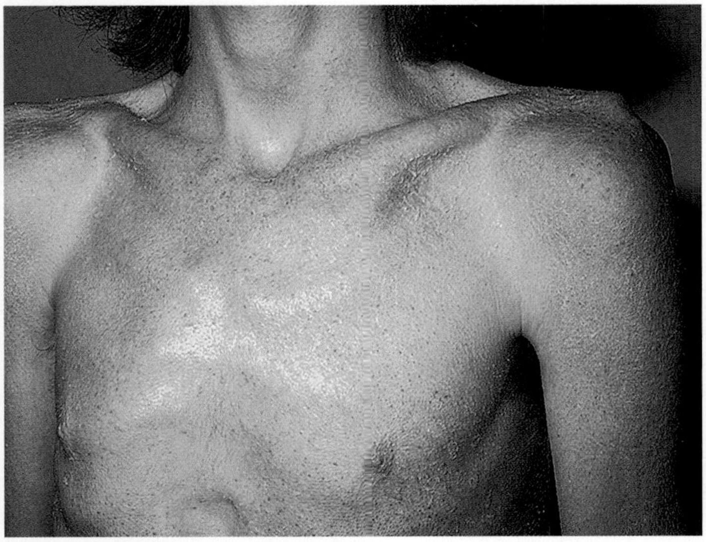

■ **Fig. 10.173** HIV wasting syndrome.

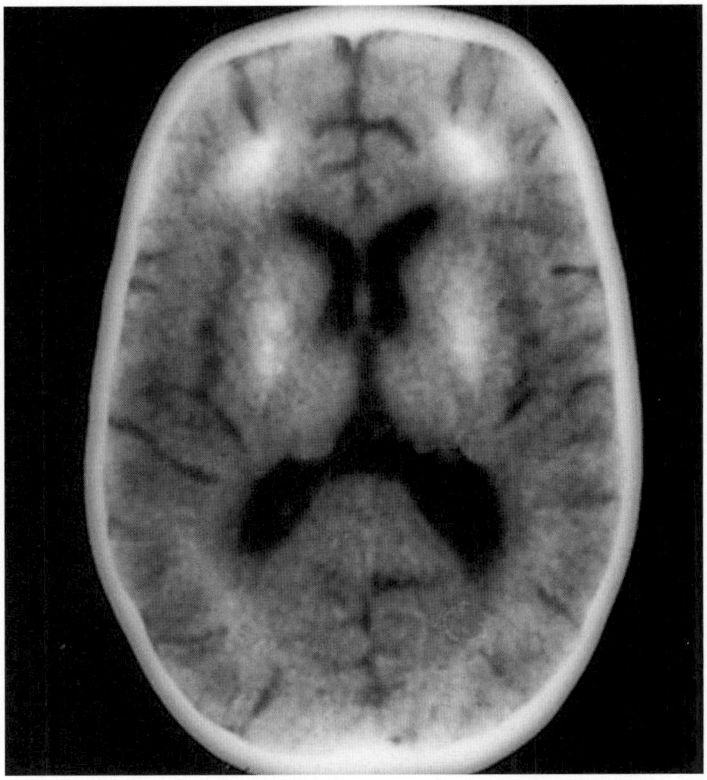

■ **Fig. 10.174** CT scan in an infant with AIDS encephalopathy showing increase in ventricular size secondary to brain atrophy and calcification in the basal ganglia and frontal lobes. (Courtesy of B. J. Zitelli and H. W. Davis.)

CMV retinitis

Indolent

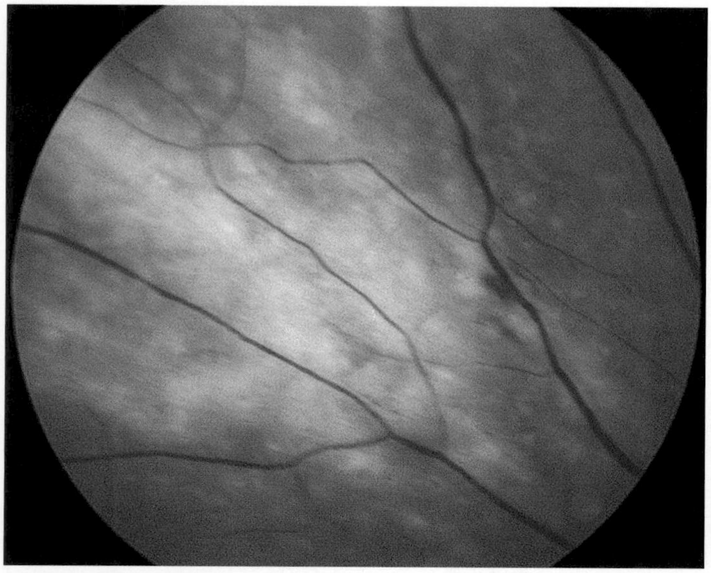

■ **Fig. 10.175** Subtle granular opacification without vasculitis, which often starts in the periphery.

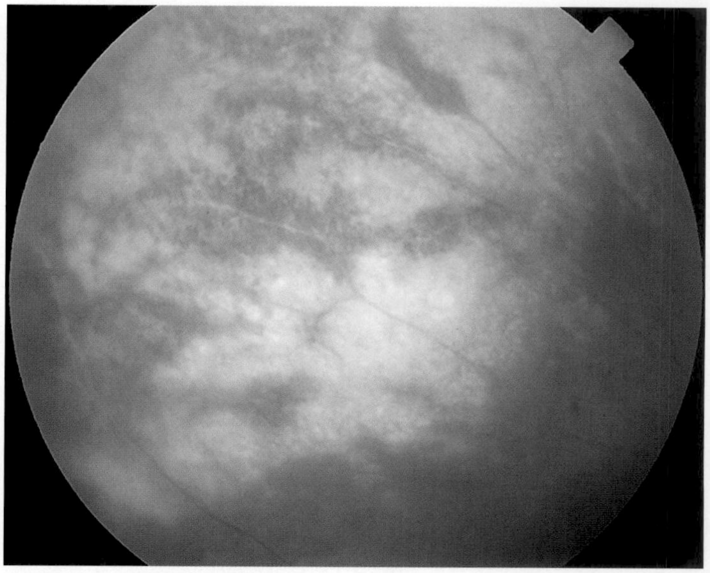

■ **Fig. 10.176** Slow progression.

Fulminating

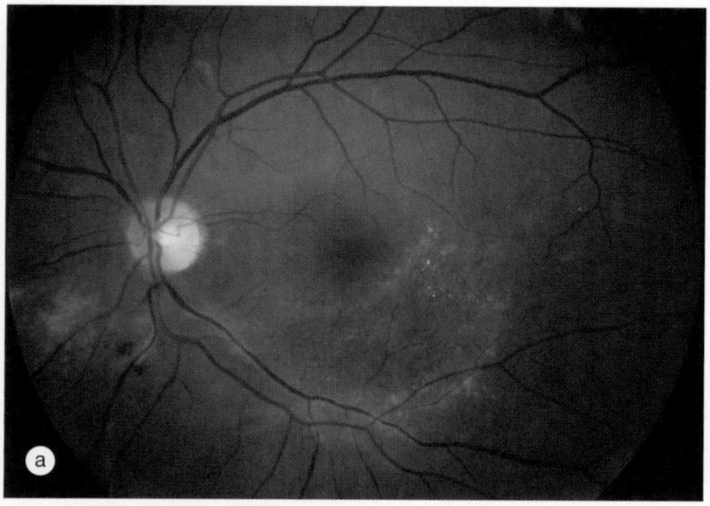

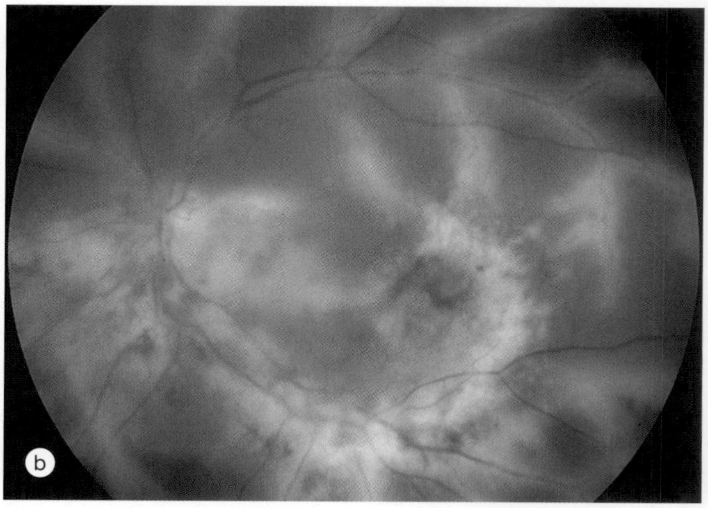

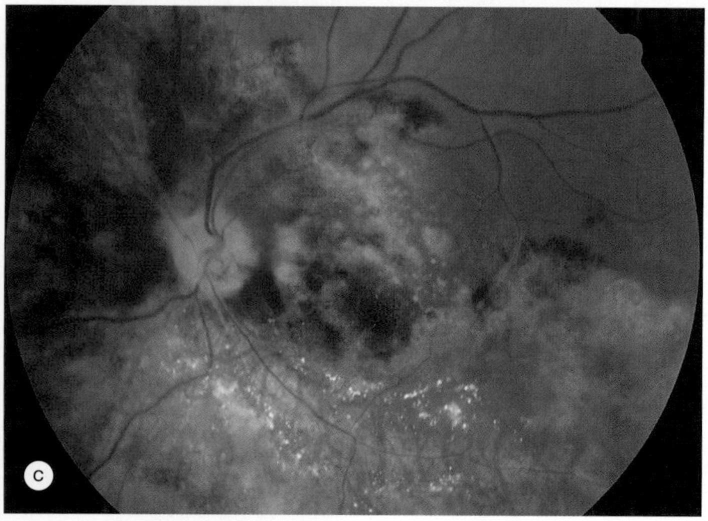

■ **Fig. 10.177** **(a)** Subtle vasculitis involving the inferotemporal arcade associated with mild opacification at the macula. **(b)** 3 weeks later there is extensive progression of vasculitis and retinal opacification. **(c)** 5 weeks later there is extensive retinal haemorrhage and severe retinal necrosis inferiorly. (Courtesy of L. Merin.)

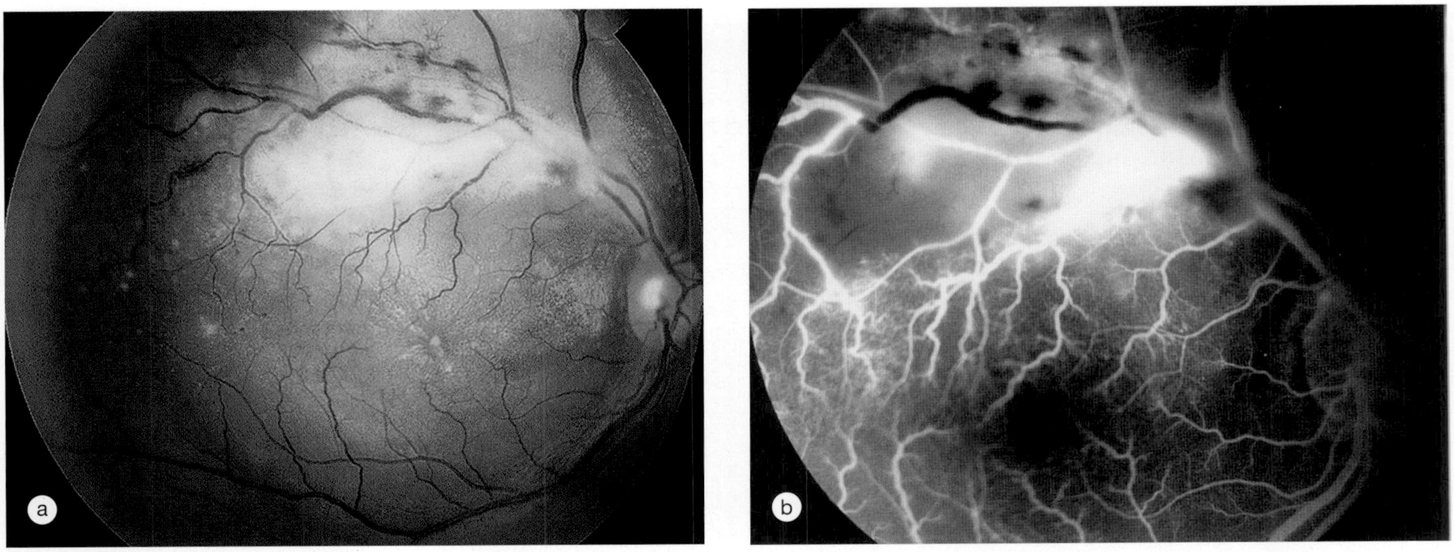

■ **Fig. 10.178** **(a)** 'Brushfire-like' extension along the superotemporal arcade. **(b)** FA shows hypofluorescence in areas of retinal necrosis. (Courtesy of S. Milewski.)

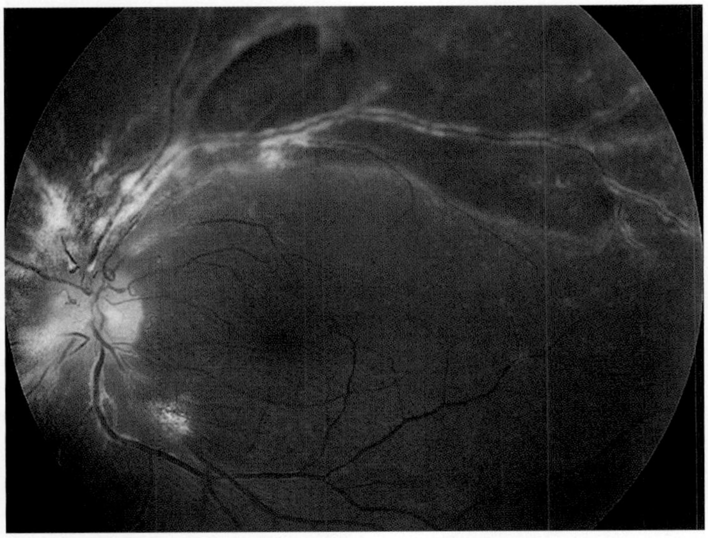

■ **Fig. 10.179** Retinal necrosis resulting in a large posterior retinal break and early retinal detachment. (Courtesy of C. Barry.)

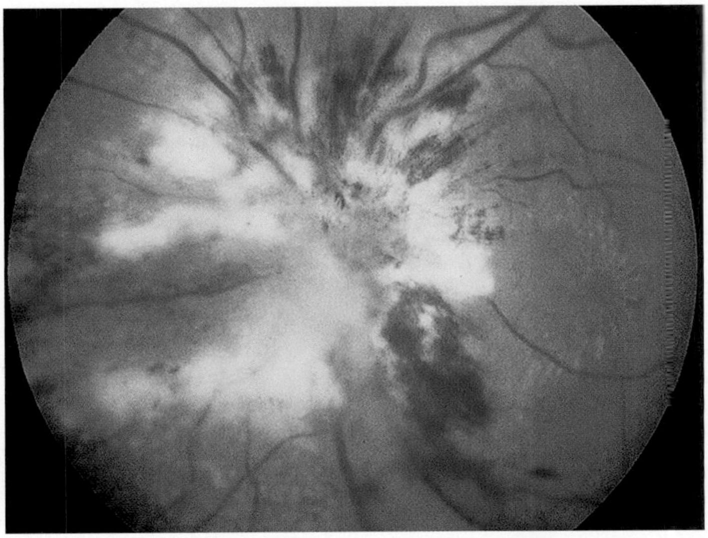

■ **Fig. 10.180** Severe retinitis with involvement of the optic nerve head. (Courtesy of S. Mitchell.)

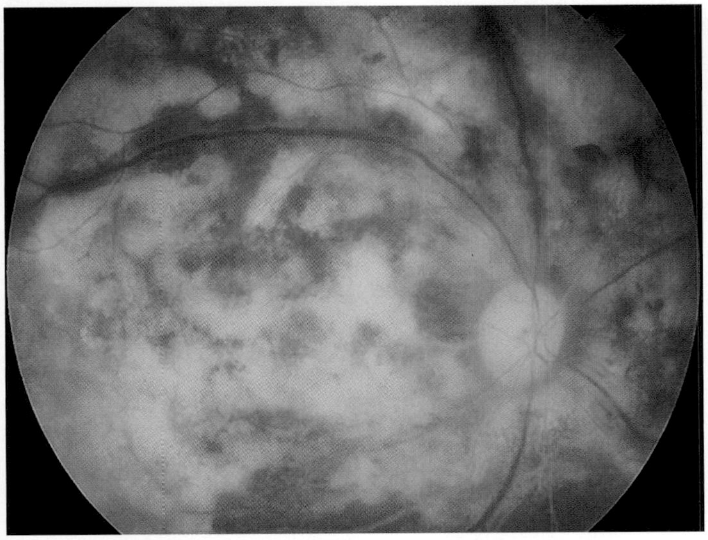

■ **Fig. 10.181** Extensive retinal necrosis and consecutive optic atrophy in end-stage disease. (Courtesy of S. Ford and R. Marsh.)

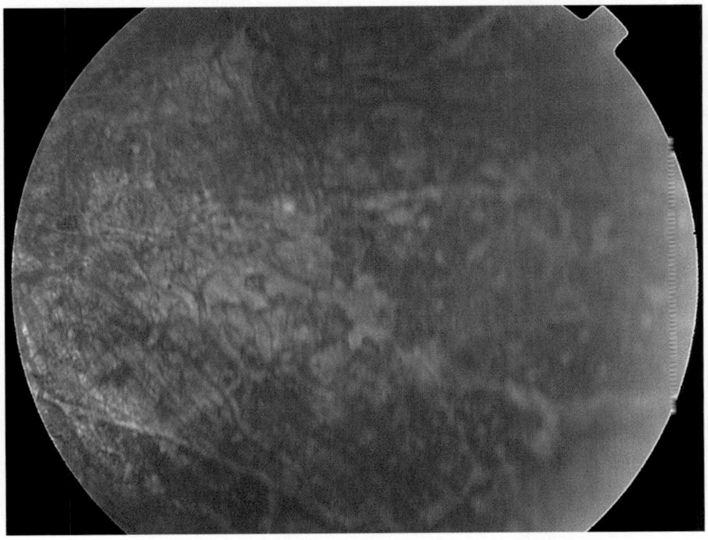

■ **Fig. 10.182** Regression is characterised by fewer haemorrhages and less opacification, followed by diffuse atrophy and mild pigmentary changes.

Progressive outer retinal necrosis (PORN)

PORN is a rare but devastating necrotising retinitis, caused by varicella zoster virus, which behaves more aggressively in patients with profound immunosuppression.

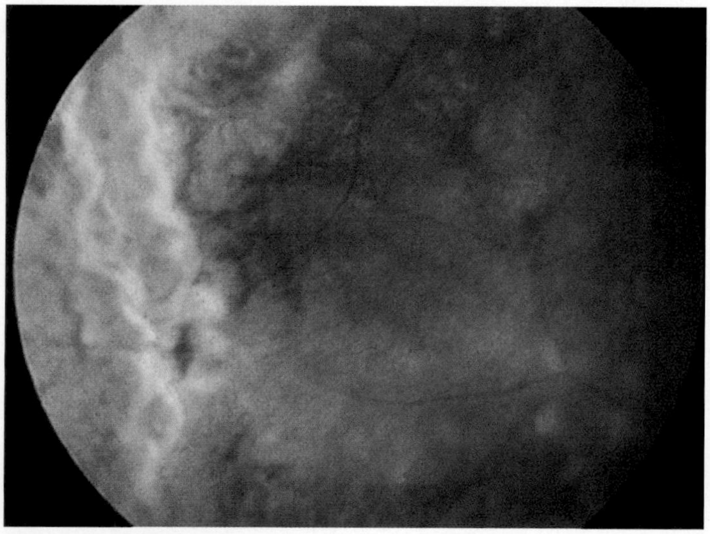

Fig. 10.183 Peripheral retinitis with minimal vitritis. (Courtesy of S. Mitchell.)

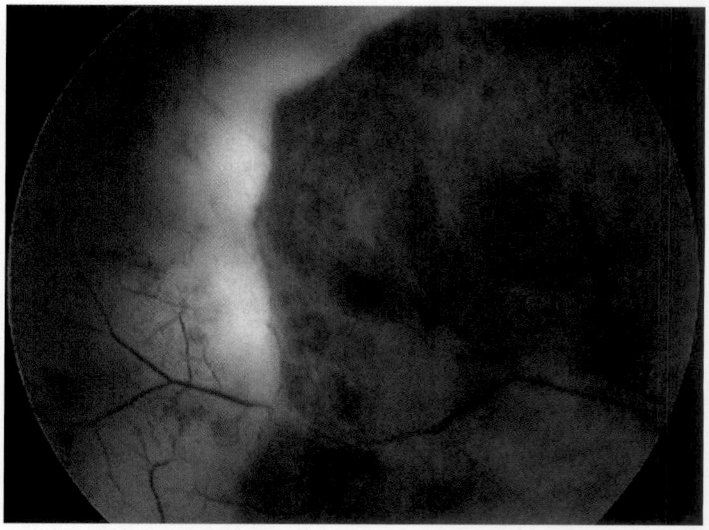

Fig. 10.184 Rapidly progressive full-thickness retinal necrosis.

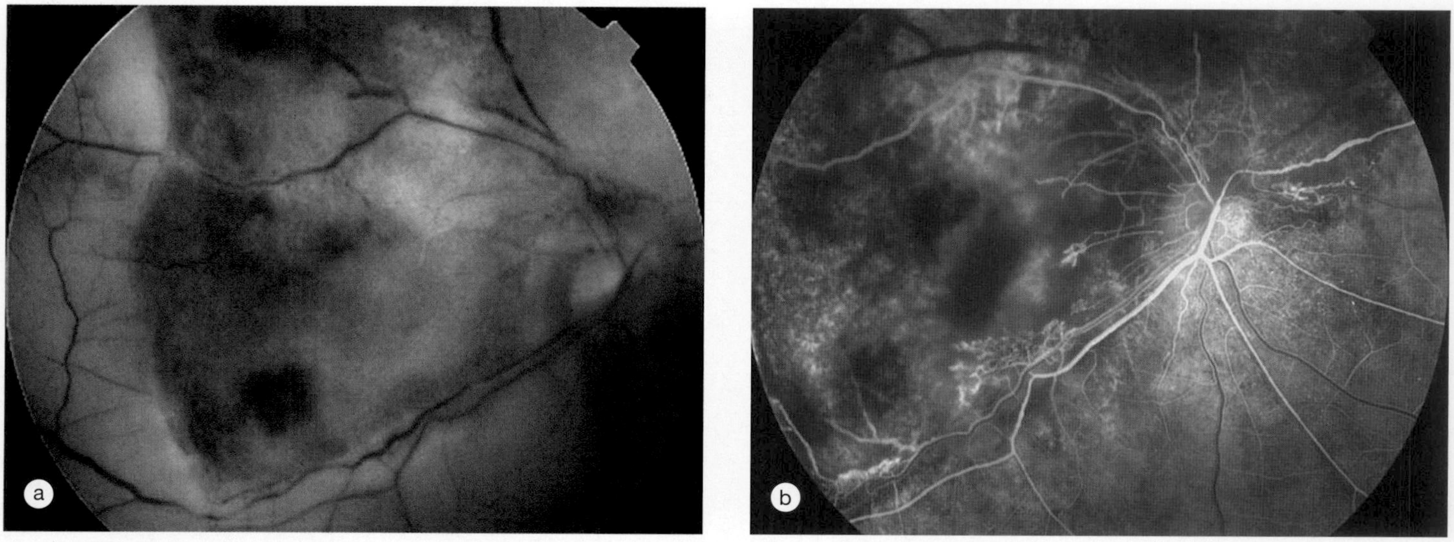

Fig. 10.185 **(a)** Early macular involvement. **(b)** FA shows severe macular non-perfusion.

Acute retinal necrosis (ARN)

ARN typically affects otherwise healthy individuals. It is caused by herpes simplex in young patients and herpes zoster in older individuals and is associated with granulomatous anterior uveitis and vitritis.

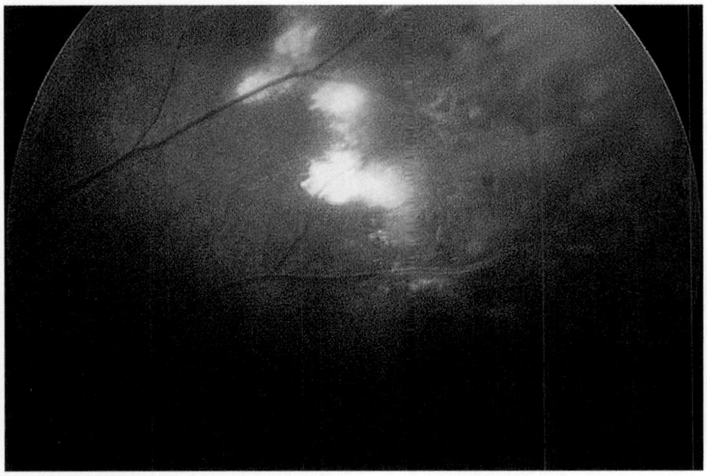

Fig. 10.186 Peripheral retinal periarteritis associated with multifocal, deep, yellow-white retinal infiltrates.

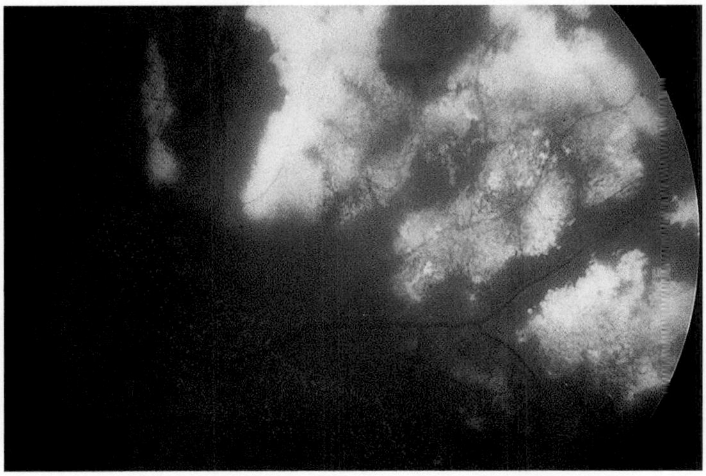

Fig. 10.187 Increase in number and gradual confluence of lesions associated with full-thickness retinal necrosis. (Courtesy of S. Ford and R. Marsh.)

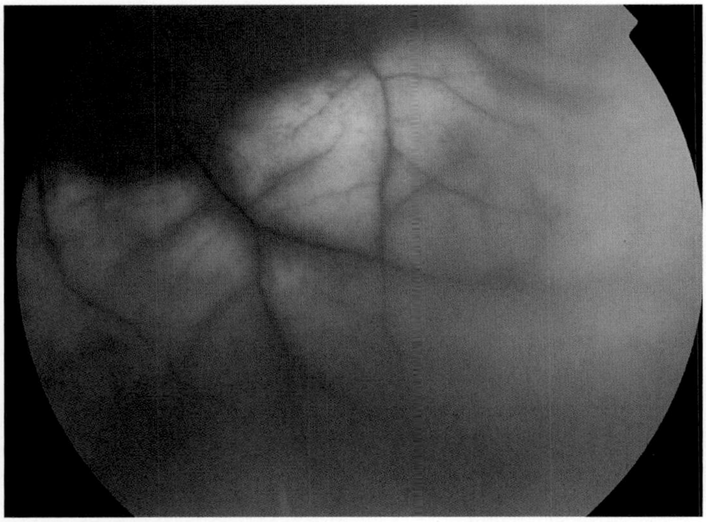

Fig. 10.188 Circumferential spread. (Courtesy of C. Pavésio.)

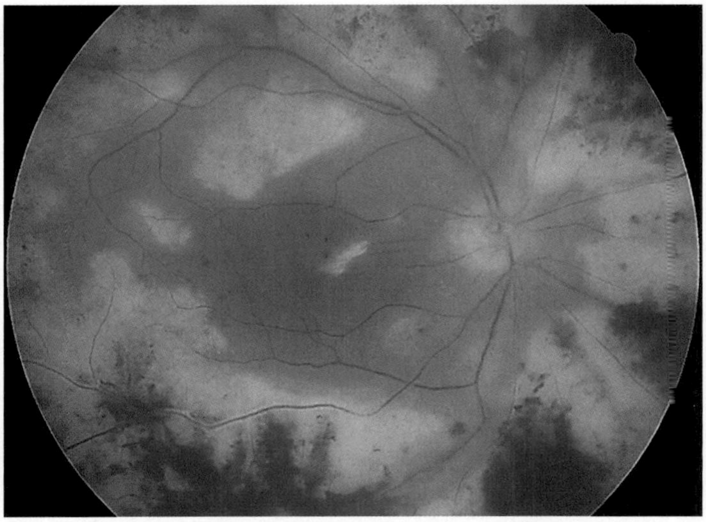

Fig. 10.189 The posterior pole is usually spared until late. (Courtesy of C. Barry.)

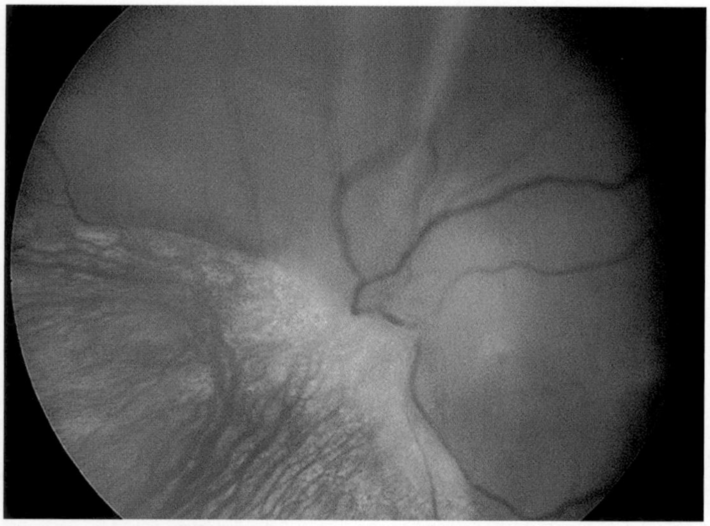

Fig. 10.190 Rhegmatogenous retinal detachment develops as a result of retinal holes at the margin of uninvolved and involved zones. (Courtesy of S. Mitchell.)

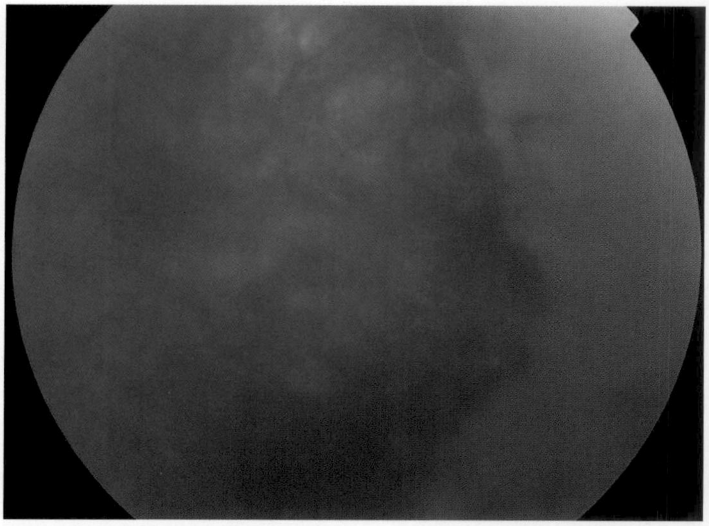

Fig. 10.191 Resolved ARN.

Subacute sclerosing panencephalitis (SSP)

SSP is a progressive neurological disease caused by chronic measles (rubeola) infection.

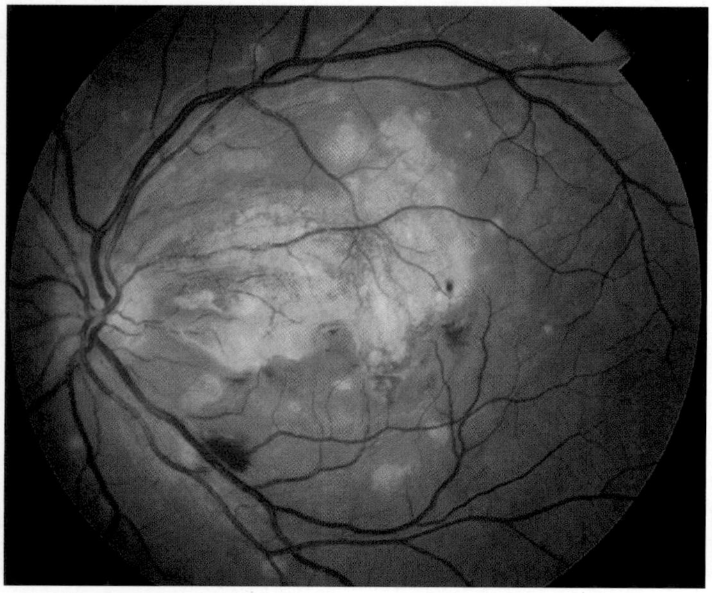

Fig. 10.192 Retinitis and mild periphlebitis involving the posterior pole and periphery, which may be associated with a cherry-red spot at the fovea. (Courtesy of Z. Bashshur.)

BACTERIAL UVEITIS

Tuberculosis

Tuberculosis is a chronic granulomatous infection caused by the tubercle bacillus, which may be bovine (*Mycobacterium bovis*) or human (*Mycobacterium tuberculosis*).

Systemic signs

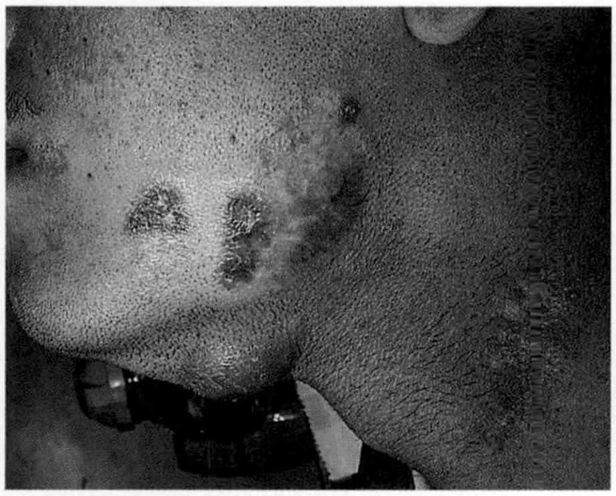

Fig. 10.193 Tuberculous cervical adenitis.

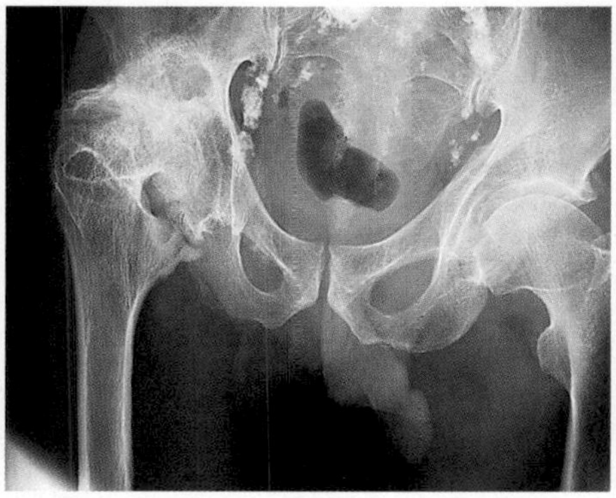

Fig. 10.194 Tuberculous involvement of the right hip.

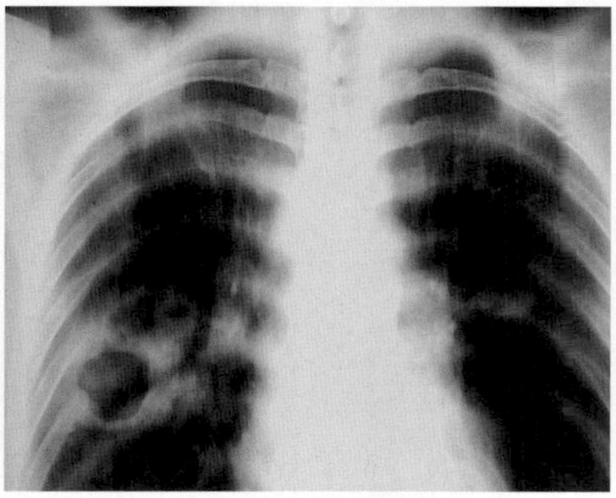

Fig. 10.195 Radiograph showing tuberculous cavitation in the right lower lobe.

Ocular signs

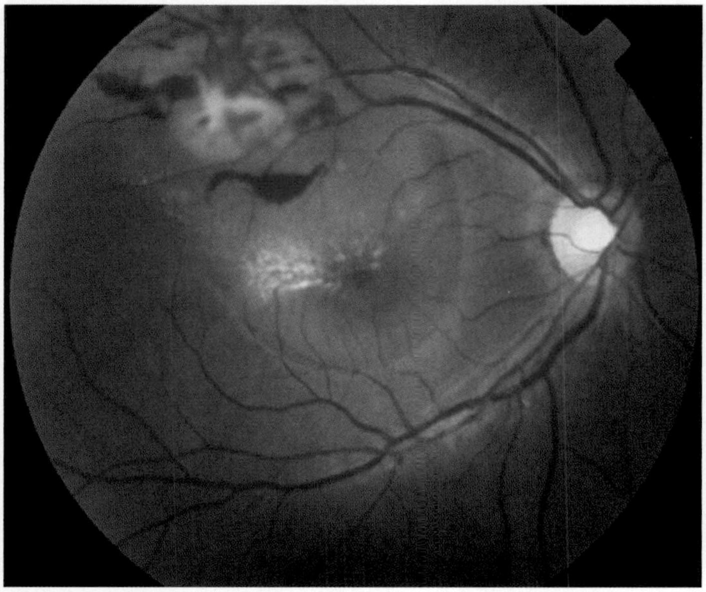

Fig. 10.196 Occlusive periphlebitis (Courtesy C. Pavesio.)

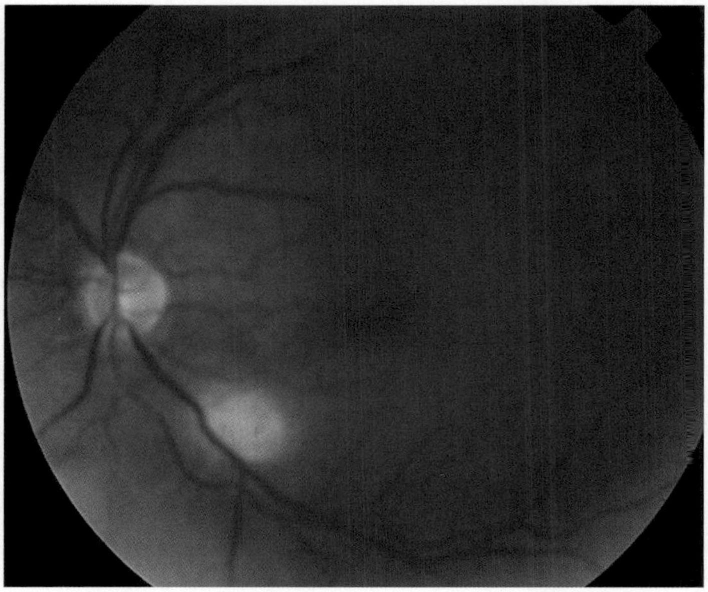

Fig. 10.197 Small choroidal tubercle. (Courtesy of A. Curi.)

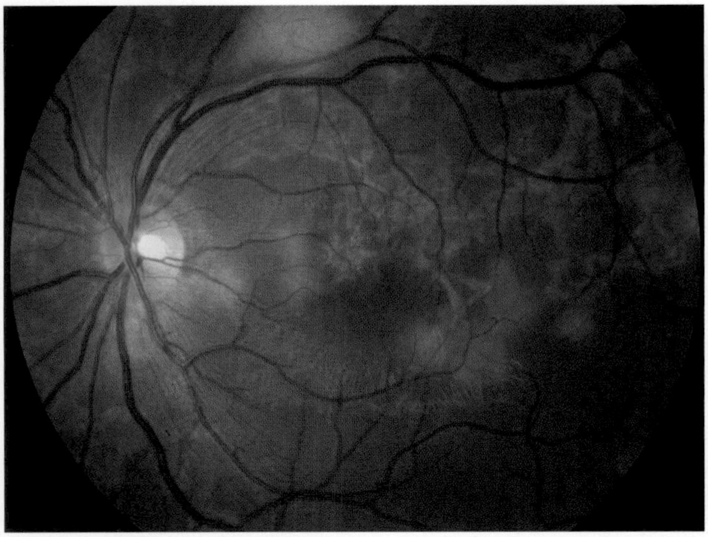

Fig. 10.198 Choroiditis resembling serpiginous choroidopathy is uncommon.

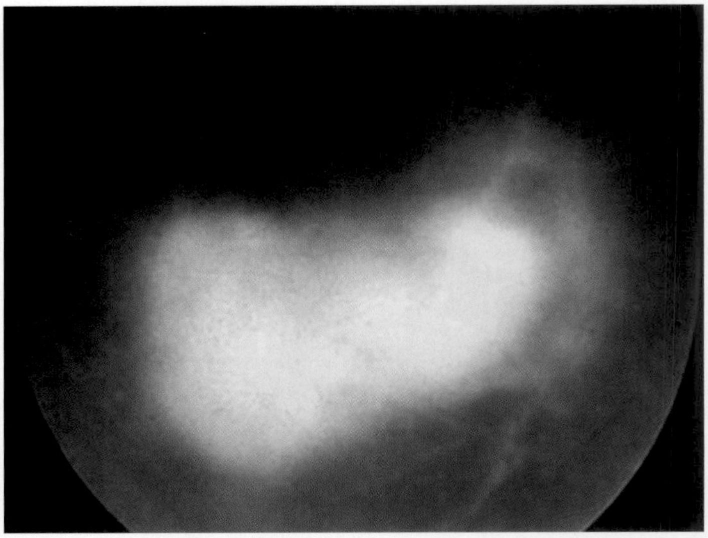

Fig. 10.199 Large, solitary choroidal tuberculoma. (Courtesy of C. de A. Garcia.)

Syphilis

Syphilis is a sexually transmitted infection caused by the spirochaete *Treponema pallidum*. Uveitis typically develops during the secondary stage.

Signs of secondary syphilis

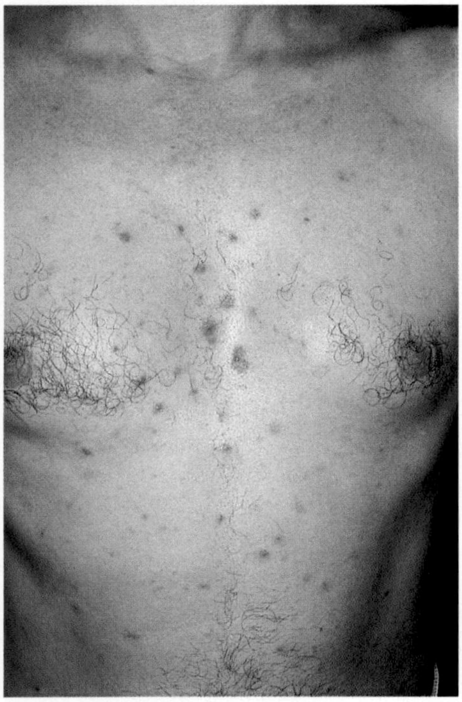

Fig. 10.200 Non-irritable maculopapular rash on the trunk.

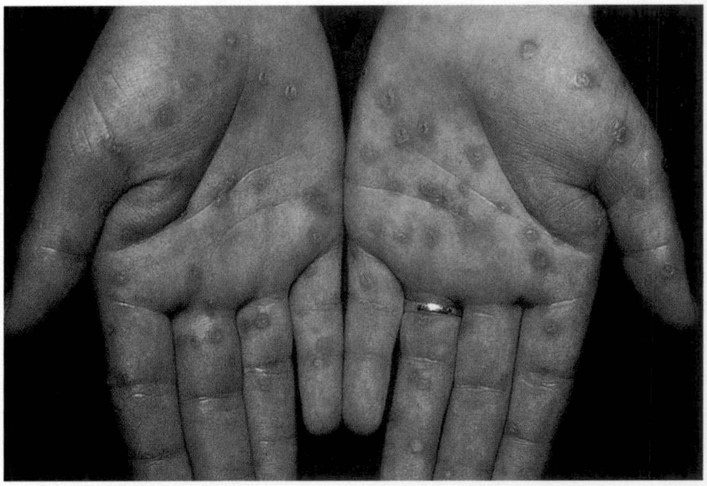

Fig. 10.201 Involvement of the palms and soles is typical. (Courtesy of M. A. Mir.)

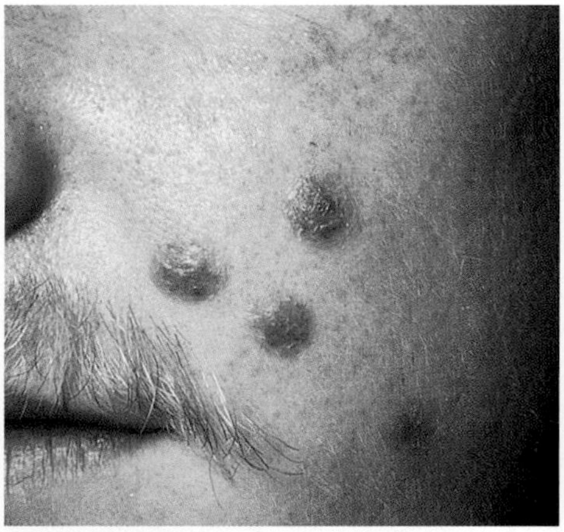

Fig. 10.202 Larger facial papules. (Courtesy of M. A. Mir.)

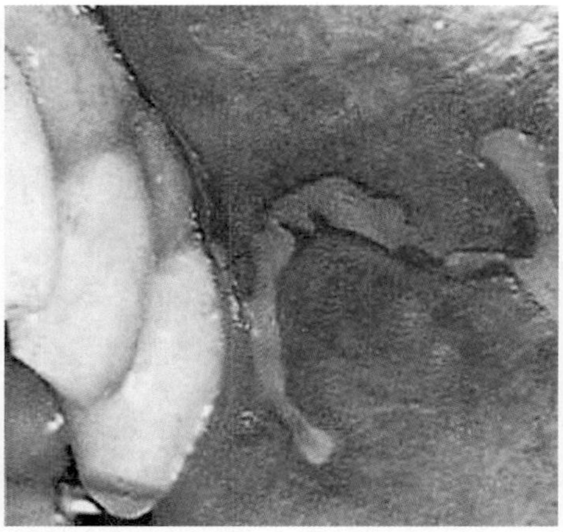

Fig. 10.203 'Snail-track' ulceration in the mouth. (Courtesy of C. D. Forbes and W. F. Jackson.)

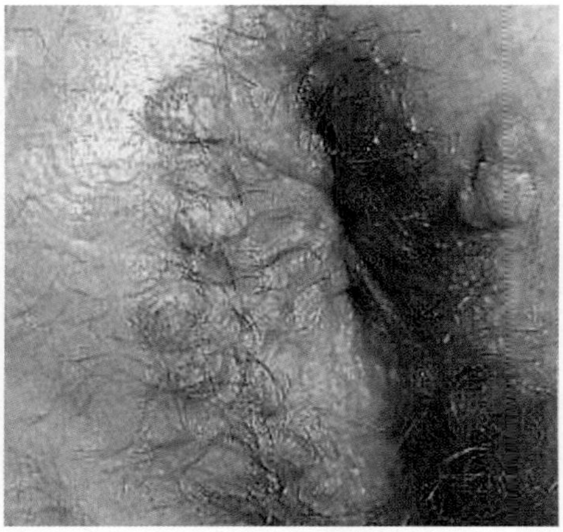

Fig. 10.204 Condylomata lata develop in moist warm sites. (Courtesy of P. C. Hayes and N. D. C. Finlayson.)

Ocular signs

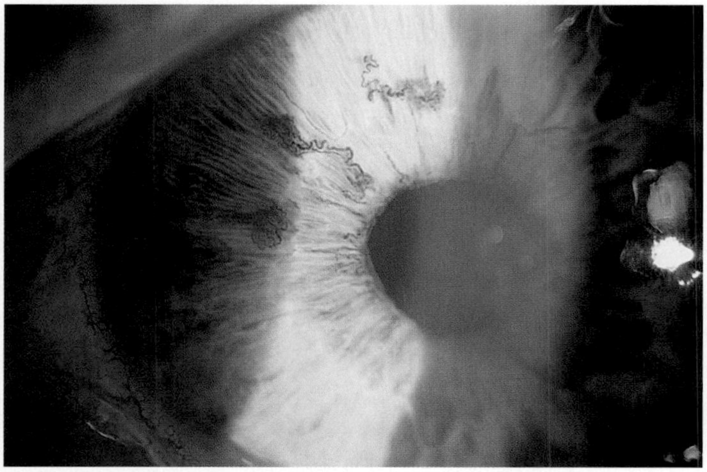

Fig. 10.205 Acute anterior uveitis may be associated with dilated iris capillaries (roseolae).

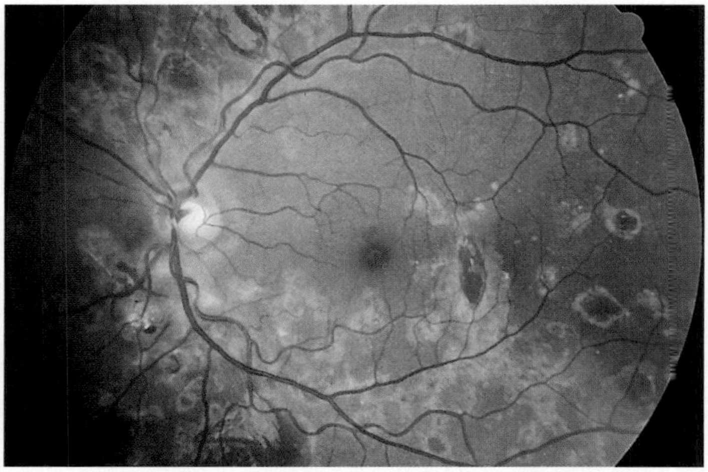

Fig. 10.206 Multifocal choroiditis, which, on healing, appears as focal areas of chorioretinal atrophy associated with hyperpigmentation. (Courtesy of J. Salmon.)

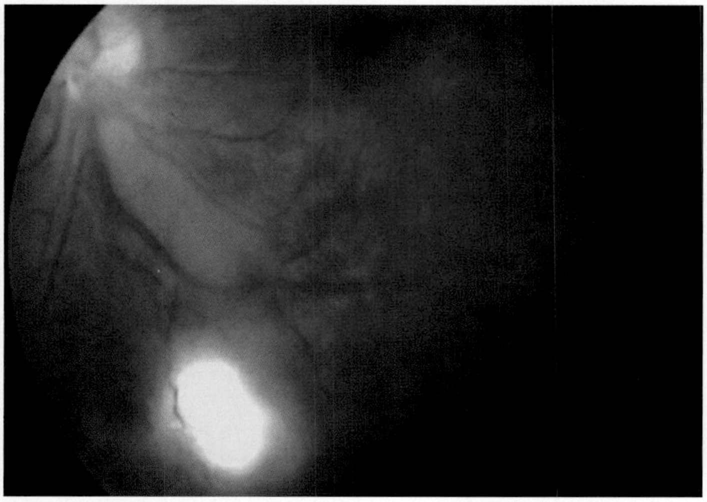

Fig. 10.207 Focal chorioretinitis is less common and frequently bilateral. (Courtesy of C. de A. Garcia.)

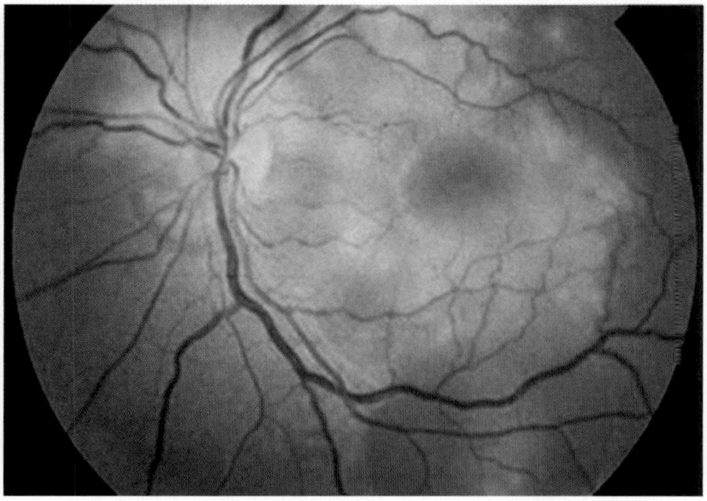

Fig. 10.208 Acute posterior placoid chorioretinitis is uncommon. (Courtesy of C. de A. Garcia.)

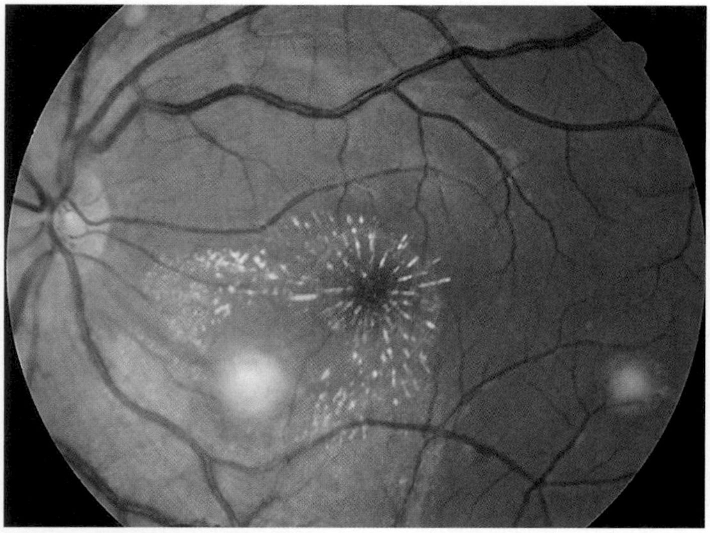

Fig. 10.209 Acute neuroretinitis (Courtesy of J. Salmon.)

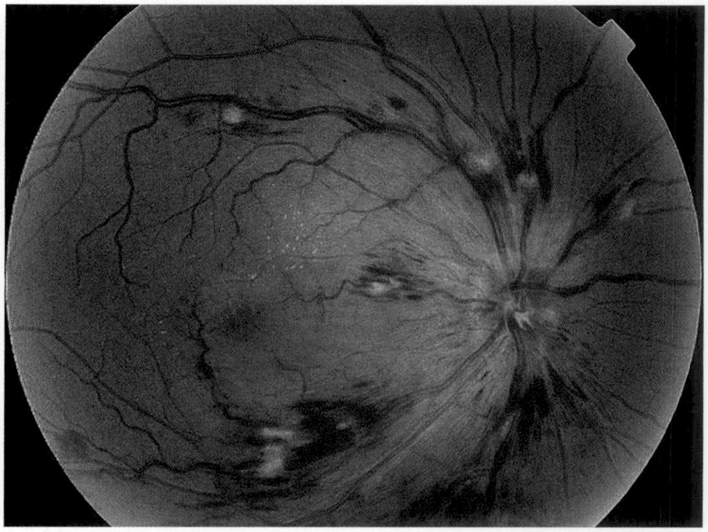

Fig. 10.210 Periphlebitis, which may be associated with central retinal vein occlusion.

Leprosy

Leprosy (Hansen disease) is a chronic granulomatous infection caused by *Mycobacterium leprae.*

Systemic signs

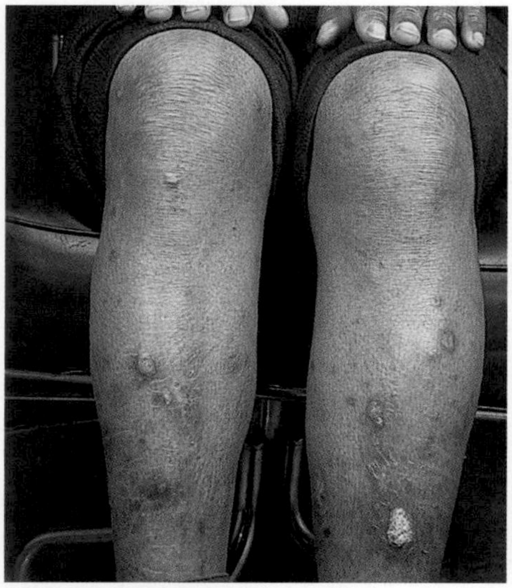

Fig. 10.211 Cutaneous plaques.

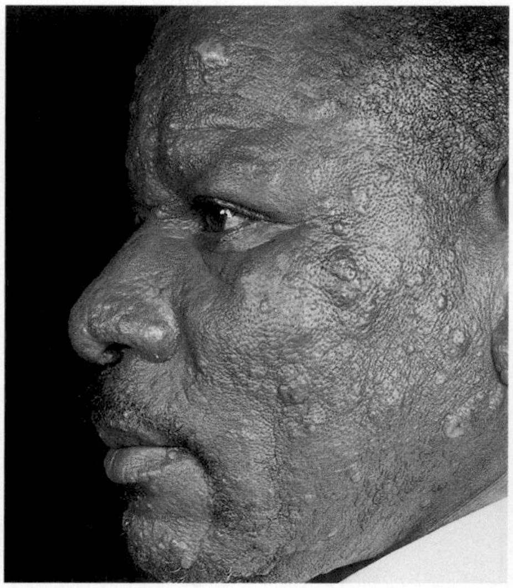

Fig. 10.212 Cutaneous nodules.

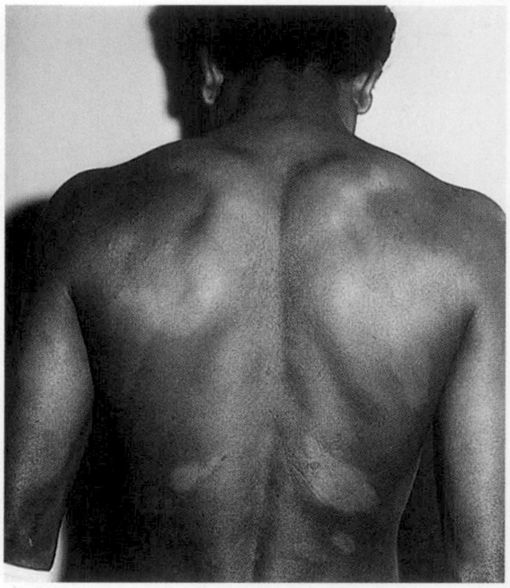

Fig. 10.213 Annular, anaesthetic, hypopigmented skin patches.

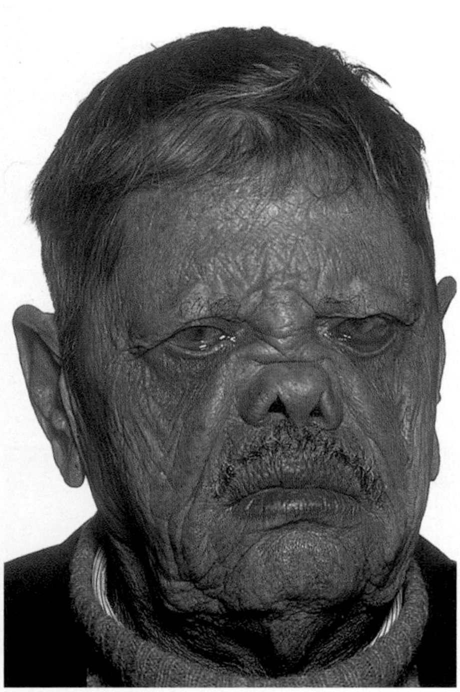

Fig. 10.214 Saddle-shaped nasal deformity; also note bilateral ectropion and corneal scarring. (Courtesy of T. ffytche.)

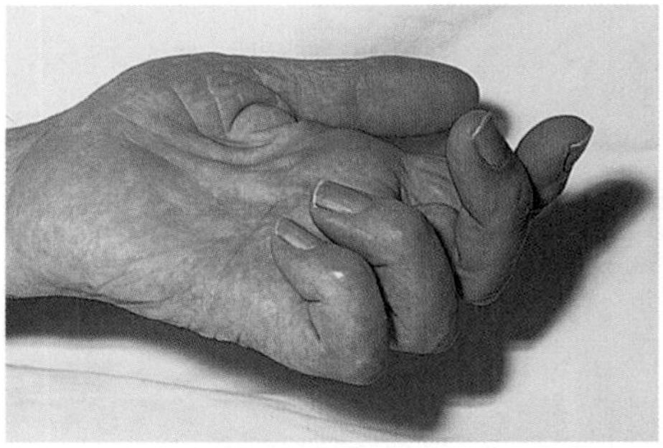

Fig. 10.215 Claw hand due to ulnar nerve palsy.

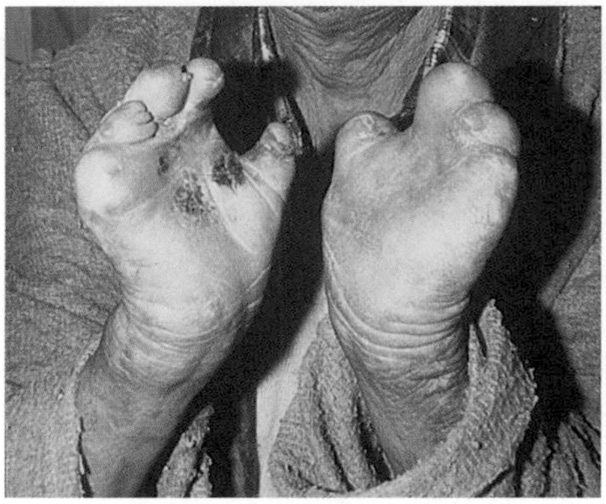

Fig. 10.216 Shortening of digits due to sensory neuropathy. (Courtesy of T. ffytche.)

Ocular signs

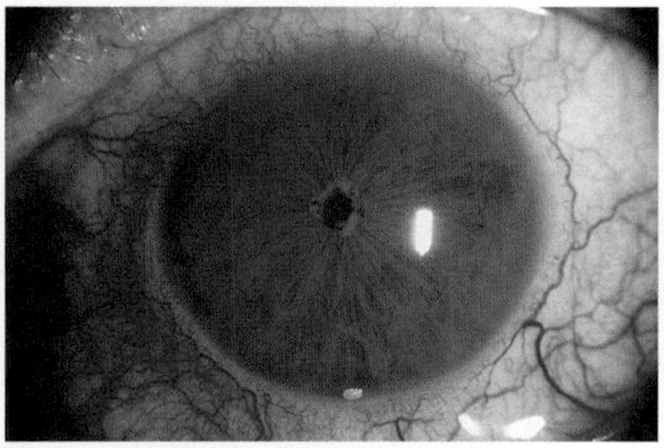

Fig. 10.217 Chronic iritis resulting in severe miosis. (Courtesy of P. Gili.)

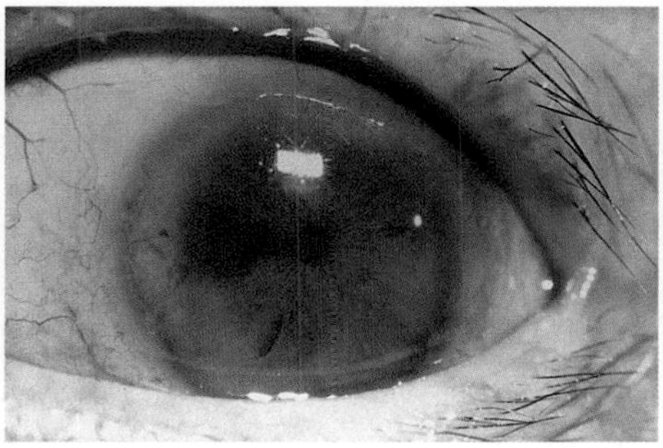

Fig. 10.218 Miosis and mild iris atrophy. (Courtesy of T. ffytche.)

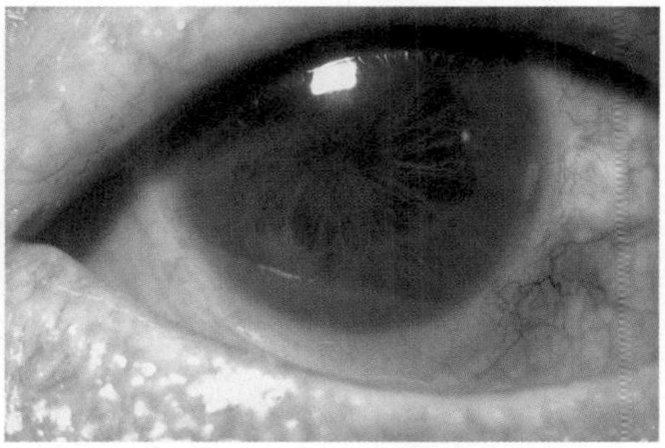

Fig. 10.219 Miosis and severe iris atrophy. (Courtesy of T. ffytche.)

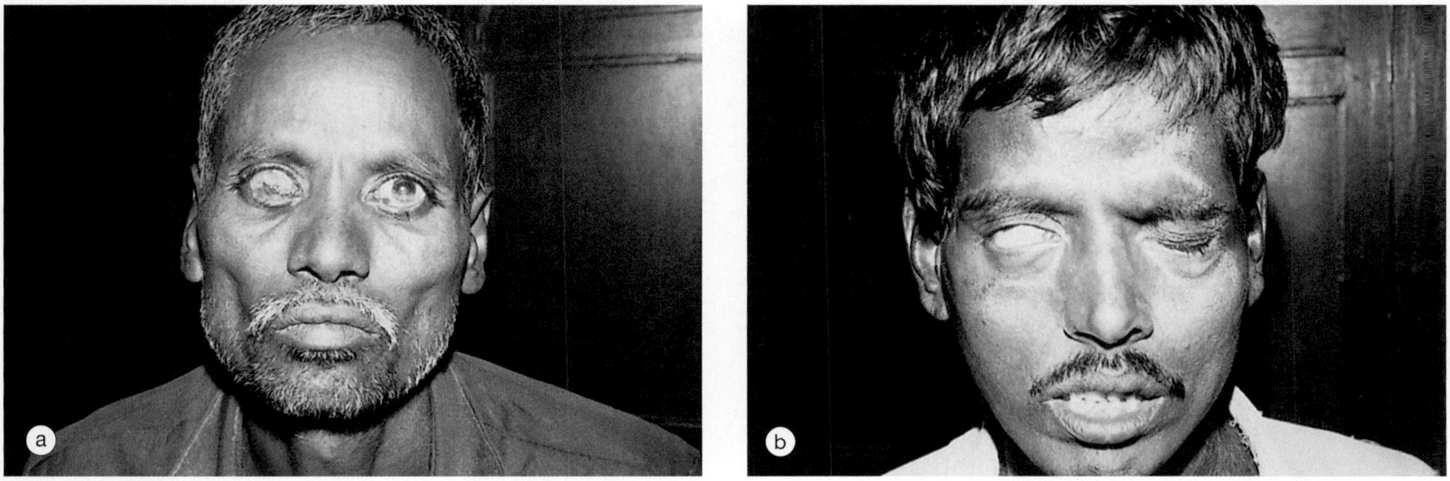

Fig. 10.220 **(a)** Severe corneal scarring. **(b)** Lagophthalmos due to facial palsy. (Courtesy of T. ffytche.)

Cat-scratch disease

Cat-scratch disease is a subacute infection of the skin, soft tissues and regional lymph nodes caused by *Bartonella henselae*.

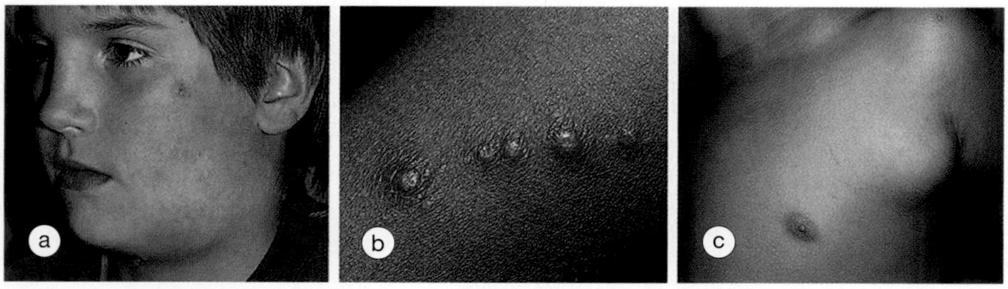

Fig. 10.221 **(a)** Scratch on the left cheek, inflicted by a cat, and cervical lymphadenopathy. **(b)** A line of papules on the forearm of another patient at the site of a cat scratch. **(c)** Ipsilateral axillary lymphadenopathy. (Courtesy of B. J. Zitelli and H. W. Davis.)

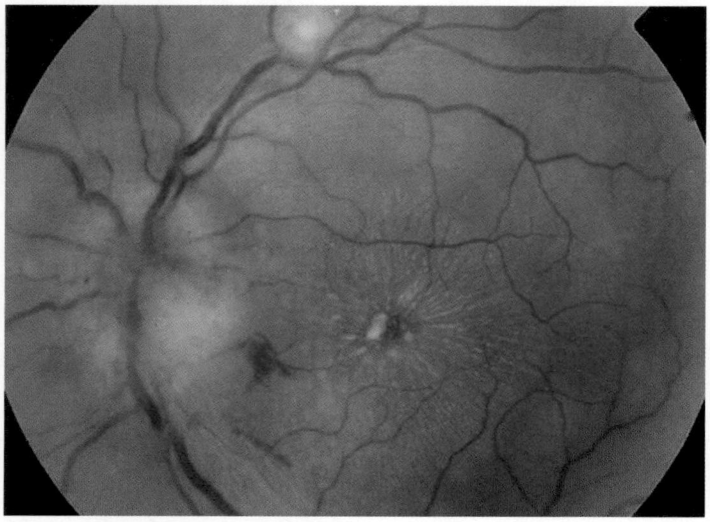

Fig. 10.222 Acute neuroretinitis. (Courtesy of P. Curi.)

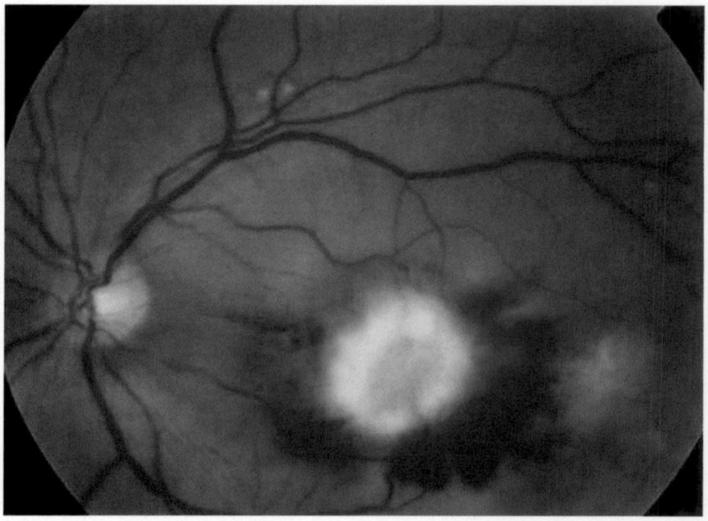

Fig. 10.223 Focal chorioretinitis is less common. (Courtesy of P. Curi.)

Nocardiosis

Nocardia asteroides, a Gram-positive, aerobic bacterium that typically causes pulmonary pseudo-tuberculosis and brain abscesses, especially in immunocompromised patients.

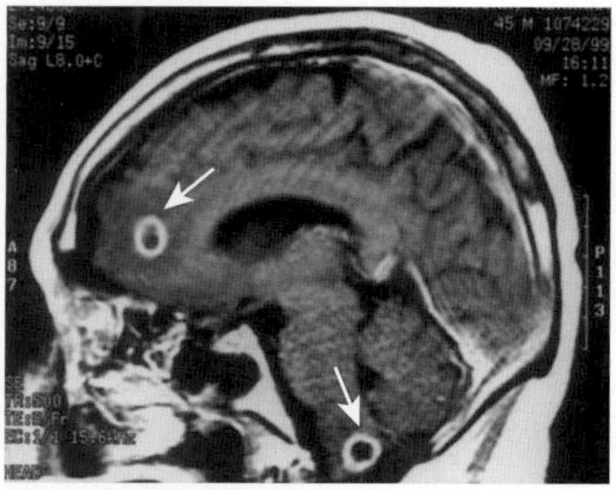

Fig. 10.224 MRI showing two gadolinium-enhanced brain lesions. (Courtesy of L. Goldman and D. Ausiello.)

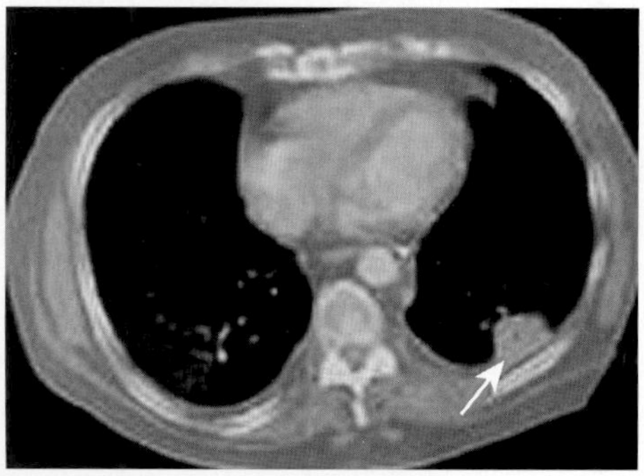

Fig. 10.225 Chest CT showing a peripheral nodule. (Courtesy of L. Goldman and D. Ausiello.)

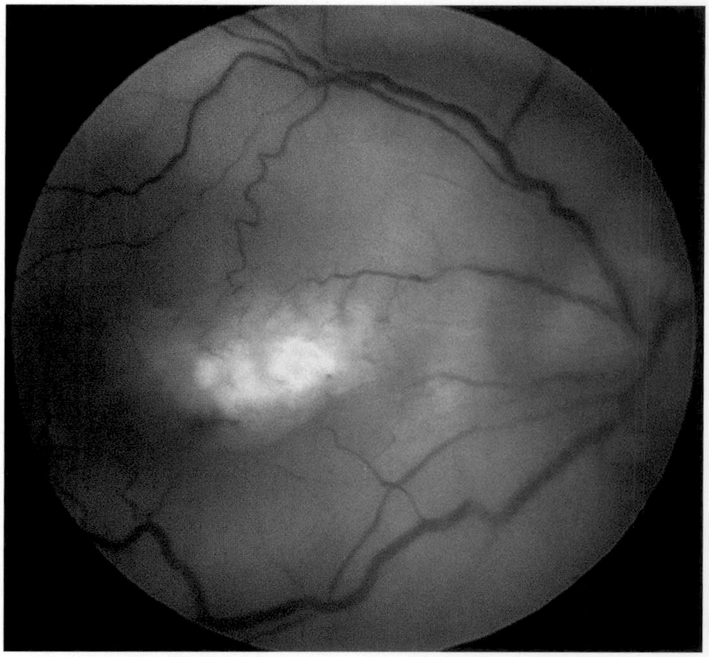

Fig. 10.226 Chorioretinitis with subretinal abscess.

FUNGAL UVEITIS

Histoplasmosis

Histoplasmosis is a fungal infection caused by *Histoplasma capsulatum*. Severe visual loss may occur as a result of exudative maculopathy secondary to choroidal neovascularisation (CNV).

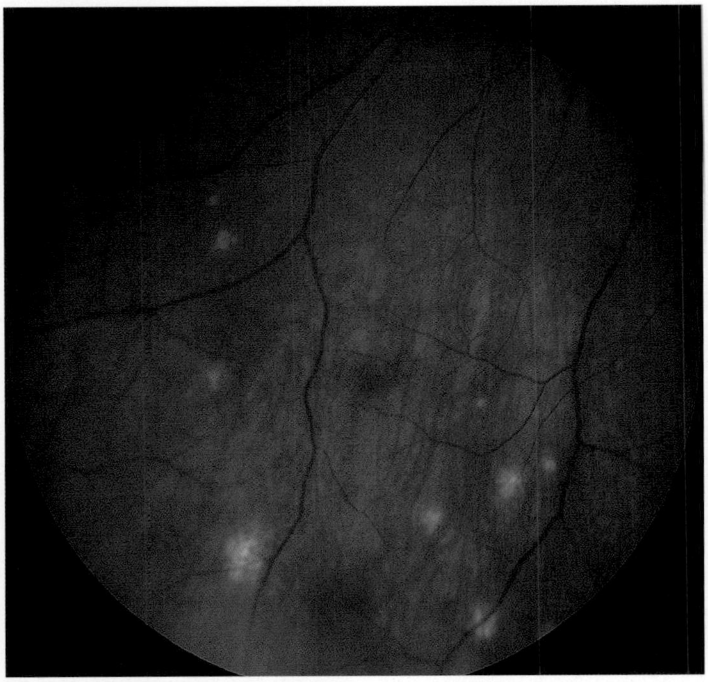

Fig. 10.227 Atrophic 'histo' spots consist of roundish, slightly irregular, yellowish-white lesions that may be associated with small pigment clumps scattered in the mid-retinal periphery.

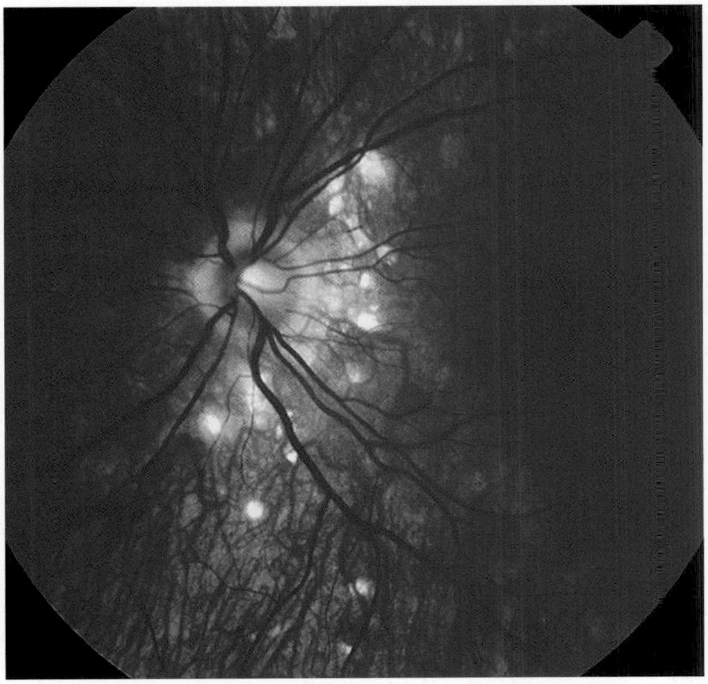

Fig. 10.228 Multiple central 'histo' spots, some of which are peripapillary.

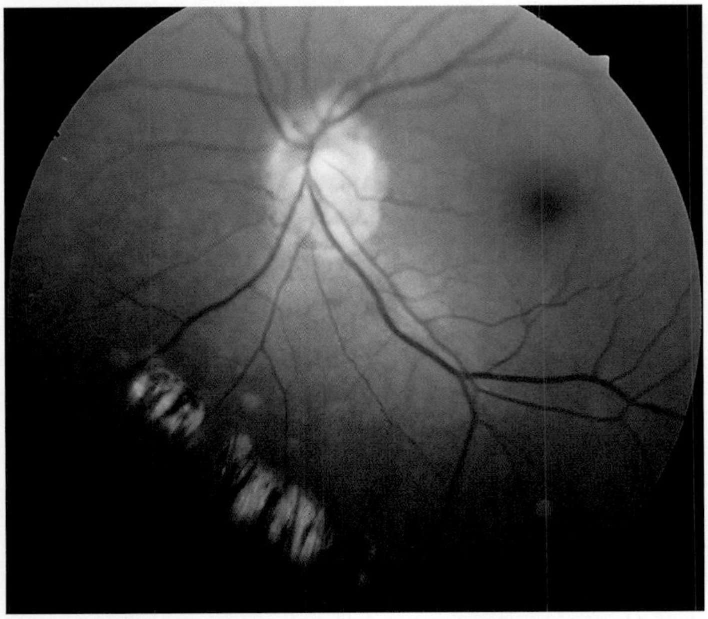

Fig. 10.229 Peripheral linear streaks of chorioretinal atrophy.

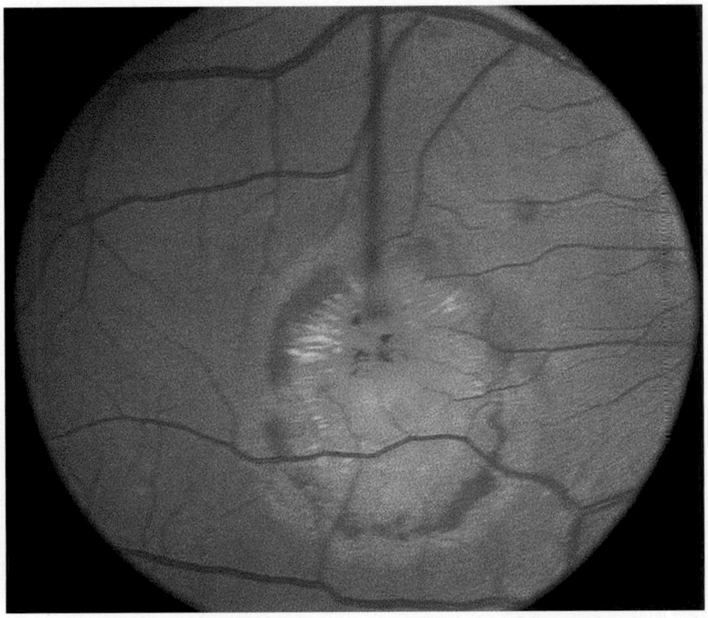

Fig. 10.230 Subretinal fluid, haemorrhage and small exudates associated with CNV at the macula.

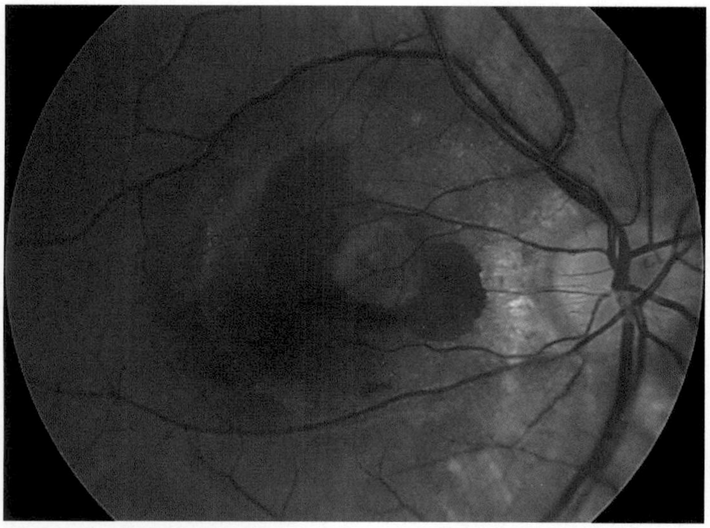

Fig. 10.231 Large subretinal haemorrhage from CNV. (Courtesy of C. Barry.)

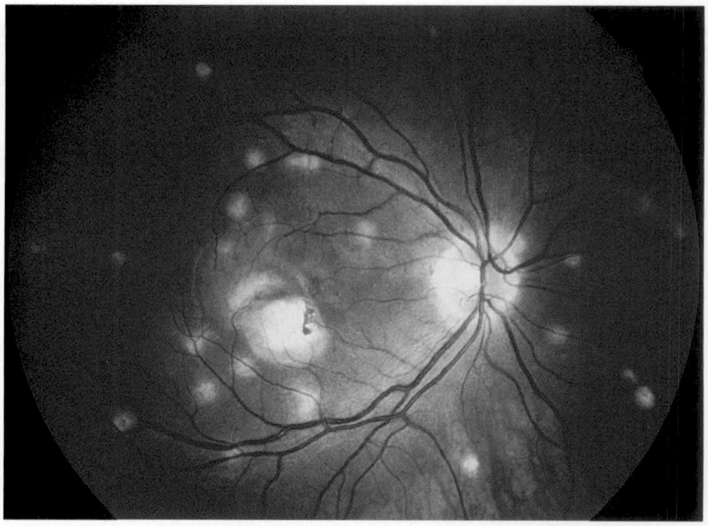

Fig. 10.232 Disciform macular scar due to CNV, and numerous 'histo' spots.

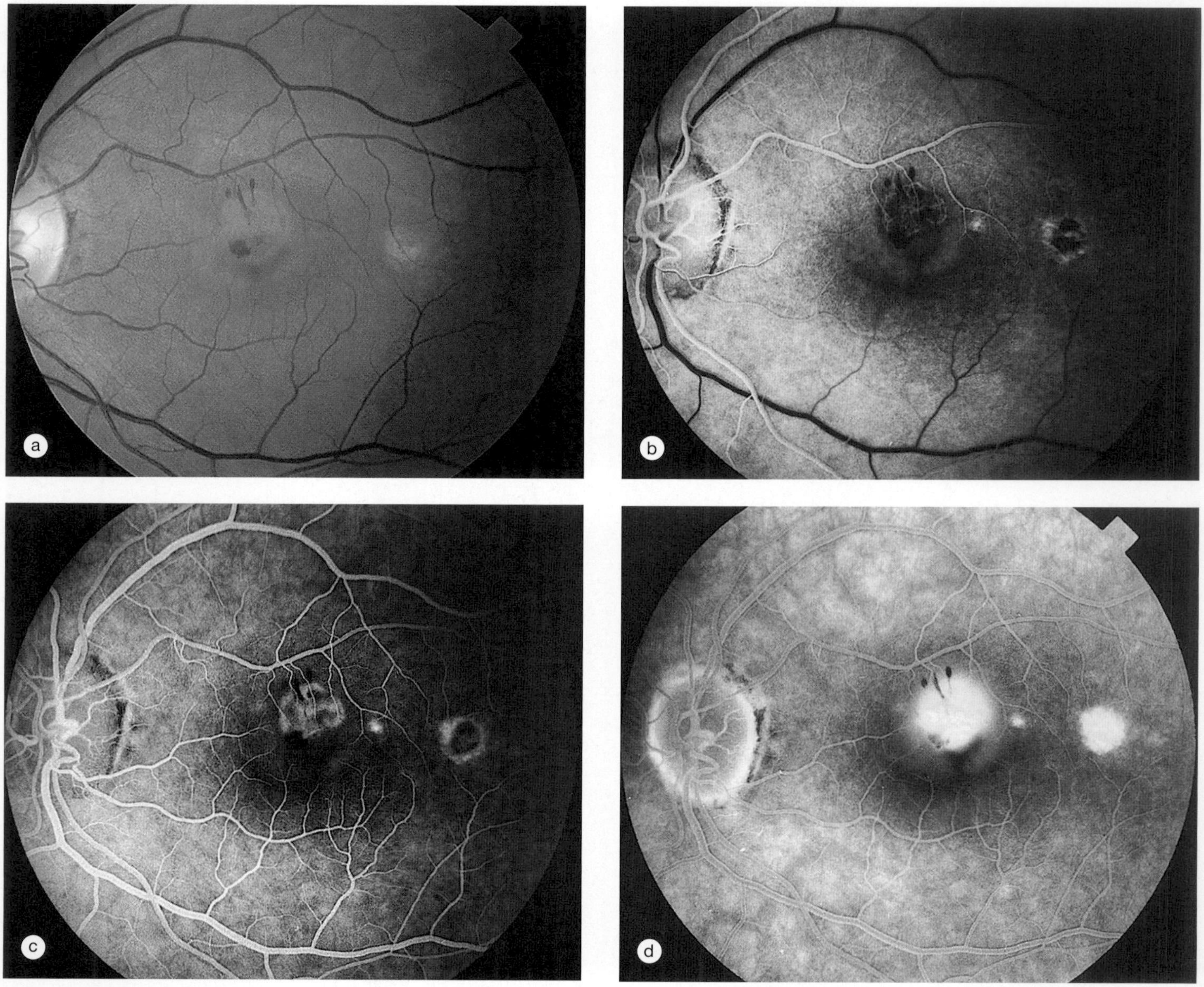

Fig. 10.233 **(a)** Foveal oedema and haemorrhage. **(b)** FA arterial phase shows juxtafoveal CNV. **(c)** Venous phase shows increasing hyperfluorescence of CNV. **(d)** Late phase shows intense hyperfluorescence due to leakage; also note two 'histo' spots temporal to the fovea. (Courtesy of S. Milewski.)

Candidiasis

Candidiasis is an opportunist infection in which the organism acquires pathogenic properties. Candidaemia, which may result in ocular involvement, occurs in injecting drug addicts and patients with long-term indwelling catheters.

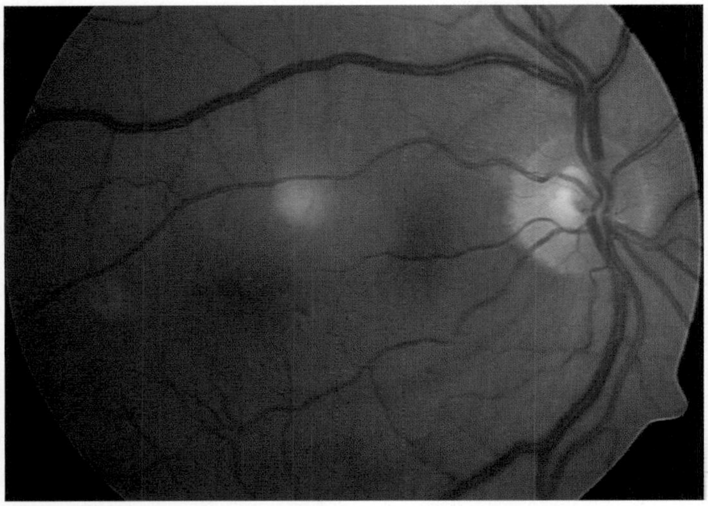

Fig. 10.234 Focal choroiditis. (Courtesy of P. Gili.)

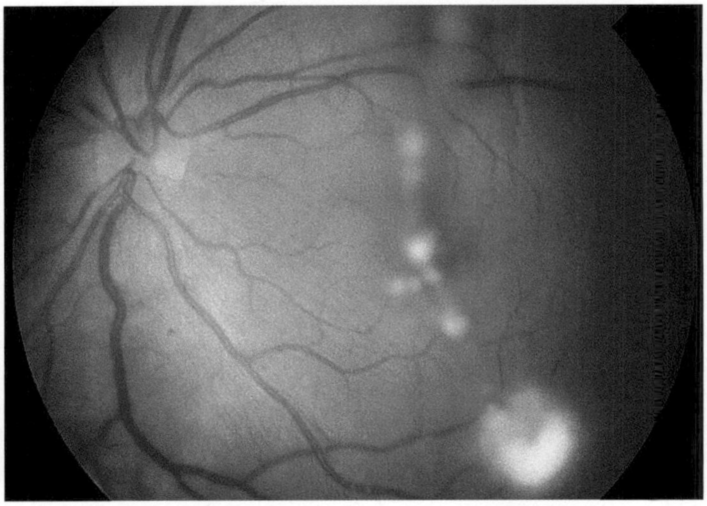

Fig. 10.235 Multifocal retinitis manifest as small, round, white, slightly elevated lesions with indistinct borders.

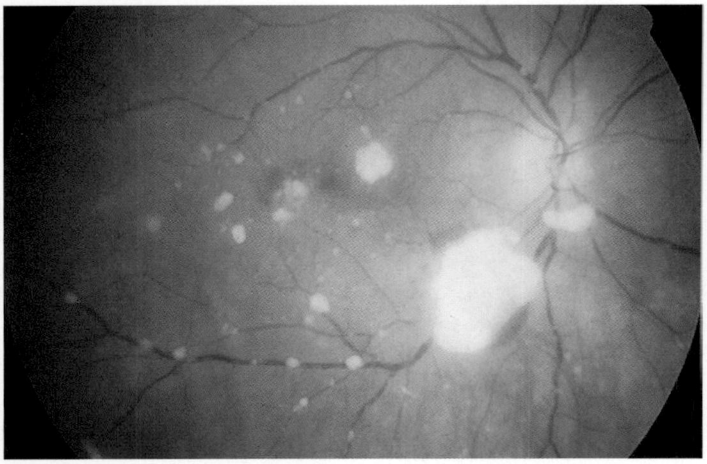

Fig. 10.236 Multifocal retinitis and vitreous 'cotton balls'.

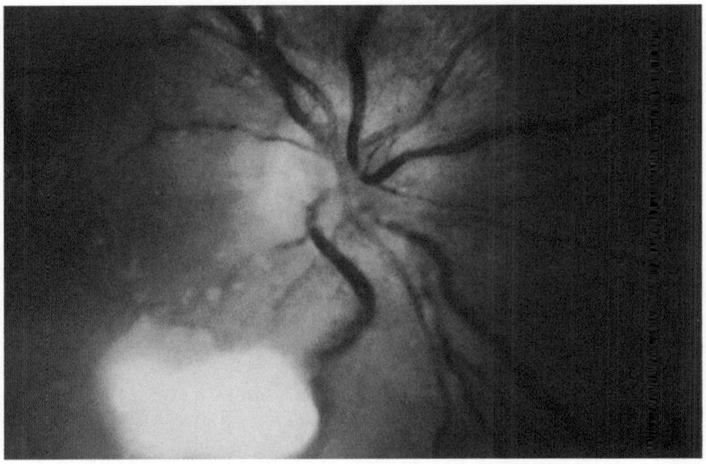

Fig.10.237 Papillitis associated with a large vitreous 'cotton ball' and smaller 'string of pearls' colonies.

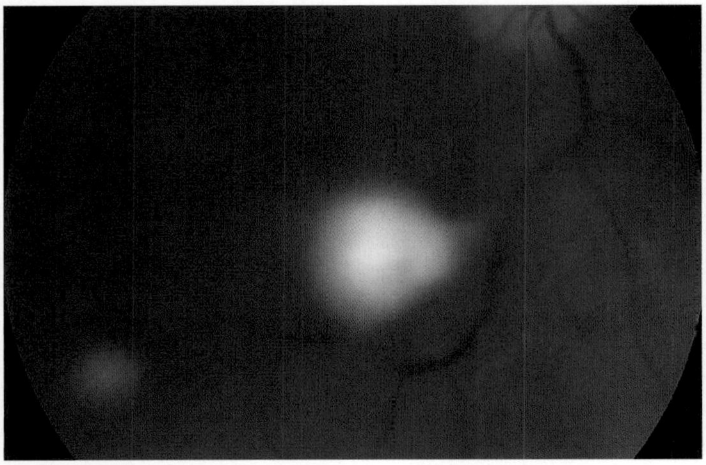

Fig. 10.238 'Cotton balls' and increasing vitreous haze.

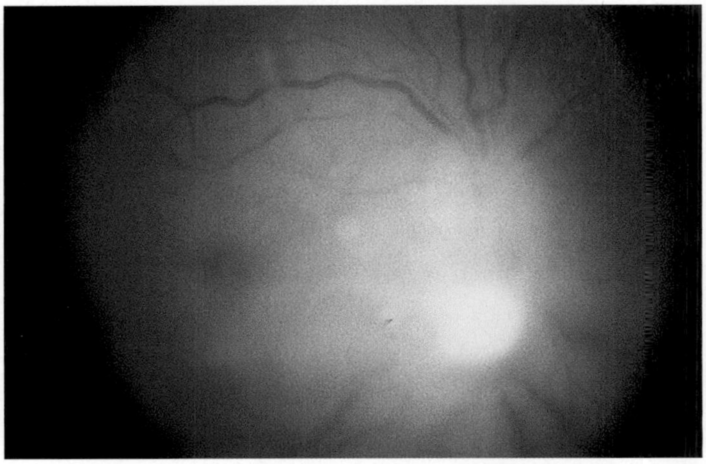

Fig. 10.239 Chronic endophthalmitis characterised by severe vitreous infiltration.

Aspergillosis

Aspergillus species are ubiquitous saprophytic moulds. Ocular infection typically affects injecting drug users and patients with immune deficiency.

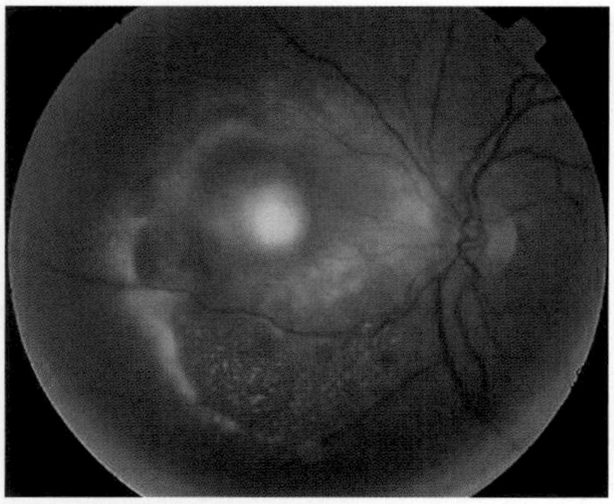

Fig. 10.240 Yellowish subretinal lesion surrounded by fluid and exudates. (Courtesy of A. Curi.)

Cryptococcosis

Cryptococcus neoformans frequently infects the central nervous system in patients with AIDS, although clinical ocular involvement is rare.

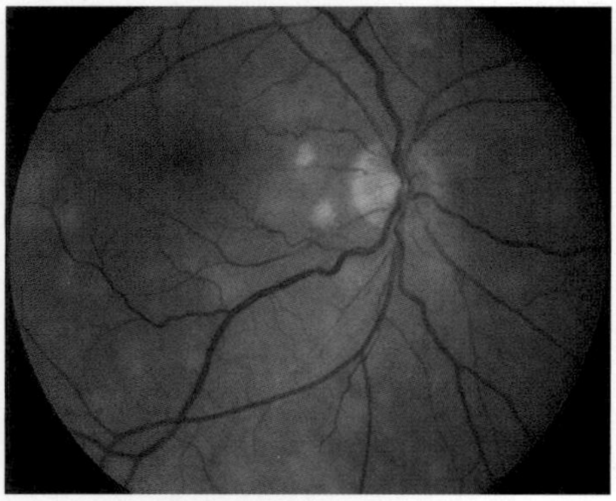

Fig. 10.241 Asymptomatic multifocal choroiditis. (Courtesy of A. Curi.)

Sporotrichosis

Sporotrichosis is caused by the common saprophytic filamentous branching fungus *Sporothrix schenckii*. Infection is usually acquired by traumatic implantation through the skin.

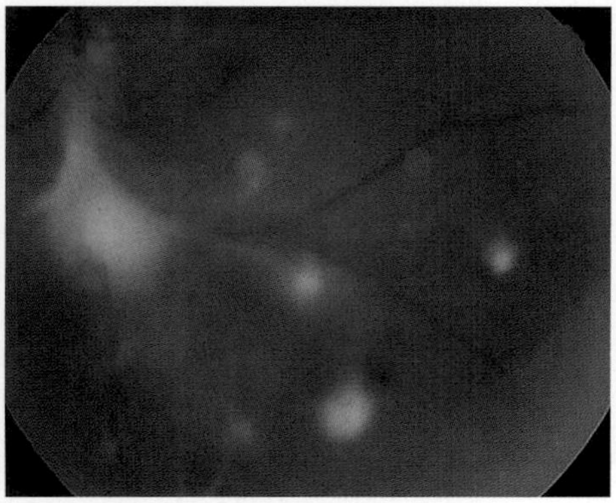

Fig. 10.242 Endophthalmitis similar to that associated with candidiasis but more resistant to treatment. Most patients also have severe anterior uveitis. (Courtesy of A. Curi.)

IDIOPATHIC MULTIFOCAL POSTERIOR UVEITIS (WHITE DOT) SYNDROMES

Acute posterior multifocal placoid pigment epitheliopathy (APMPPE)

APMPPE is a usually bilateral, self-limiting condition that typically affects healthy young adults.

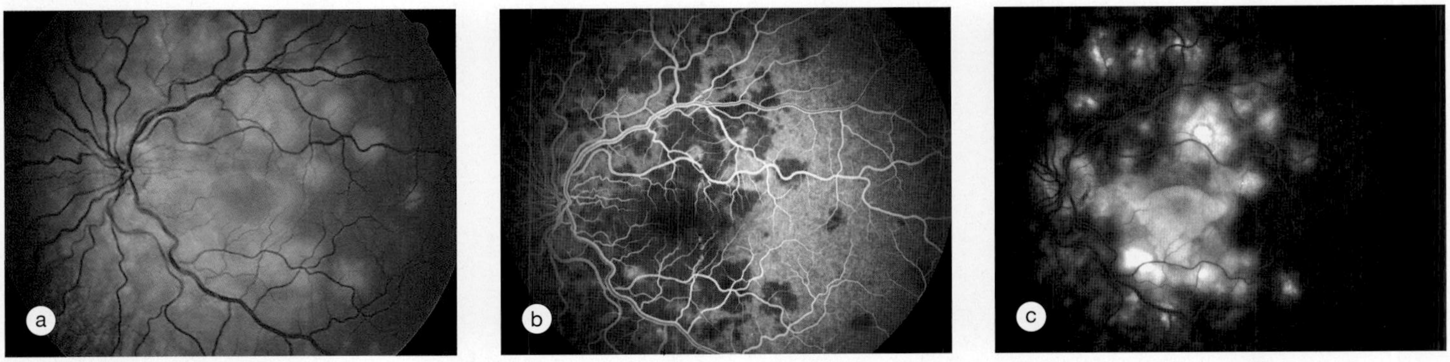

■ **Fig. 10.243** **(a)** Multiple large, cream-coloured or greyish-white, subretinal plaque-like lesions. **(b)** FA shows early dense hypofluorescence due to non-perfusion of the choriocapillaris. **(c)** Late hyperfluorescence due to staining. (Courtesy of C. Barry.)

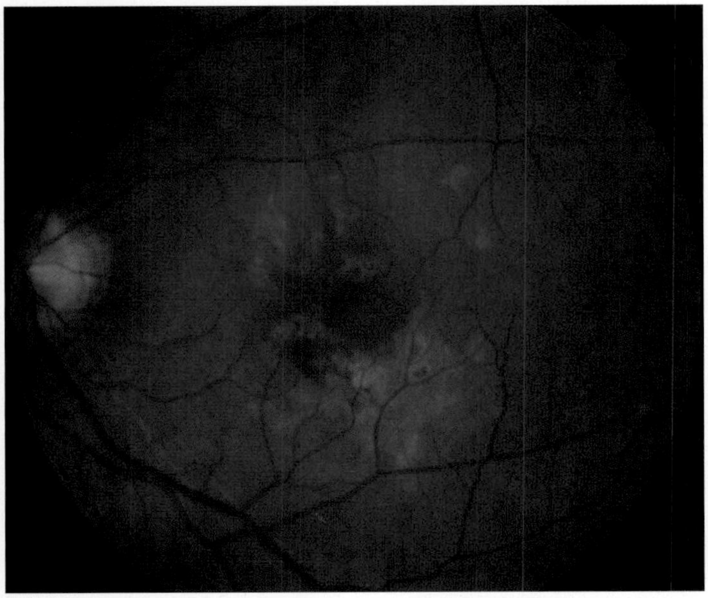

■ **Fig. 10.244** After a few weeks the lesions fade leaving variable residual multifocal areas of depigmentation and clumping of the RPE. (Courtesy of Moorfields Eye Hospital.)

Serpiginous choroidopathy

Serpiginous choroidopathy is a serious progressive, usually bilateral, disease which typically affects patients between the fourth and sixth decade of life.

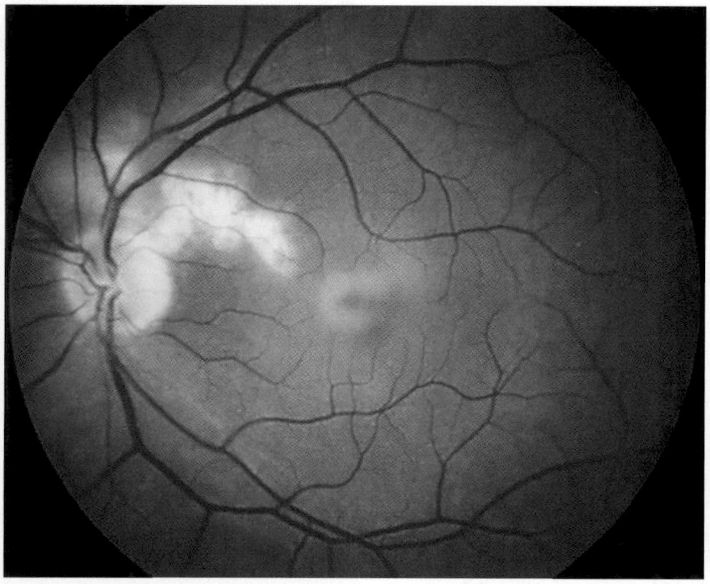

■ **Fig. 10.245** Active lesions consist of grey-white to yellow-white subretinal lesions with hazy borders that typically start around the optic disc.

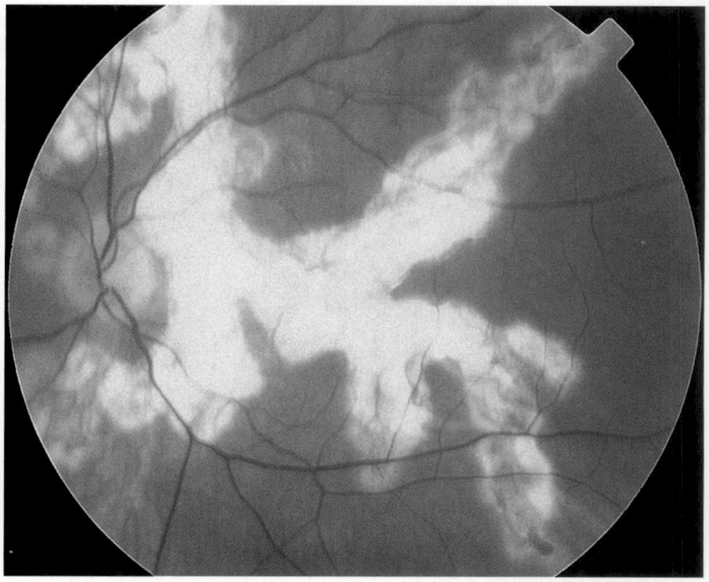

■ **Fig. 10.246** Gradual spread outwards in a snake-like manner. (Courtesy of S. Milewski.)

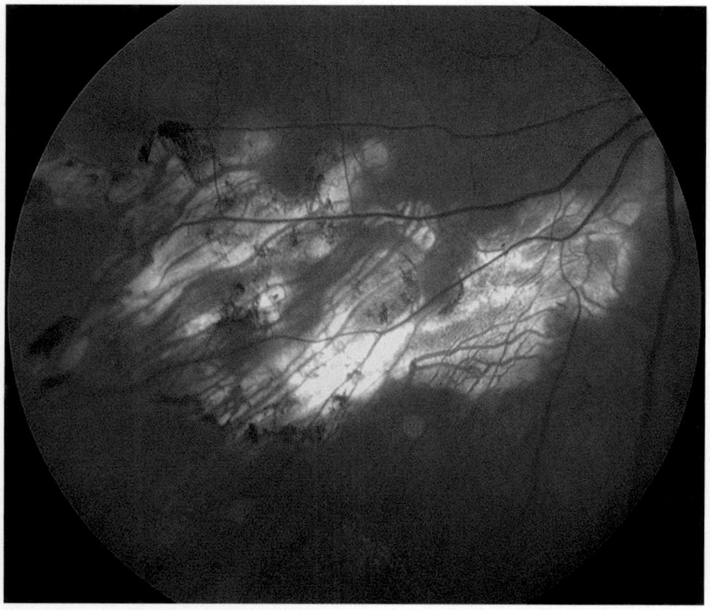

■ **Fig. 10.247** Inactive lesions are characterised by scalloped, atrophic, 'punched-out' areas of choroidal atrophy associated with RPE changes.

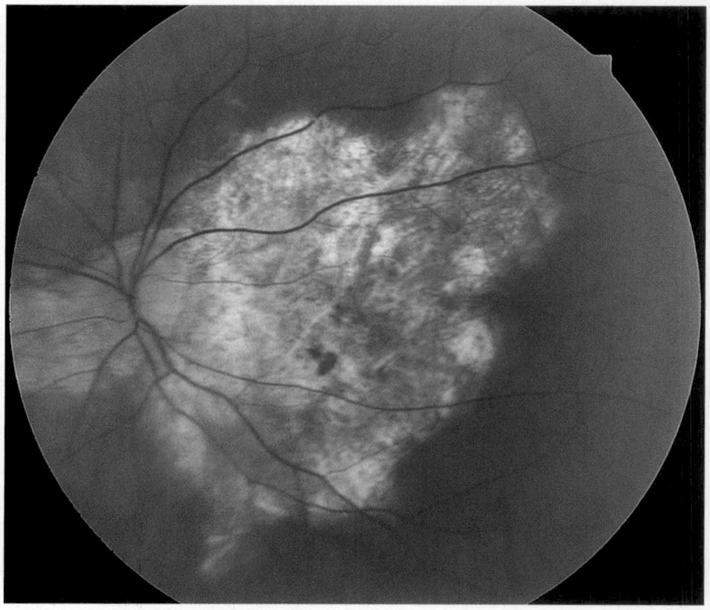

■ **Fig. 10.248** Extensive involvement of the posterior pole.

Birdshot retinochoroidopathy

Birdshot retinochoroidopathy is a serious bilateral, chronic disease that typically affects middle-aged individuals.

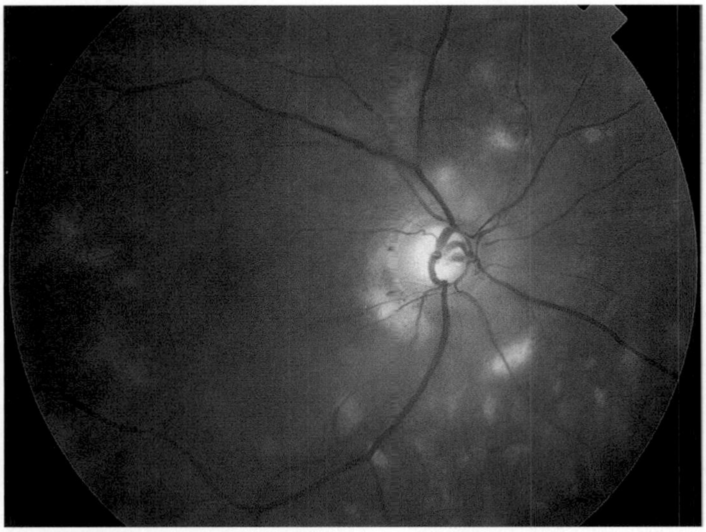

Fig. 10.249 Subretinal, poorly defined, cream-coloured ovoid spots.

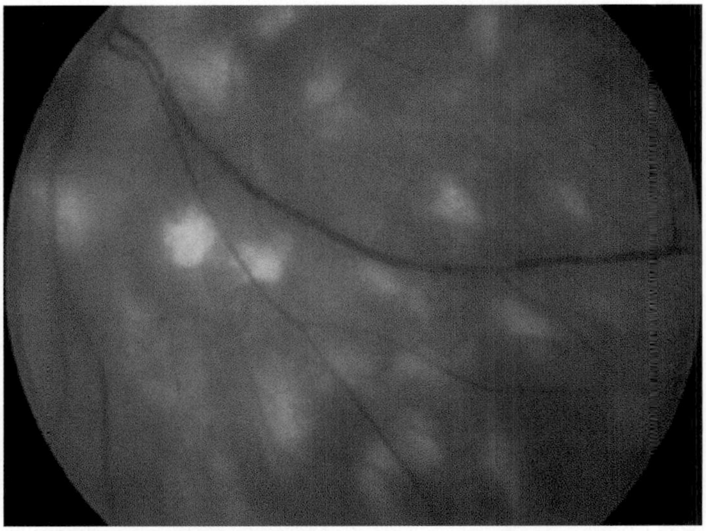

Fig. 10.250 Peripheral lesions.

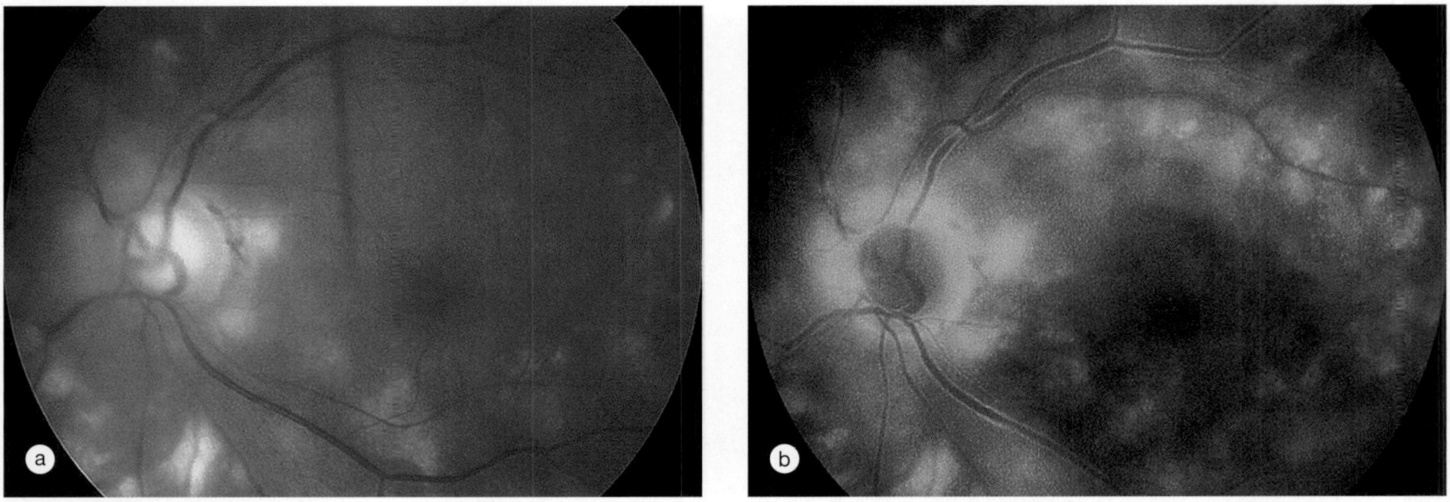

Fig. 10.251 **(a)** Active birdshot retinochoroidopathy. **(b)** FA shows late staining. (Courtesy of S. Milewski.)

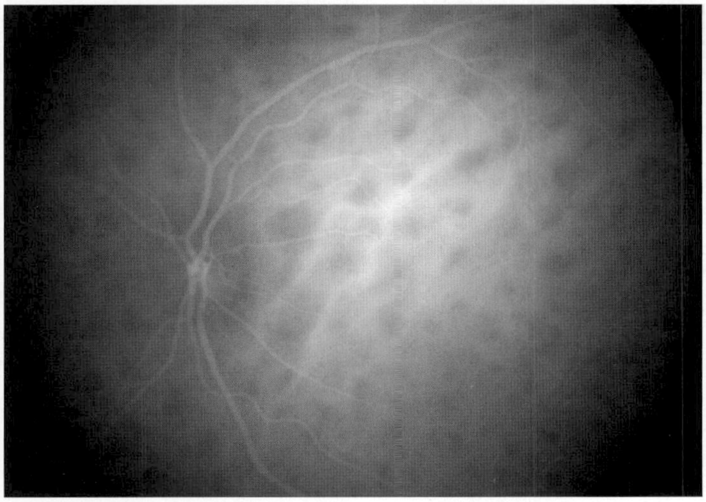

Fig. 10.252 ICG shows hypofluorescence. (Courtesy of P. Gili.)

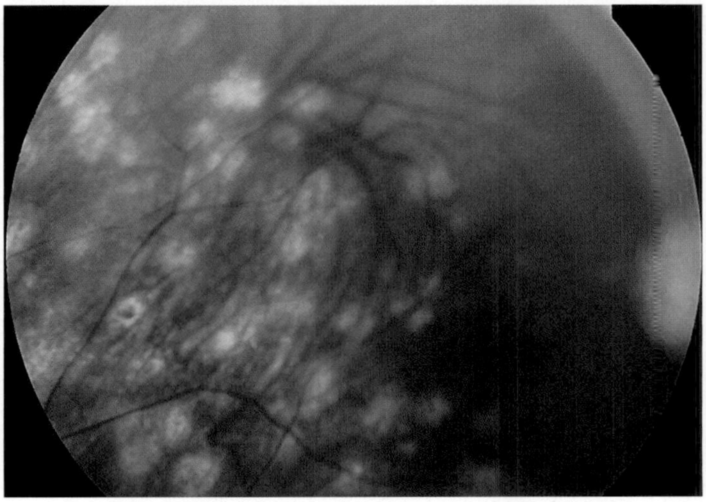

Fig. 10.253 Inactive lesions consist of well-delineated, white atrophic spots.

Punctate inner choroidopathy (PIC)

PIC typically affects both eyes of young myopic women.

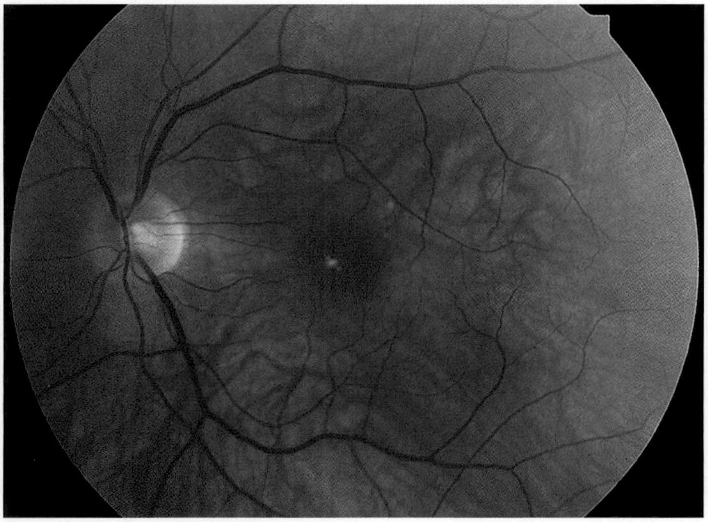

Fig. 10.254 Small, yellow-white spots with fuzzy borders at the level of the inner choroid.

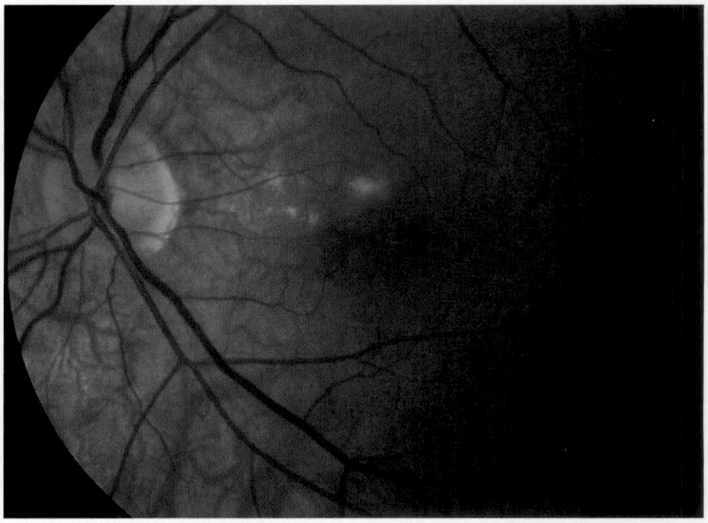

Fig. 10.255 The lesions are all of the same age and principally involve the posterior pole. (Courtesy of Moorfields Eye Hospital.)

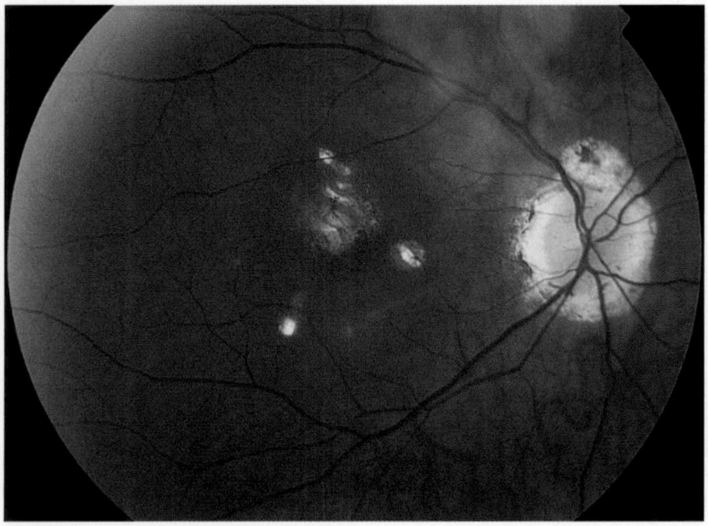

Fig. 10.256 Larger PIC lesions. (Courtesy of Moorfields Eye Hospital.)

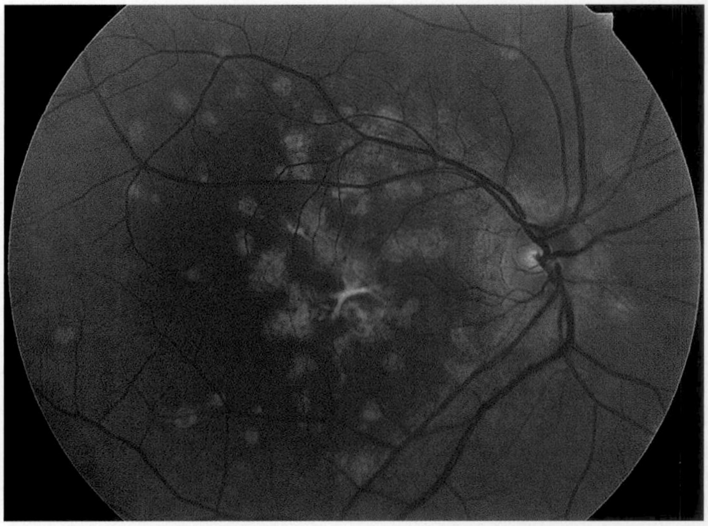

Fig. 10.257 Inactive lesions consist of sharply demarcated atrophic scars.

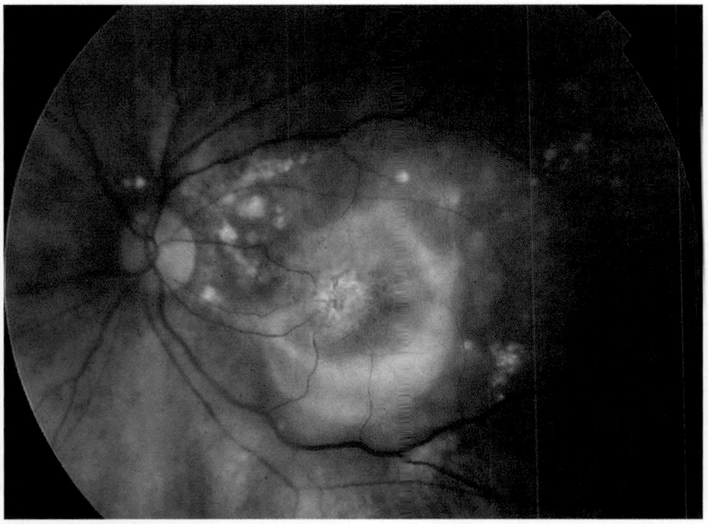

Fig. 10.258 Serous macular elevation due to leakage from secondary CNV.

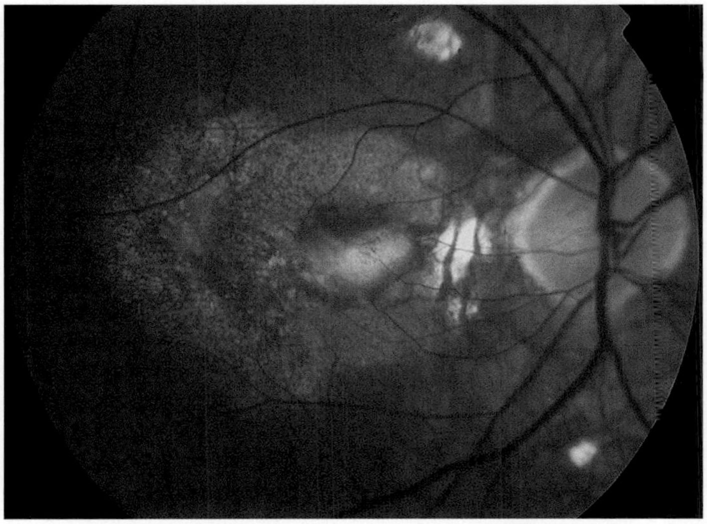

Fig. 10.259 Extensive scarring at the posterior pole resulting from CNV. (Courtesy of Moorfields Eye Hospital.)

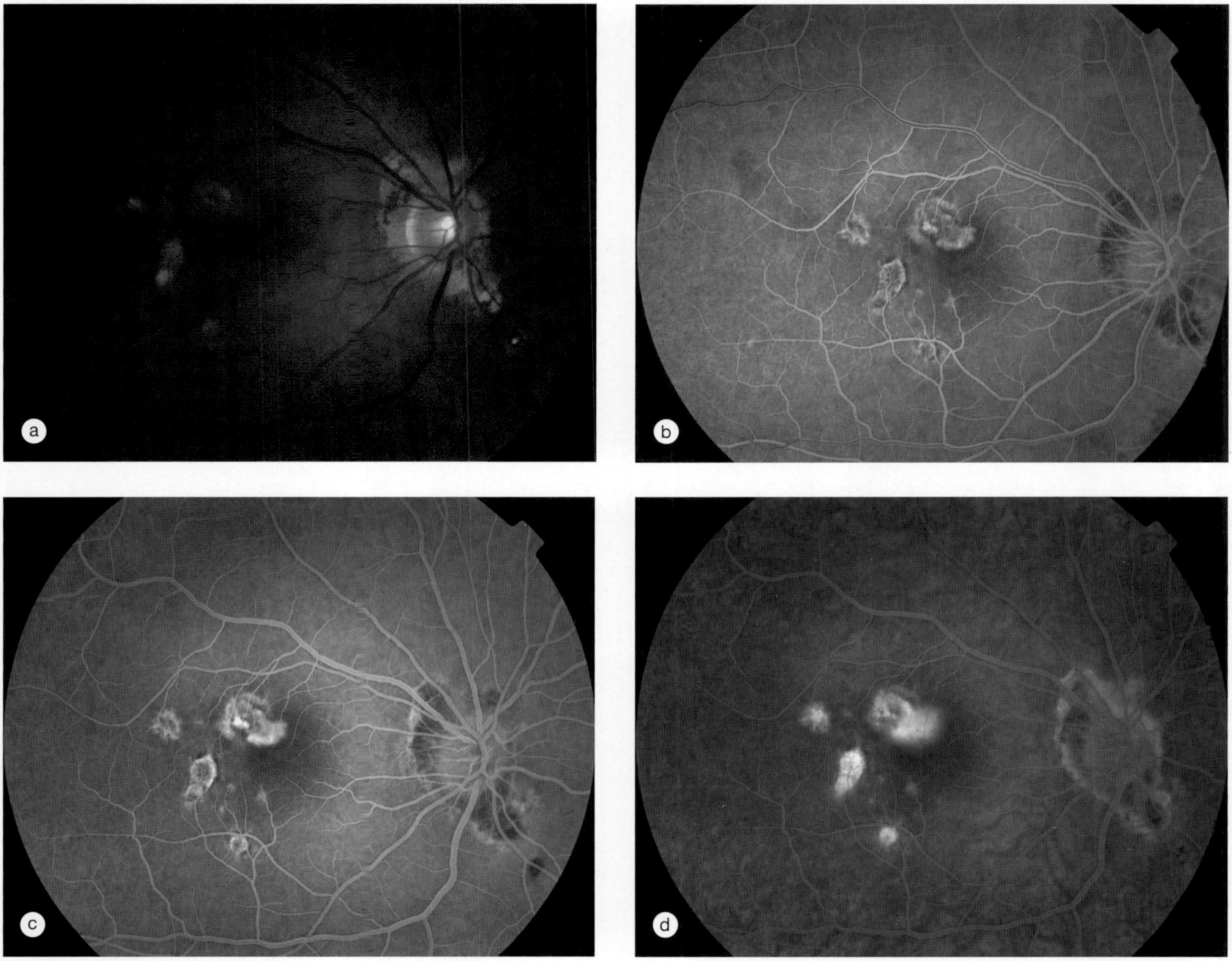

Fig. 10.260 **(a)** Multifocal CNV in PIC. **(b)** FA early venous phase shows hyperfluorescence: **(c)** Mid-venous phase shows increasing hyperfluorescence. **(d)** Late phase shows intense hyperfluorescence due to staining. (Courtesy of Moorfields Eye Hospital.)

Multifocal choroiditis with panuveitis (MCPU)

MCPU is a usually bilateral, recurrent disease which is associated with anterior uveitis and vitritis.

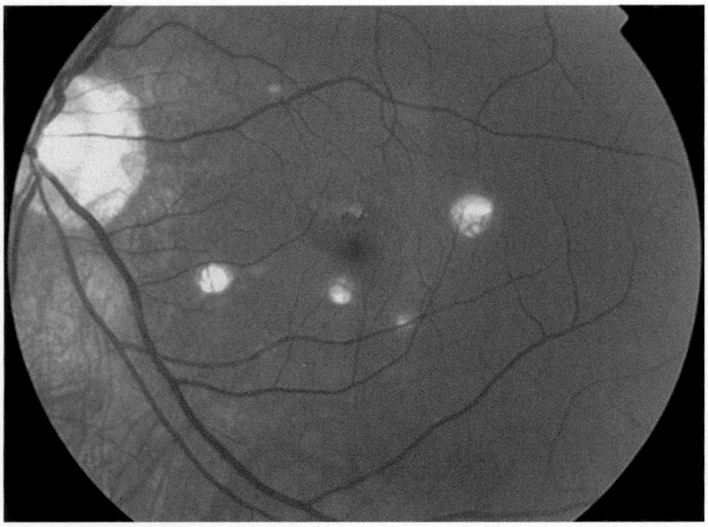

Fig. 10.261 Bilateral, multiple, discrete, round or ovoid, yellowish-grey lesions at the level of the RPE and choriocapillaris at the posterior pole and periphery. (Courtesy of Moorfields Eye Hospital.)

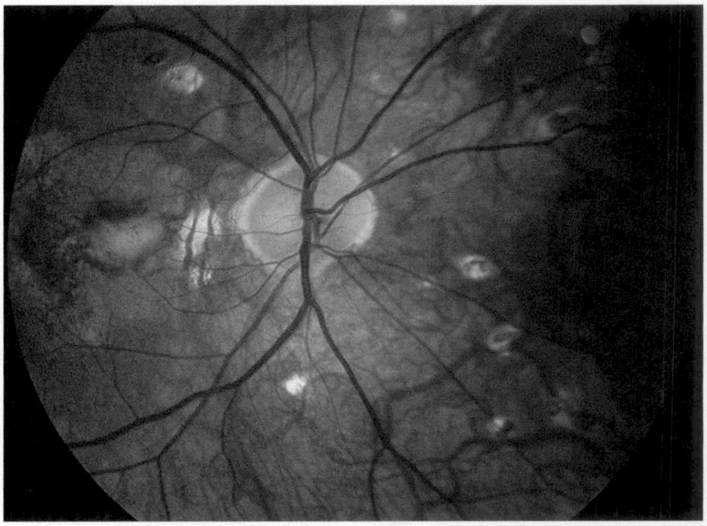

Fig. 10.262 Inactive lesions have sharp, 'punched-out' margins and pigmented borders.

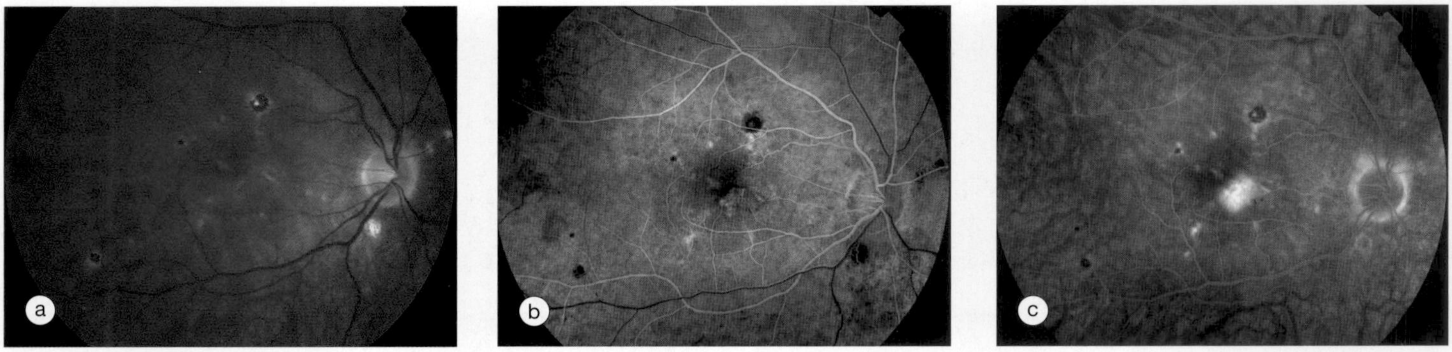

Fig. 10.263 **(a)** CNV in inactive MCPU. **(b)** FA early venous phase shows hypofluorescence of lesions and lacy hyperfluorescence at the fovea due to CNV. **(c)** Late phase shows more intense hyperfluorescence at the fovea due to staining. (Courtesy of Moorfields Eye Hospital.)

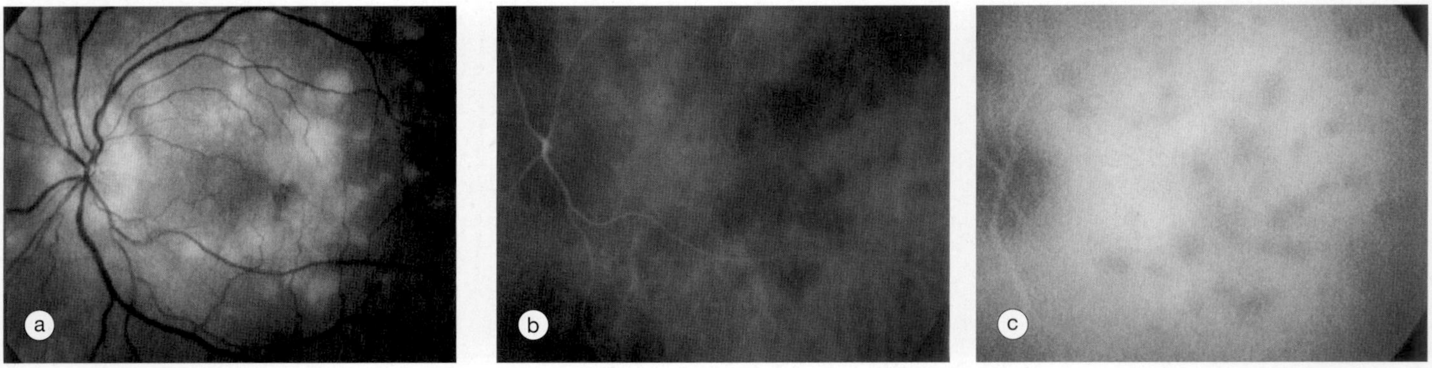

Fig. 10.264 **(a)** Red-free image of inactive MCPU. **(b, c)** IGC shows persistent hypofluorescence of the lesions. (Courtesy of S. Milewski.)

Multiple evanescent white dot syndrome (MEWDS)

MEWDS is a usually unilateral, self-limiting disease that typically affects healthy young individuals, particularly females.

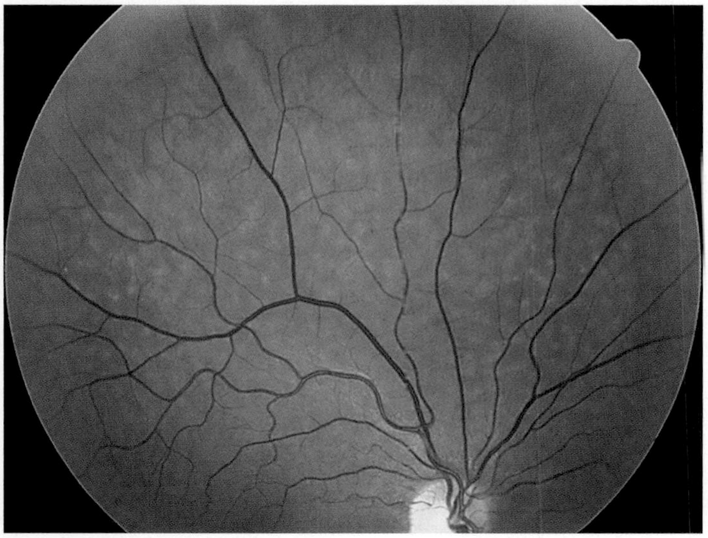

Fig. 10.265 Numerous very small, white dots at the level of the deep retina and RPE. (Courtesy of C. Barry.)

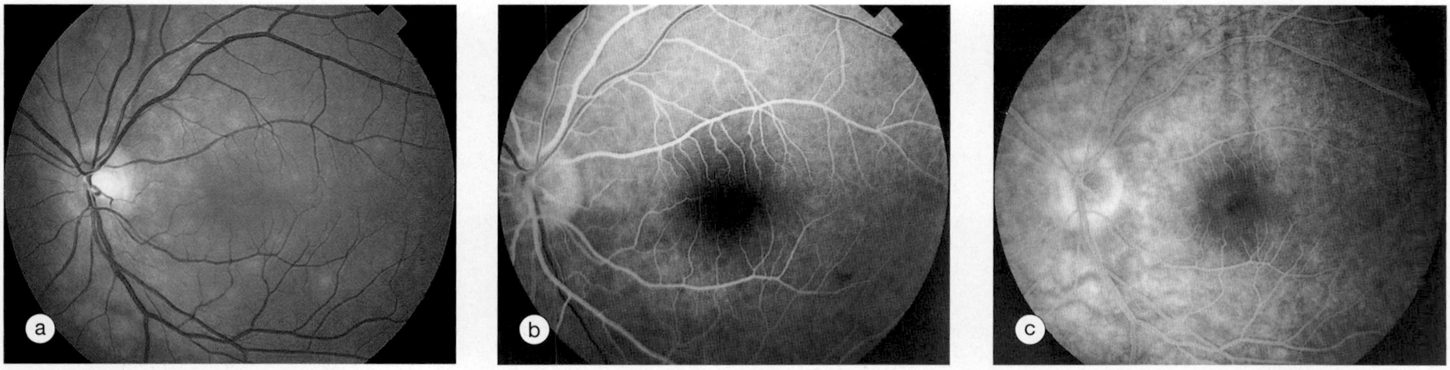

Fig.10.266 **(a)** More subtle lesions at the posterior pole that spare the fovea, which has a granular appearance with an absent foveal reflex. **(b)** FA arteriovenous phase is normal. **(c)** Late phase shows hyperfluorescence of the disc and lesions. (Courtesy of S. Milewski.)

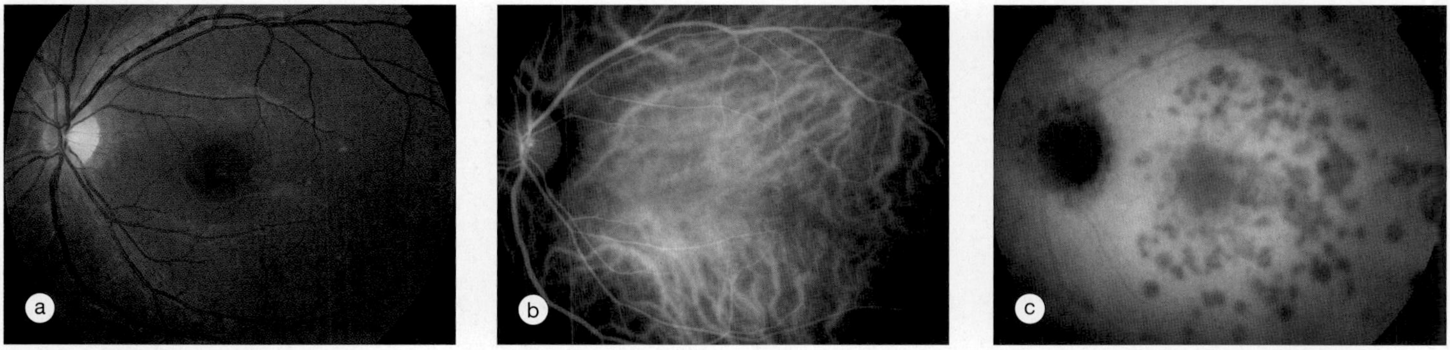

Fig. 10.267 **(a)** Active MEWDS. **(b)** ICG early phase is normal. **(c)** Late phase shows striking hypofluorescence of the lesions. (Courtesy of Moorfields Eye Hospital.)

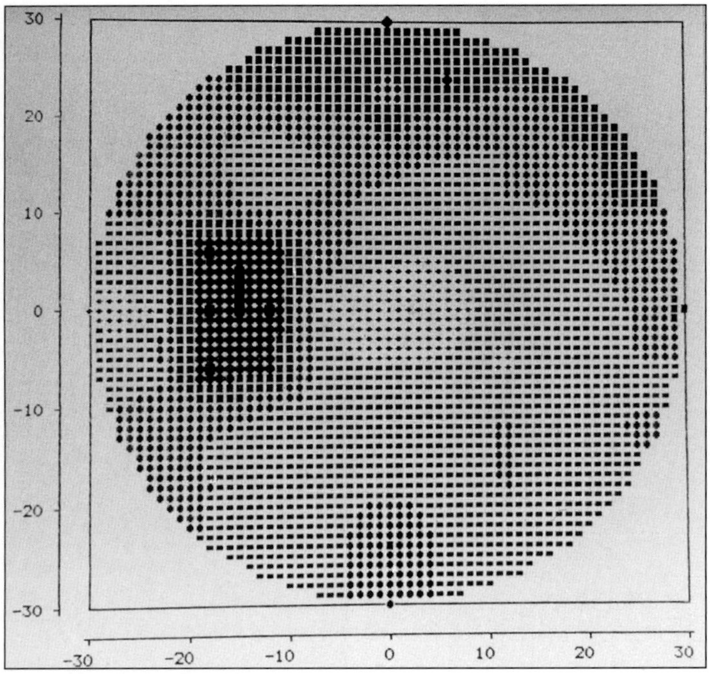

■ **Fig. 10.268** The blind spot is enlarged.

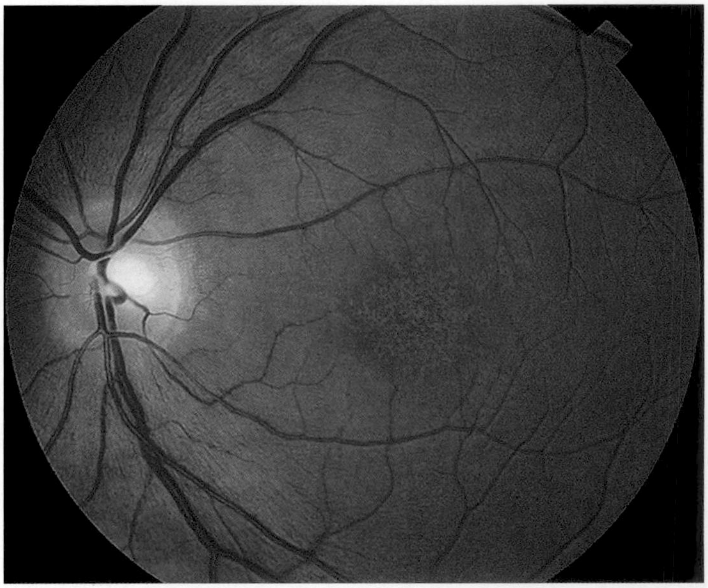

■ **Fig. 10.269** The spots gradually fade but the fovea remains abnormal. (Courtesy of S. Milewski.)

Acute retinal pigment epitheliitis

Acute retinal pigment epitheliitis is an often unilateral, self-limiting condition involving the macula.

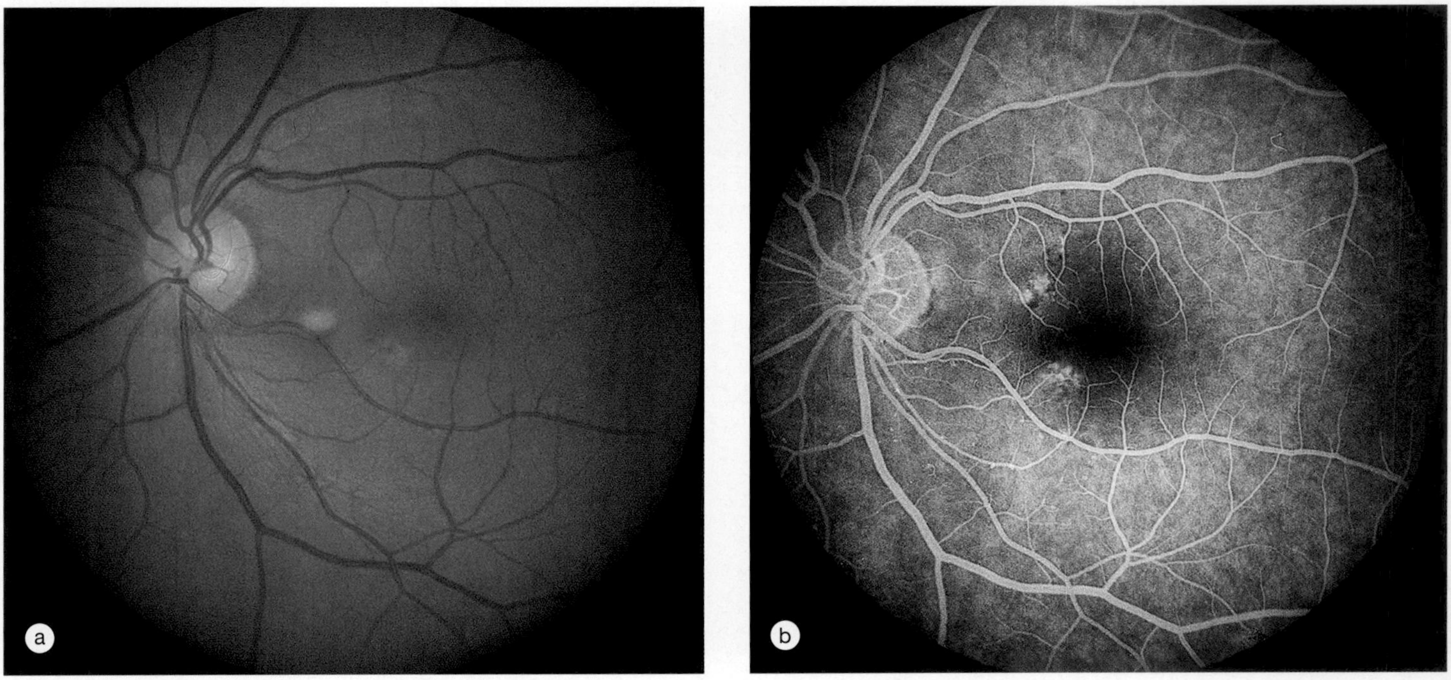

■ **Fig. 10.270** **(a)** The fovea shows a blunted reflex with discrete clusters of a few, subtle, small, brown or grey spots at the level of the RPE that may be surrounded by hypopigmented yellow halos. **(b)** FA venous phase shows small hyperfluorescent dots with hypofluorescent centres ('honeycomb' appearance) without leakage. (Courtesy of M. Prost.)

MISCELLANEOUS UVEITIS

Sympathetic ophthalmitis

Sympathetic ophthalmitis is a rare, bilateral granulomatous panuveitis associated with penetrating trauma.

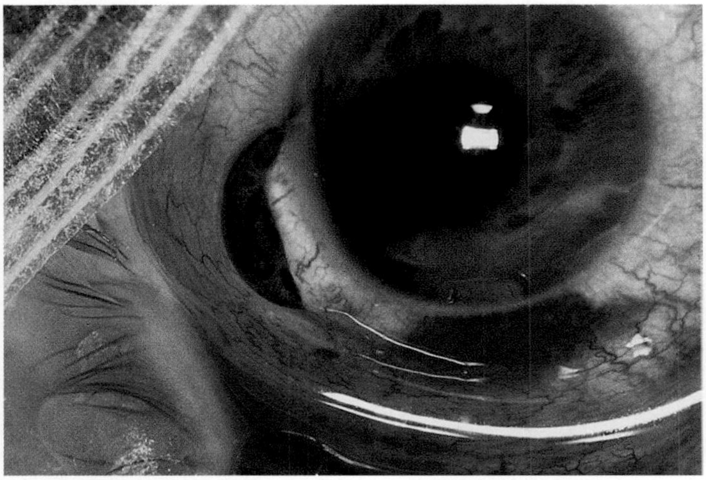

Fig. 10.271 Uveitis typically develops after penetrating trauma, often associated with uveal prolapse (Courtesy of Wilmer Institute.)

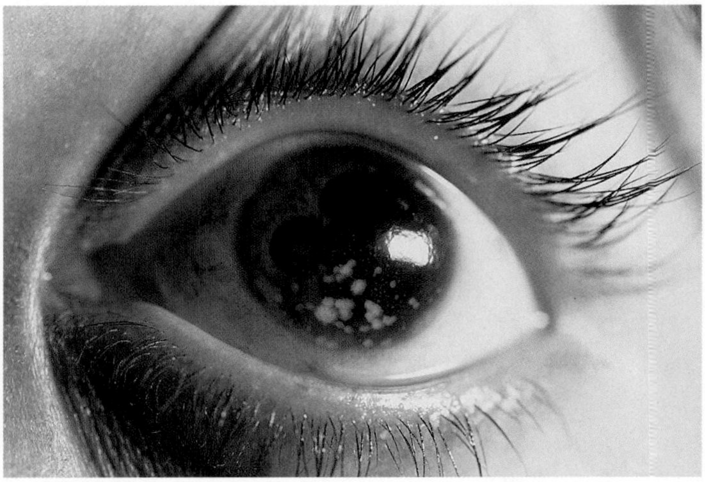

Fig. 10.272 Bilateral granulomatous anterior uveitis. (Courtesy of U. Raina.)

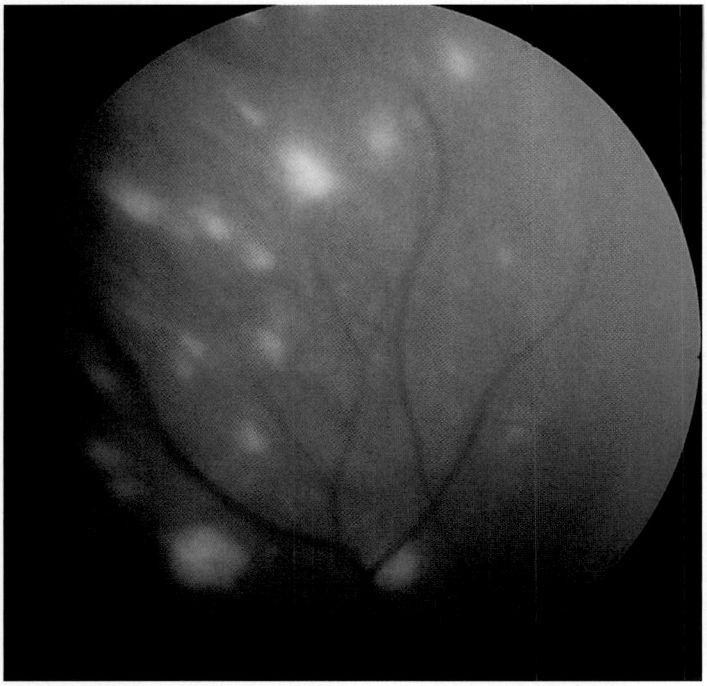

Fig. 10.273 Multifocal choroiditis. (Courtesy of J. Salmon.)

Acute macular neuroretinopathy

Acute macular neuroretinopathy is a predominantly bilateral but self-limiting condition that typically affects healthy females between the second and fourth decade of life.

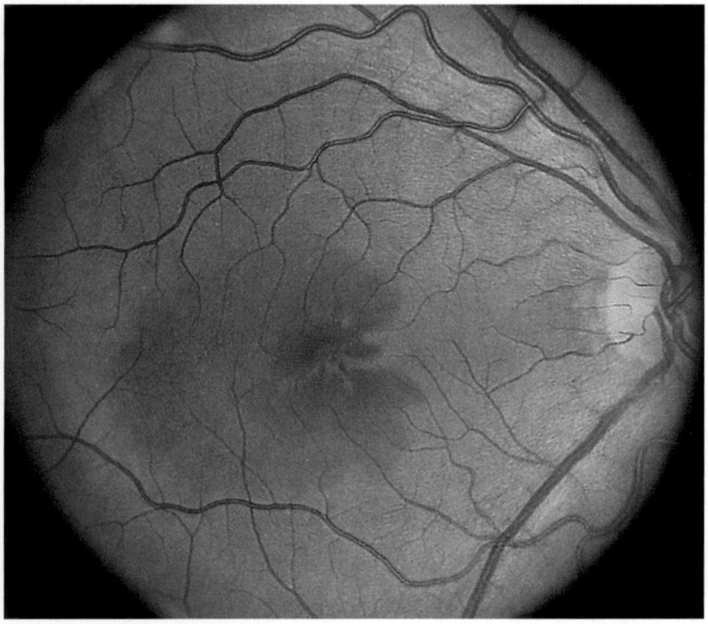

■ **Fig. 10.274** Darkish, brown-red, wedge-shaped lesions in a flower-petal arrangement around the centre of the macula. (Courtesy of J. D. M. Gass.)

Acute idiopathic maculopathy

Acute idiopathic maculopathy is a usually unilateral, self-limiting condition that typically affects young adults.

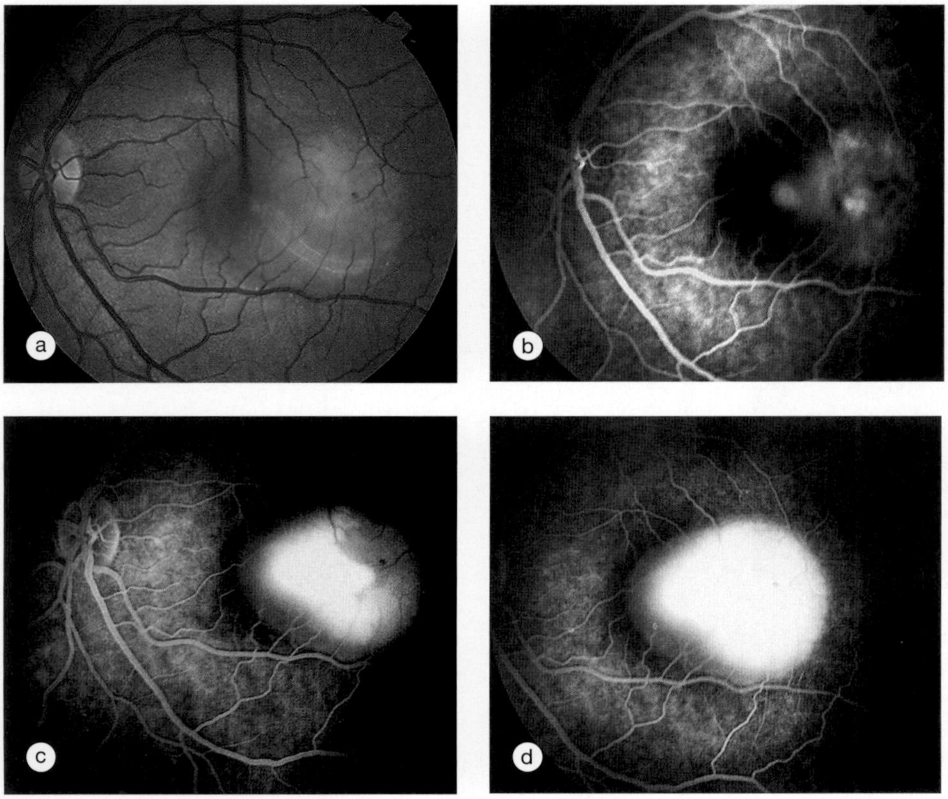

■ **Fig. 10.275** **(a)** Detachment of the sensory retina at the macula with an irregular outline. **(b)** FA early venous phase shows minimal subretinal hypofluorescence as well as hyperfluorescence beneath the sensory retinal detachment. **(c)** The mid-venous phases show two levels of hyperfluorescence, one from staining of the subretinal thickening at the level of the RPE and the second due to pooling of dye within the subretinal space. **(d)** The late phase shows complete staining of the overlying sensory retinal detachment. (Courtesy of S. Milewski.)

Acute multifocal retinitis

Acute multifocal retinitis is a frequently bilateral, self-limiting condition that typically affects healthy, young to middle-aged adults.

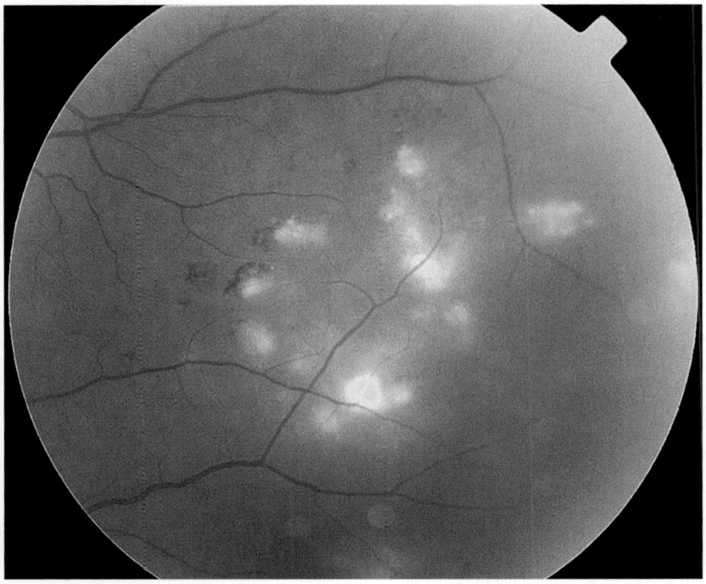

■ **Fig. 10.276** Several, transient, white retinal infiltrates of variable size. (Courtesy of S. Milewski.)

Subretinal fibrosis and uveitis syndrome

The progressive subretinal fibrosis and uveitis syndrome is a serious, bilateral condition which typically affects healthy young adult females.

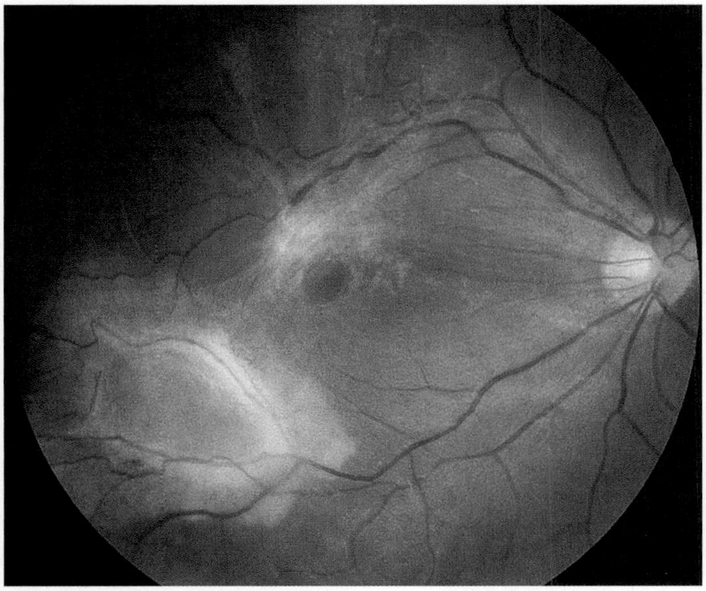

■ **Fig. 10.277** Yellow, indistinct subretinal lesions that coalesce into dirty yellow mounds.

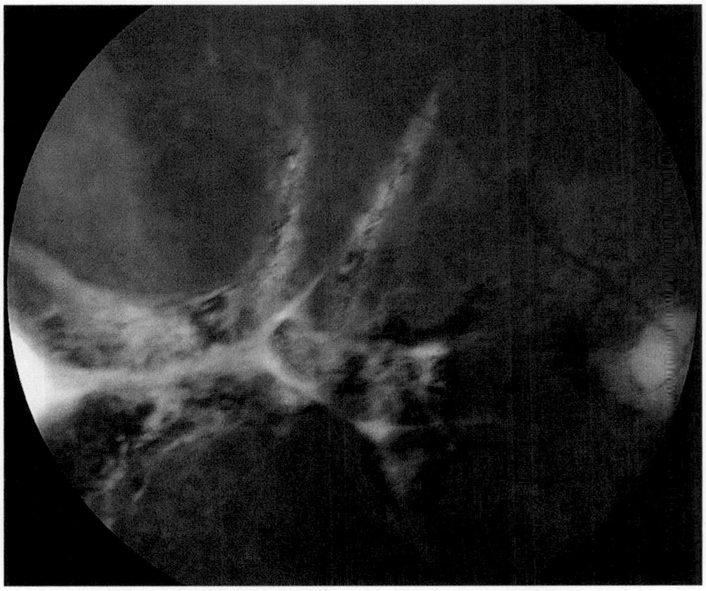

■ **Fig. 10.278** The prognosis is poor because of subretinal opaque bands and RPE changes at the macula.

Solitary idiopathic choroiditis

Solitary idiopathic choroiditis is a distinct clinical entity that may give rise to diagnostic problems as it may simulate other pathology, particularly amelanotic tumours.

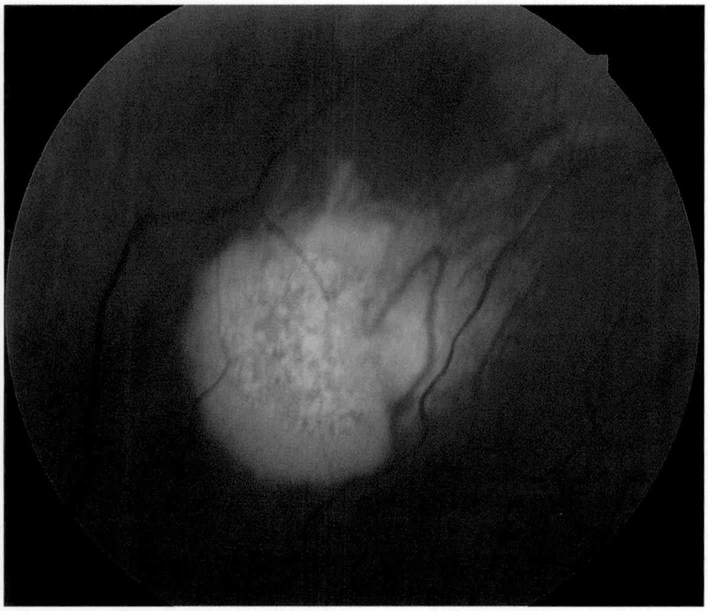

Fig. 10.279 A postequatorial, dull yellow choroidal lesion with an ill-defined margin and localised subretinal fluid.

Primary frosted branch angiitis

Primary frosted branch angiitis is a very rare condition that predominantly affects the young and healthy.

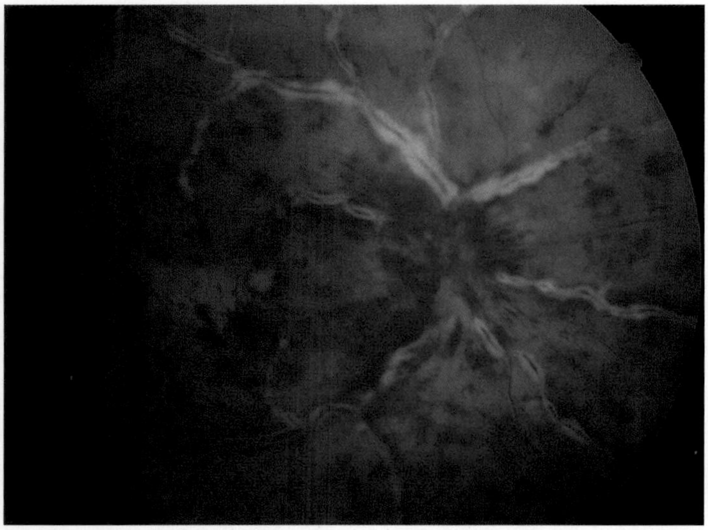

Fig. 10.280 Florid perivascular sheathing of arteries and veins, disc and macular oedema, retinal haemorrhages and variable uveitis. (Courtesy of C. Barry.)

Idiopathic retinal vasculitis aneurysms and neuroretinitis (IRVAN)

IRVAN is a rare entity characterised by bilateral arteritis, numerous aneurysmal dilatations of the retinal and optic nerve head arteries, neuroretinitis and uveitis.

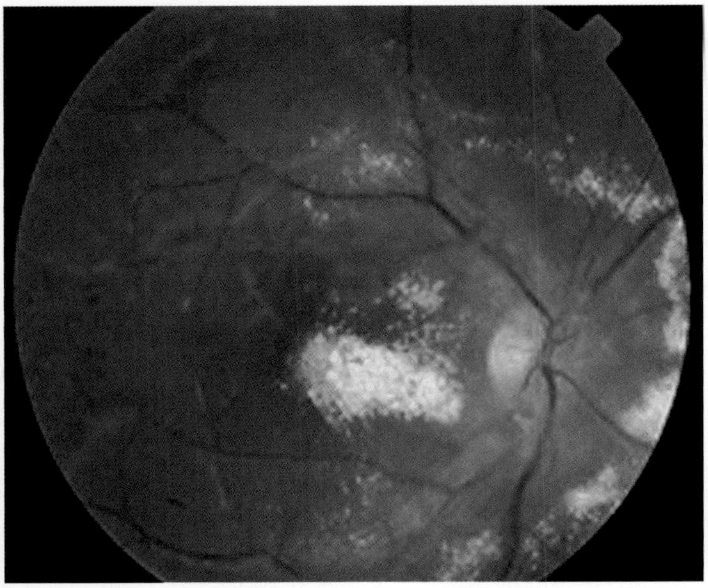

Fig. 10.281 Extensive peripapillary and macular lipid, and aneurysmal dilatation along the retinal arteries. (Courtesy of A. Abu El-Asrar.)

CHAPTER 11

RETINAL DETACHMENT

PERIPHERAL RETINAL DEGENERATIONS

Benign degenerations

Oral pigmentary degeneration

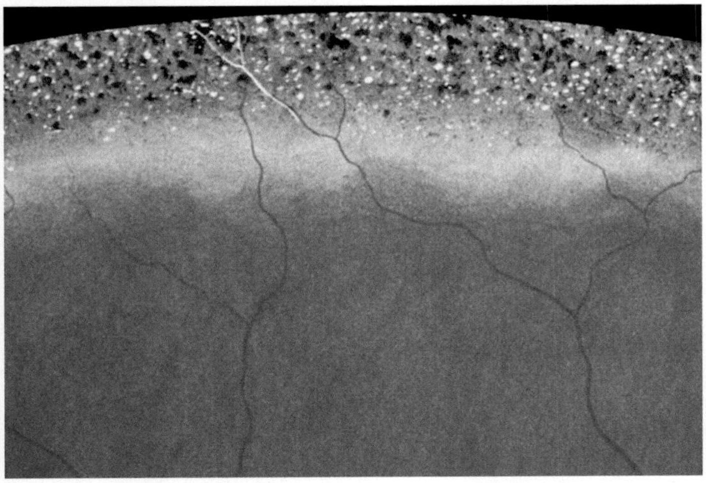

Fig. 11.1 An age-related change consisting of a hyperpigmented band running adjacent to the ora serrata.

Honeycomb (reticular) degeneration

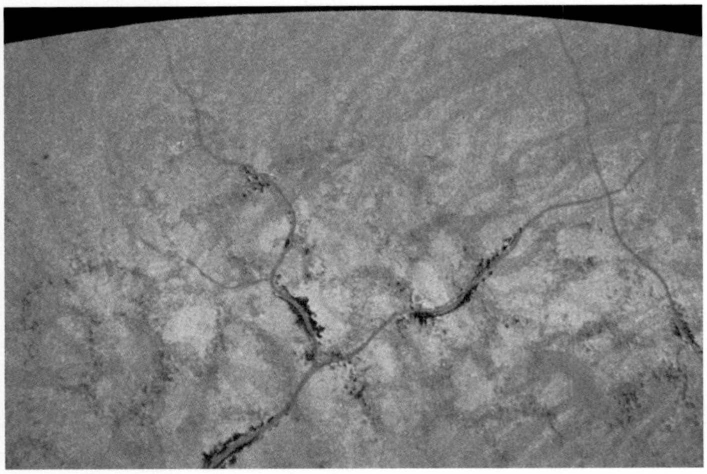

Fig. 11.2 An age-related change characterised by a fine network of perivascular pigmentation, which may extend posterior to the equator.

Snowflake degeneration

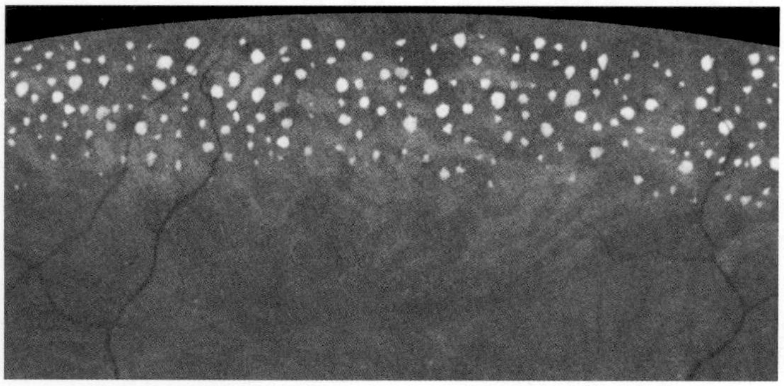

Fig. 11.3 Minute, glistening, yellow-white dots scattered diffusely in the peripheral fundus.

Microcystoid degeneration

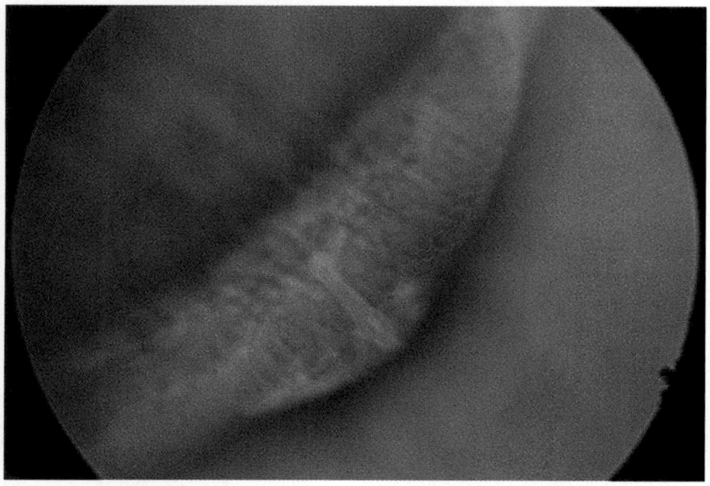

Fig. 11.4 Tiny vesicles with indistinct boundaries on a greyish-white background. (Courtesy of N. E. Byer.)

Pavingstone degeneration

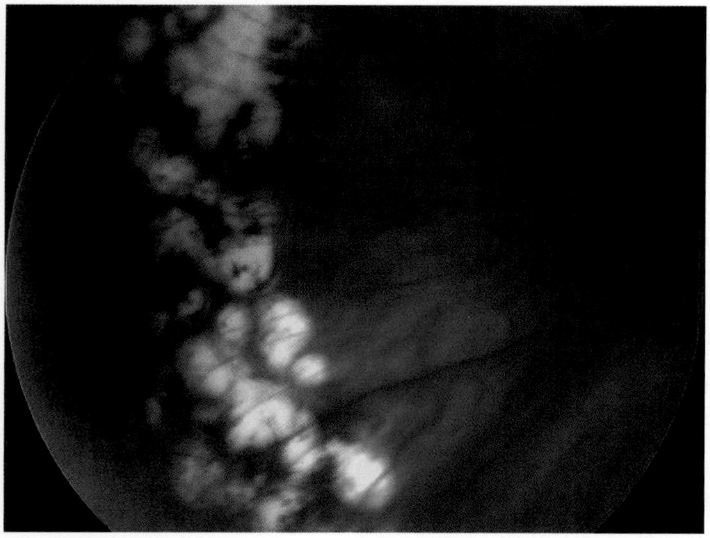

Fig. 11.5 Discrete, yellow-white patches of focal chorioretinal atrophy that are present, to some extent, in 25% of normal eyes.

Predisposing degenerations

Lattice degeneration

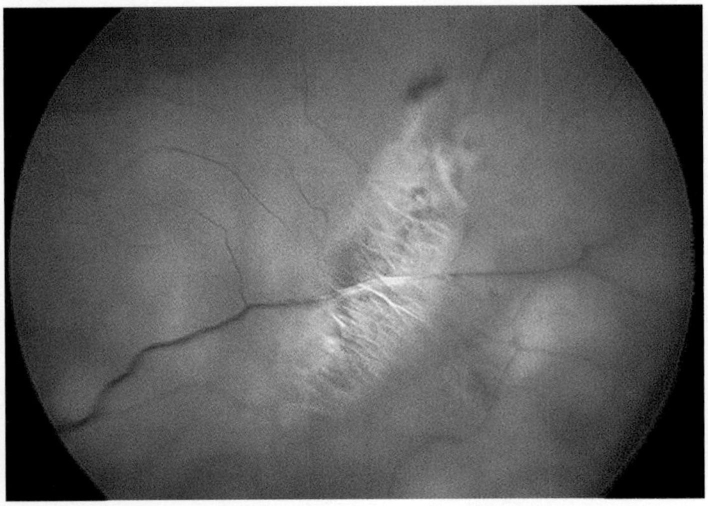

Fig. 11.6 Sharply demarcated, spindle-shaped areas of retinal thinning associated with an arborising network of white lines. (Courtesy of P. Morse.)

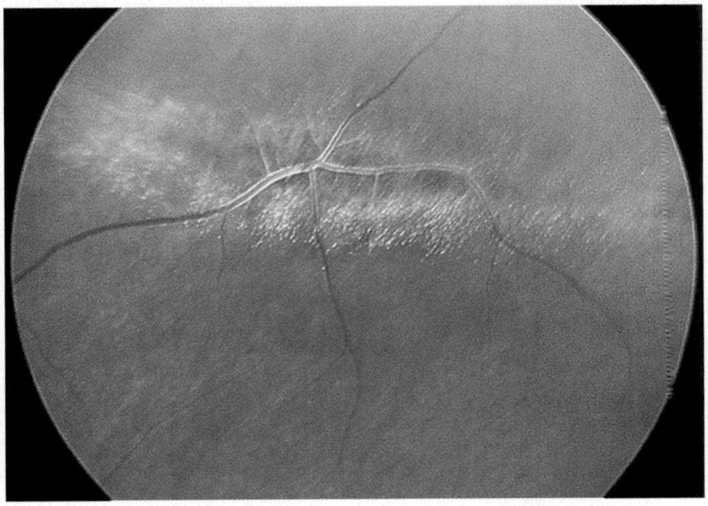

Fig. 11.7 Lattice associated with 'snowflakes'. (Courtesy of N. E. Byer.)

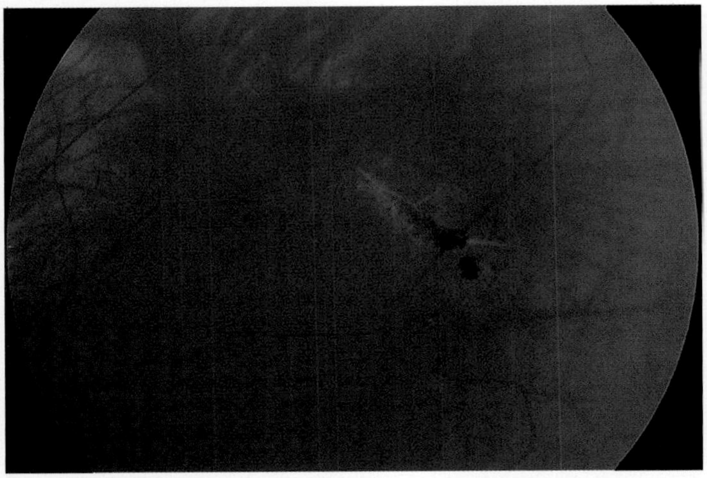

Fig. 11.8 A small island of lattice associated with hyperplasia of the RPE and less conspicuous white lines.

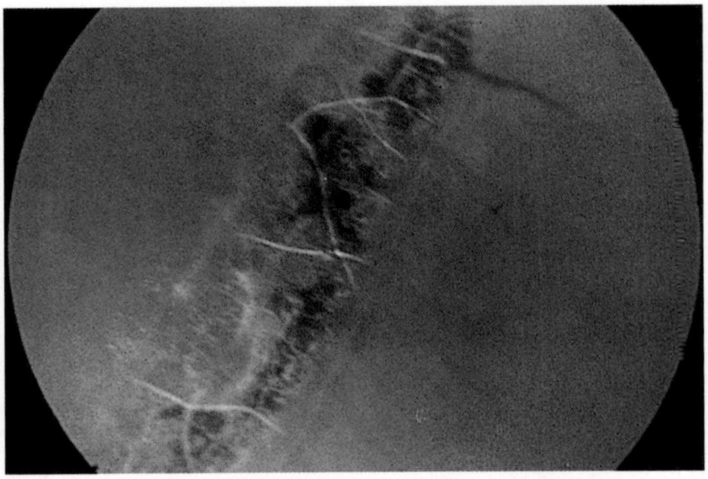

Fig. 11.9 Lattice with characteristic white lines and RPE hyperplasia.

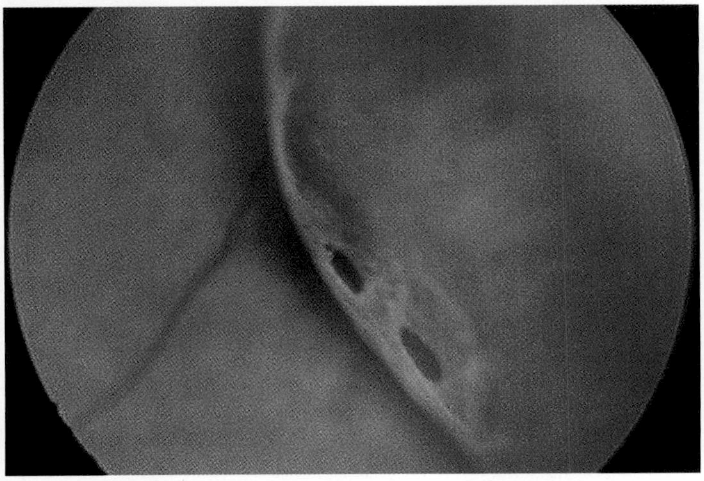

Fig. 11.10 Small holes within the lattice lesions are common and usually innocuous. (Courtesy of N. E. Byer.)

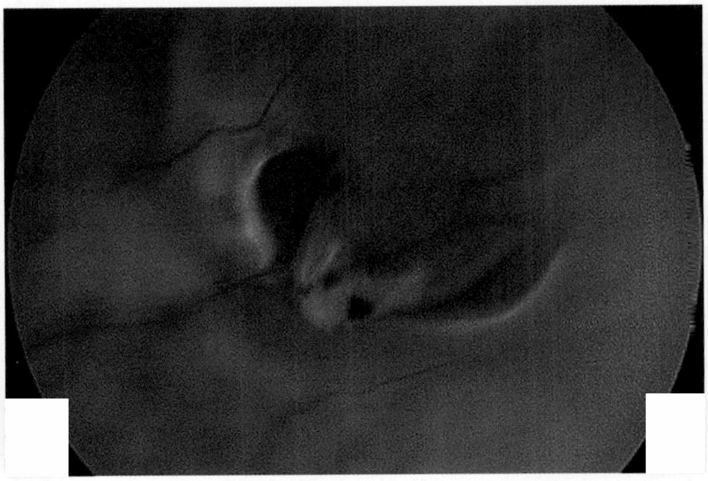

Fig. 11.11 U-shaped tear with lattice on its flap is much more dangerous. (Courtesy of N. E. Bye.)

Snailtrack degeneration

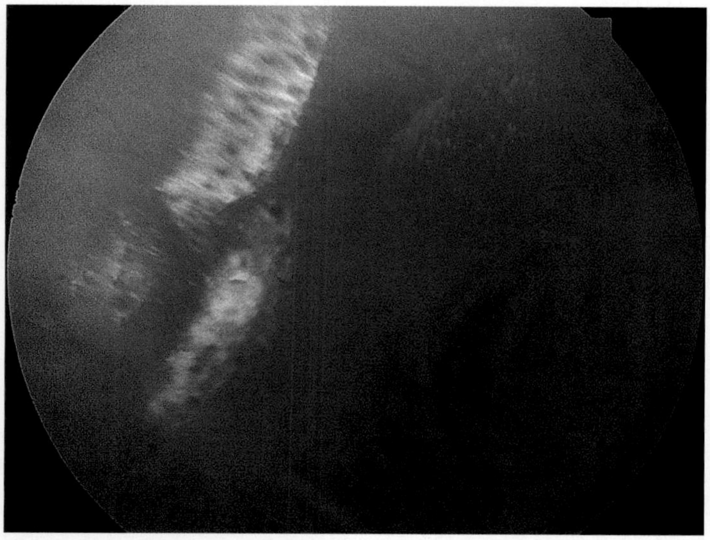

■ **Fig. 11.12** Sharply demarcated bands of tightly packed 'snowflakes', which give the peripheral retina a white frost-like appearance.

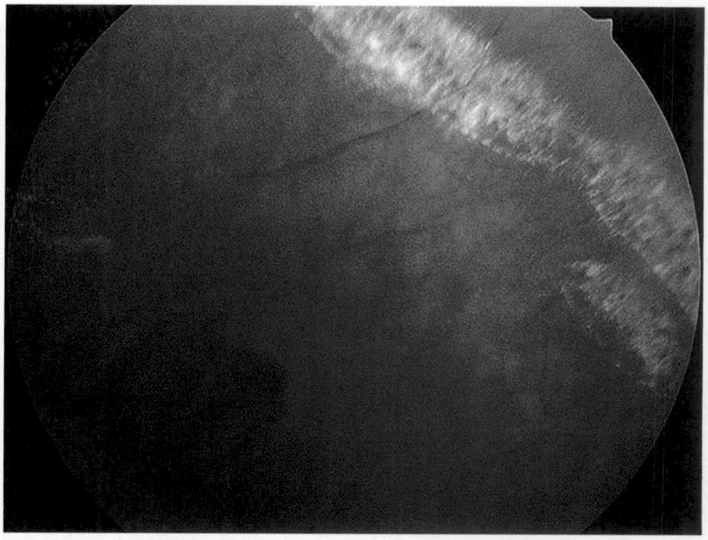

■ **Fig. 11.13** The lesions are often longer than islands of lattice and may be associated with small, round holes.

Degenerative retinoschisis

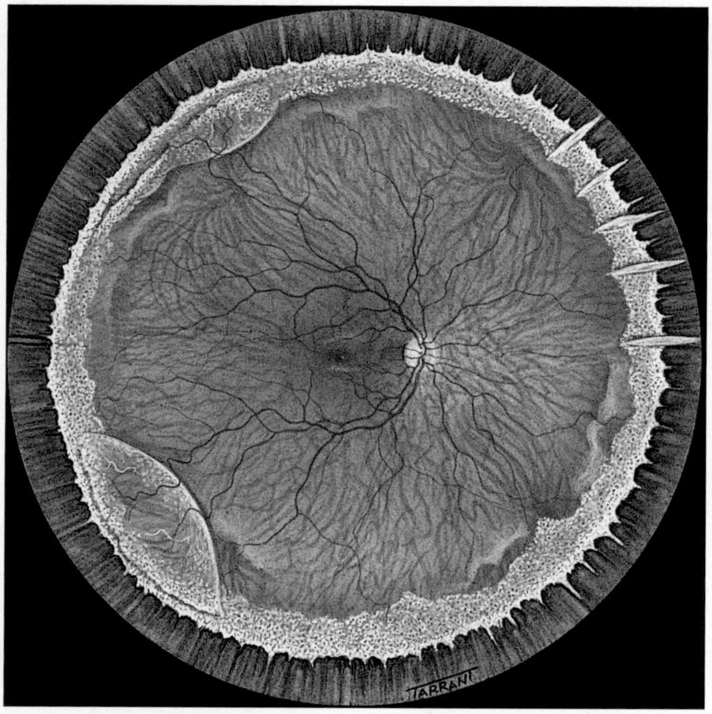

■ **Fig. 11.14** Early retinoschisis usually involves the extreme inferotemporal periphery of both fundi, appearing as an exaggeration of microcystoid degeneration with a smooth elevation of the retina.

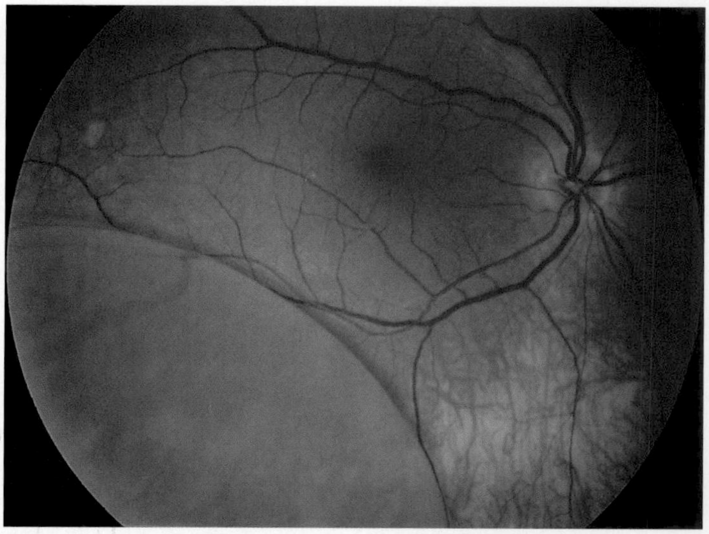

■ **Fig. 11.15** The reticular form of retinoschisis may rarely spread beyond the equator.

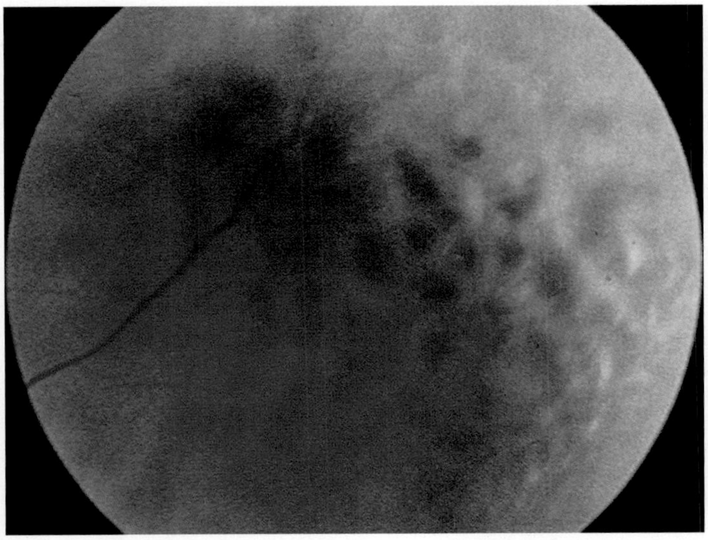

■ **Fig. 11.16** The outer layer has a 'beaten metal' appearance and shows the phenomenon of 'white-with-pressure' (see below).

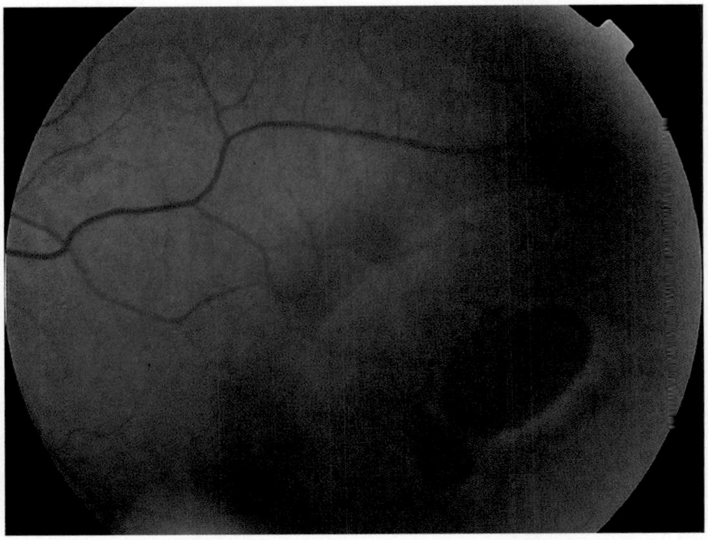

■ **Fig. 11.17** Retinoschisis with two outer layer breaks, which are typically large and have rolled edges.

'White-with-pressure'

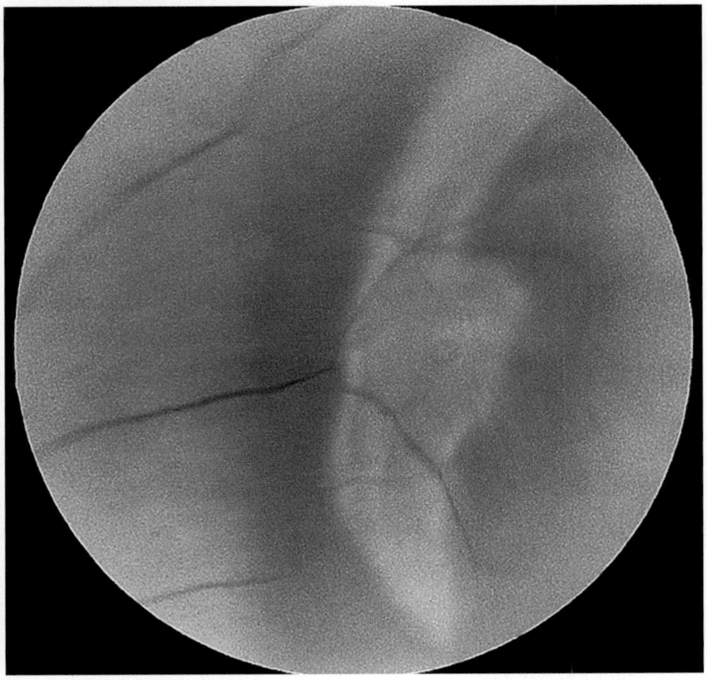

■ **Fig. 11.18** A translucent grey appearance of the retina, induced by indenting the sclera. (Courtesy of N. E. Byer.)

'White-without-pressure'

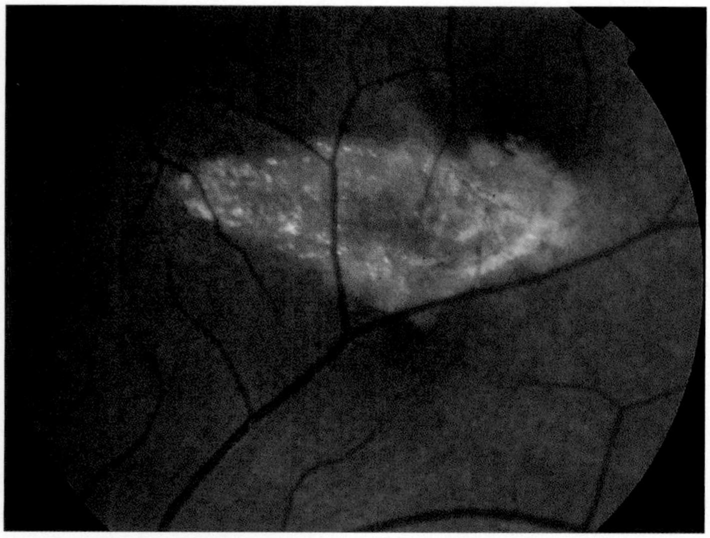

■ **Fig. 11.19** The same appearance as 'white-with-pressure' but present without scleral indentation.

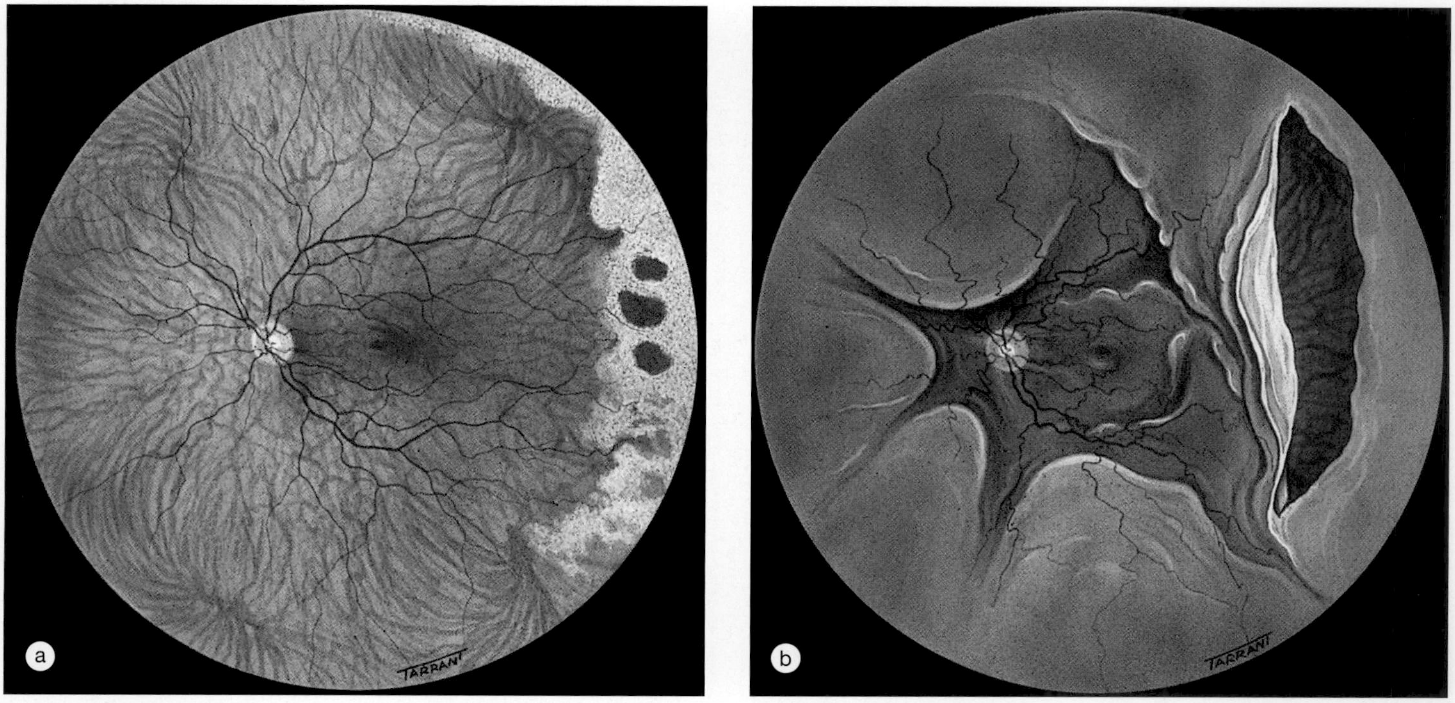

■ **Fig. 11.20** **(a)** On cursory examination a normal area of retina surrounded by white-without-pressure may be mistaken for a flat retinal hole. **(b)** Giant tears occasionally develop along the posterior border of white-without-pressure.

RHEGMATOGENOUS RETINAL DETACHMENT

A rhegmatogenous retinal detachment is caused by a retinal break, which may be a tear or hole.

Retinal breaks

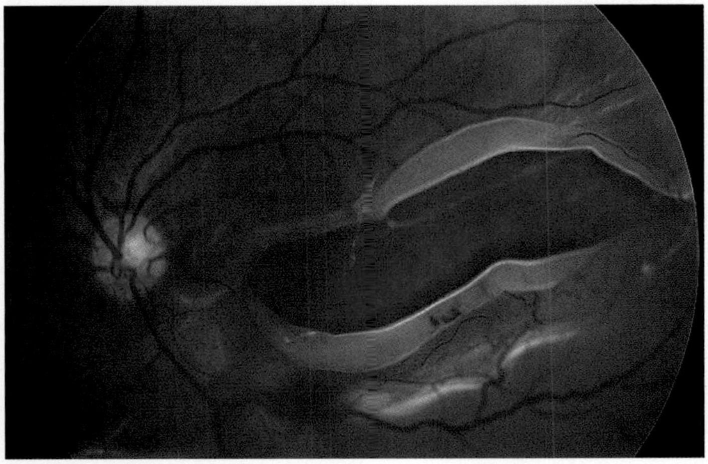

Fig. 11.21 Very large linear tear with rolled edges at the posterior pole. (Courtesy of C. Barry.)

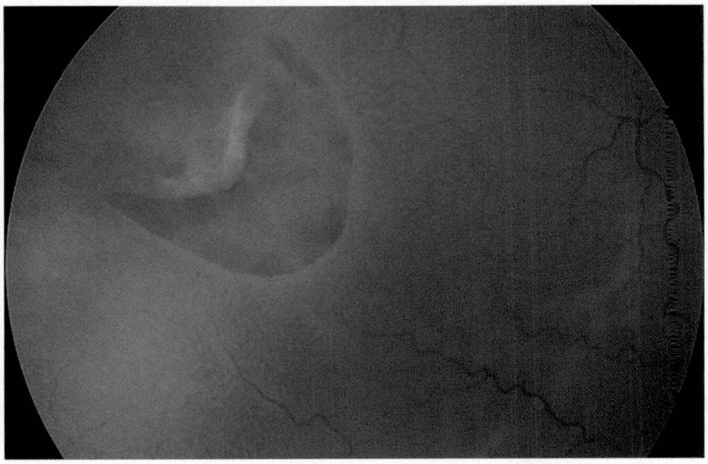

Fig. 11.22 U-tear resulting in retinal detachment. (Courtesy of P. Gili.)

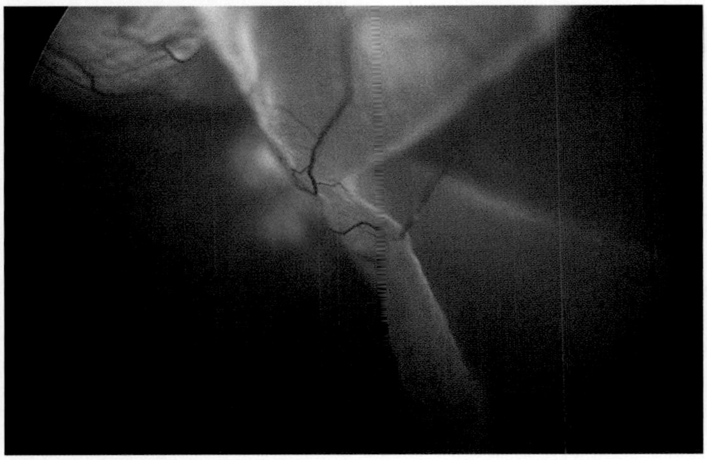

Fig. 11.23 A giant tear involves 90° or more of the circumference of the globe. (Courtesy of C. Barry.)

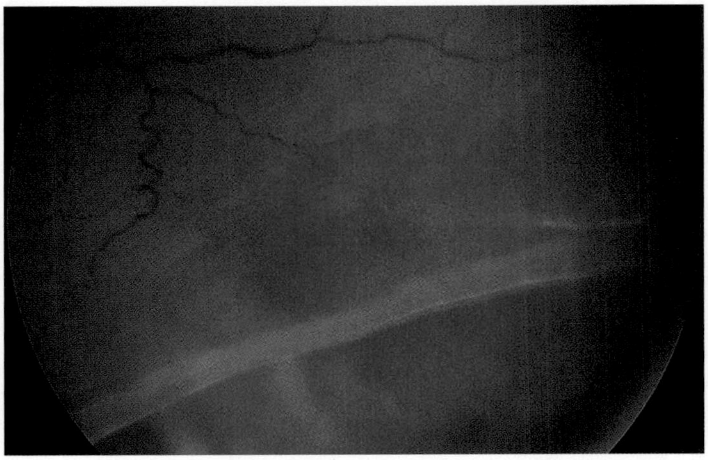

Fig. 11.24 Circumferential tear along the ora serrata (dialysis). (Courtesy of C. Barry.)

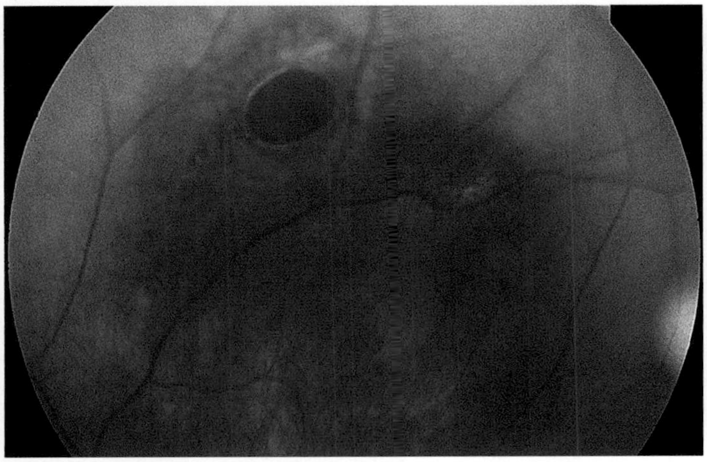

Fig. 11.25 Retinal hole in flat retina.

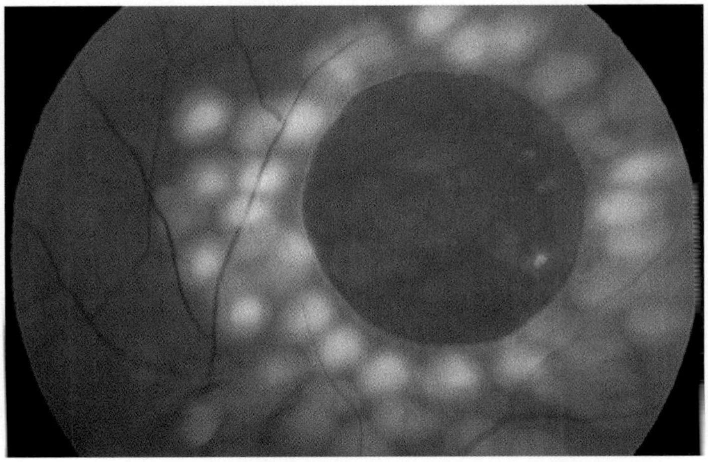

Fig. 11.26 Large hole surrounded by laser burns.

Fresh retinal detachment

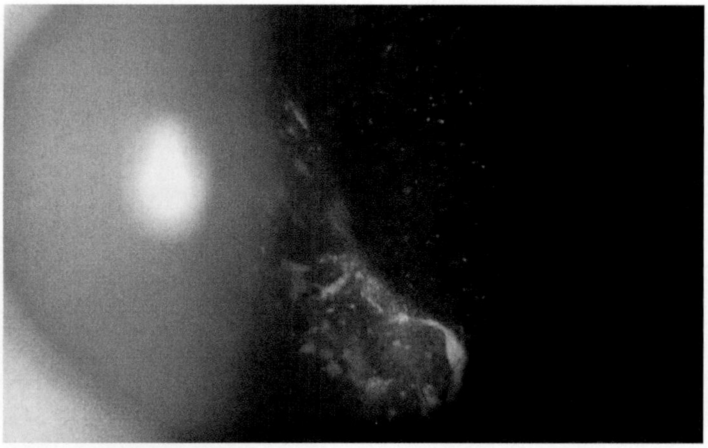

Fig. 11.27 Pigment particles ('tobacco dust') in the anterior vitreous are very suggestive of the presence of a retinal tear. (Courtesy of V. Tanner.)

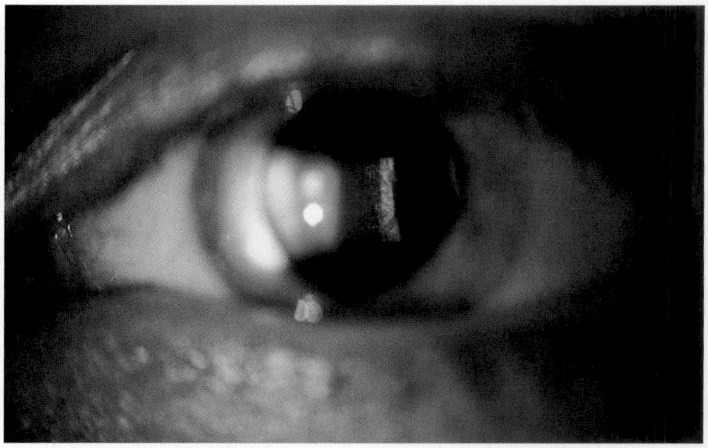

Fig. 11.28 'Tobacco dust' and posterior vitreous detachment.

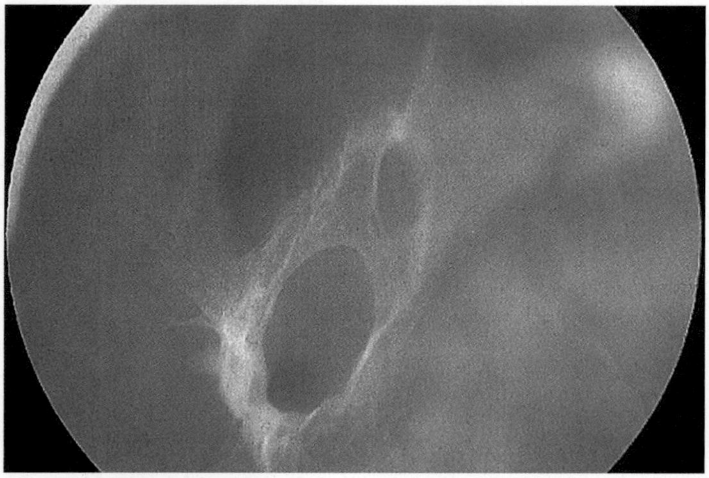

Fig. 11.29 A Weiss ring is a solitary floater consisting of the detached annular attachment of vitreous to the margin of the optic disc. (Courtesy of V. Tanner.)

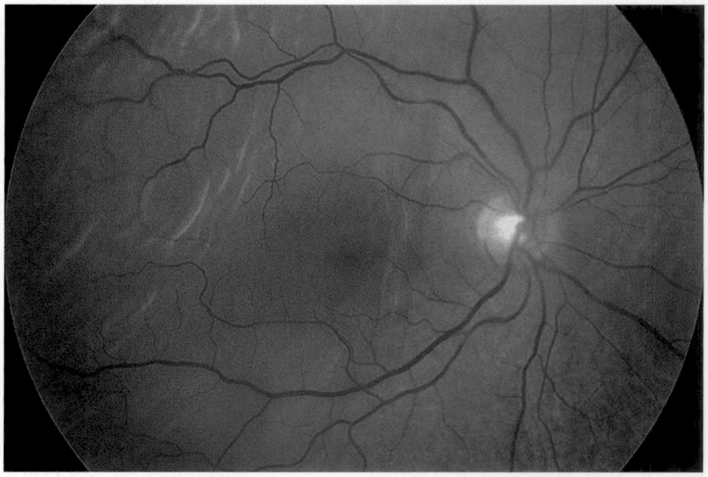

Fig. 11.30 Shallow superotemporal retinal detachment. The detached retina has a convex configuration and a slightly opaque and corrugated appearance as a result of intraretinal oedema. (Courtesy of C. Barry.)

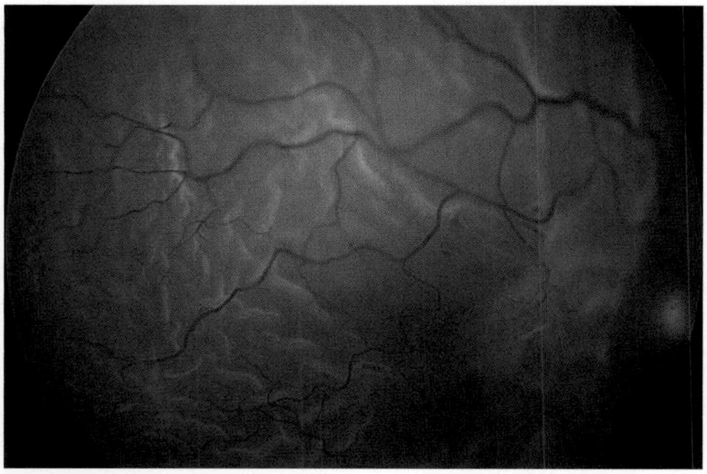

Fig. 11.31 Extensive retinal detachment in which the retinal blood vessels appear darker than in flat retina, so the colour contrast between veins and arteries is less apparent. (Courtesy of L. Merin.)

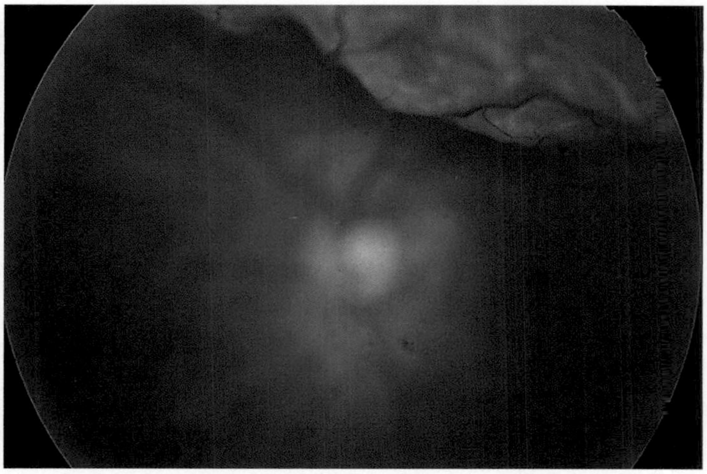

Fig. 11.32 Superior bullous retinal detachment. (Courtesy of C. Barry.)

Long-standing retinal detachment

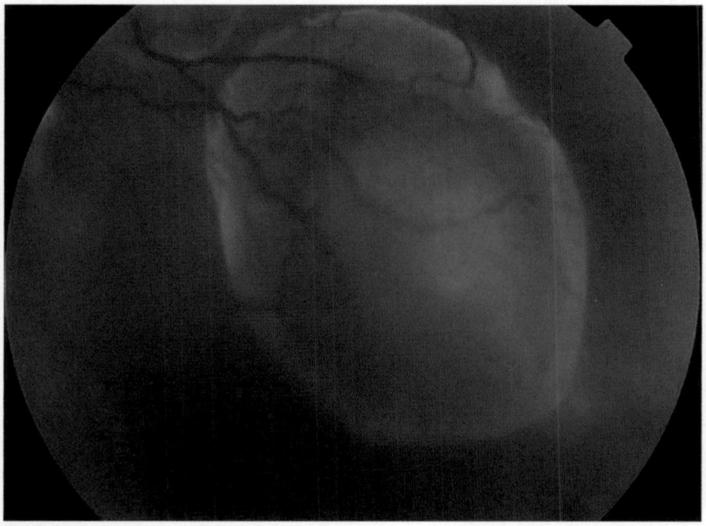

Fig. 11.33 Thin retina with a secondary intraretinal cyst.

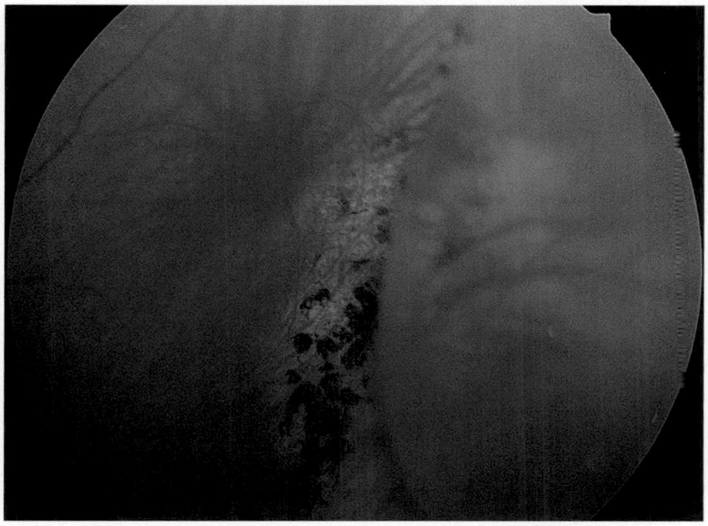

Fig. 11.34 Pigmented subretinal demarcation lines (high water marks) form at the junction of flat and detached retina and are convex with respect to the ora serrata.

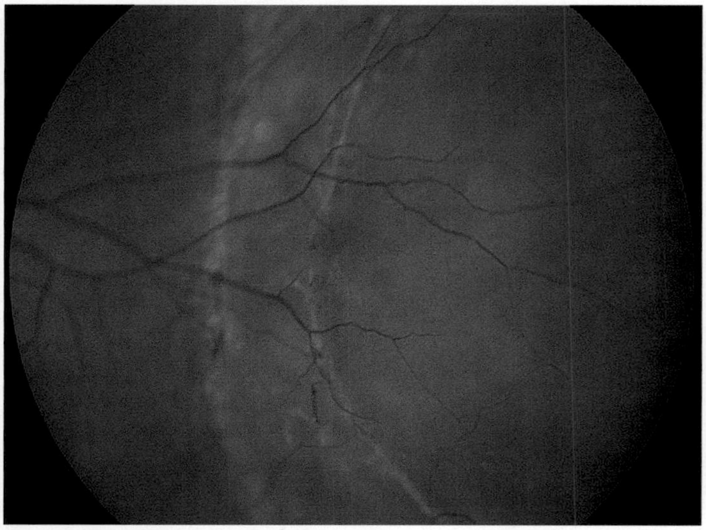

Fig. 11.35 Two thin demarcation lines that have not prevented spread of subretinal fluid.

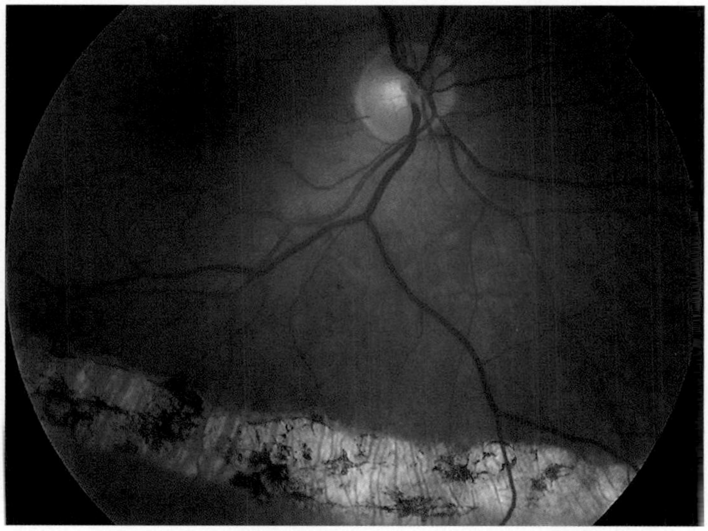

Fig. 11.36 Very broad demarcation line.

Proliferative vitreoretinopathy (PVR)

PVR typically occurs following retinal surgery and is characterised by the proliferation of retinal membranes.

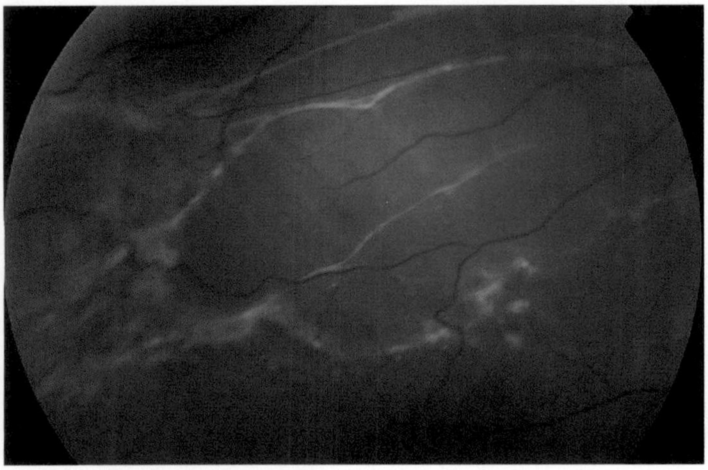

Fig. 11.37 Subretinal bands.

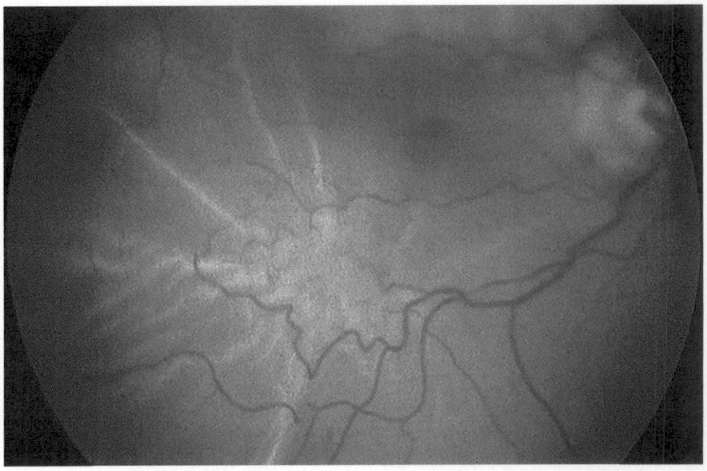

Fig. 11.38 Wrinkling of the inner retinal surface and tortuosity of blood vessels.

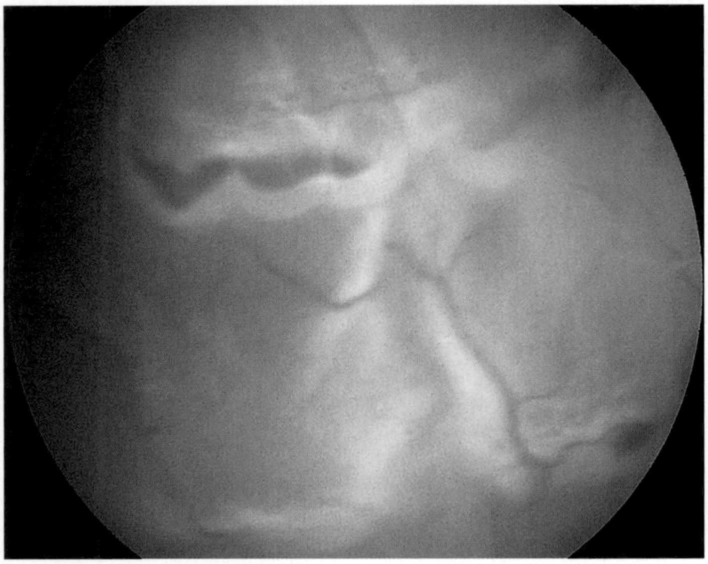

Fig. 11.39 Retinal stiffness and rolled and irregular edges of retinal breaks.

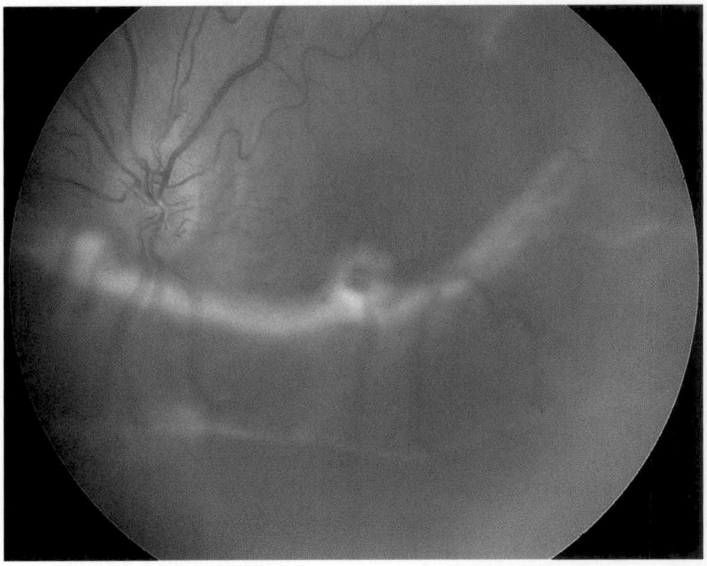

Fig. 11.40 Dense subretinal band.

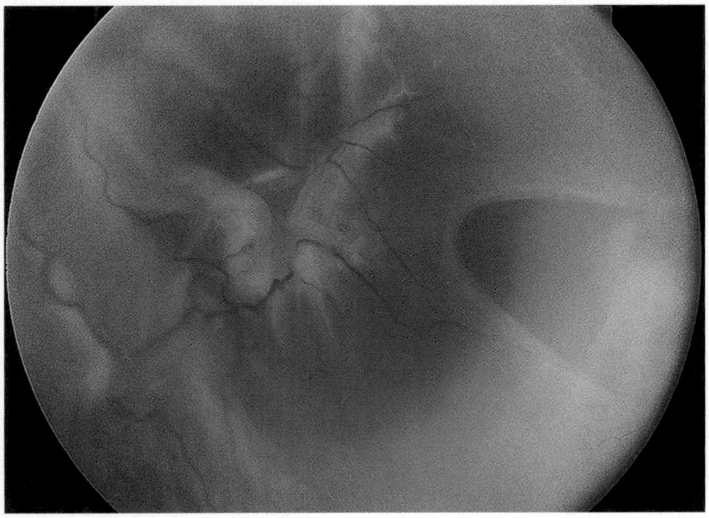

Fig. 11.41 Focal retinal fold and opening of a previously closed retinal tear.

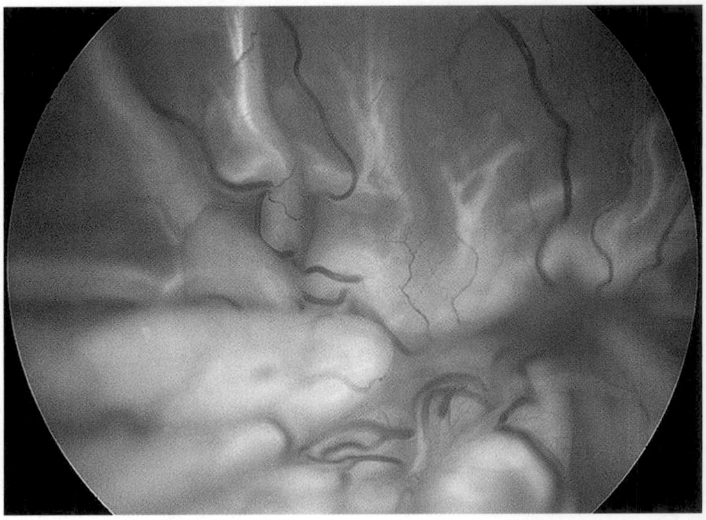

Fig. 11.42 End-stage PVR.

Differential diagnosis

Tractional retinal detachment

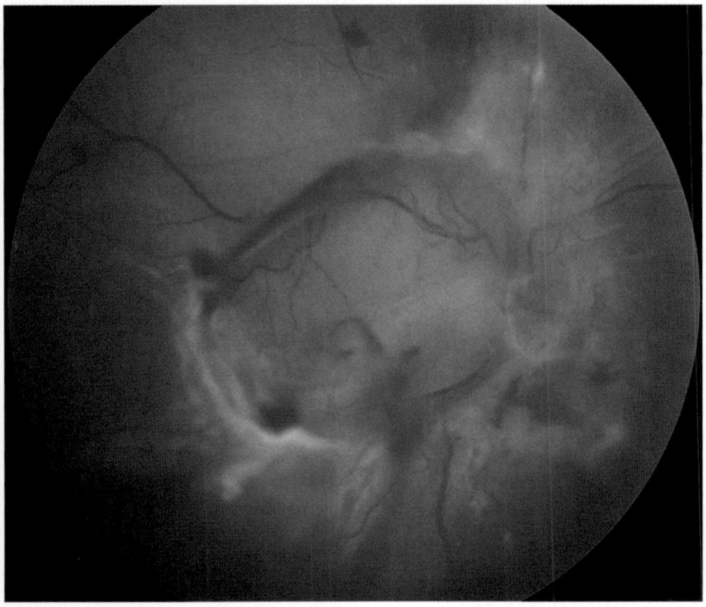

Fig. 11.43 The elevation is concave, shallow and immobile, with absence of retinal breaks.

Exudative retinal detachment

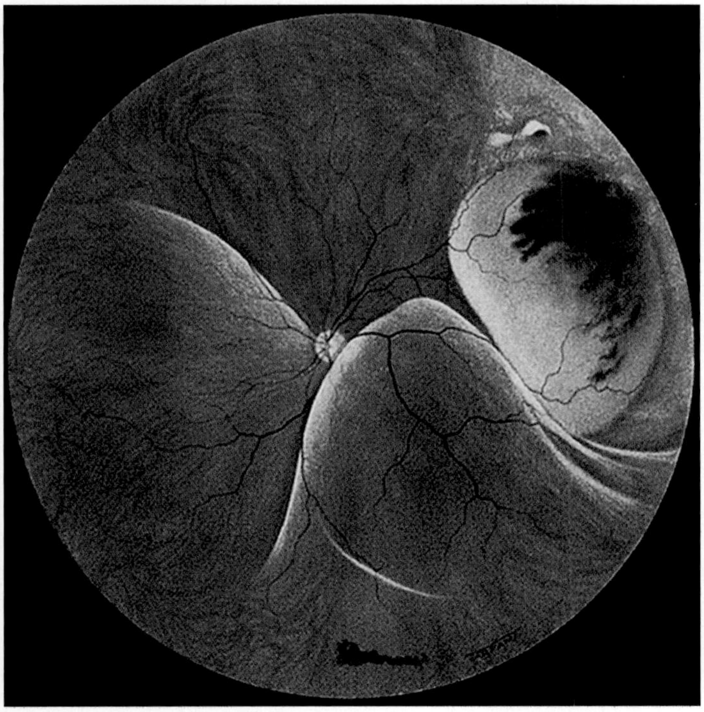

Fig. 11.44 The elevation is convex, often very deep and mobile, with absence of retinal breaks; in this case it is caused by a choroidal mass.

Degenerative retinoschisis

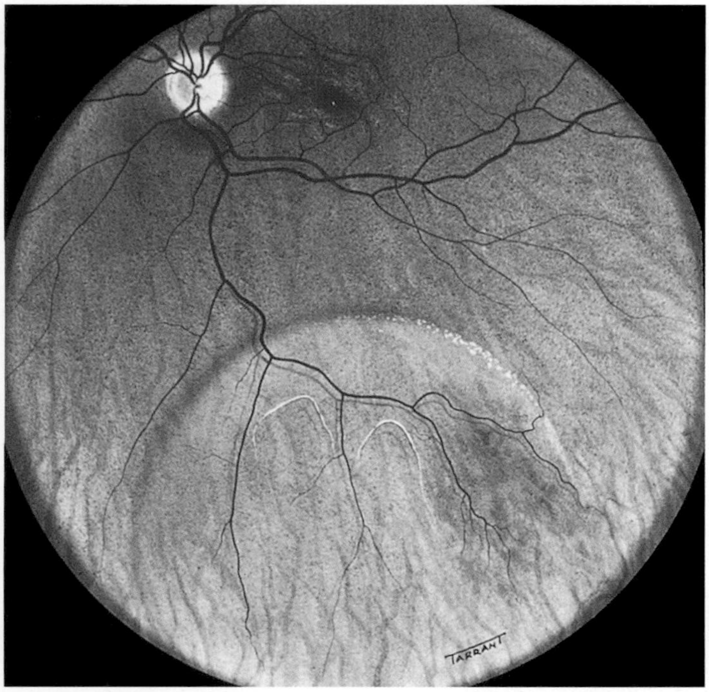

■ **Fig. 11.45** The elevation is convex, smooth, thin and relatively immobile. Two breaks are present in the inner layer which also shows snowflakes.

Choroidal detachment

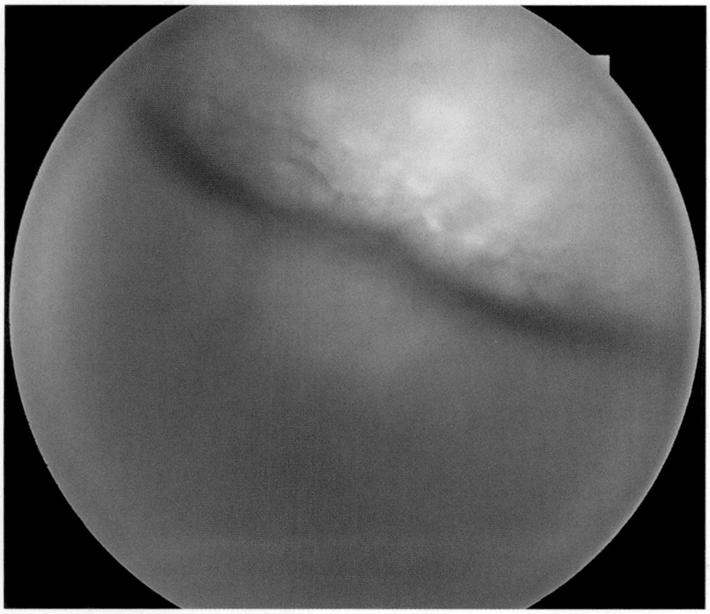

■ **Fig. 11.46** The elevation is peripheral, brown, convex, smooth and relatively immobile.

Uveal effusion syndrome

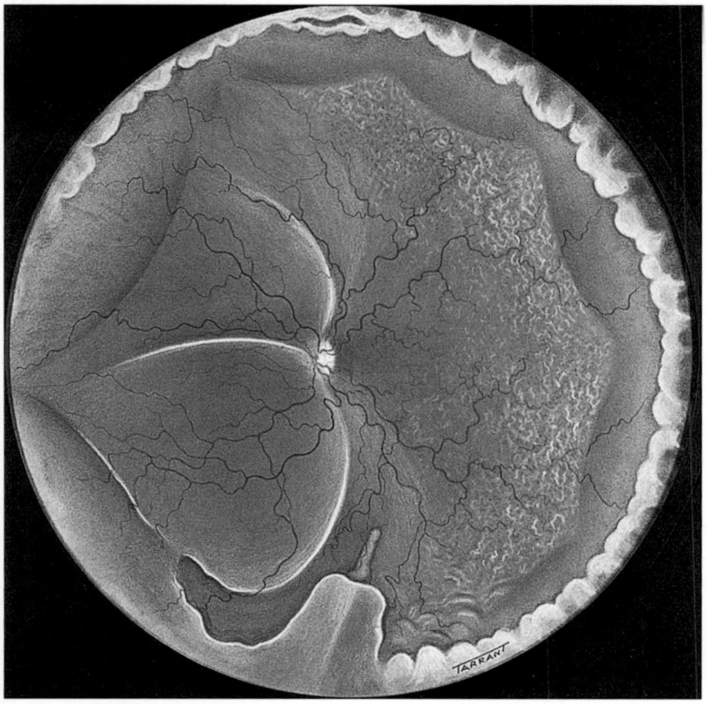

Fig. 11.47 Ciliochoroidal detachment followed by exudative retinal detachment, which may be bilateral.

Complications of surgery

Operative

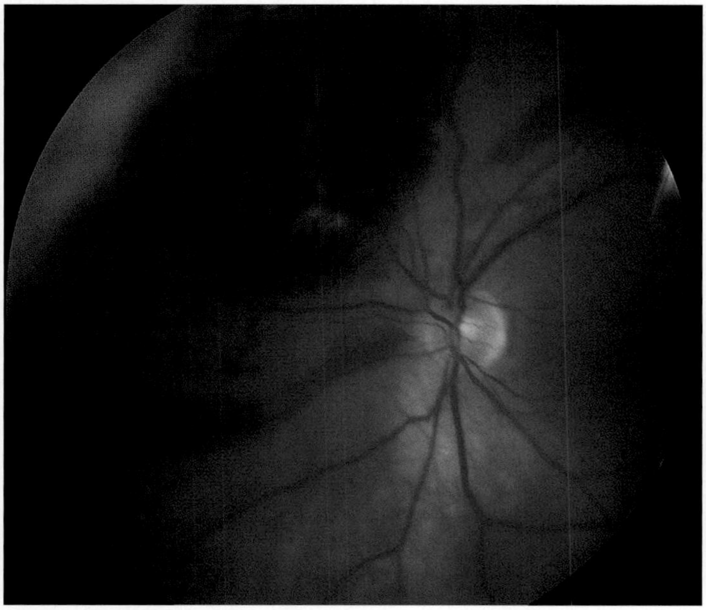

Fig. 11.48 Subretinal haemorrhage associated with drainage of subretinal fluid.

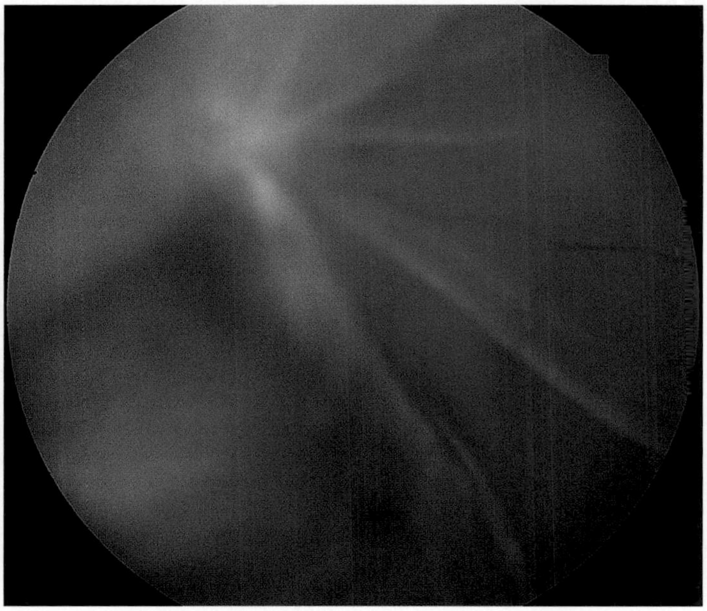

Fig. 11.49 Retinal incarceration into the drainage site.

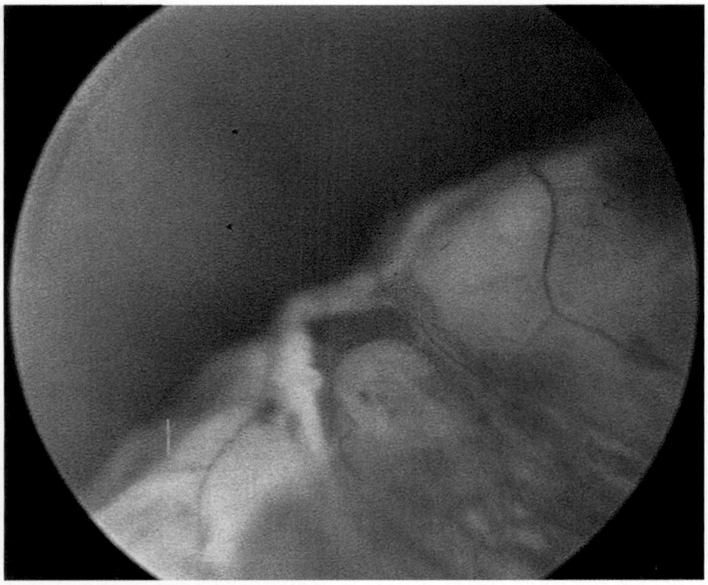

Fig. 11.50 'Fish-mouthing' of a retinal tear.

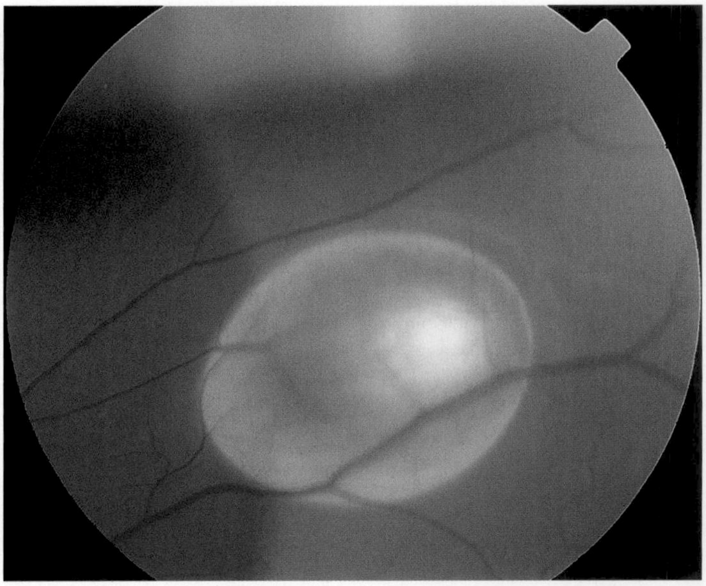

Fig. 11.51 Accidental subretinal injection of gas.

Postoperative

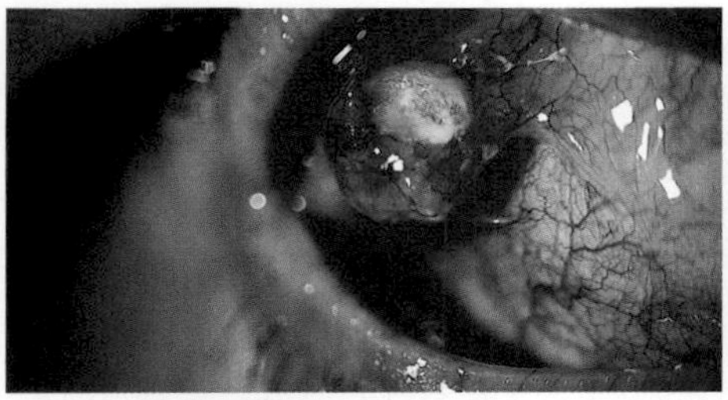

Fig. 11.52 Infection and extrusion of an explant.

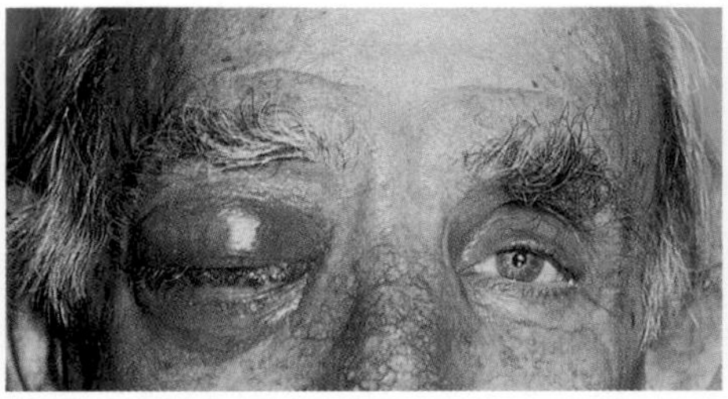

Fig. 11.53 Orbital cellulitis.

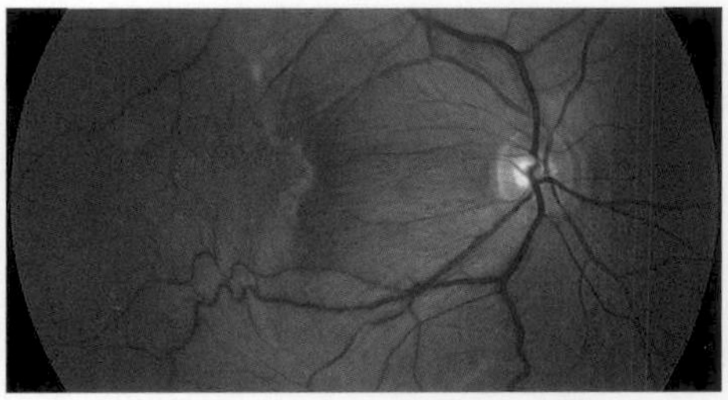

Fig. 11.54 Macular pucker. (Courtesy of C. Barry.)

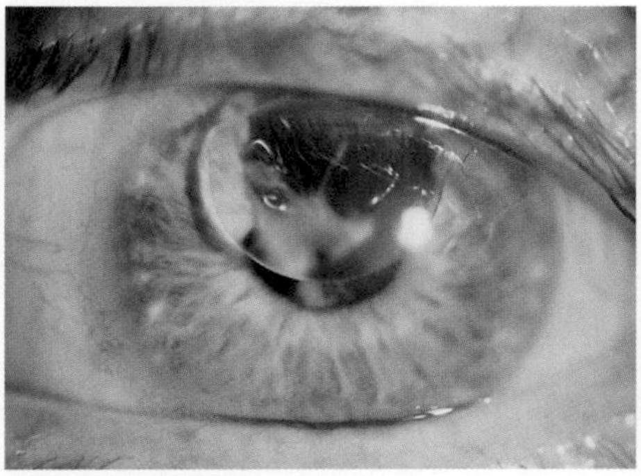

Fig. 11.55 Migration of silicone oil into the anterior chamber.

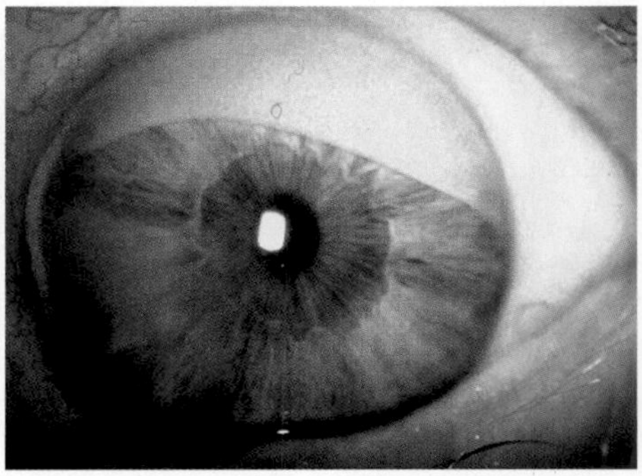

Fig. 11.56 Emulsified silicone oil in the anterior chamber forming a pseudohypopyon. (Courtesy of S. Ford and R. Marsh.)

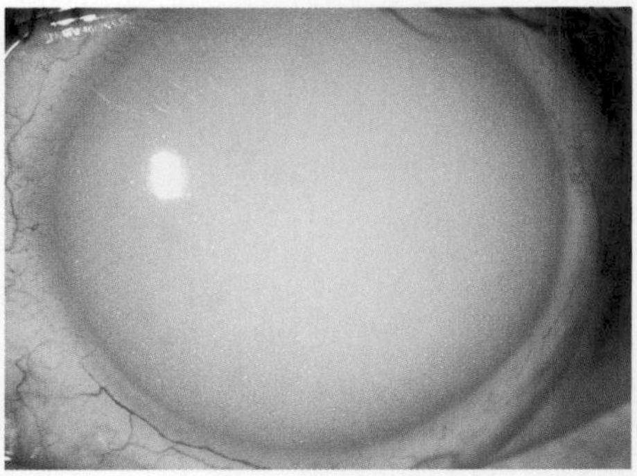

Fig. 11.57 The anterior chamber is full of emulsified silicone oil.

Postoperative appearances

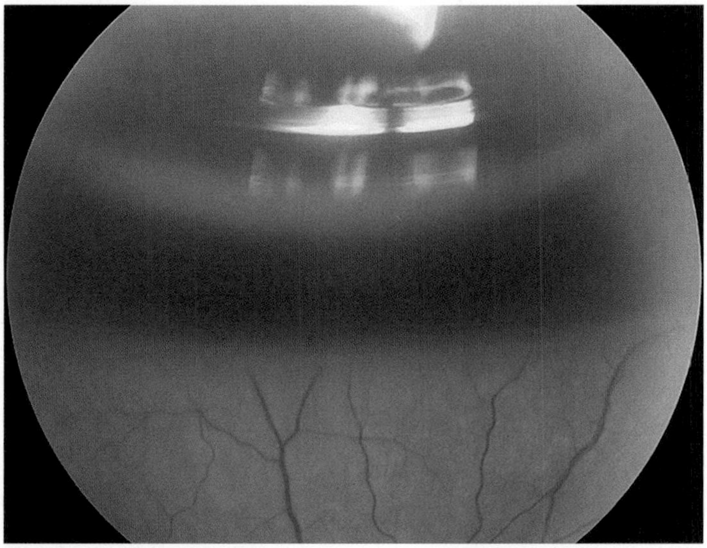

■ **Fig. 11.58** Gas bubble in the vitreous. (Courtesy of C. Barry.)

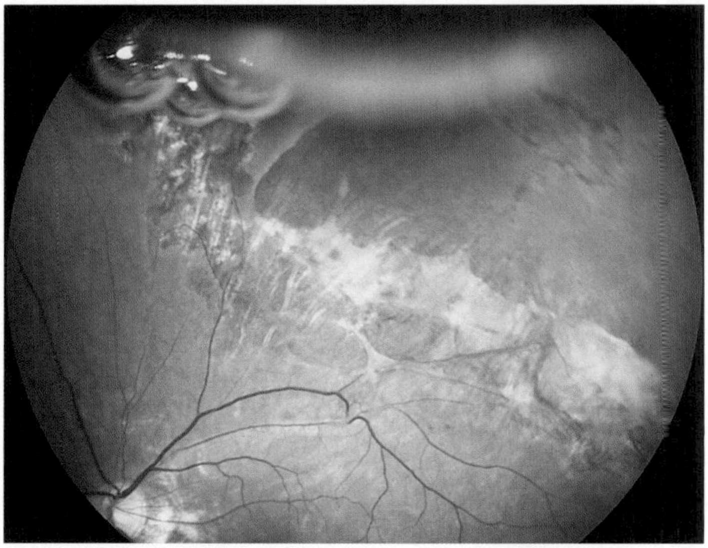

■ **Fig. 11.59** Gas bubble tamponading a giant retinal tear. (Courtesy of C. Barry.)

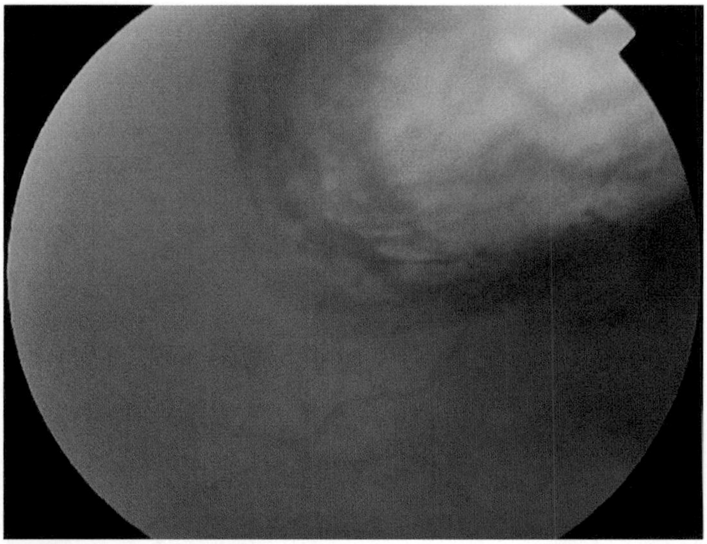

■ **Fig. 11.60** Local buckle with flat retina.

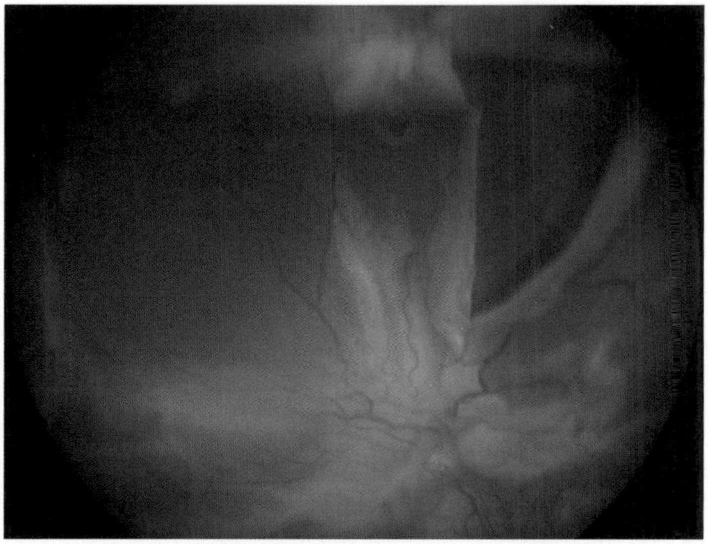

■ **Fig. 11.61** Circumferential buckle with PVR and a large open tear.

CHAPTER 12

RETINAL VASCULAR DISEASE

DIABETIC RETINOPATHY

Signs associated with diabetes mellitus

Hands

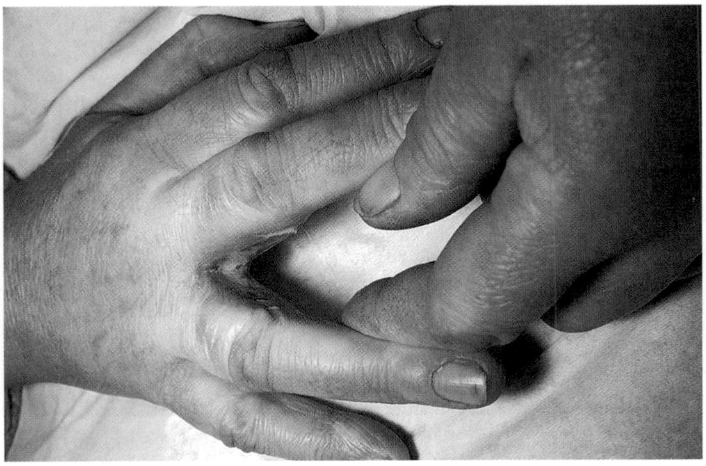

Fig. 12.1 Monilial infection between the fingers.

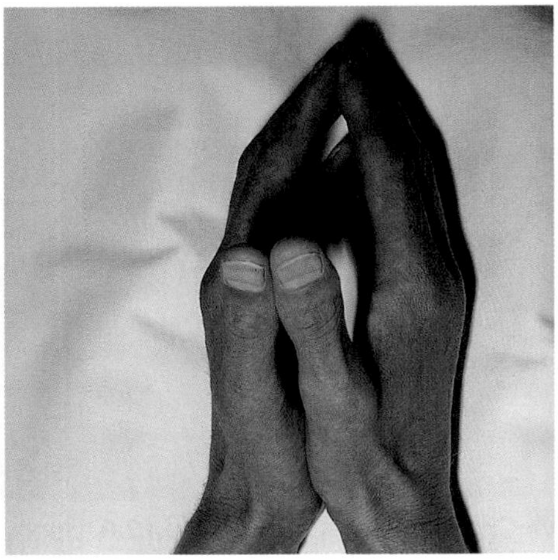

Fig. 12.2 Painless stiffness of the hands (cheiroarthropathy), which can be demonstrated by the 'prayer sign'. There is also muscle wasting as a result of symmetrical sensory polyneuropathy.

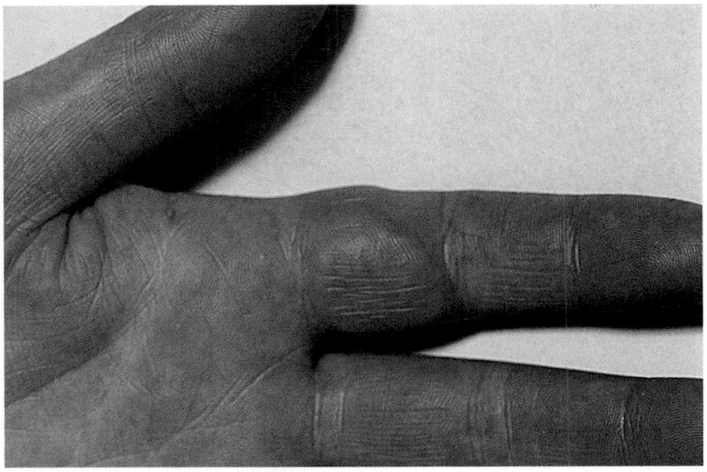

Fig. 12.3 Smooth annular plaques on the fingers (granuloma annulare) are weakly associated with diabetes as they may also develop in non-diabetic individuals.

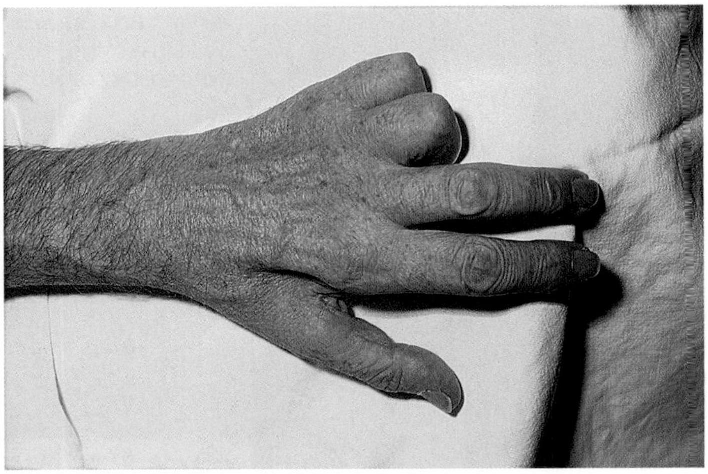

Fig. 12.4 Ulnar nerve palsy due to mononeuropathy.

Background diabetic retinopathy (BDR)

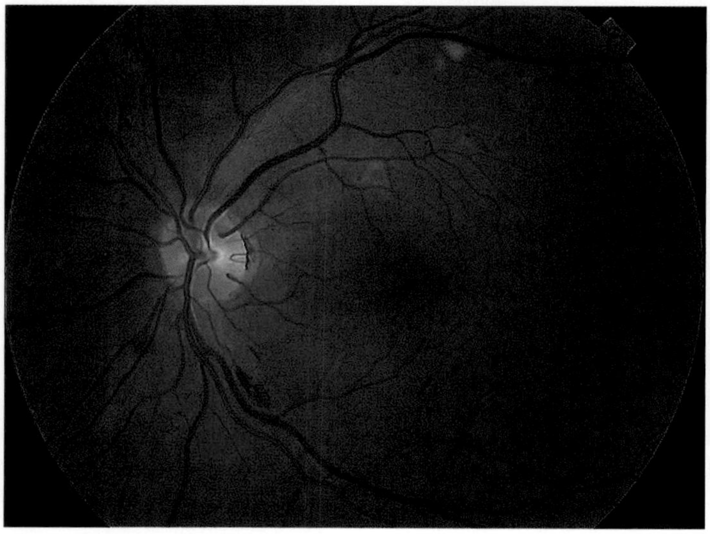

Fig. 12.19 Early BDR with scattered microaneurysms, dot haemorrhages, and a small flame-shaped haemorrhage.

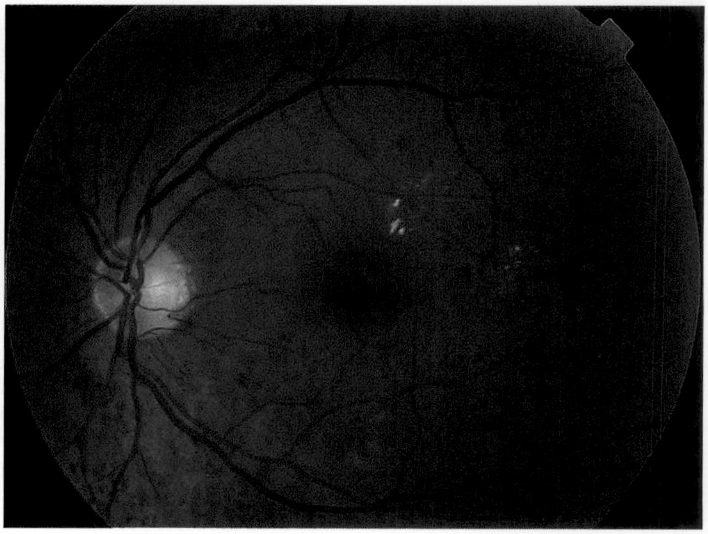

Fig. 12.20 BDR with microaneurysms, dot haemorrhages and a few small hard exudates at the macula.

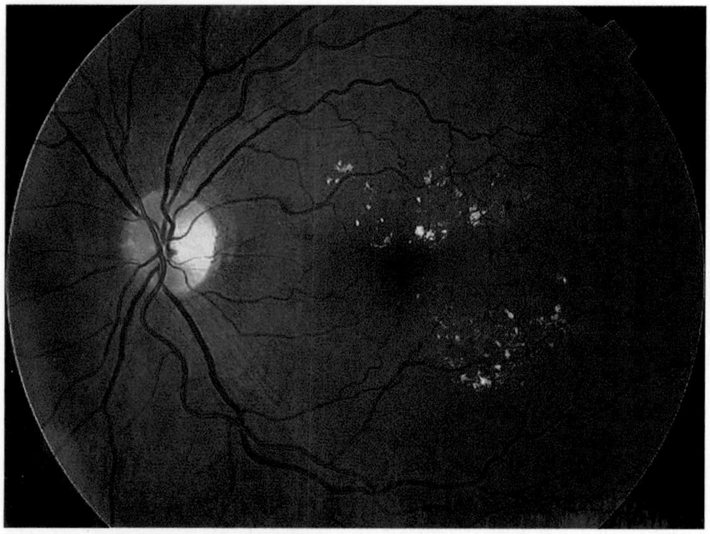

Fig. 12.21 More hard exudates but fewer microaneurysms.

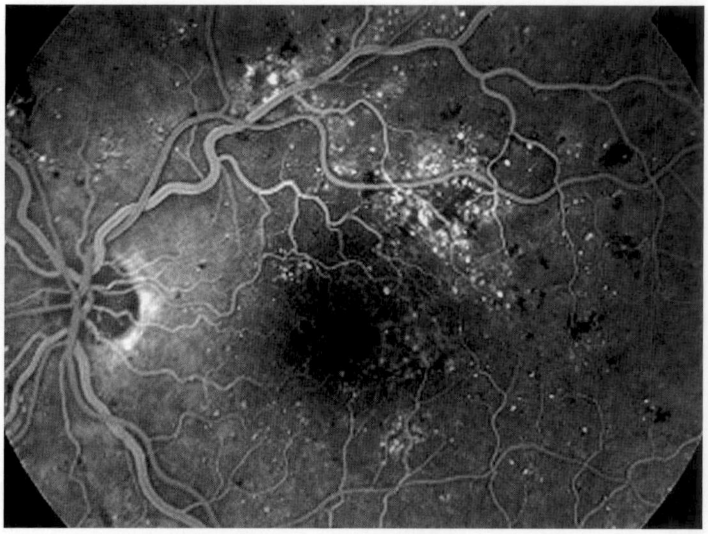

Fig. 12.22 FA shows spotty hyperfluorescence of microaneurysms and blockage by haemorrhages.

Diabetic maculopathy

Focal maculopathy

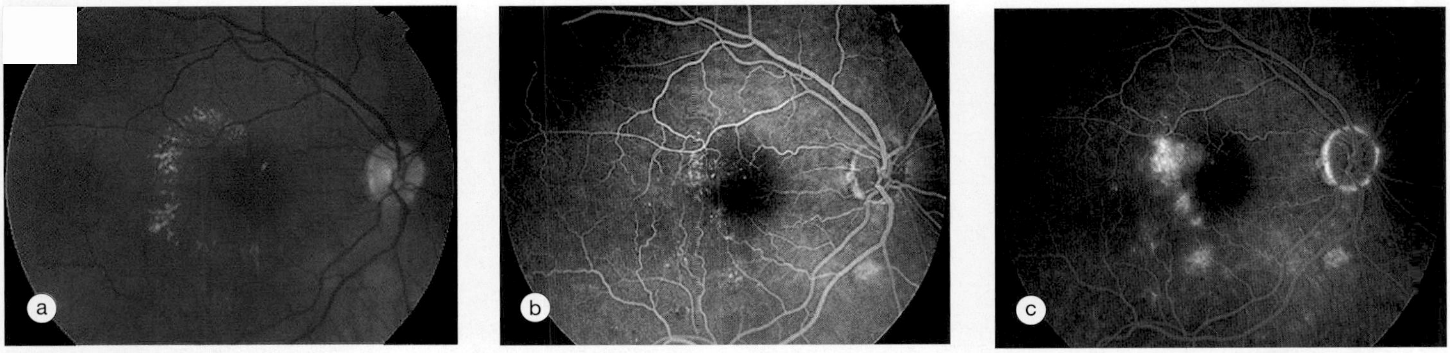

■ **Fig. 12.23** **(a)** Well-circumscribed retinal thickening associated with complete or incomplete rings of perifoveal hard exudates. **(b)** FA venous phase shows spotty hyperfluorescence of microaneurysms. **(c)** Late phases show focal hyperfluorescence due to leakage but good macular perfusion.

Diffuse maculopathy

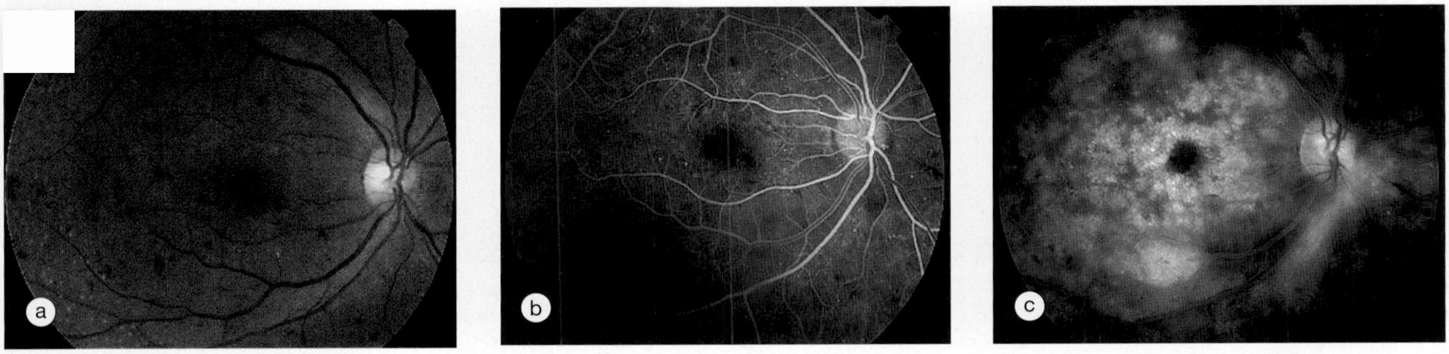

■ **Fig. 12.24** **(a)** Diffuse retinal thickening due to severe oedema. **(b)** FA early venous phase shows spotty hyperfluorescence of microaneurysms. **(c)** Late phase shows diffuse hyperfluorescence, which has a flower-petal pattern at the fovea due to cystoid macular oedema (CMO).

Ischaemic maculopathy

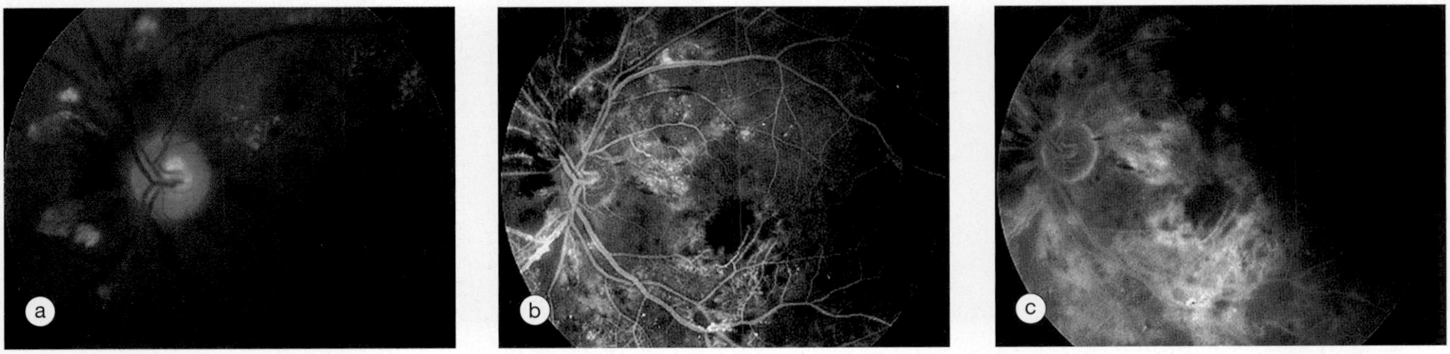

■ **Fig. 12.25** **(a)** Many flame-shaped and dark blot haemorrhages, cotton-wool spots and scattered hard exudates. **(b, c)** FA shows hyperfluorescence due to leakage but hypofluorescence at the fovea due to capillary non-perfusion.

Preproliferative diabetic retinopathy (PPDR)

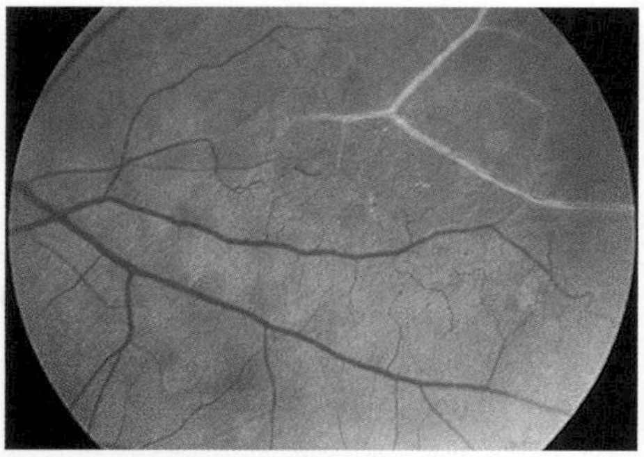

Fig 12.26 Peripheral arterial occlusion.

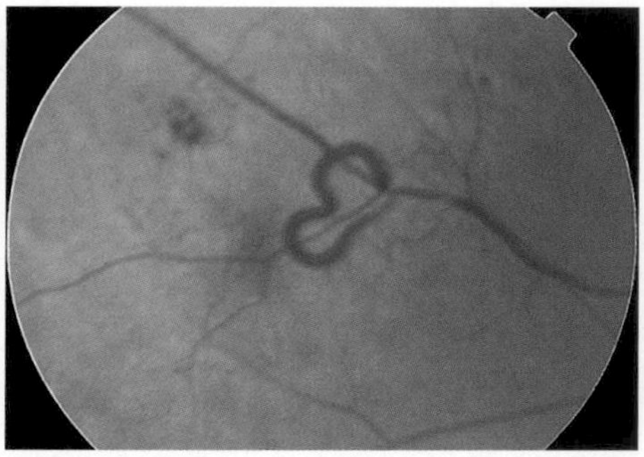

Fig. 12.27 Venous looping.

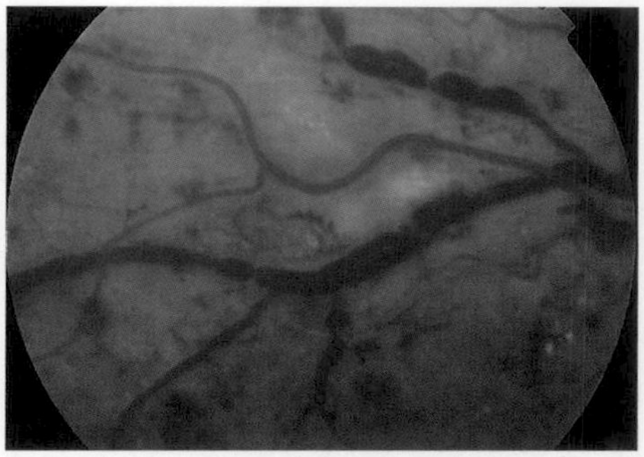

Fig. 12.28 Severe venous dilatation and sausage-like segmentation.

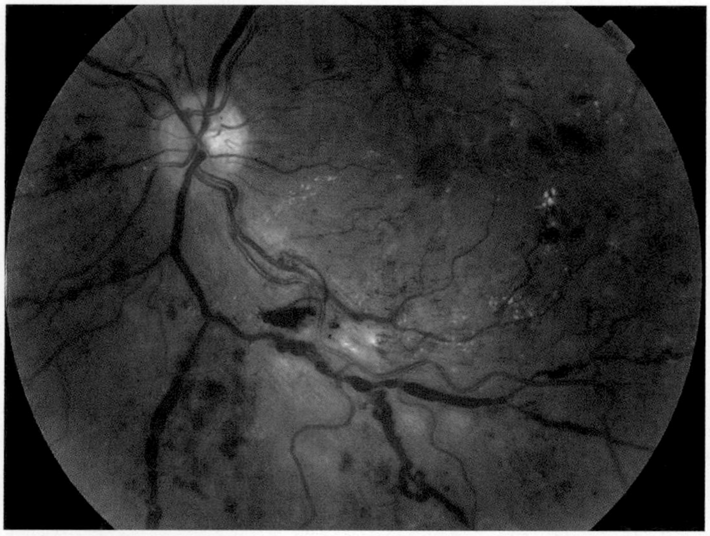

Fig. 12.29 Cotton-wool spot, severe venous changes and dark blot haemorrhages.

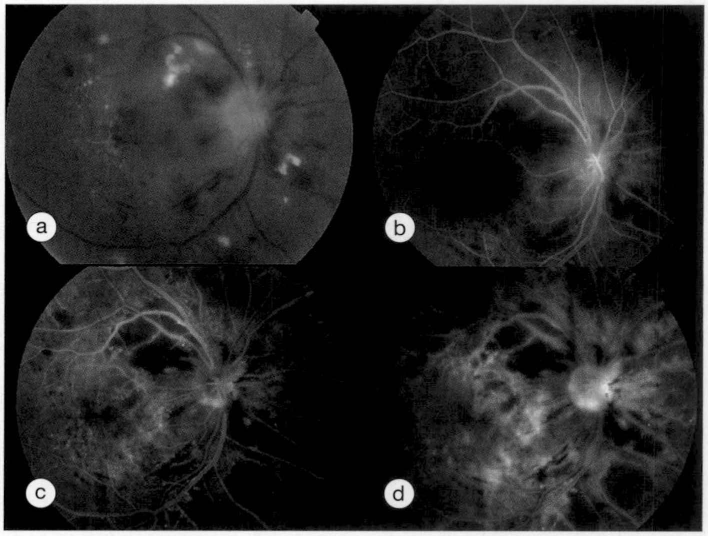

Fig. 12.30 **(a)** Flame-shaped haemorrhages, cotton-wool spots and scattered small hard exudates. **(b–d)** FA shows multiple areas of hypofluorescence due to retinal capillary non-perfusion.

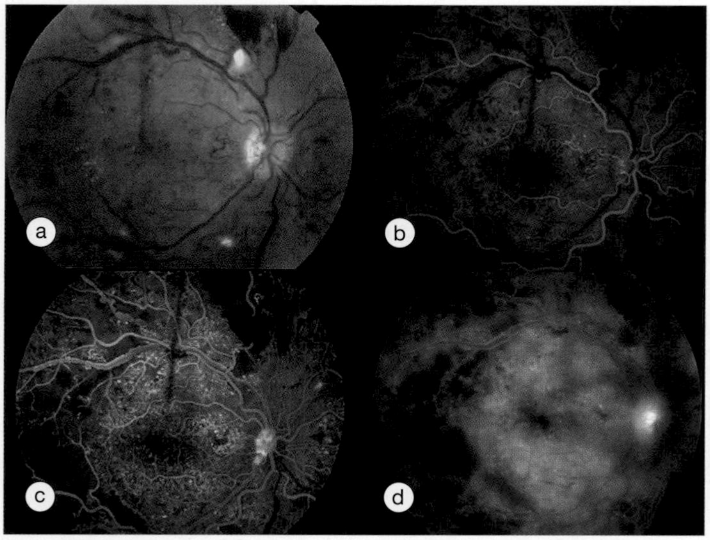

Fig. 12.31 **(a)** PPDR **(b)** FA arterial phase shows mild, spotty hyperfluorescence temporal to the disc and hypofluorescence corresponding to haemorrhages. **(c)** Venous phase highlights the venous changes and shows extensive areas of capillary non-perfusion. **(d)** Late phase shows extensive diffuse hyperfluorescence; note focal hyperfluorescence at the disc, indicative of early new vessel formation.

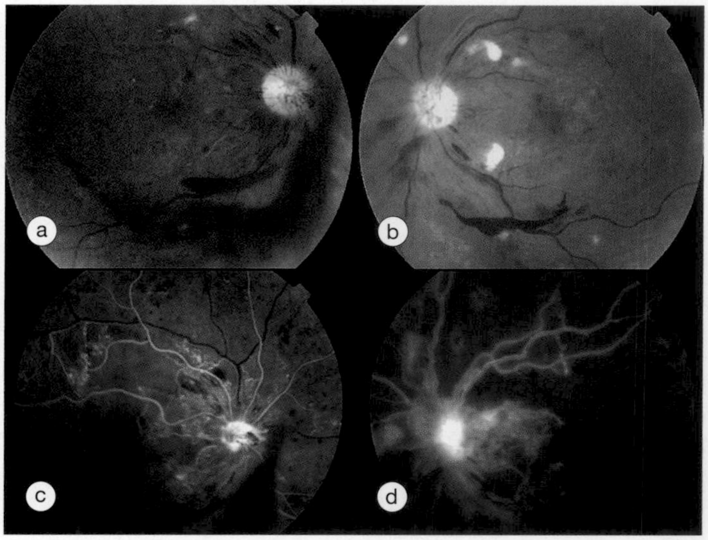

Fig. 12.32 (**a, b**) Bilateral PPDR. (**c, d**) FA shows extensive hypofluorescence due to capillary non-perfusion.

Proliferative diabetic retinopathy (PDR)

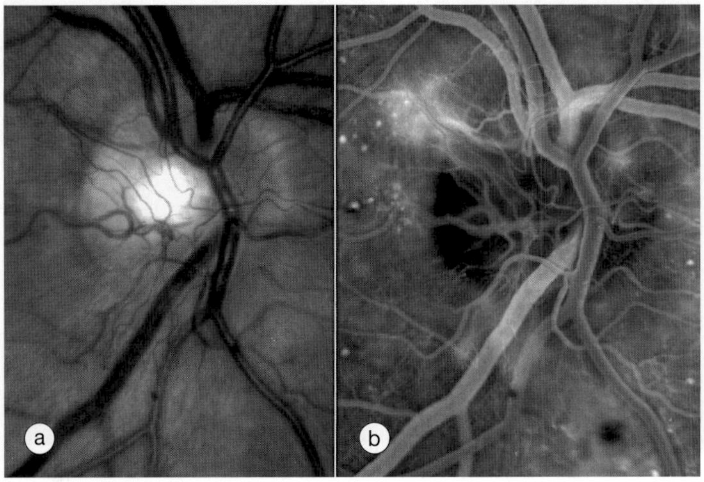

Fig. 12.33 **(a)** Red-free image showing fine disc vessels (NVD). **(b)** FA highlights the vessels and shows early leakage. (Courtesy of P. Gili.)

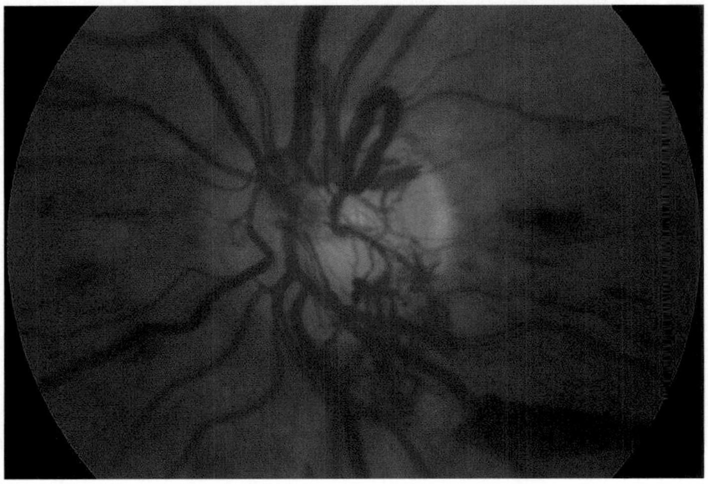

Fig. 12.34 Severe NVD with haemorrhage.

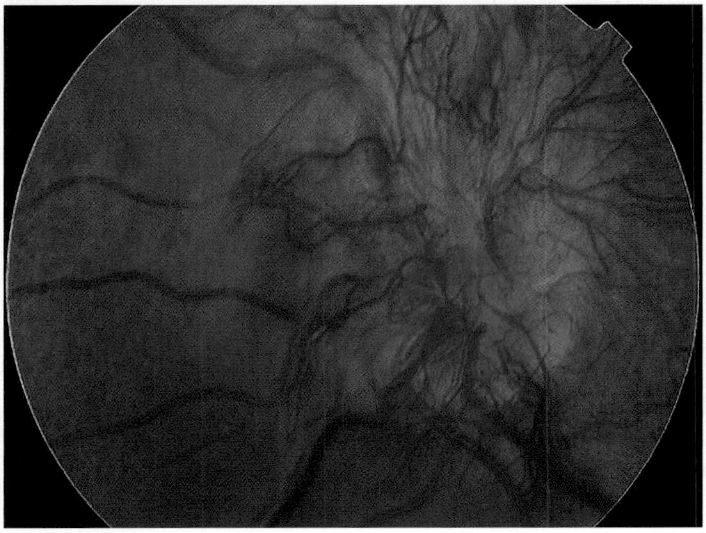

Fig. 12.35 Very severe NVD extending on to adjacent retina.

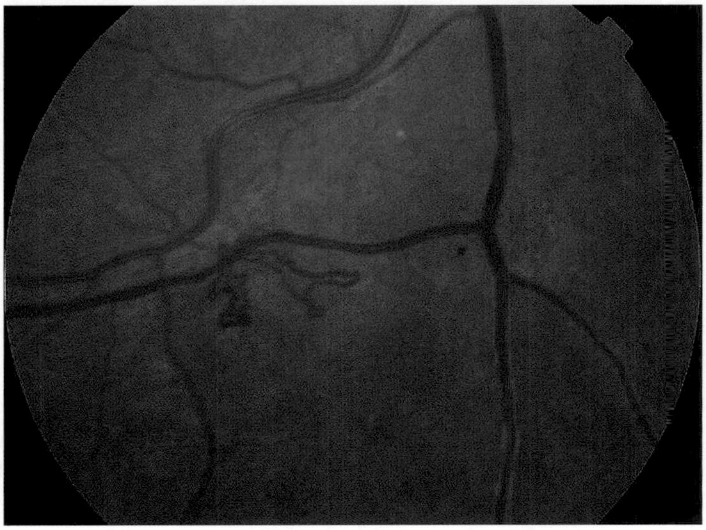

Fig. 12.36 Early new vessels everywhere (NVE).

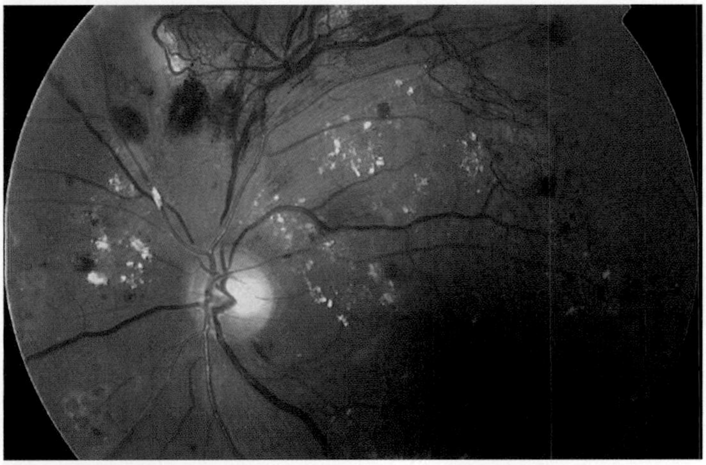

Fig. 12.37 Severe flat NVE; also note embolus in the superonasal artery.

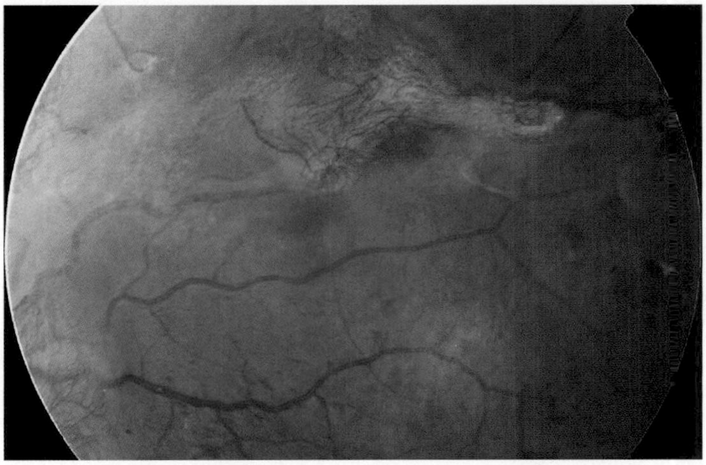

Fig. 12.38 NVE with fibrosis.

RETINAL VENOUS OCCLUSIVE DISEASE

Branch retinal vein occlusion (BRVO)

BRVO is a common condition often associated with hypertension.

Signs

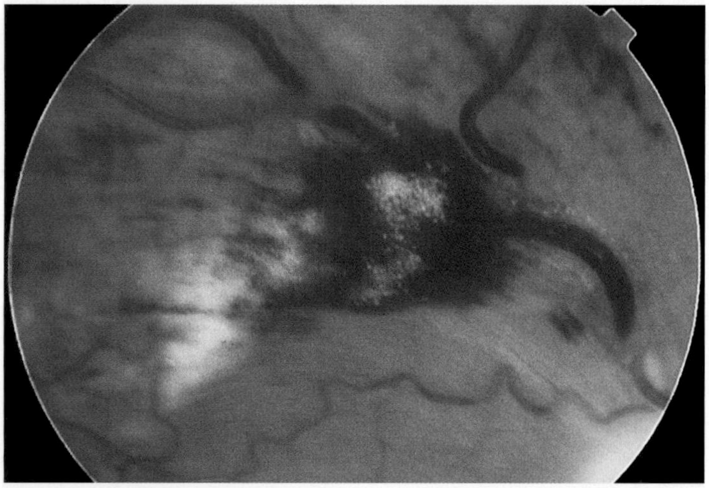

Fig. 12.49 Dilatation and tortuosity of the venous segment distal to the site of occlusion and attenuation proximal to the occlusion. Flame-shaped and dot–blot haemorrhages, retinal oedema and cotton-wool spots affecting the sector of the retina drained by the obstructed vein.

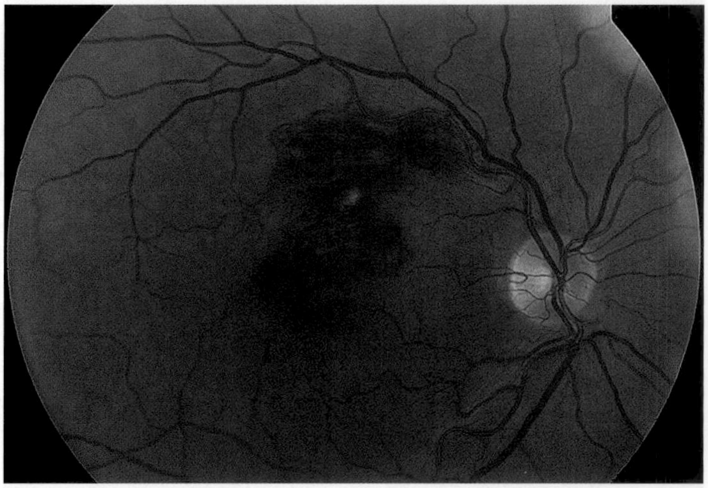

Fig. 12.50 Occlusion of a first-order temporal branch away from the disc but involving branches to the macula.

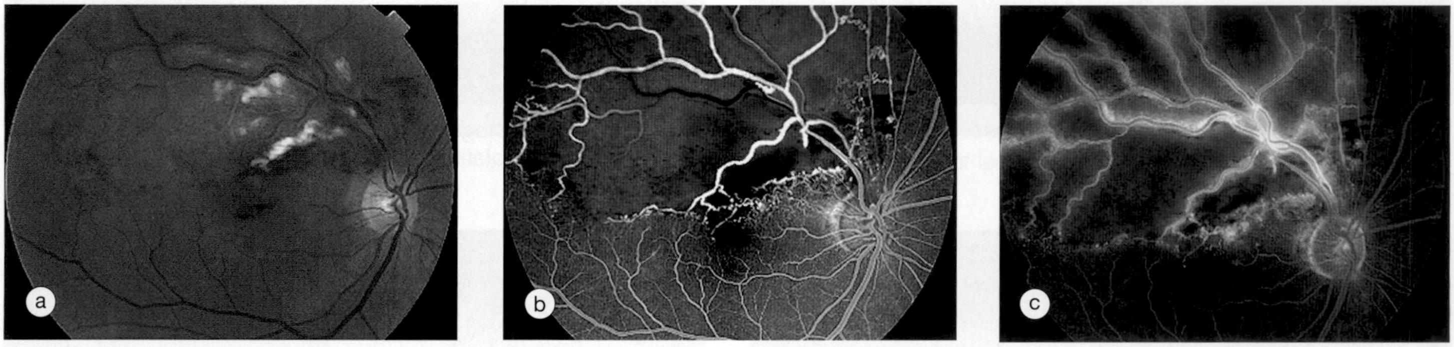

Fig. 12.51 (a) BRVO. **(b)** FA venous phase of the affected area shows delayed venous filling, extensive hypofluorescence due to capillary droop out and 'pruning' of vessels. **(c)** Late phase shows persistent hypofluorescence with perivascular hyperfluorescence due to staining.

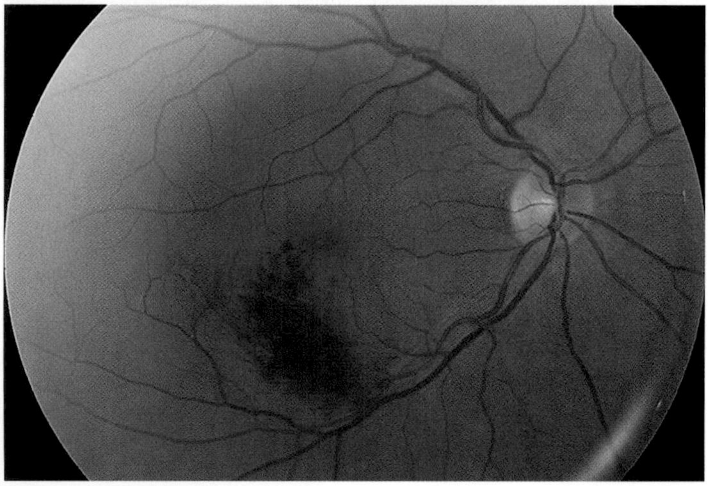

Fig. 12.52 Minor macular BRVO.

Sequelae

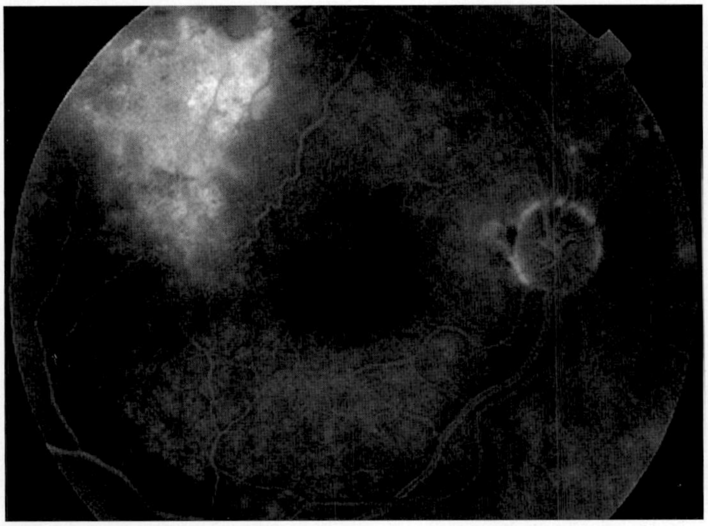

■ **Fig. 12.53** FA late phase shows hyperfluorescence due to leakage but good macular perfusion.

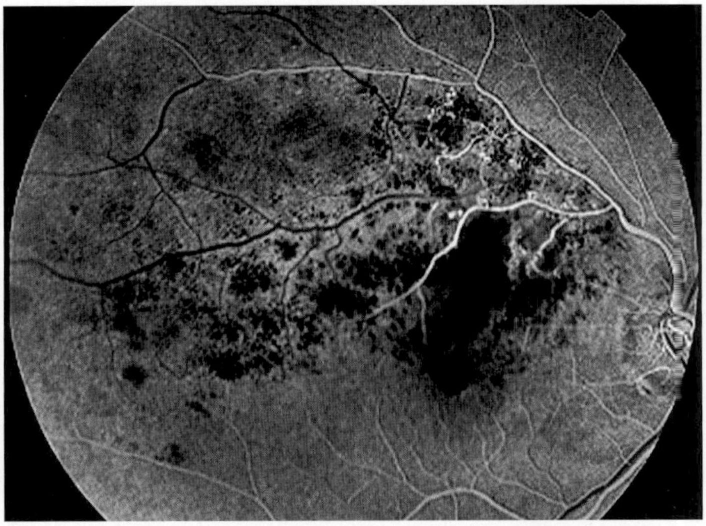

■ **Fig. 12.54** FA mid-venous phase shows delayed venous filling and macular hypofluorescence due to capillary non-perfusion.

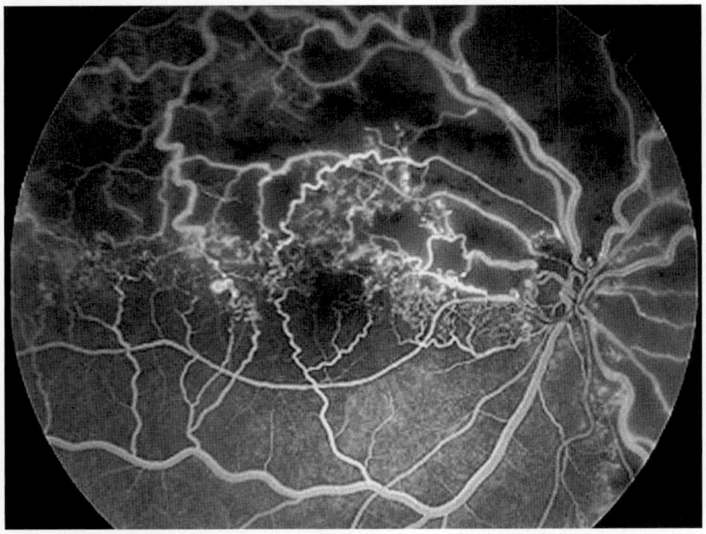

■ **Fig. 12.55** FA venous phase shows extensive hypofluorescence due to capillary non-perfusion and dilated, slightly tortuous collateral venous channels at the junction of ischaemic and normal retina.

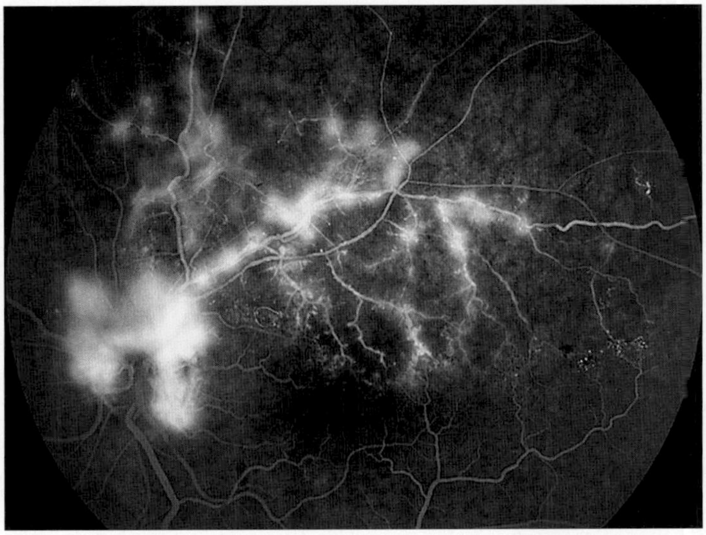

■ **Fig. 12.56** FA late phase shows hyperfluorescence at the disc and elsewhere due to new vessel formation. (Courtesy of C. Barry)

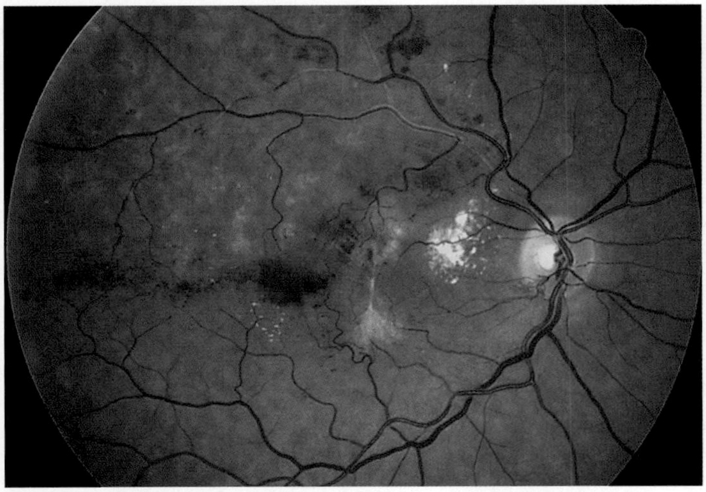

■ **Fig. 12.57** Old superotemporal BRVO showing residual haemorrhages, macular hard exudates, sheathing of the obstructed vein, collaterals along the horizontal raphe and hard exudates. (Courtesy of C. Barry.)

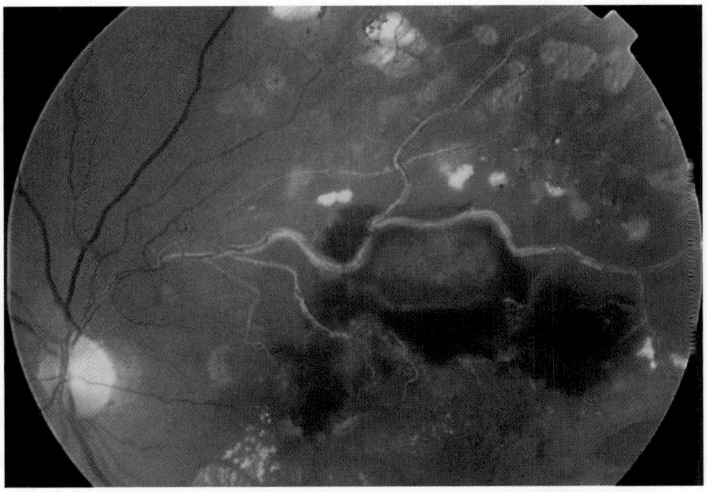

■ **Fig. 12.58** Old superotemporal BRVO showing striking sclerosis of the obstructed vein, preretinal haemorrhages and old laser burns.

Non-ischaemic central retinal vein occlusion (CRVO)

Non-ischaemic CRVO is characterised by venous dilatation and tortuosity, haemorrhages in all quadrants, variable cotton-wool spots, and oedema of the retina and disc.

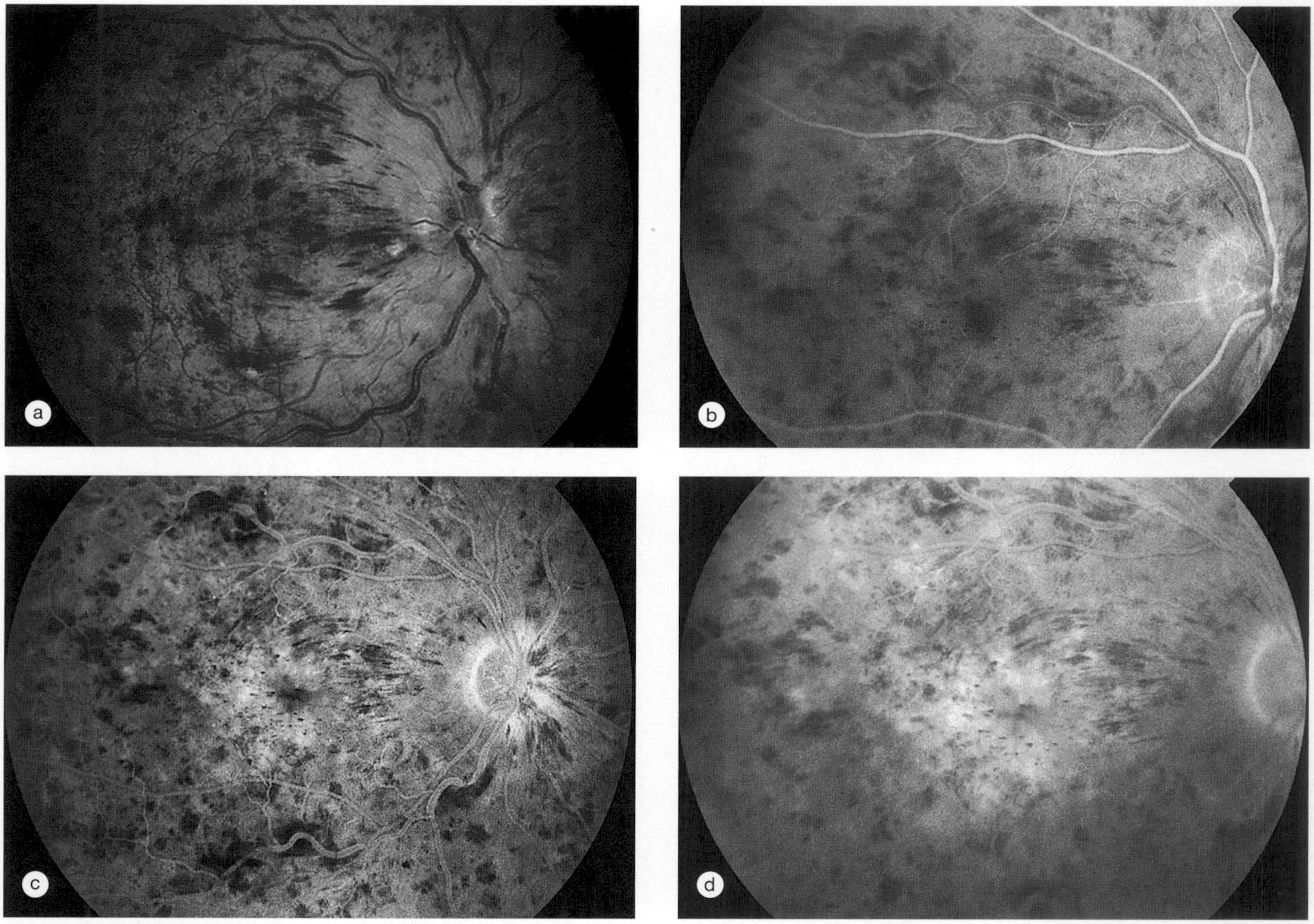

Fig. 12.59 **(a)** Non-ischaemic CRVO. **(b)** FA arteriovenous phase shows blockage by haemorrhages. **(c)** Late venous phase shows early hyperfluorescence at the macula due to leakage. **(d)** Late phase shows more extensive hyperfluorescence but good retinal perfusion. (Courtesy of S. Milewski.)

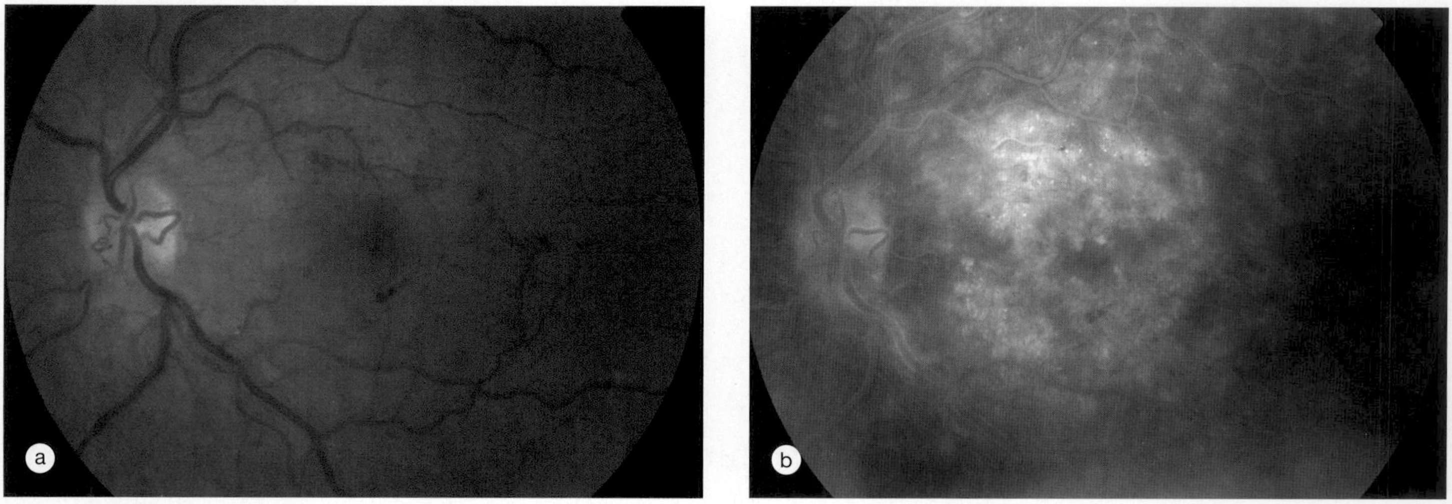

Fig. 12.60 **(a)** Old non-ischaemic CRVO with disc collaterals. **(b)** FA late phase shows diffuse hyperfluorescence at the posterior pole due to leakage and CMO. (Courtesy of Moorfields Eye Hospital.)

Ischaemic central retinal vein occlusion

Ischaemic CRVO is characterised by rapid-onset venous obstruction resulting in decreased retinal perfusion, capillary closure and retinal hypoxia. Rubeosis iridis is a serious complication.

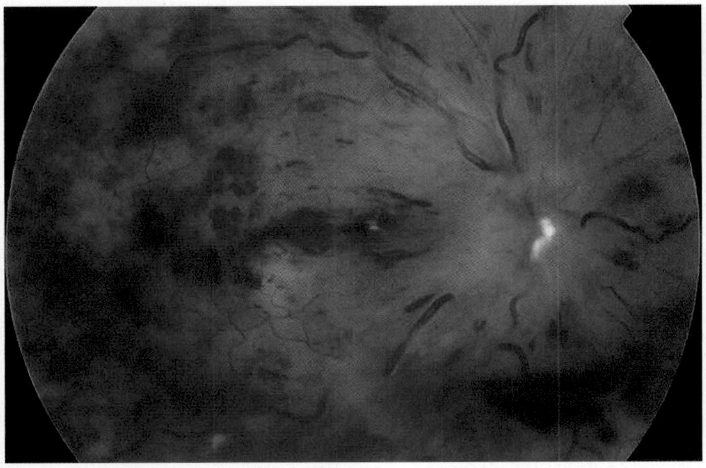

■ **Fig. 12.61** Severe tortuosity and engorgement of all branches of the central retinal vein, extensive dot–blot and flame-shaped haemorrhages involving the peripheral retina and posterior pole, cotton-wool spots, macular haemorrhage and severe disc oedema.

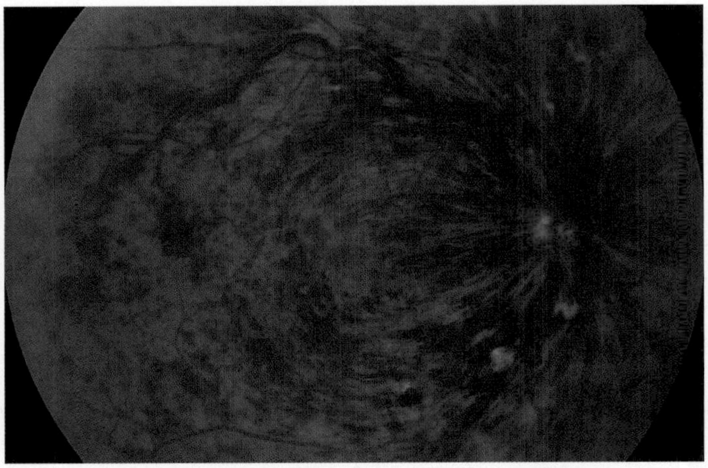

■ **Fig. 12.62** Very severe ischaemic CRVO with extensive haemorrhage. (Courtesy of L. Merin.)

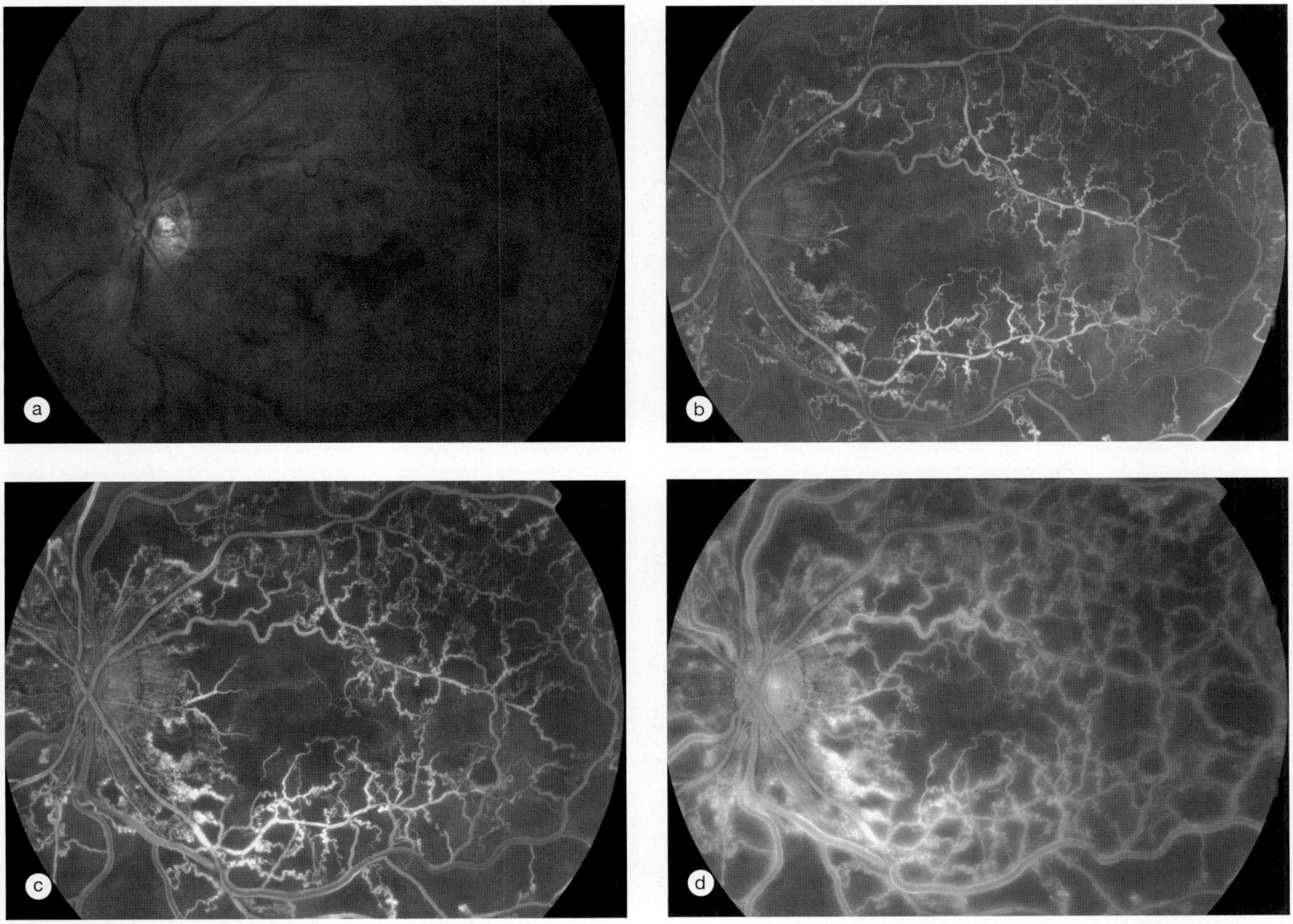

■ **Fig. 12.63** **(a)** Old ischaemic CRVO. **(b, c)** FA early phase shows many microvascular abnormalities and extensive hypofluorescence, particularly at the macula, due to retinal capillary non-perfusion. **(d)** Late phase shows perivascular staining. (Courtesy of Moorfields Eye Hospital.)

Papillophlebitis

Papillophlebitis (optic disc vasculitis) is an uncommon condition which typically affects otherwise healthy individuals under the age of 50 years.

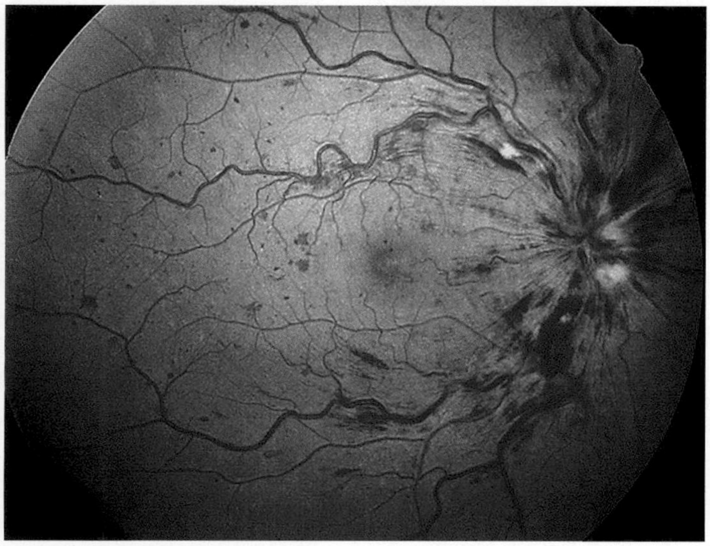

■ **Fig. 12.64** Severe disc oedema associated with peripapillary flame-shaped haemorrhages, a few cotton-wool spots, venous tortuosity and mild venous dilatation.

Hemiretinal vein occlusion

Hemiretinal vein occlusion involves the superior or inferior branch of the CRV.

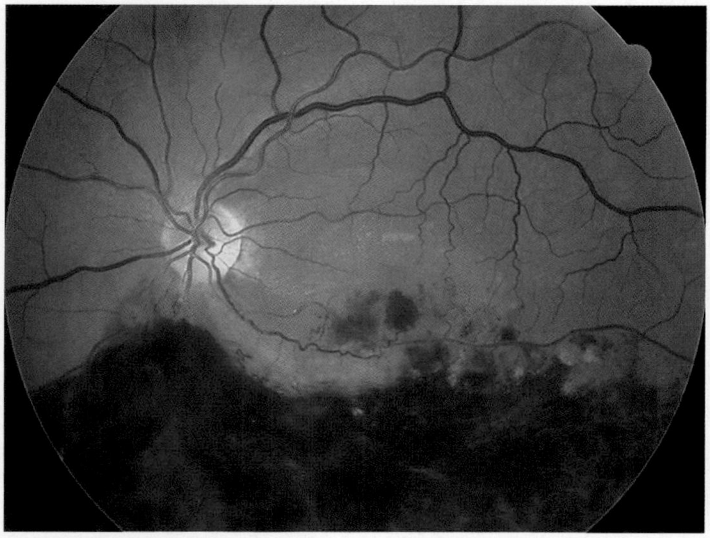

■ **Fig. 12.65** Extensive haemorrhages involving the inferior nasal and temporal fundus. (Courtesy of C. Barry.)

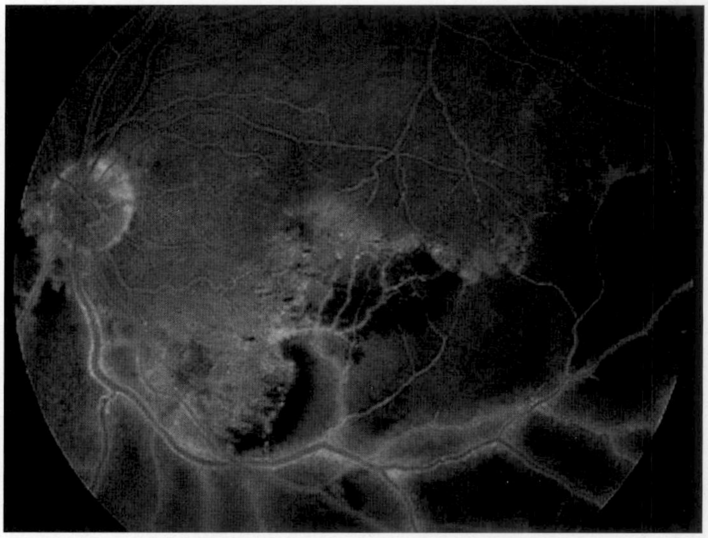

■ **Fig. 12.66** Late phase shows extensive hypofluorescence due to retinal capillary non-perfusion and mild perivascular hyperfluorescence.

RETINAL ARTERIAL OCCLUSIVE DISEASE

Branch retinal artery occlusion (BRAO)

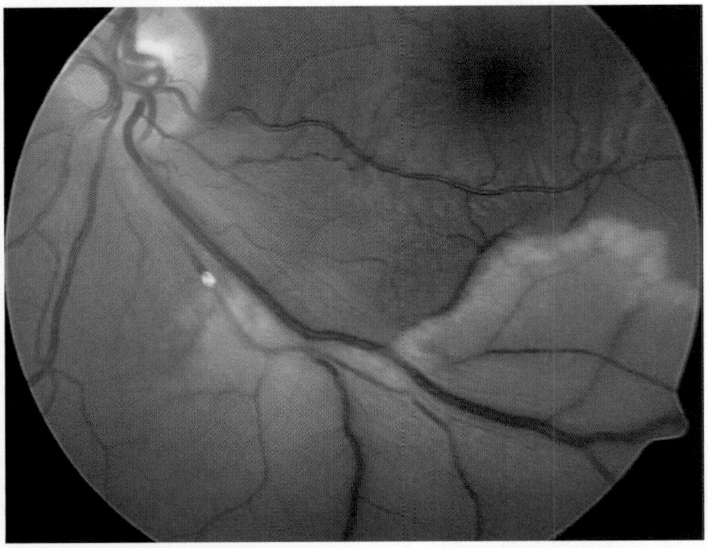

Fig. 12.67 Inferotemporal BRAO due to a calcific embolus in a patient with a calcified cardiac valve. The affected artery is attenuated and the corresponding area of retinal ischaemia is cloudy. (Courtesy of P. Gili.)

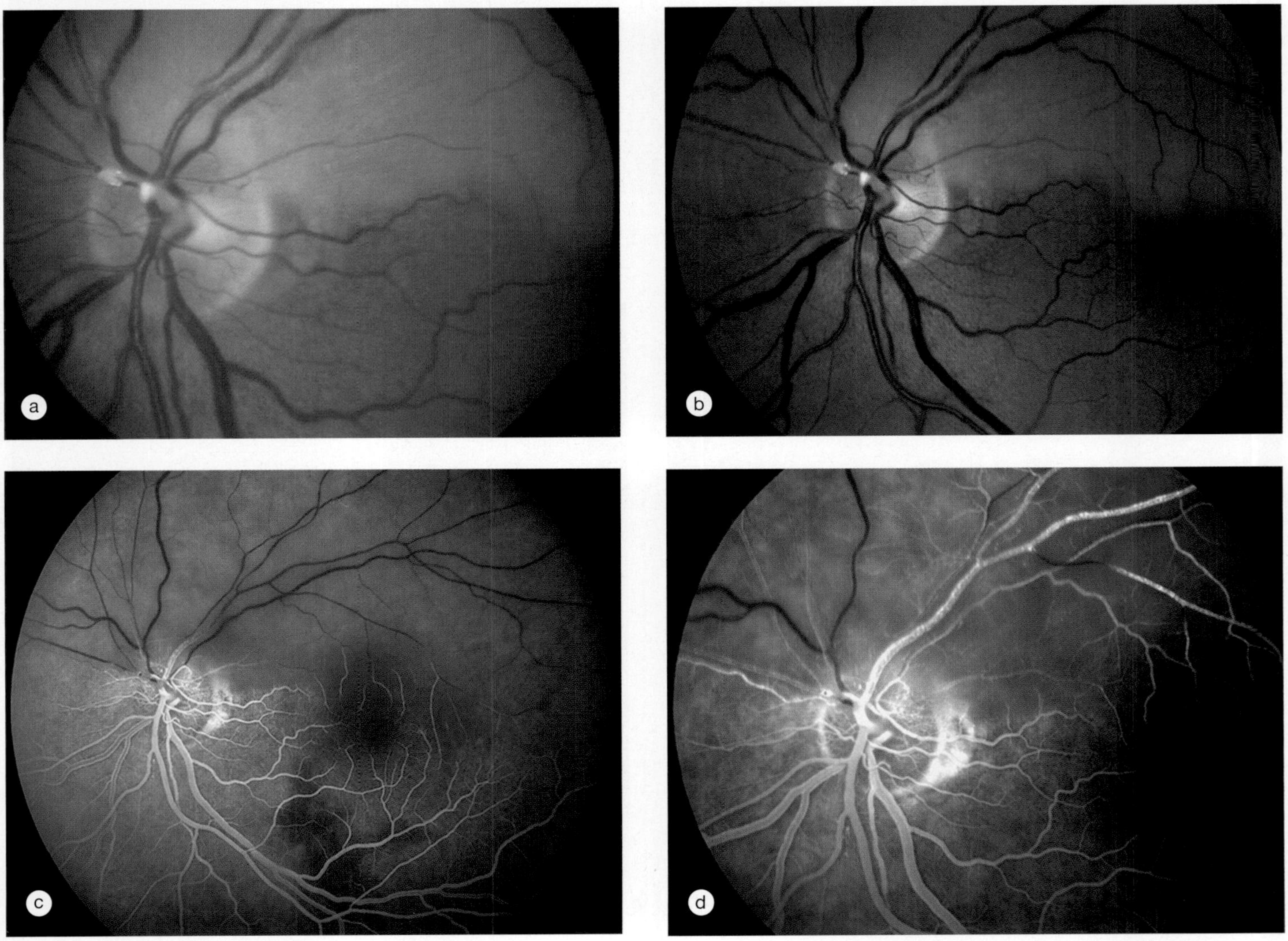

Fig. 12.68 **(a)** Superior BRAO due to an embolus at the disc. **(b)** Red-free image shows the embolus more clearly. **(c, d)** FA shows delay in arterial filling and masking of background fluorescence by retinal swelling confined to the involved sector. (Courtesy of P. Gili.)

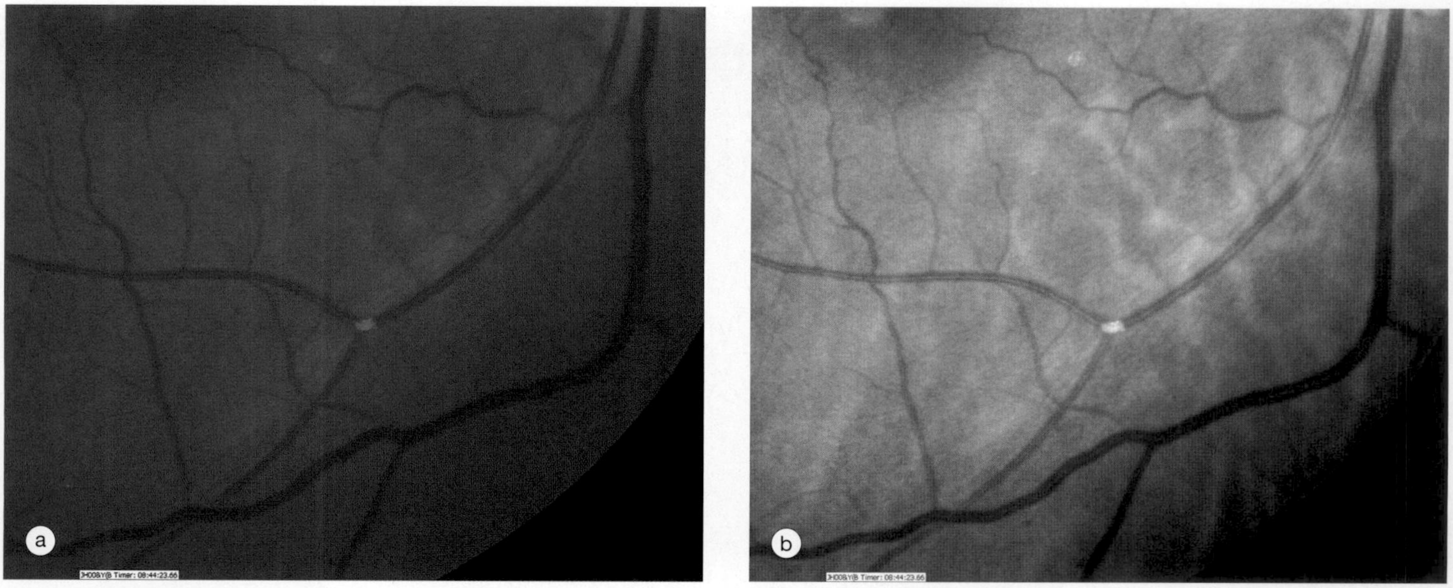

Fig. 12.69 **(a)** Cholesterol embolus (Hollenhorst plaque) at a bifurcation. **(b)** Red-free image. (Courtesy of L. Merin.)

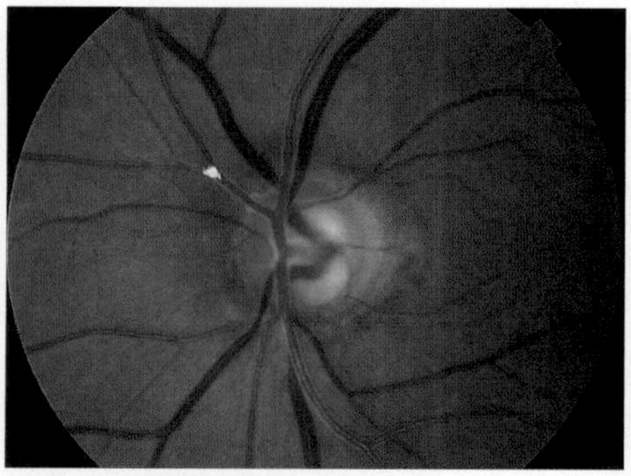

Fig. 12.70 Hollenhorst plaque in a patient with carotid stenosis.

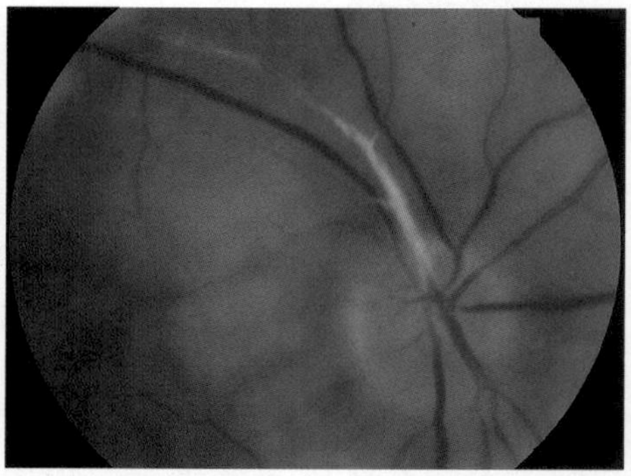

Fig. 12.71 Multiple fibrinoplatelet emboli in a patient with carotid stenosis.

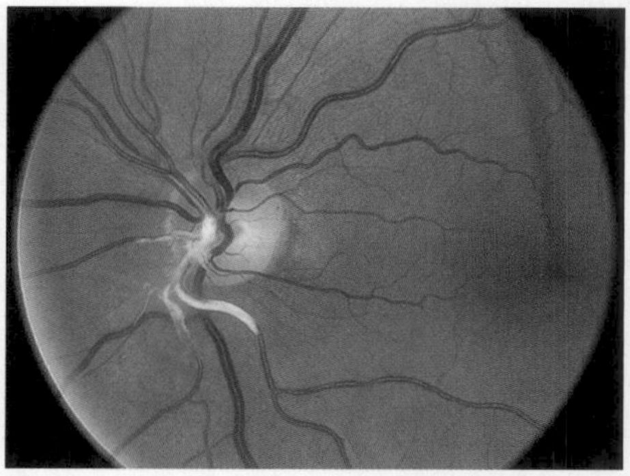

Fig. 12.72 Fibrinoplatelet emboli extending from the disc to involve three branches.

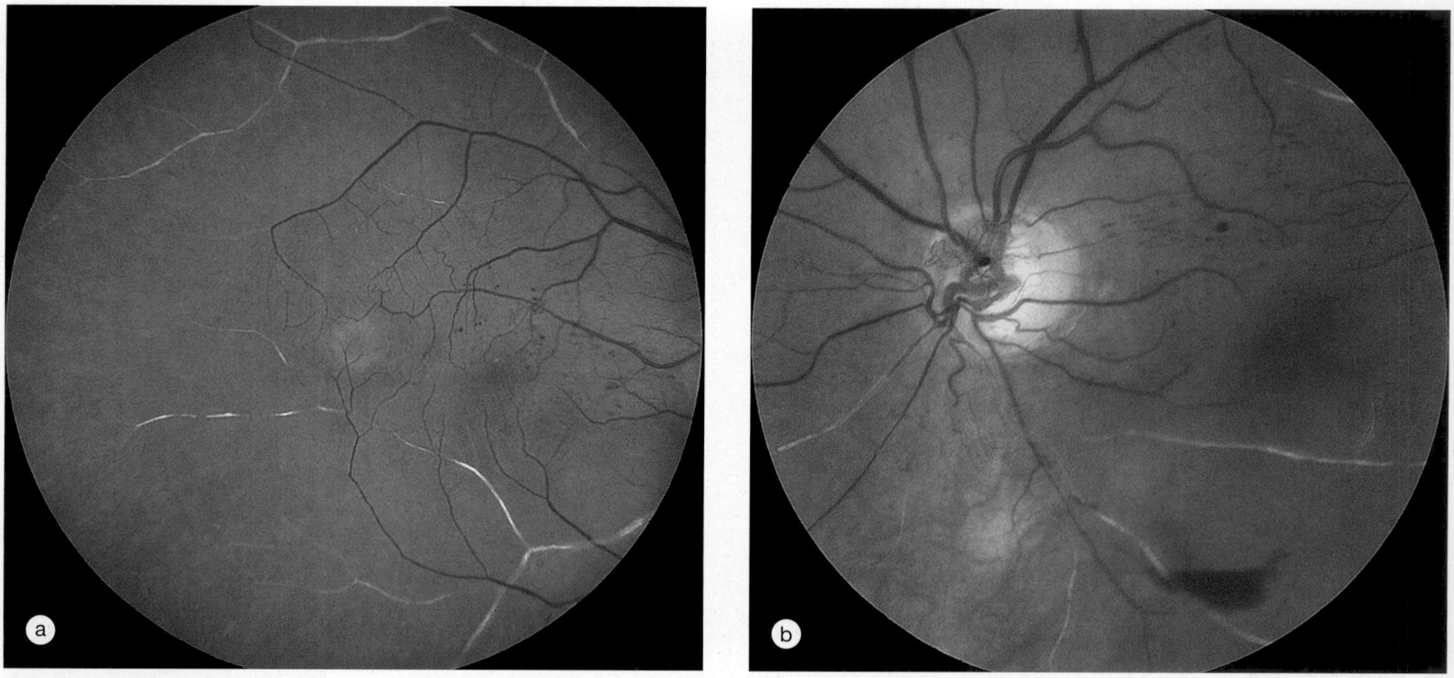

Fig. 12.73 **(a)** Multiple BRAO in a patient with polyarteritis nodosa. **(b)** NVD has developed several weeks later.

Central retinal artery occlusion (CRAO)

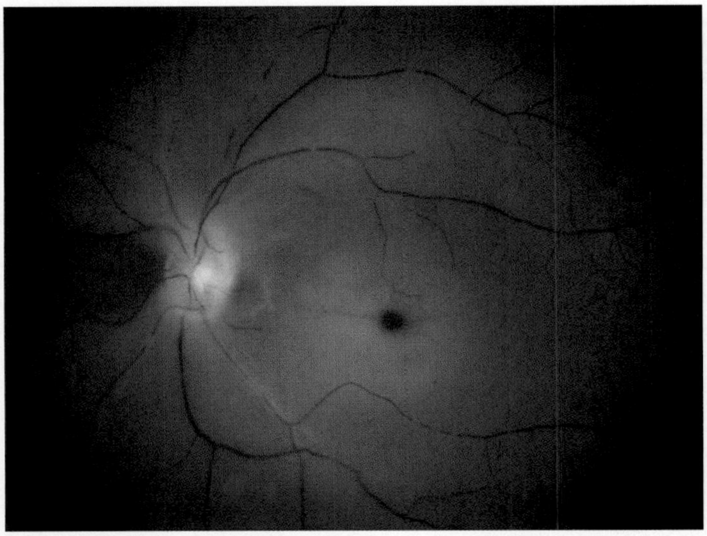

Fig. 12.74 Attenuation of arteries and veins with segmentation of the blood column ('cattle-trucking'), extensive retinal cloudiness and a 'cherry-red' spot at the fovea. (Courtesy of L. Merin.)

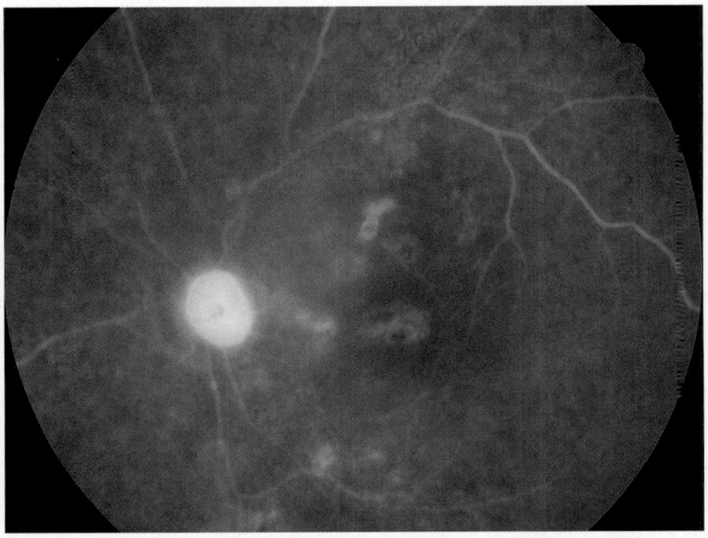

Fig. 12.75 Subsequently the attenuated retinal vessels become sclerosed and consecutive optic atrophy ensues.

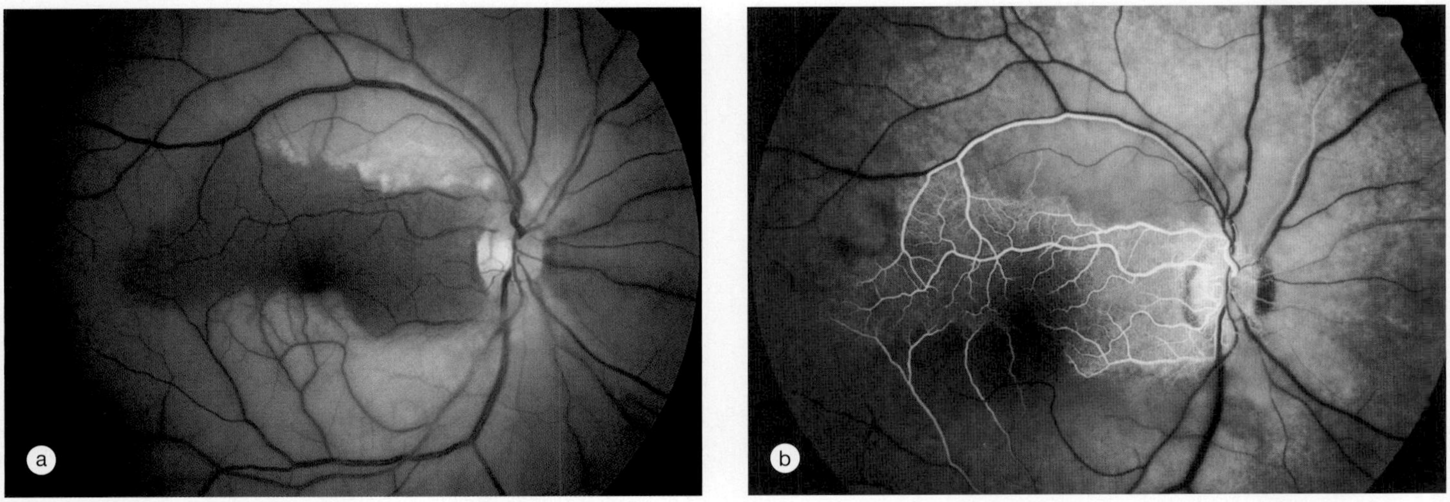

Fig. 12.76 **(a)** CRAO with a patent cilioretinal artery. **(b)** FA shows masking of background choroidal fluorescence by retinal swelling but normal perfusion at the posterior pole. (Courtesy of L. Merin.)

Cilioretinal artery occlusion (CIRAO)

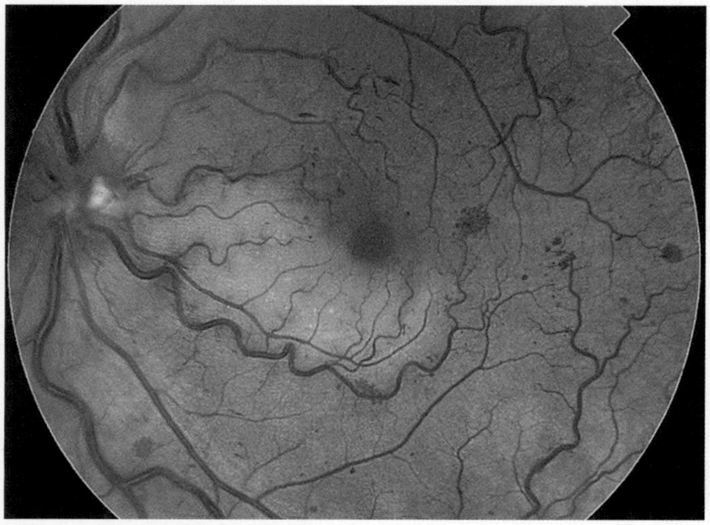

■ **Fig. 12.77** Isolated CIRAO typically affects young patients with associated systemic vasculitis. (Courtesy of S. Milewski.)

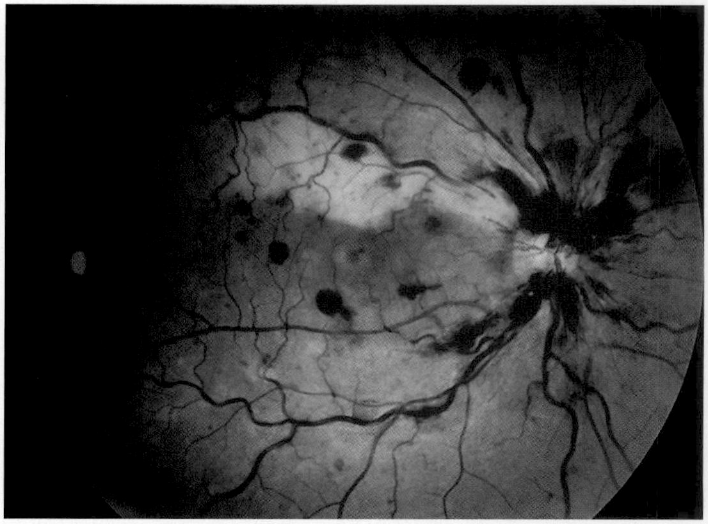

■ **Fig. 12.78** CIRAO combined with CRVO.

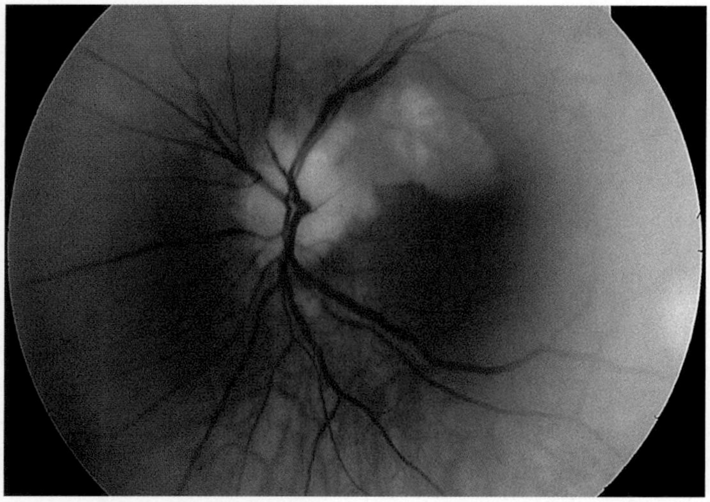

■ **Fig. 12.79** CIRAO combined with anterior ischaemic optic neuropathy typically affects patients with giant cell arteritis.

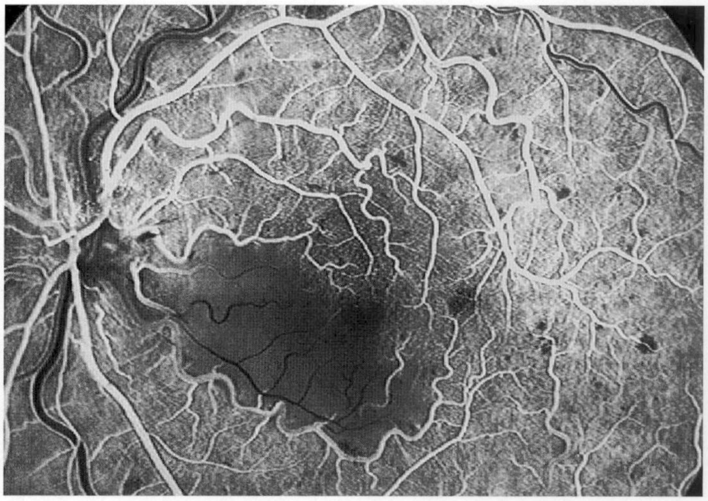

■ **Fig. 12.80** FA of isolated CIRAO showing hypofluorescence at the macula due to lack of filling and blockage by retinal swelling. (Courtesy of S. Milewski.)

Ocular ischaemic syndrome

Ocular ischaemic syndrome is an uncommon condition that is the result of chronic ocular hypoperfusion.

Causes

Ipsilateral atherosclerotic carotid stenosis

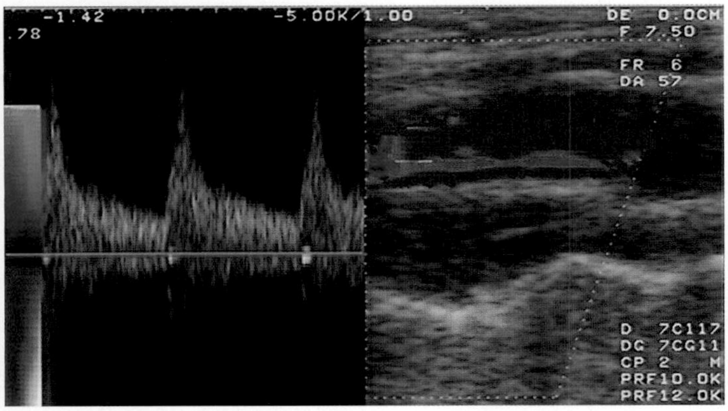

■ **Fig. 12.81** Carotid Doppler shows carotid stenosis.

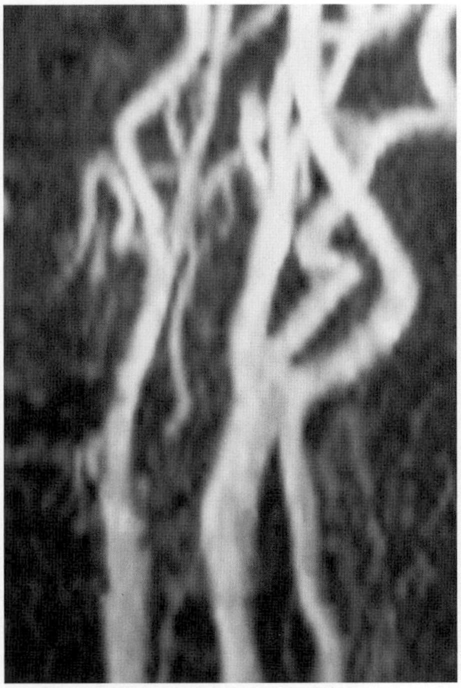

■ **Fig. 12.82** Magnetic resonance angiogram shows severe stenosis of the right internal carotid artery. (Courtesy of D. Thomas.)

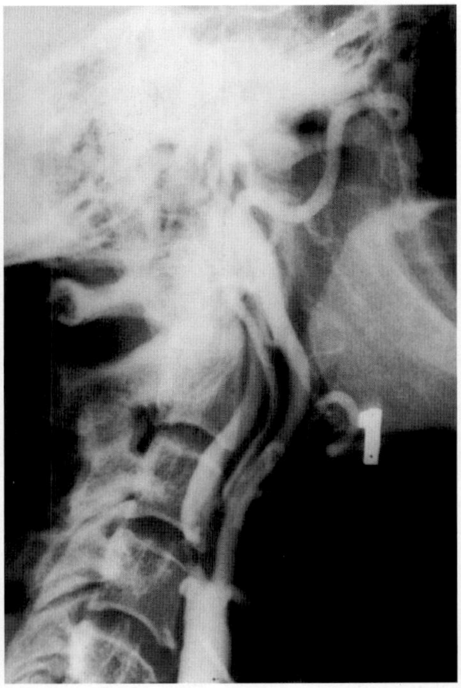

■ **Fig. 12.83** Conventional intra-arterial angiogram shows severe stenosis of the right internal carotid. (Courtesy of D. Thomas.)

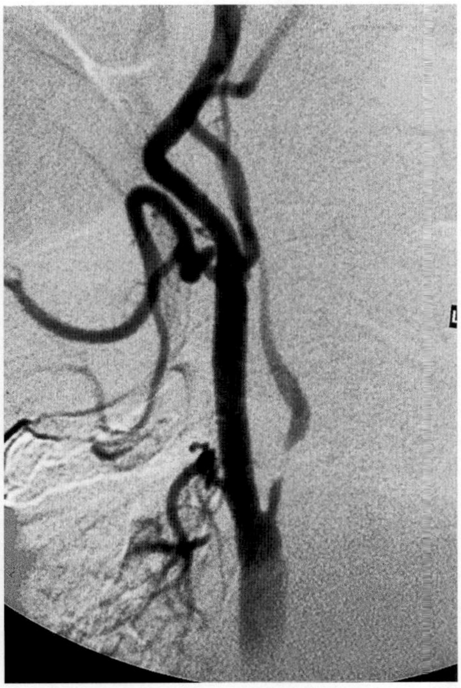

■ **Fig. 12.84** Digital subtraction arteriogram shows severe stenosis of the right internal carotid artery. (Courtesy of D. Thomas.)

Takayasu (pulseless) disease

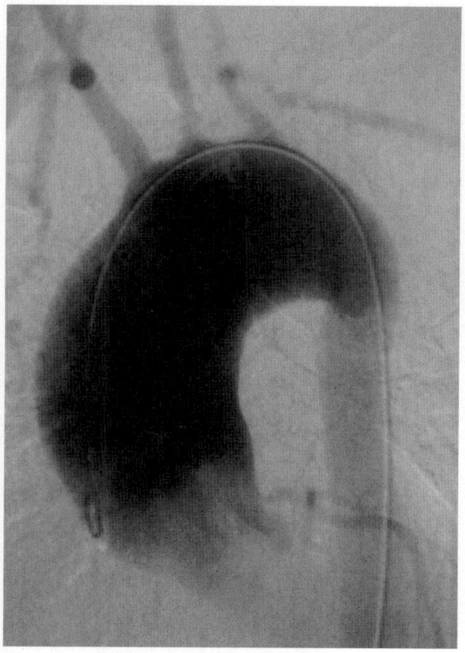

Fig. 12.85 Aortic arch angiogram showing dilatation of the ascending aorta and aortic arch and stenosis near the origin of the left common carotid artery. (Courtesy of L. Goldman and D. Ausiello.)

Signs

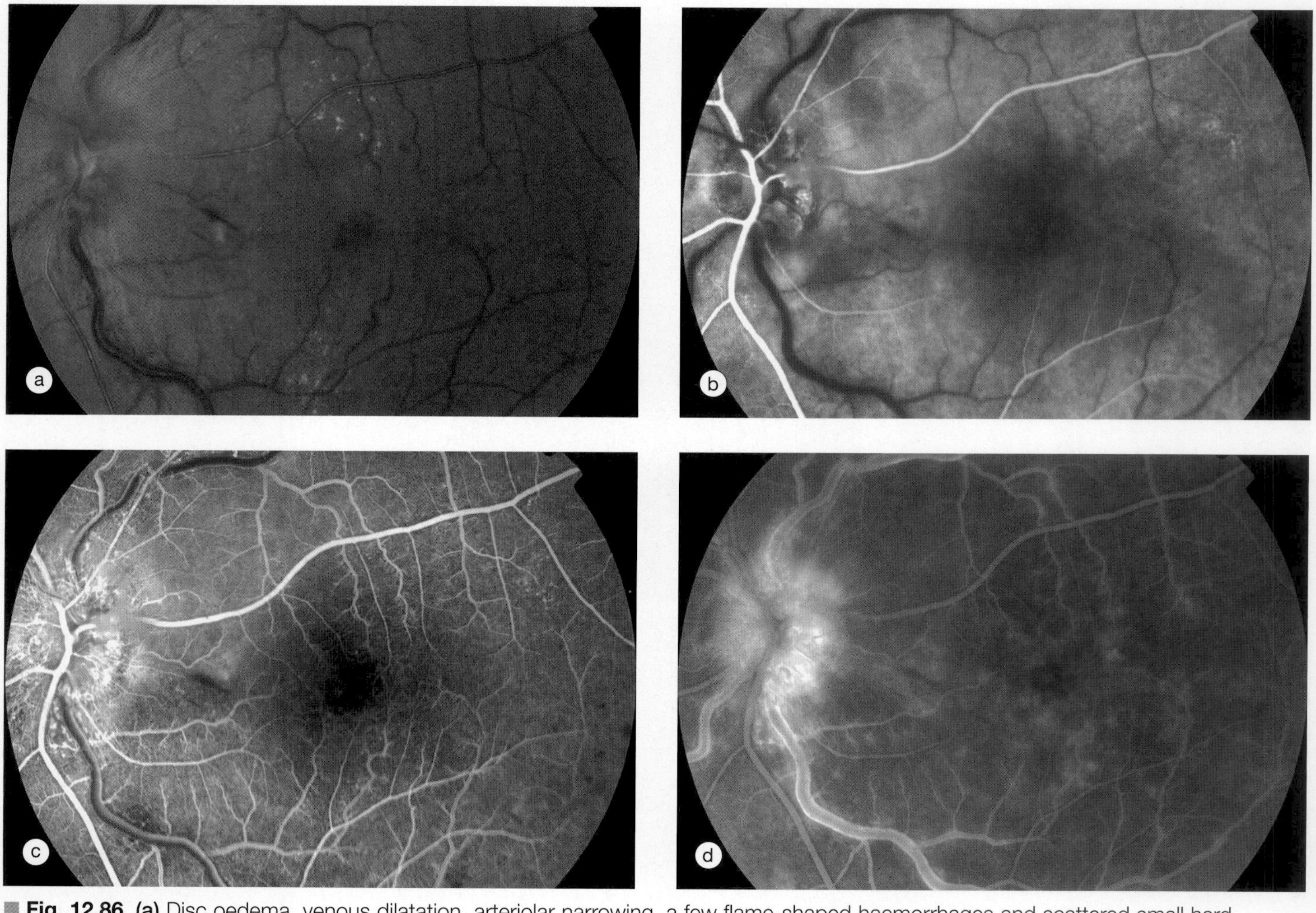

Fig. 12.86 **(a)** Disc oedema, venous dilatation, arteriolar narrowing, a few flame-shaped haemorrhages and scattered small hard exudates. **(b–d)** FA shows delayed and patchy choroidal filling, prolonged arteriovenous transit time and late leakage from the disc.

HYPERTENSIVE DISEASE

Hypertension

Hypertension is defined as blood pressure >140/90 mmHg.

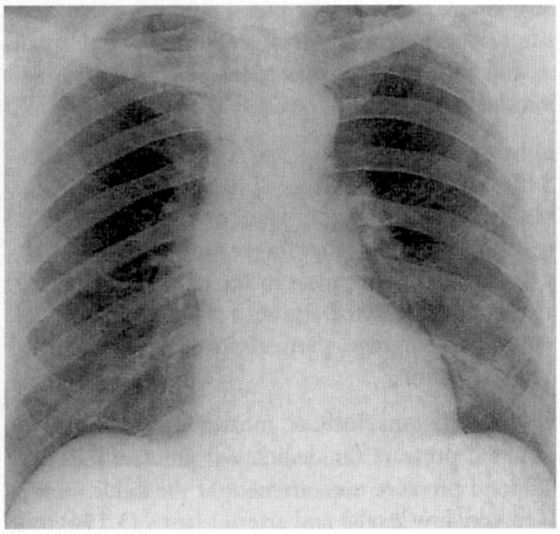

Fig. 12.87 Plain chest radiograph showing left ventricular hypertrophy. (Courtesy of C. D. Forbes and W. F. Jackson.)

Hypertensive retinopathy

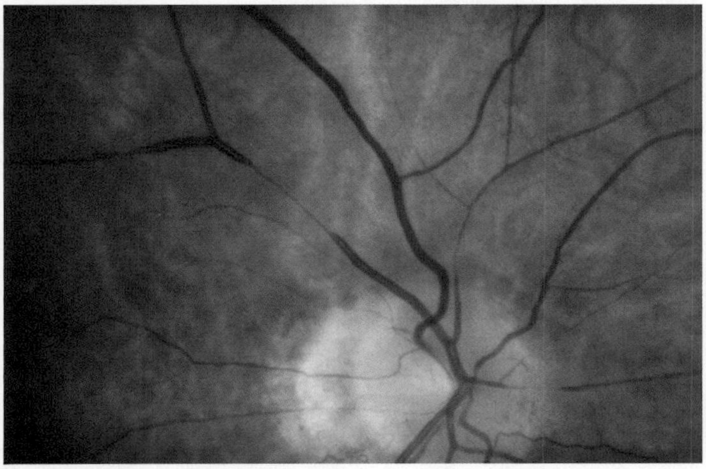

Fig. 12.88 Focal and generalised arterial narrowing resulting in an increased ratio between the diameters of arteries and veins.

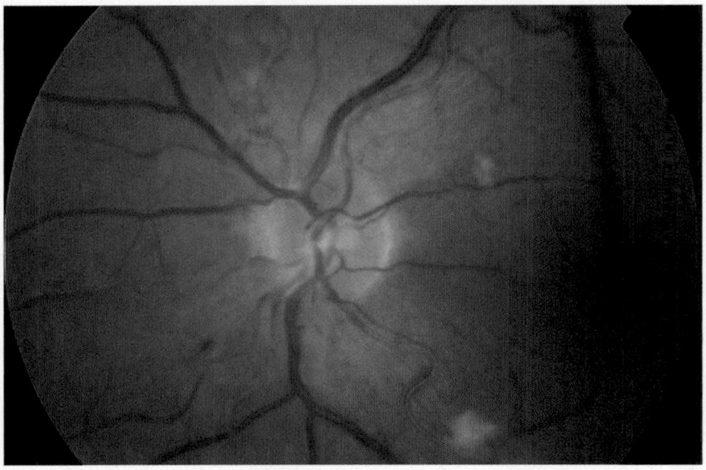

Fig. 12.89 Cotton-wool spots.

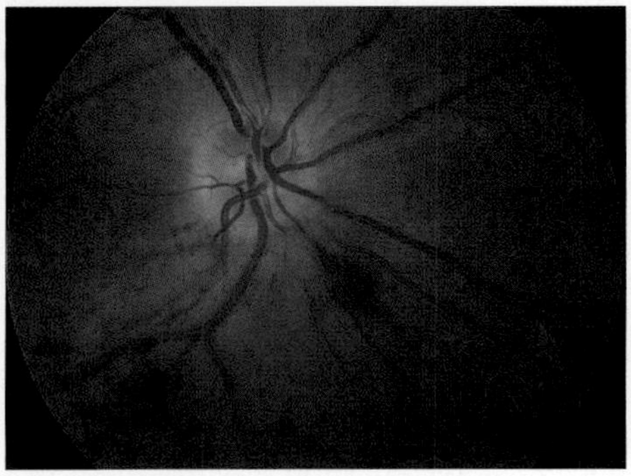

Fig. 12.90 Flame-shaped retinal haemorrhages.

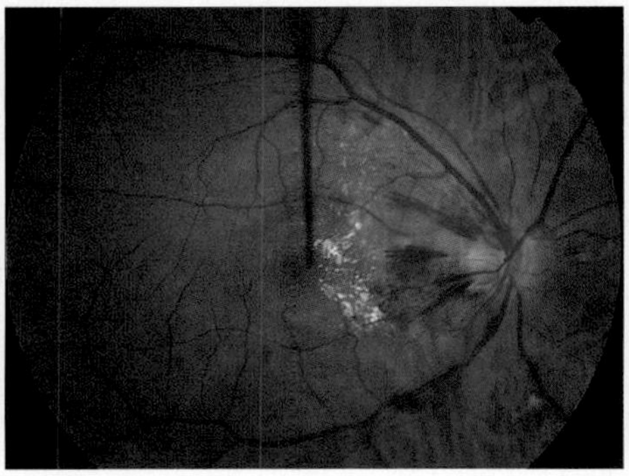

Fig. 12.91 Flame-shaped haemorrhages and small hard exudates at the macula.

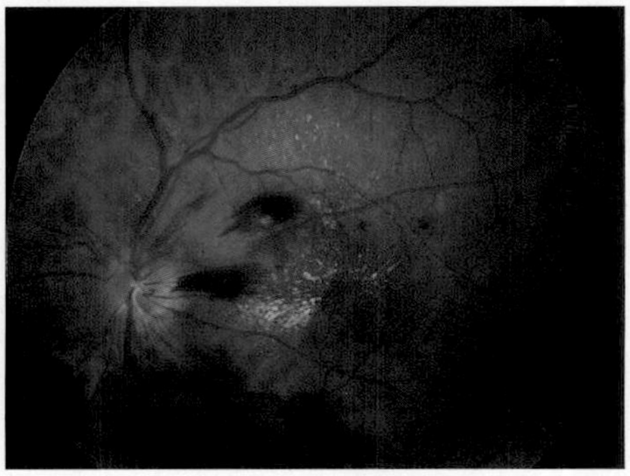

Fig. 12.92 Extensive flame-shaped haemorrhages and hard exudates at the macula forming an incomplete star figure.

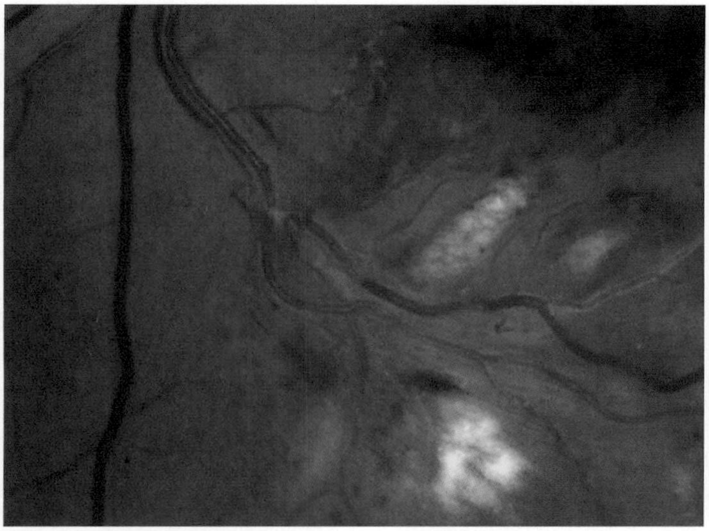

Fig. 12.93 Compression of veins at arteriovenous crossings, due to arteriolosclerosis, and cotton-wool spots.

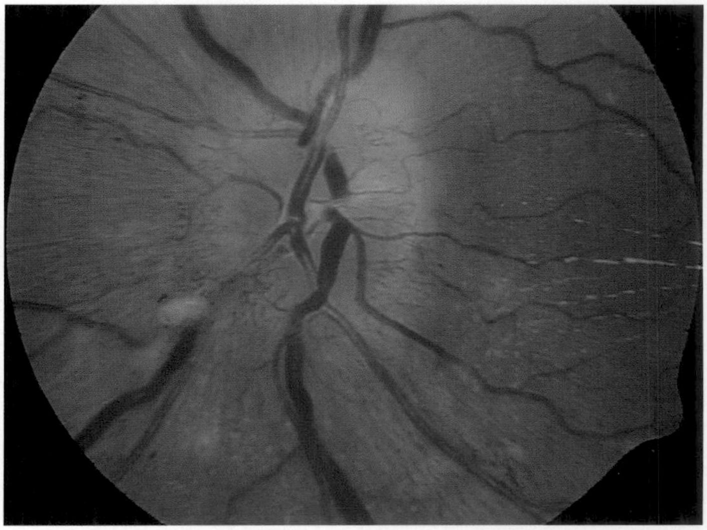

Fig. 12.94 Mild disc oedema, which is the hallmark of malignant hypertension. (Courtesy of P. Gili.)

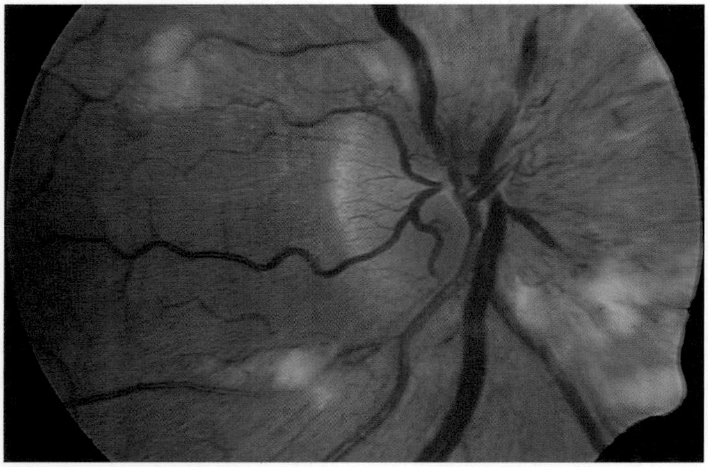

Fig. 12.95 More severe disc oedema and multiple cotton-wool spots. (Courtesy of P. Gili.)

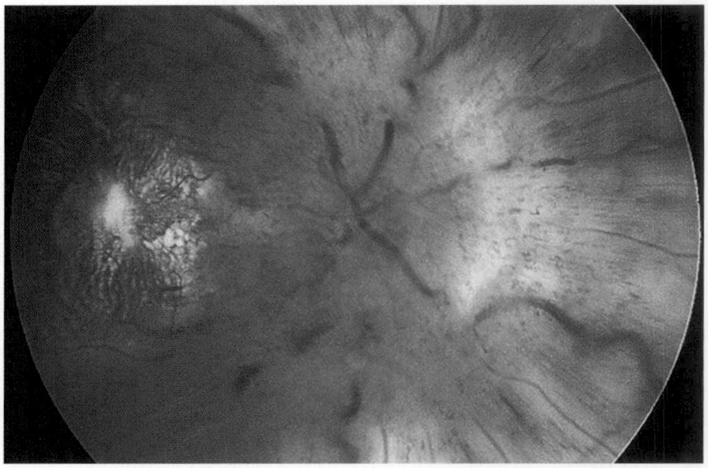

Fig. 12.96 Severe disc oedema and a macular star.

Hypertensive choroidopathy

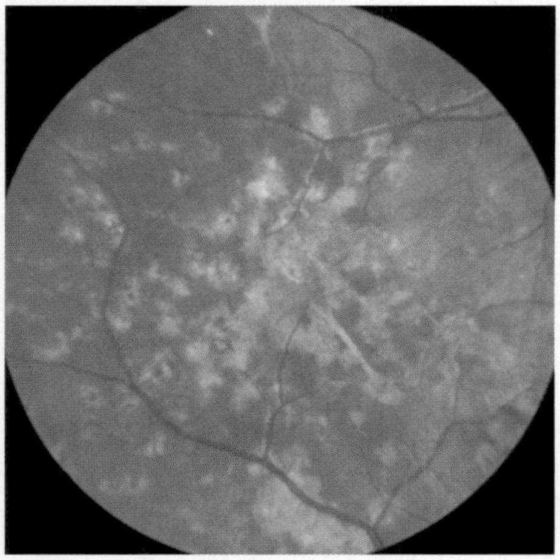

Fig. 12.97 Elschnig spots are small, black spots surrounded by yellow halos that represent focal choroidal infarcts.

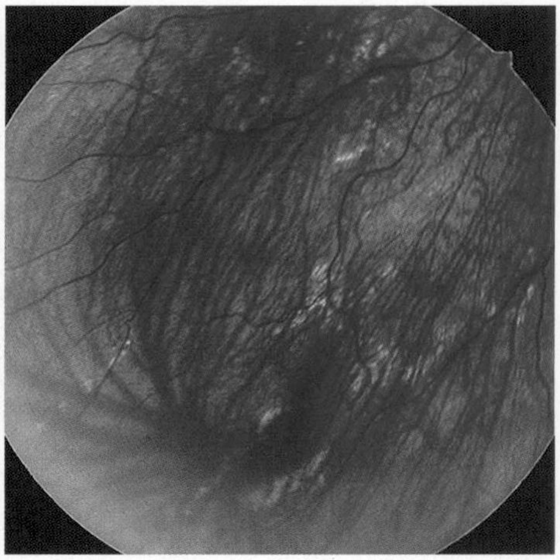

Fig. 12.98 Siegrist streaks are flecks arranged linearly along choroidal vessels that are indicative of fibrinoid necrosis associated with malignant hypertension.

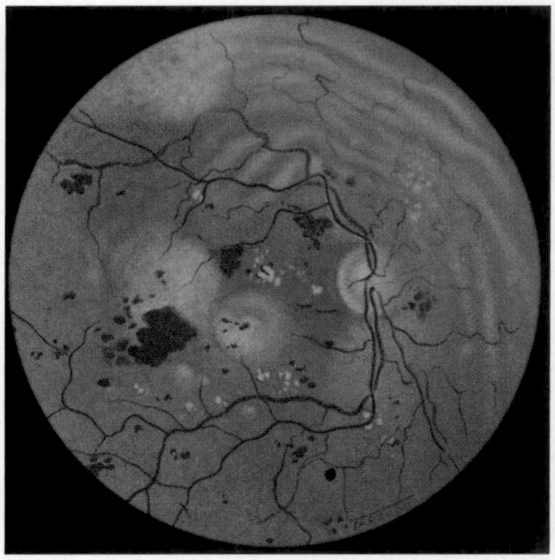

Fig. 12.99 Exudative retinal detachment, sometimes bilateral, may occur in severe acute hypertension such as that associated with toxaemia of pregnancy.

HAEMATOLOGICAL DISEASE

Sickle cell disease

Systemic signs

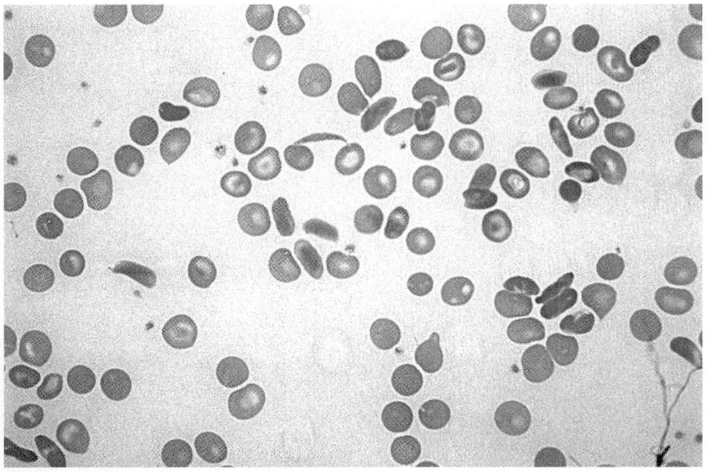

Fig. 12.100 Peripheral blood smear showing scattered sickle cells.

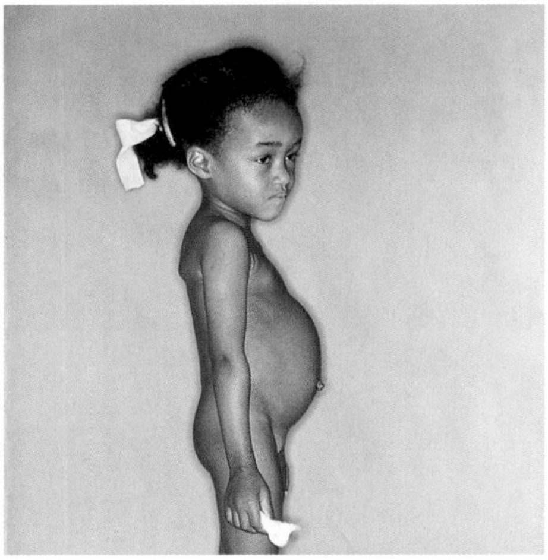

Fig. 12.101 Hepatosplenomegaly.

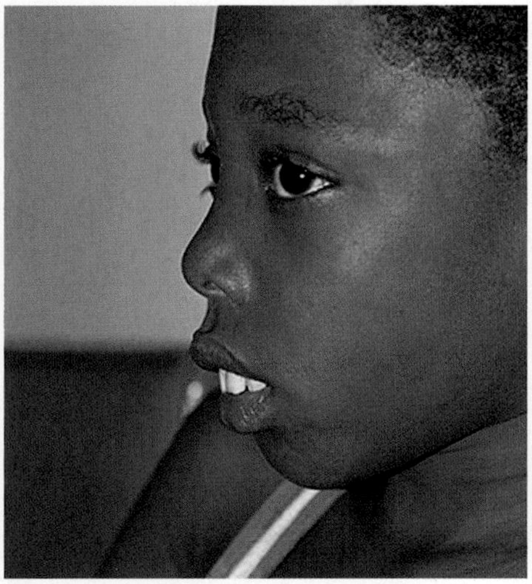

Fig. 12.102 Sickle cell facies with maxillary hyperplasia. (Courtesy of B. J. Zitelli and H. W. Davis.)

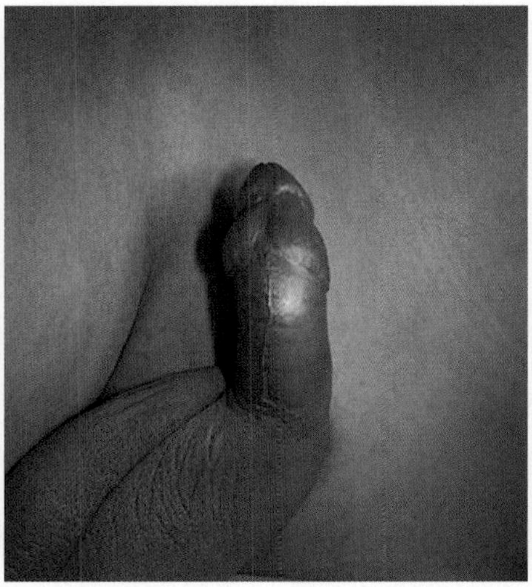

Fig. 12.103 Painful priapism associated with vaso-occlusive crisis. (Courtesy of B. J. Zitelli and H. W. Davis.)

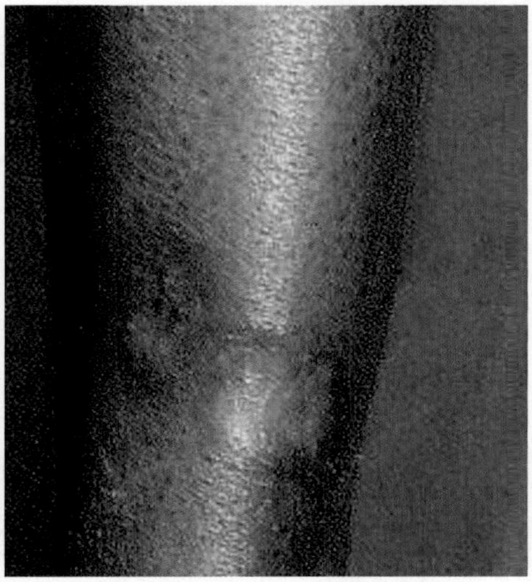

Fig. 12.104 Skin ulceration and scarring. (Courtesy of J. M. H. Moll.)

Retinopathy

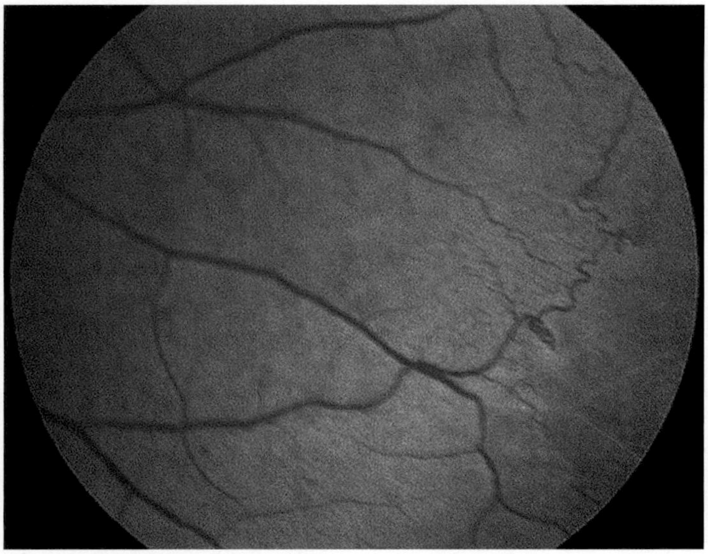

Fig. 12.105 Peripheral arteriolar occlusion. (Courtesy of R. Marsh.)

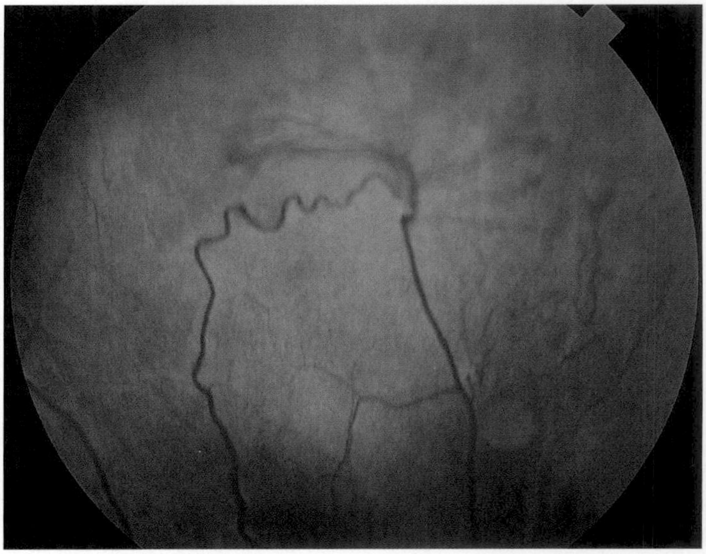

Fig. 12.106 Arteriovenous anastomoses at the junction of perfused and non-perfused retina. (Courtesy of R. Marsh.)

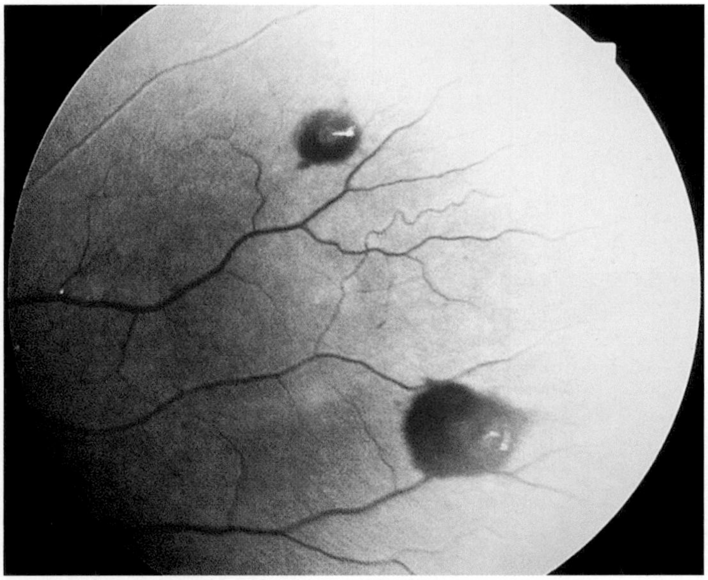

Fig. 12.107 'Salmon patch' haemorrhage at the site of arteriovenous anastomosis. (Courtesy of K. Nischal.)

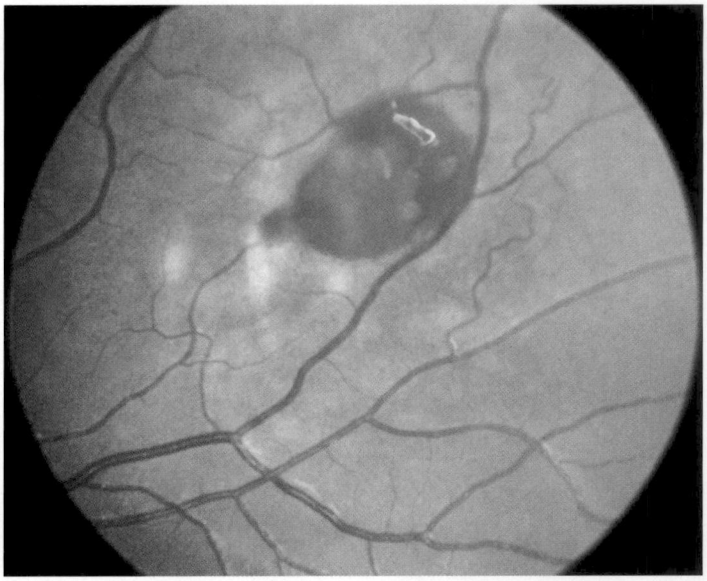

Fig. 12.108 Magnified view of a 'salmon patch'. (Courtesy of R. Marsh.)

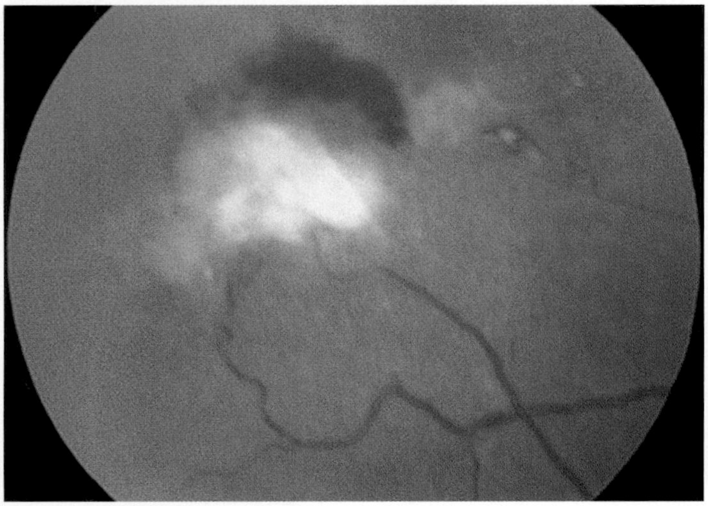

Fig. 12.109 Partially resorbed 'salmon patch'. (Courtesy of R. Marsh.)

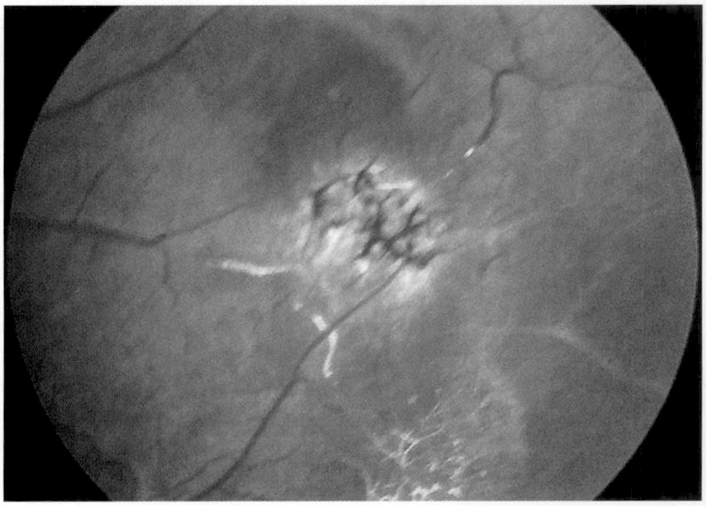

Fig. 12.110 Iridescent area following resorption of a 'salmon patch'.

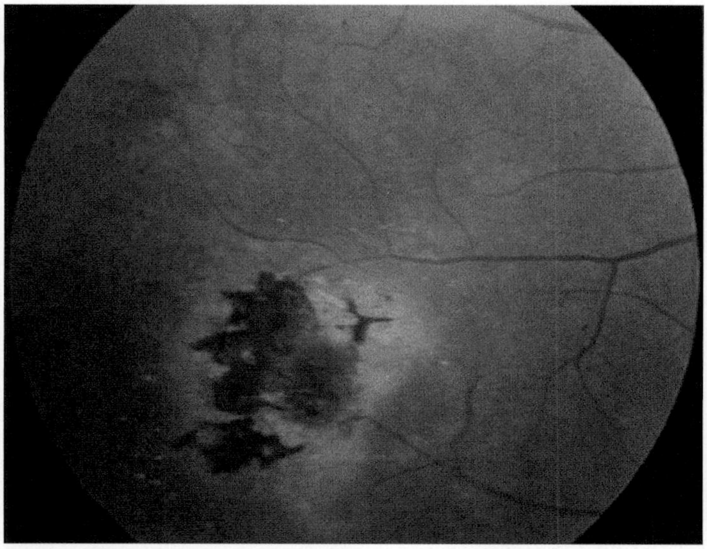

Fig. 12.111 Oval patches of RPE hyperplasia ('black sunbursts') may also develop following resorption of a 'salmon patch'.

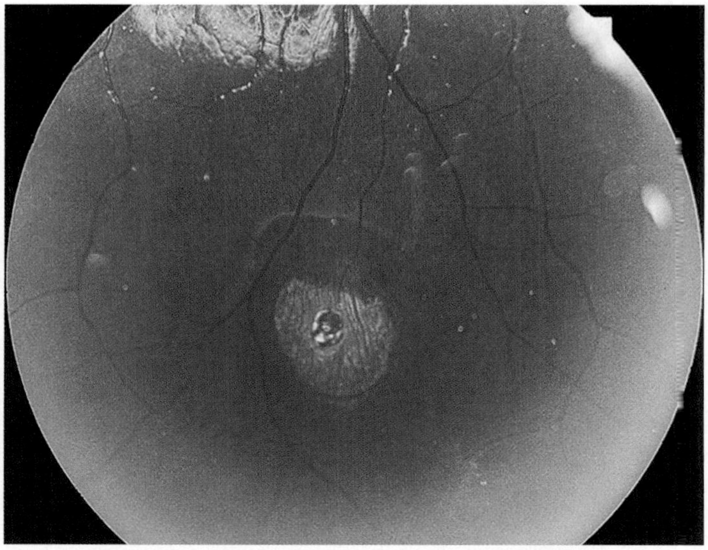

Fig. 12.112 Peripheral retinal holes and areas of whitening similar to 'white-without-pressure' are occasionally seen.

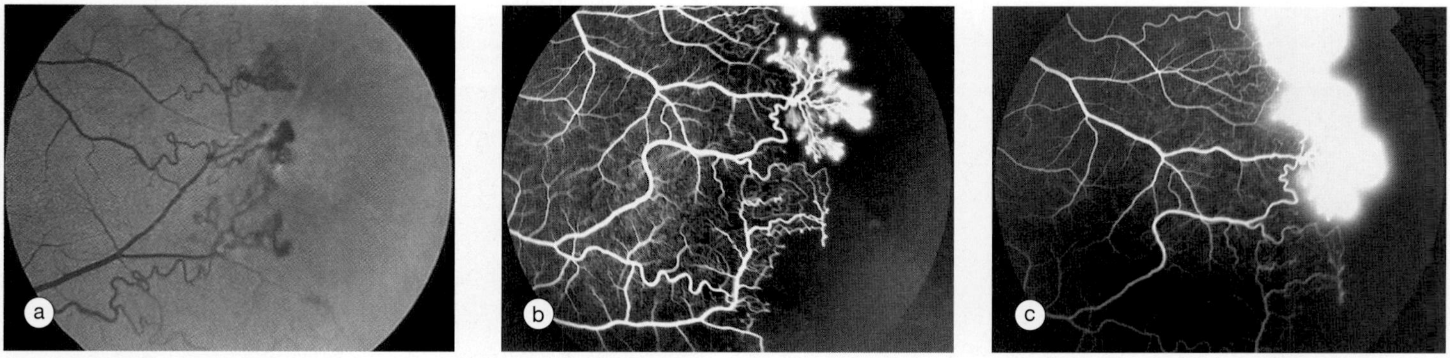

Fig. 12.113 **(a)** New vessel formation from the anastomoses ('sea-fans'). **(b)** FA early phase shows filling of vessels and extensive peripheral retinal capillary non-perfusion. **(c)** Late phase shows leakage from new vessels.

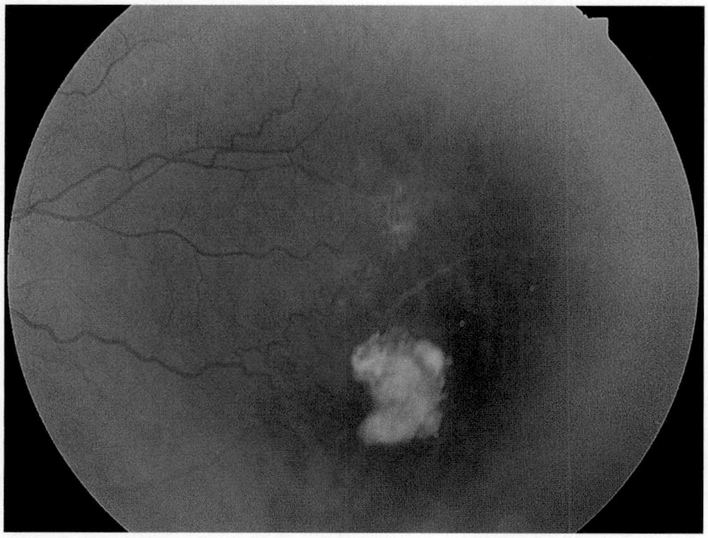

Fig. 12.114 'Sea-fans' often spontaneously involute as a result of autoinfarction and appear as greyish fibrovascular lesions.

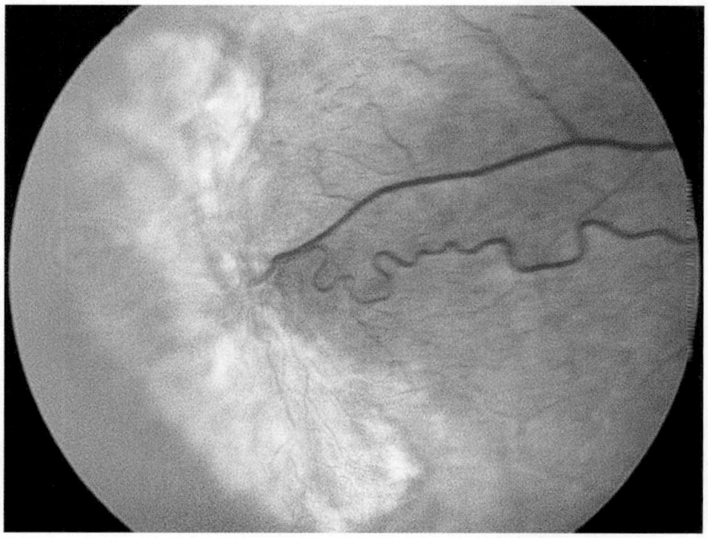

Fig. 12.115 In other cases the neovascular tufts continue to proliferate. (Courtesy of R. Marsh.)

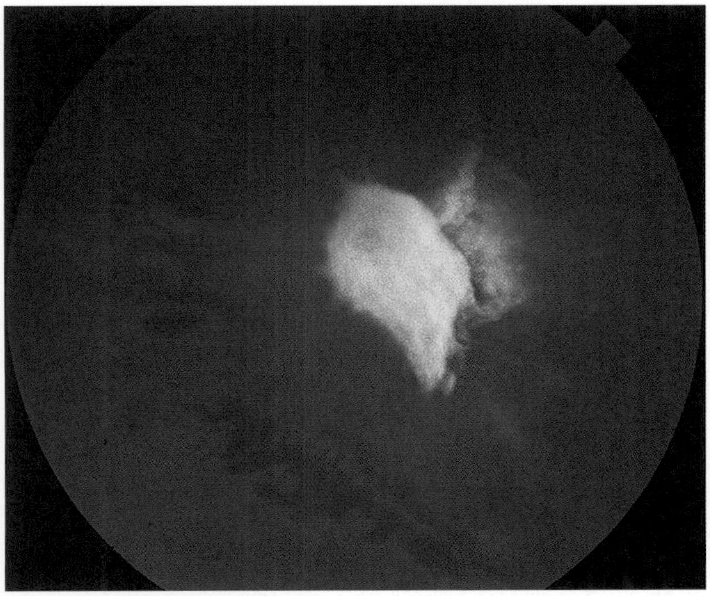

Fig.12.116 Bleeding from new vessels.

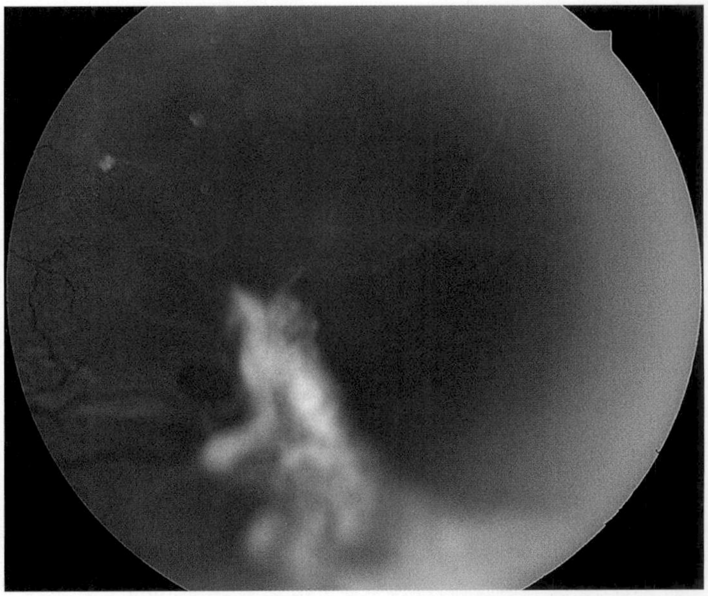

Fig. 12.117 Localised rhegmatogenous retinal detachment associated with a small tractional retinal hole adjacent to fibrovascular proliferation.

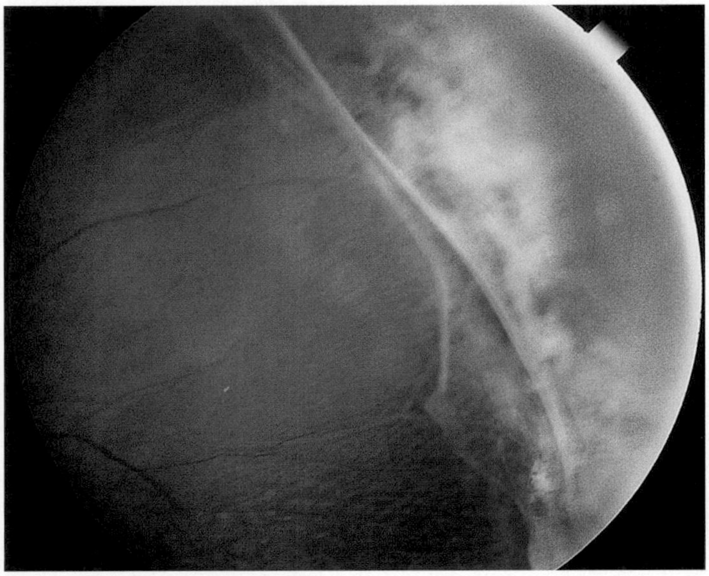

Fig. 12.118 Very severe fibrovascular proliferation, which may result in tractional retinal detachment. (Courtesy to R. Marsh.)

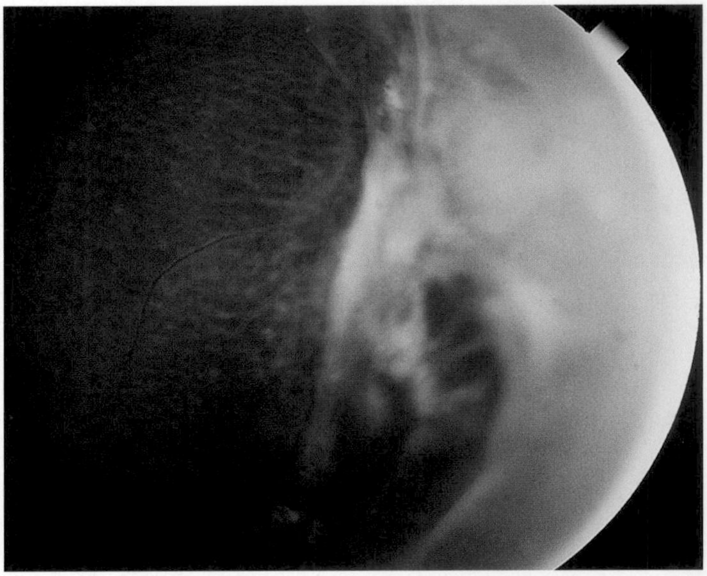

Fig. 12.119 End-stage disease. (Courtesy of R. Marsh.)

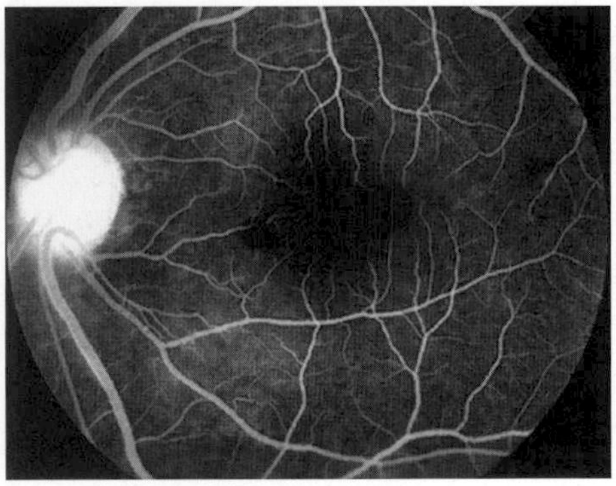

Fig. 12.120 FA showing macular ischaemia.

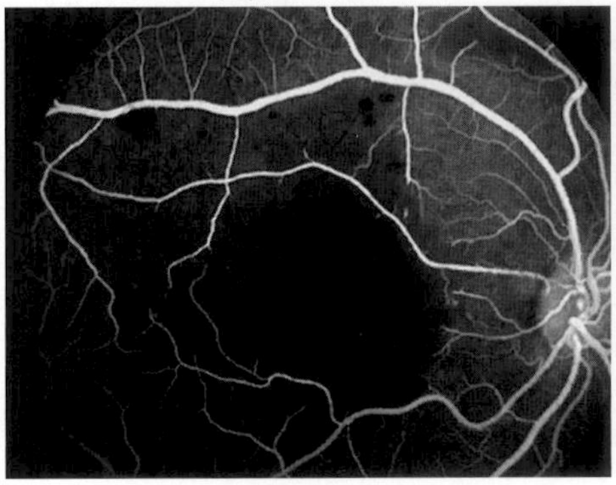

Fig. 12.121 FA showing gross ischaemia of the posterior pole.

Acute leukaemia

Systemic signs

The clinical features are the result of bone marrow failure, invasion of normal organs by leukaemic cells and opportunistic infection.

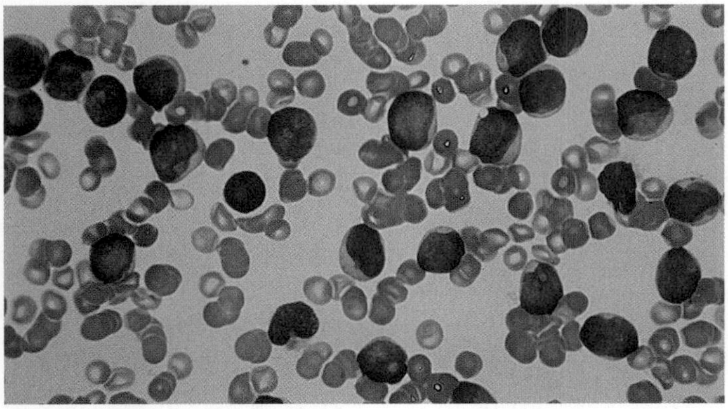

Fig. 12.122 Marrow aspirate in acute myeloid leukaemia showing many immature blast cells.

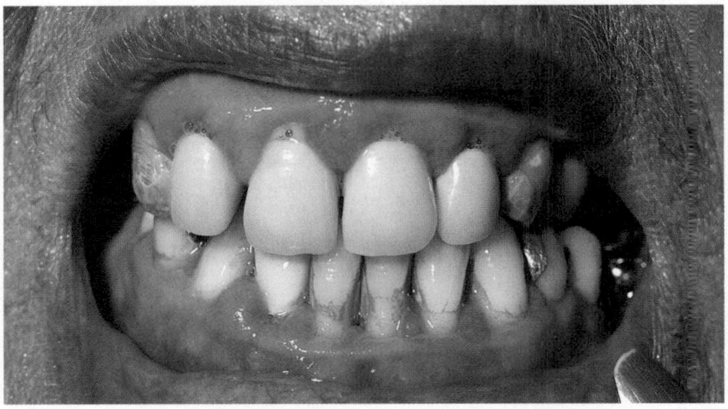

Fig. 12.123 Gingival hypertrophy and bleeding.

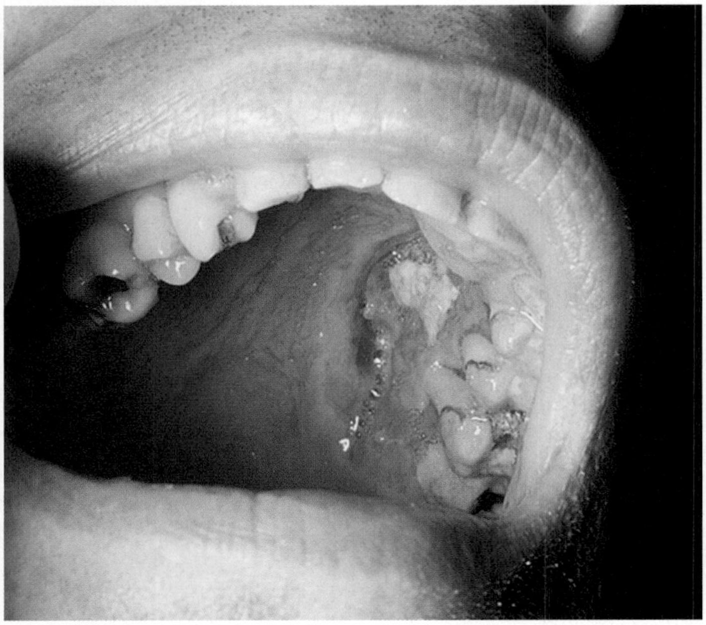

Fig. 12.124 Blood blisters and ulceration on the palate.

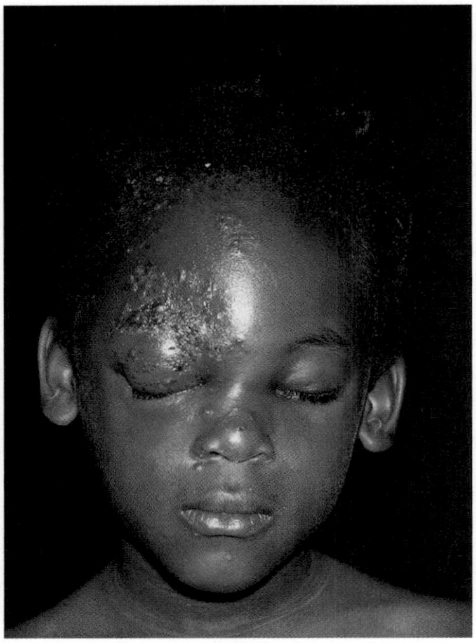

Fig. 12.125 Severe shingles. (Courtesy of R. Marsh.)

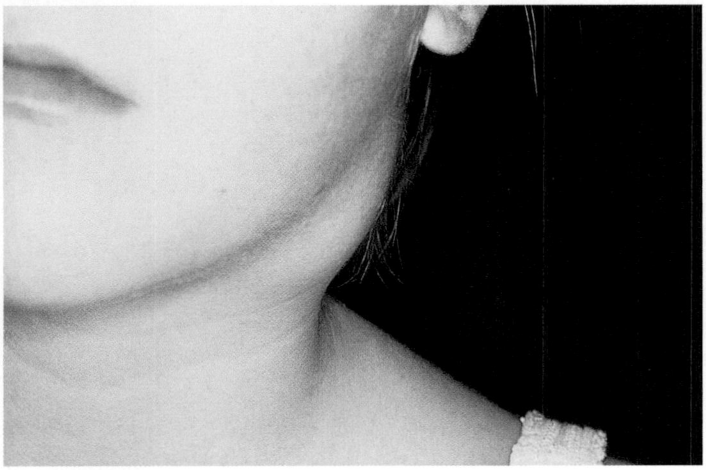

Fig. 12.126 Lymphadenopathy.

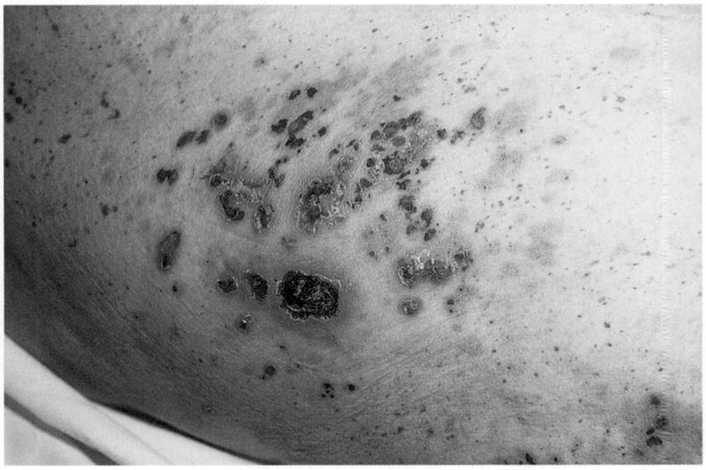

Fig. 12.127 Purpura and easy bruising.

Ocular signs

Retinopathy

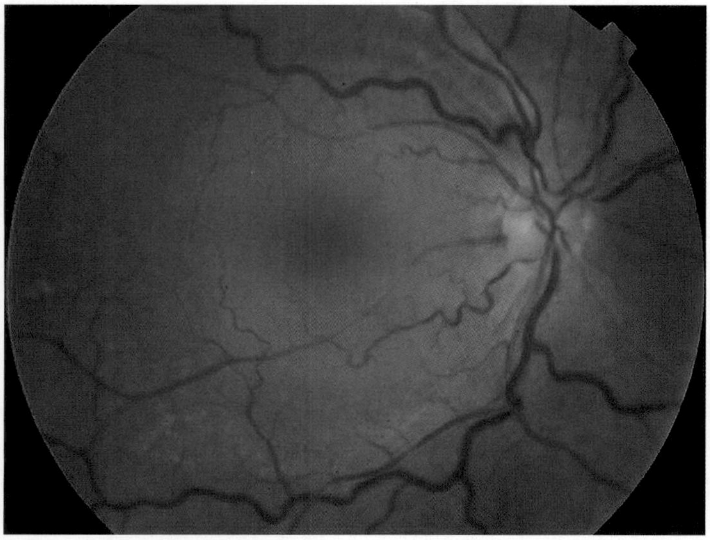

Fig. 12.128 Venous dilatation and tortuosity.

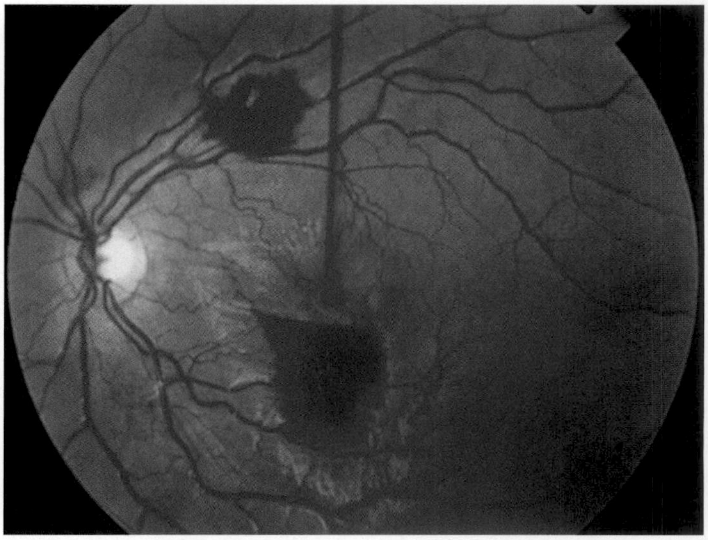

Fig. 12.129 Preretinal haemorrhage at the macula and an intraretinal haemorrhage with a white centre (Roth spot) along the superotemporal arcade. (Courtesy of S. Milewski.)

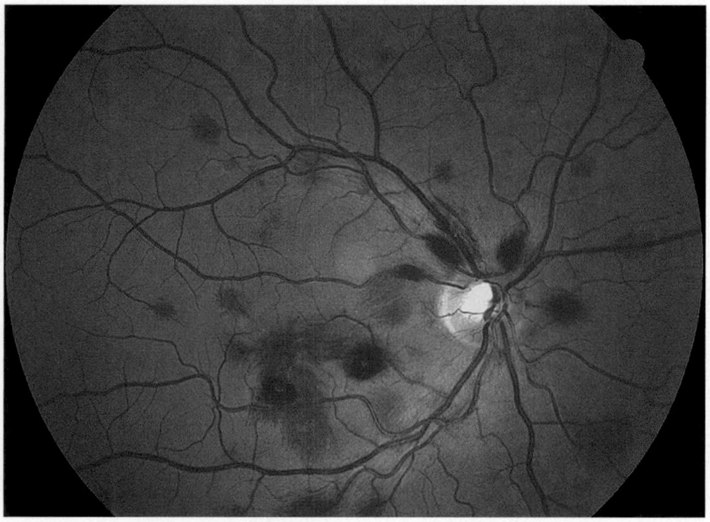

Fig. 12.130 Scattered flame-shapes haemorrhages and Roth spots.

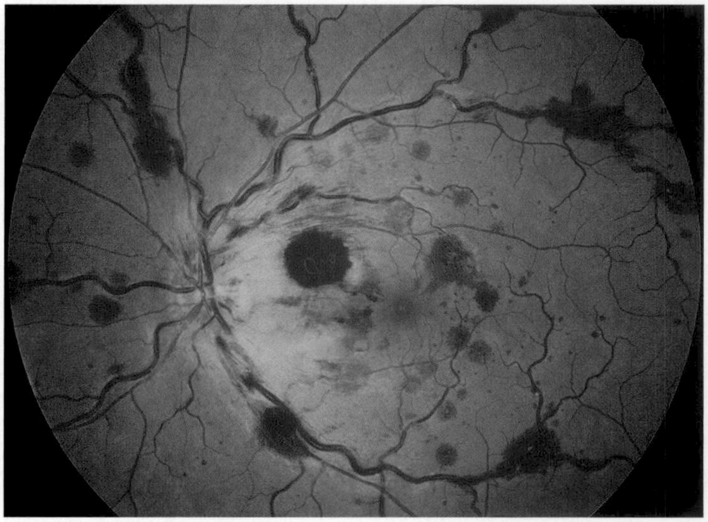

Fig. 12.131 Venous tortuosity and multiple haemorrhages at different levels in the retina. (Courtesy of C. Barry.)

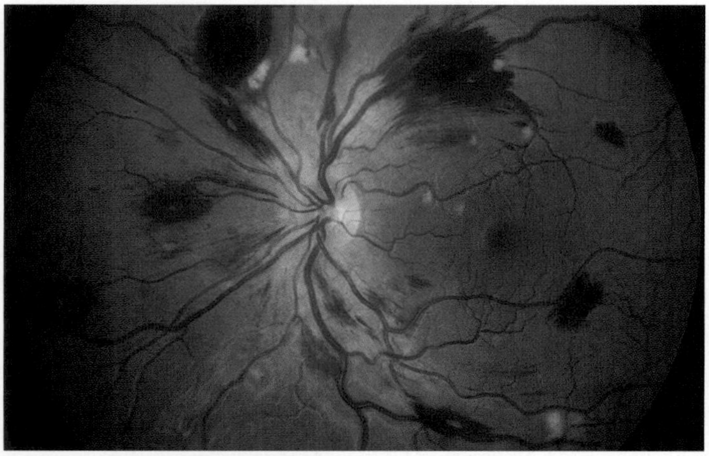

Fig. 12.132 Roth spots and small cotton-wool spots. (Courtesy of P. Saine.)

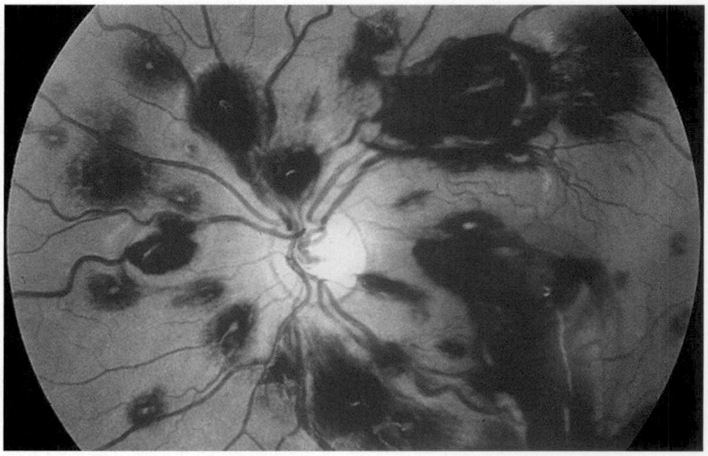

Fig. 12.133 Extensive Roth spots. (Courtesy of S. Milewski.)

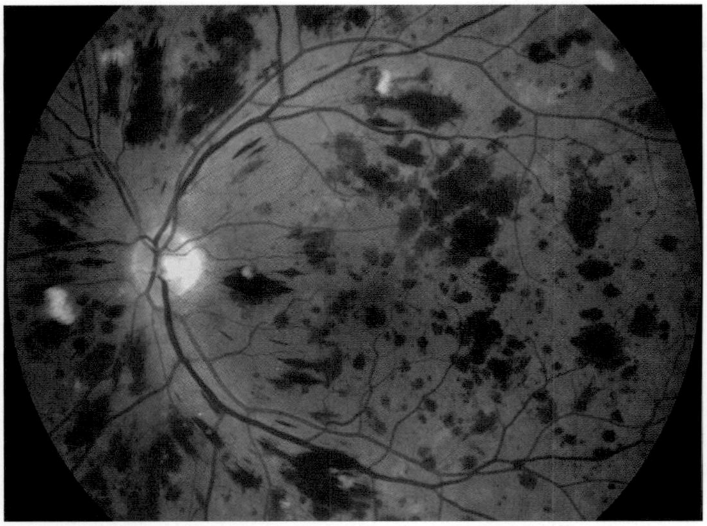

■ **Fig. 12.134** Extensive haemorrhages and a few Roth spots and cotton-wool spots. (Courtesy of C. Barry.)

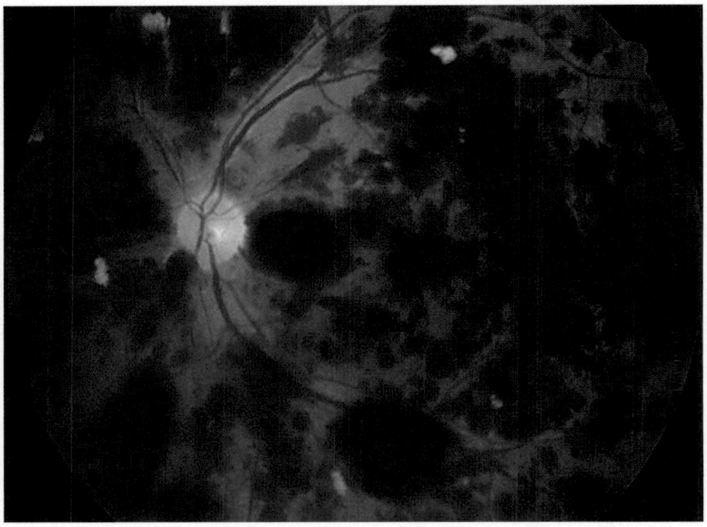

■ **Fig. 12.135** Very severe haemorrhagic retinopathy. (Courtesy of C. Barry.)

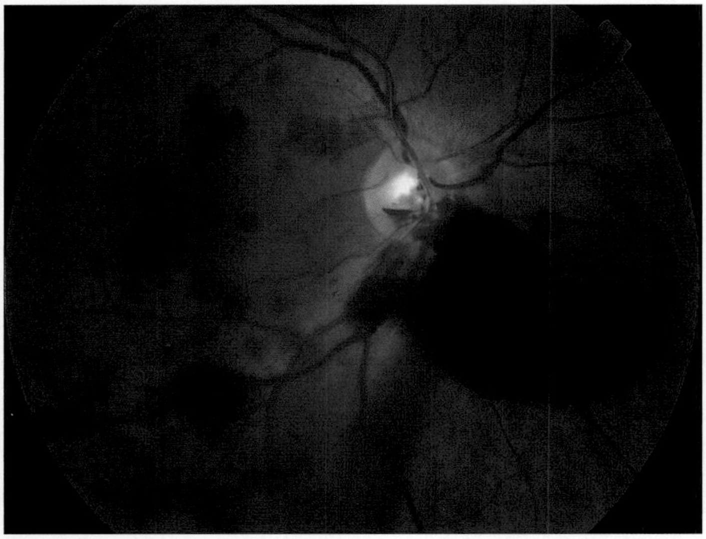

■ **Fig. 12.136** Vitreous haemorrhage.

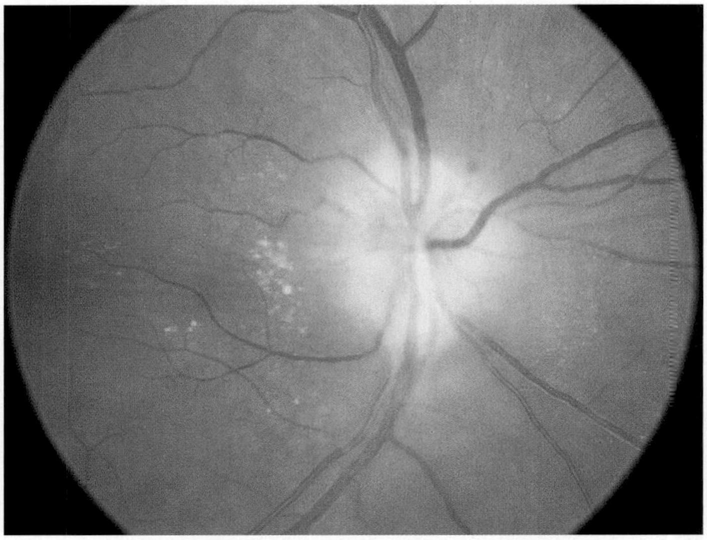

■ **Fig. 12.137** Infiltration of the optic nerve head.

Other signs

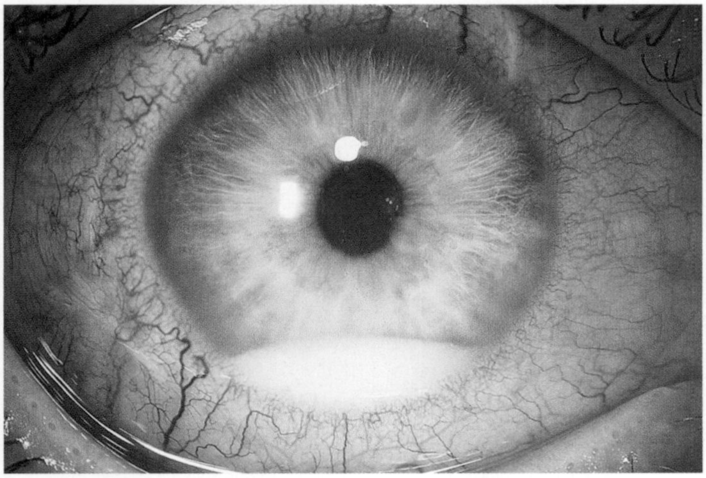

■ **Fig. 12.138** Infiltration of the iris and aqueous giving rise to a pseudohypopyon.

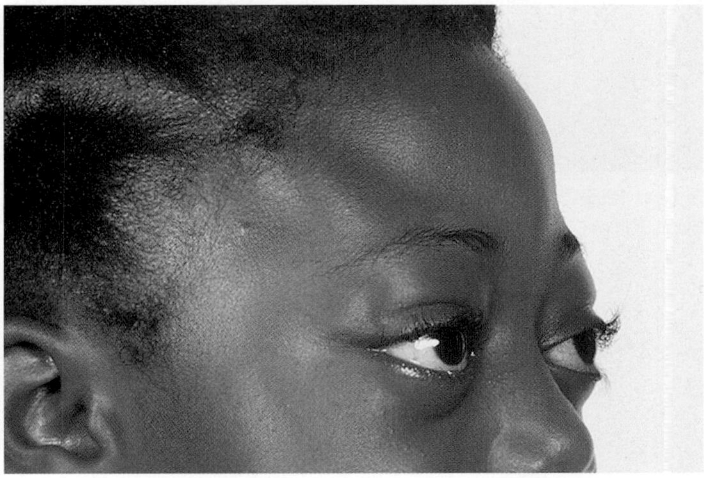

■ **Fig. 12.139** Orbital involvement, particularly in children with myeloid leukaemia.

Chronic leukaemia

Systemic signs

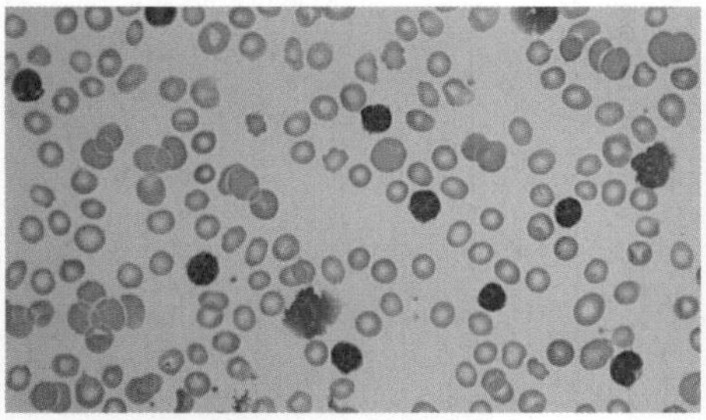

Fig. 12.140 Blood smear in chronic lymphocytic leukaemia, showing that virtually all white cells are mature lymphocytes.

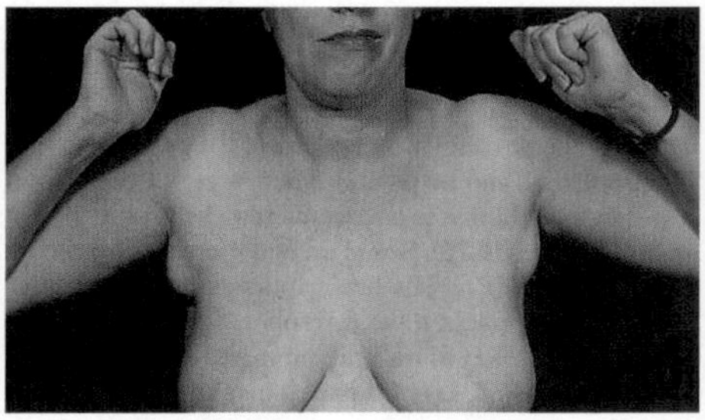

Fig. 12.141 Painless generalised lymphadenopathy. (Courtesy of C. D. Forbes and W. F. Jackson.)

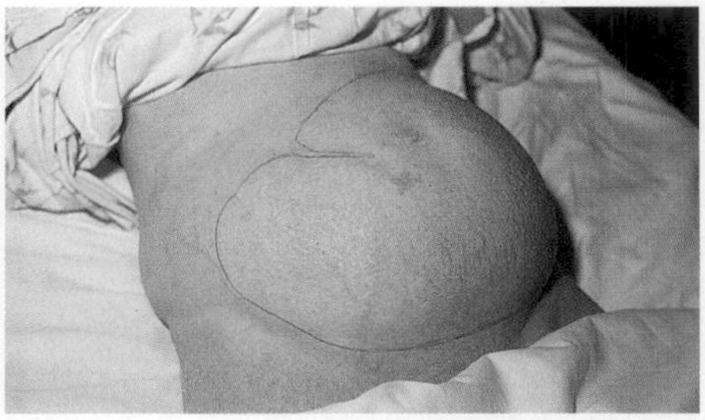

Fig. 12.142 Massive splenomegaly.

Fundus signs

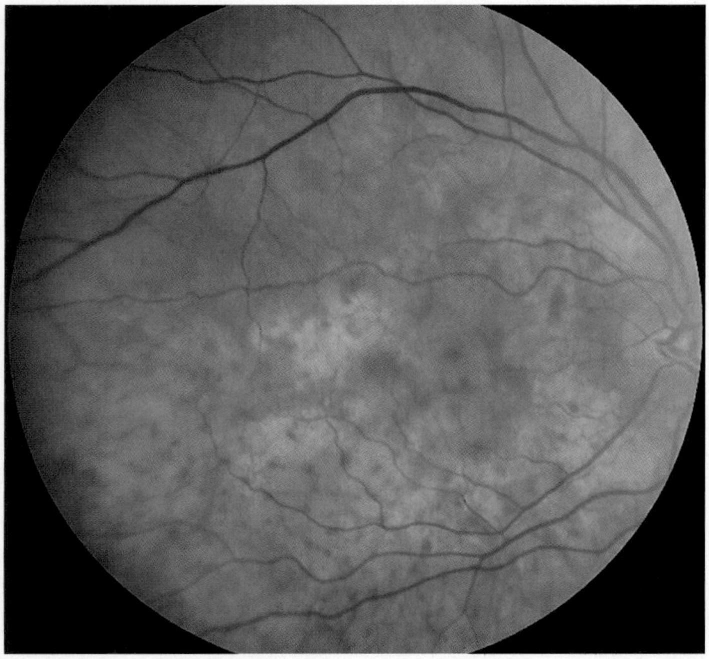

Fig. 12.143 Choroidal deposits may cause a 'leopard skin' RPE appearance.

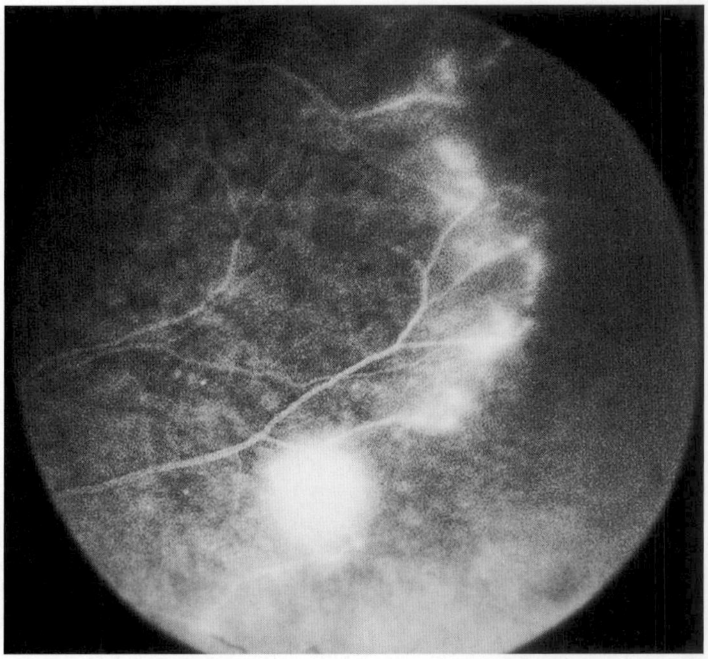

Fig. 12.144 FA shows leakage from peripheral retinal new vessels. (Courtesy of R. Marsh.)

Hyperviscosity

Causes

Multiple myeloma

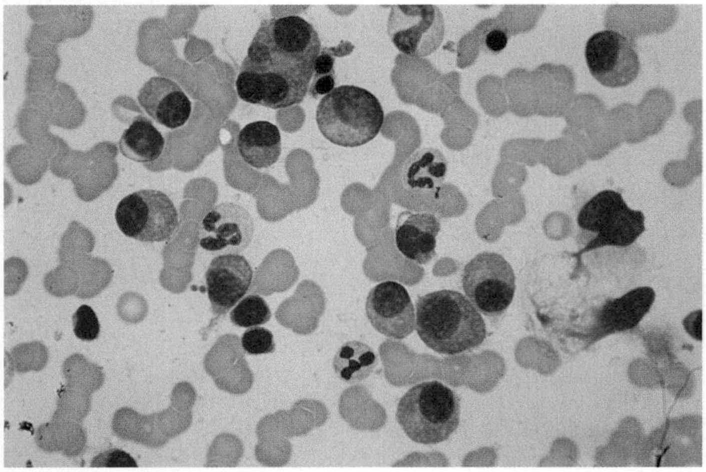

■ **Fig. 12.145** Marrow aspirate showing large plasma cells with eccentric nuclei and deep blue cytoplasm.

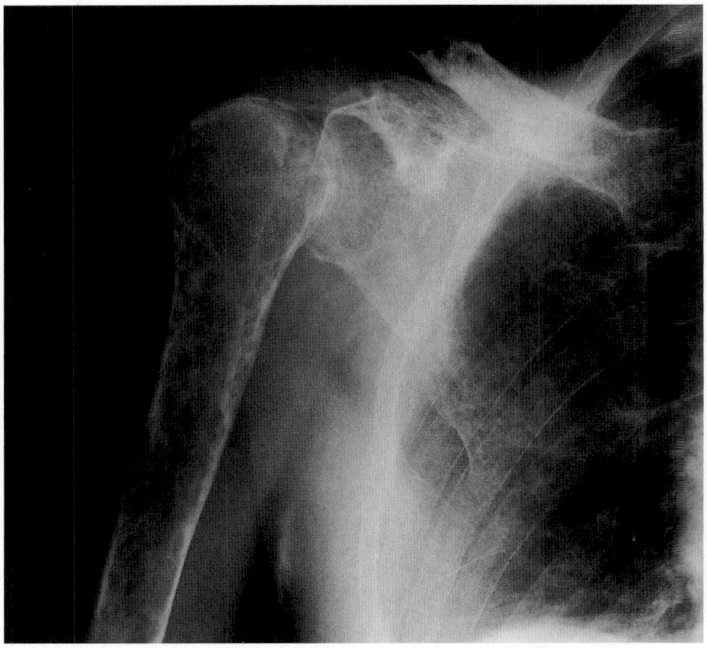

■ **Fig. 12.146** Myeloma lesions in the humerus, scapula and clavicle.

Waldenström macroglobulinaemia

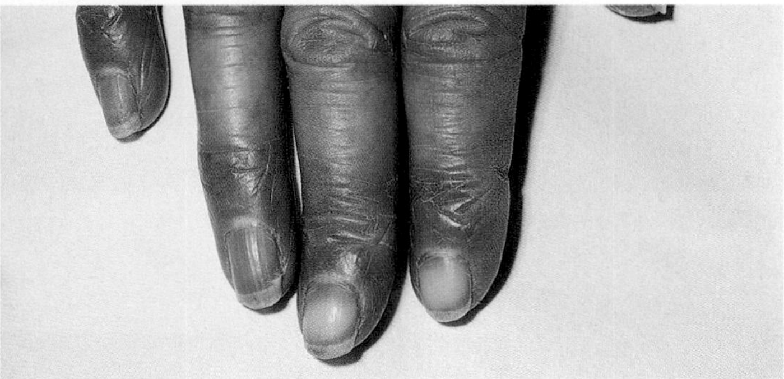

■ **Fig. 12.147** Raynaud phenomenon.

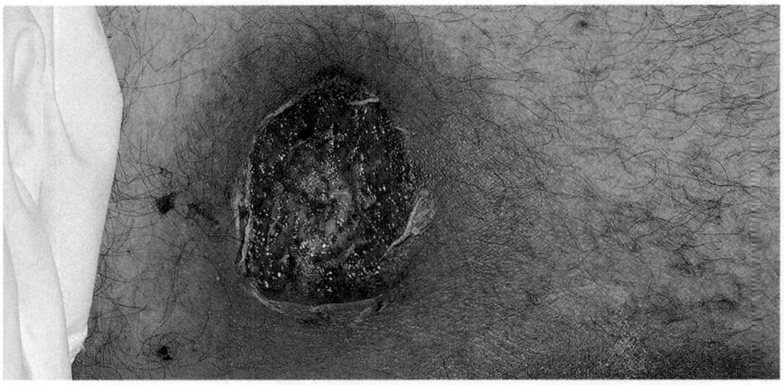

■ **Fig. 12.148** Pyoderma gangrenosum.

Cryoglobulinaemia

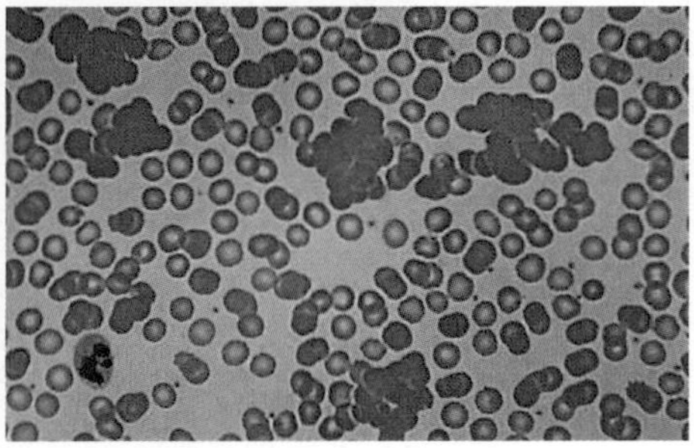

■ **Fig. 12.149** Cryoglobulins are circulating globulins that precipitate out on cooling. (Courtesy of P.-M. Bouloux.)

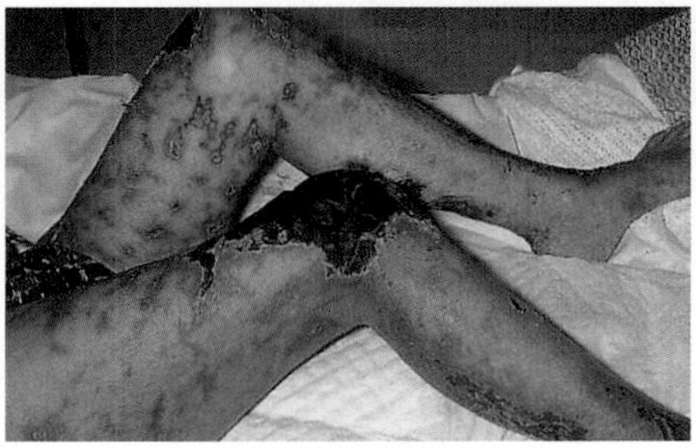

■ **Fig. 12.150** Cutaneous ulceration and necrosis. (Courtesy of C. D. Forbes and W. F. Jackson.)

Polycythaemia

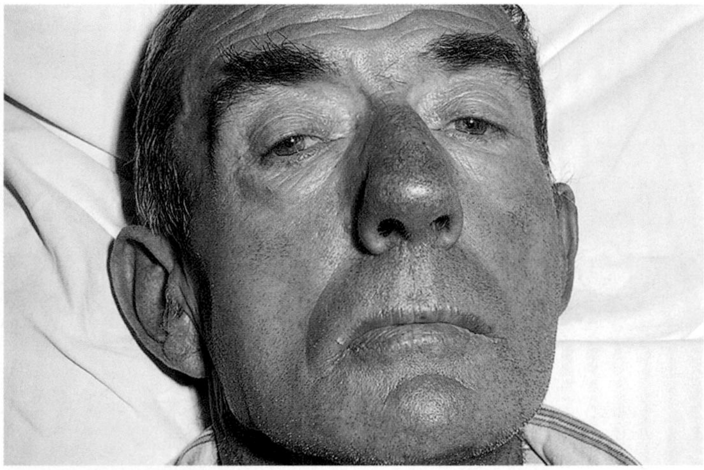

Fig. 12.151 Facial plethora.

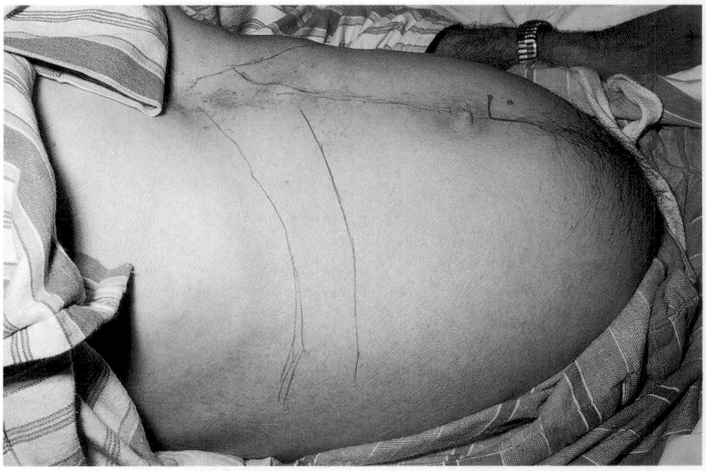

Fig. 12.152 Hepatomegaly is common.

Ocular signs

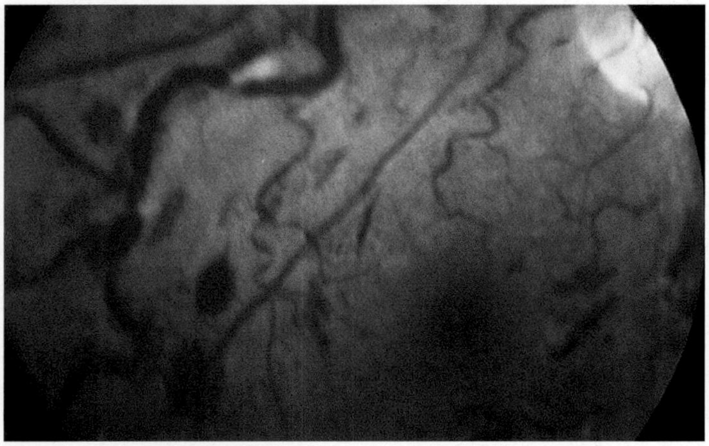

Fig. 12.153 Retinal venous dilatation, segmentation tortuosity, and haemorrhages.

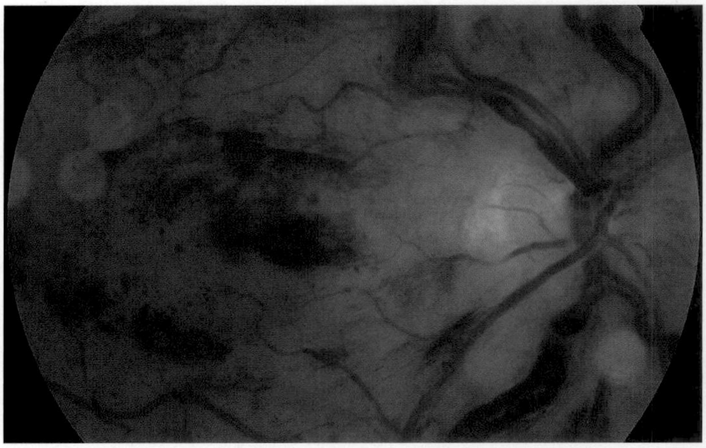

Fig. 12.154 Severe venous changes.

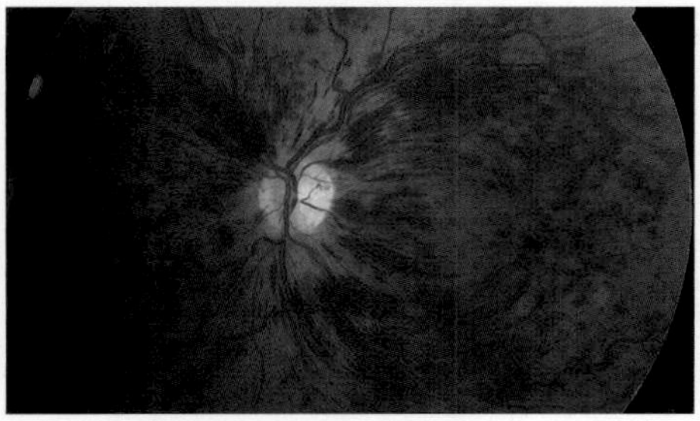

Fig. 12.155 Retinal venous occlusion is uncommon.

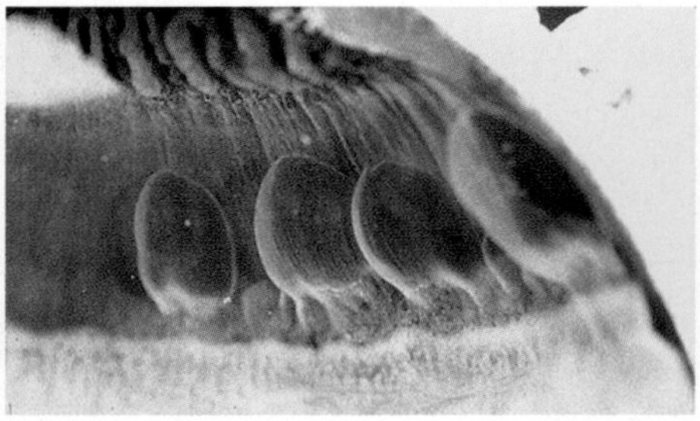

Fig. 12.156 Pars plana cysts may be found post-mortem in patients with multiple myeloma.

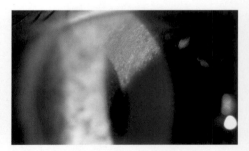

Fig. 12.157 Corneal crystals may occasionally be seen in association with paraproteinaemia.

RETINOPATHY OF PREMATURITY (ROP)

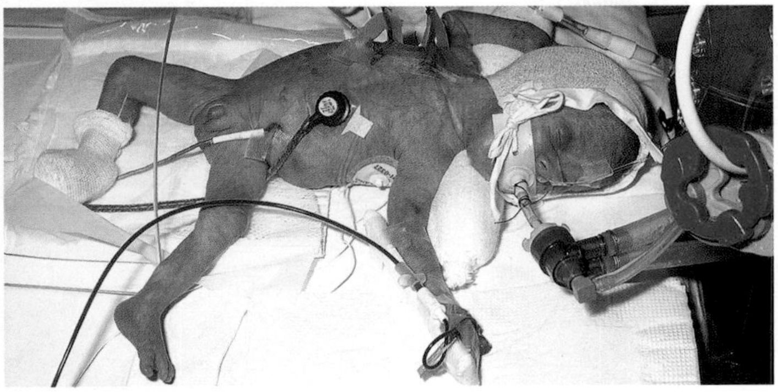

Fig. 12.158 ROP is a proliferative retinopathy affecting premature infants of very low birth weight exposed to high ambient oxygen concentrations.

Acute ROP

Stage 1

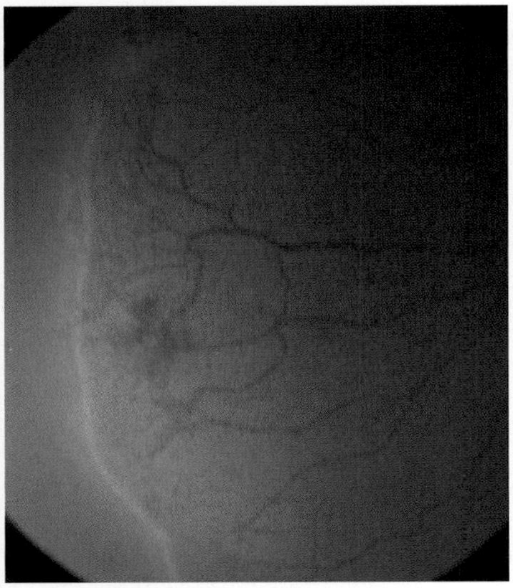

Fig. 12.159 A thin, tortuous, grey-white line runs roughly parallel with the ora serrata and separates avascular immature peripheral retina from vascularised posterior retina. (Courtesy of L. MacKeen.)

Stage 2

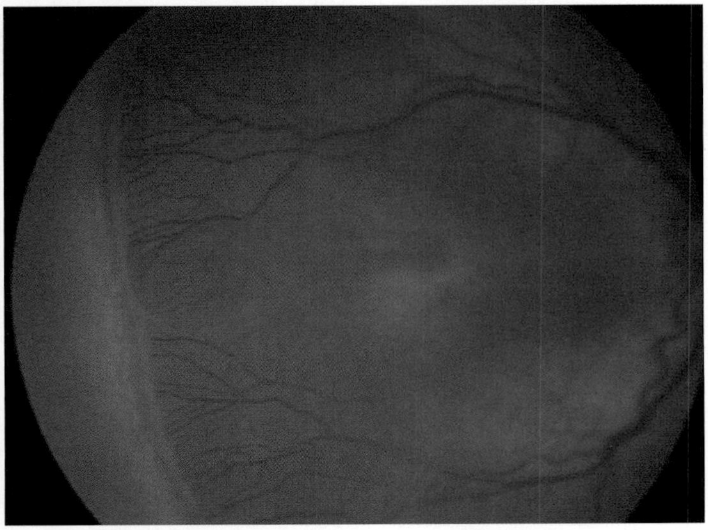

Fig. 12.160 The demarcation line develops into an elevated ridge, which represents a mesenchymal shunt joining arteries with veins. (Courtesy of P. Watts.)

Stage 3

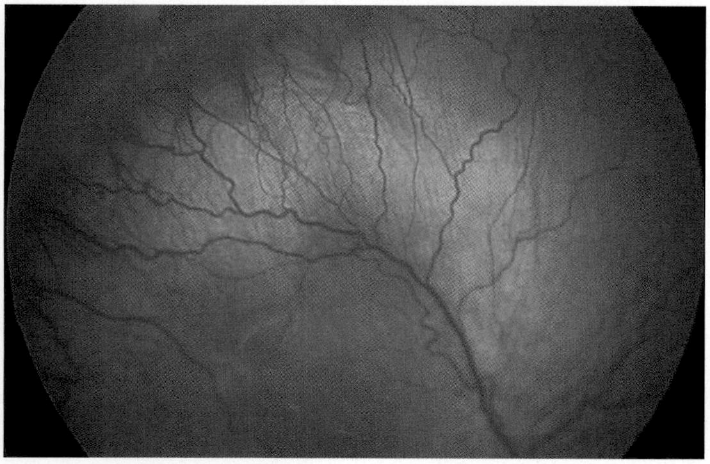

Fig. 12.161 Ridge associated with fibrovascular proliferation that grows along the surface of the retina and into the vitreous. (Courtesy of L. MacKeen.)

Stage 4

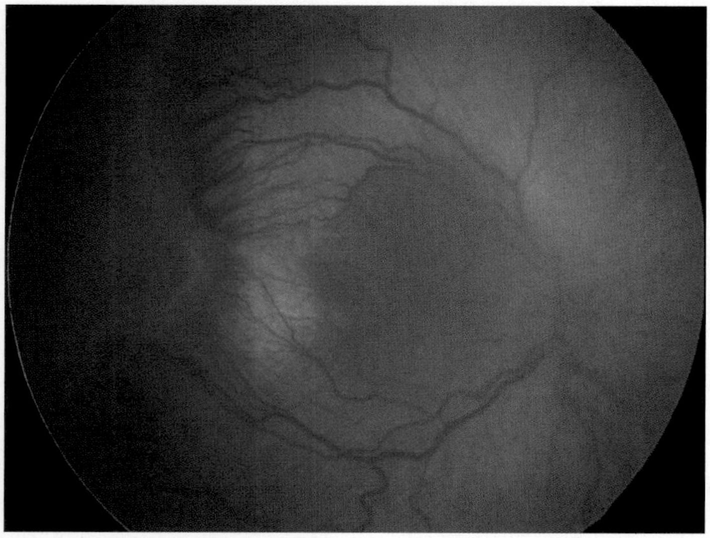

Fig. 12.162 Partial retinal detachment. (Courtesy of L. MacKeen.)

Stage 5

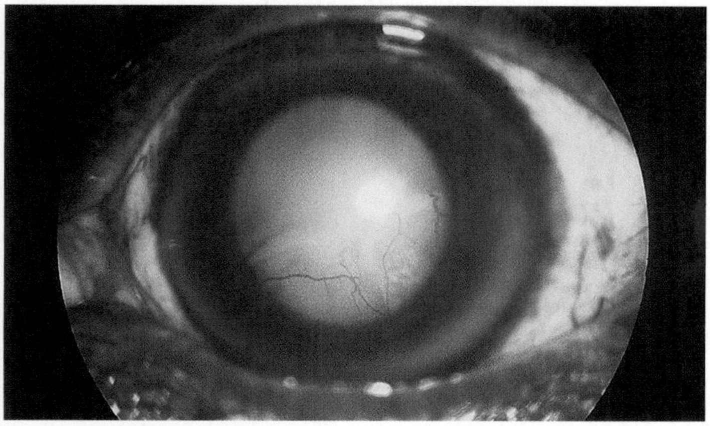

Fig. 12.163 Total retinal detachment.

Plus disease

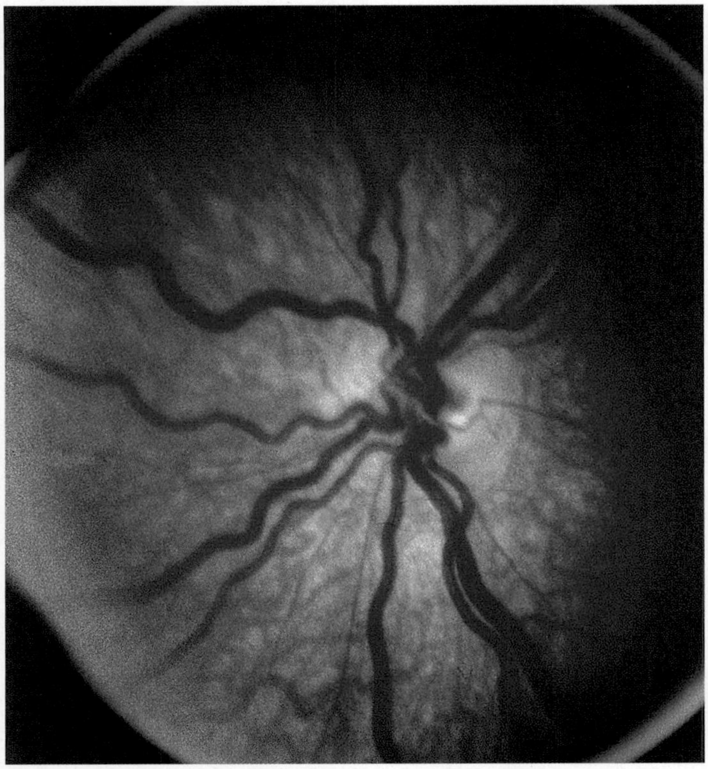

■ **Fig. 12.164** Vitreous haze associated with dilatation of veins and tortuosity of arteries in the posterior fundus.

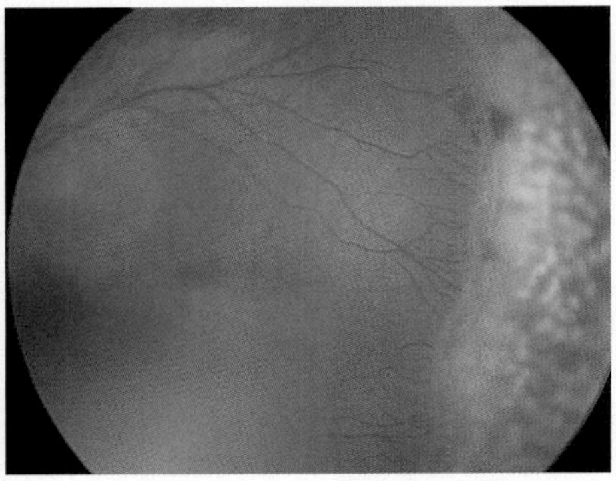

■ **Fig. 12.165** Appearance immediately after laser treatment. (Courtesy of P. Watts.)

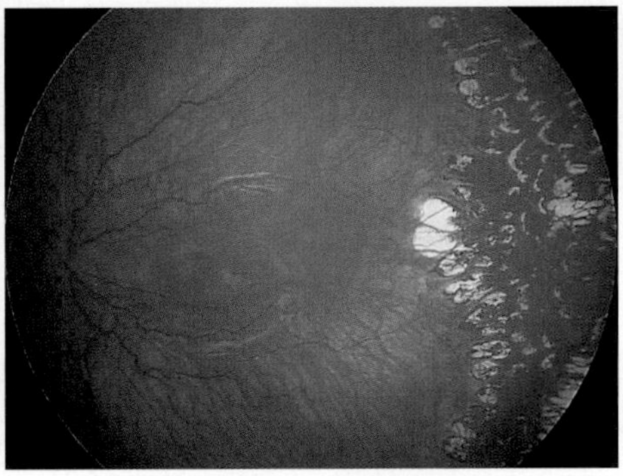

■ **Fig. 12.166** Appearance several weeks after treatment. (Courtesy of L. MacKeen.)

Cicatricial ROP

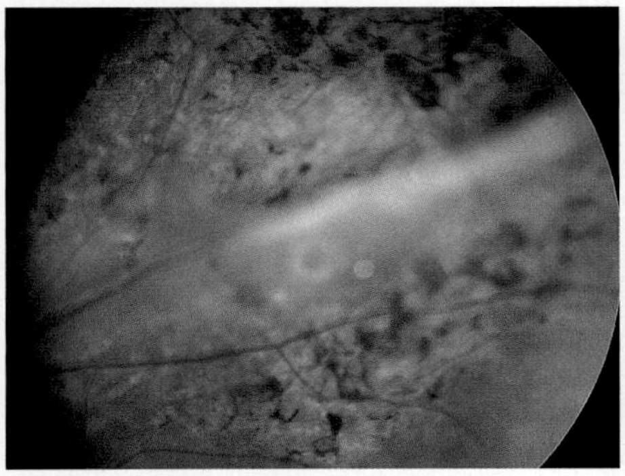

■ **Fig. 12.167** Myopia associated with peripheral retinal pigmentary disturbance.

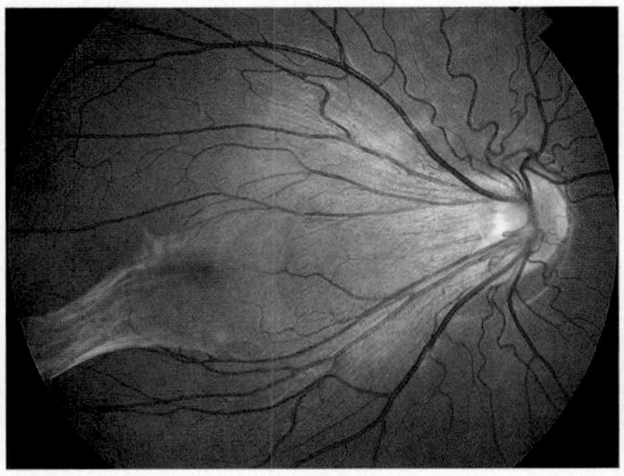

■ **Fig. 12.168** Temporal vitroretinal fibroses with 'dragging' of the macula and disc.

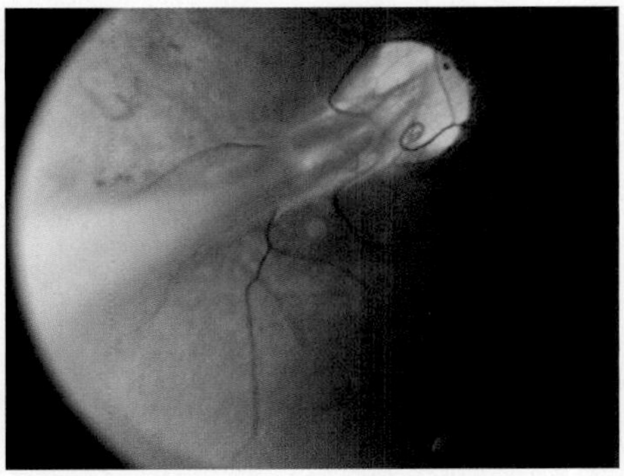

■ **Fig. 12.169** Very severe dragging associated with a falciform fold.

PRIMARY RETINAL TELANGIECTASIA

Idiopathic juxtafoveolar retinal telangiectasia

This comprises a group of rare, idiopathic, congenital or acquired retinal vascular abnormalities of varying severity.

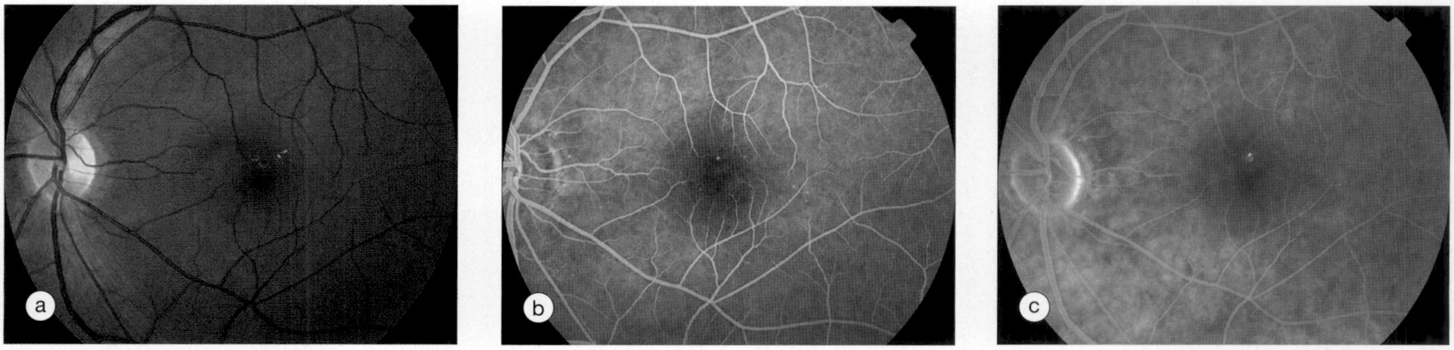

Fig. 12.170 **(a)** Unilateral telangiectasia confined to one clock hour at the edge of the foveal avascular zone (FAZ). **(b, c)** FA shows absence of leakage. (Courtesy of Moorfields Eye Hospital.)

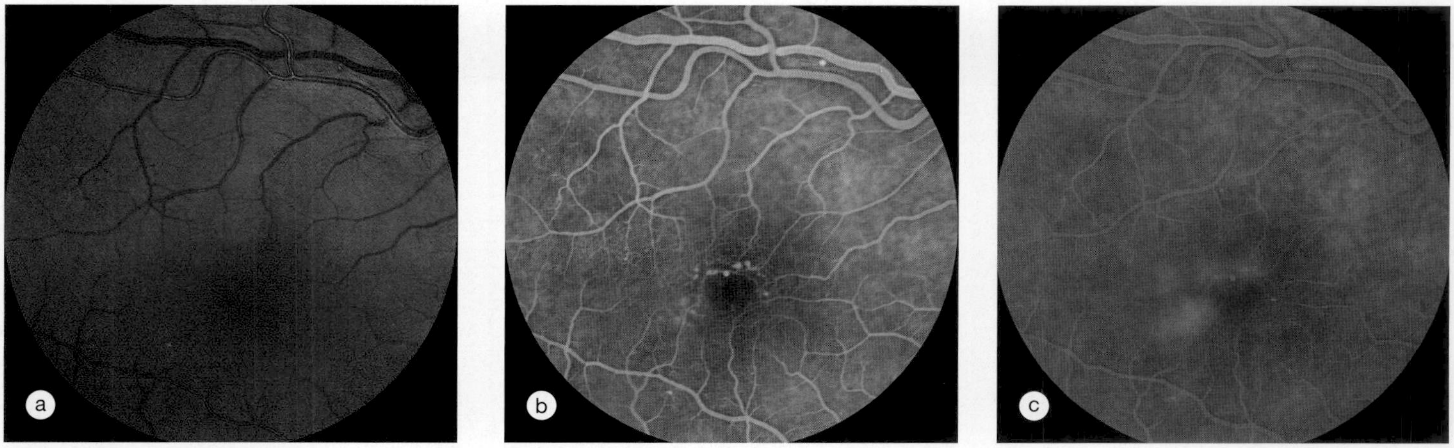

Fig. 12.171 **(a)** Unilateral very subtle perifoveolar telangiectasia. **(b)** FA venous phase highlights the lesions. **(c)** Late phase shows leakage. (Courtesy of P. Saine.)

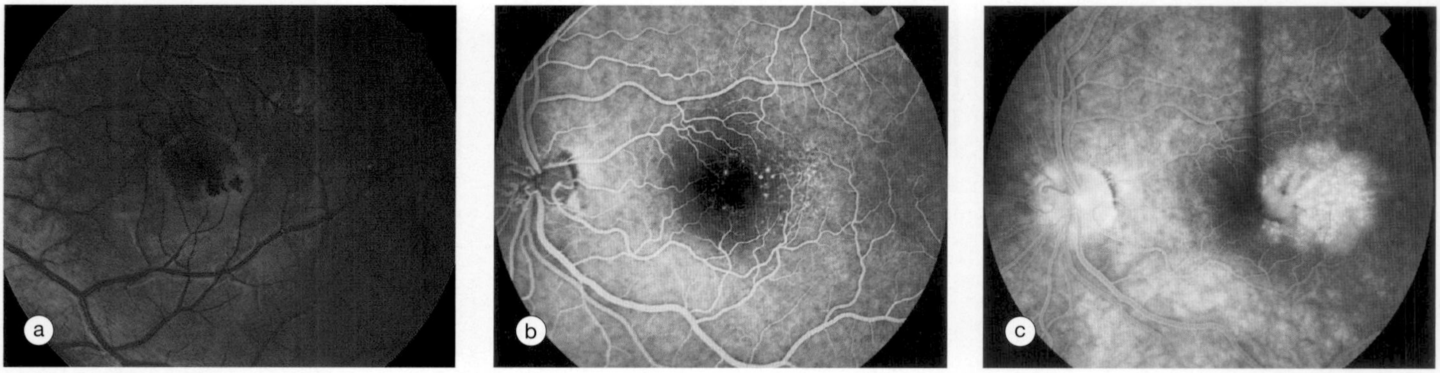

Fig. 12.172 **(a)** Parafoveal telangiectasia without hard exudates. **(b)** FA venous phase shows capillary dilatation outside the FAZ. **(c)** Late phase shows extensive leakage.

Coats disease

Coats disease typically involves one eye of a young boy.

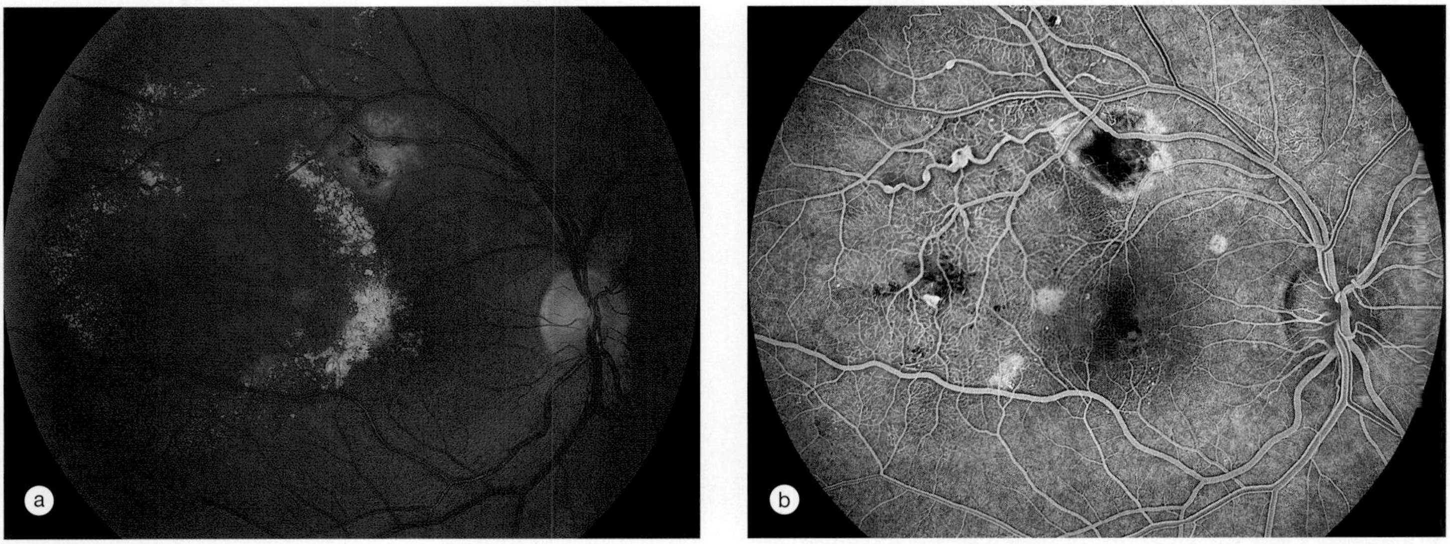

Fig. 12.173 **(a)** Intraretinal and subretinal yellowish exudation, often affecting areas remote from the vascular abnormalities, particularly the macula. **(b)** FA early venous phase highlights the lesions along the superotemporal arcade. (Courtesy of P. Saine.)

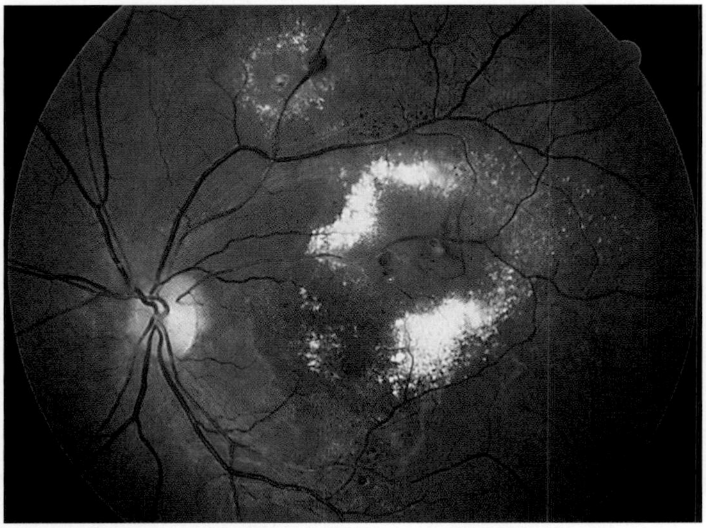

Fig. 12.174 Increase in subretinal exudate deposition and peripheral telangiectatic foci. (Courtesy of C. Barry.)

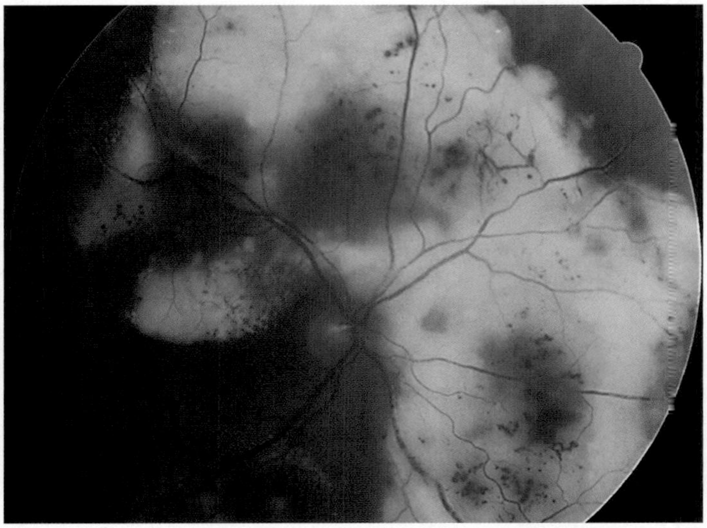

Fig. 12.175 Massive subretinal exudation. (Courtesy of C. Barry.)

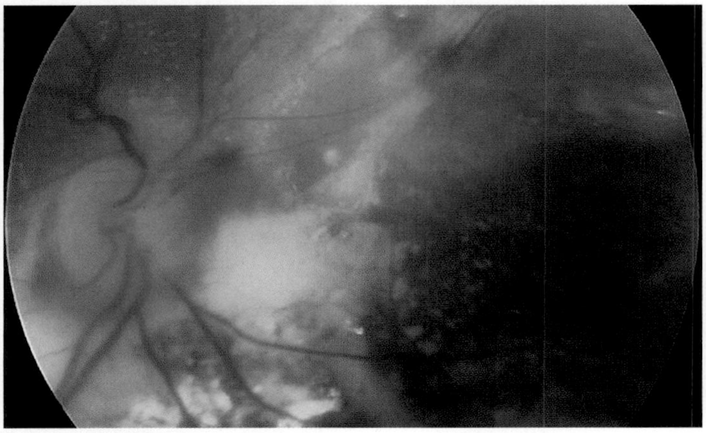

Fig. 12.176 Shallow exudation retinal detachment.

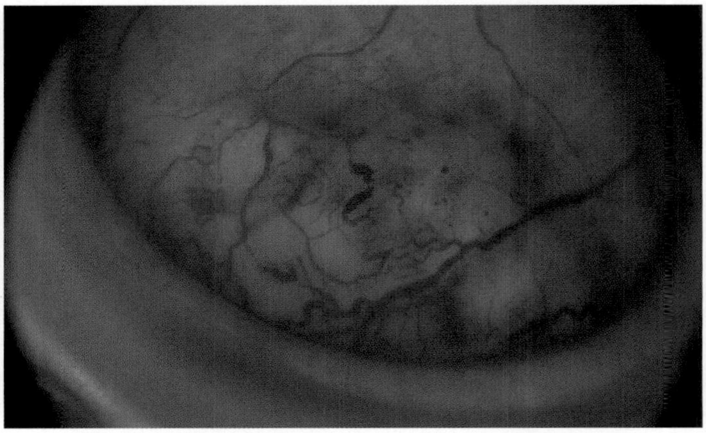

Fig. 12.177 Deeper exudative retinal detachment. (Courtesy of L. MacKeen.)

MISCELLANEOUS VASCULAR DISORDERS

Retinal artery macroaneurysm

Macroaneurysms typically effect elderly hypertensive women.

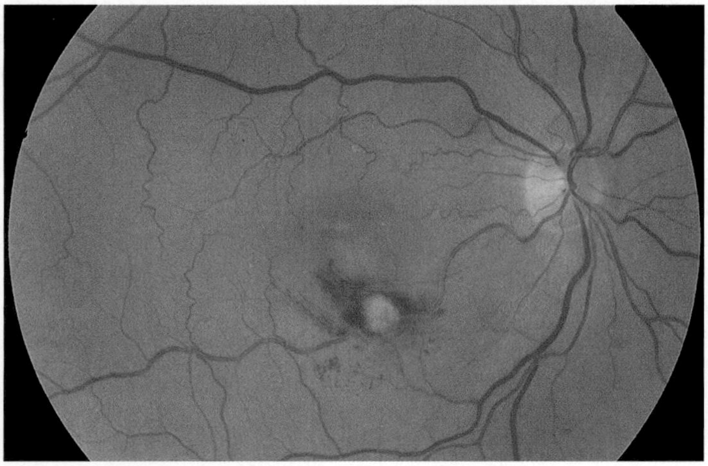

Fig. 12.178 A saccular or fusiform arteriolar dilatation, most frequently occurring at a bifurcation or an arteriovenous crossing along the temporal vascular arcades, often associated with retinal haemorrhage.

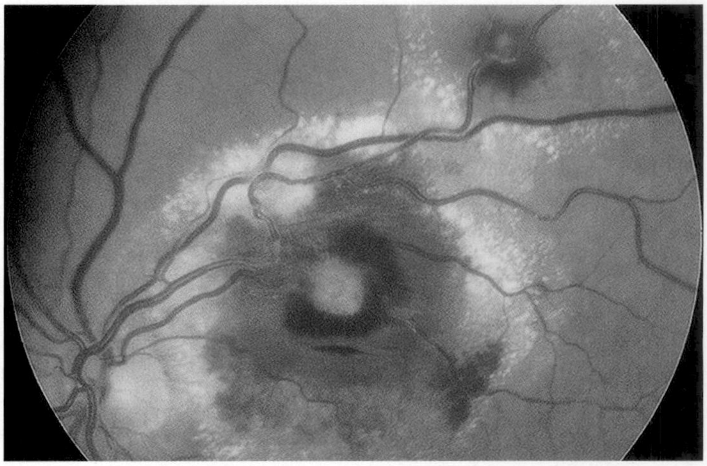

Fig. 12.179 Multiple macroaneurysms along the same or different arterioles may occasionally be present.

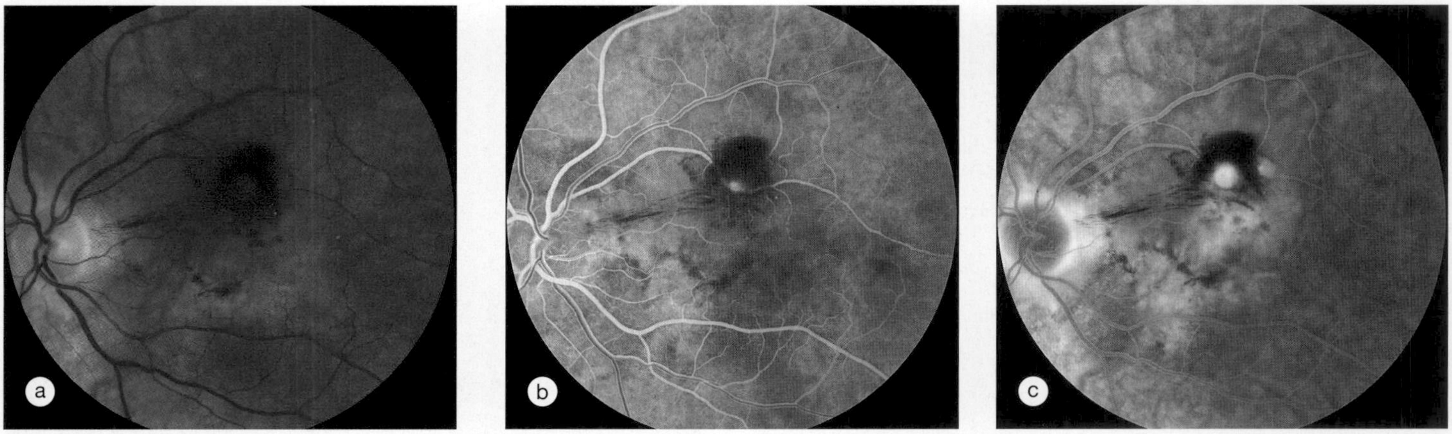

Fig. 12.180 **(a)** Retinal artery macroaneurysm surrounded by haemorrhage. **(b)** FA early venous phase shows hyperfluorescence of the macroaneurysm with surrounding hypofluorescence due to blockage by blood. **(c)** Late phase shows increased hyperfluorescence of the macroaneurysm. (Courtesy of P. Saine.)

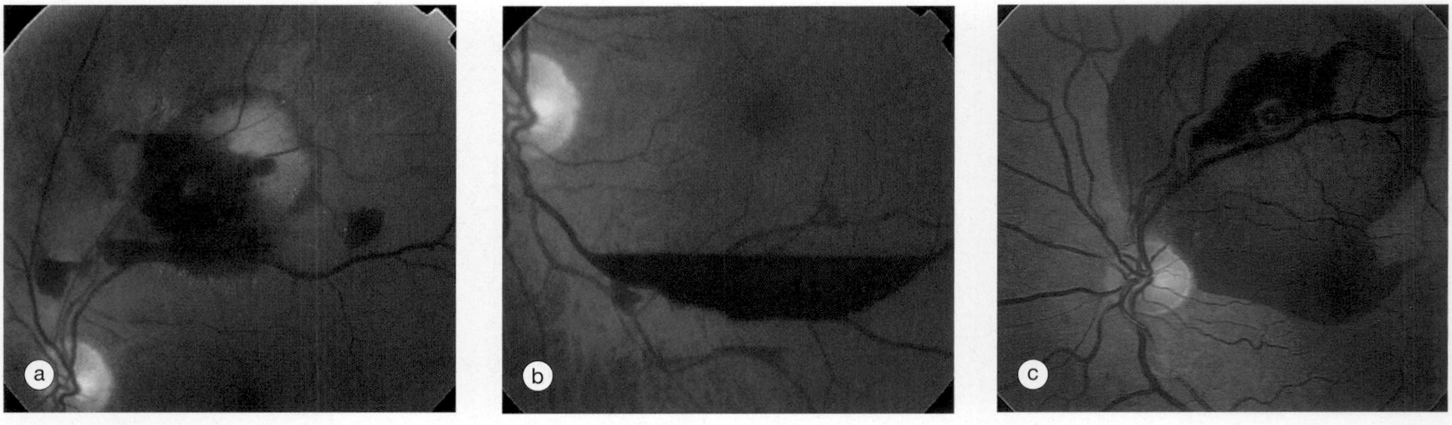

Fig. 12.181 Bleeding macroaneurysm. **(a)** Intraretinal haemorrhage. **(b)** Preretinal haemorrhage. **(c)** Very large subretinal haemorrhage is uncommon. (Courtesy of P. Gili.)

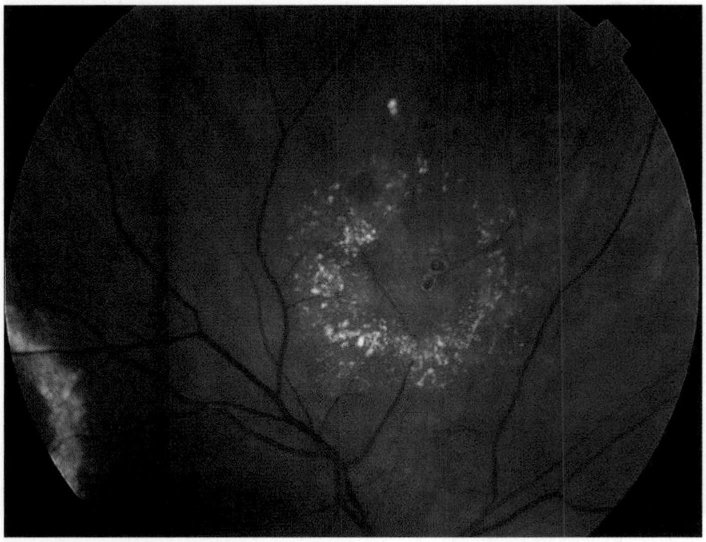

Fig. 12.182 A small incomplete ring of hard exudates surrounding retinal oedema due to a leaking macroaneurysm.

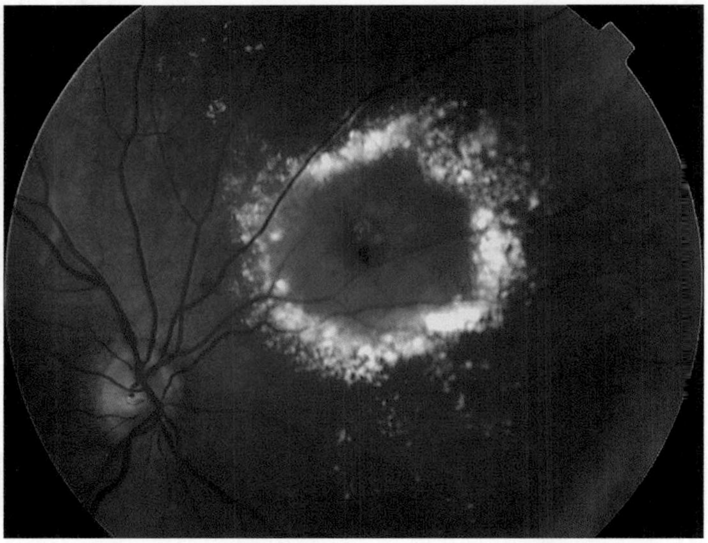

Fig. 12.183 A large complete ring of hard exudates associated with chronic leakage.

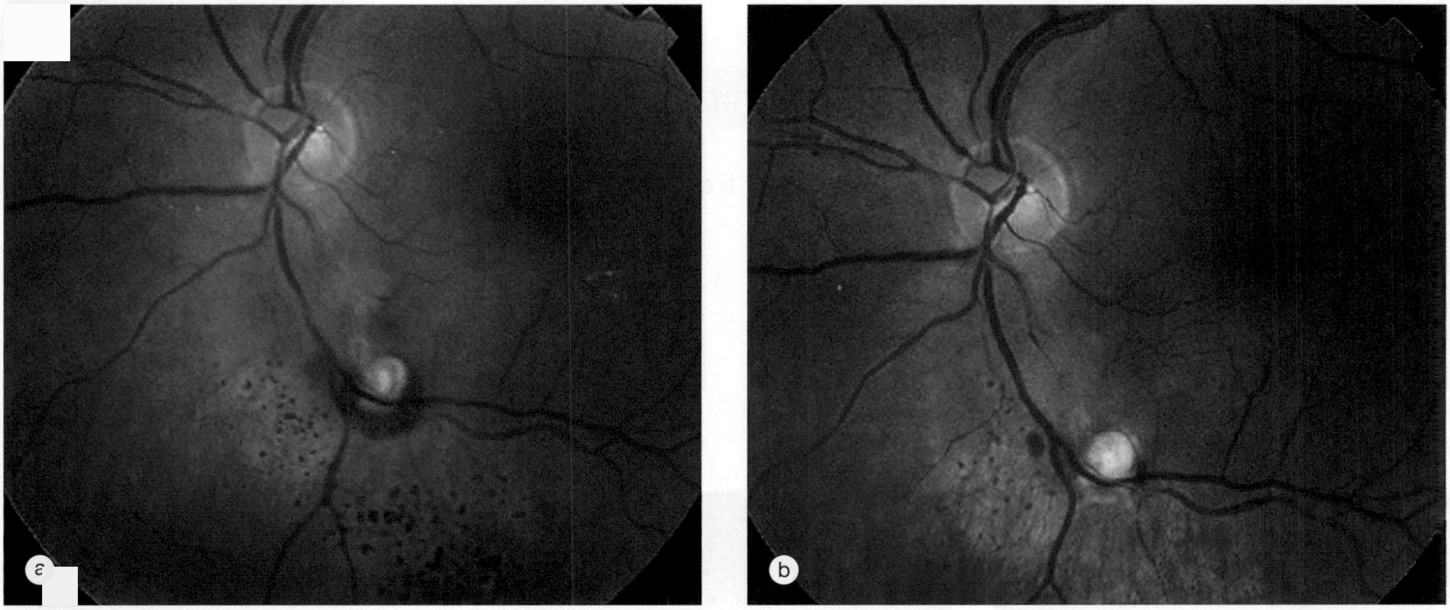

Fig. 12.184 Laser treatment of a leaking macroaneurysm. **(a)** A few weeks after treatment. **(b)** Several months after treatment the macroaneurysm is white and fibrotic.

CHAPTER 13

ACQUIRED MACULAR DISORDERS

AGE-RELATED MACULAR DEGENERATION

Age-related macular degeneration (AMD) is the most common cause of visual loss in the developed world in individuals over 50 years of age.

Drusen

Drusen consist of discrete deposits of abnormal material between the basal lamina of the RPE and the inner collagenous layer of Bruch membrane.

Hard drusen

Hard drusen occasionally precede the development of AMD.

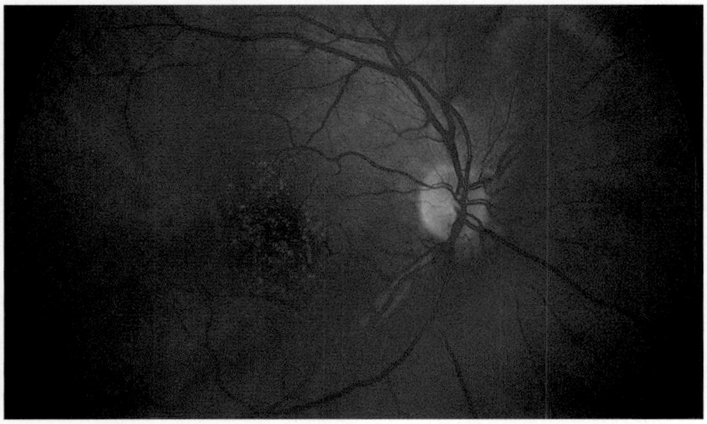

Fig. 13.1 Small, round, discrete, yellow-white spots at the posterior pole that appear in old age.

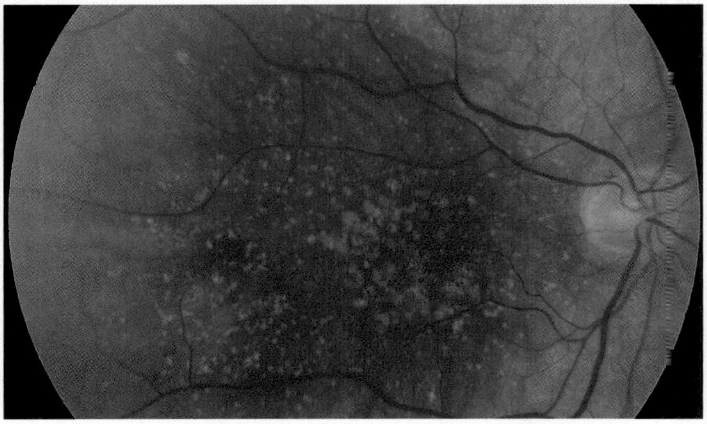

Fig. 13.2 More numerous and slightly larger hard drusen.

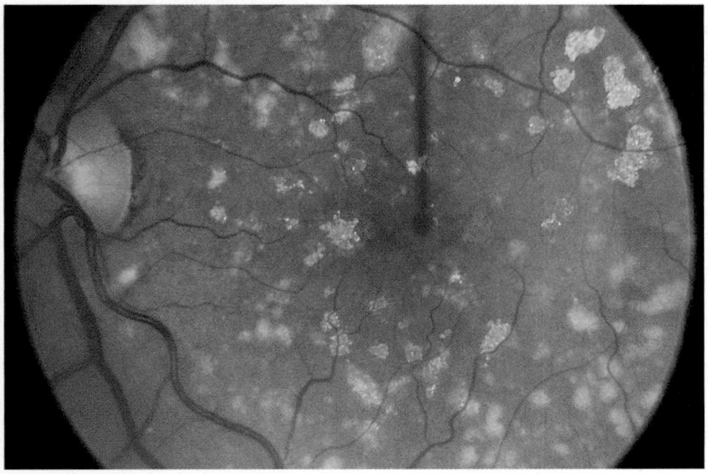

Fig. 13.3 Drusen may undergo secondary dystrophic calcification and acquire a glistening appearance.

Soft drusen

Soft drusen are frequent precursors of AMD.

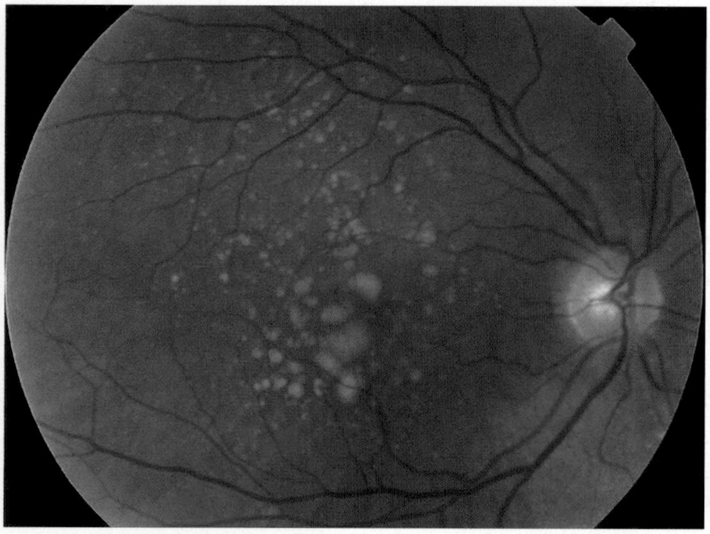

■ **Fig. 13.4** Larger, greyish-white or pale yellow nodules with indistinct margins.

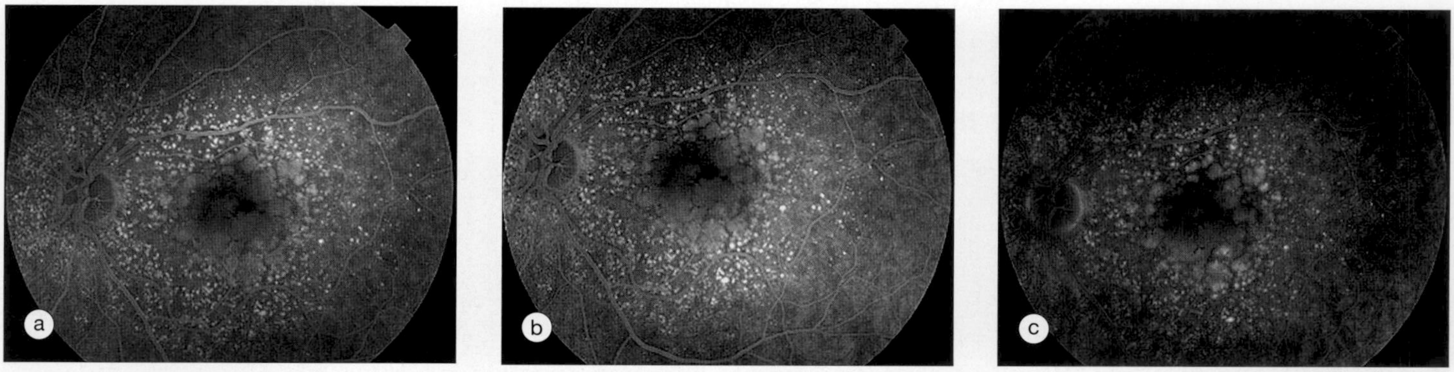

■ **Fig. 13.5 (a, b)** FA venous phase shows hyperfluorescent due to window defects. **(c)** Late phase shows persistent hyperfluorescence due to staining. The centre of the macula also shows a 'drusenoid' detachment of the RPE due to coalescence of soft drusen.

Atrophic (dry) age-related macular degeneration

Atrophic AMD is a slowly progressive condition which is more common than the exudative type.

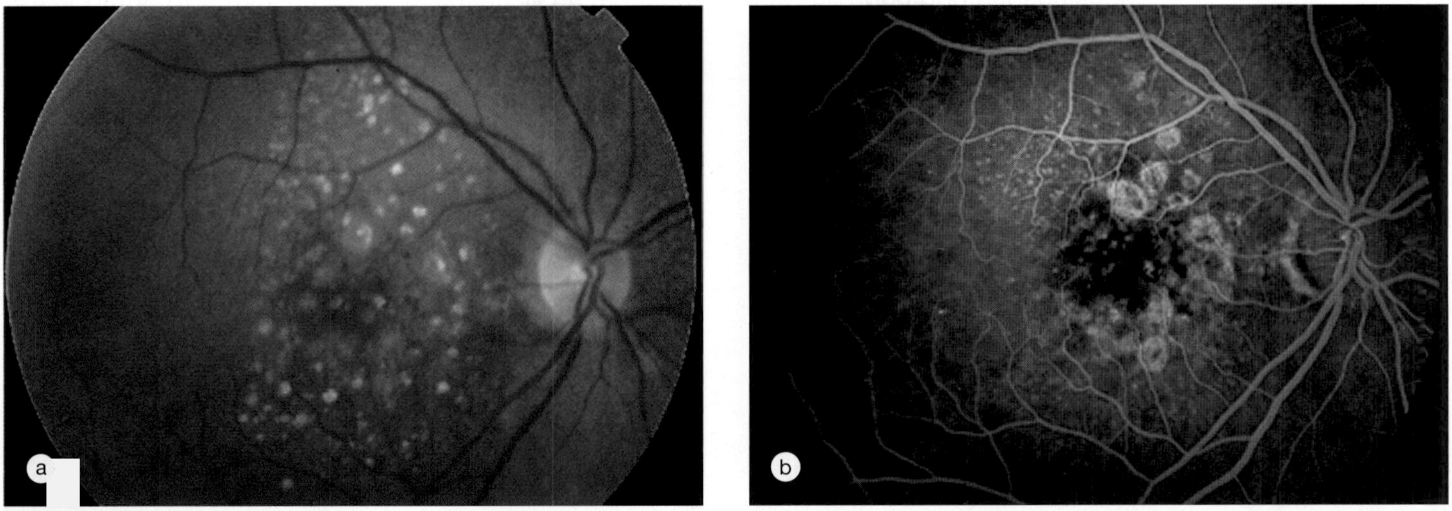

Fig. 13.6 **(a)** Focal atrophy of the RPE in association with macular drusen. **(b)** FA venous phase shows corresponding hyperfluorescence due to window defects.

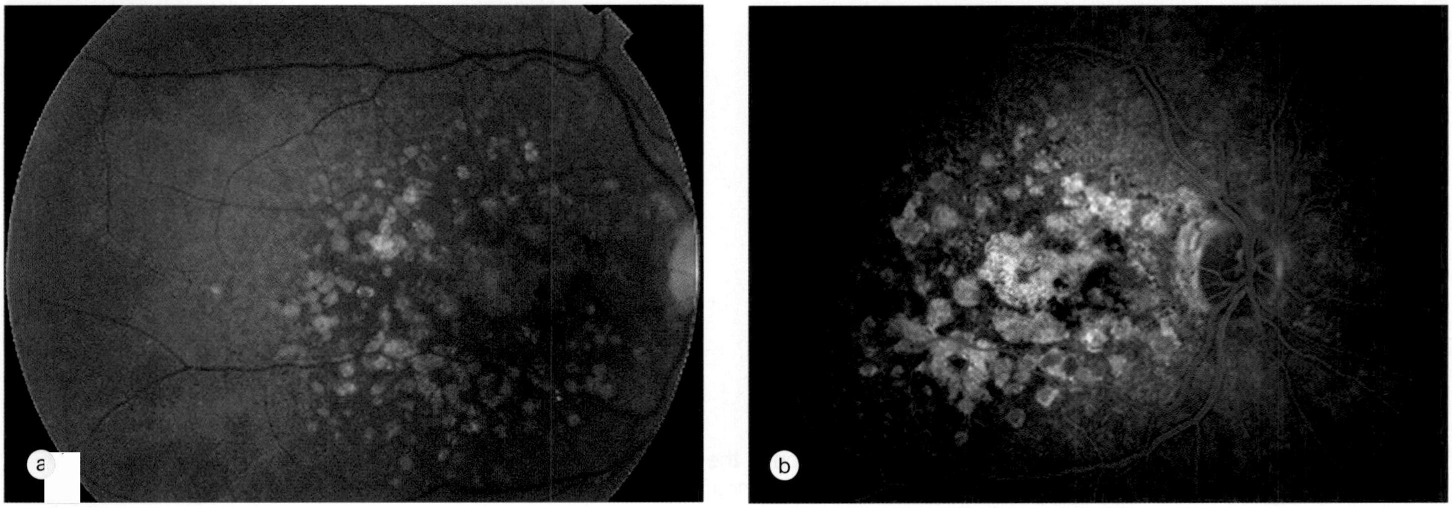

Fig. 13.7 **(a)** Coalescence of atrophic areas. **(b)** FA late venous phase shows increased areas of hyperfluorescence.

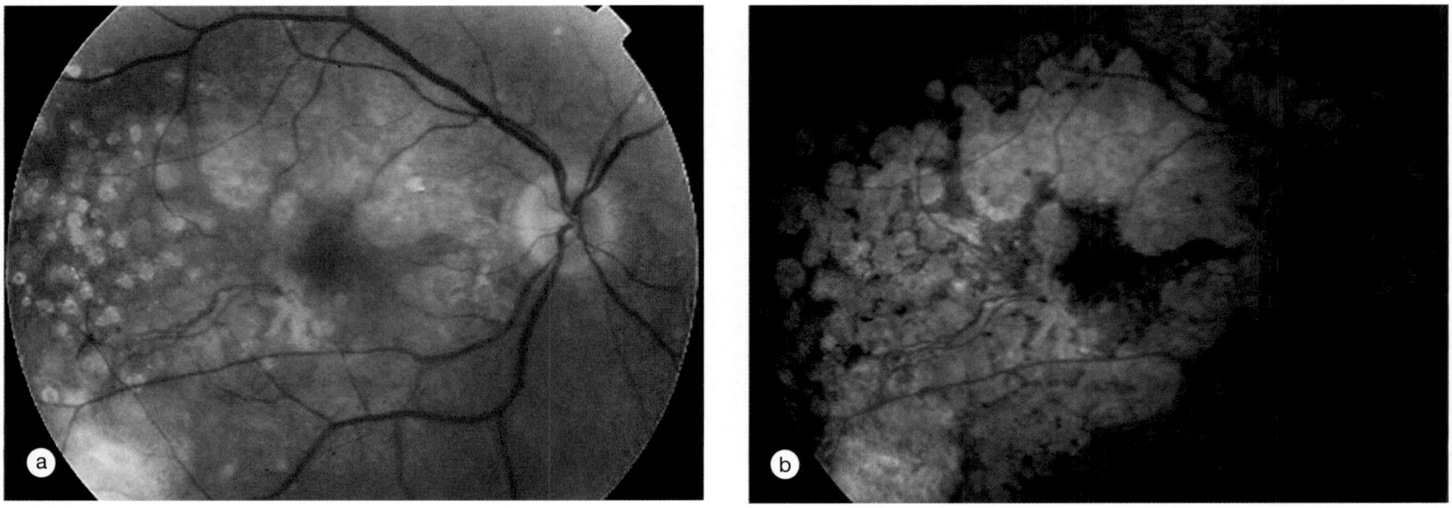

Fig. 13.8 **(a)** Further enlargement of the atrophic areas (geographic atrophy). **(b)** FA late phase shows hyperfluorescence due to staining of the exposed sclera.

Exudative (wet) age-related macular degeneration

Exudative AMD is caused by choroidal neovascularisation (CNV), which grows through defects in Bruch membrane.

Classic CNV

Classic CNV is a well-defined membrane with a characteristic appearance during early phase FA.

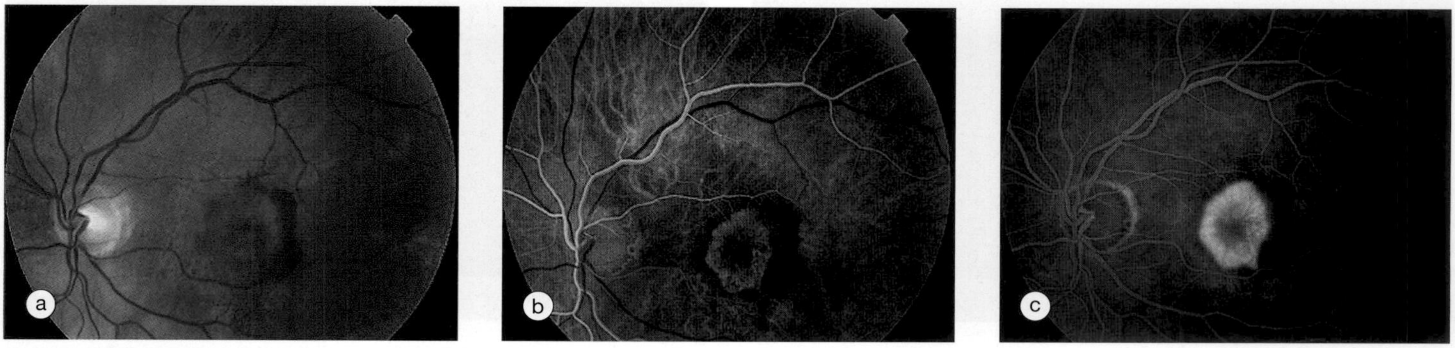

Fig. 13.11 Classic subfoveal CNV. **(a)** Crescent-shaped subretinal haemorrhage temporal to the macula. **(b)** FA arterial phase shows well-defined hyperfluorescence at the macula and blockage by blood of background choroidal fluorescence. **(c)** Late venous phase shows more intense hyperfluorescence due to leakage around the CNV and into the subretinal space.

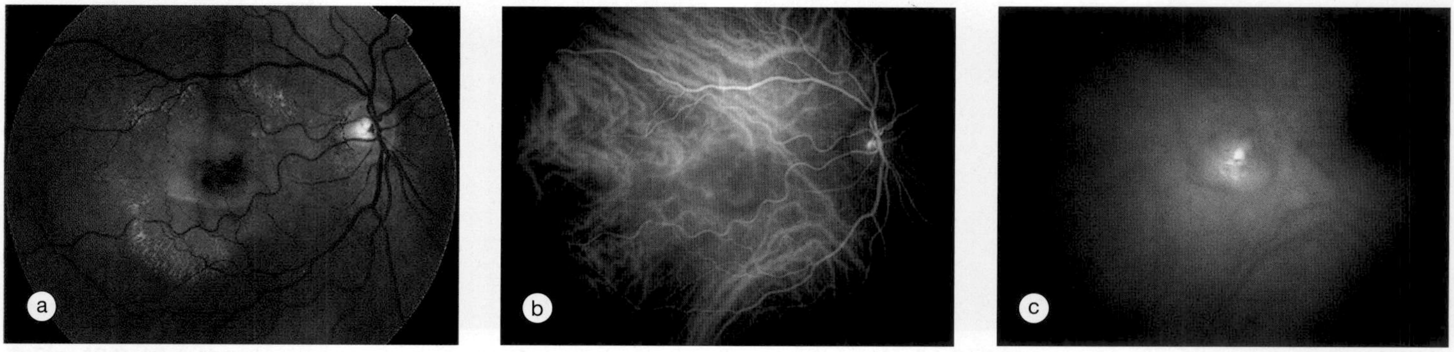

Fig. 13.12 Subfoveal CNV. **(a)** Blood and fluid at the macula surrounded by a ring of hard exudates. (**b, c**) ICG shows a small area of increasing hyperfluorescence (hot spot) due to underlying CNV.

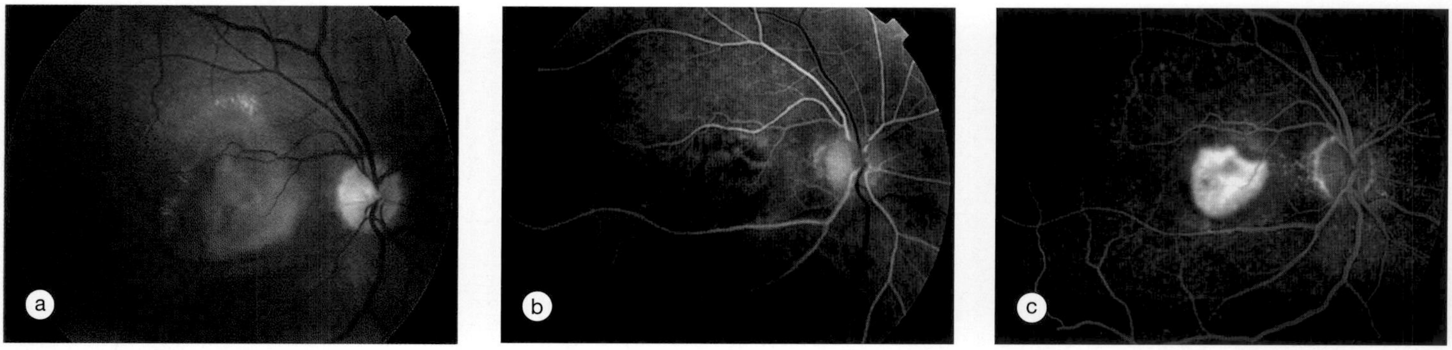

Fig. 13.13 Larger classic subfoveal CNV. **(a)** Serous macular elevation with small hard exudates above. **(b)** FA arteriovenous phase shows lacy hyperfluorescence. **(c)** Late venous phase shows dense hyperfluorescence at the macula and scattered spotty hyperfluorescence of associated drusen.

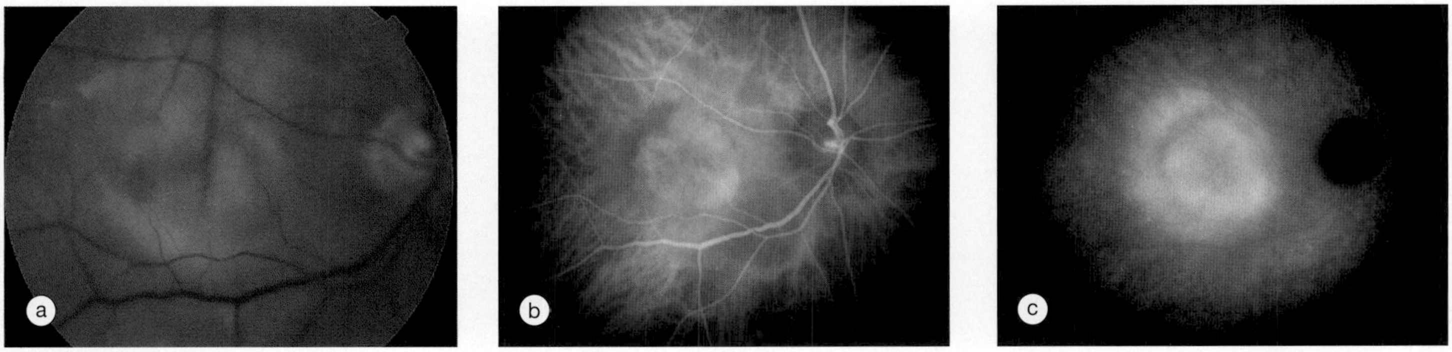

Fig. 13.14 Large subfoveal CNV. **(a)** Fluid at the posterior pole. **(b)** ICG shows a round area of hyperfluorescence. **(c)** Late phase shows extension of hyperfluorescence due to leakage.

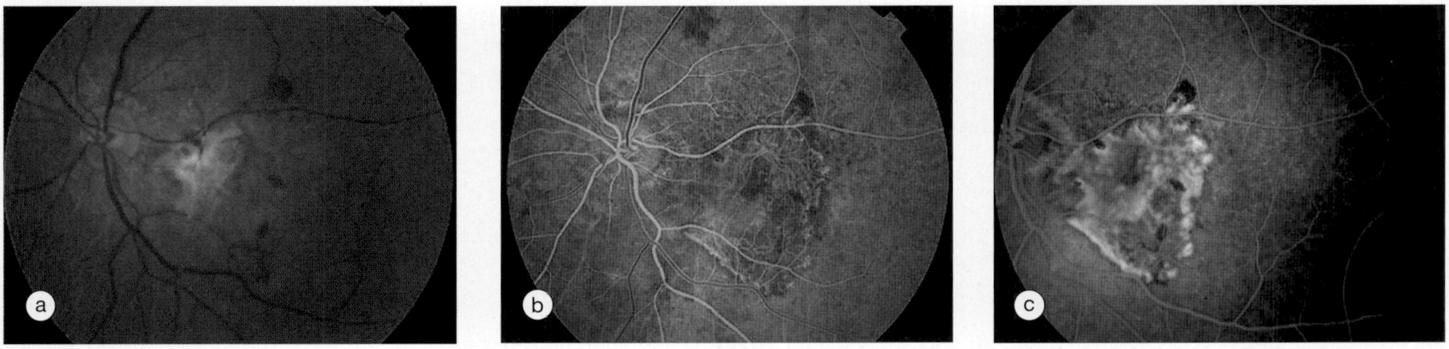

Fig. 13.15 Very large classic subfoveal CNV. **(a)** Small subretinal scar and scattered haemorrhages. **(b)** FA early venous phase shows a very large area of lacy hyperfluorescence at the posterior pole. **(c)** Late venous phase shows increased hyperfluorescence.

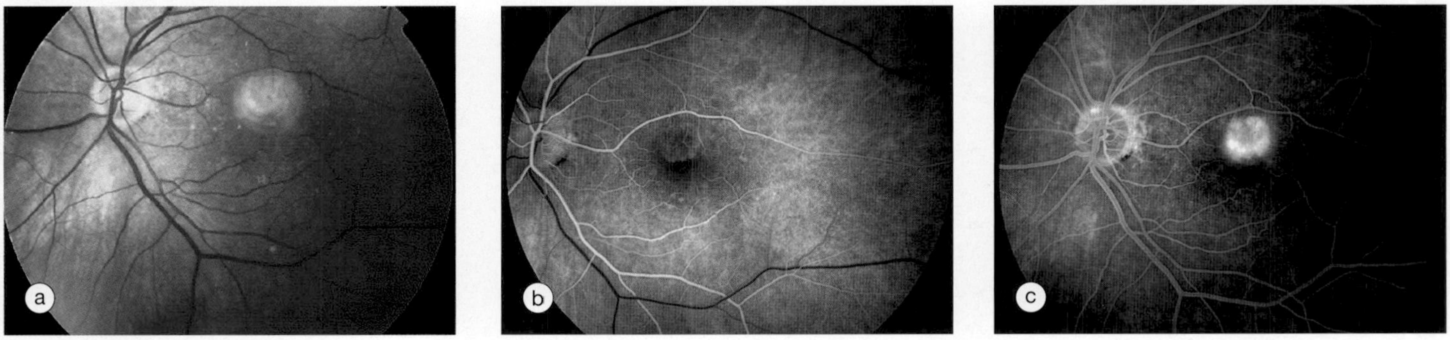

Fig. 13.16 Small classic juxtafoveal CNV. **(a)** Small yellowish retinal elevation above the fovea. **(b)** FA arterial phase shows hyperfluorescence that is closer than 200 μm from the centre of the foveal avascular zone (FAZ) but does not involve it. **(c)** Hyperfluorescence remains juxtafoveal.

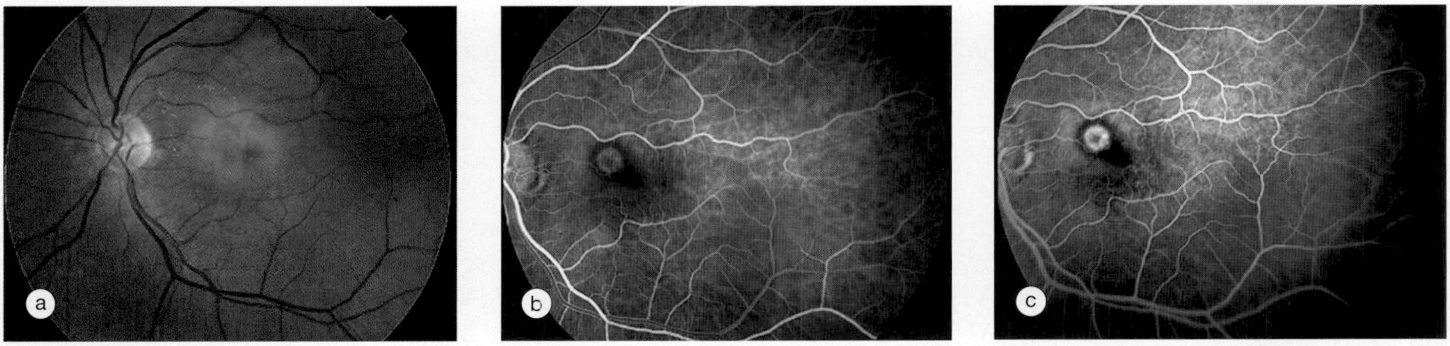

Fig. 13.17 Small classic extrafoveal CNV. **(a)** Shallow serous macular elevation associated with a few peripheral hard exudates. **(b)** FA arteriovenous phase shows hyperfluorescence that is more than 200 μm from the centre of the FAZ. **(c)** Early venous phase shows more intense hyperfluorescence.

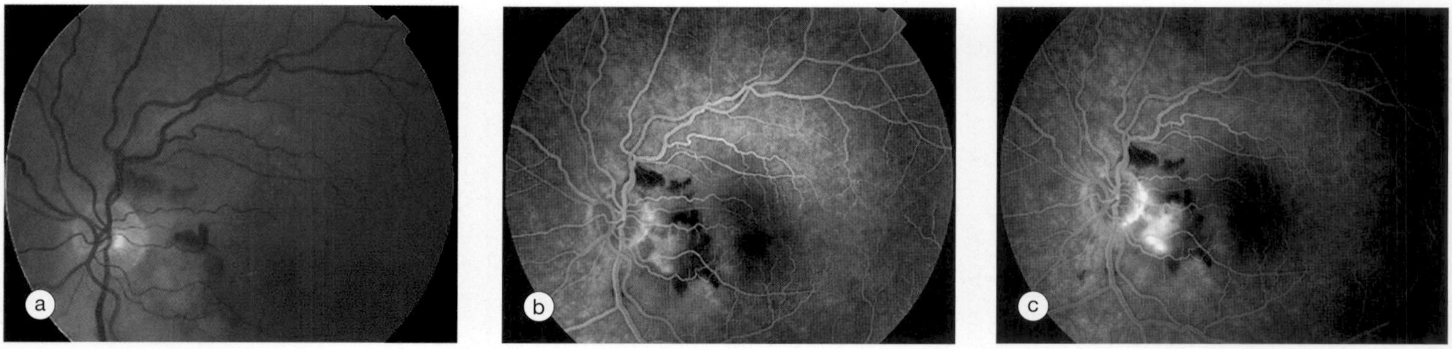

■ **Fig. 13.18** Classic juxtapapillary CNV. **(a)** Blood between the macula and disc. **(b)** FA early venous phase shows blockage by blood and an area of hyperfluorescence at the temporal edge of the disc. **(c)** Late venous phase shows more intense hyperfluorescence.

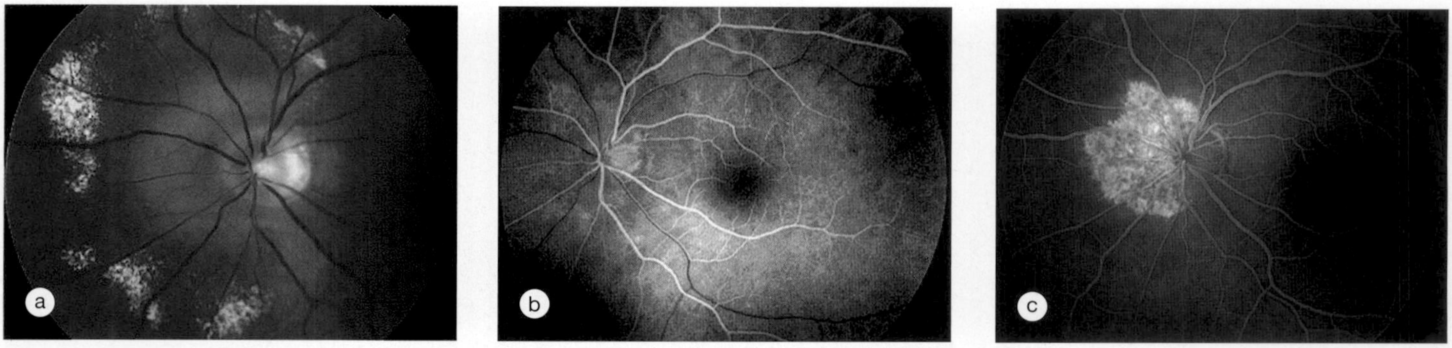

■ **Fig. 13.19** Large classic juxtapapillary CNV. **(a)** Serous retinal elevation and hard exudates nasal to the disc. **(b)** FA arteriovenous phase shows very early lacy juxtapapillary hyperfluorescence. **(c)** Late phases show increasing hyperfluorescence.

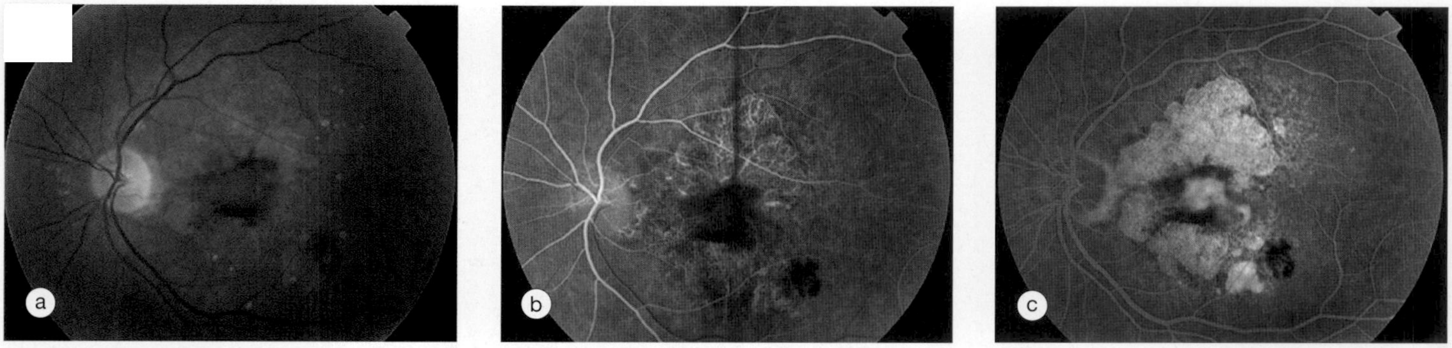

■ **Fig. 13.20** Combined dry AMD and CNV. **(a)** Geographic atrophy and haemorrhage at the macula. **(b)** FA arteriovenous phase shows unmasking of larger choroidal vessels at the posterior pole due to RPE atrophy; the macula shows hypofluorescence due to blockage by blood with very early lacy central hyperfluorescence at the fovea. **(c)** Late venous phase shows marked hyperfluorescence at the fovea.

Occult CNV

Occult CNV is a poorly defined membrane with imprecise features during early phase FA.

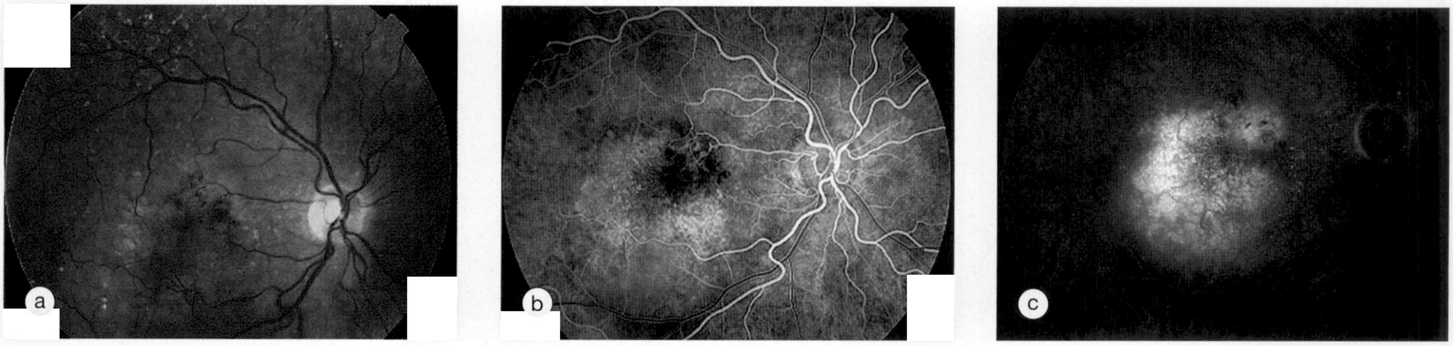

■ **Fig. 13.21** **(a)** Fluid and spotty haemorrhage at the macula. **(b)** FA arteriovenous phase shows diffuse hyperfluorescence without precise features. **(c)** Late phases show increasing diffuse hyperfluorescence.

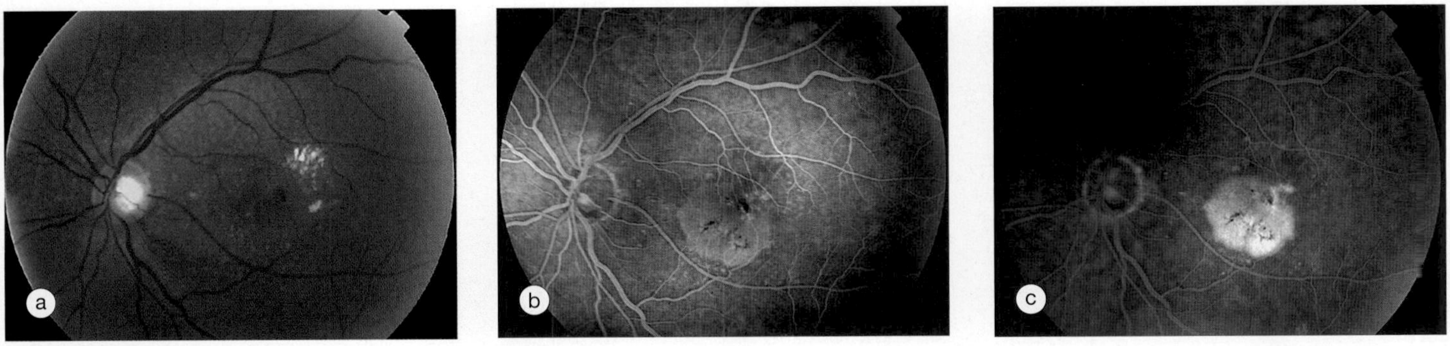

■ **Fig. 13.22** **(a)** PED and a few small hard exudates at its temporal edge suggestive of chronic leakage from CNV. **(b, c)** FA shows a round area of hyperfluorescence that increases in intensity but not in dimension and a smaller area of hyperfluorescence at the temporal edge of the PED that could possible represent occult CNV.

Fibrovascular PED

This is a combination of CNV and PED.

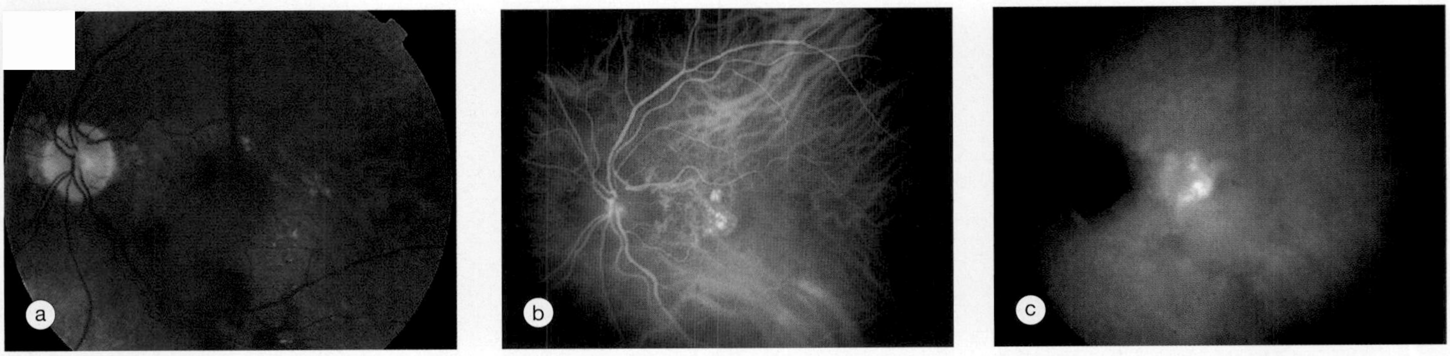

■ **Fig. 13.23** **(a)** PED with blood inferiorly. **(b)** ICG shows hypofluorescence of PED and two small areas of hyperfluorescence (hot spots) from CNV underlying the PED. **(c)** Late phase shows extension of hyperfluorescence due to leakage.

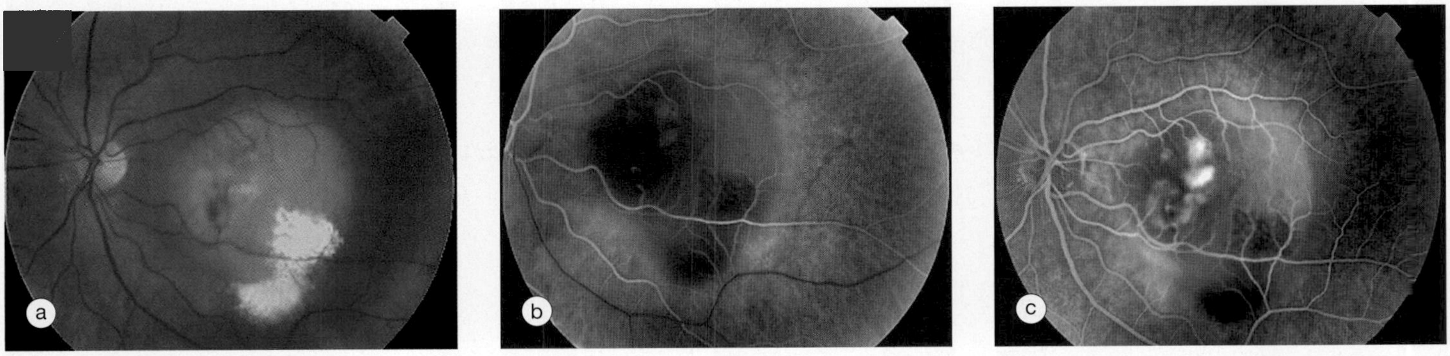

■ **Fig. 13.24** **(a)** PED with a plaque of subretinal exudate due to chronic leakage from CNV. **(b)** FA arteriovenous phase shows blockage corresponding to the plaque and two small areas of subtle hyperfluorescence superonasal to the fovea due to CNV. **(c)** Venous phase shows increase in hyperfluorescence of the CNV and PED.

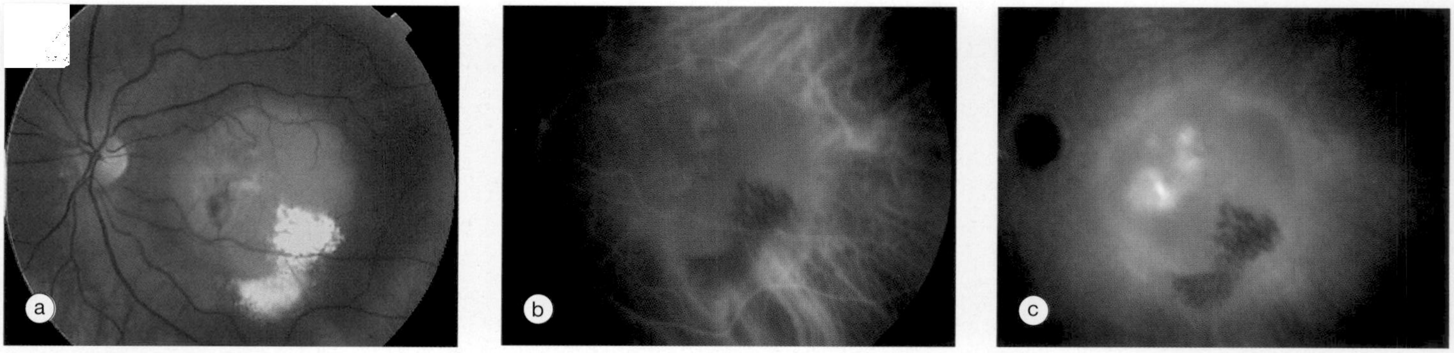

Fig. 13.25 **(a)** Same eye as in Fig. 13.24. **(b, c)** ICG shows blockage by hard exudate, hyperfluorescence of CNV and hypofluorescence of PED.

Advanced disease

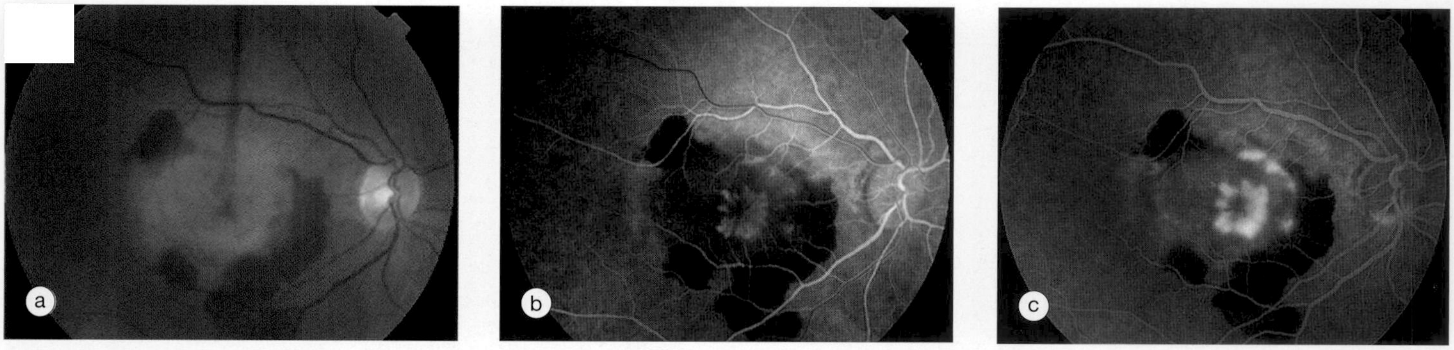

Fig. 13.26 **(a)** Subretinal haemorrhage from CNV. (**b, c**) FA shows blockage by blood and hyperfluorescence of CNV.

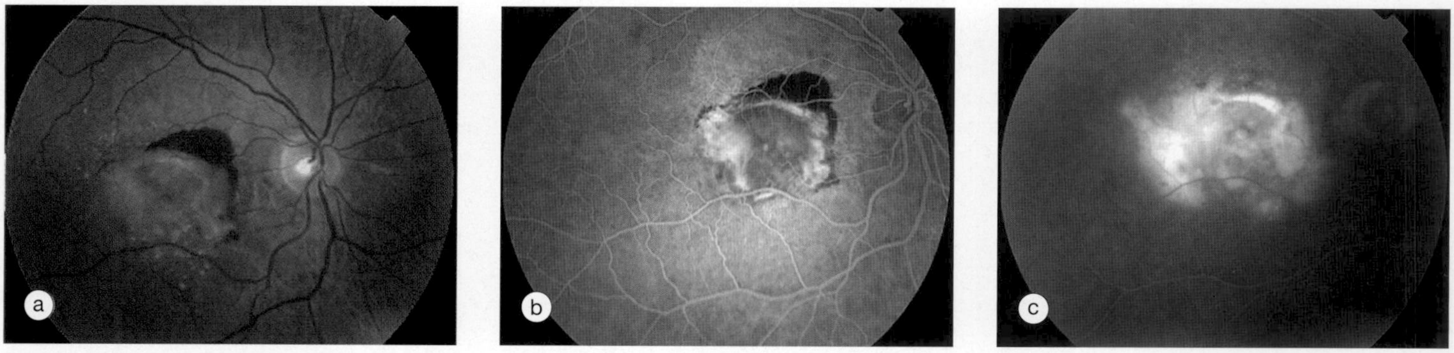

Fig. 13.27 **(a)** Subretinal scarring with adjacent haemorrhage. (**b, c**) FA shows blockage by blood and progressive hyperfluorescence of scar tissue.

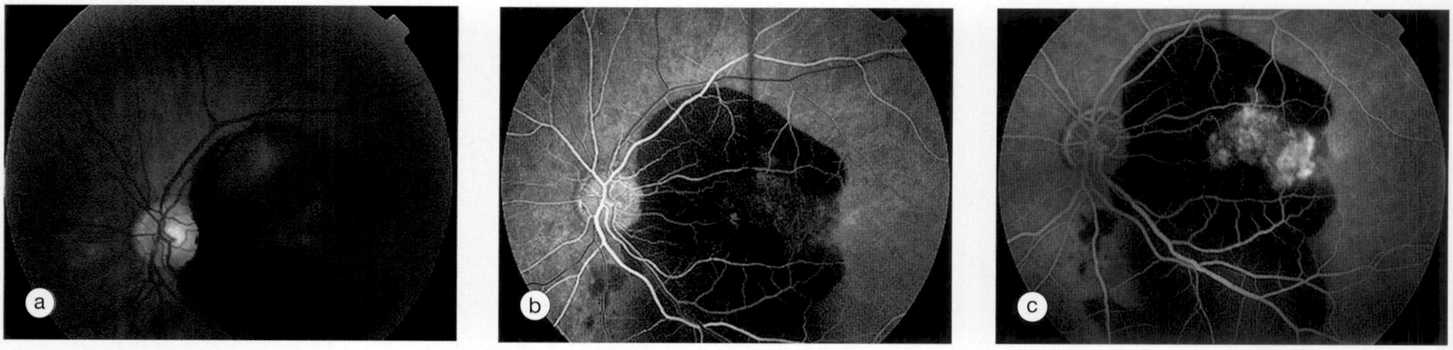

Fig. 13.28 **(a)** Extensive subretinal haemorrhage. (**b, c**) FA shows blockage by blood and hyperfluorescence of scar tissue.

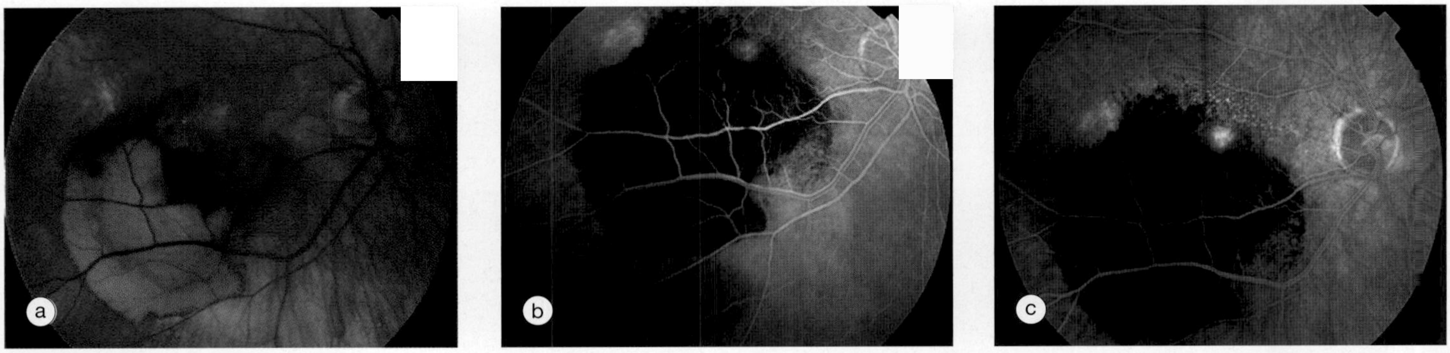

■ **Fig. 13.29** **(a)** Haemorrhagic PED caused by rupture of blood vessels within the CNV appears as a dark elevated mound. **(b, c)** FA shows blockage of background choroidal fluorescence and two hypofluorescent spots above the haemorrhage.

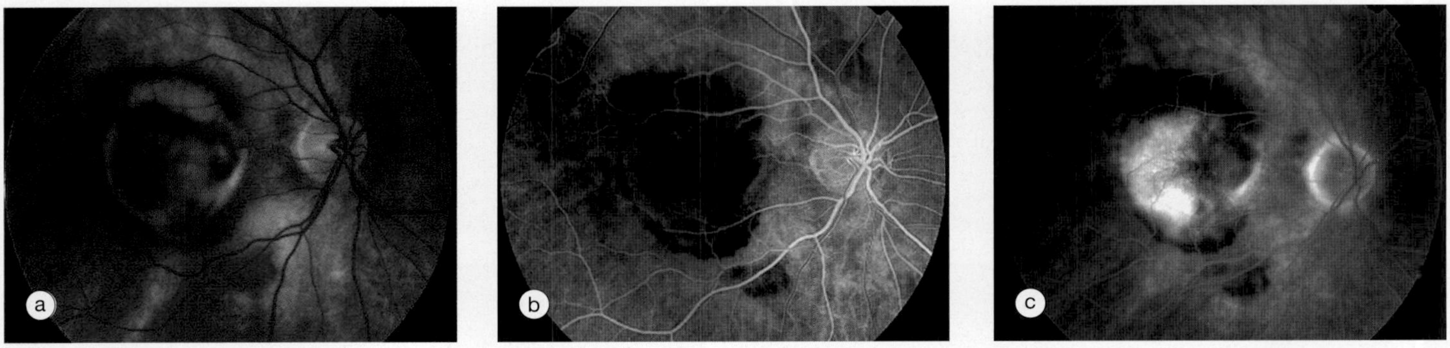

■ **Fig. 13.30** **(a)** Haemorrhagic PED and severe subretinal (disciform) scarring. **(b)** FA arteriovenous phase shows blockage by blood. **(c)** Late phase shows staining of scar tissue.

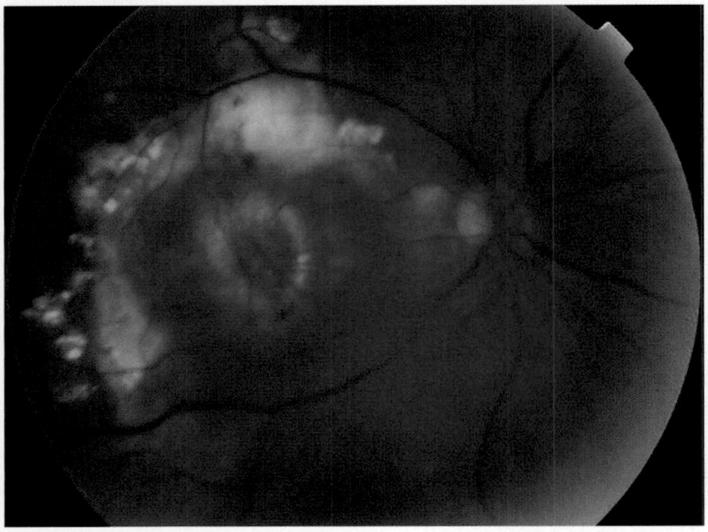

■ **Fig. 13.31** Massive exudation, both intra- and subretinal, may develop in some eyes with disciform scars as a result of chronic leakage from CNV.

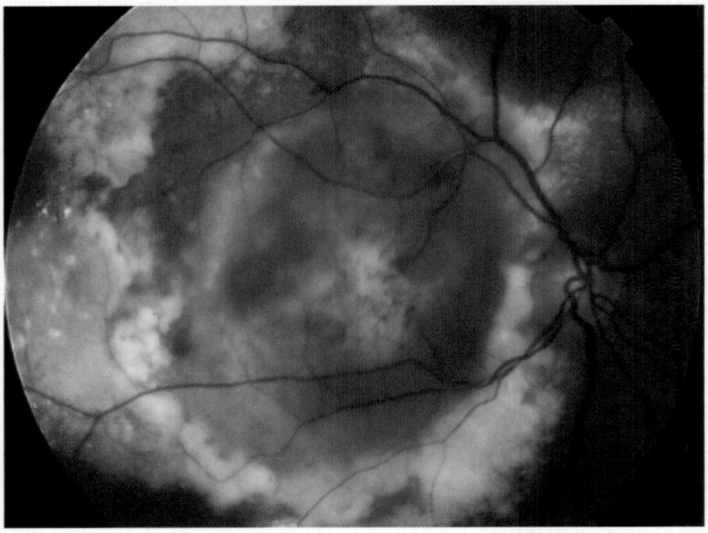

■ **Fig. 13.32** The subretinal fluid may spread beyond the macula and destroy peripheral vision.

Retinal angiomatous proliferation (RAP)

RAP is a variant of exudative AMD which is characterised by fronds of intraretinal neovascularisation rather than CNV.

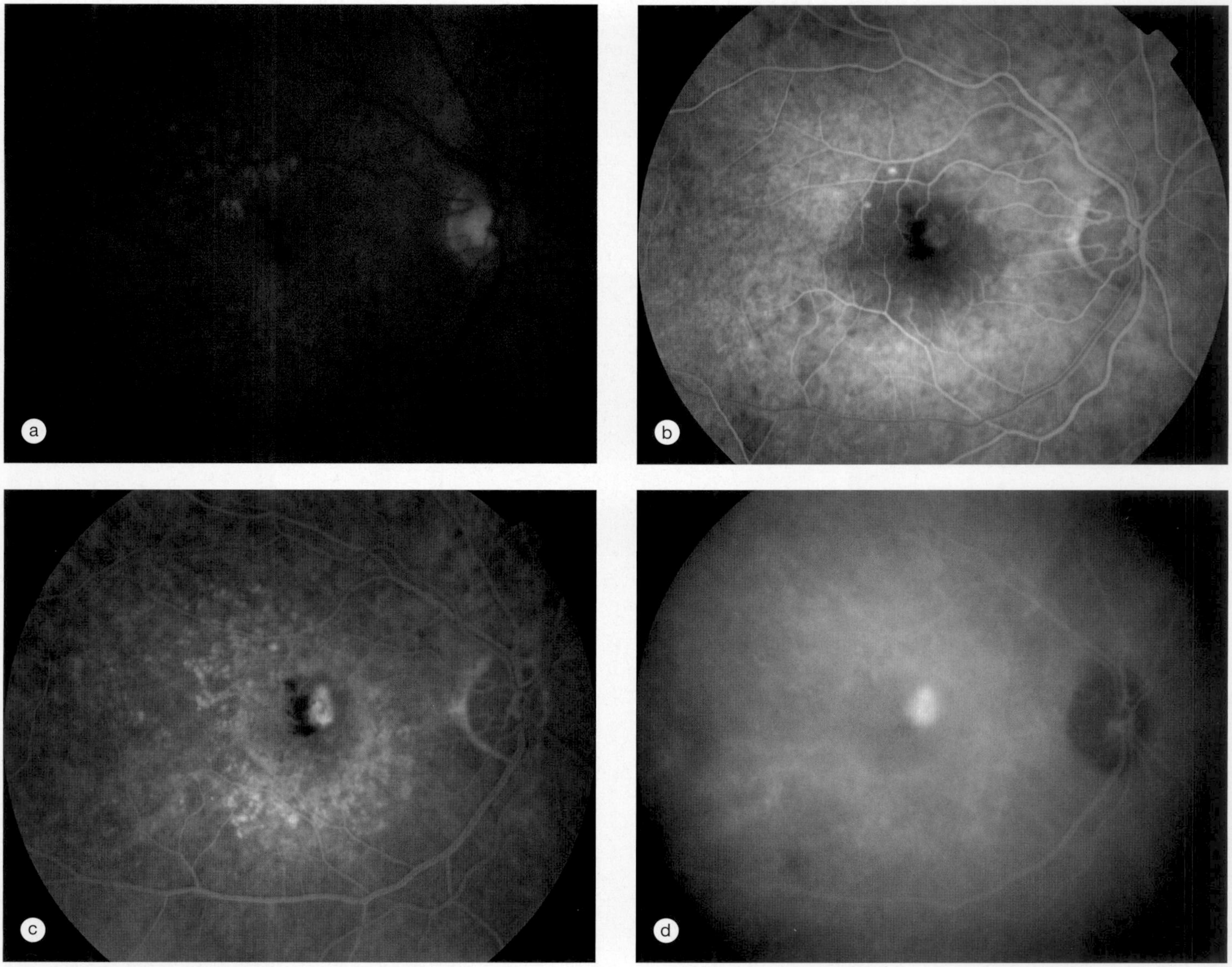

Fig. 13.33 **(a)** Drusen associated with a small intraretinal haemorrhage at the fovea. **(b)** FA early venous phase shows faint hyperfluorescence at the fovea due to a small frond of intraretinal neovascularisation. **(b)** Late venous phase shows more intense hyperfluorescence with adjacent blockage by blood. **(d)** ICG shows hyperfluorescence of the frond. (Courtesy of Moorfields Eye Hospital.)

MISCELLANEOUS MACULAR DISORDERS

Polypoidal choroidal vasculopathy (PCV)

PCV is characterised by a delicate network of dilated inner choroidal vessels with multiple terminal aneurysmal protuberances that have a polypoidal configuration.

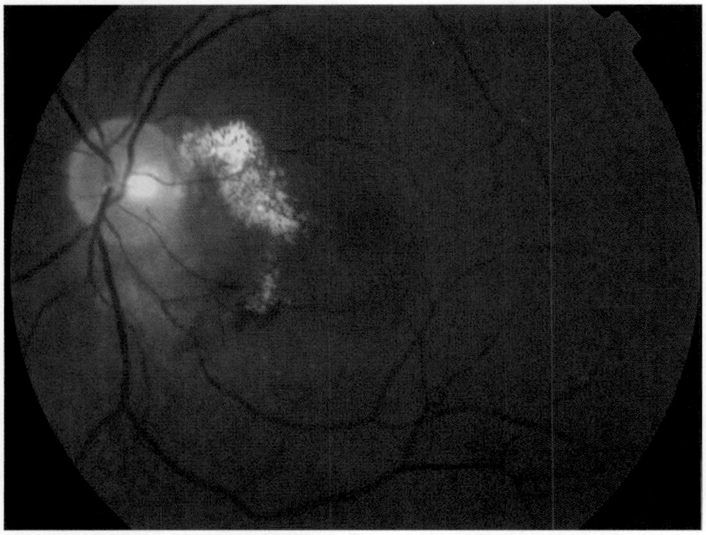

■ **Fig. 13.34** Exudative pattern PCV is characterised by serous PED and serous retinal detachment associated with intraretinal lipid deposits in the macula. (Courtesy of Moorfields Eye Hospital.)

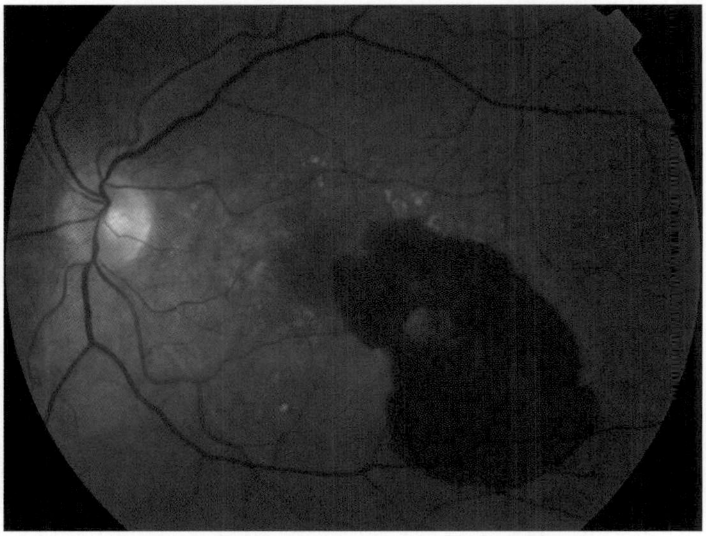

■ **Fig. 13.35** Haemorrhagic pattern is characterised by haemorrhagic PED and subretinal haemorrhage in the macula. (Courtesy of Moorfields Eye Hospital.)

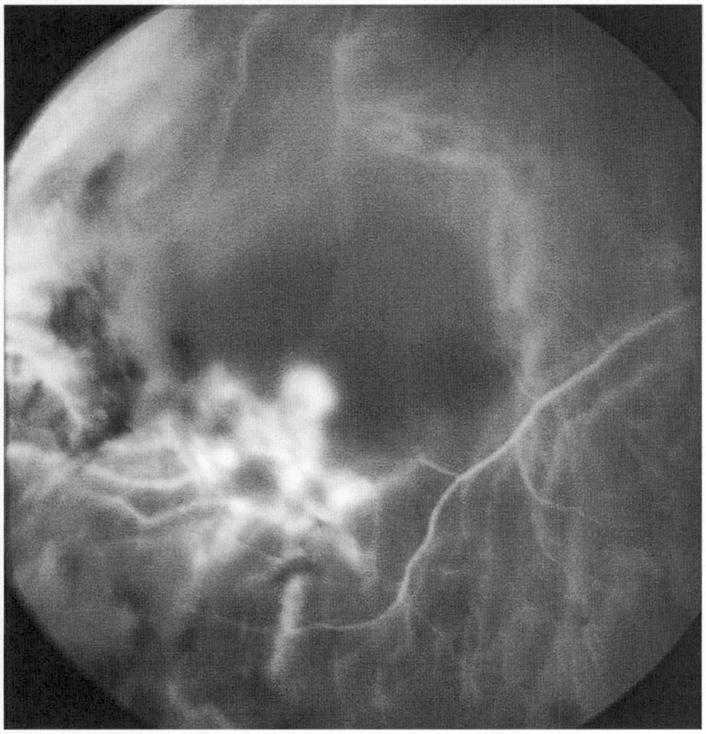

■ **Fig. 13.36** ICG shows a branching vascular network from the choroidal circulation with polypoidal and aneurysmal dilatations at the terminals of the branching vessels that fill slowly and then leak intensely. (Courtesy of V. Tanner.)

Age-related macular hole

Macular hole is a relatively common cause of loss of central vision in elderly patients.

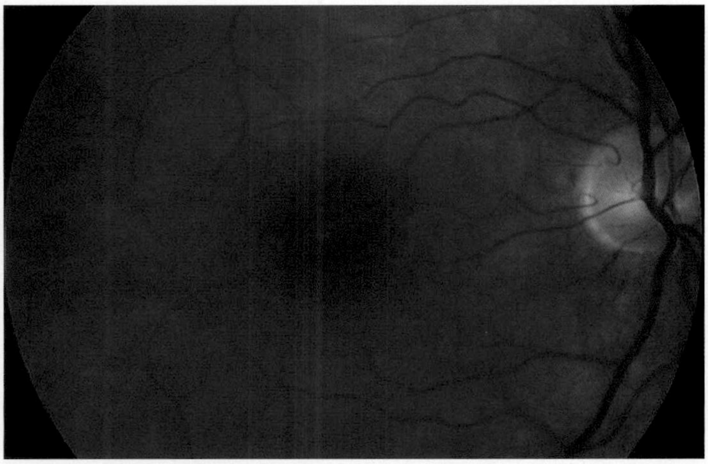

Fig. 13.37 Impending macular hole (stage 1a) is characterised by a yellow spot at the foveola with loss at the foveolar reflex which represents a foveal cyst. Stage 1b (occult) macular hole is characterised by a yellow ring with a bridging interface of vitreous cortex.

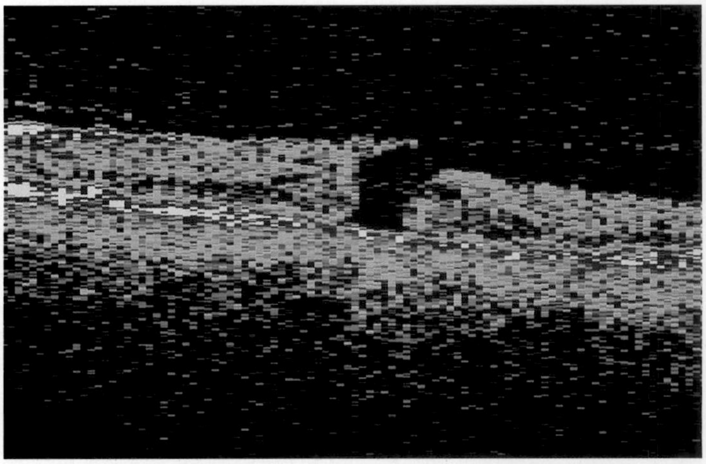

Fig. 13.38 Early full-thickness macular hole (FTMH) (stage 2) is characterised by an eccentric, oval, crescentic or horseshoe-shaped retinal defect less than 400 μm in diameter with or without an overlying prefoveal opacity (pseudo-operculum). (Courtesy of V. Tanner.)

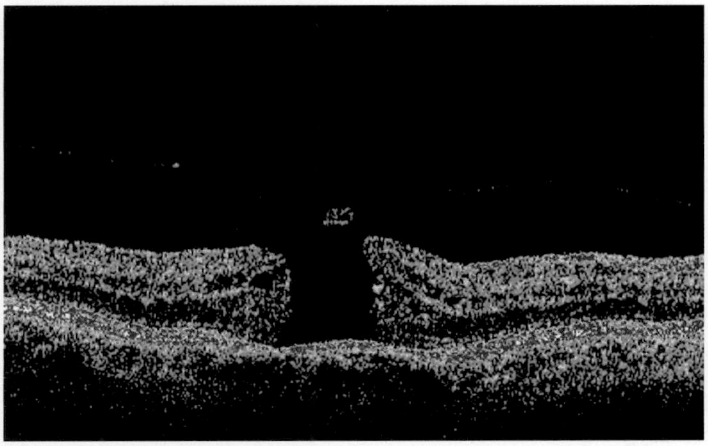

Fig. 13.39 Established FTMH (stage 3) is characterised by a round retinal defect with an attached posterior vitreous face with or without an overlying pseudo-operculum. (Courtesy of C. Barry.)

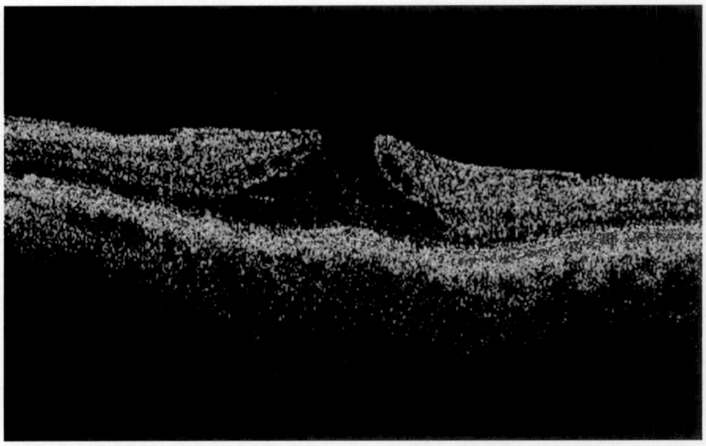

Fig. 13.40 Stage 4 FTMH is characterised by a round retinal defect surrounded by a cuff of subretinal fluid and associated with complete separation of the posterior vitreous. (Courtesy of C. Barry.)

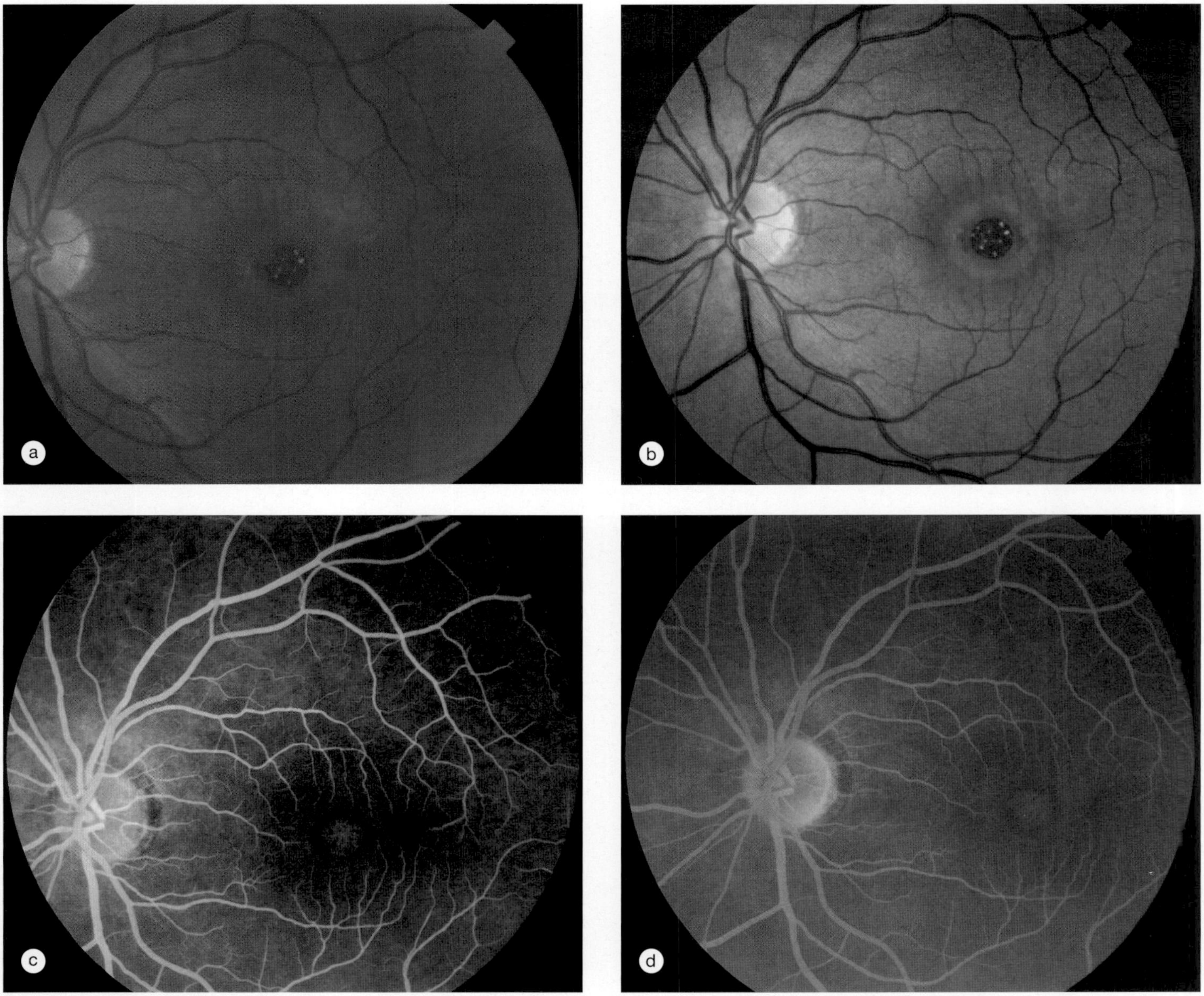

■ **Fig. 13.41 (a)** Stage 4 FTMH with a small cuff of surrounding subretinal fluid and tiny yellowish deposits at the base of the crater. **(b)** Red-free image. **(c, d)** FA shows a round area of hyperfluorescence resulting from unmasking of background choroidal fluorescence caused by a defect in xanthophyll due to centrifugal displacement. (Courtesy of A. Frohlichstein.)

Central serous retinopathy (CSR)

CSR, also known as central serous chorioretinopathy, is a sporadic, self-limited disease typically affecting young or middle-aged men with type A personality.

Typical CSR

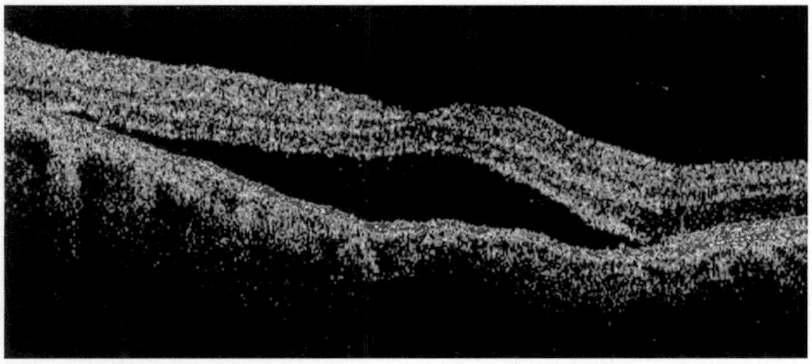

Fig. 13.42 OCT shows localised separation of the sensory retina from the RPE at the macula. (Courtesy of C. Barry.)

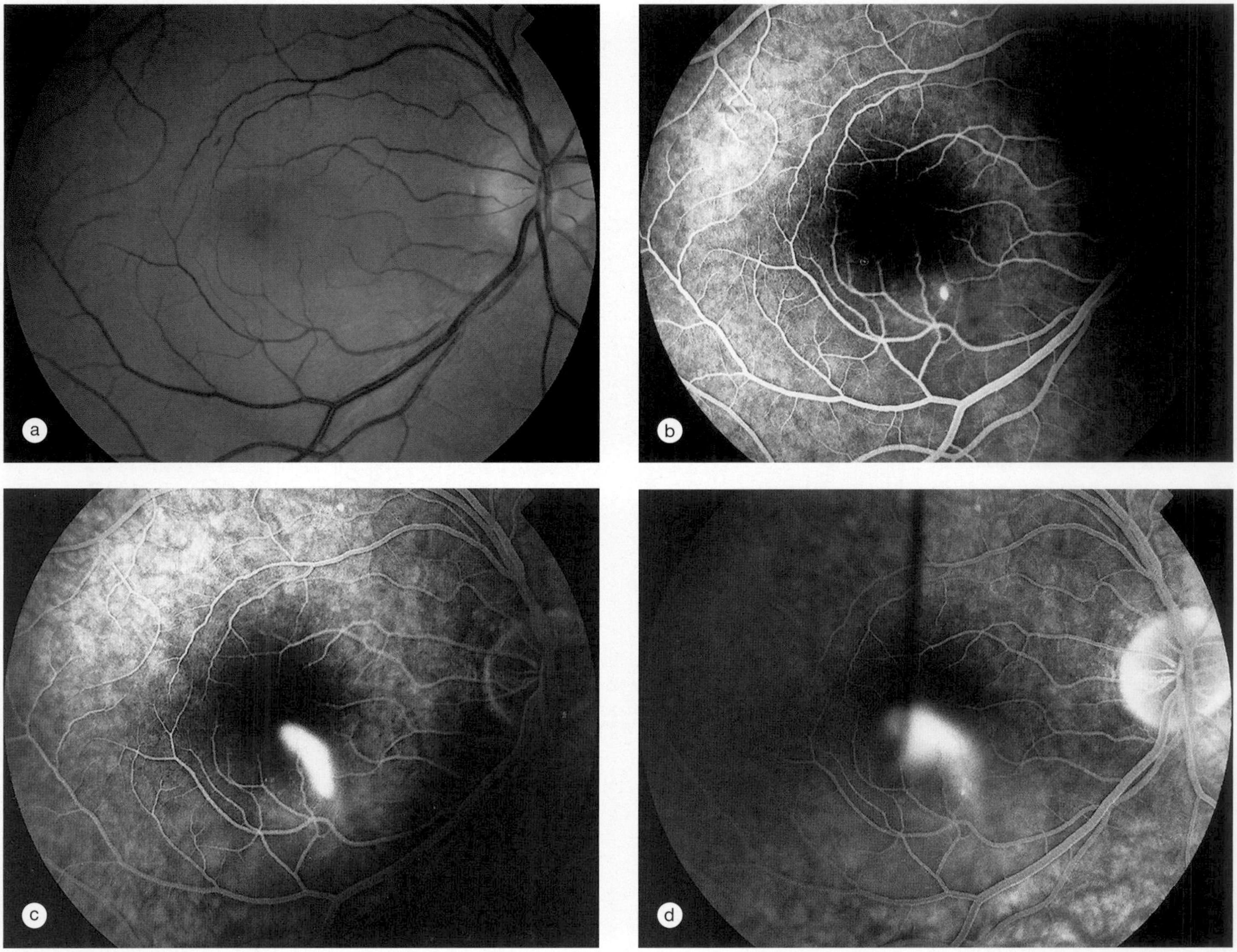

Fig. 13.43 CSR. **(a)** Oval elevation of the sensory retina at the macula. **(b)** FA early venous phase shows a small hyperfluorescent spot due to leakage of dye through the RPE. **(c)** During the late venous phase, fluorescein passes into the subretinal space and ascends vertically (like a smoke stack) from the point of leakage. **(d)** The dye then spreads laterally, taking on a 'mushroom' or 'umbrella' configuration until the entire area of detachment is filled (smoke-stack appearance). (Courtesy of S. Milewski.)

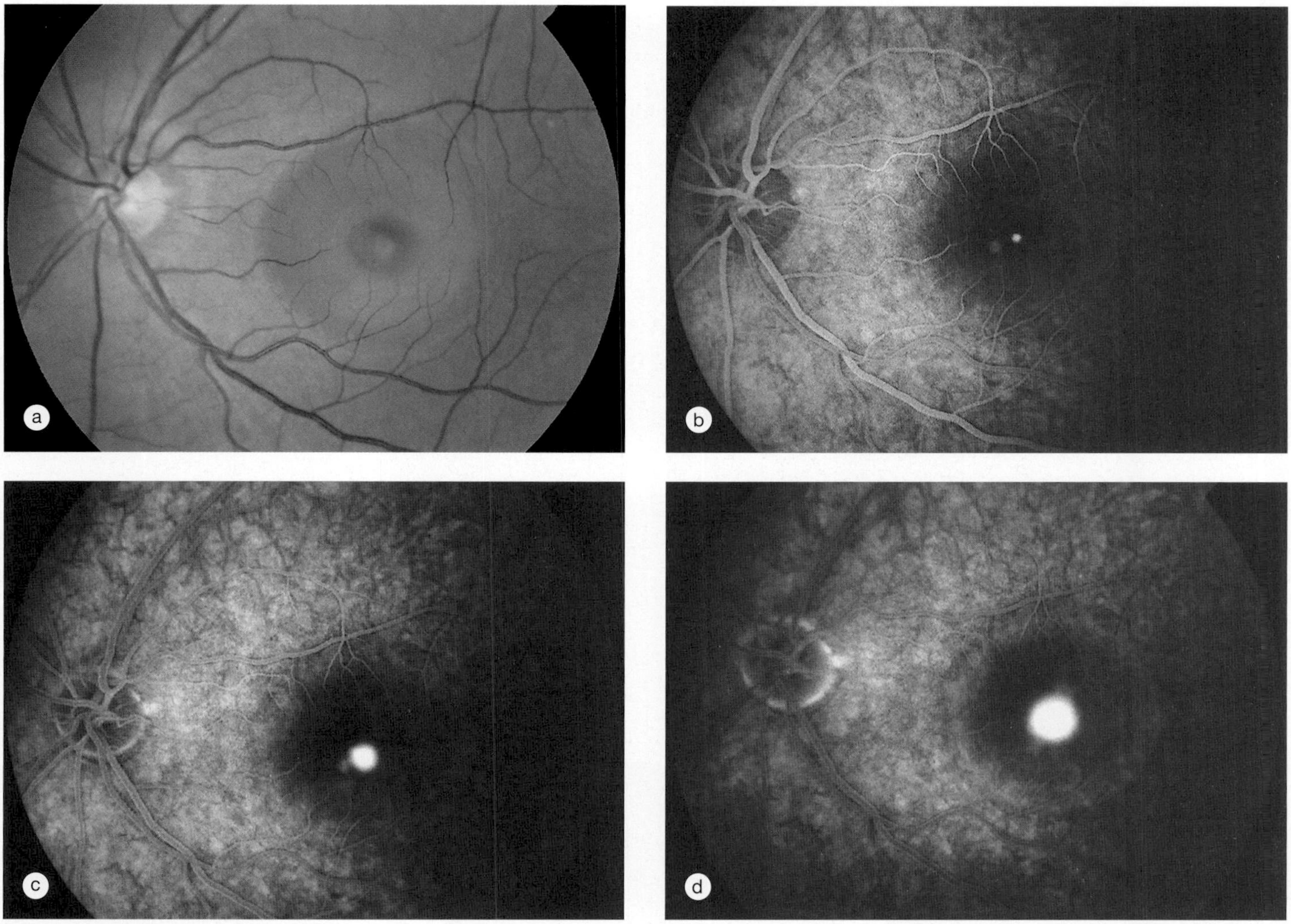

■ **Fig. 13.44** **(a)** CSR. **(b)** FA venous phase shows a small hyperfluorescent spot. **(c, d)** The spot gradually enlarges centrifugally until the entire detachment is filled (ink-blot appearance). (Courtesy of S. Milewski.)

Chronic CSR

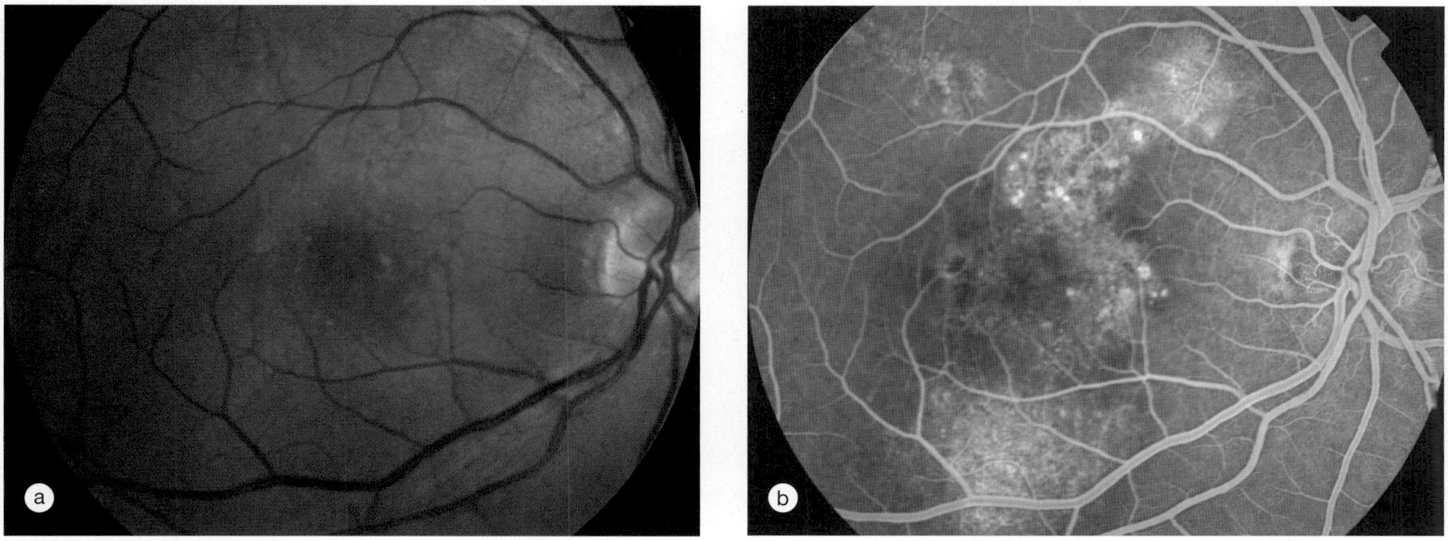

■ **Fig. 13.45** **(a)** Mild diffuse RPE changes. **(b)** FA shows granular hyperfluorescence. (Courtesy of Moorfields Eye Hospital.)

Cystoid macular oedema (CMO)

CMO is the result of accumulation of fluid in the outer plexiform and inner nuclear layers of the retina with the formation of fluid-filled-cyst-like changes.

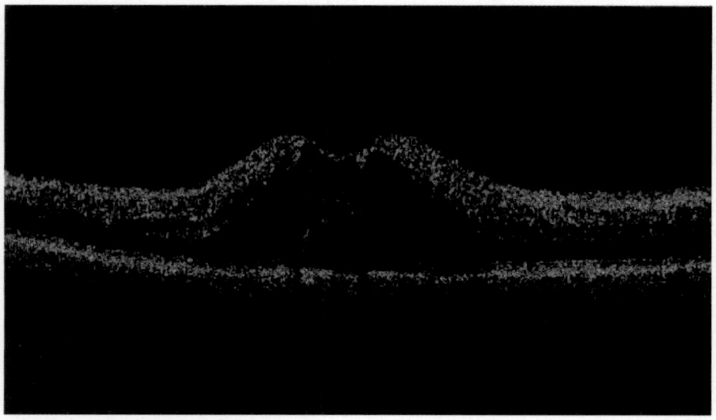

■ **Fig. 13.46** OCT of CMO.

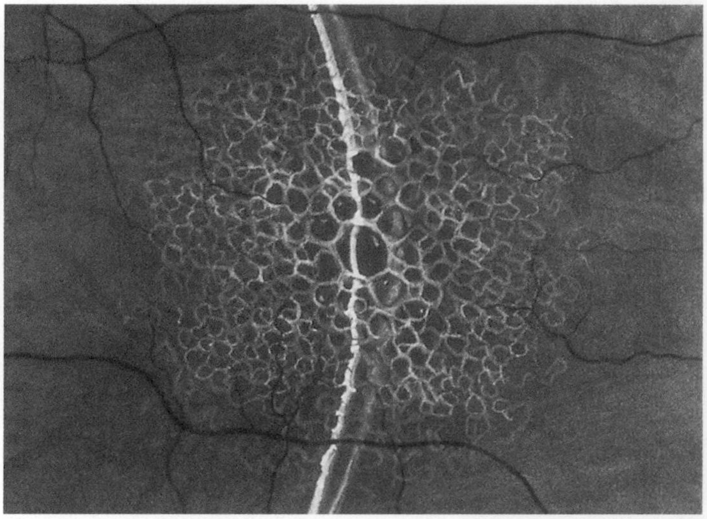

■ **Fig. 13.47** Loss of the foveal depression, thickening of the retina and multiple cystoid areas in the sensory retina.

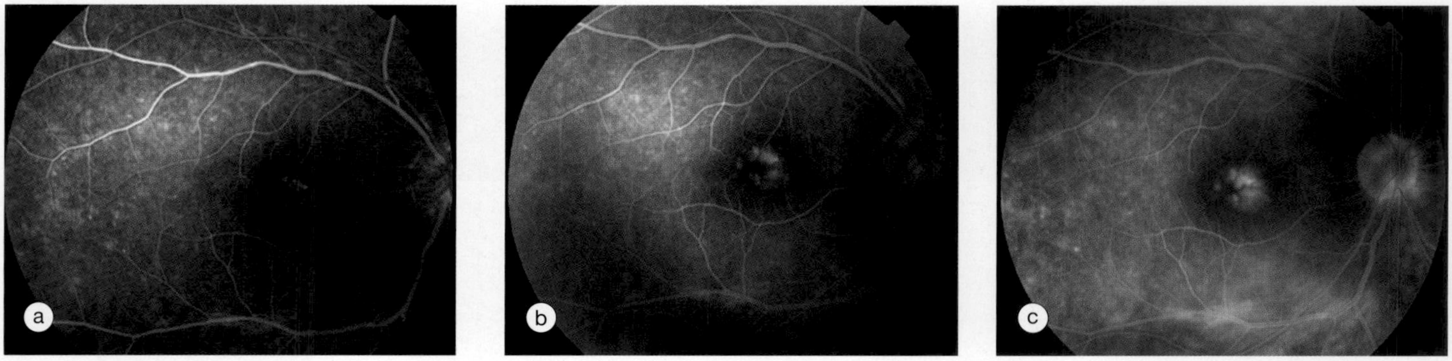

■ **Fig. 13.48** Mild CMO. **(a)** FA early venous phase shows small hyperfluorescent spots due to early leakage. **(b, c)** Late phase shows increasing hyperfluorescence and coalescence of the focal leaks in a 'flower-petal' pattern caused by accumulation of dye within microcystic spaces in the outer plexiform layer of the retina, with its radial arrangement of fibres about the centre of the foveola (Henle layer).

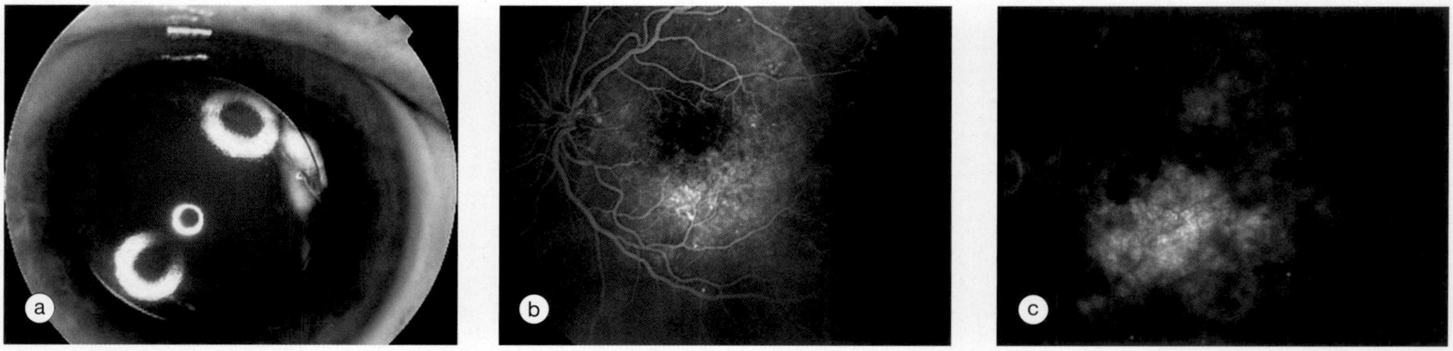

■ **Fig. 13.49** **(a)** Intraocular implant and defect in the posterior capsule resulting from inadvertent capsular rupture during cataract surgery. **(b, c)** Very severe CMO.

Macular epiretinal membrane

Macular epiretinal membrane formation is caused by proliferation of glial tissue at the vitreoretinal interface.

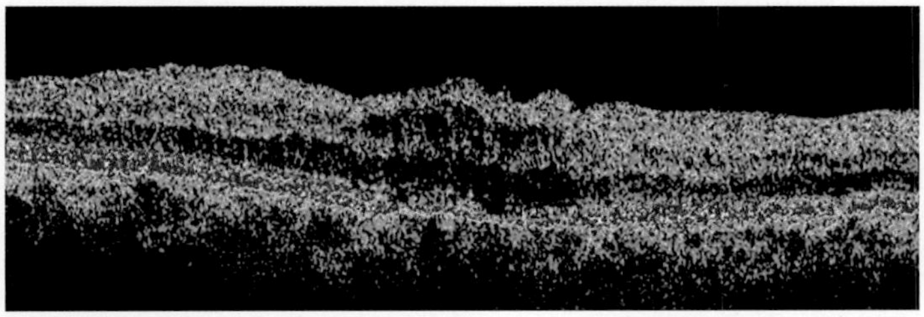

■ **Fig. 13.50** OCT shows contraction of the membrane causing mild puckering of the retinal surface. (Courtesy of C. Barry.)

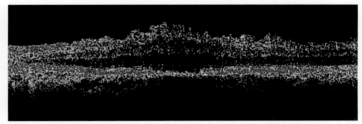

■ **Fig. 13.51** OCT of more severe retinal puckering. (Courtesy of C. Barry.)

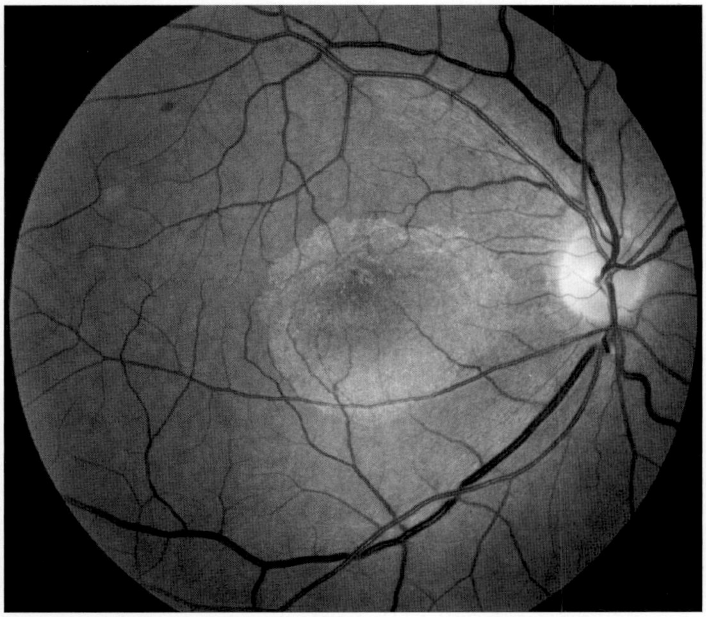

■ **Fig. 13.52** A very mild translucent epimacular membrane (cellophane maculopathy) is best detected by using red-free light. (Courtesy of L. Merin.)

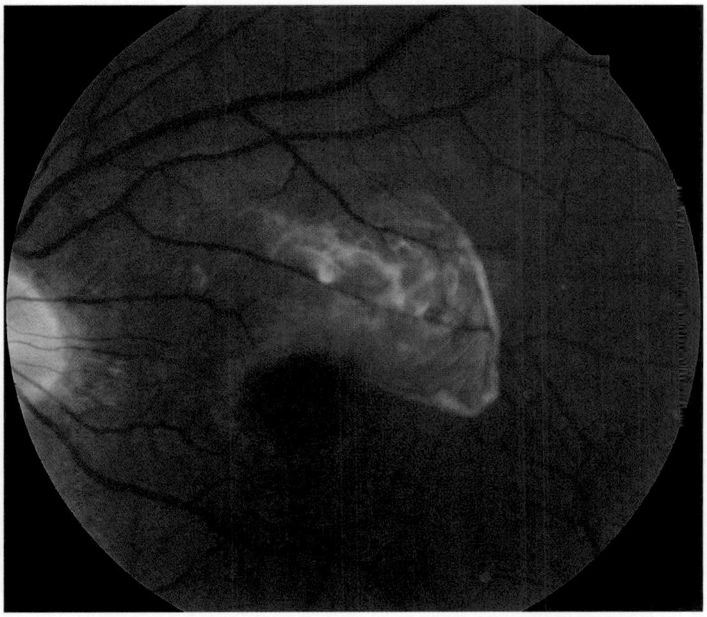

■ **Fig. 13.53** A slightly thicker epimacular membrane with minimal distortion.

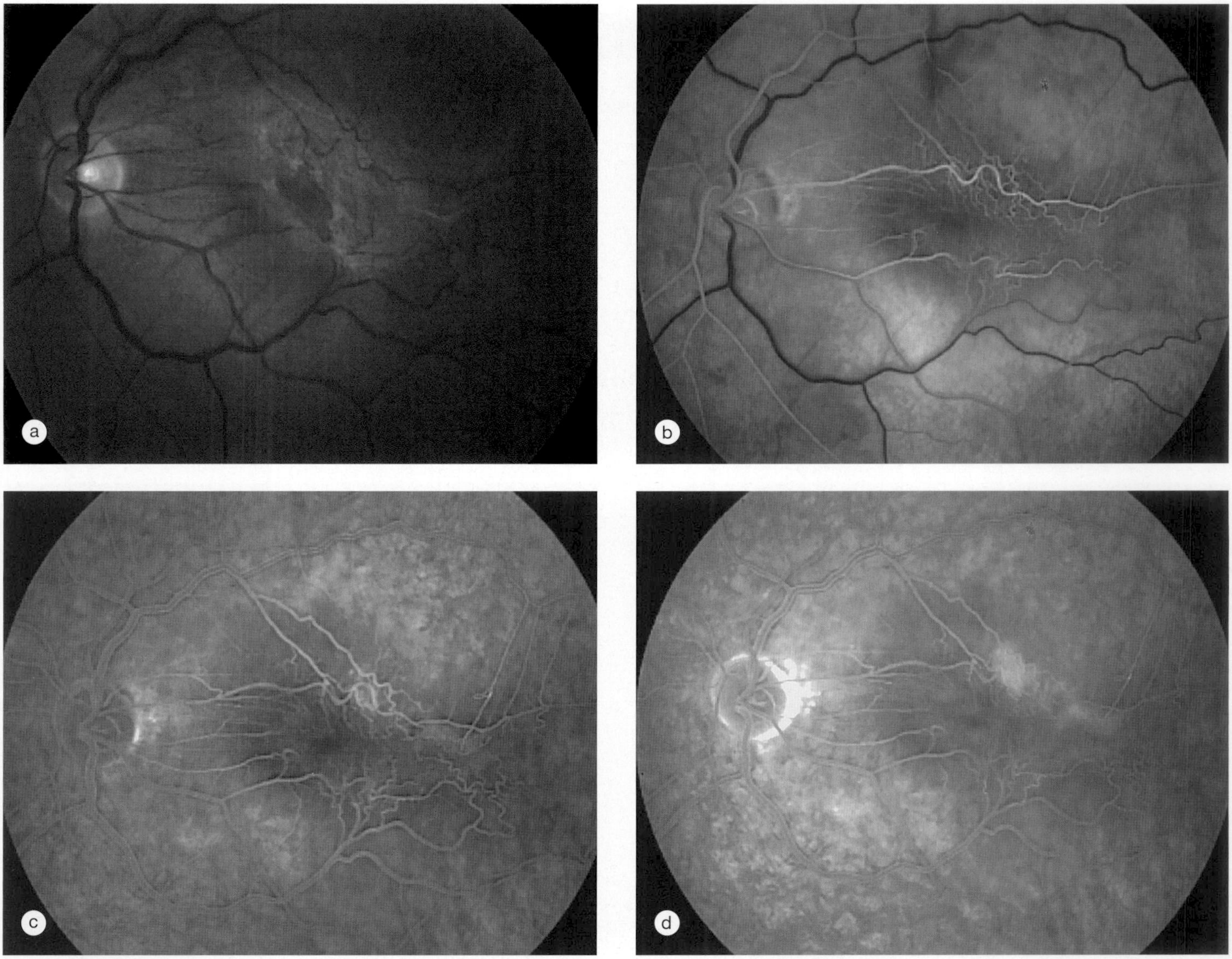

■ **Fig. 13.54** **(a)** Severe epiretinal membrane (macular pucker). **(b)** Arterial phase shows vascular tortuosity at the macula. **(c, d)** Late phase shows hyperfluorescence due to leakage. (Courtesy of S. Milewski.)

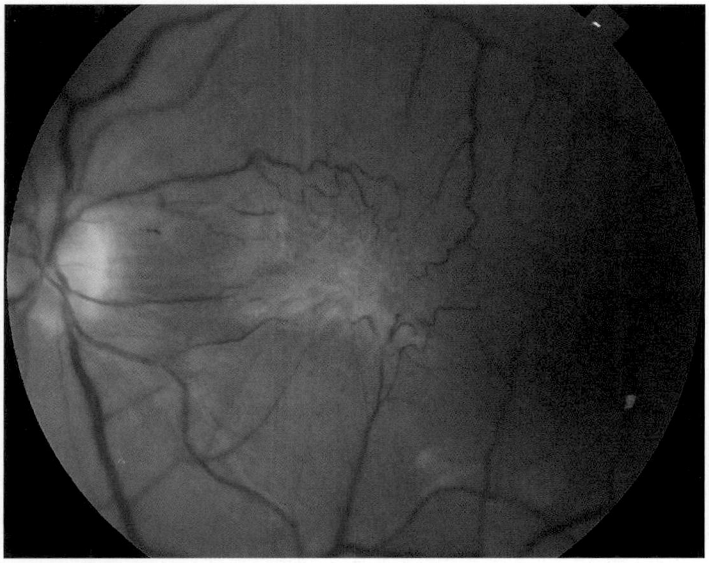

■ **Fig. 13.55** Very severe macular pucker.

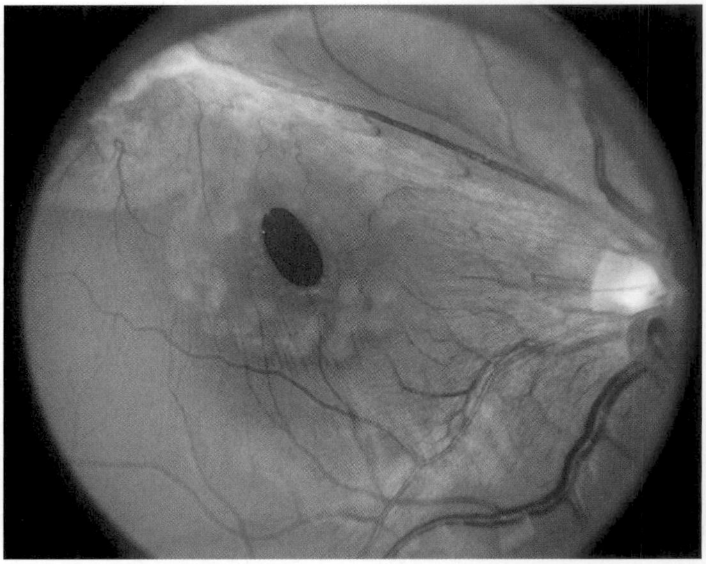

■ **Fig. 13.56** Very dense epiretinal membrane with a macular pseudohole.

Choroidal folds

Choroidal folds are grooves involving the inner choroid, Bruch membrane, RPE and occasionally the outer sensory retina.

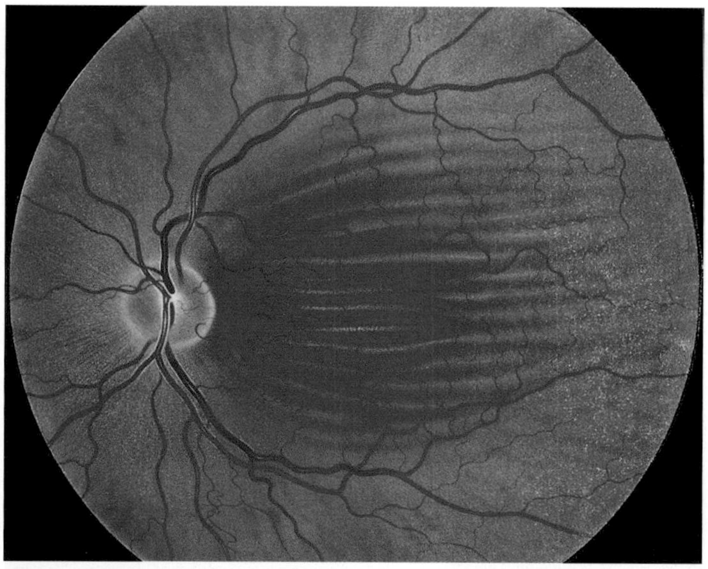

■ **Fig. 13.57** Parallel lines typically located at the posterior pole. The crest (elevated portion) of a fold is yellow and less pigmented as a result of stretching and thinning of the RPE and the trough is darker because of compression of the RPE.

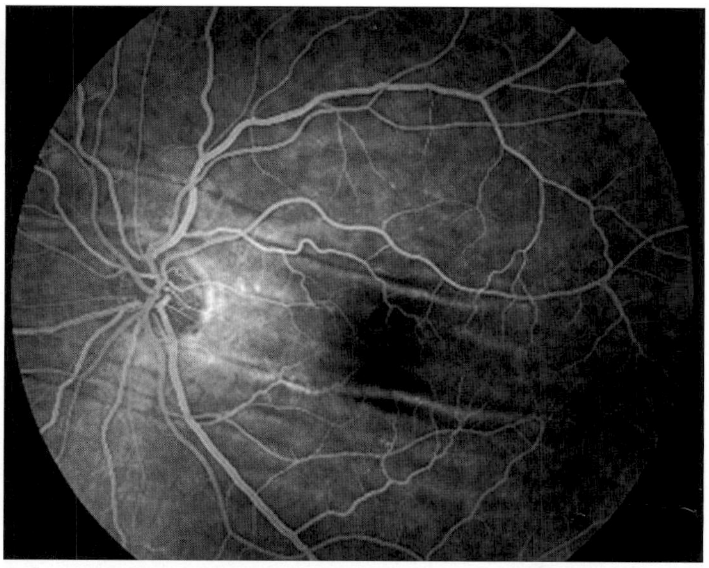

■ **Fig. 13.58** FA shows alternating hyperfluorescent and hypofluorescent streaks. The hyperfluorescence corresponds to the crests as a result of increased background choroidal fluorescence showing through the stretched and thinned RPE and the hypofluorescence corresponds to the troughs due to blockage of choroidal fluorescence by the compressed and thickened RPE.

Hypotony maculopathy

This is most frequently the result of low intraocular pressure following glaucoma filtration surgery.

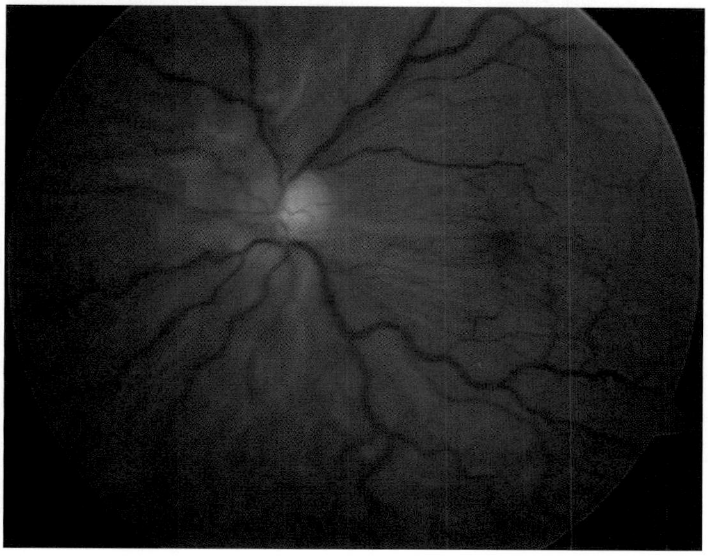

■ **Fig. 13.59** Extensive choroidal folds and macular striae. (Courtesy of P. Gili.)

Maculopathy

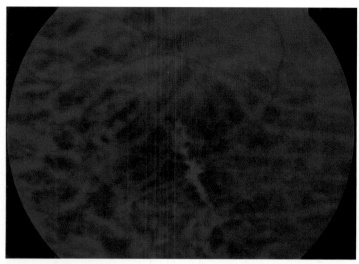

■ **Fig. 13.68** A fine irregular yellow line (lacquer crack) represents a break in Bruch membrane, which predisposes to CNV.

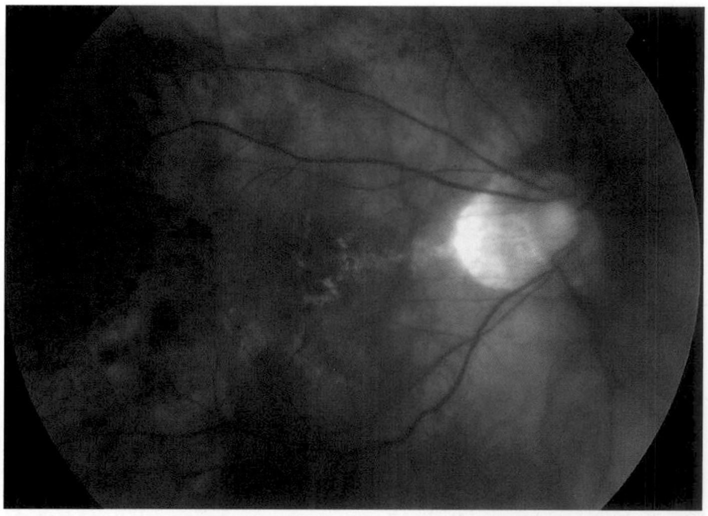

■ **Fig. 13.69** More extensive lacquer cracks.

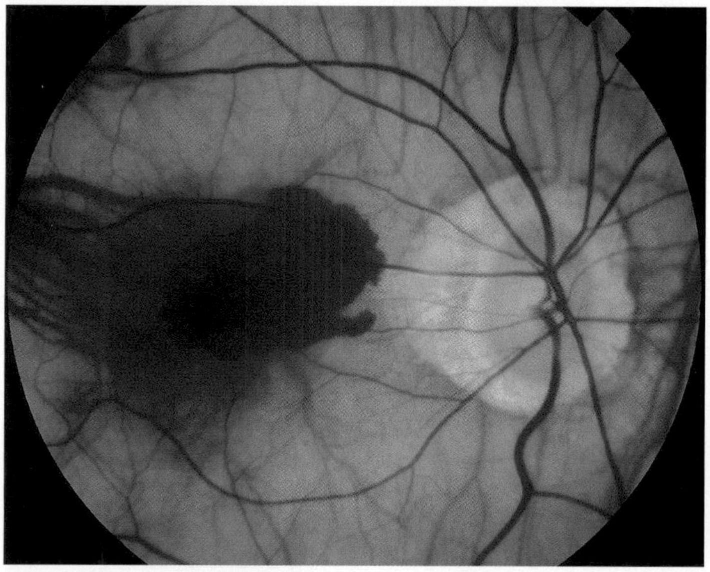

■ **Fig. 13.70** Subretinal haemorrhage at the macula due to CNV, which may be associated with a lacquer crack. (Courtesy of S. Ford and R. Marsh.)

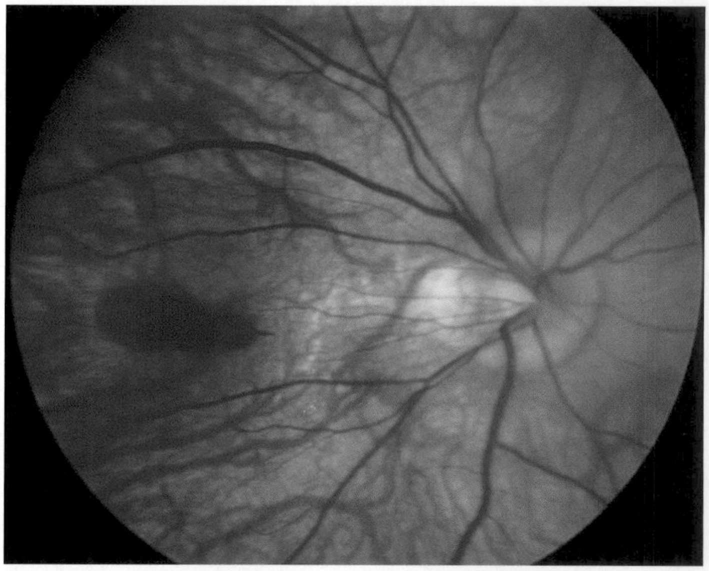

■ **Fig. 13.71** Small subretinal 'coin' haemorrhage may develop from lacquer cracks in the absence of CNV. (Courtesy of P. Morse.)

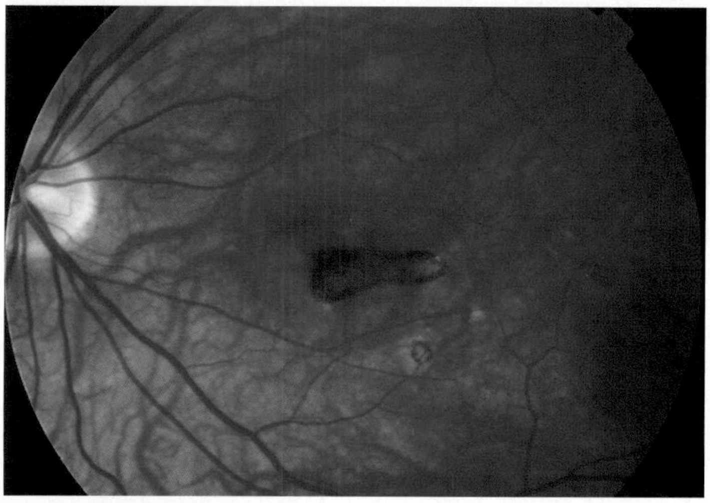

■ **Fig. 13.72** A raised, circular, pigmented lesion (Foerster–Fuchs spot) may develop after a macular haemorrhage has absorbed.

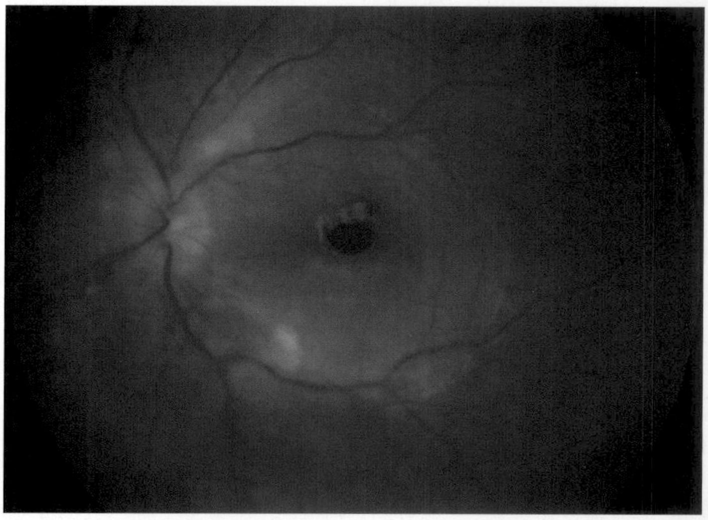

■ **Fig. 13.73** Shallow retinal detachment confined to the posterior pole resulting from a macular hole. (Courtesy of M. Khairallah.)

ANGIOID STREAKS

Angioid streaks are the result of crack-like dehiscences in thickened, calcified and abnormally brittle collagenous and elastic portions of Bruch membrane with secondary changes in the RPE and choriocapillaris.

Signs

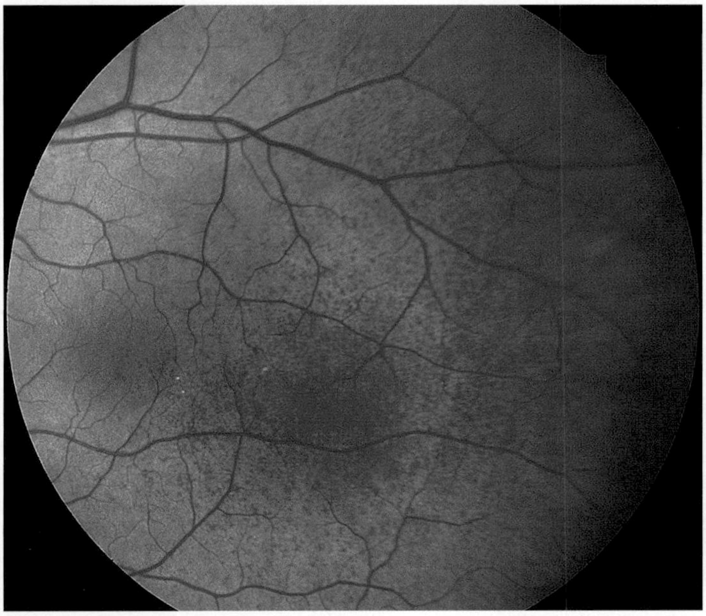

Fig. 13.74 'Peau d'orange' (orange skin), consisting of mottled pigmentation of the posterior pole, may occasionally antedate the appearance of angioid streaks.

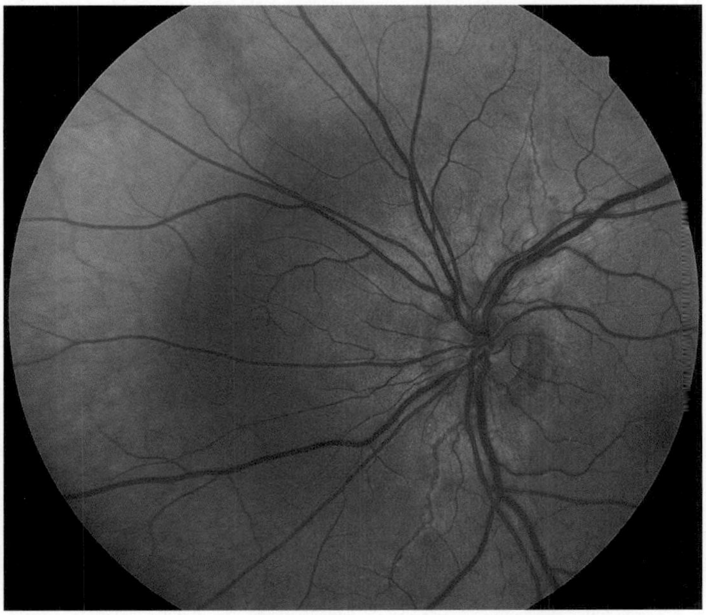

Fig. 13.75 Very subtle angioid streaks inferior to the disc.

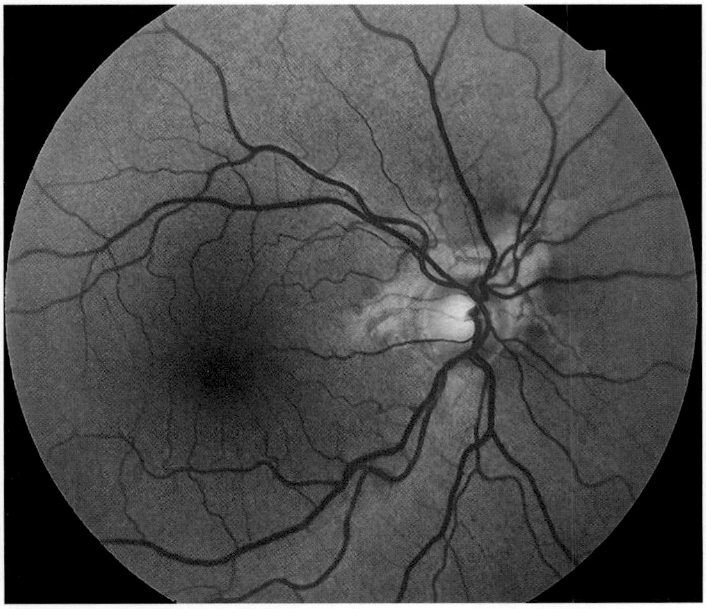

Fig. 13.76 'Peau d'orange' and mild angioid streaks emanating radially from the disc.

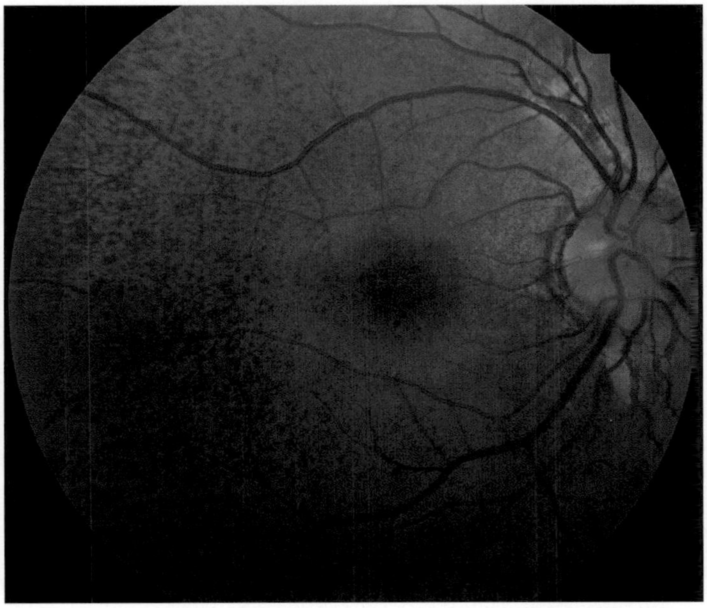

Fig. 13.77 More pigmented 'peau d'orange' and thicker angioid streaks near the optic disc.

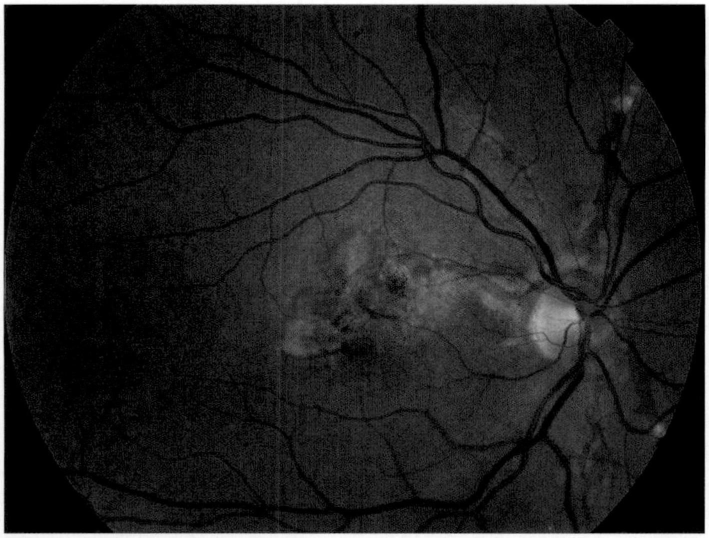

Fig. 13.78 Advanced angioid streaks extending into the fovea.

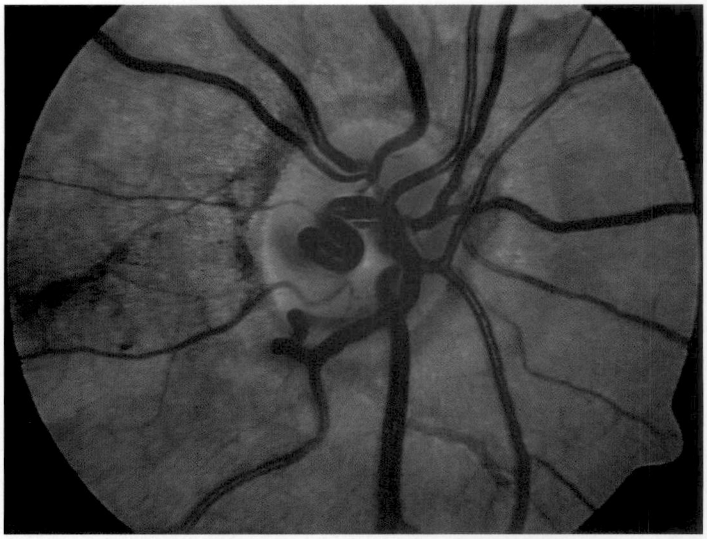

Fig. 13.79 Mild peripapillary angioid streaks associated with a congenital vascular anomaly on the disc. (Courtesy of P. Gili.)

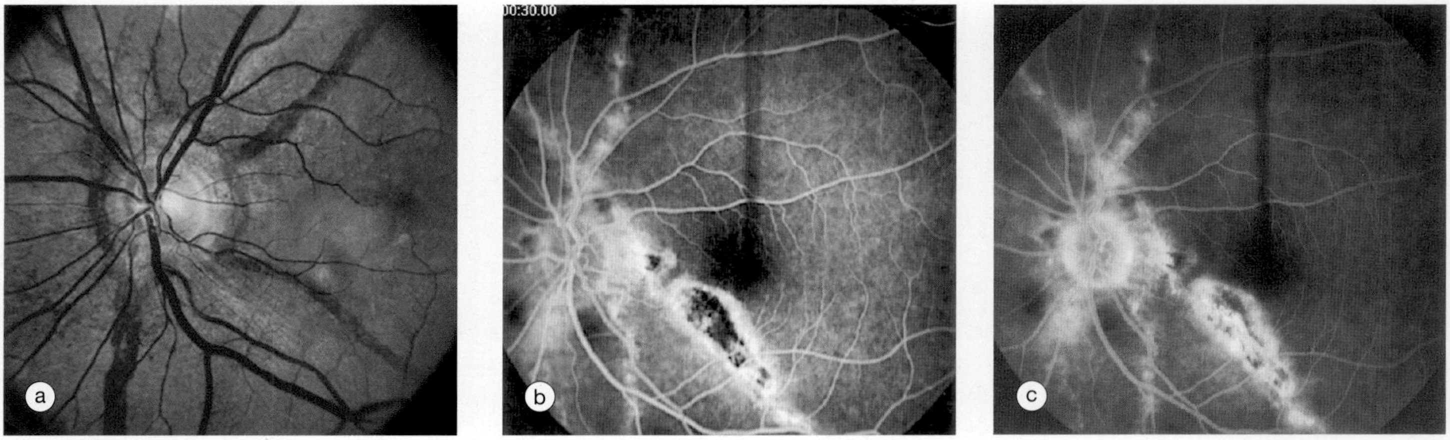

Fig. 13.80 **(a)** Angioid streaks. **(b, c)** FA shows hyperfluorescence caused by RPE window defects over the streaks, associated with variable hypofluorescence corresponding to RPE hyperplasia.

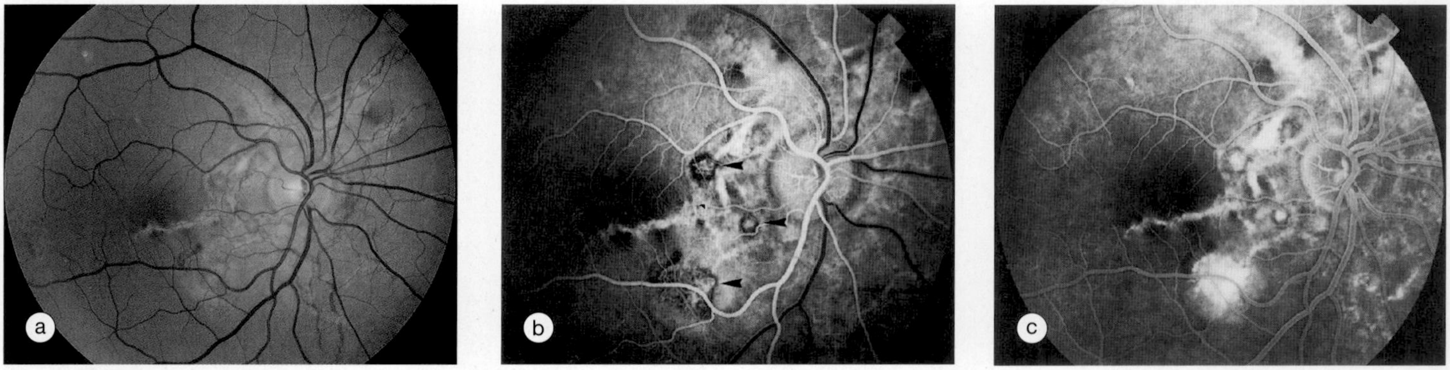

Fig. 13.81 **(a)** Angioid streaks and CNV. **(b)** FA arterial phase shows three round areas of hyperfluorescence (arrows) associated with CNV. **(c)** Venous phase shows more intense hyperfluorescence due to leakage from CNV. (Courtesy of S. Milewski.)

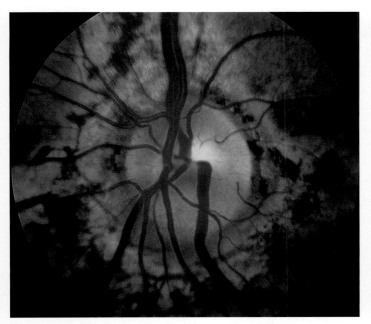

■ **Fig. 13.82** Advanced peripapillary angioid streaks and a large anomalous vein emanating from the disc.

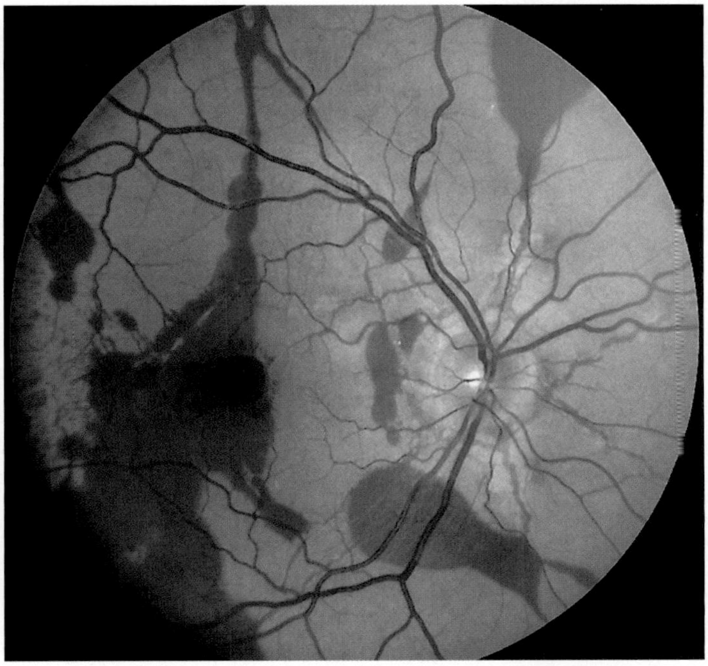

■ **Fig. 13.83** Choroidal rupture may occur following relatively trivial ocular trauma.

Systemic associations

Systemic associations are present in approximately 50% of patients with angioid streaks.

Pseudoxanthoma elasticum

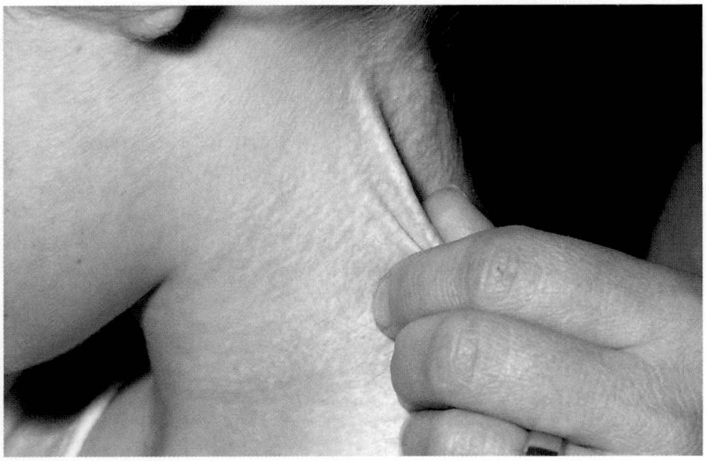

■ **Fig. 13.84** Yellow papules arranged in a linear or reticulate pattern, giving rise to a 'chicken-skin' appearance that is associated with fragility and looseness.

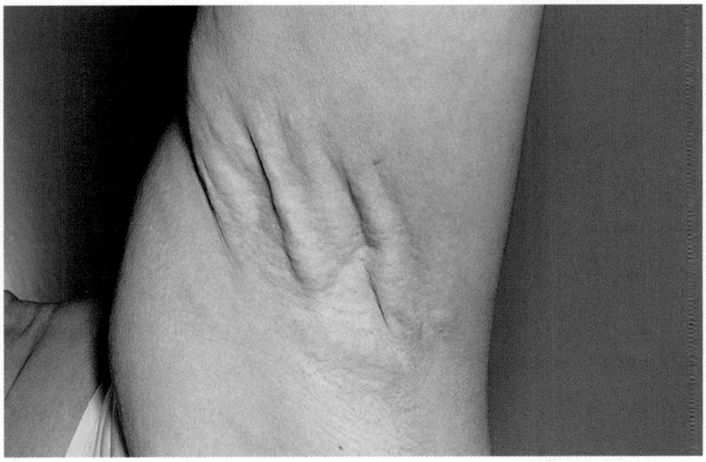

■ **Fig. 13.85** Axillary involvement is common.

Ehlers–Danlos syndrome type 6

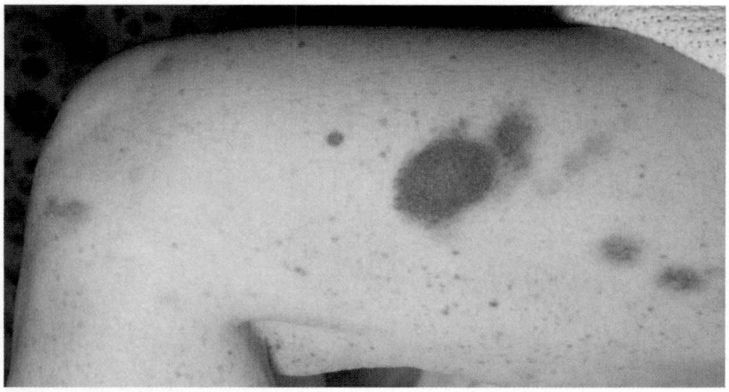

Fig. 13.86 Cutaneous fragility resulting in easy bruising and poor healing. (Courtesy of J. M. H. Moll.)

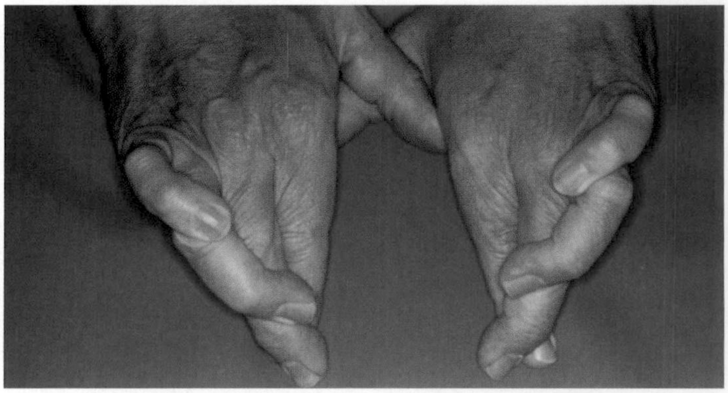

Fig. 13.87 Joint hyperextensibility. (Courtesy of J. M. H. Moll.)

Paget disease

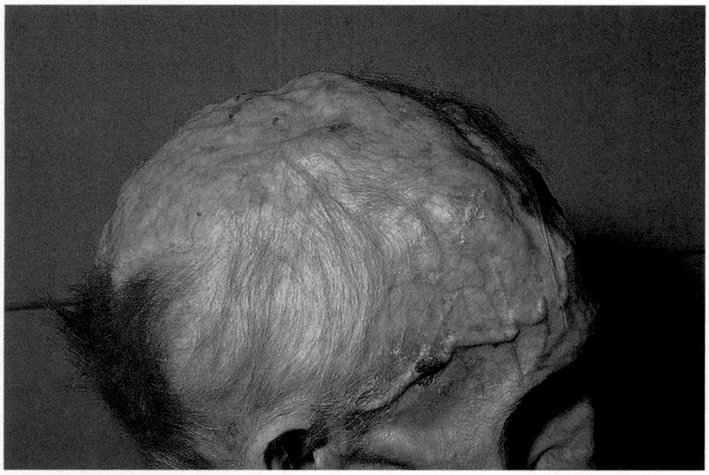

Fig. 13.88 Enlargement of the skull.

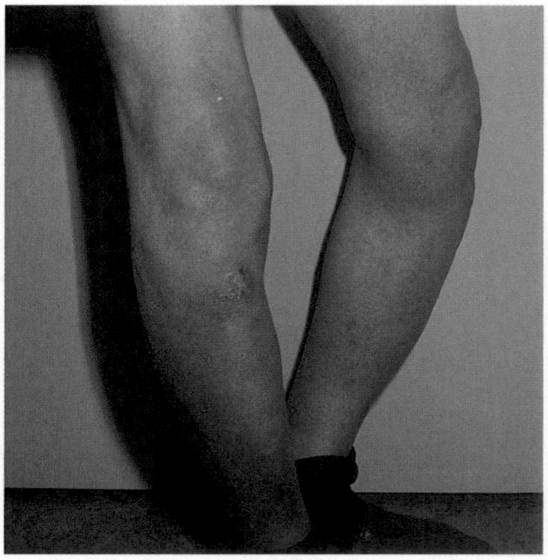

Fig. 13.89 Anterior bowing of the tibias and arthropathy.

Haemogobinopathies

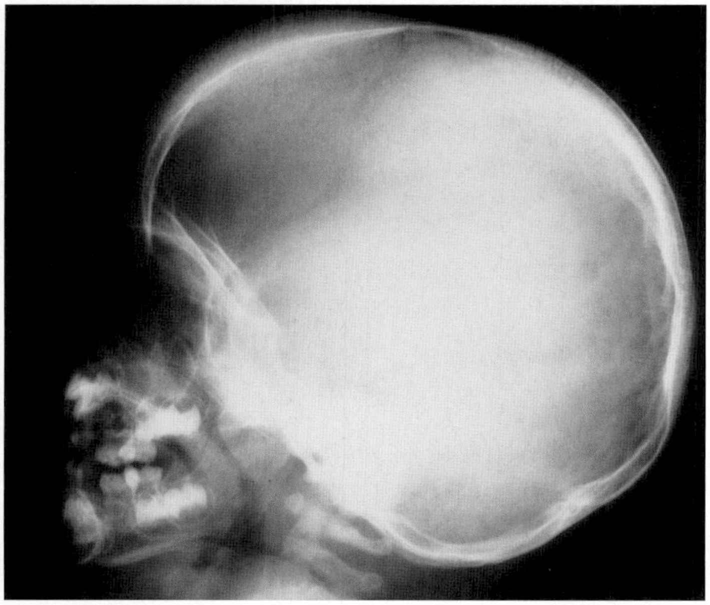

Fig. 13.90 Frontal bossing and 'hair on end' appearance of the skull caused by hyperplasia of bone marrow in thalassaemia. (Courtesy of S. Ghiacy.)

TOXIC RETINOPATHIES

Antimalarials

Chloroquine and hydroxychloroquine are used in the prophylaxis and treatment of malaria as well as in the treatment of certain rheumatological diseases.

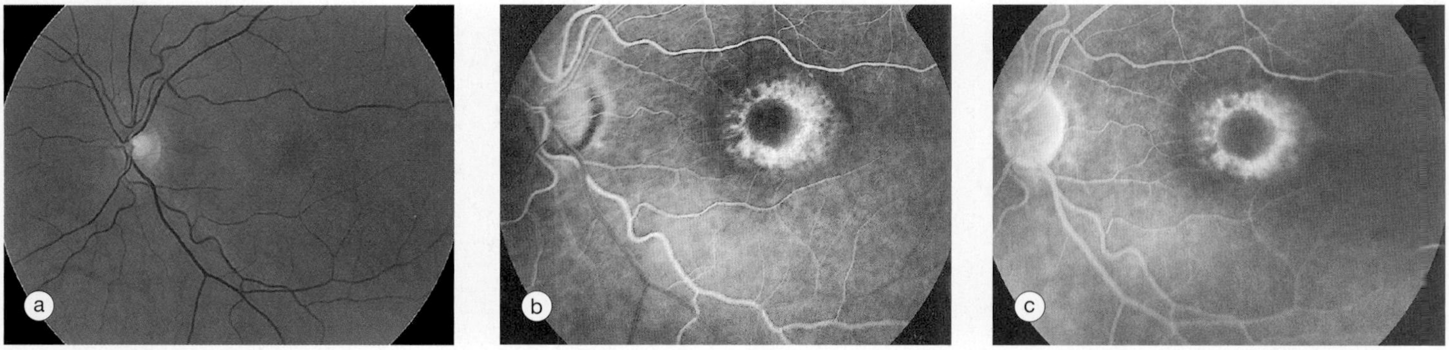

Fig. 13.91 **(a)** Subtle 'bull's eye' macular lesion characterised by central foveolar pigmentation surrounded by a depigmented zone of RPE atrophy that is itself encircled by a hyperpigmented ring. **(b, c)** FA shows a hyperfluorescent ring due to a window defect corresponding to RPE atrophy. (Courtesy of S. Milewski.)

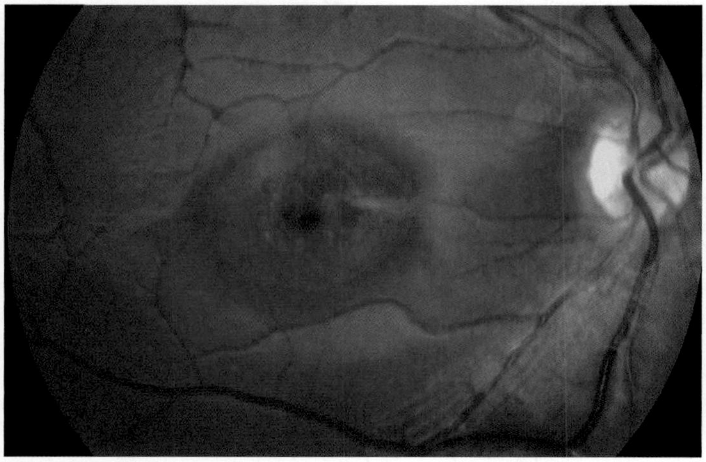

Fig. 13.92 A more obvious 'bull's eye' macular lesion. (Courtesy of Moorfields Eye Hospital.)

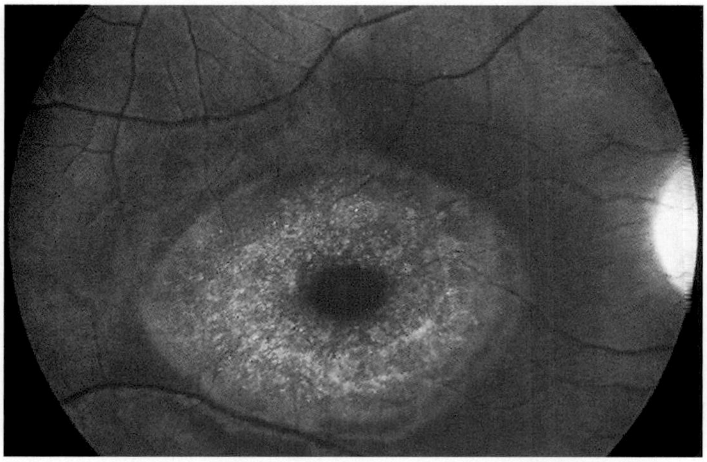

Fig. 13.93 Widespread RPE atrophy surrounding the fovea.

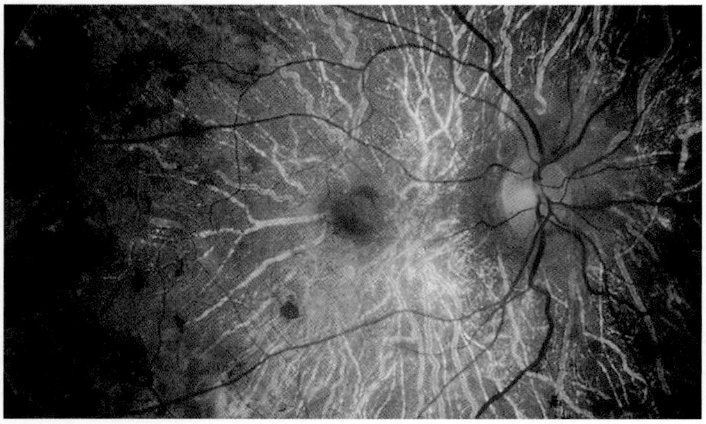

Fig. 13.94 Severe atrophy of the RPE with unmasking of the larger choroidal blood vessels, arteriolar attenuation and pigment clumping. (Courtesy of J. Salmon.)

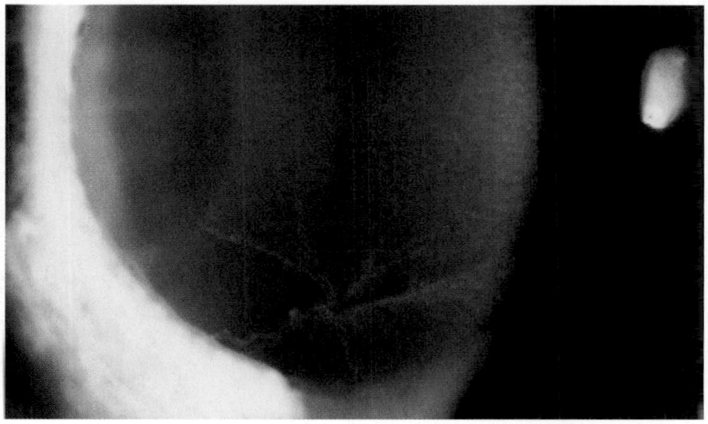

Fig. 13.95 Vortex keratopathy is common but innocuous.

Thioridazine

Thioridazine is used in the treatment of psychoses.

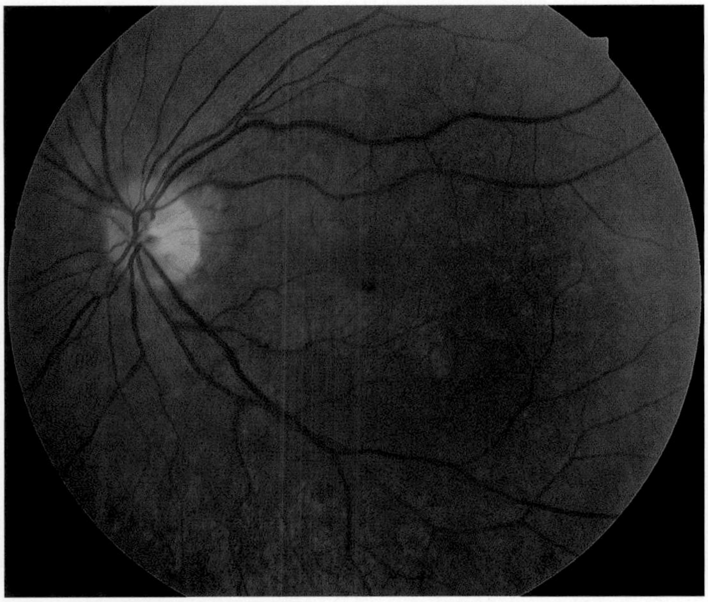

Fig. 13.96 Mild non-specific pigmentary disturbance involving the mid-periphery and posterior pole.

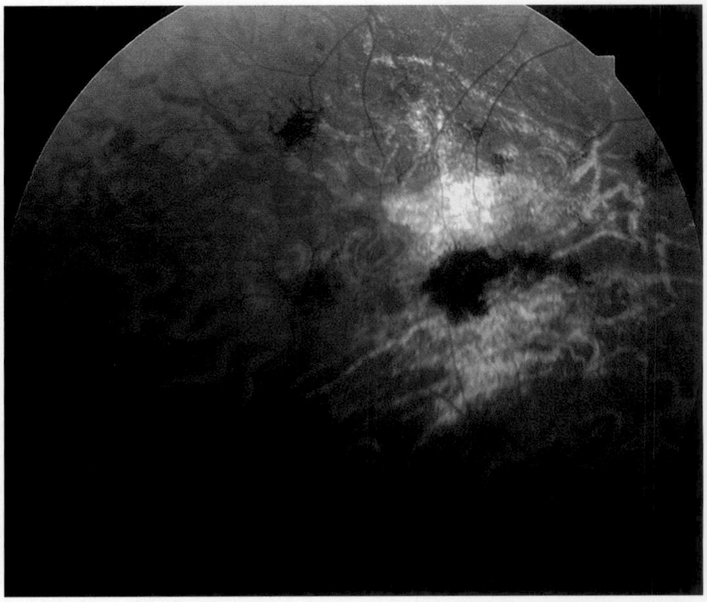

Fig. 13.97 Plaque-like pigmentation and focal loss of the RPE and choriocapillaris.

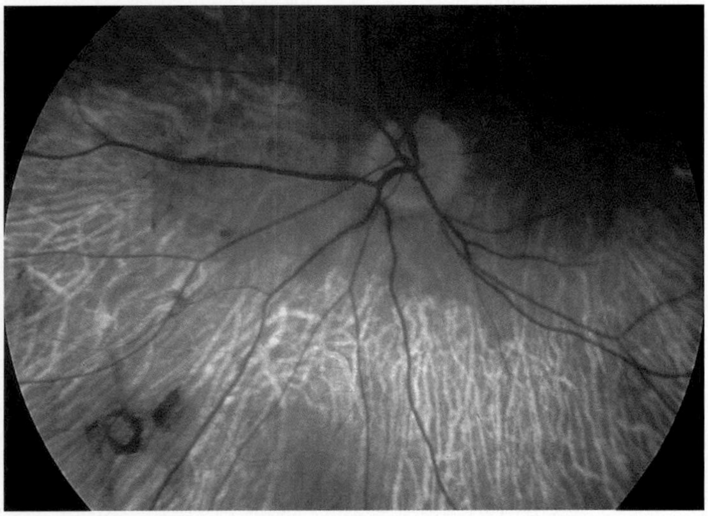

Fig. 13.98 Diffuse loss of the RPE and choriocapillaris.

Tamoxifen

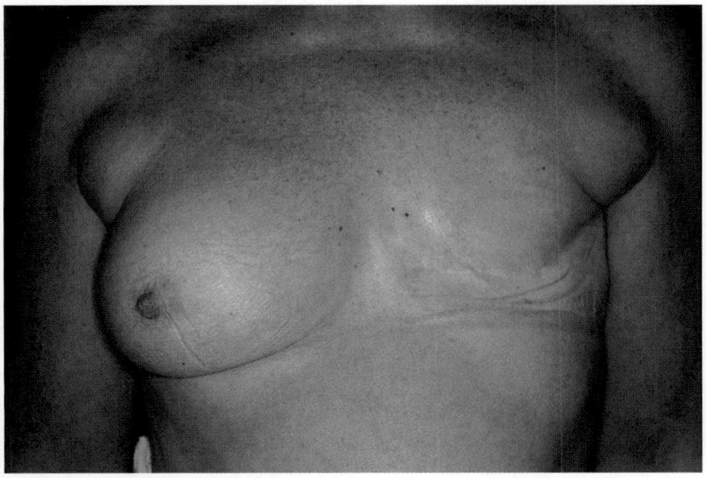

■ **Fig. 13.99** Tamoxifen is used in the treatment of breast cancer.

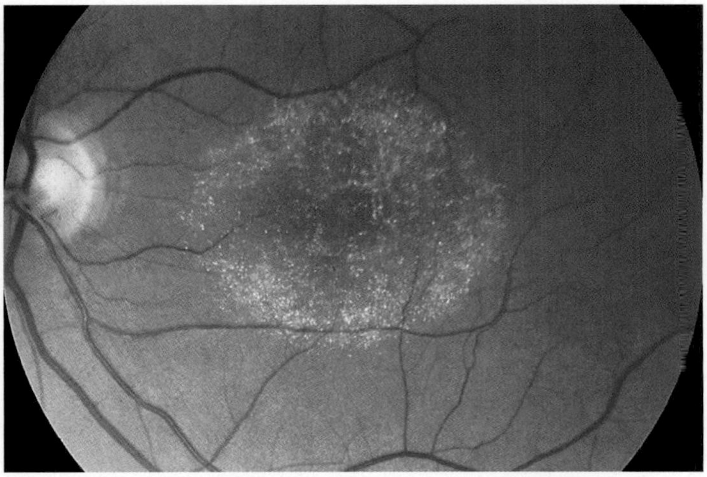

■ **Fig. 13.100** Bilateral, yellow, crystalline, ring-like macular deposits.

Canthaxanthin

Canthaxanthin is used to enhance sun tanning.

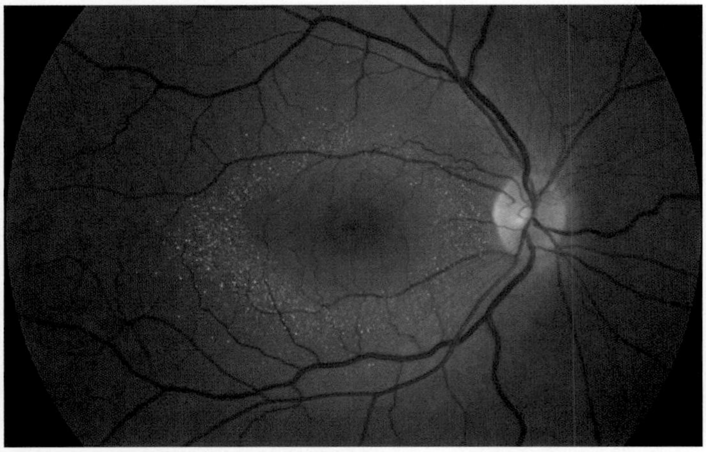

■ **Fig. 13.101** Bilateral, tiny, glistening, yellow deposits arranged symmetrically in a doughnut shape at the posterior poles. (Courtesy of L. Merin.)

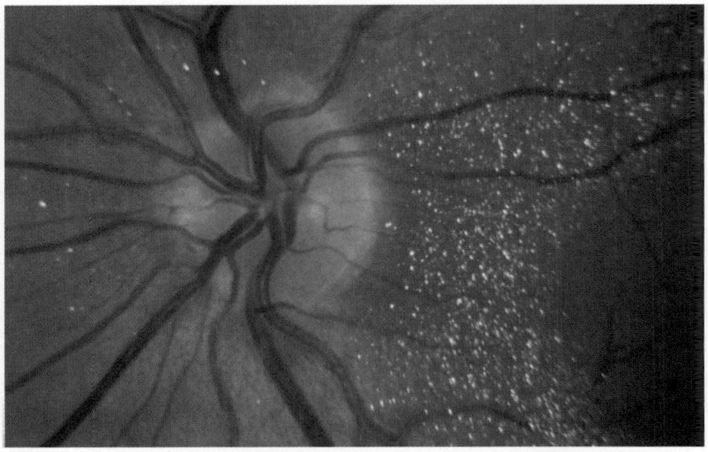

■ **Fig. 13.102** Magnified view in another patient. (Courtesy of W. Lisch.)

Interferon alpha

Interferon alpha is used in a variety of conditions, including malignancies and chronic hepatitis C.

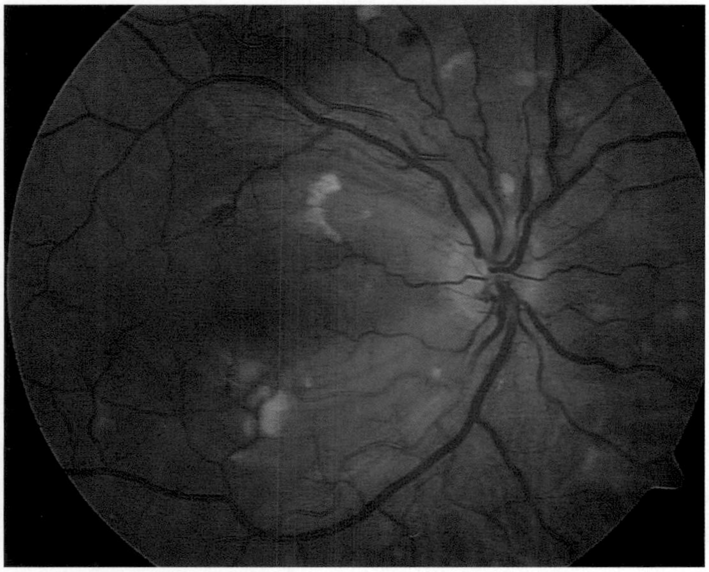

■ **Fig. 13.103** Cotton-wool spots and intraretinal haemorrhages may develop in some patients, particularly those on high-dose therapy. (Courtesy of P. Gili.)

Gentamicin

Gentamicin may cause severe retinal ischaemia when injected intravitreally for the treatment of bacterial endophthalmitis. Rarely, retinal toxicity may result from periocular injection.

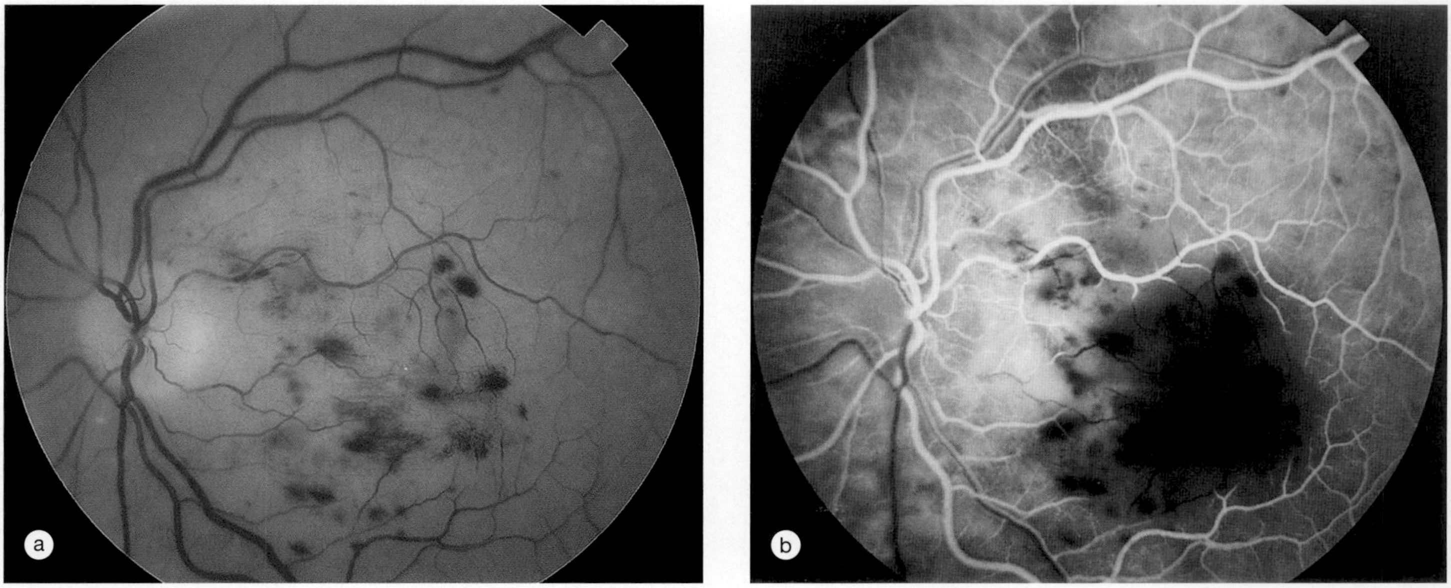

■ **Fig. 13.104** **(a)** Pallor and haemorrhages at the posterior pole. **(b)** FA early venous phase shows gross hypofluorescence due to ischaemia. (Courtesy of S. Milewski.)

Carbon monoxide retinopathy

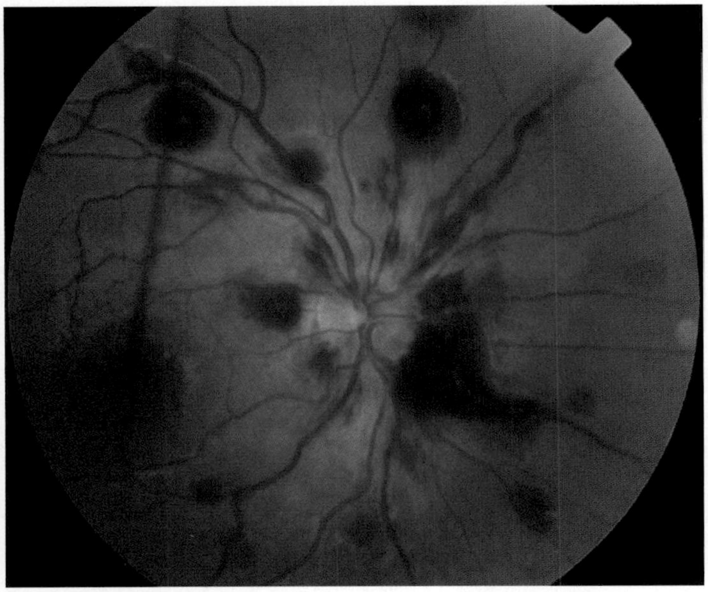

■ **Fig. 13.105** Multiple intraretinal, flame-shaped and preretinal haemorrhages. (Courtesy of R. Curtis.)

Oxalosis

Oxalosis is the deposition of calcium salts in body tissues, which may be the result of an inborn error of metabolism or a toxic reaction to ethylene glycol or methoxyflurane general anaesthesia.

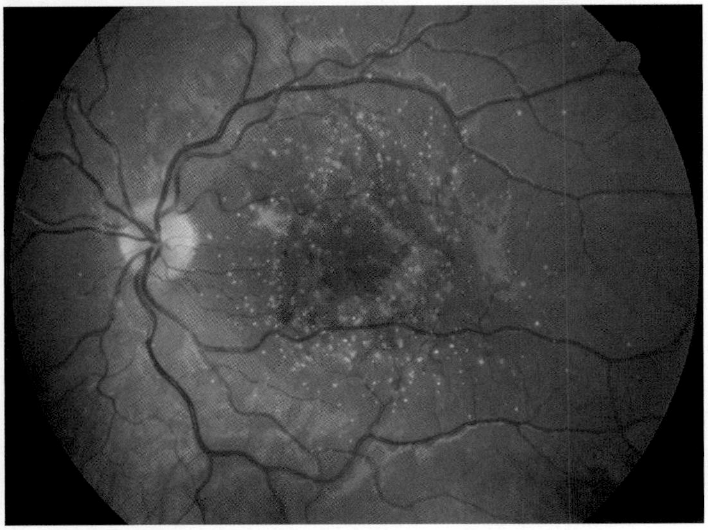

■ **Fig. 13.106** Numerous punctate crystalline spots scattered diffusely throughout the posterior pole and mid-periphery. (Courtesy of L. Merin.)

PARANEOPLASTIC RETINOPATHY

Cancer-associated retinopathy (CAR)

CAR is a very rare condition that primarily occurs in patients with small-cell bronchial carcinoma.

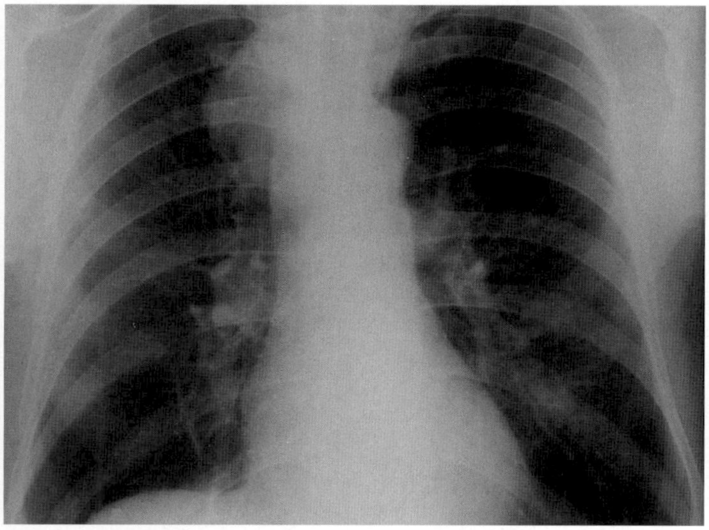

Fig. 13.107 Radiograph showing bronchial carcinoma.

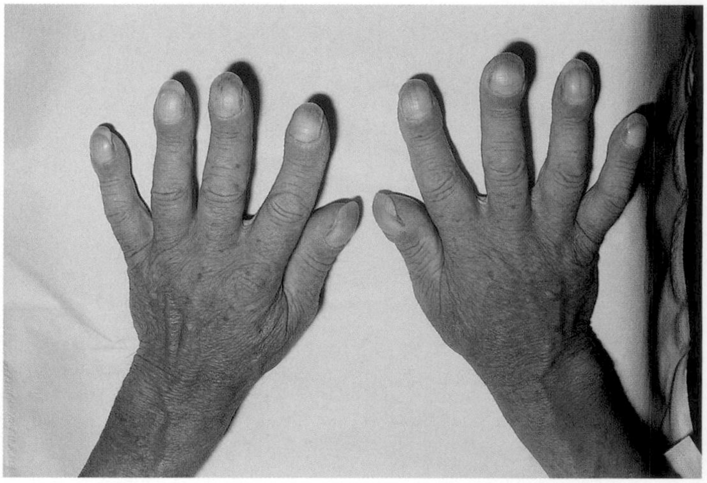

Fig. 13.108 Finger clubbing in bronchial carcinoma.

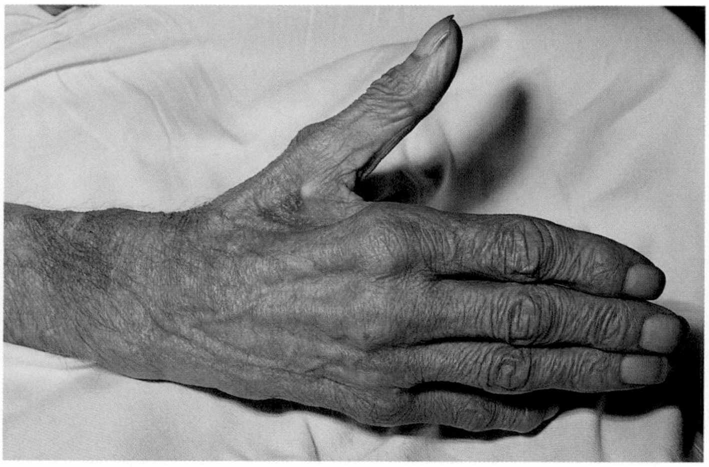

Fig. 13.109 Wasting of the small muscles of the hand supplied by the ulnar nerve resulting from invasion of the brachial plexus by an apical (Pancoast) tumour.

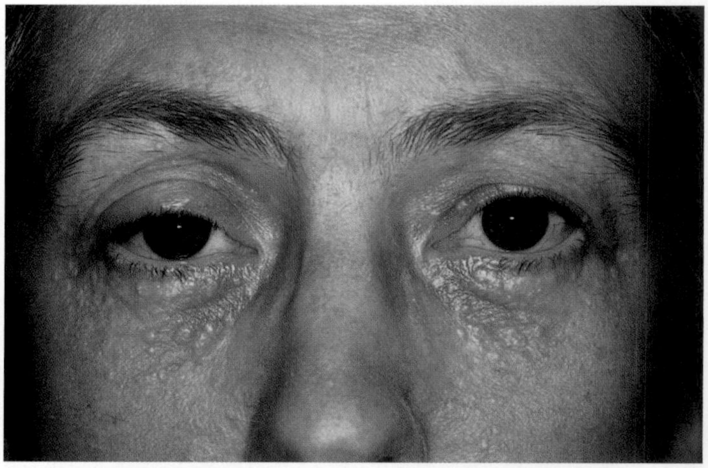

Fig. 13.110 Right Horner syndrome due to invasion of the sympathetic chain by a Pancoast tumour.

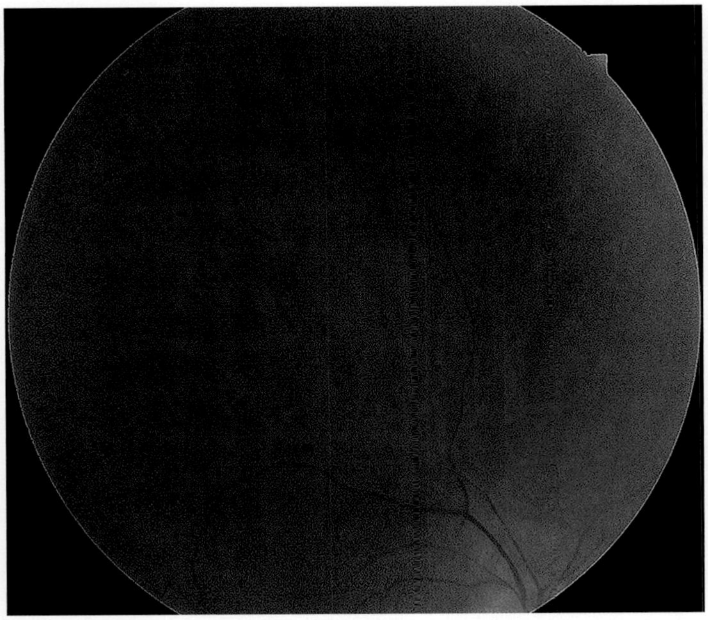

■ **Fig. 13.111** Arteriolar attenuation, which is bilateral.

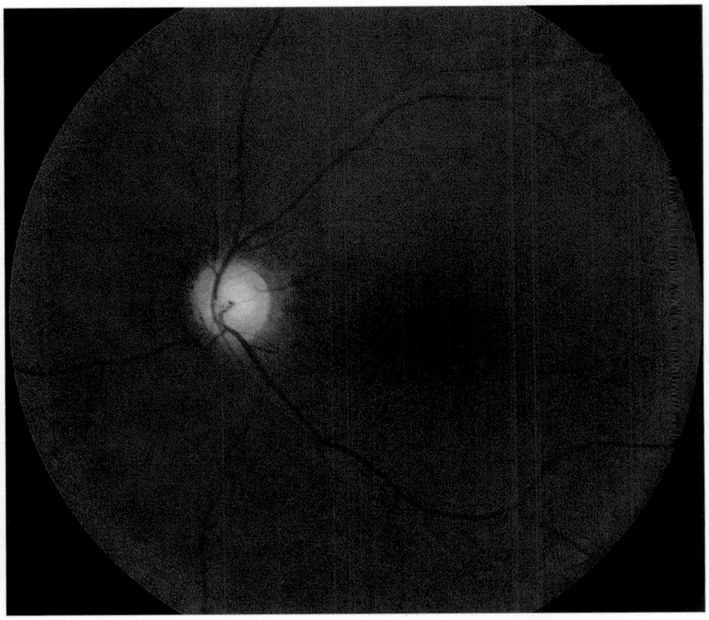

■ **Fig. 13.112** Severe arteriolar attenuation and optic atrophy.

Melanoma-associated retinopathy (MAR)

MAR is a similar condition except that it tends to occur years after treatment of cutaneous melanoma and is usually associated with clinical metastatic disease.

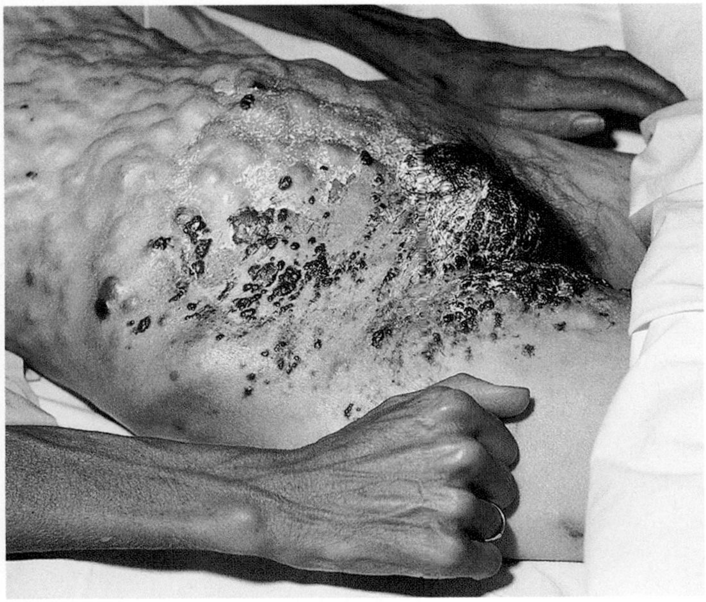

■ **Fig. 13.113** Advanced melanomatosis.

CHAPTER 14

FUNDUS DYSTROPHIES

RETINAL DYSTROPHIES

Retinitis pigmentosa (RP)

RP is a diffuse retinal dystrophy predominantly affecting rod photoreceptor cells.

Typical RP

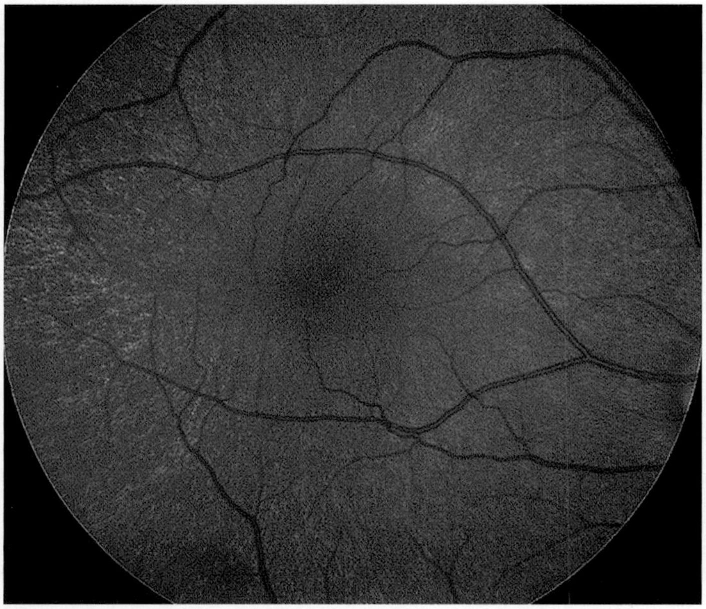

Fig. 14.1 Scintillating golden reflex in a carrier of XL disease.

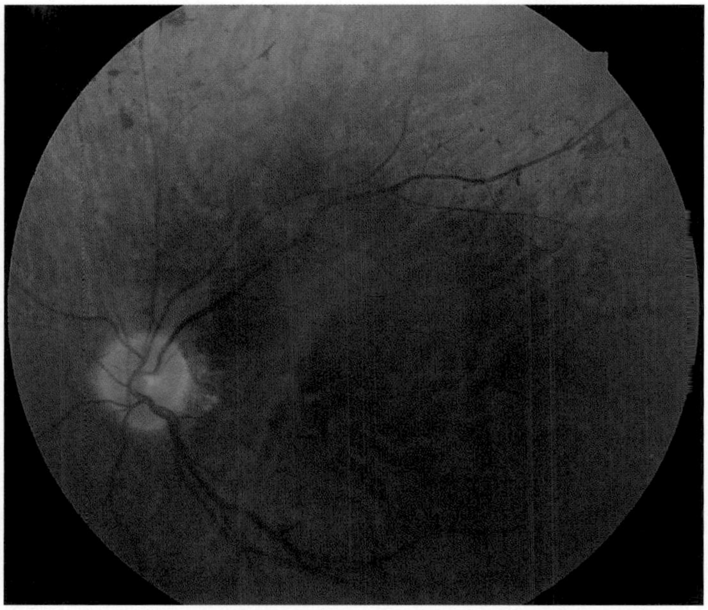

Fig. 14.2 Arteriolar narrowing and sparse pigmentary changes.

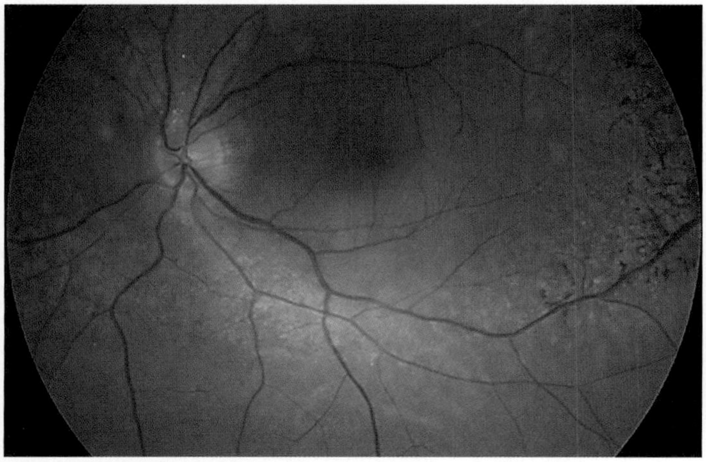

Fig. 14.3 Mid-peripheral, coarse, perivascular 'bone-spicule' pigmentary changes. (Courtesy of C. Barry.)

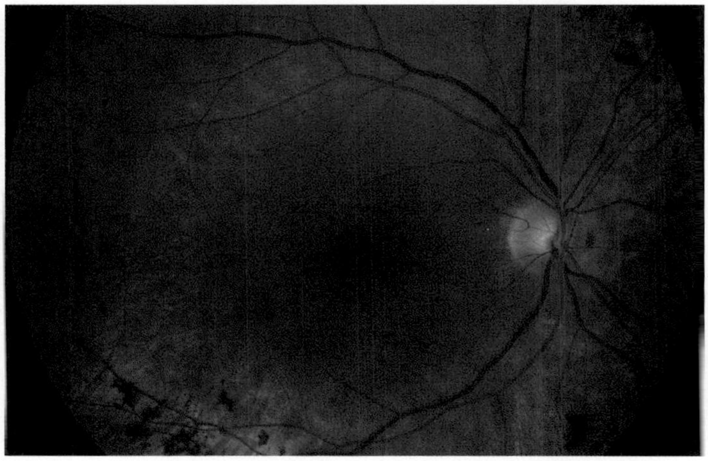

Fig. 14.4 Gradual increase in density of pigmentary changes with spread anteriorly and posteriorly. (Courtesy of P. Saine.)

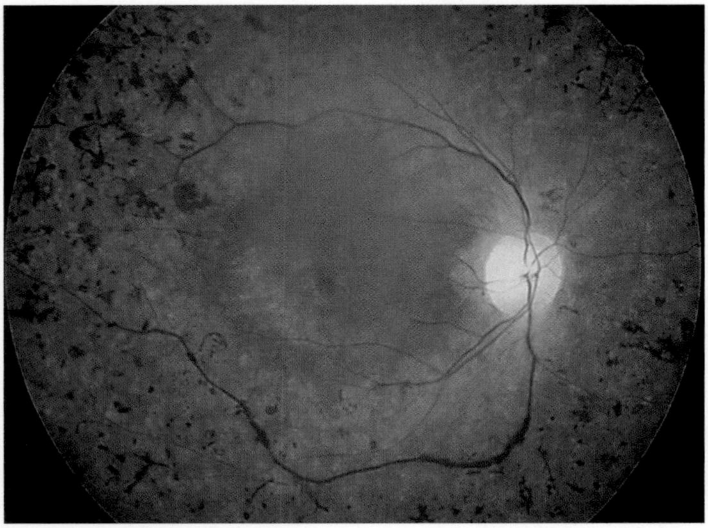

Fig. 14.5 Severe arteriolar attenuation and waxy disc pallor in advanced disease. (Courtesy of C. Barry.)

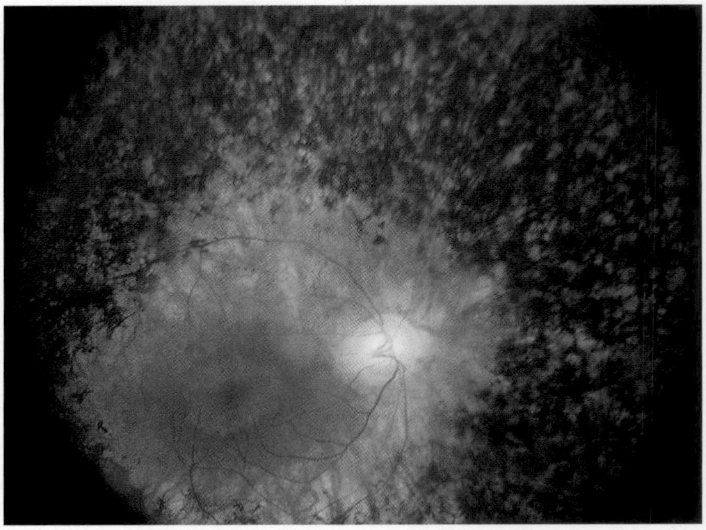

Fig. 14.6 Extensive pigmentary changes and bull's eye maculopathy in end-stage disease.

Atypical RP

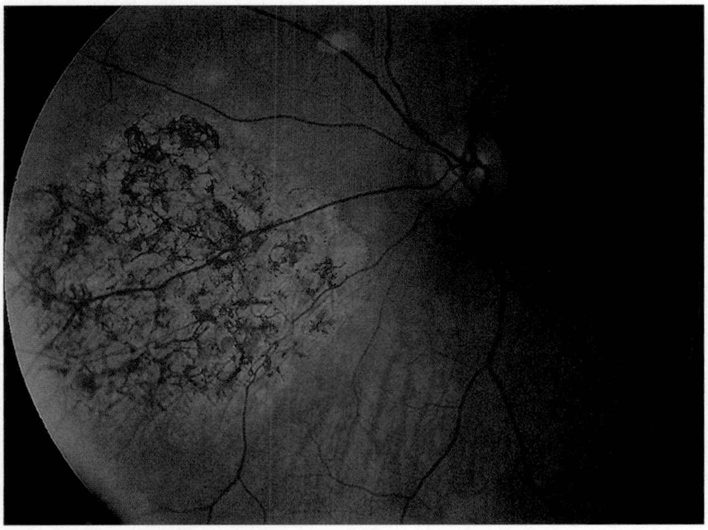

Fig. 14.7 Sector RP in which the abnormalities are confined to one quadrant (usually nasal) or one half (usually inferior).

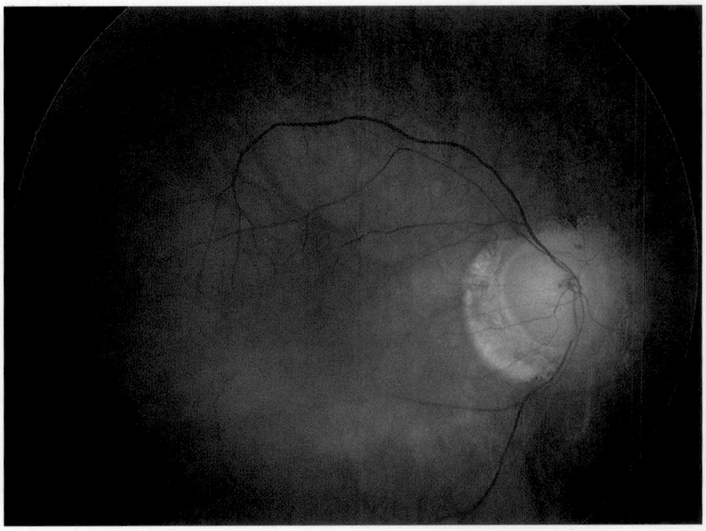

Fig. 14.8 RP sine pigmento is characterised by arteriolar attenuation and optic atrophy but absence of pigmentary changes.

Ocular associations

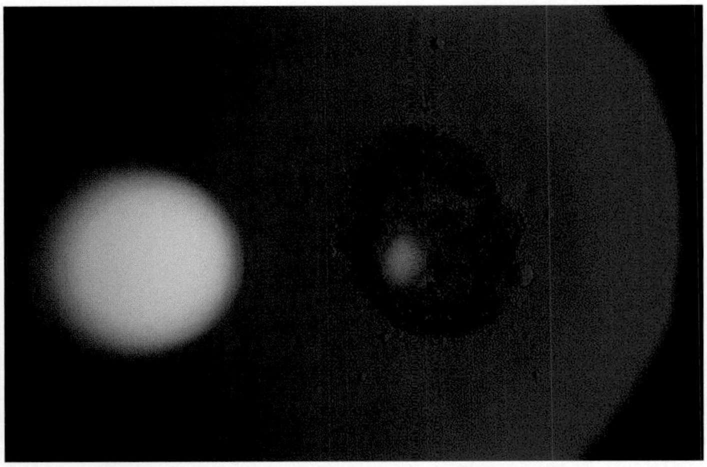

■ **Fig. 14.9** Posterior subcapsular cataracts are common.

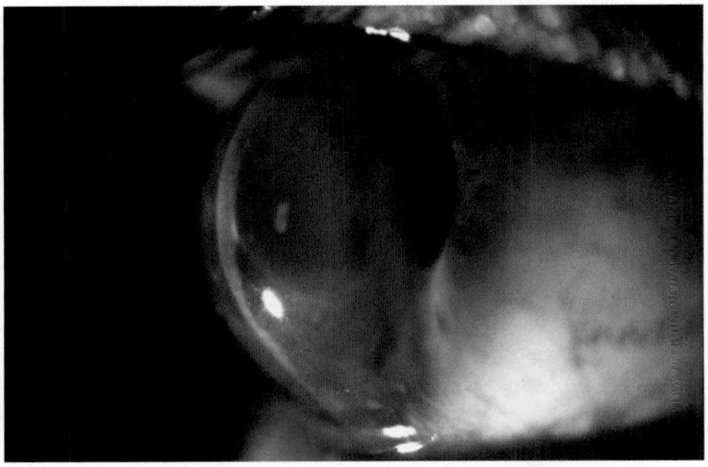

■ **Fig. 14.10** Keratoconus is uncommon. (Courtesy of P. Gili.)

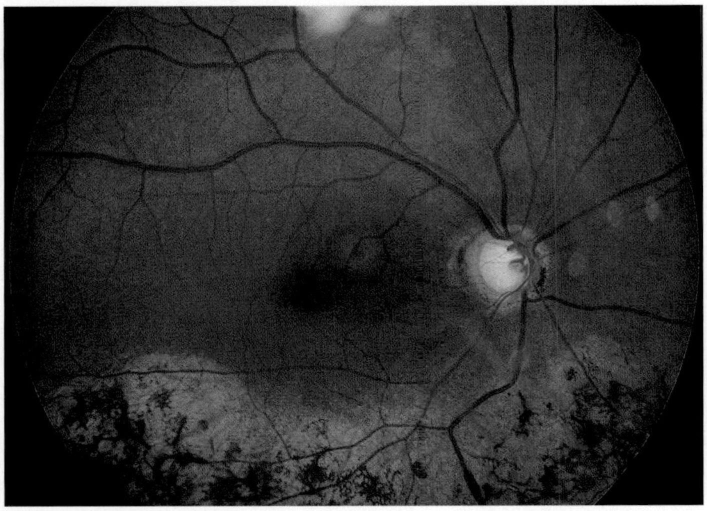

■ **Fig. 14.11** Open-angle glaucoma affects about 3% of patients; note the glaucomatous cupping.

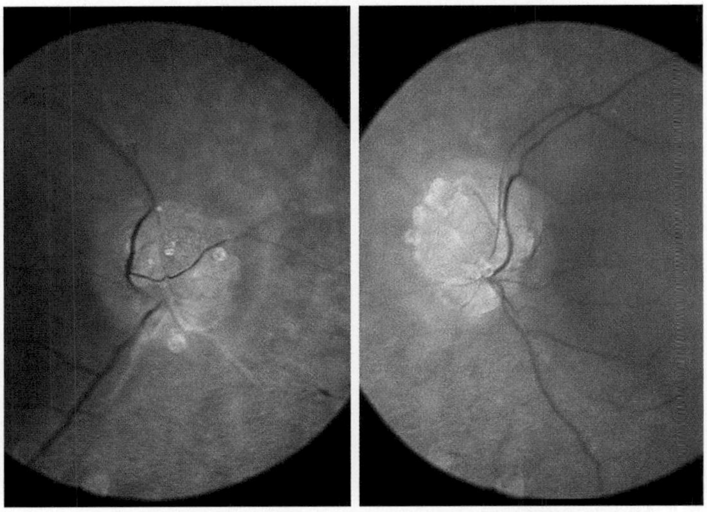

■ **Fig. 14.12** Optic disc drusen occur more frequently than in normals.

Progressive cone–rod dystrophy

Most cases are sporadic. Of the remainder the most frequent inheritance pattern is AD and a small proportion may be AR or XL. Presentation is in the first to second decade with impairment of central and colour vision.

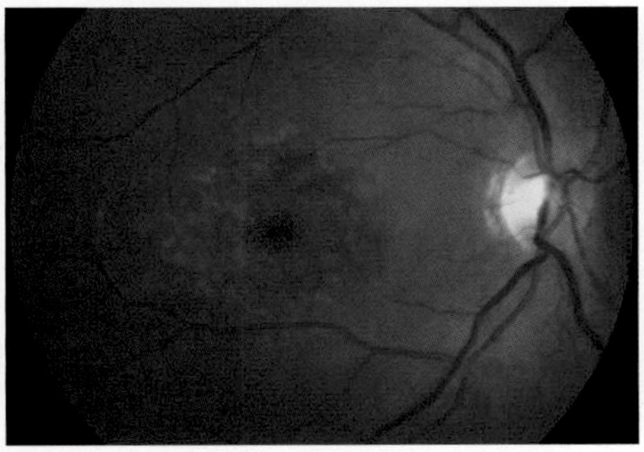

■ **Fig. 14.13** RPE mottling with an early bull's eye pattern. (Courtesy of Moorfields Eye Hospital.)

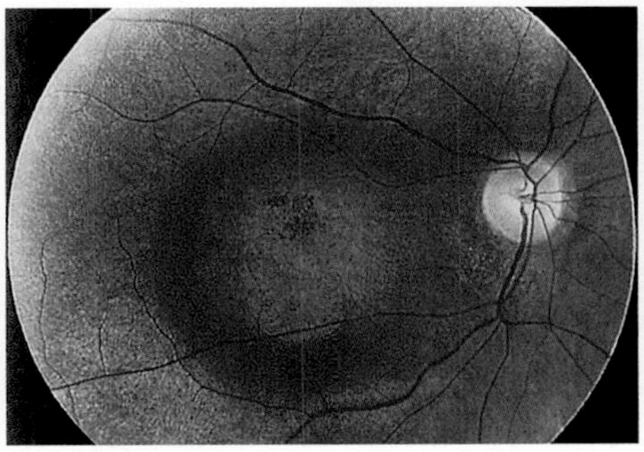

■ **Fig. 14.14** Established bull's eye maculopathy.

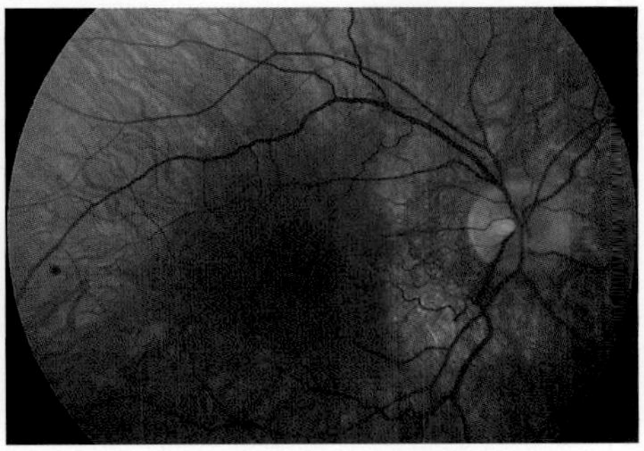

■ **Fig. 14.15** Mid-peripheral 'bone-spicule' pigmentation, arteriolar attenuation and temporal disc pallor develops in some cases.

Systemic association of rod–cone dystrophies

Kearns–Sayre syndrome

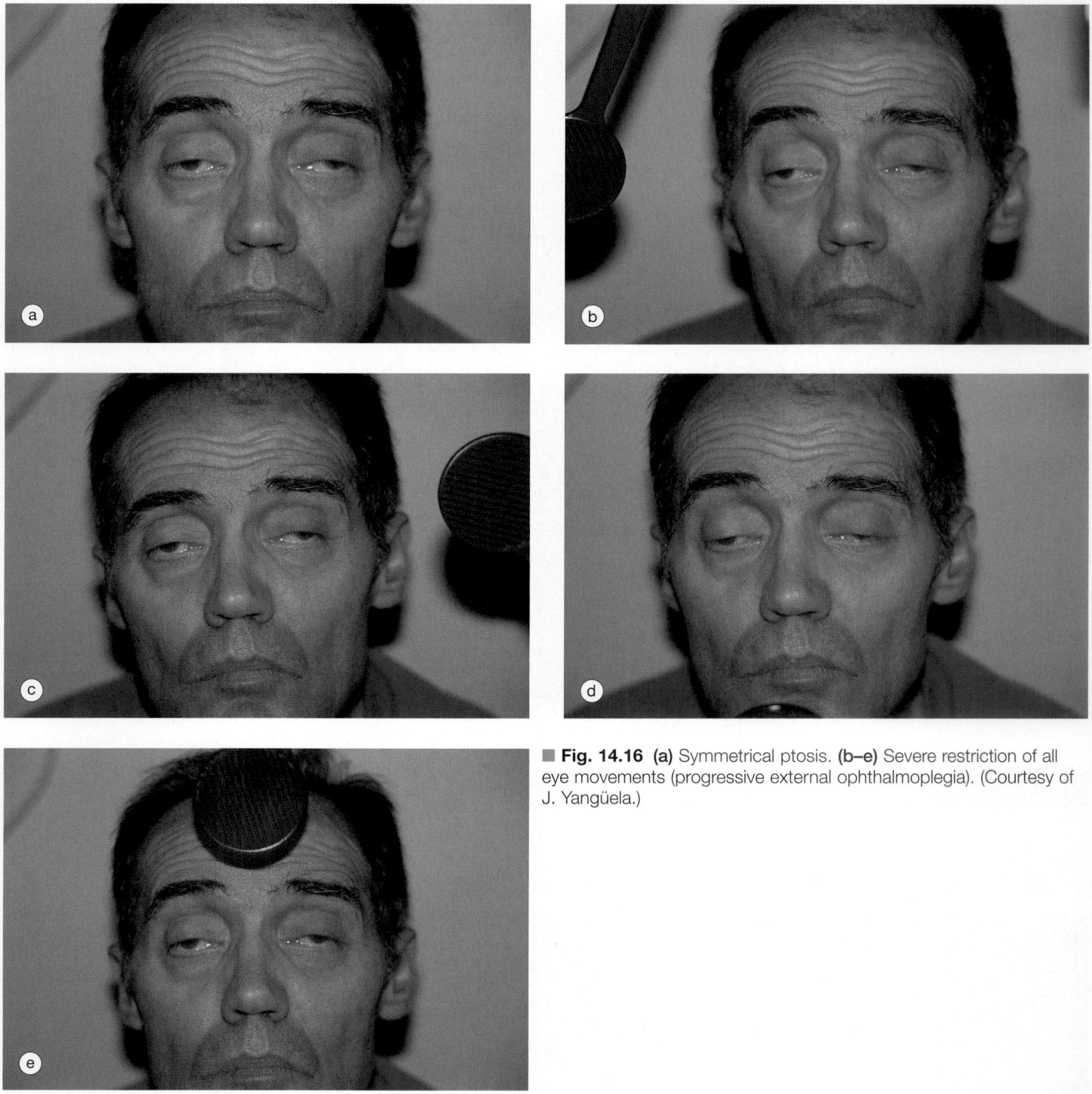

■ **Fig. 14.16** **(a)** Symmetrical ptosis. **(b–e)** Severe restriction of all eye movements (progressive external ophthalmoplegia). (Courtesy of J. Yangüela.)

Bardet–Biedl syndrome

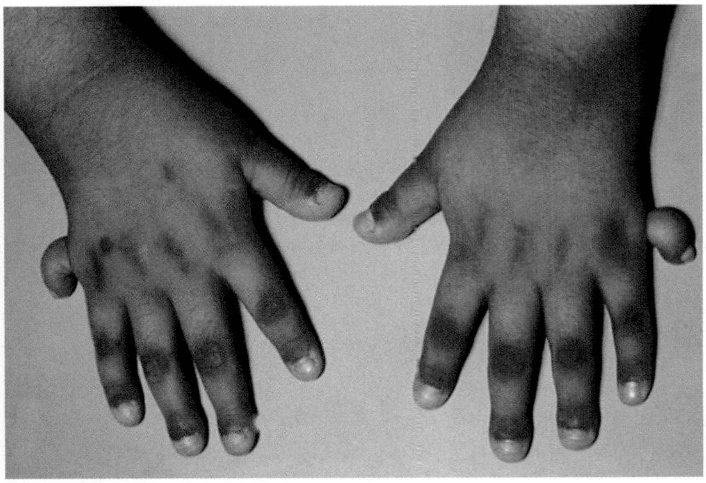

■ **Fig. 14.17** Polydactyly; also obesity, hypogenitalism and mental handicap. Laurence–Moon syndrome is similar but without obesity and polydactyly.

Bassen–Kornzweig syndrome

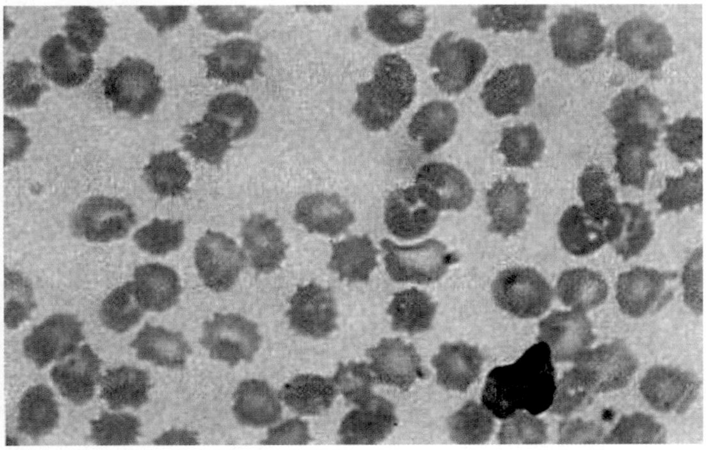

■ **Fig. 14.18** Acanthocytosis (spur cells) in peripheral blood; also malabsorption, spinocerebellar ataxia, ptosis and progressive external ophthalmoplegia.

Refsum disease

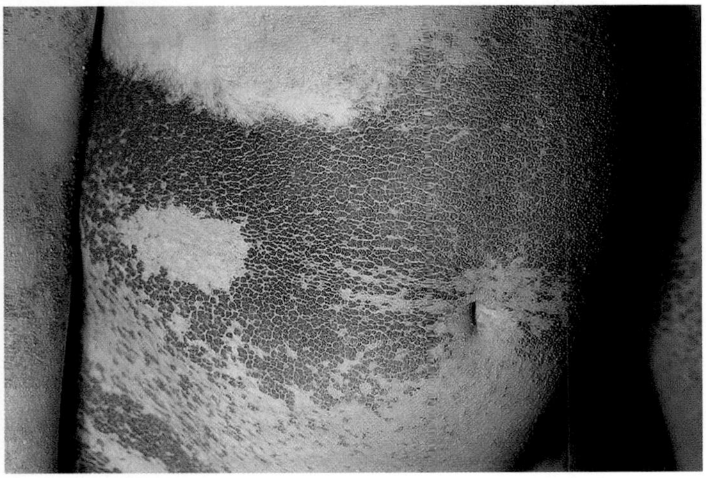

■ **Fig. 14.19** Ichthyosis; also polyneuropathy, cerebellar ataxia and cardiac disease.

Mucopolysaccharidoses (except Morquio syndrome)

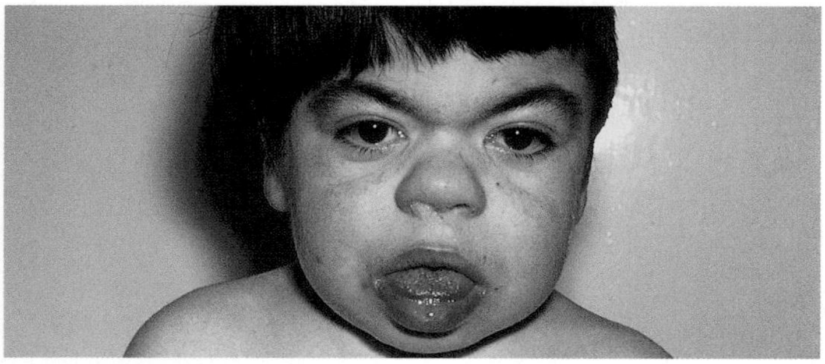

Fig. 14.20 Coarse facial features and macroglossia in Hurler syndrome; also mental retardation, stunted growth, hepatosplenomegaly and corneal clouding.

Zellweger (hepatocerebrorenal) syndrome

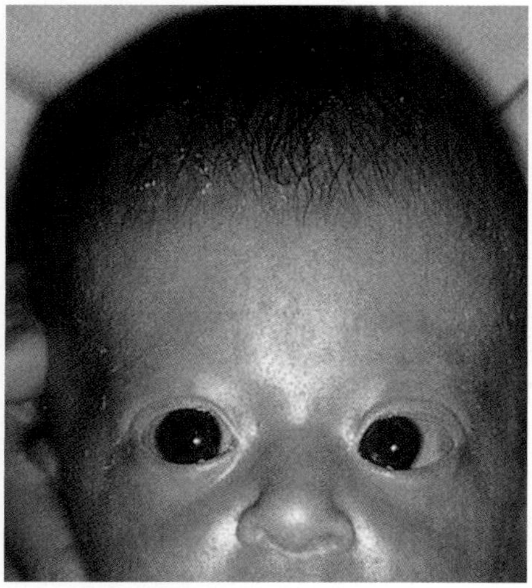

Fig. 14.21 Long, narrow head, high forehead and shallow supraorbital ridges; also hypotonia, seizures, delayed development, hepatomegaly, renal cysts and early demise. (Courtesy of D. M. Albert and F. A. Jakobiec.)

Jeune syndrome

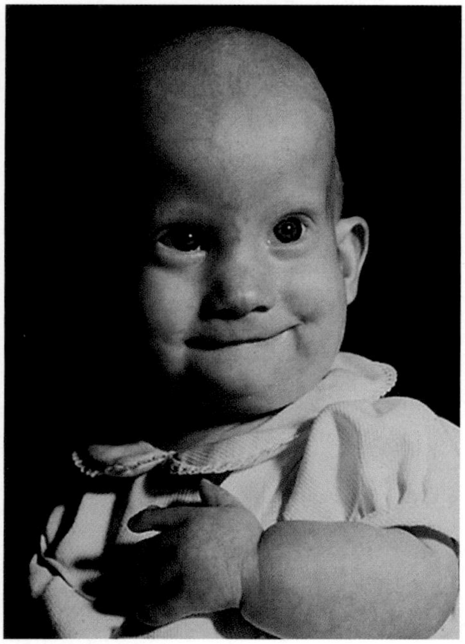

Fig. 14.22 Brachycephaly, short stubby fingers, alopecia and short stature. (Courtesy of B. J. Zitelli and H. W. Davis.)

Albinism

Albinism is a genetically determined, heterogeneous group of disorders of melanin synthesis in which either the eyes alone (ocular albinism) or the eyes, skin and hair (oculocutaneous albinism) may be affected. The latter may be either tyrosinase-positive or tyrosinase-negative.

Oculocutaneous albinism

Tyrosinase-negative (complete)

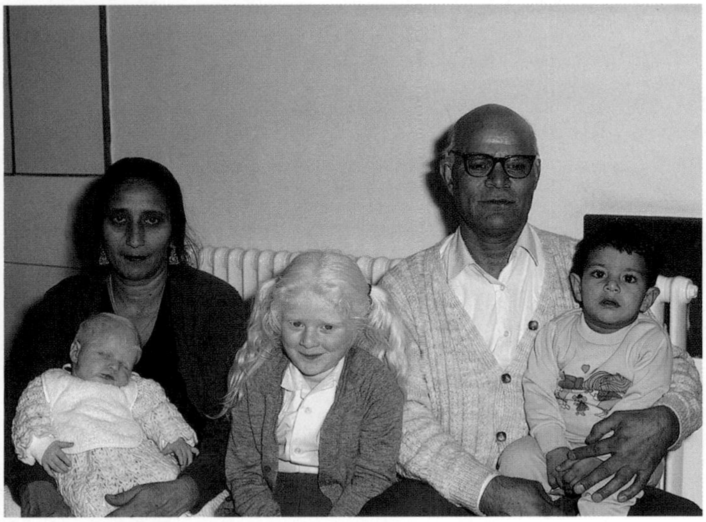

Fig. 14.23 Inheritance may by AD or AR.

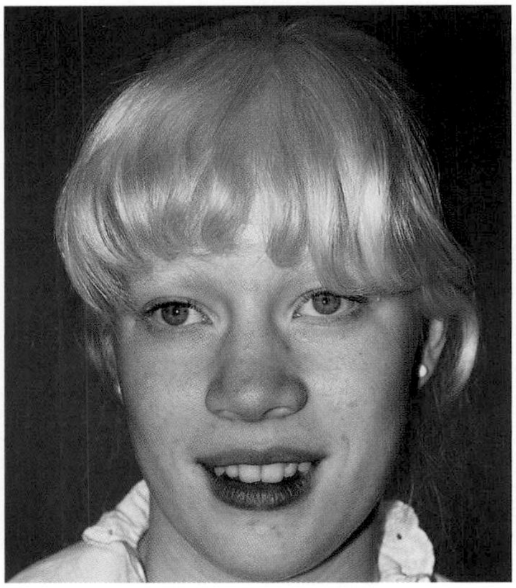

Fig. 14.24 Platinum blond hair, very pale skin and a 'pink-eyes' appearance.

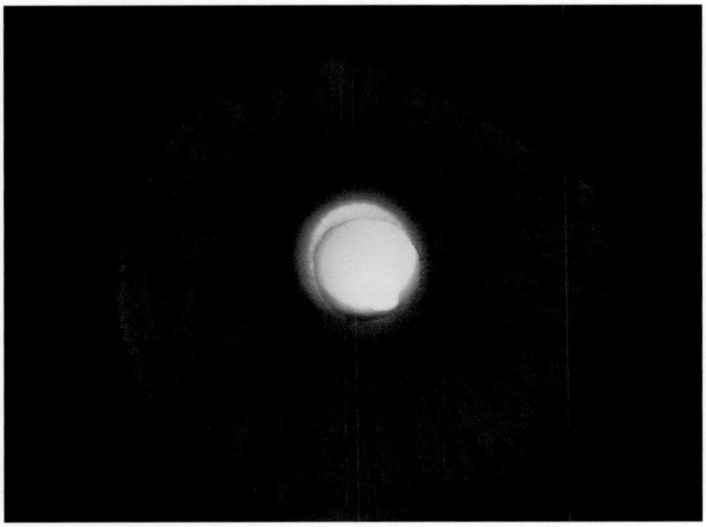

Fig. 14.25 Diaphanous and translucent irides.

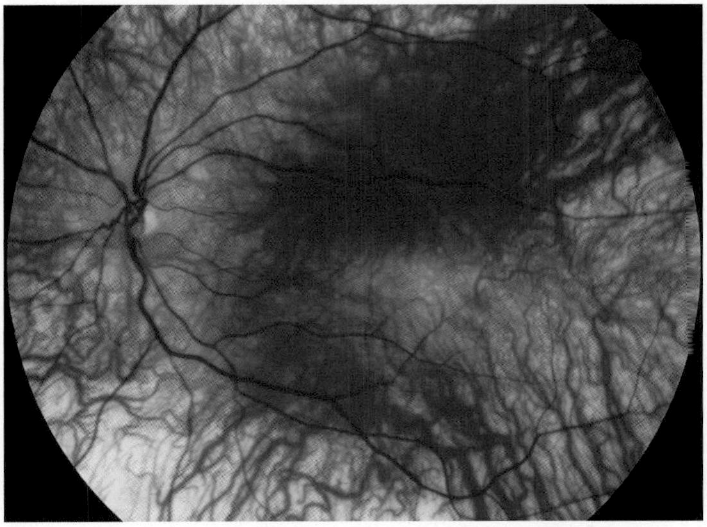

Fig. 14.26 The fundus shows lack of pigment with conspicuously large choroidal vessels, foveal hypoplasia with absence of the foveal pit, and lack of vessels forming the perimacular arcades. (Courtesy of L. Merin.)

Tyrosinase-positive (incomplete)

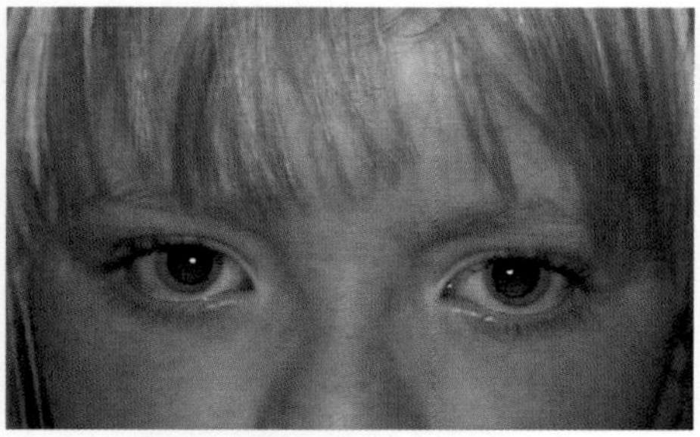

■ **Fig. 14.27** The hair may be white, yellow or red and darkens with age, as does the skin. (Courtesy of M. Parulekar.)

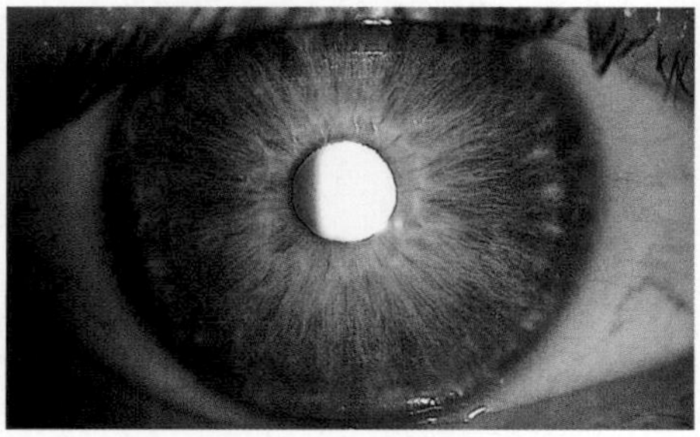

■ **Fig. 14.28** The iris may be blue or dark brown and variably translucent.

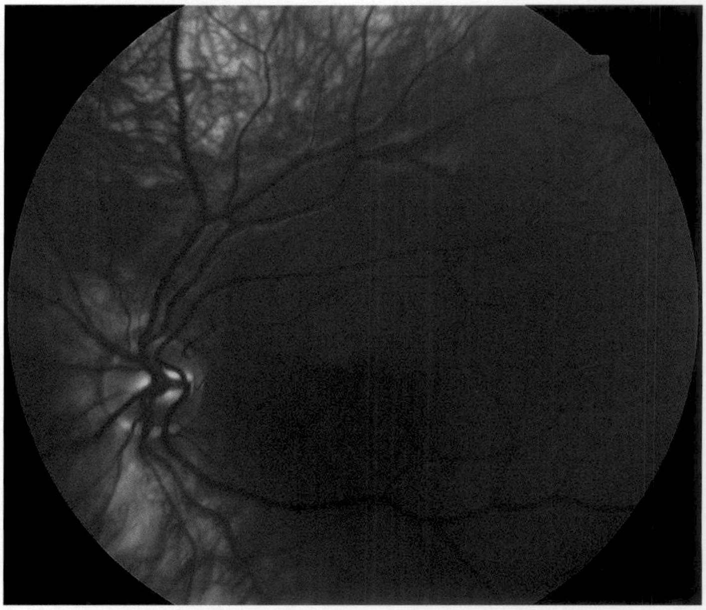

■ **Fig. 14.29** The fundus shows less hypopigmentation and a normal macula.

Ocular albinism

Involvement is predominantly ocular with normal skin and hair. Inheritance is usually XL.

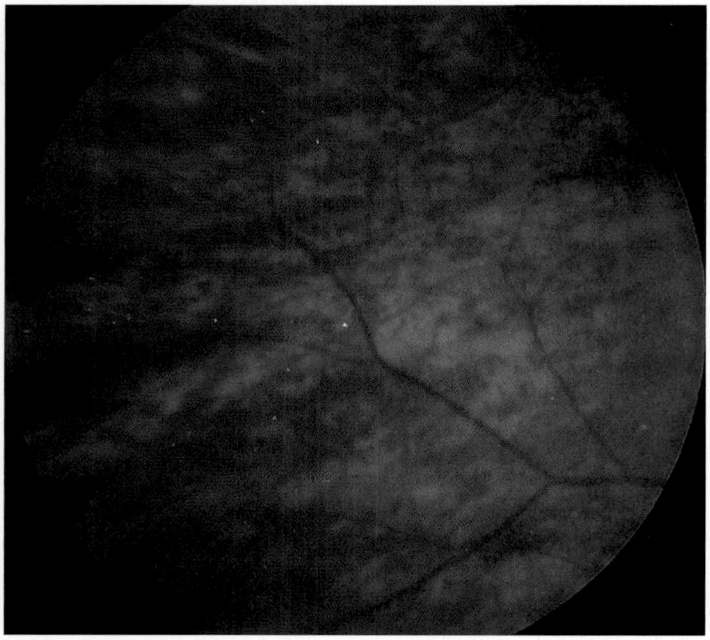

■ **Fig. 14.30** Female carrier: macular stippling and mid-peripheral scattered areas of depigmentation and granularity.

Stargardt disease and fundus flavimaculatus

Stargardt disease (juvenile macular dystrophy) and fundus flavimaculatus are regarded as variants of the same disease despite presenting at different times and carrying different prognoses.

Stargardt disease

Presentation of this AR condition is during the first or second decade.

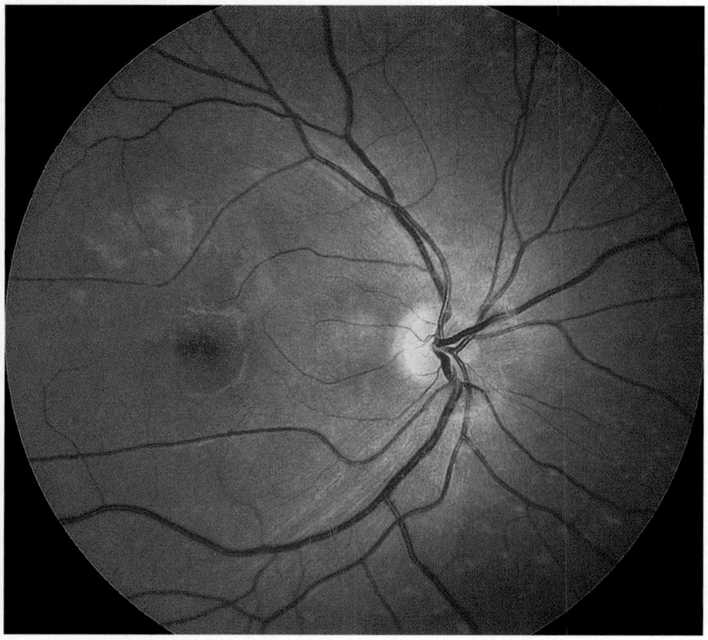

Fig. 14.31 The fovea may be normal or show non-specific mottling and a subtle 'snail-slime' appearance.

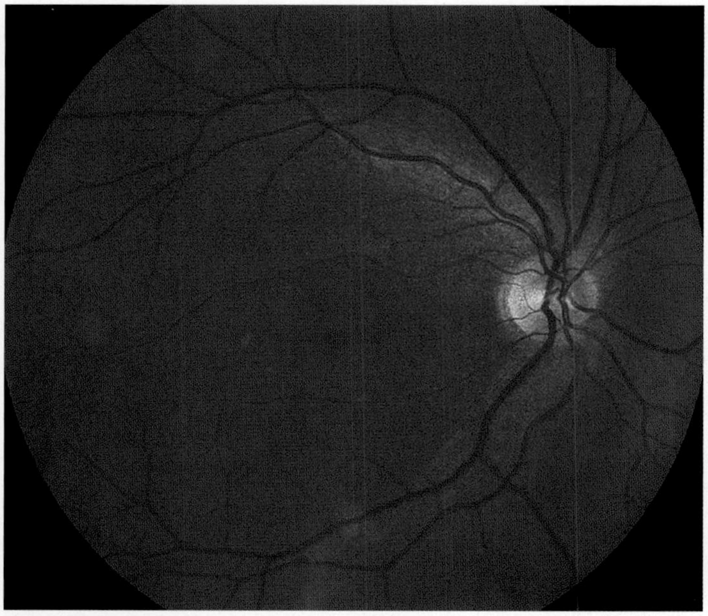

Fig. 14.32 The fovea has a 'beaten bronze' appearance surrounded by yellow-white flecks.

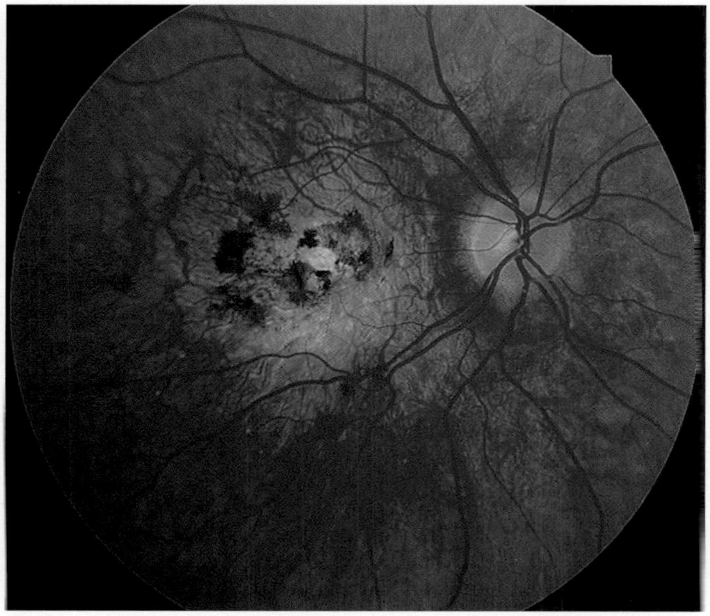

Fig. 14.33 End-stage geographic atrophy, which may have a slight bull's eye configuration.

Fundus flavimaculatus

Presentation of this AR disease is in adult life, although in the absence of macular involvement the condition may be asymptomatic.

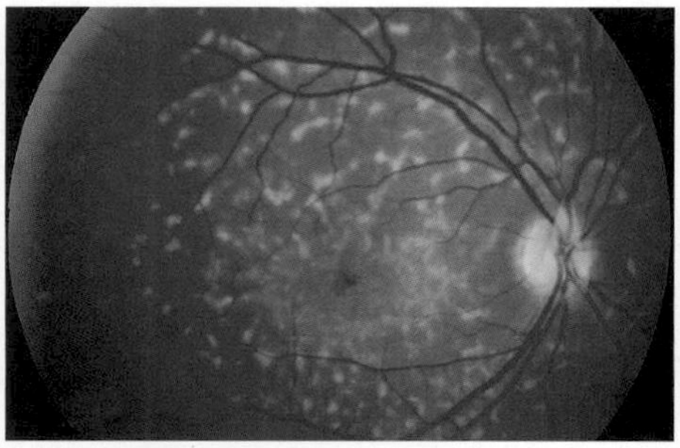

■ **Fig. 14.34** Innumerable yellow-white flecks scattered throughout the posterior pole and mid-periphery; the fundus has a vermilion colour in about 50% of cases. (Courtesy of S. Milewski.)

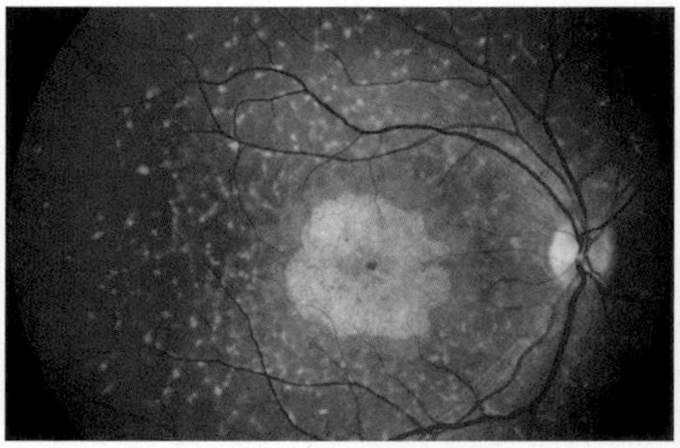

■ **Fig. 14.35** Early geographic atrophy. (Courtesy of S. Milewski.)

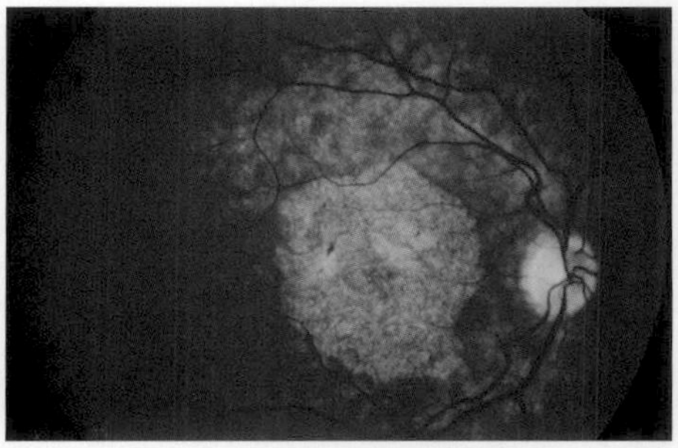

■ **Fig. 14.36** Advanced geographic atrophy with fading flecks. (Courtesy of J. Salmon.)

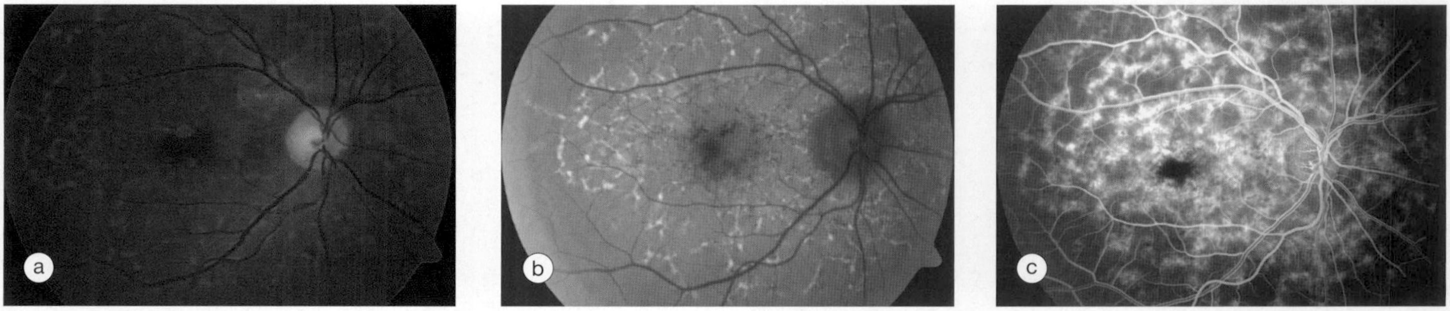

■ **Fig. 14.37** **(a)** Fundus flavimaculatus. (**b**) Autofluorescence of flecks. **(c)** FA early venous phase shows a 'dark choroid' and hyperfluorescence of flecks. (Courtesy of P. Gili.)

Juvenile Best macular dystrophy

Inheritance is AD with variable penetrance and expressivity.

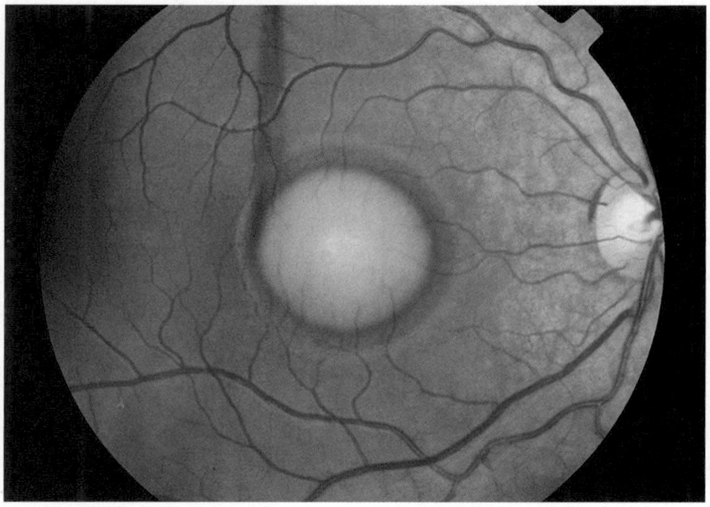

■ **Fig. 14.38** Round, egg-yolk ('sunny side up') macular lesion consisting of accumulation of lipofuscin within the RPE that develops in childhood.

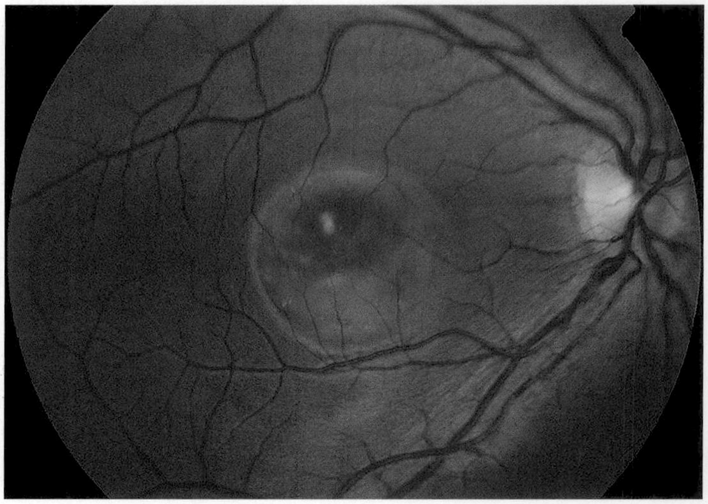

■ **Fig. 14.39** Part of the lesion is beginning to absorb. (Courtesy of S. Milewski.)

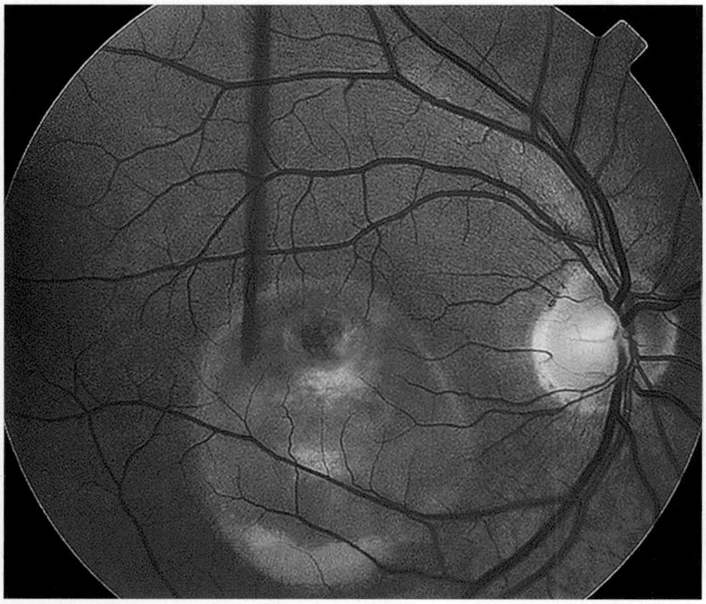

■ **Fig. 14.40** In some cases absorption continues and becomes complete. (Courtesy of S. Milewski.)

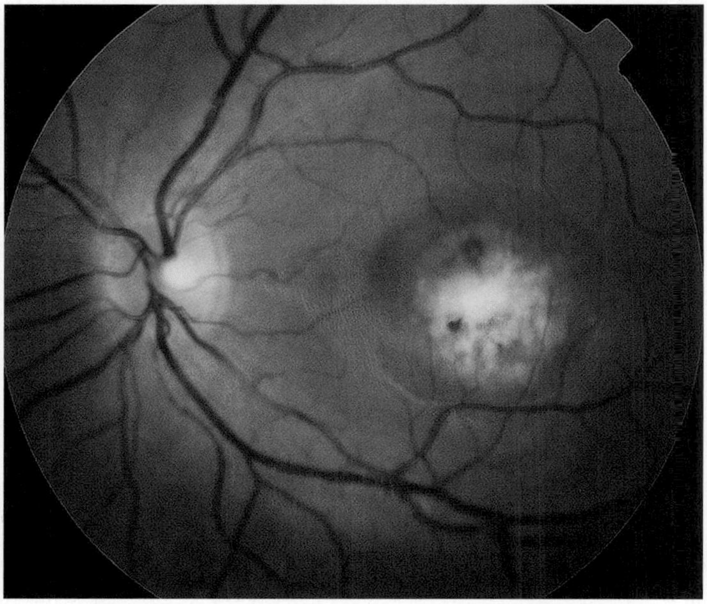

■ **Fig. 14.41** Rupture and scrambling of the lesion is serious because it may result in visual loss, which may be associated with choroidal neovascularisation (CNV).

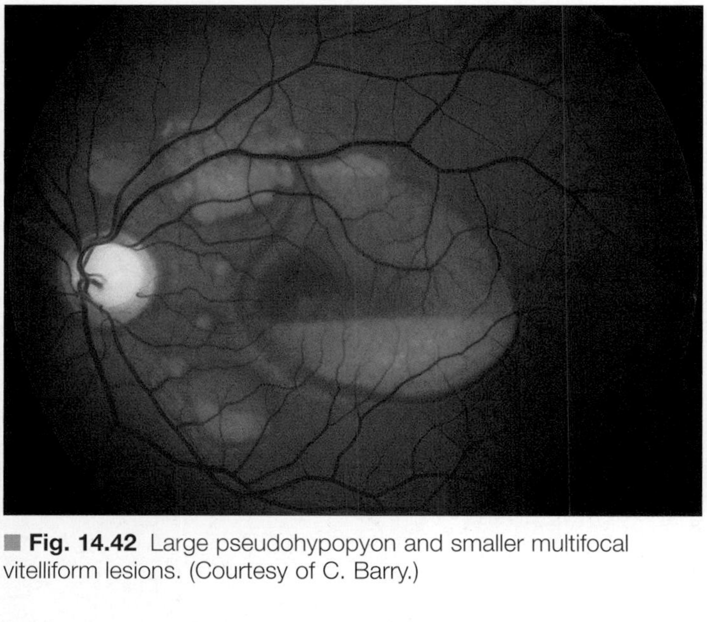

■ **Fig. 14.42** Large pseudohypopyon and smaller multifocal vitelliform lesions. (Courtesy of C. Barry.)

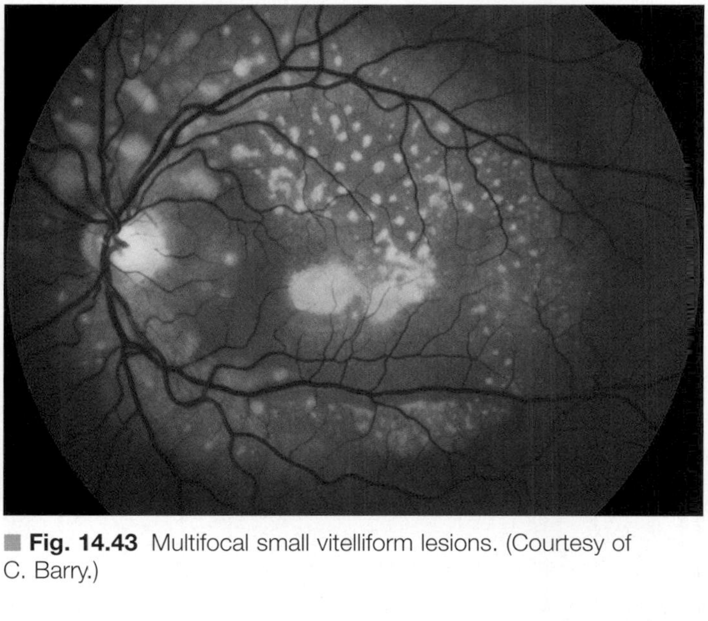

■ **Fig. 14.43** Multifocal small vitelliform lesions. (Courtesy of C. Barry.)

Acute exudative polymorphous vitelliform maculopathy disease

This is a very rare, sporadic condition that develops in adult life.

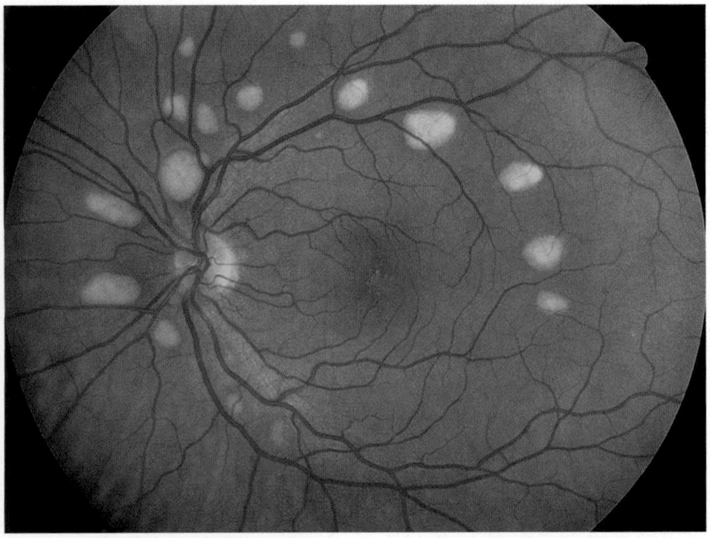

■ **Fig. 14.44** Sudden onset of bilateral, multifocal vitelliform lesions. (Courtesy of C. Barry.)

Congenital retinoschisis

Presentation of this XL condition is during the first decade with slowly progressive decrease in central vision. Foveal retinoschisis is universal but peripheral involvement is present in only 50% of cases.

Foveal schisis

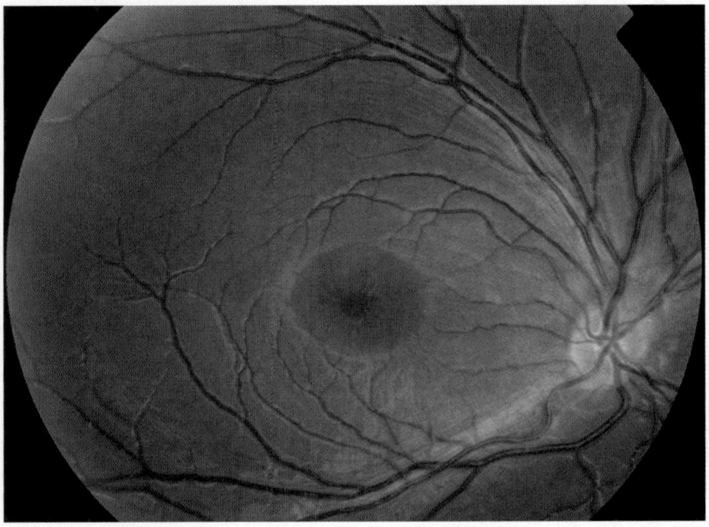

■ **Fig. 14.45** Foveal schisis is characterised by tiny cystoid spaces with a 'bicycle-wheel' pattern of radial striae. (Courtesy of G-C. Sarra.)

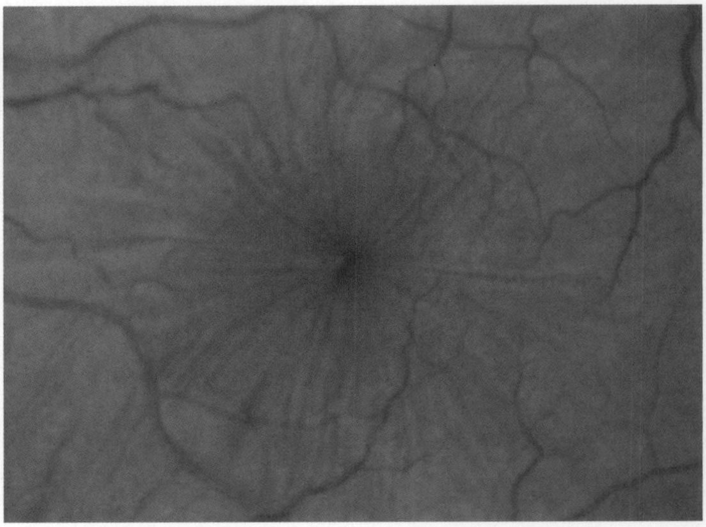

■ **Fig. 14.46** Magnified view. (Courtesy of Moorfields Eye Hospital.)

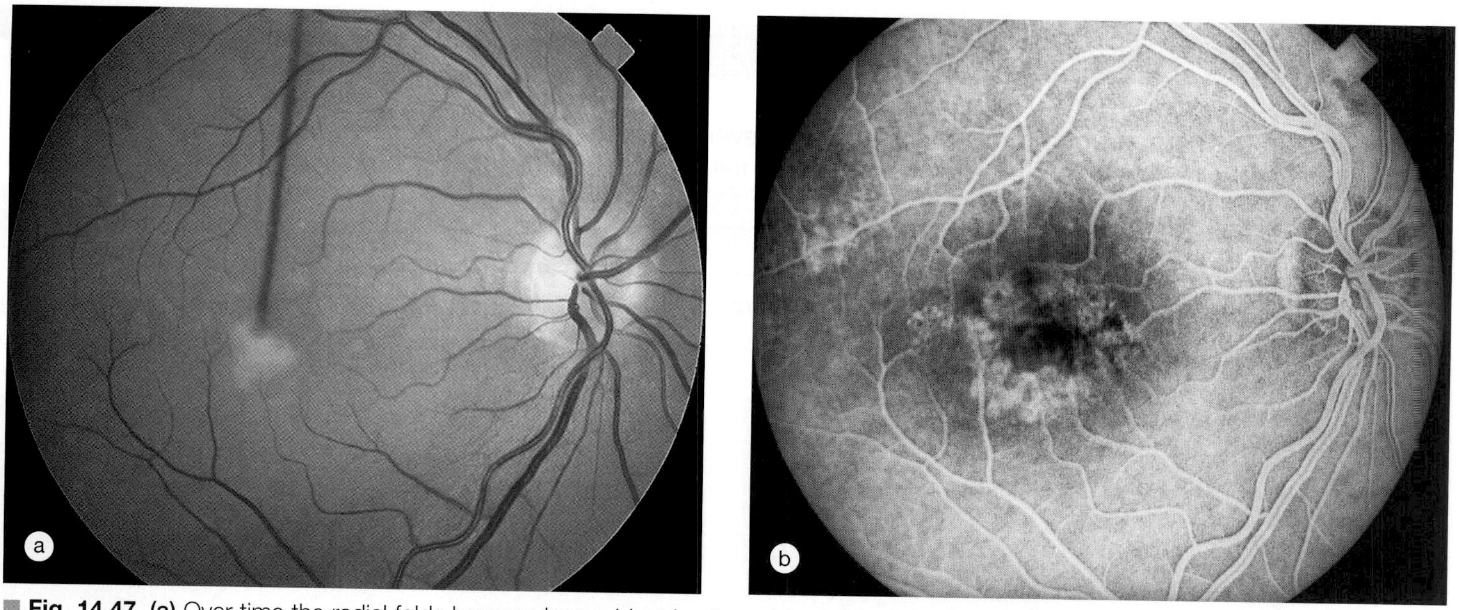

■ **Fig. 14.47** **(a)** Over time the radial folds become less evident leaving a blunted foveal reflex. **(b)** FA venous phase shows hyperfluorescence due to window defects. (Courtesy of S. Milewski.)

Peripheral schisis

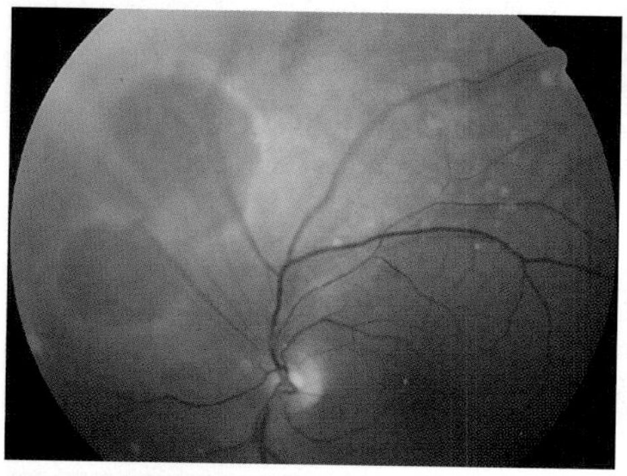

■ **Fig. 14.48** Two large defects in the inner leaf of retinoschisis. (Courtesy of C. Barry.)

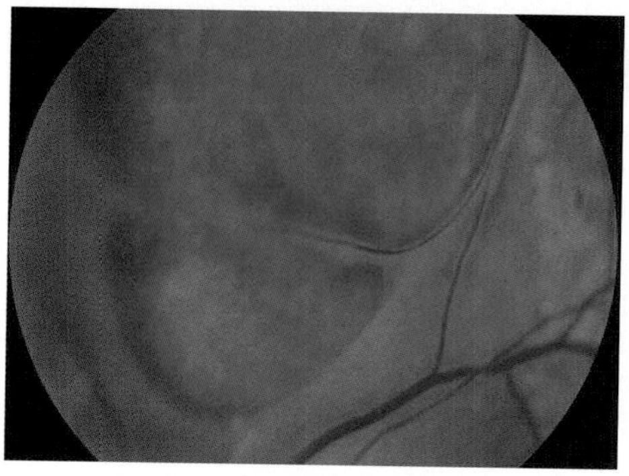

■ **Fig. 14.49** Coalescence of inner leaf defects leaving only retinal blood vessels floating in the vitreous ('vitreous veils'). (Courtesy of C. Barry.)

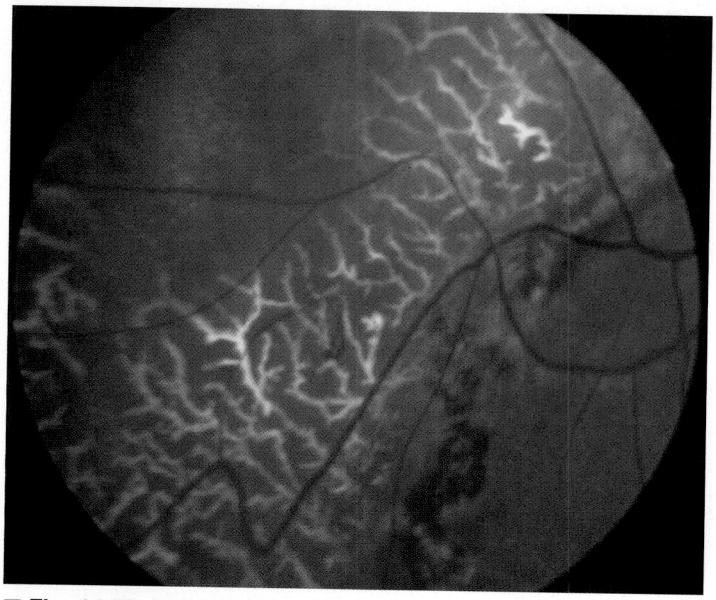

■ **Fig. 14.50** Peripheral dendritiform lesions consisting of sheathed and occluded vessels. (Courtesy of Moorfields Eye Hospital.)

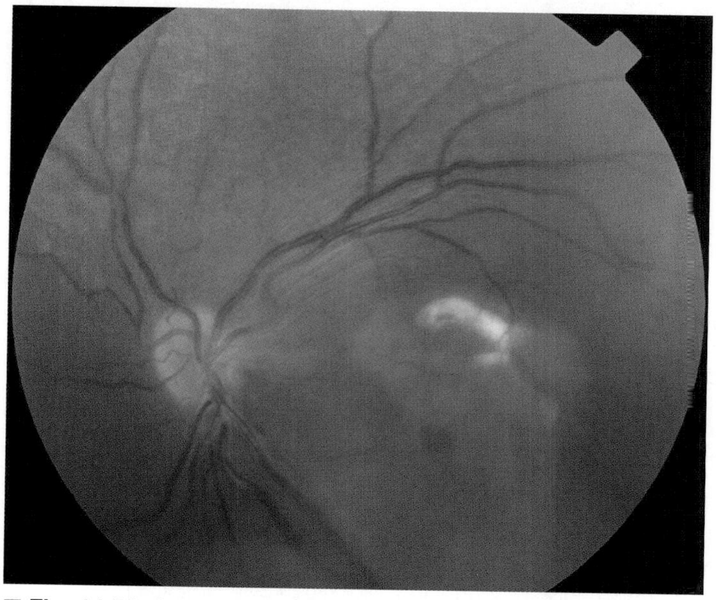

■ **Fig. 14.51** Subretinal exudation is uncommon. (Courtesy of G-C. Sarra.)

■ **Fig. 14.60** Macular coloboma-like atrophy. (Courtesy of A. Moore.)

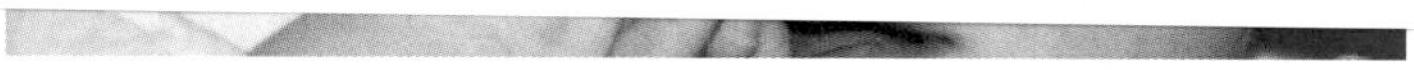

■ **Fig. 14.61** Oculodigital syndrome in which constant rubbing of the eyes by the child causes enophthalmos as a result of resorption of orbital fat. (Courtesy of M. Szreter.)

Adult-onset foveomacular vitelliform dystrophy

Presentation is in middle age with mild visual impairment. Inheritance is probably AD.

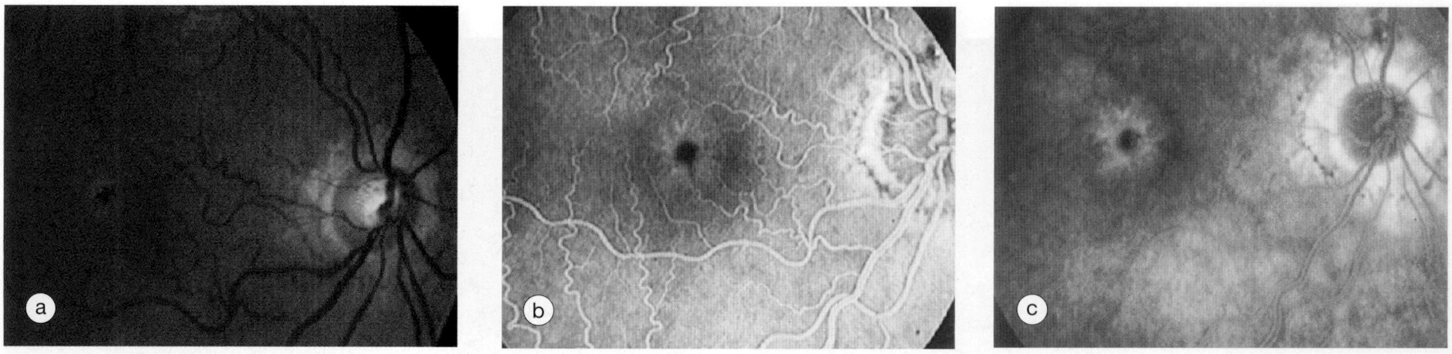

■ **Fig. 14.70** **(a)** Bilateral, symmetrical, round or oval, slightly elevated, yellowish subfoveal deposits, about one-third of a disc diameter in size, often centred on a pigmented spot. **(b)** FA venous phase shows early central hypofluorescence surrounded by a small irregular hyperfluorescent ring. **(c)** Late phase shows persistent hyperfluorescence.

Butterfly-shaped macular dystrophy

Presentation is in the second to fifth decade usually by chance and occasionally because of mild visual symptoms. Inheritance is probably AD.

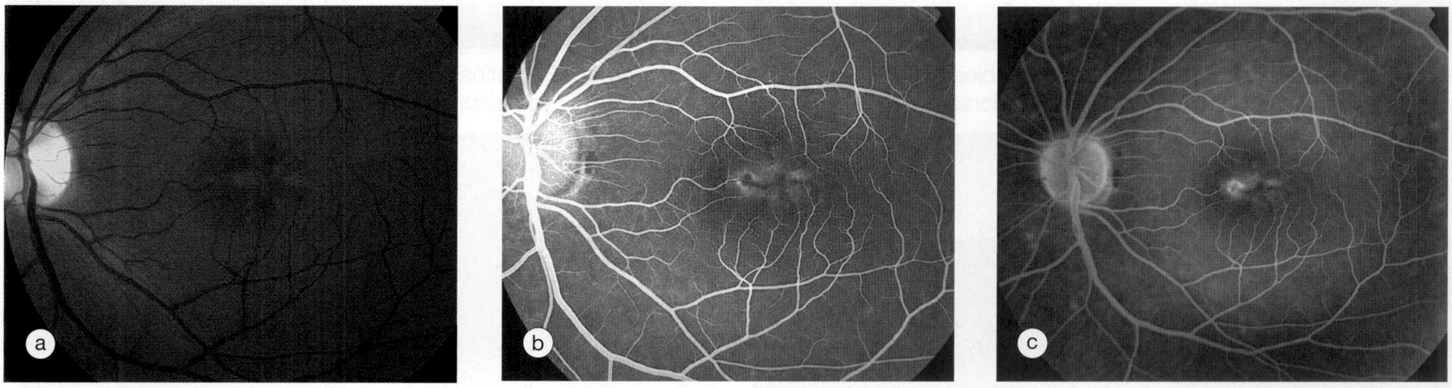

■ **Fig. 14.71** **(a)** Yellow pigment at the fovea arranged in a triradiate manner. **(b)** FA venous phase shows hyperfluorescence of the lesions. **(c)** Late phase shows persistent hyperfluorescence. (Courtesy of Moorfields Eye Hospital.)

Multifocal pattern dystrophy simulating fundus flavimaculatus

Presentation of this AD disease is in the fourth decade with mild visual impairment.

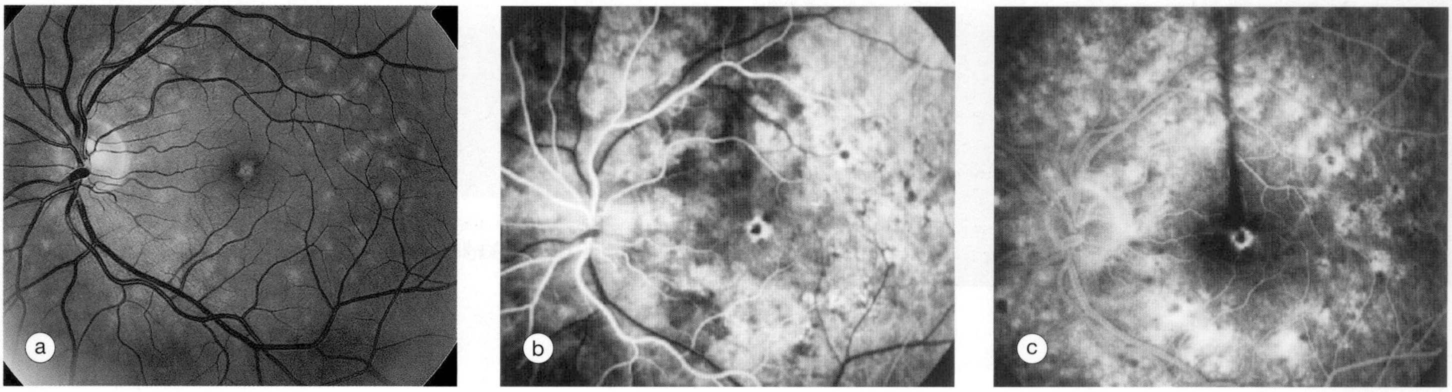

■ **Fig. 14.72** **(a)** Widely scattered, irregular, yellow lesions that may be similar to those seen in fundus flavimaculatus. **(b)** FA arterial phase shows hyperfluorescence of flecks but the choroid is not dark. **(c)** Late phase shows persistent hyperfluorescence. (Courtesy of S. Milewski.)

Dominant macular oedema

Presentation of this AD condition is in the first to second decade with gradual bilateral impairment of central vision.

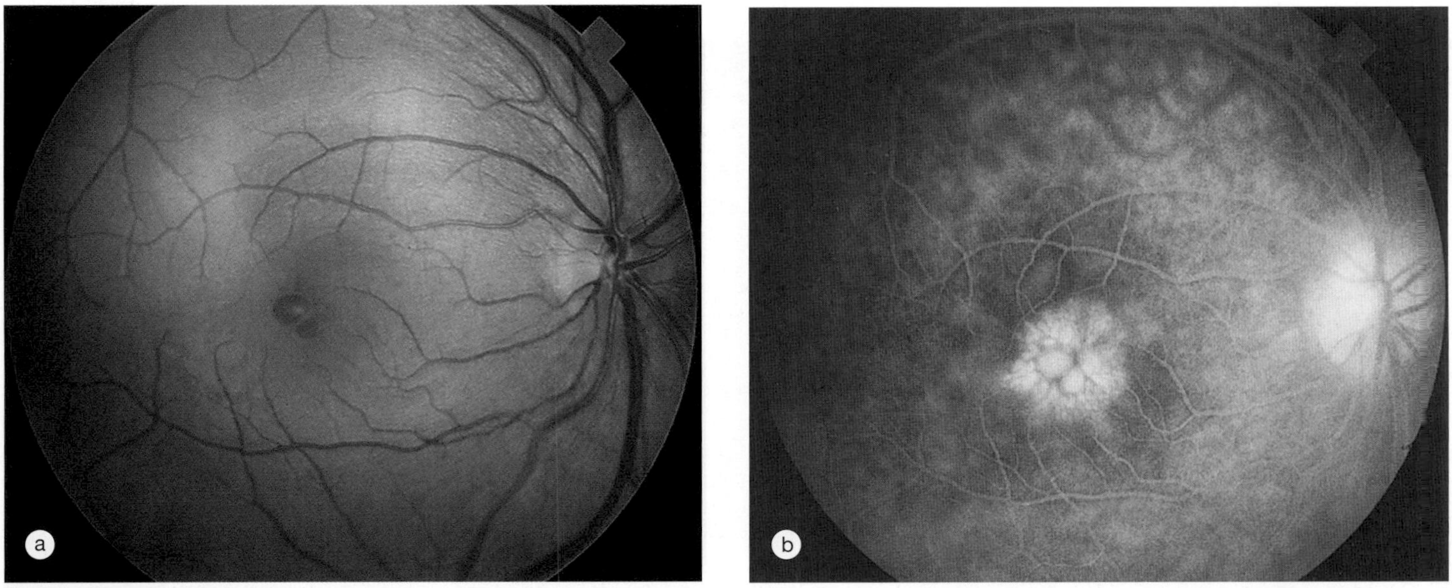

Fig. 14.73 **(a)** CMO. **(b)** FA late phase shows hyperfluorescence, which has a 'flower-petal' pattern.

Bietti crystalline dystrophy

Presentation is in the third decade with slowly progressive visual loss. Inheritance is usually AR and occasionally AD or XL.

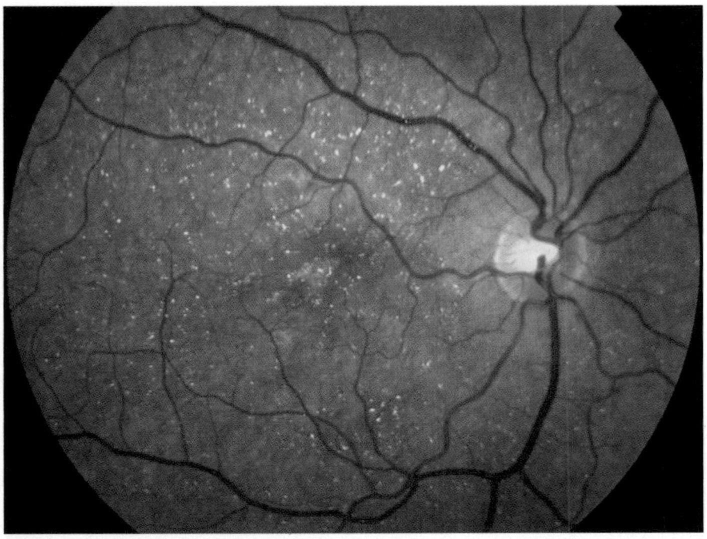

Fig. 14.74 Numerous, fine, glistening, yellow-white crystals scattered throughout the posterior fundus followed by geographic atrophy.

Benign concentric annular macular dystrophy

Presentation of this AD condition is in adult life with very mild impairment of central vision.

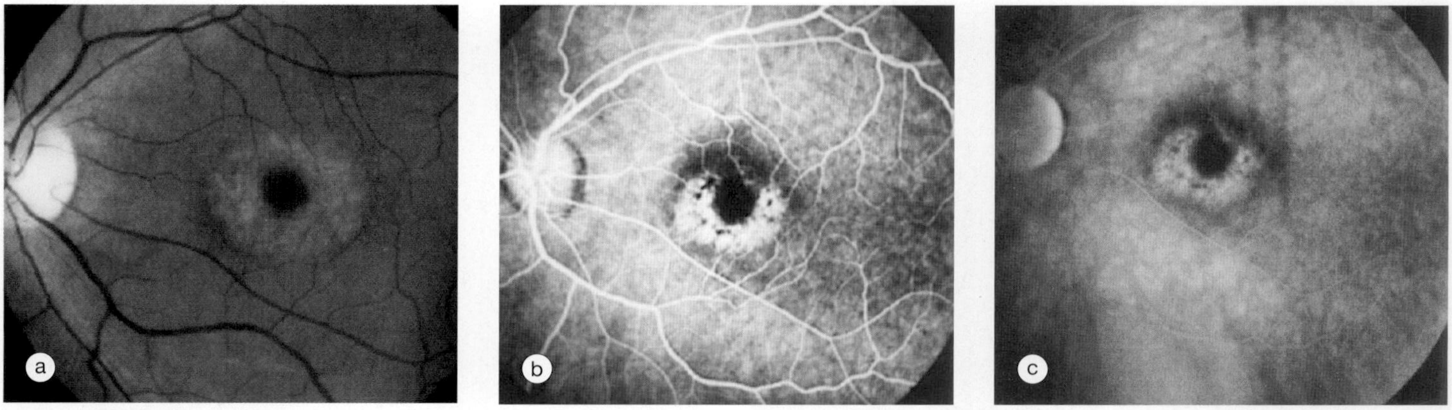

Fig. 14.82 **(a)** Bull's eye maculopathy. **(b)** FA venous phase shows an annular RPE window defect. **(c)** Late phase shows less fluorescence. (Courtesy of S. Milewski.)

Oguchi disease

Oguchi disease is an AR condition characterised by stationary night blindness.

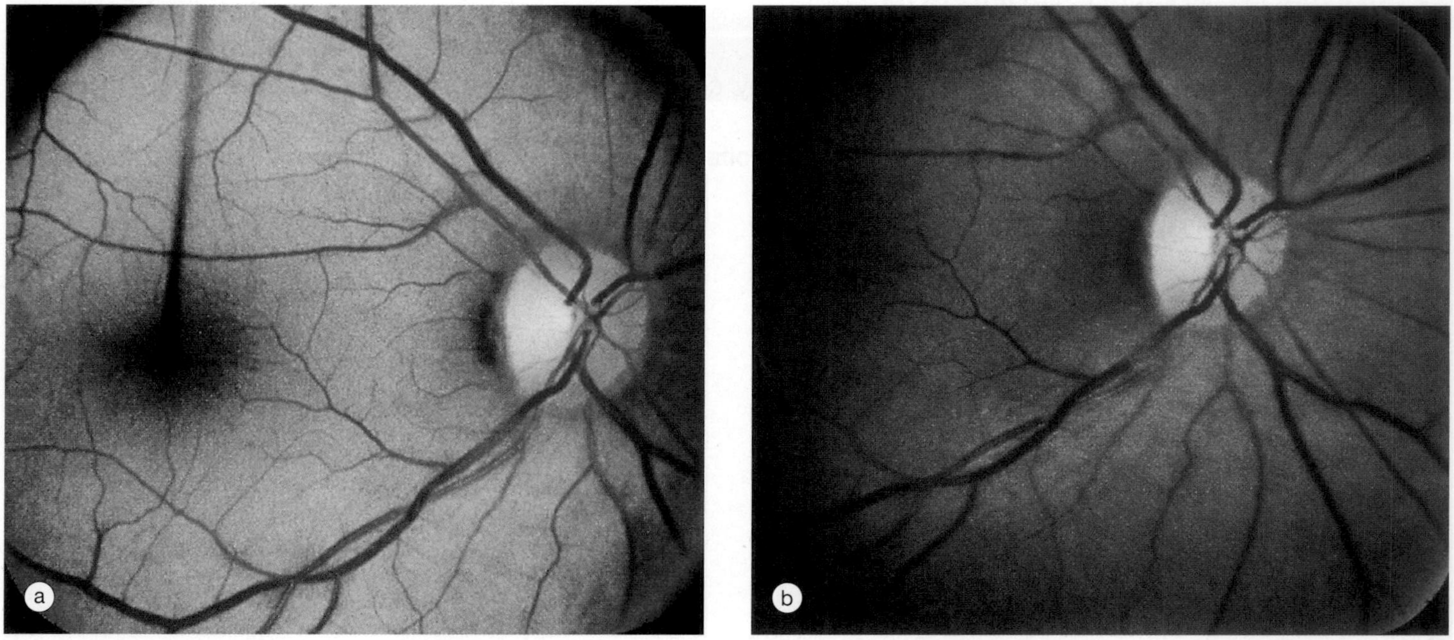

Fig. 14.83 Mizuo phenomenon. **(a)** Golden-brown fundus in the light-adapted state. **(b)** Normal colour in the dark-adapted state. (Courtesy of J. D. M. Gass.)

Fundus albipunctatus

Fundus albipunctatus is an AR condition characterised by stationary night blindness.

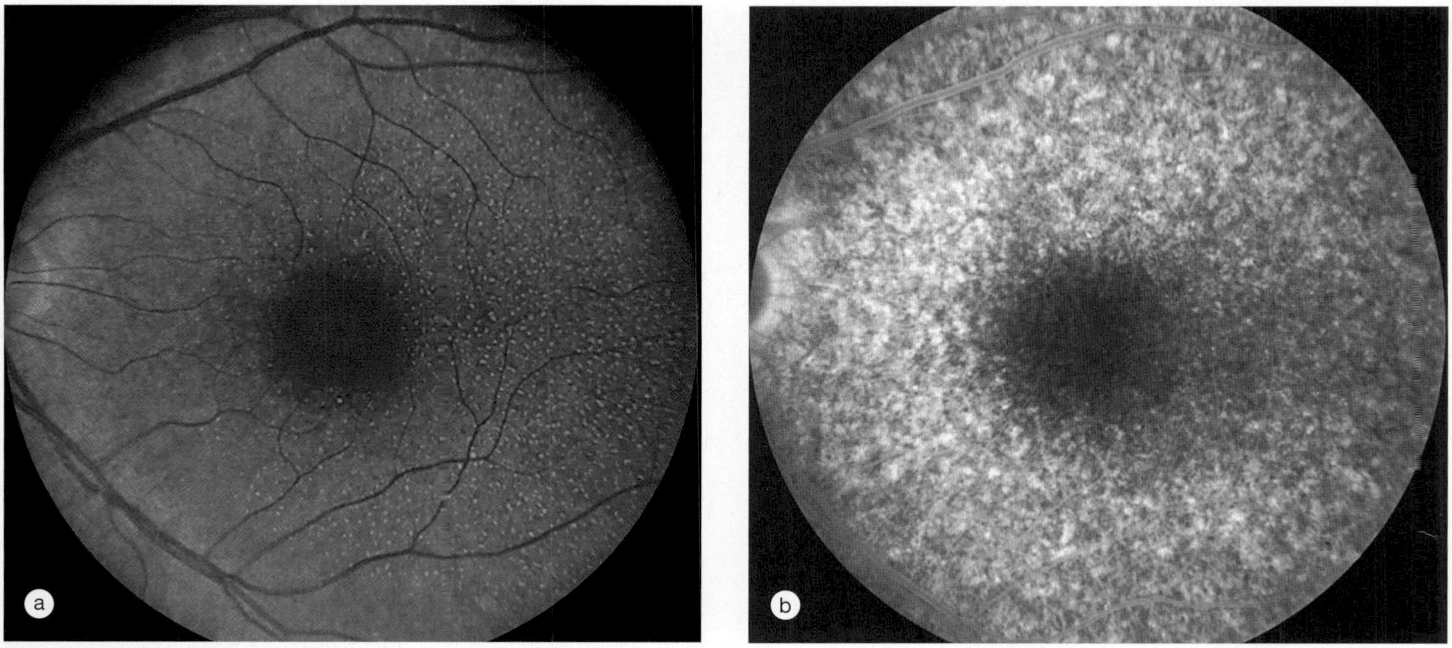

Fig. 14.84 (a) A multitude of tiny, yellow-white spots at the posterior pole, sparing the fovea. **(b)** FA shows corresponding hyperfluorescence. (Courtesy of C. Barry.)

Cherry-red spot at macula

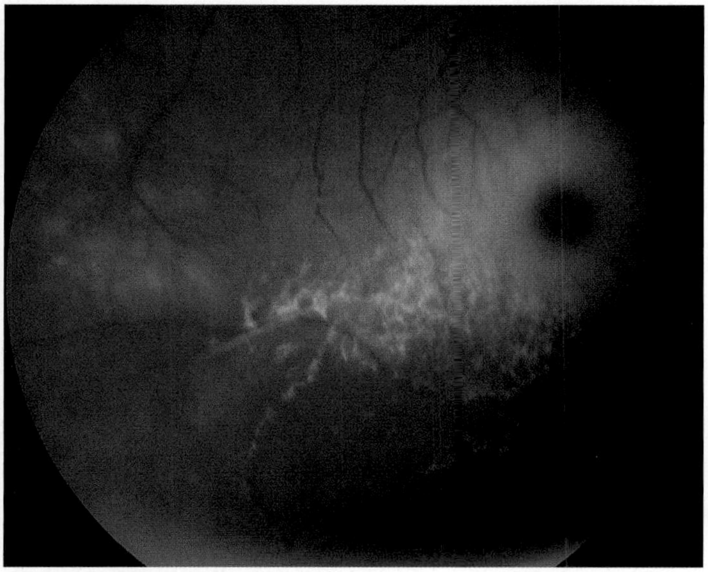

Fig. 14.85 The cherry-red spot at the macula is caused by accumulation of sphingolipids in retinal ganglion cells in the parafoveal area. The fovea itself retains its normal colour because it is devoid of ganglion cells. The two most common underlying systemic diseases are Tay–Sachs and Niemann–Pick. (Courtesy of S. Ford and R Marsh.)

VITREORETINOPATHIES

Stickler syndrome (hereditary arthro-ophthalmopathy)

Inheritance is AD with complete penetrance but variable expressivity.

Systemic signs

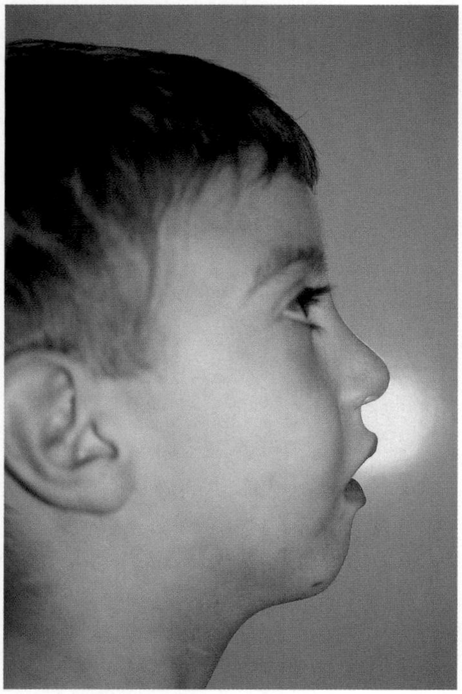

Fig. 14.86 Flat nasal bridge, maxillary hypoplasia, micrognathia and small tongue.

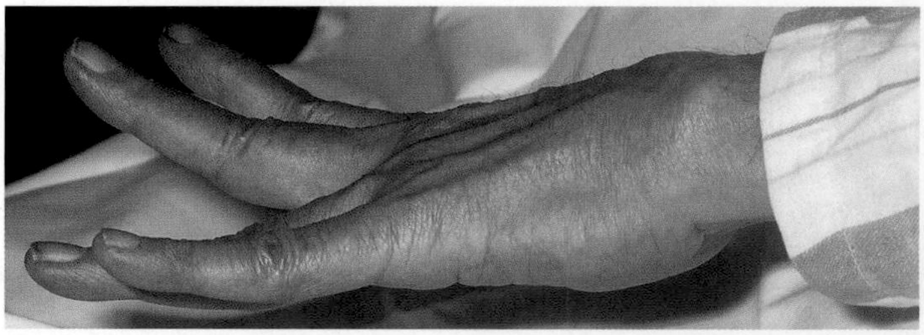

Fig. 14.87 Arachnodactyly and joint hyperextensibility.

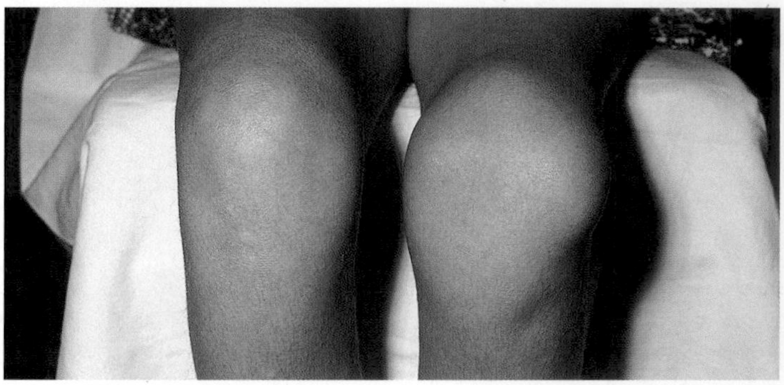

Fig. 14.88 Arthropathy.

Eye signs

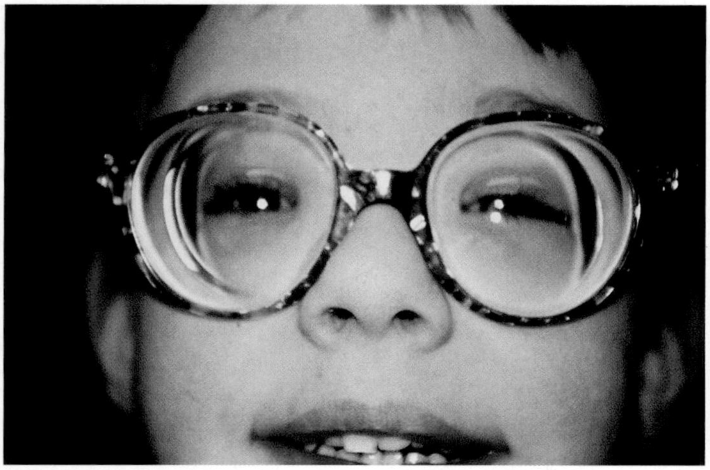

Fig. 14.89 High myopia. (Courtesy of K. Nischal.)

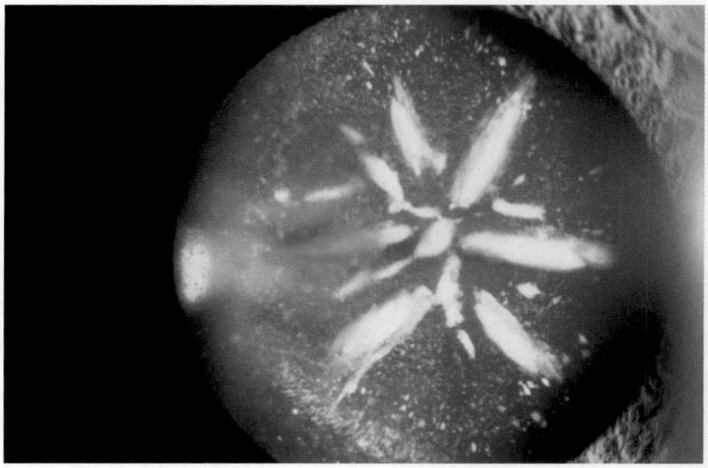

Fig. 14.90 Non-progressive lens opacities are common.

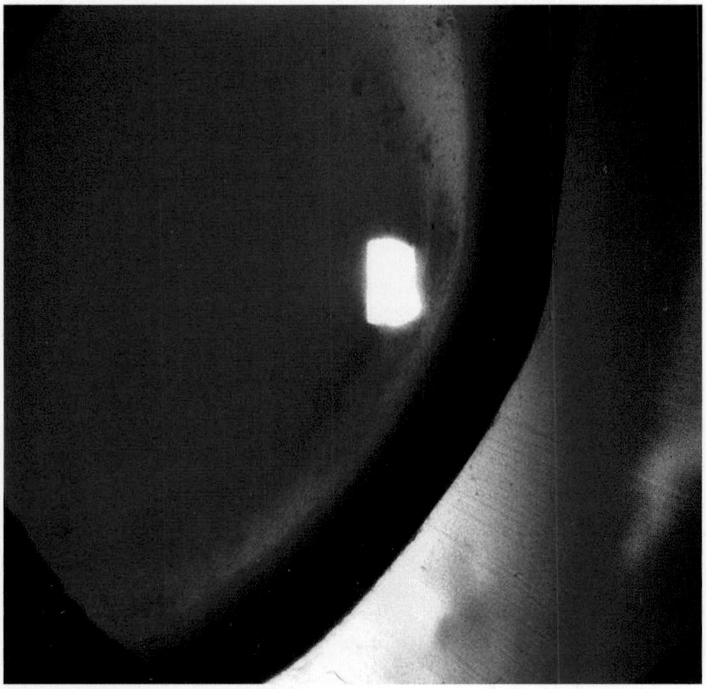

■ **Fig. 14.91** Ectopia lentis is uncommon.

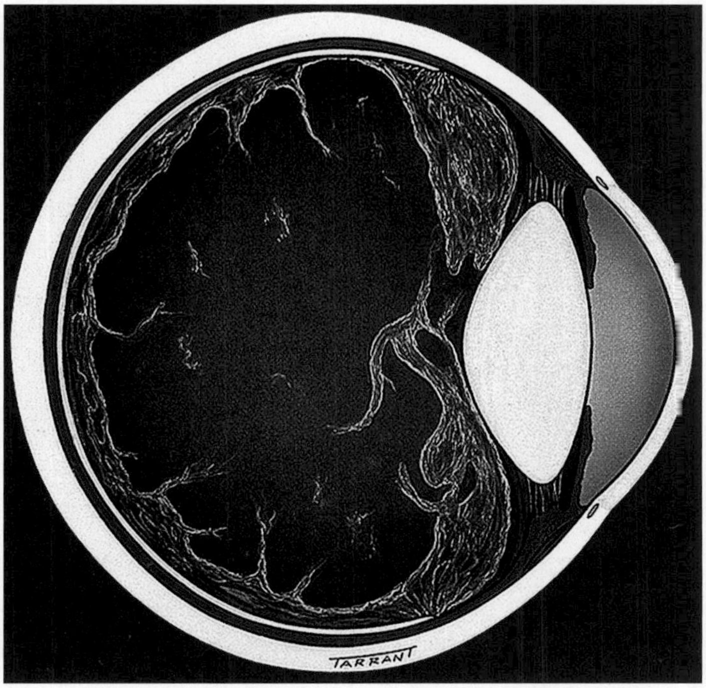

■ **Fig. 14.92** An optically empty central vitreous cavity due to liquefaction and syneresis (contraction) associated with circumferential, equatorial membranes extending a short way into the vitreous cavity.

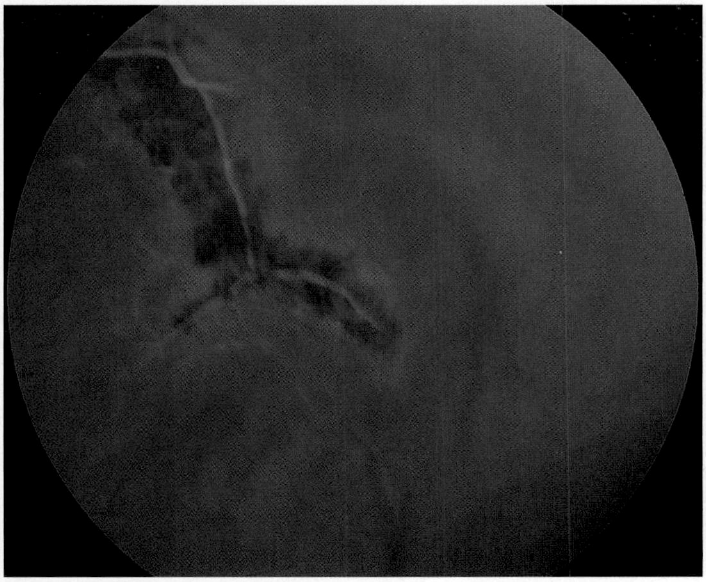

■ **Fig. 14.93** Radial lattice-like degeneration associated with RPE hyperplasia, vascular sheathing and sclerosis.

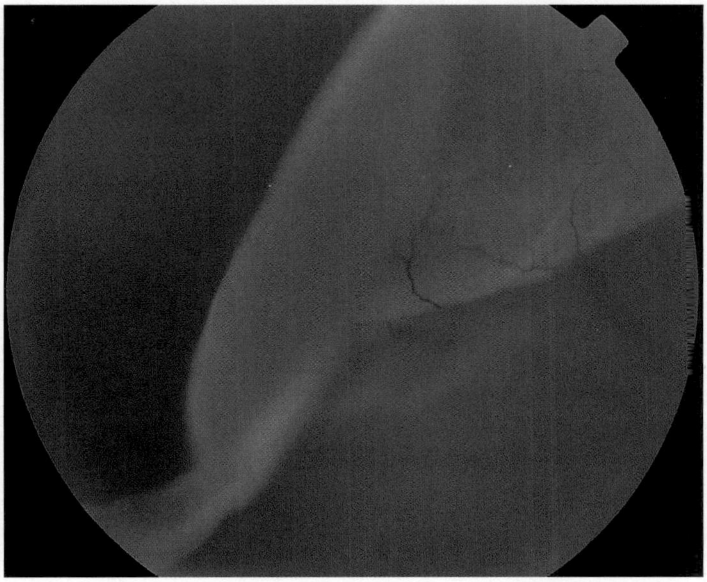

■ **Fig. 14.94** Retinal detachment, often as a result of giant tears, develops in approximately 30% of patients in the first decade of life.

Wagner syndrome

Inheritance is AD.

Fig. 14.95 Vitreous liquefaction with complete absence of normal scaffolding. (Courtesy of E. Messmer.)

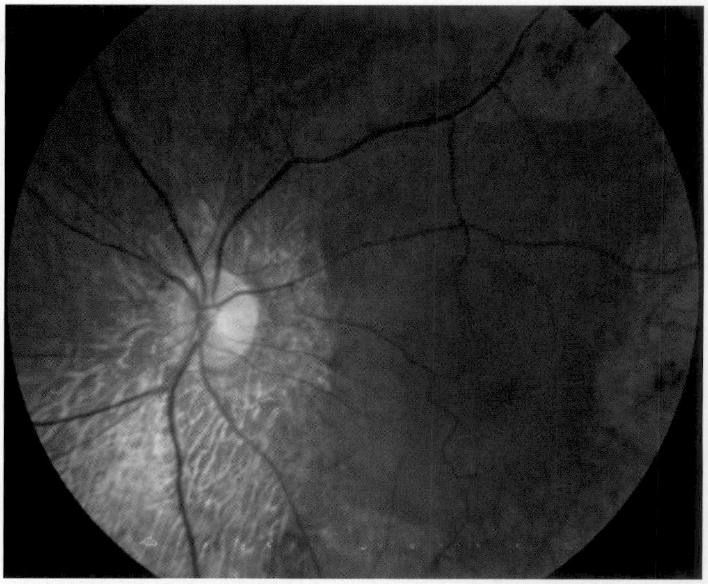

Fig. 14.96 Progressive chorioretinal atrophy. (Courtesy of E. Messmer.)

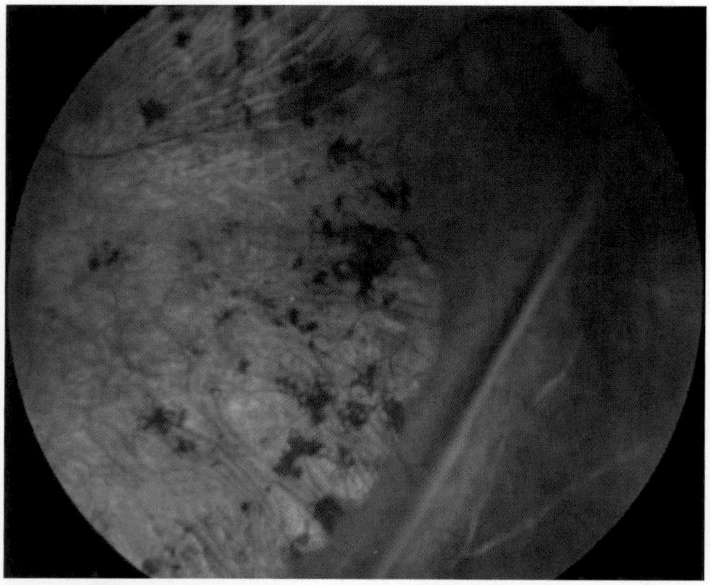

Fig. 14.97 Peripheral chorioretinal atrophy, avascularity and preretinal greyish-white membranes. (Courtesy of E. Messmer.)

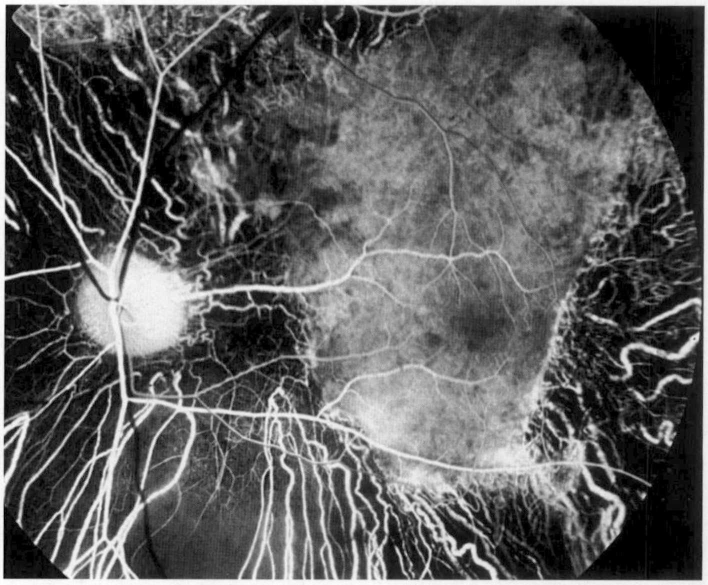

Fig. 14.98 FA shows gross loss of the choriocapillaris. (Courtesy of E. Messmer.)

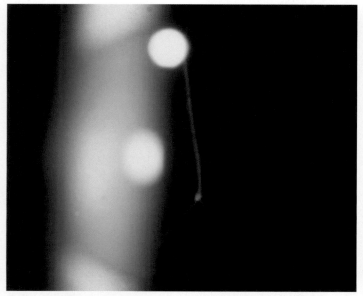

Familial exudative vitreoretinopathy (Criswick–Schepens syndrome)

Inheritance is AD and rarely X-linked recessive (XLR) with high penetrance and variable expressivity. Presentation is in late childhood.

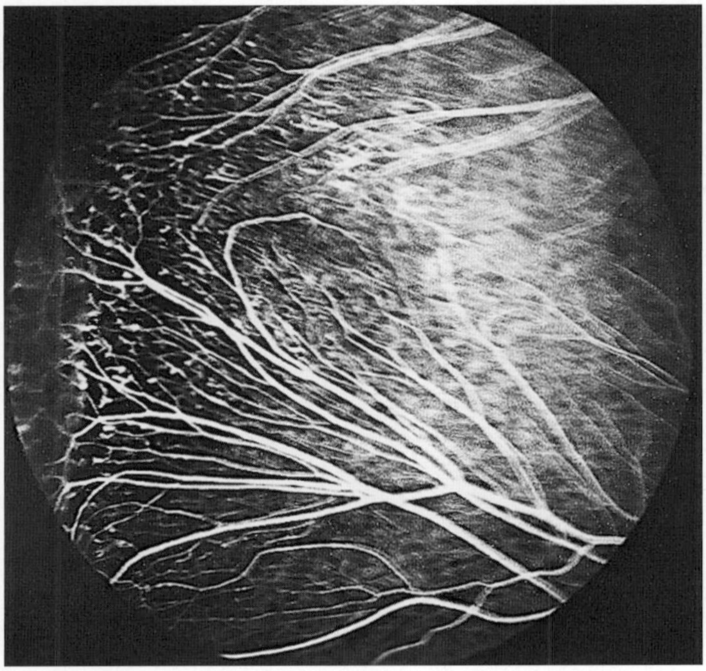

Fig. 14.99 FA shows peripheral non-perfusion with abrupt termination and straightening of vessels.

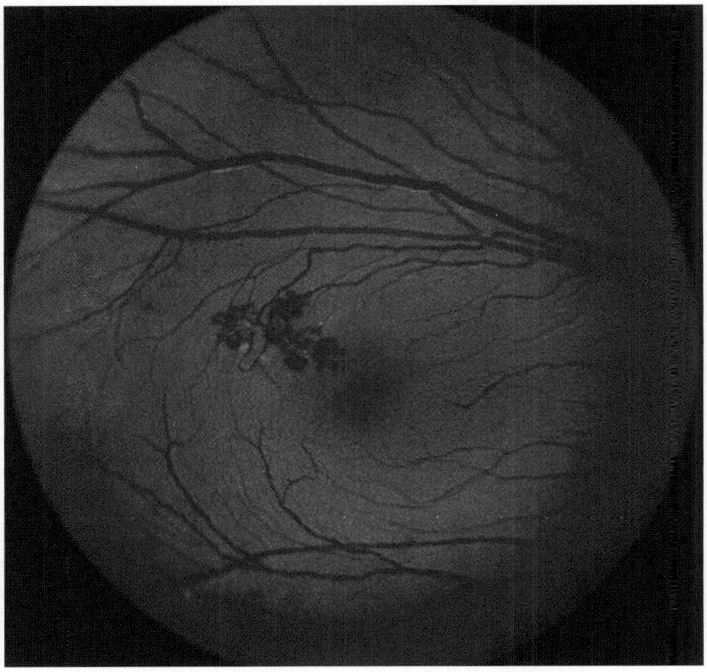

Fig. 14.100 Early peripheral retinal telangiectasis.

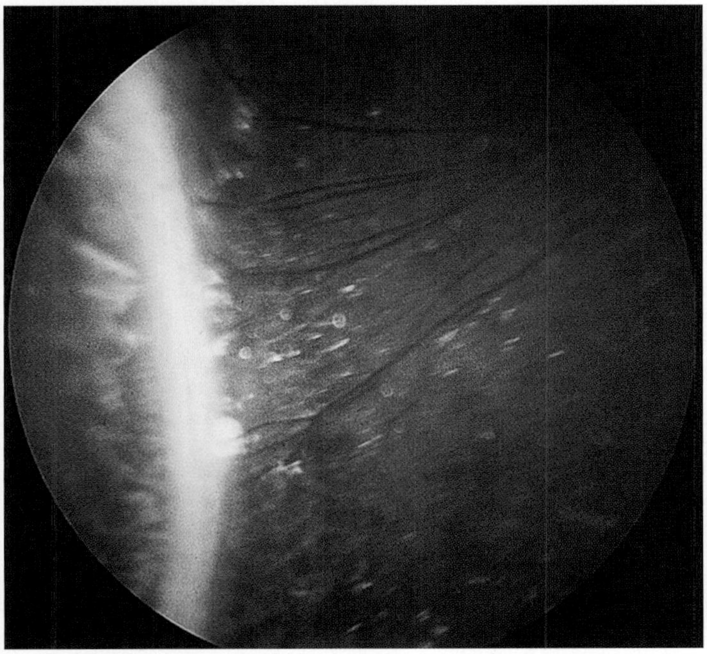

Fig. 14.101 Fibrovascular proliferation and vitreoretinal traction resulting in ridge formation.

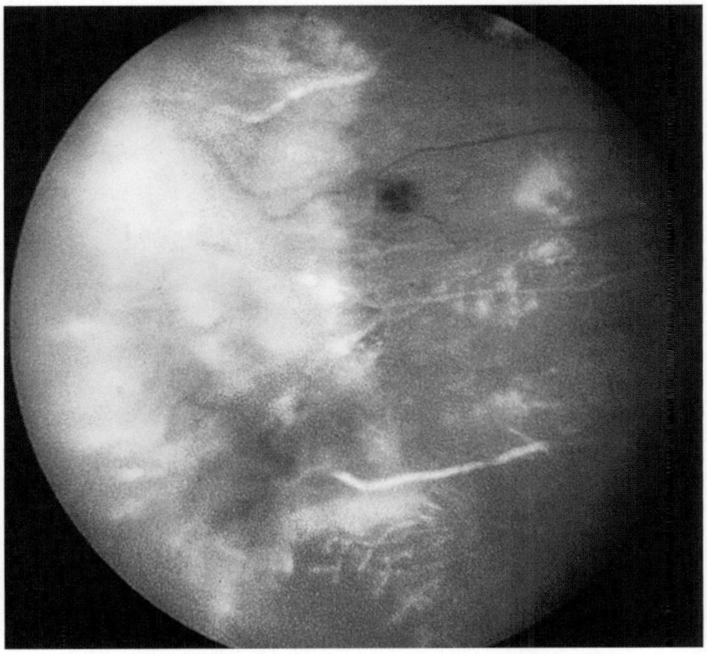

Fig. 14.102 Severe peripheral fibrovascular proliferation.

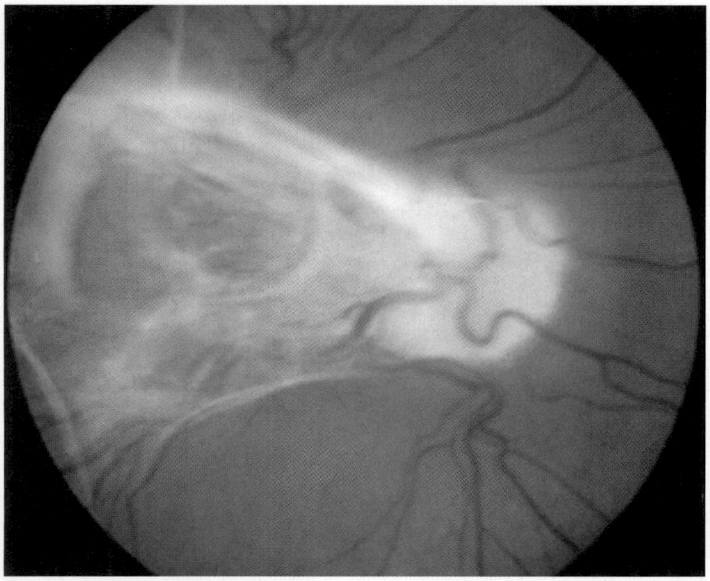

■ **Fig. 14.103** Temporal 'dragging' of the macula and disc by fibrous tissue.

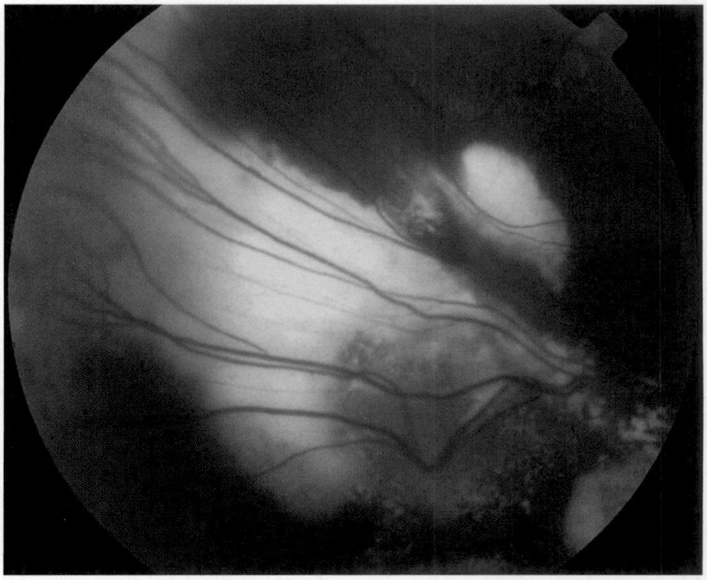

■ **Fig. 14.104** Massive subretinal exudation is uncommon. (Courtesy of C. Hoyng.)

Snowflake vitreoretinal degeneration

Inheritance is AD.

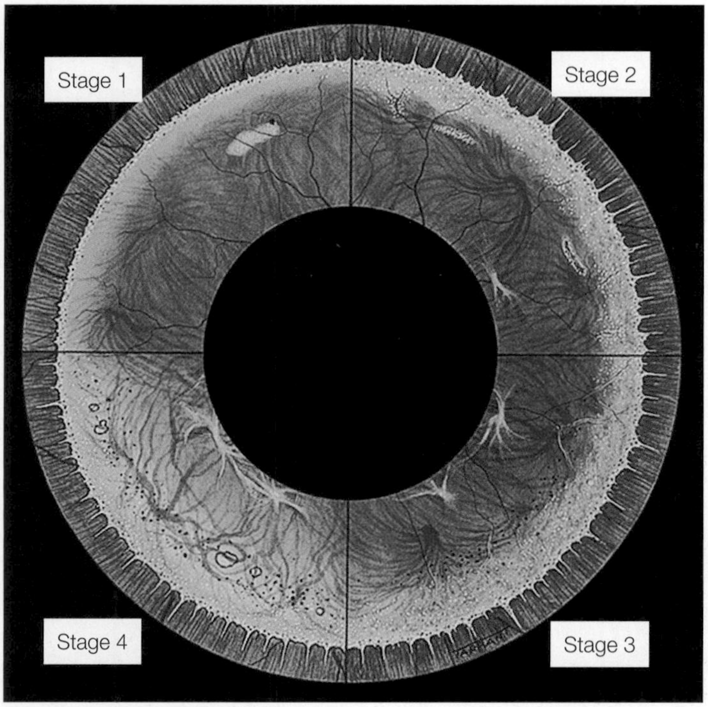

■ **Fig. 14.105** Stage 1 – extensive areas of 'white-without-pressure' in patients under the age of 15 years; stage 2 – snowflake-like, yellow-white spots in areas of 'white-with-pressure' between 15 and 25 years; stage 3 – vascular sheathing and pigmentation posterior to the area of snowflake degeneration between 25 and 50 years; stage 4 – increased pigmentation, gross vascular attenuation, areas of chorioretinal atrophy and less apparent snowflakes over the age of 60 years.

CHOROIDAL DYSTROPHIES

Choroideraemia

Presentation of this XLR condition is in the first decade with nyctalopia.

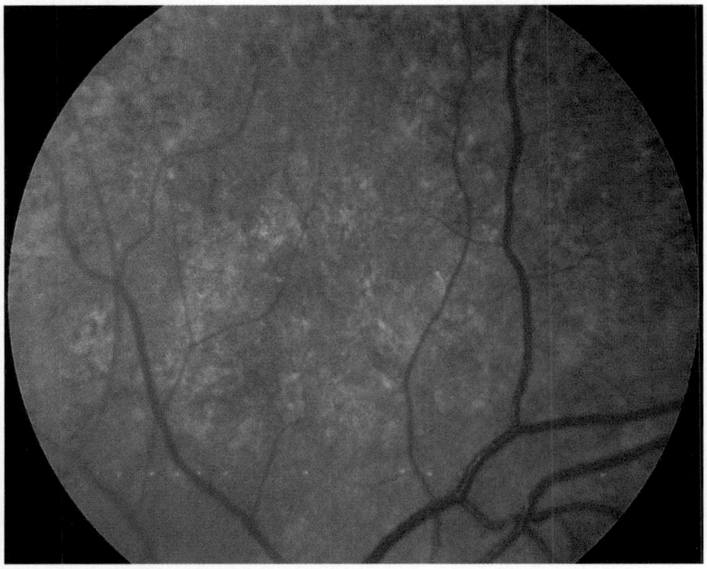

Fig. 14.106 Peripheral pigmentary changes in a female carrier of choroideraemia.

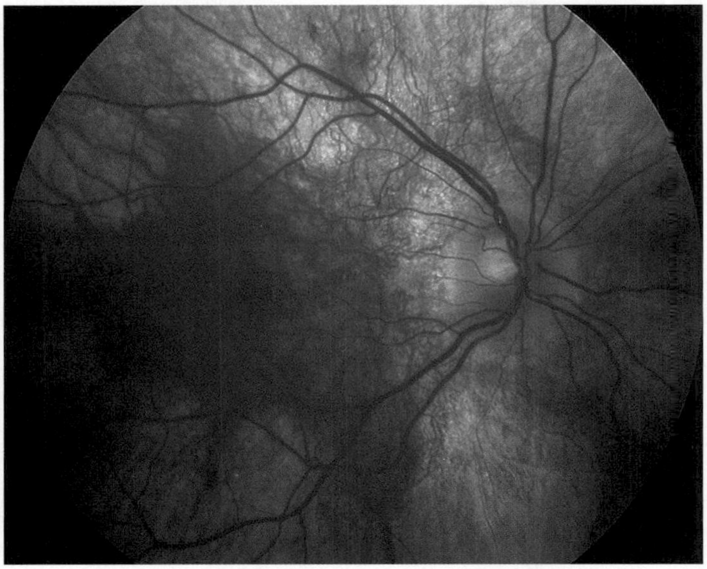

Fig. 14.107 Mid-peripheral patches of choroidal and RPE atrophy.

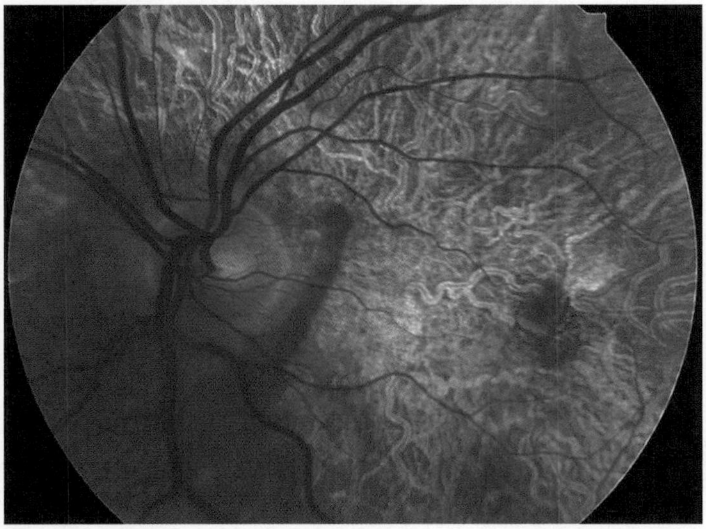

Fig. 14.108 Diffuse atrophy of the choriocapillaris and RPE with preservation of the intermediate and large choroidal vessels.

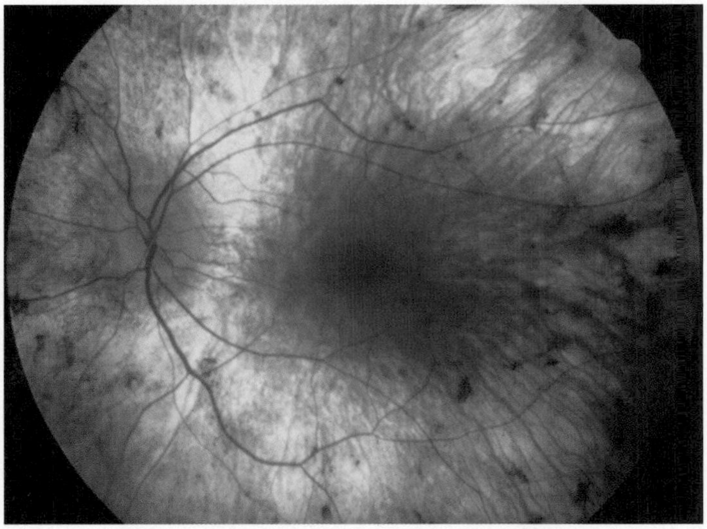

Fig. 14.109 Advanced disease with visibility of the sclera except at the posterior pole. (Courtesy of L. Merin.)

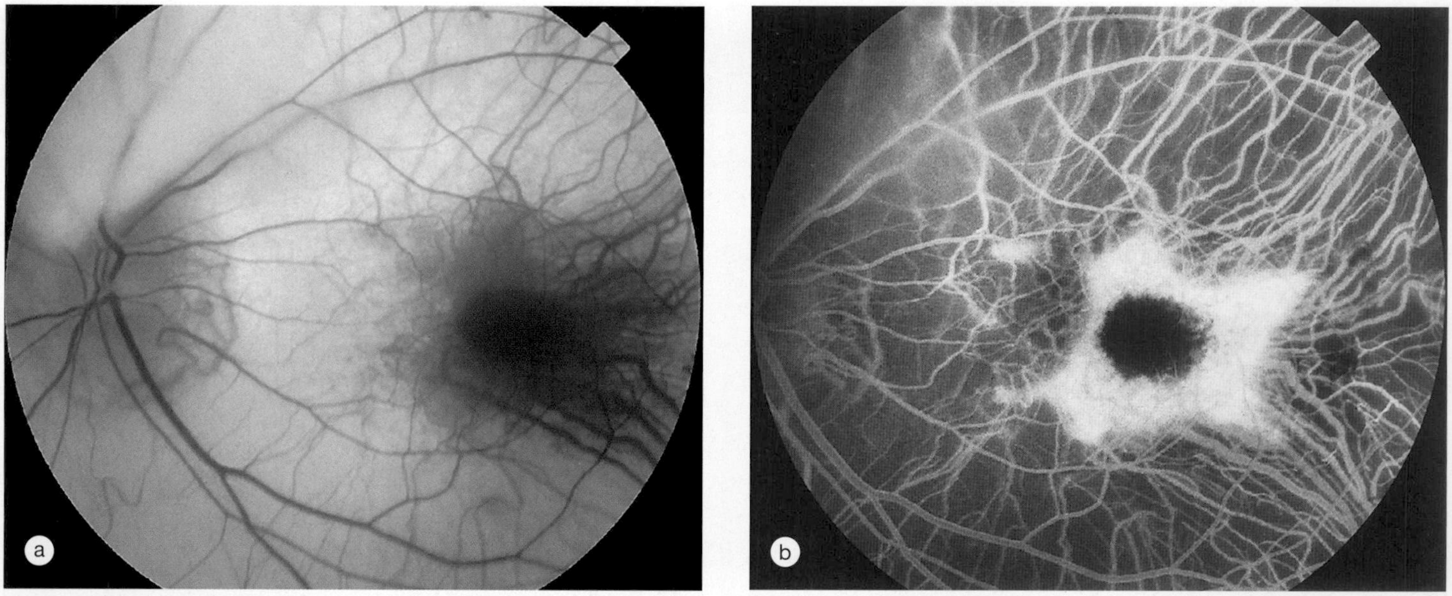

■ **Fig. 14.110** **(a)** Very advanced with preservation of the fovea. **(b)** FA shows filling of the retinal and large choroidal vessels but not of the choriocapillaris. There is also hypofluorescence corresponding to the intact fovea and a surrounding area of hyperfluorescence due to a window defect. (Courtesy of S. Milewski.)

Gyrate atrophy

Presentation of this AR disease is in the first decade with axial myopia and reduction of peripheral vision, often associated with nyctalopia.

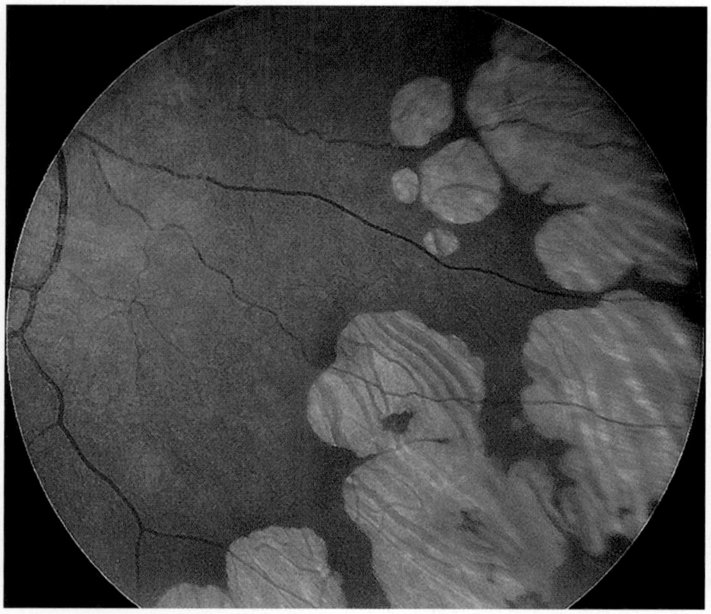

■ **Fig. 14.111** Peripheral patches of chorioretinal atrophy.

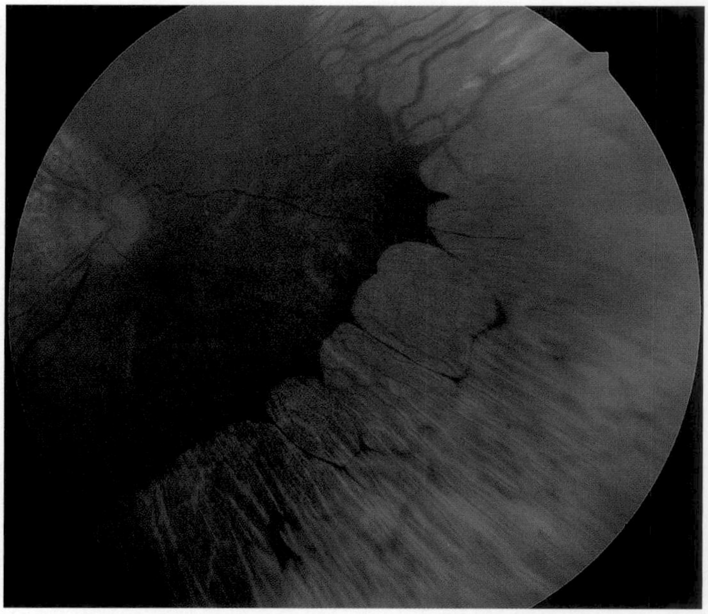

■ **Fig. 14.112** Increase in size and number of the lesions with coalescence forming a scalloped posterior border with subsequent gradual central spread.

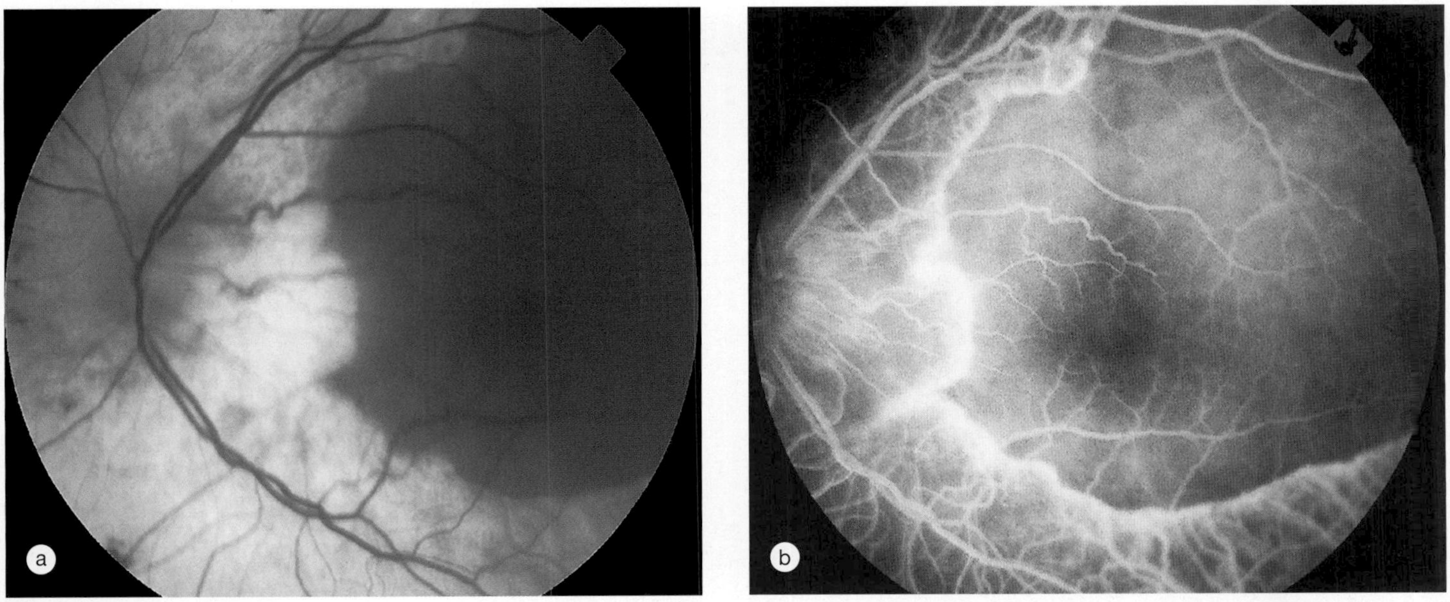

■ **Fig. 14.113** **(a)** Gyrate atrophy. **(b)** FA shows the sharp contrast between normal and atrophic areas. (Courtesy of S. Milewski.)

Central areolar choroidal dystrophy

Presentation of this AD condition is in the third to fourth decade with gradual impairment of central vision.

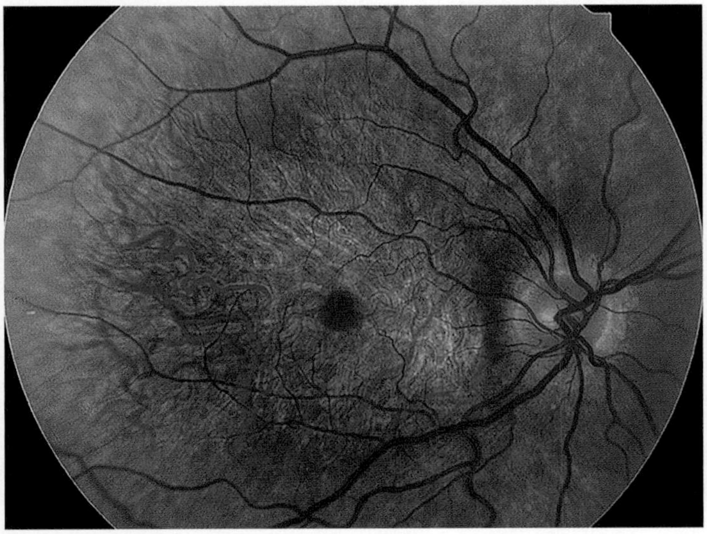

■ **Fig. 14.114** Circumscribed RPE atrophy and loss of the choriocapillaris at the macula.

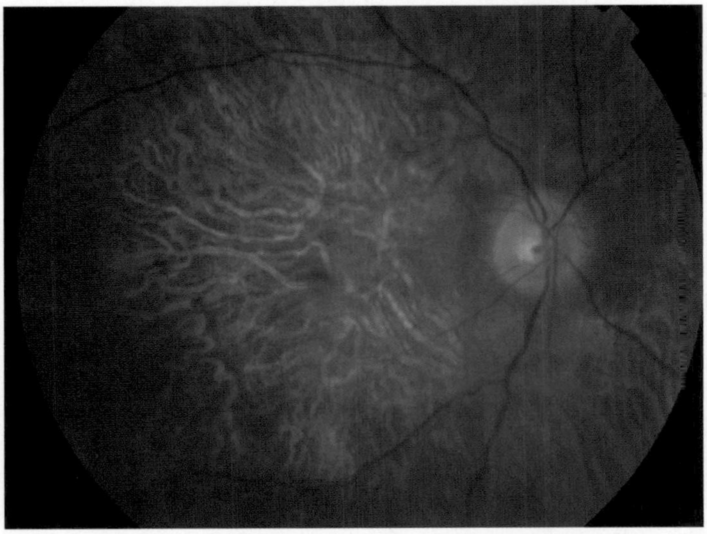

■ **Fig. 14.115** Slowly expanding geographic atrophy within which the larger choroidal vessels are prominent. (Courtesy of Moorfields Eye Hospital.)

Diffuse choroidal atrophy

Presentation of this AD condition is in the fourth to fifth decade with impairment of central vision or nyctalopia.

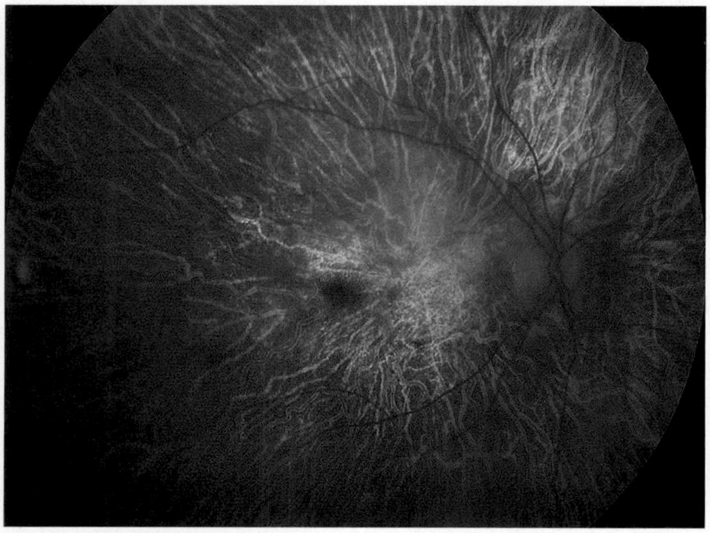

Fig. 14.116 Diffuse atrophy of the RPE and choriocapillaris.

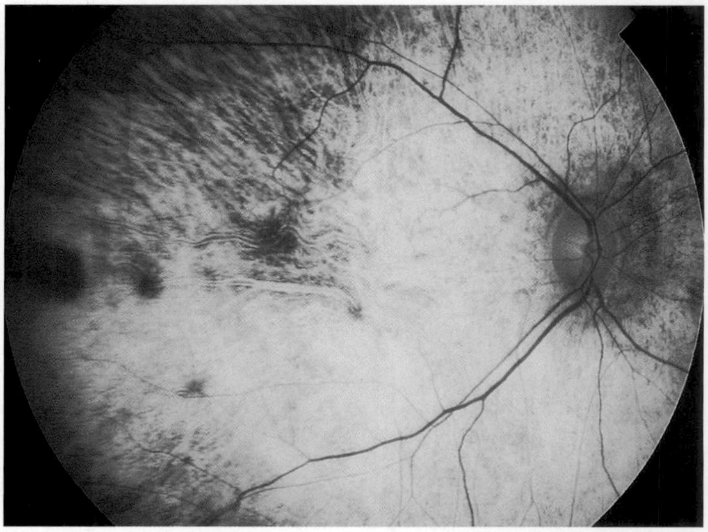

Fig. 14.117 Atrophy of most of the larger choroidal vessels with scleral exposure.

Pigmented paravenous retinochoroidal atrophy

Presentation is often by chance because the condition is usually asymptomatic. Inheritance is uncertain.

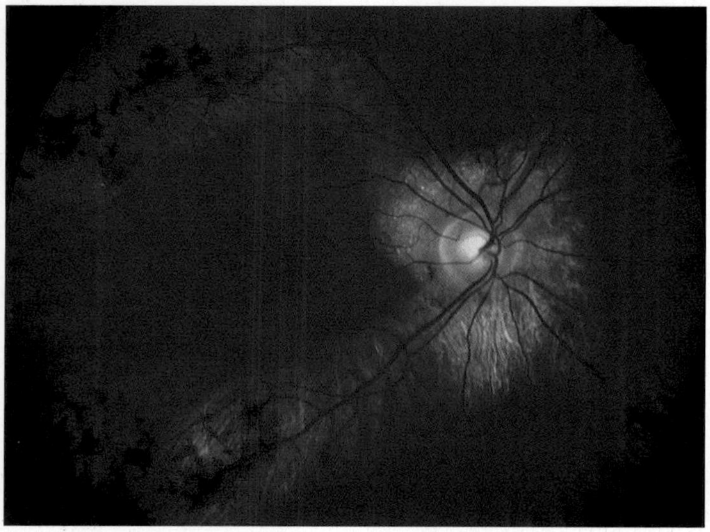

Fig. 14.118 Paravenous zones of chorioretinal atrophy associated with bone-spicule pigmentation. (Courtesy of C. Barry.)

Progressive bifocal chorioretinal atrophy

Presentation of this very rare AD condition is at birth.

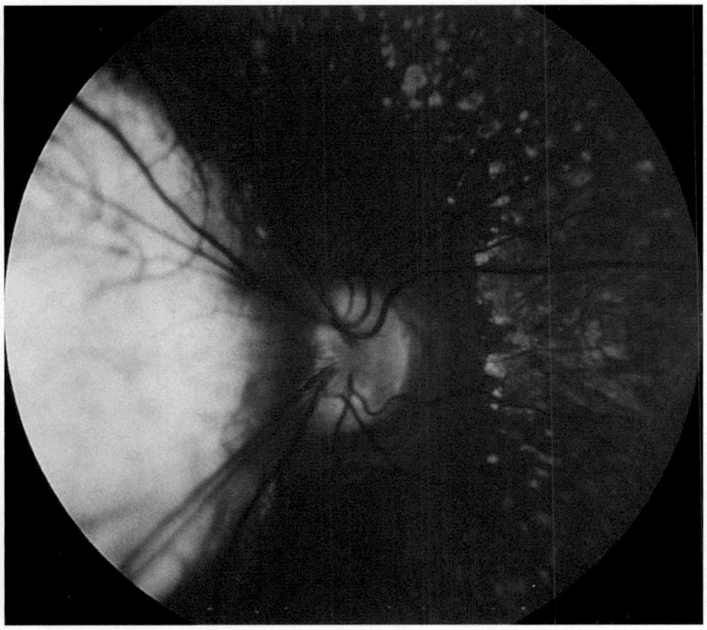

Fig. 14.119 A focus of chorioretinal atrophy temporal to the disc that extends in all directions. A similar lesion develops nasally. The end result manifests two separate areas of chorioretinal atrophy separated by a normal segment. (Courtesy of Moorfields Eye Hospital.)

CHAPTER 15

CONGENITAL ANOMALIES OF THE POSTERIOR SEGMENT

RETINA AND CHOROID

Retinochoroidal coloboma

A retinochoroidal coloboma is the result of incomplete closure of the embryonic fissure.

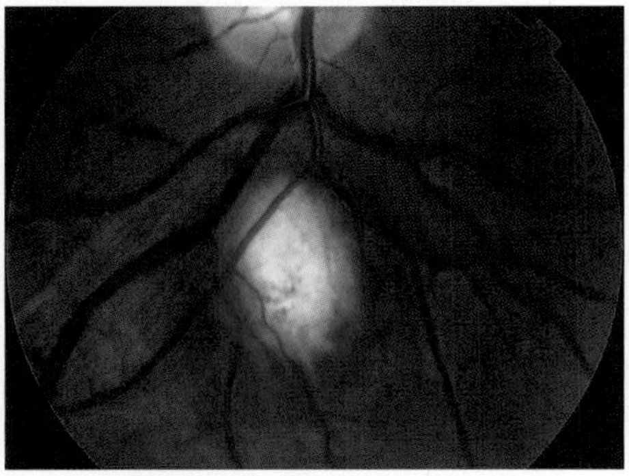

■ **Fig. 15.1** Sharply circumscribed, white area, devoid of blood vessels, in the inferior fundus.

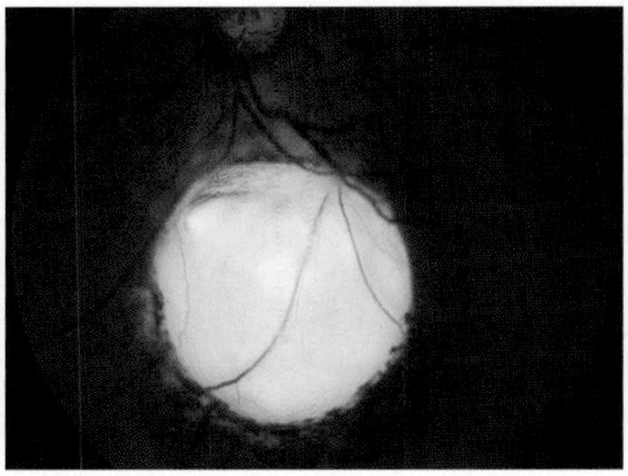

■ **Fig. 15.2** Larger circumscribed coloboma.

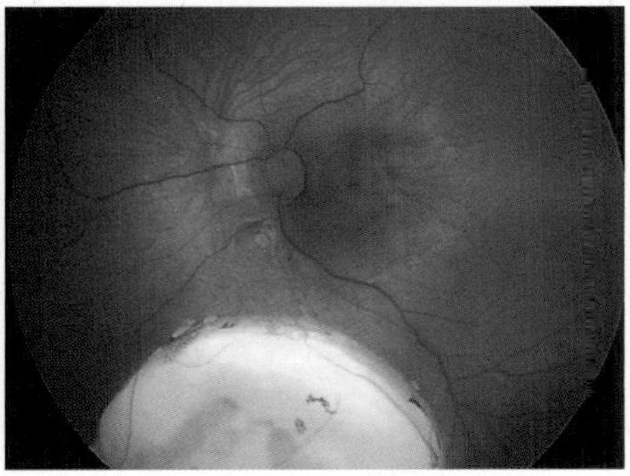

■ **Fig. 15.3** Large inferior coloboma. (Courtesy of L. MacKeen.)

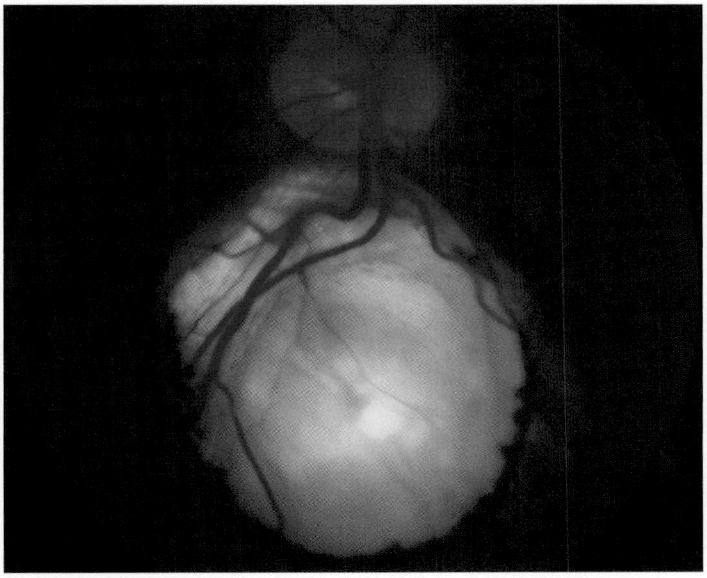

■ **Fig. 15.4** A very circumscribed large coloboma touching the disc. (Courtesy of P. Gili.)

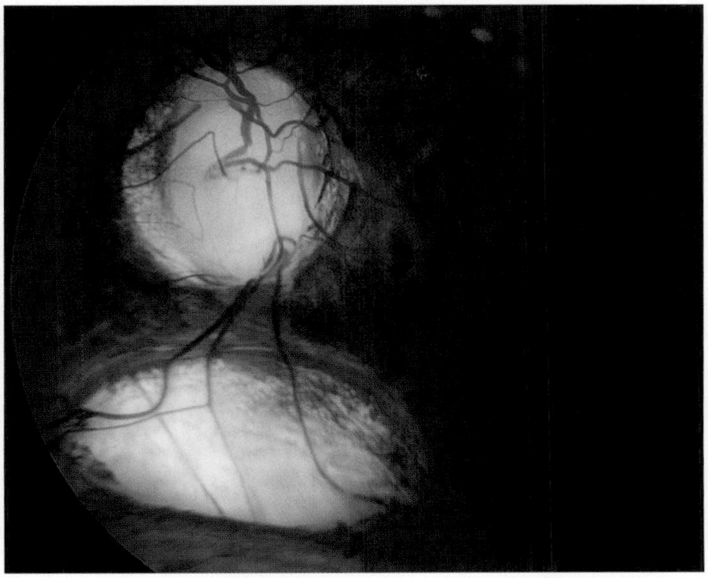

■ **Fig. 15.5** A circumscribed retinochoroidal coloboma and optic disc coloboma.

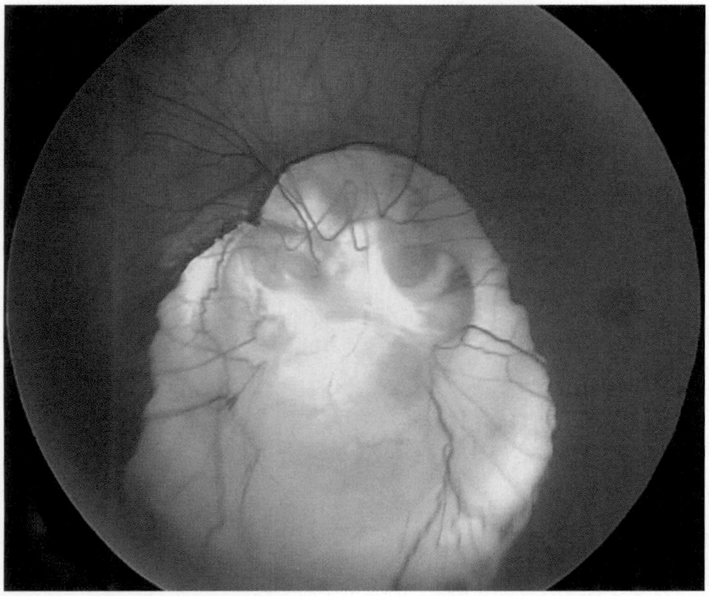

Fig. 15.6 Large coloboma with disc involvement. (Courtesy of L. MacKeen.)

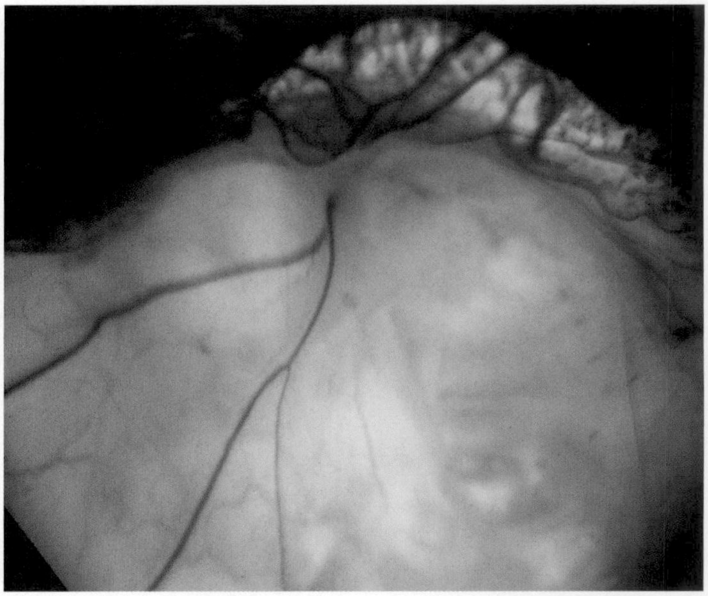

Fig. 15.7 An extremely large coloboma with gross distortion of the disc.

Ocular associations

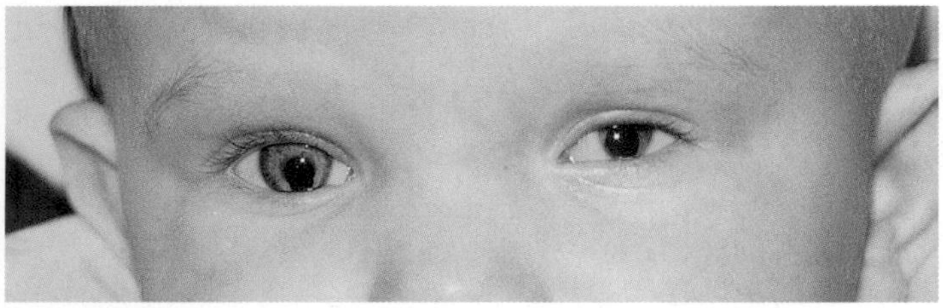

Fig. 15.8 Iris colobomas and microphthalmos may be present in some cases.

Systemic associations

Trisomy 13 (Patau syndrome)

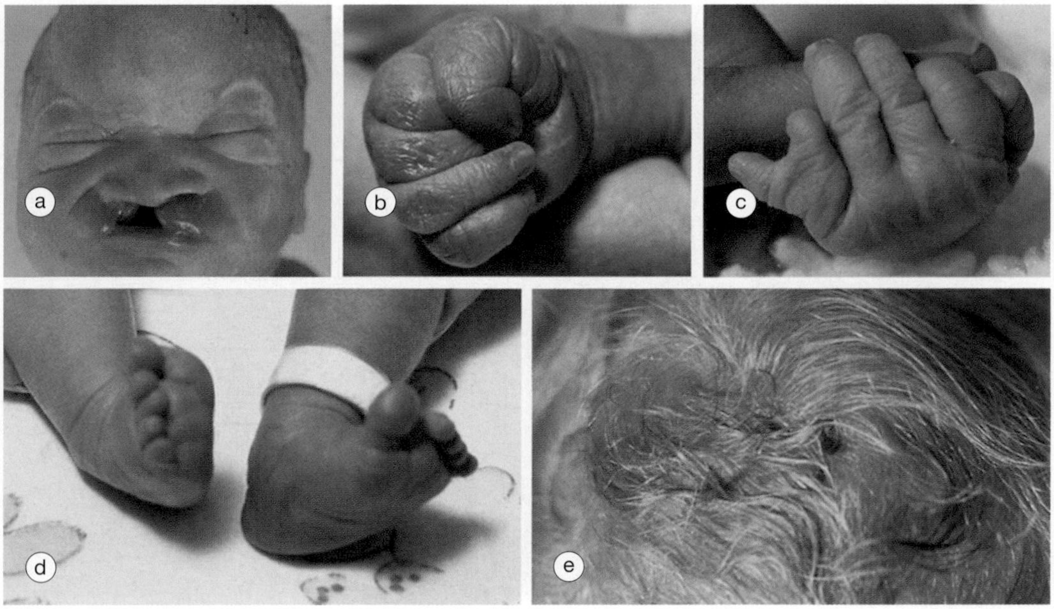

Fig. 15.9 **(a)** Hair lip and cleft palate. **(b)** Clenched hand with overlapping fingers. **(c)** Postaxial polydactyly. **(d)** Equinovarus deformity. **(e)** Punched-out scalp lesions. (Courtesy of B. J. Zitelli and H. W. Davis.)

Trisomy 18 (Edward syndrome)

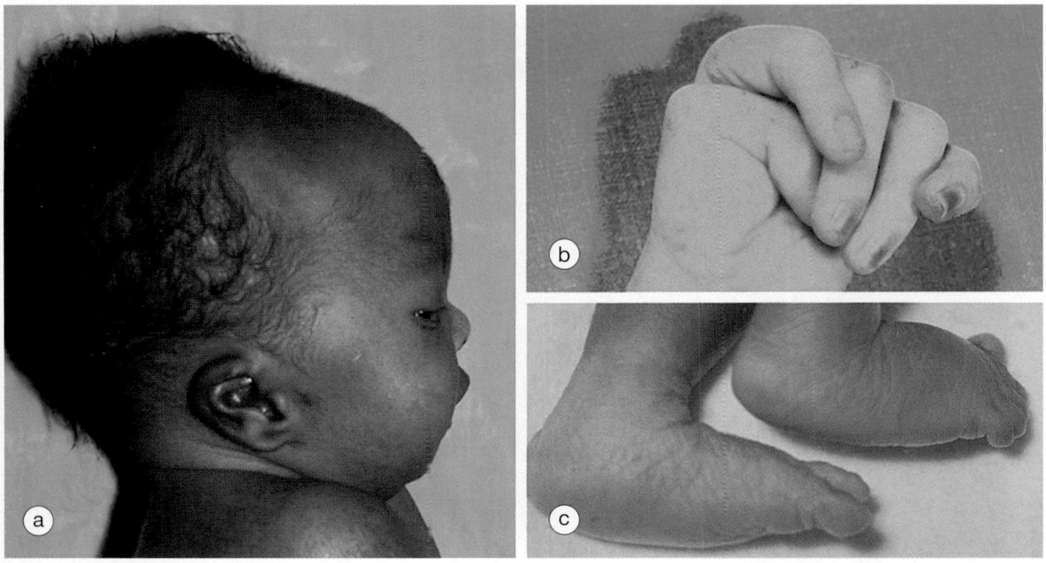

■ **Fig. 15.10** **(a)** Prominent occiput and malformed ears. **(b)** Clenched hand with overlapping fingers. **(c)** Rocker-bottom feet. (Courtesy of B. J. Zitelli and H. W. Davis.)

*'CHARGE' association (**C**oloboma, **H**eart defects, choanal **A**tresia, **R**etarded growth and **G**enital and **E**ar anomalies)*

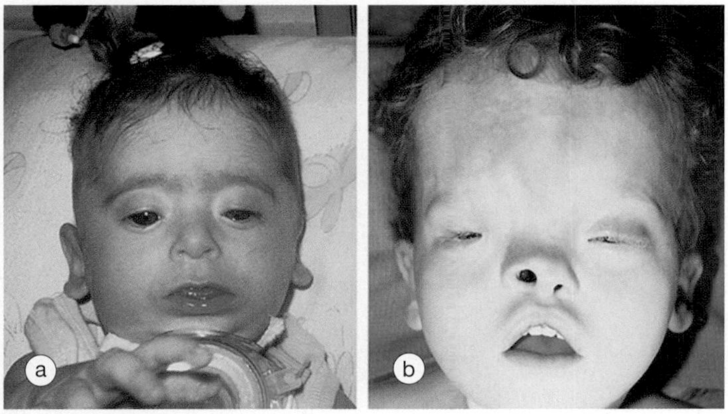

■ **Fig. 15.11** **(a)** Short palpebral fissures and ptosis, low-set dysplastic ears, small chin, tracheostomy because of choanal atresia. **(b)** Prominent forehead, hypertelorism, small palpebral fissures and ptosis, hypoplasia of the left naris, low-set ears and a Cupid-bow mouth. (Courtesy of B. J. Zitelli and H. W. Davis.)

Goldenhar syndrome

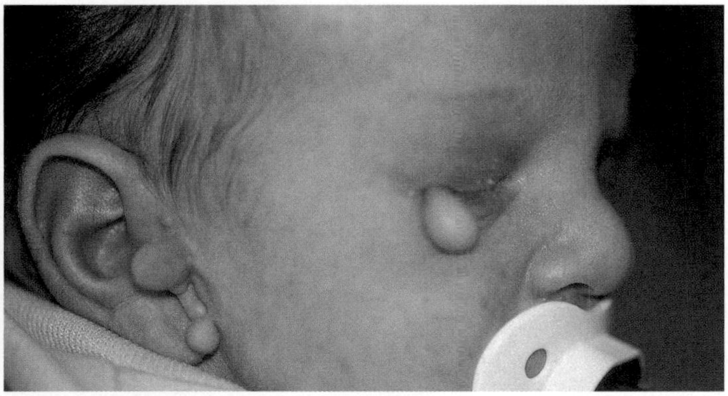

■ **Fig. 15.12** Preauricular appendages and limbal dermoid.

Aicardi syndrome

Inheritance is X-linked dominant (XLD); the condition is lethal in utero for males.

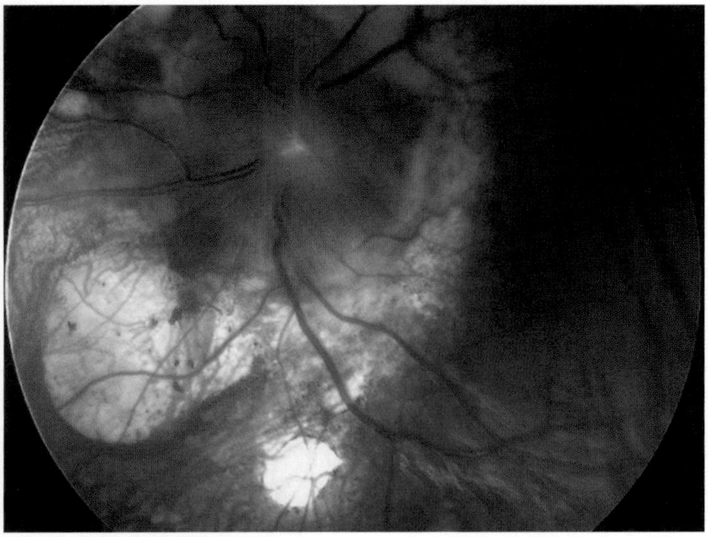

■ **Fig. 15.13** Multiple depigmented 'chorioretinal lacunae' clustered around a pigmented dysplastic disc.

Myelinated nerve fibres

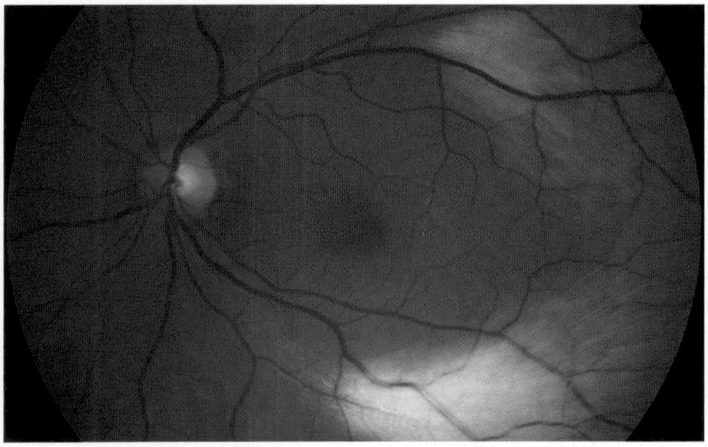

■ **Fig. 15.14** White feathery streaks running within the retinal nerve fibre layer towards the disc. (Courtesy of L. Merin.)

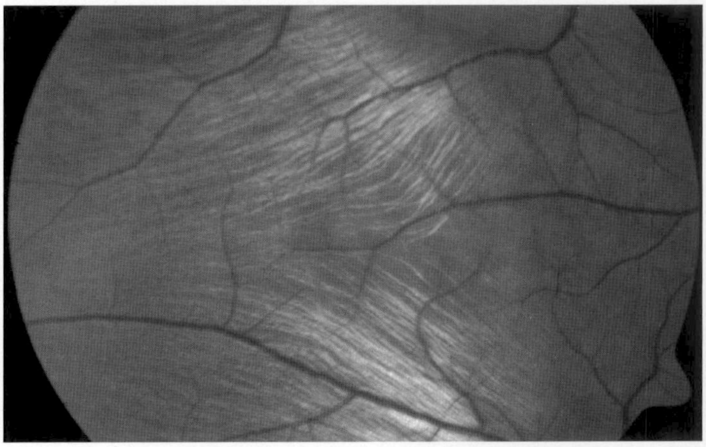

■ **Fig. 15.15** Retinal demyelination seen with a blue filter. (Courtesy of P. Gili.)

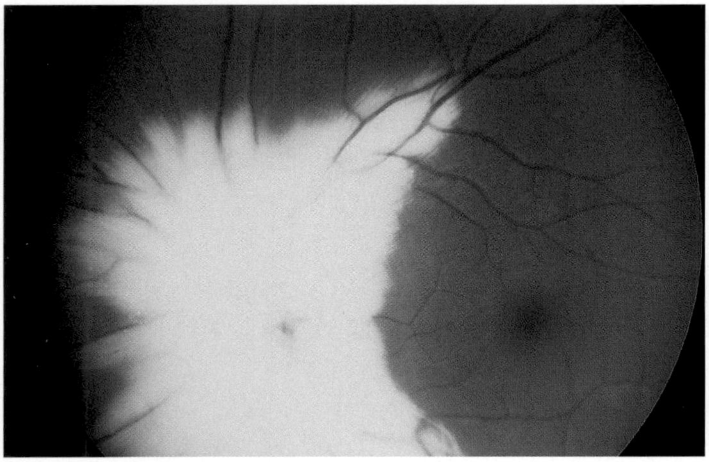

■ **Fig. 15.16** Severe myelination obscuring the disc.

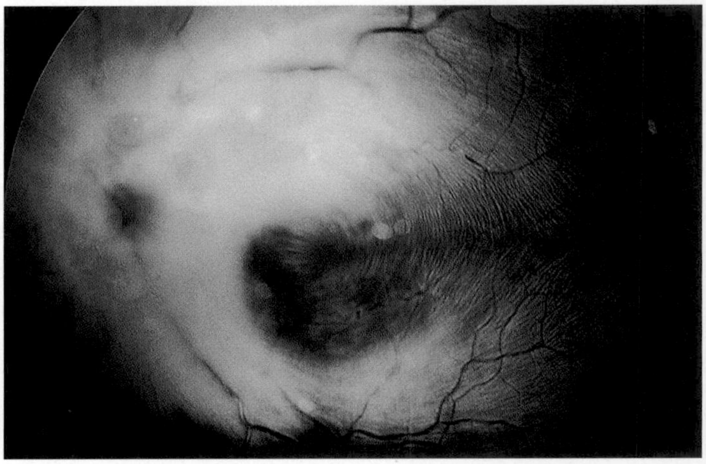

■ **Fig. 15.17** Very extensive myelination.

Macular hypoplasia

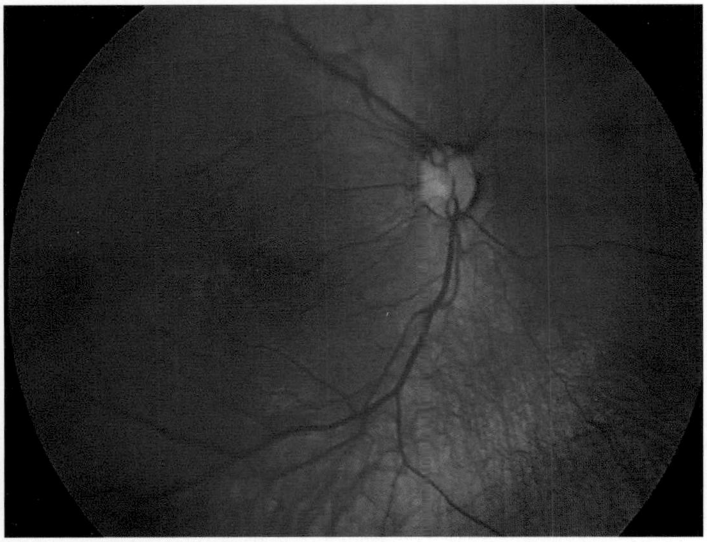

Fig. 15.18 Lack of differentiation of the fovea often associated with aniridia. (Courtesy of L. MacKeen.)

Vascular anomalies

Retinal macrovessel

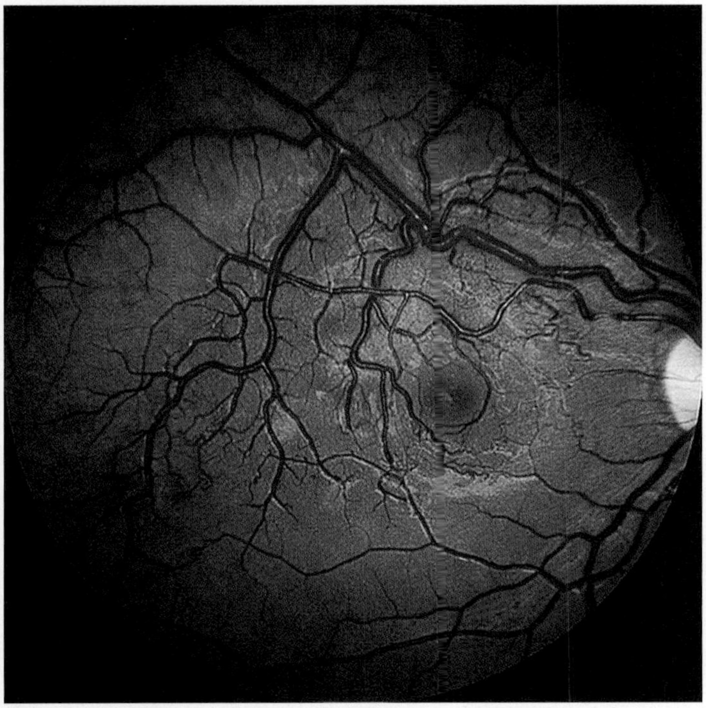

Fig. 15.19 A large, aberrant retinal vessel is present in the posterior pole; its two branches cross the horizontal raphe.

Familial retinal arteriolar tortuosity

Inheritance is AD.

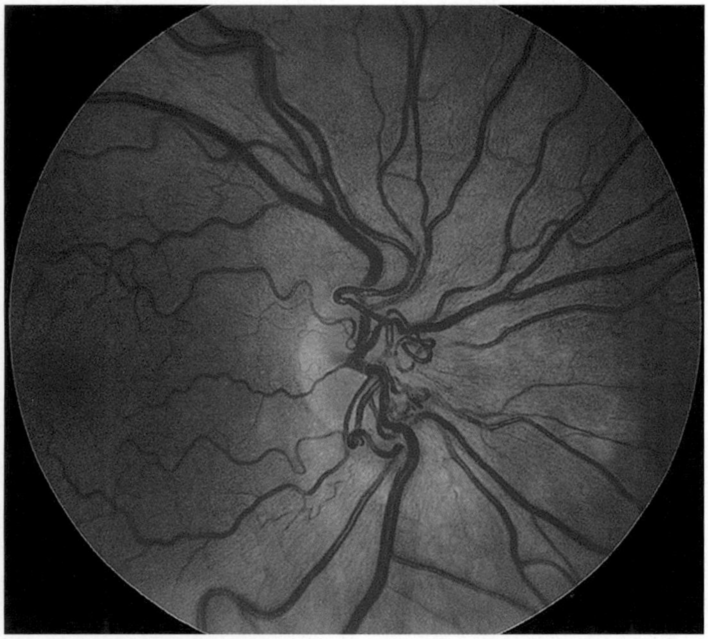

Fig. 15.20 Tortuous small retinal arterioles but normal venules.

Arteriovenous malformation

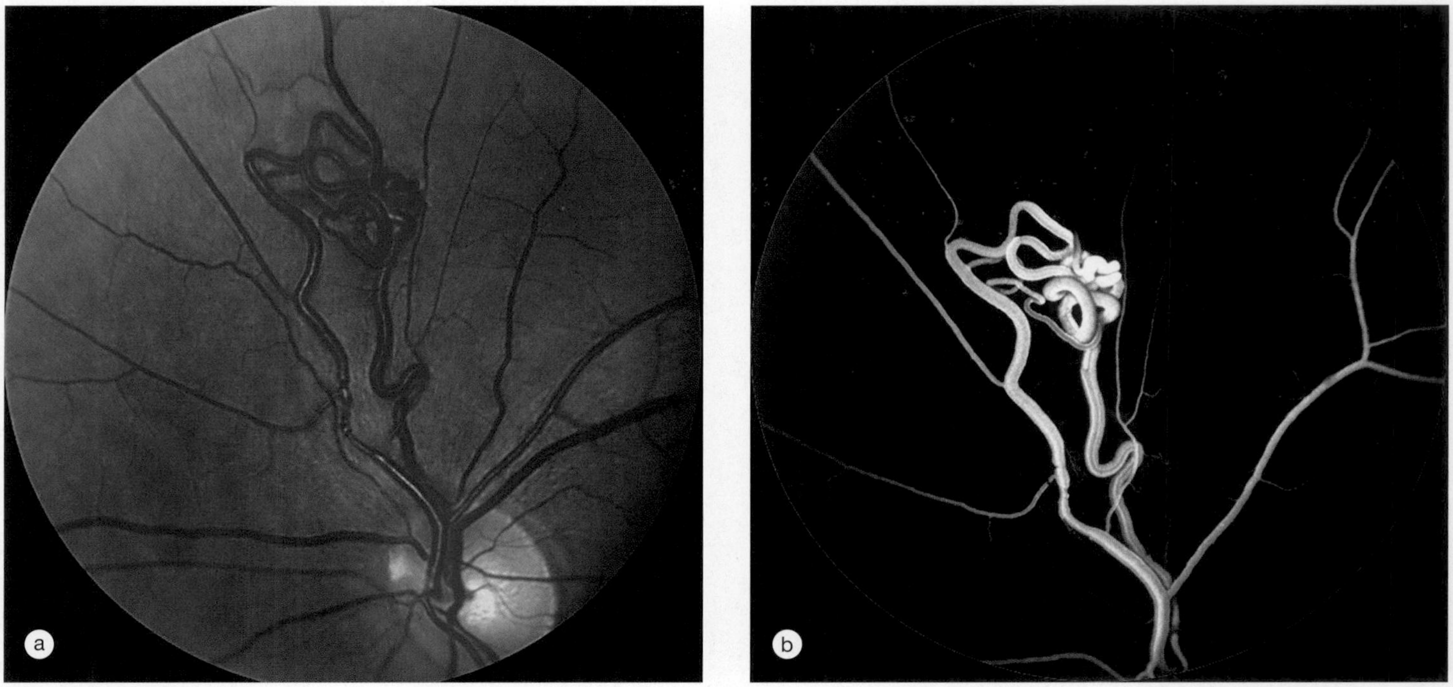

Fig. 15.21 **(a)** Connection between a large vein and artery both of which are dilated. **(b)** FA shows hyperfluorescence of the malformation but lack of leakage. (Courtesy of C. Barry.)

OPTIC DISC

Prepapillary loop

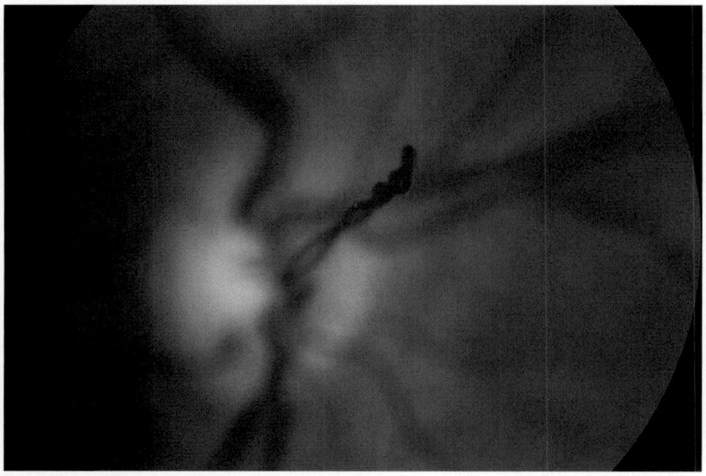

Fig. 15.22 A unilateral, vascular loop extending from the disc into the vitreous cavity and then back.

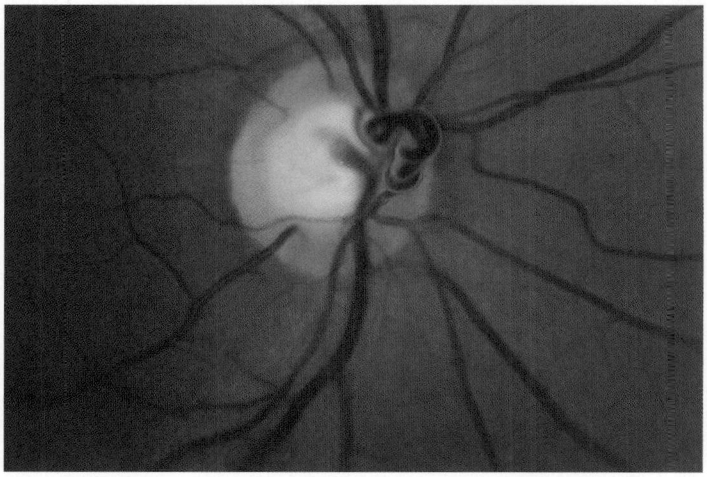

Fig. 15.23 A larger prepapillary loop.

Bergmeister papilla

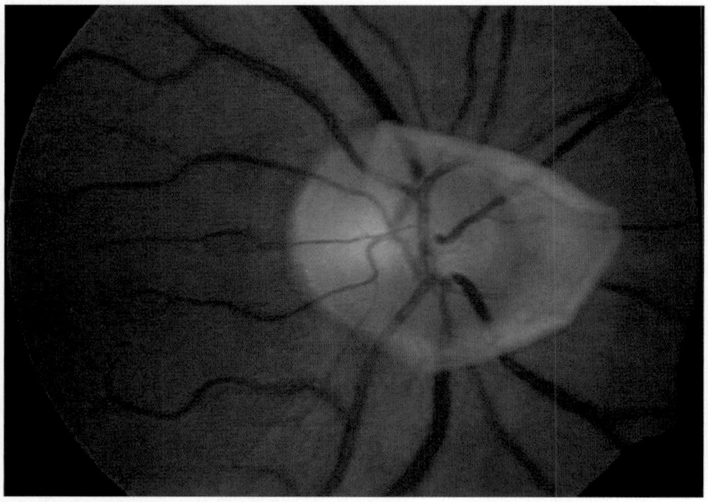

Fig. 15.24 Raised glial tissue on the disc surface. (Courtesy of P. Gili.)

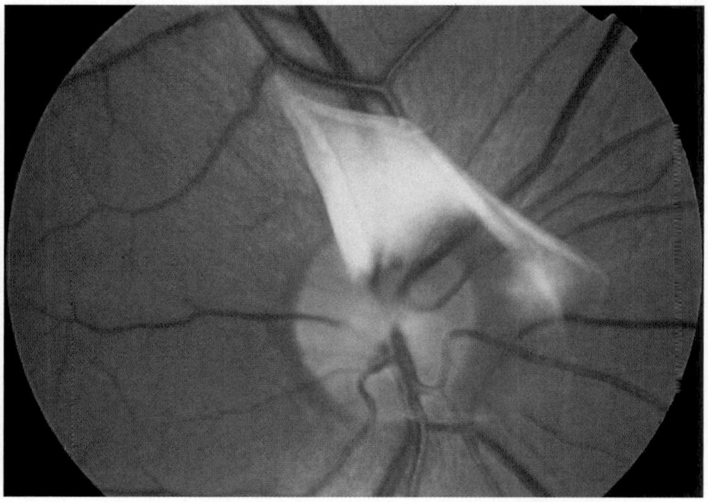

Fig. 15.25 A larger and more opaque Bergmeister papilla.

Tilted disc

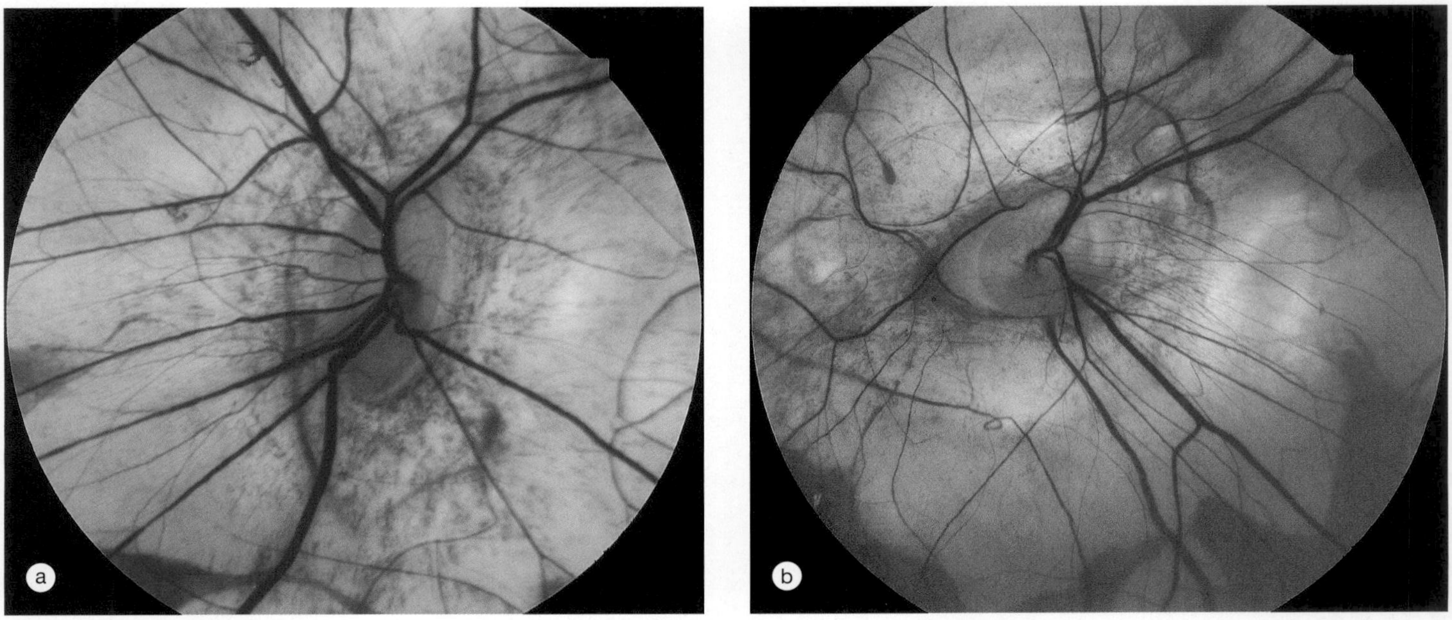

Fig. 15.26 Bilateral tilted discs in a highly myopic patient. **(a)** The right disc has a vertical axis. **(b)** The left disc has an oblique axis.

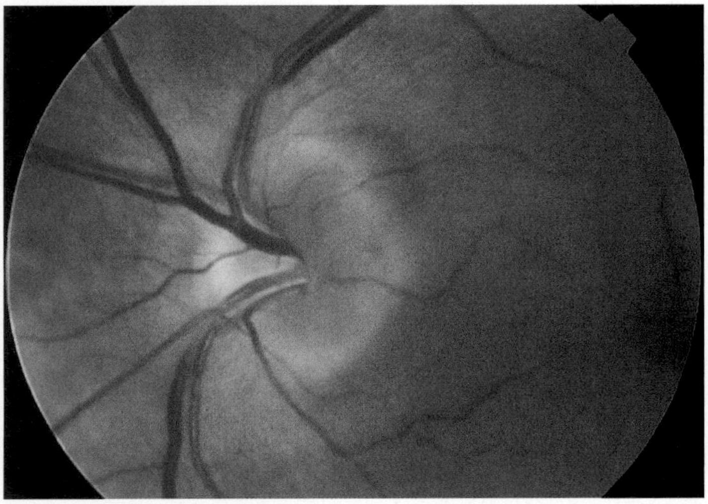

Fig. 15.27 Small, oval or D-shaped disc with an indistinct margin and situs inversus in which the temporal vessels deviate nasally before turning temporally.

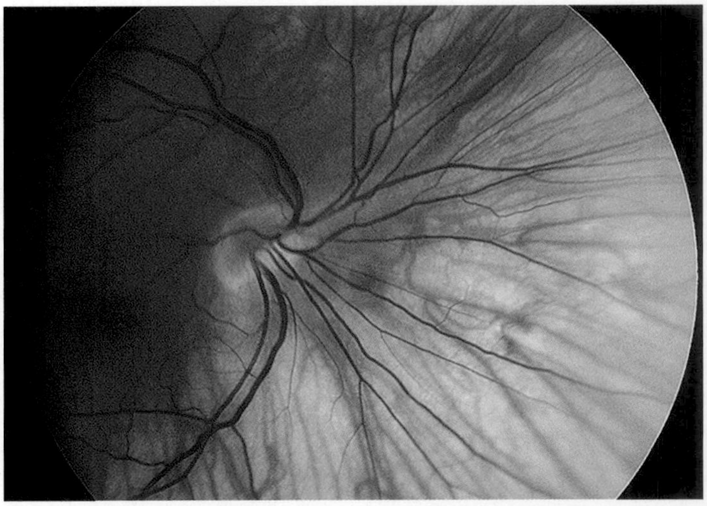

Fig. 15.28 Inferonasal chorioretinal thinning may be associated with a superotemporal visual field defect.

Optic disc pit

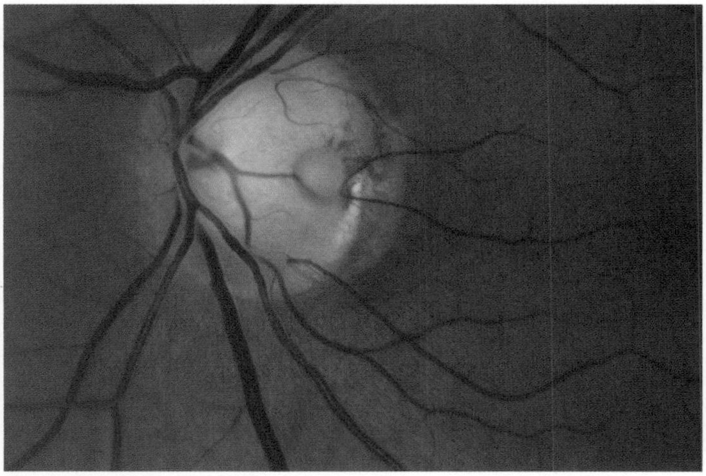

■ **Fig. 15.29** The disc is larger than normal and contains a round or oval pit, which is usually located in the temporal aspect of the disc.

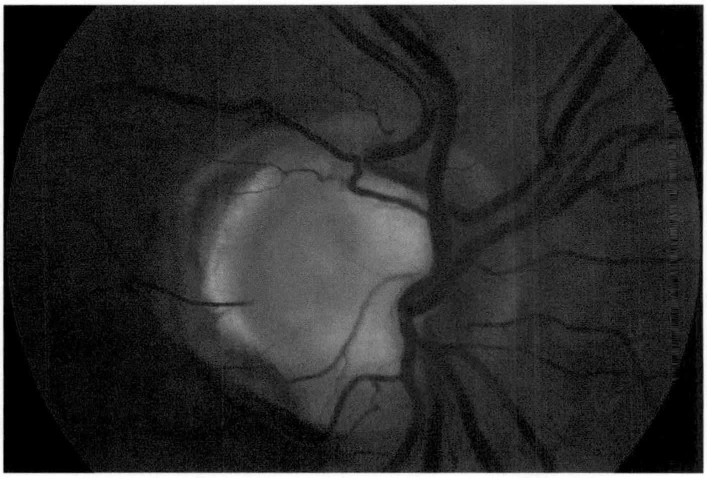

■ **Fig. 15.30** Large optic disc pit.

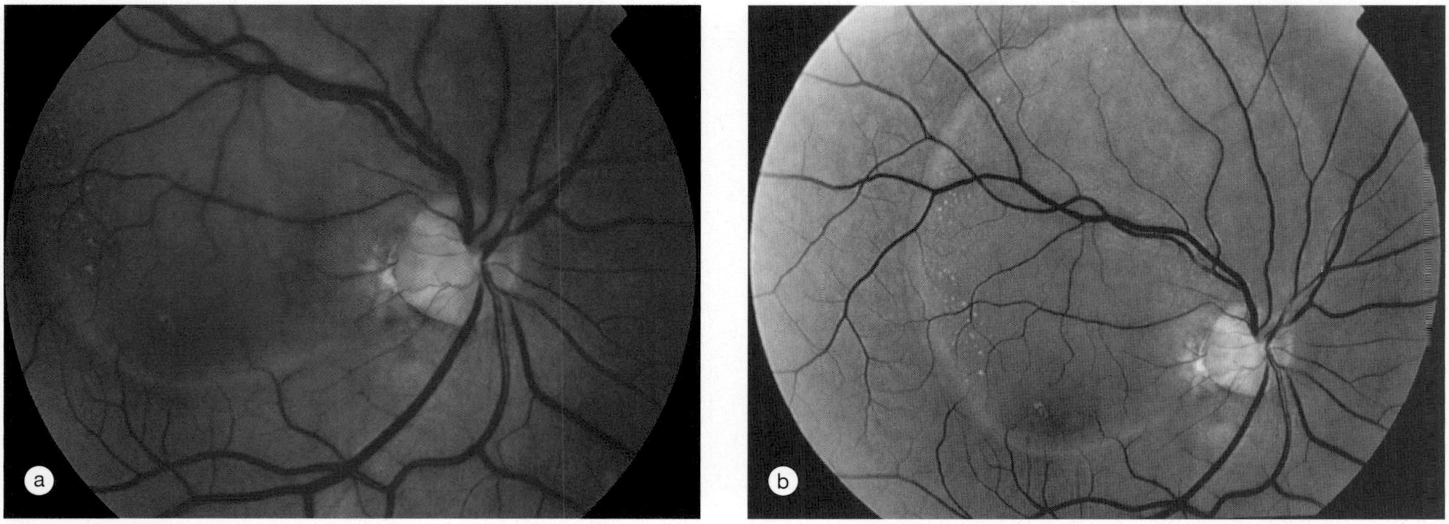

■ **Fig. 15.31** **(a)** Serous detachment at the macula with a few small subretinal deposits. **(b)** Red-free image. (Courtesy of P. Gili.)

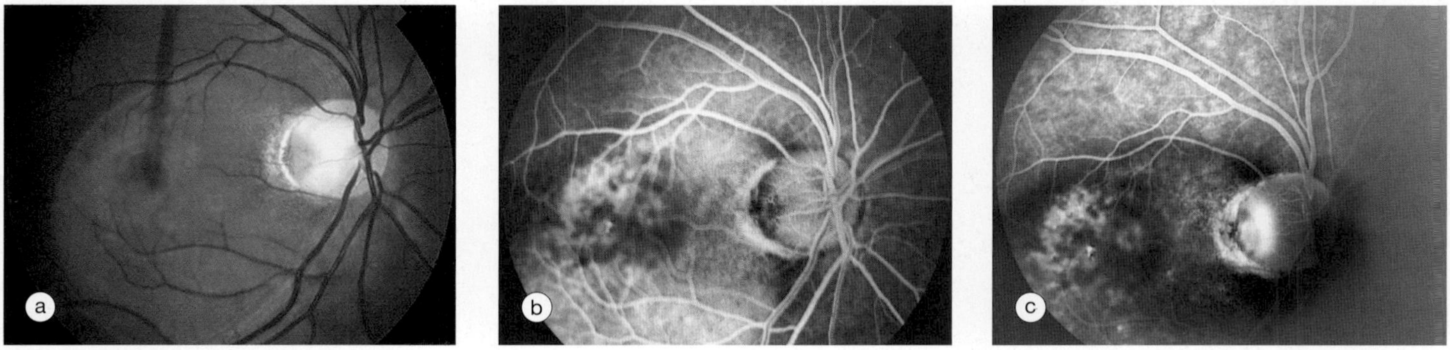

■ **Fig. 15.32** **(a)** Optic disc pit. **(b)** FA early phase shows hypofluorescence of the pit. **(c)** Late phase shows hyperfluorescence. There is also spotty hyperfluorescence at the posterior pole due to RPE atrophy associated with previous serous macular detachment. (Courtesy of S. Milewski.)

Optic disc drusen

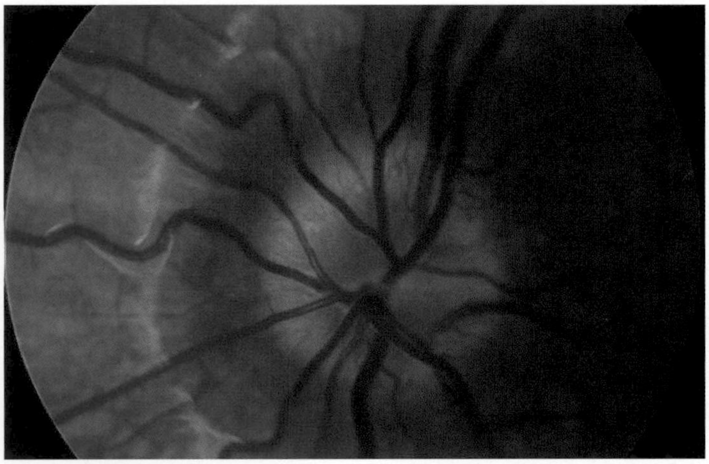

Fig. 15.33 Buried drusen characterised by an elevated disc with a scalloped margin without a physiological cup and an anomalous vascular pattern including early branching, increased number of major retinal vessels and vascular tortuosity.

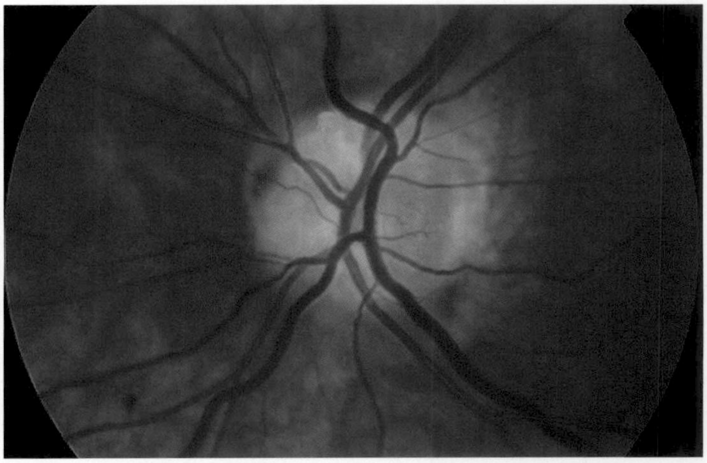

Fig. 15.34 Small, waxy, pearl-like irregularity at the disc margin at 11 o'clock indicative of exposed drusen.

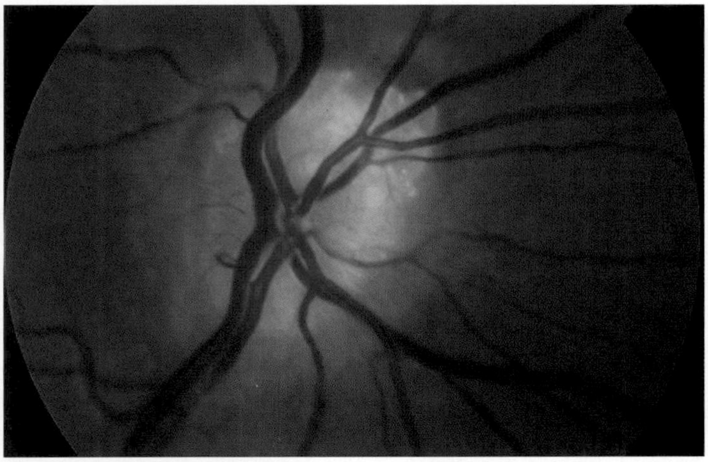

Fig. 15.35 More extensive exposed drusen between 1 and 2 o'clock.

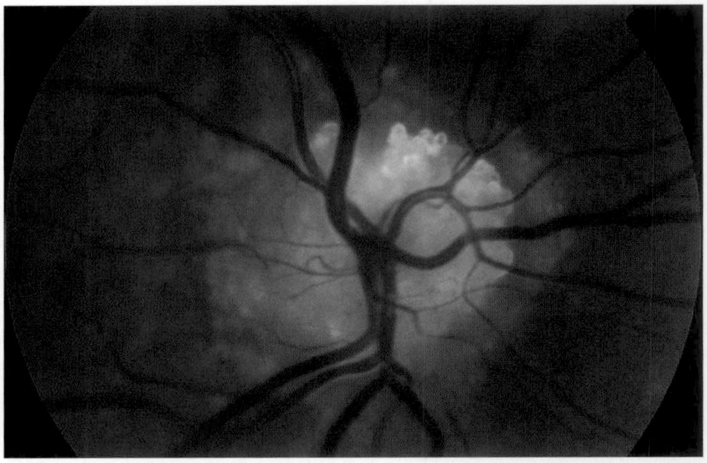

Fig. 15.36 Exposed drusen involving the upper half of the disc.

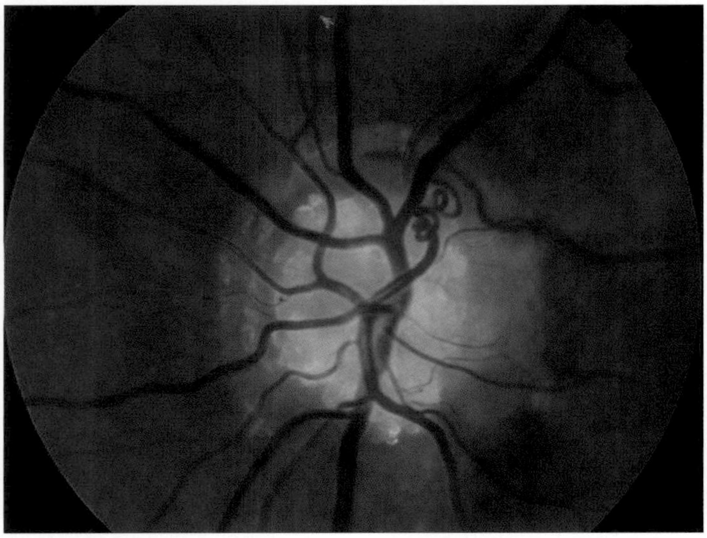

Fig. 15.37 Exposed drusen involving the entire disc.

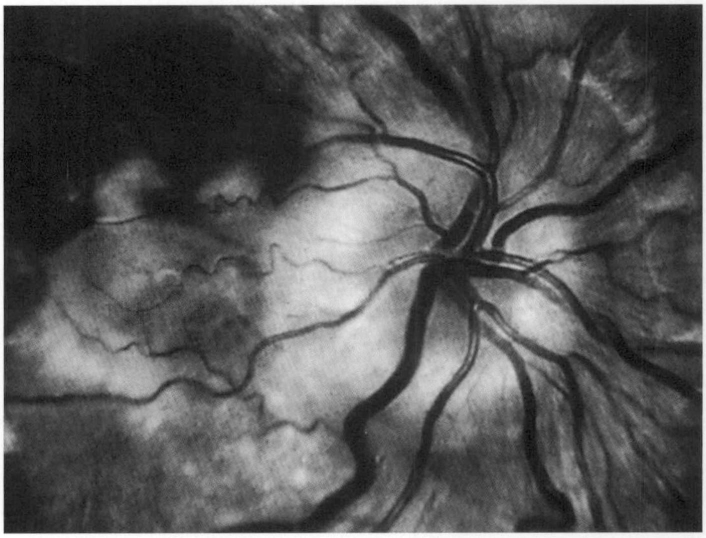

Fig. 15.38 Buried drusen and peripapillary haemorrhage due to choroidal neovascularisation.

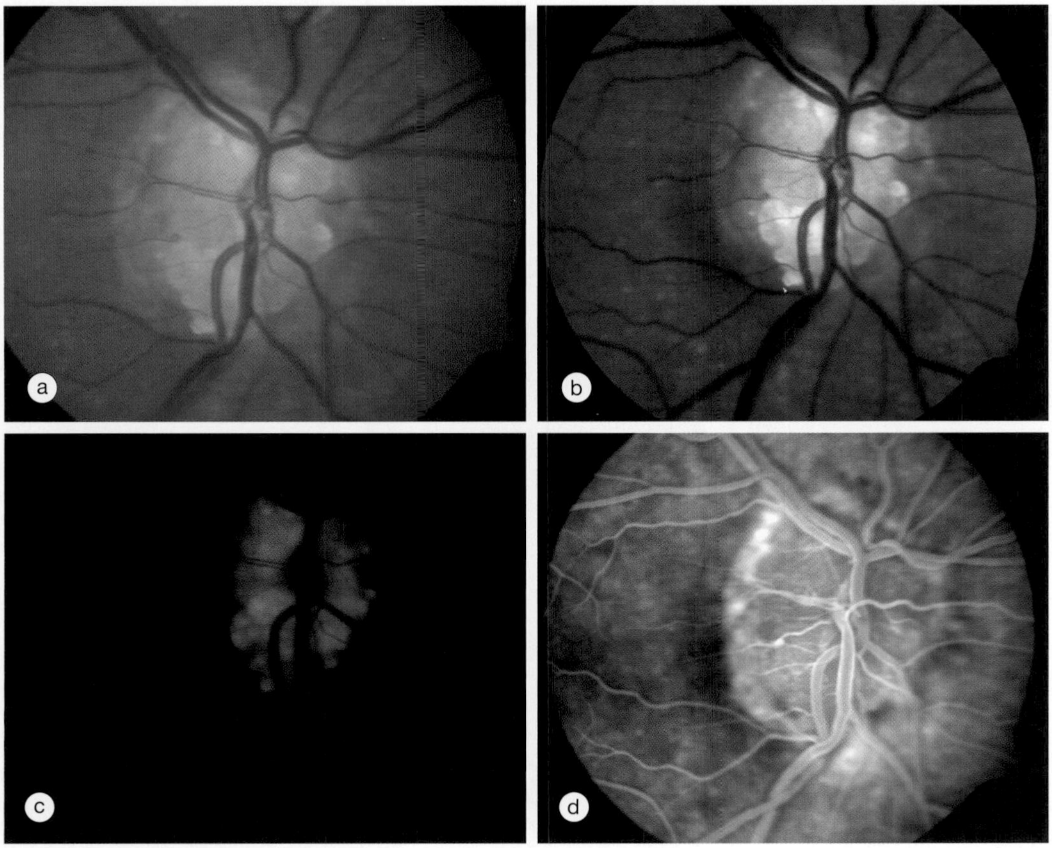

Fig. 15.39 **(a)** Exposed drusen. **(b)** Red-free image. **(c)** Autofluorescence prior to injection of fluorescein. **(d)** FA shows lack of leakage. (Courtesy of P. Gili.)

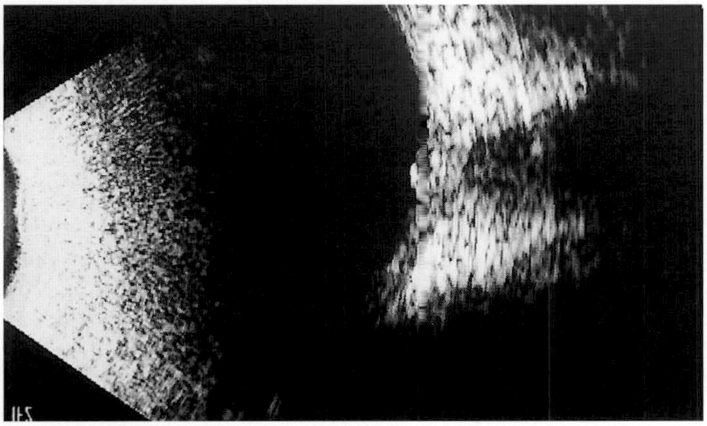

Fig. 15.40 US shows high acoustic reflectivity of drusen.

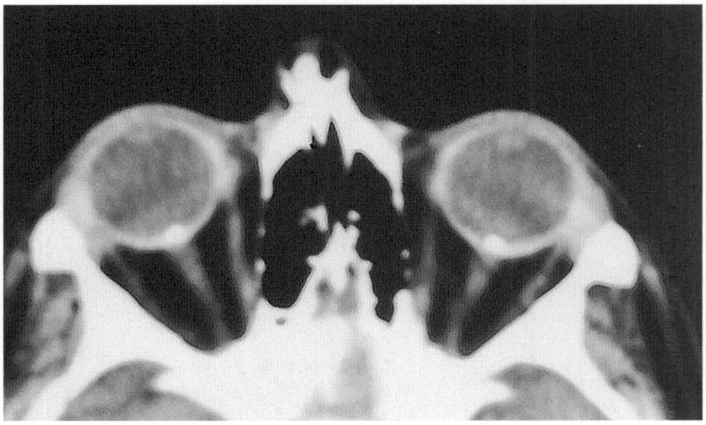

Fig. 15.41 CT is less sensitive than ultrasonography and may miss small drusen.

Ocular associations

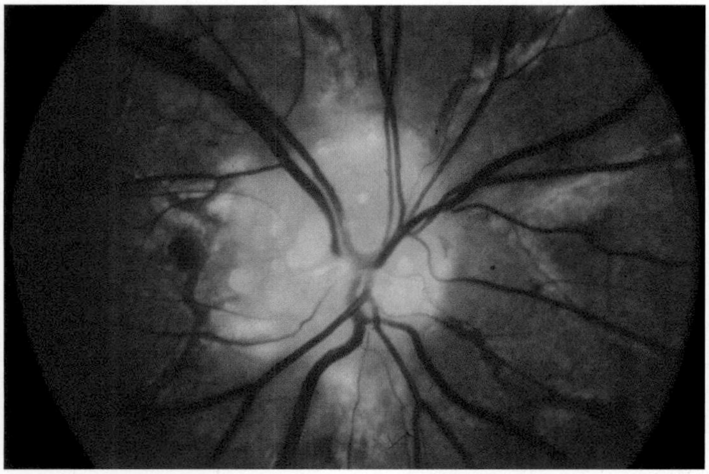

Fig. 15.42 Angioid streaks. (Courtesy of S. Ford and R. Marsh.)

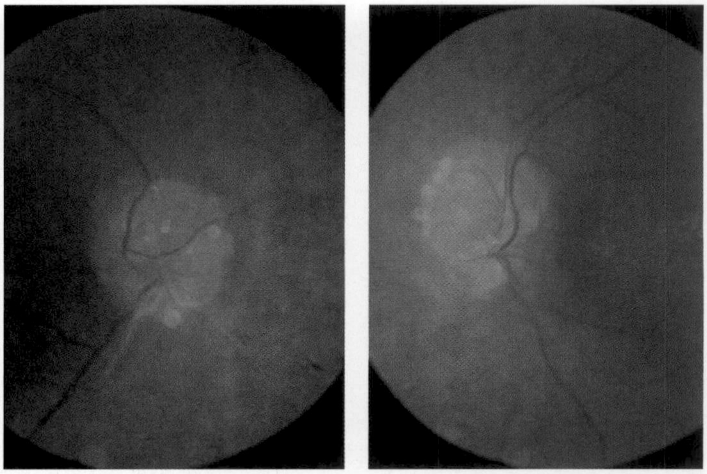

Fig. 15.43 Retinitis pigmentosa. (Courtesy of S. Ford and R. Marsh.)

Systemic association

Alagille syndrome (arteriohepatic dysplasia).

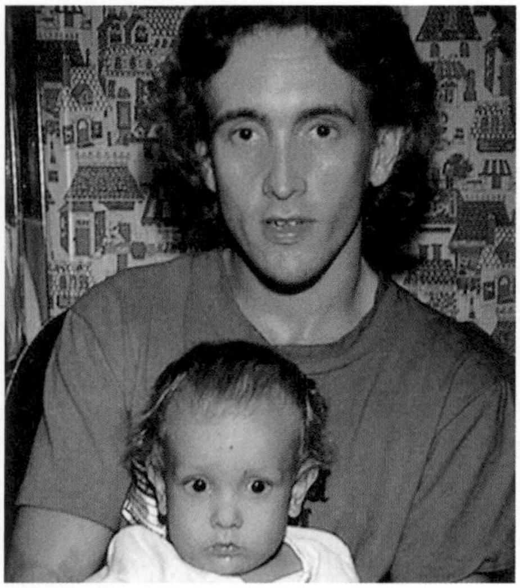

Fig. 15.44 The child has biliary hypoplasia, butterfly vertebrae and pulmonary stenosis. The father has pulmonary stenosis, deep-set eyes and a thin face with a pointed chin. (Courtesy of B. J. Zitelli and H. W. Davis.)

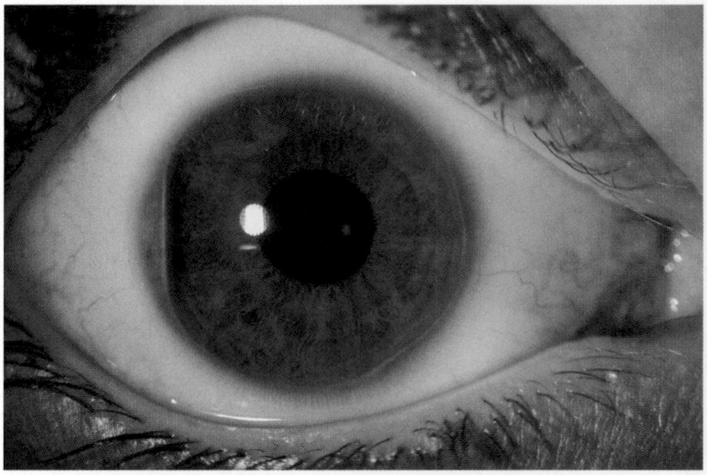

Fig. 15.45 Posterior embryotoxon is common.

Optic disc coloboma

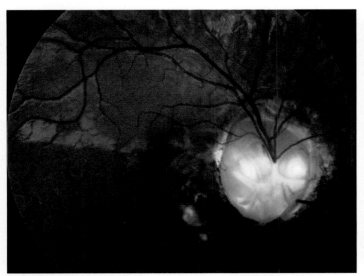

Fig. 15.46 Glistening, white, bowl-shaped excavation, decentred inferiorly with an absent inferior neuroretinal rim and normal disc tissue; retinal nerve fibres are confined to a superior wedge.

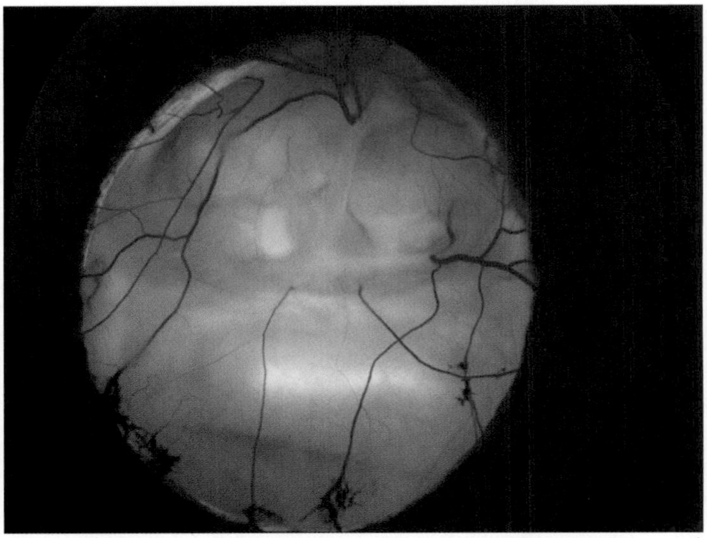

Fig. 15.47 Very large coloboma. (Courtesy of P. Gili.)

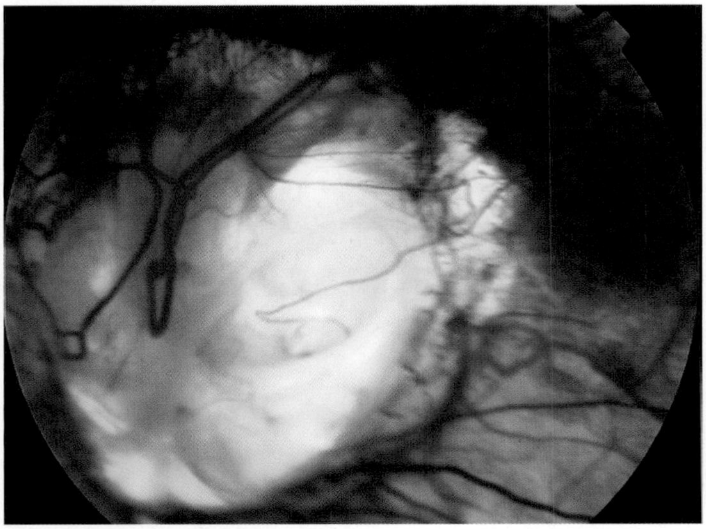

Fig. 15.48 Extremely large coloboma.

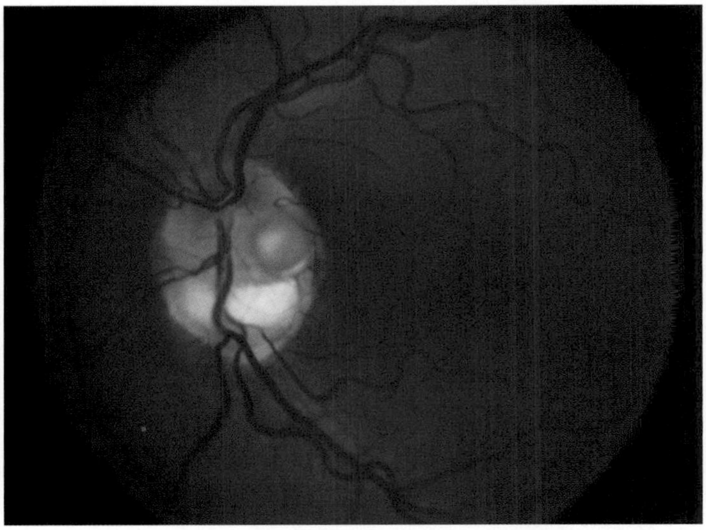

Fig. 15.49 Optic disc pit and a small coloboma. (Courtesy of L. Merin.)

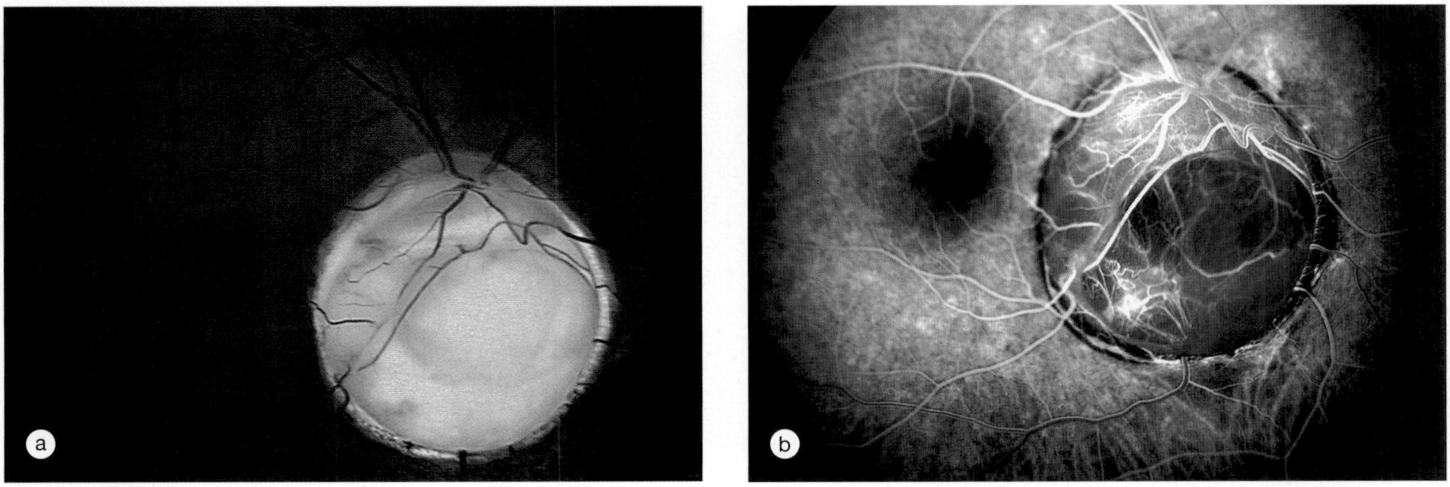

Fig. 15.50 **(a)** Optic disc coloboma. **(b)** FA early venous phase shows hypofluorescence of the coloboma. (Courtesy of P. Gili.)

Morning glory anomaly

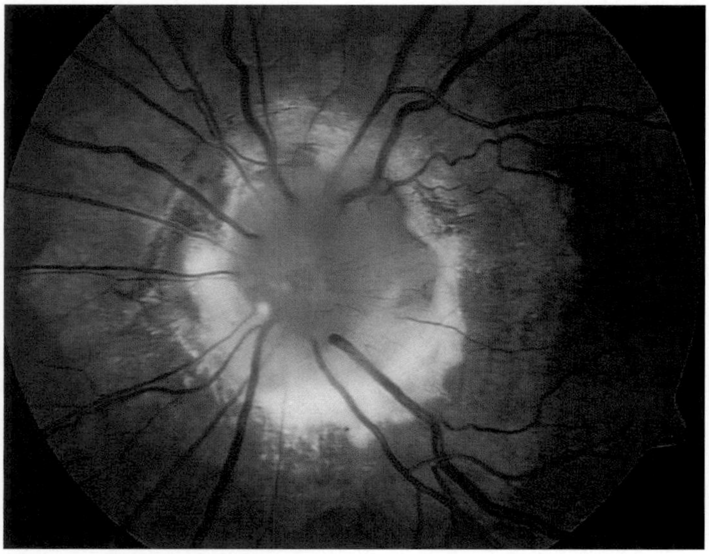

Fig. 15.51 A large excavation surrounded by an elevated annulus of chorioretinal pigmentary disturbance. (Courtesy of P. Gili.)

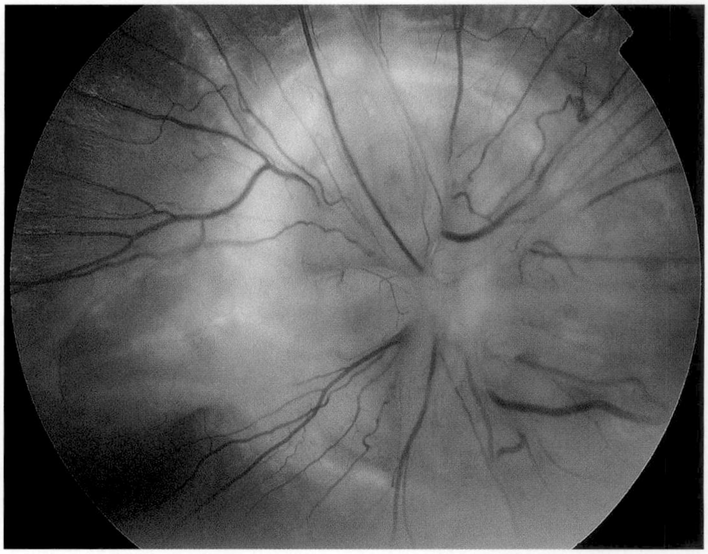

Fig. 15.52 The blood vessels emerge from the rim of the excavation in a radial pattern like the spokes of a wheel. They are increased in number and it is difficult to distinguish arteries from veins.

Systemic association

Frontonasal dysplasia

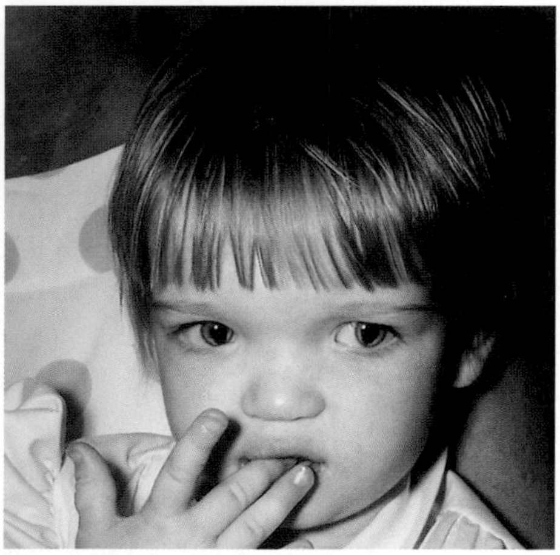

Fig. 15.53 Hypertelorism and depressed nasal bridge; note bilateral iris colobomas.

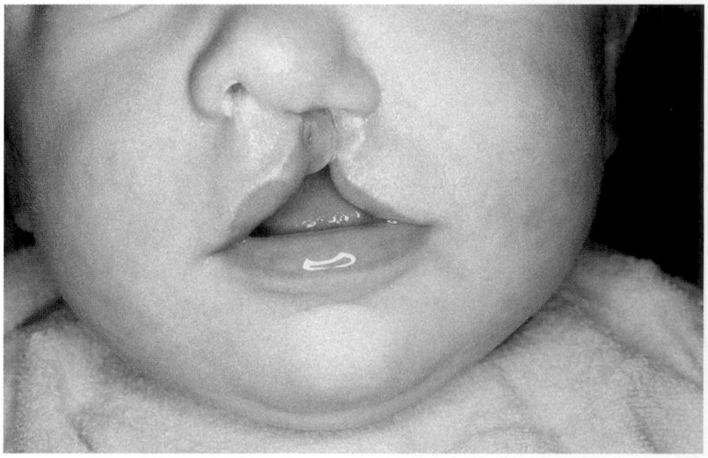

Fig. 15.54 Hare lip and cleft palate.

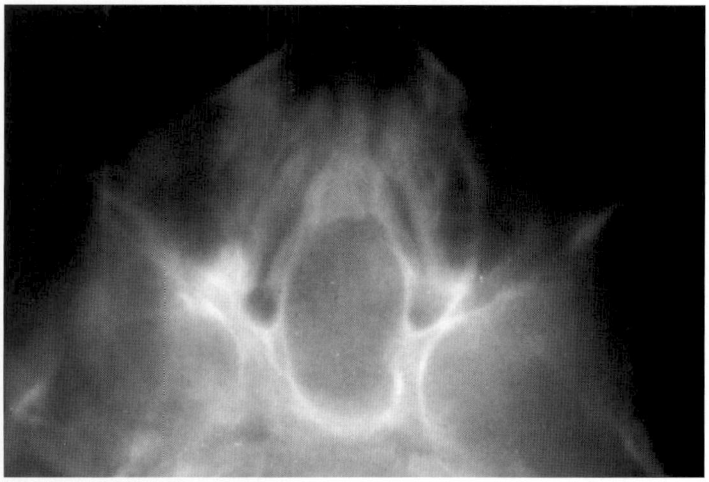

Fig. 15.55 Defect in the base of the skull resulting in basal encephalocele. (Courtesy of Moorfields Eye Hospital.)

Optic nerve hypoplasia

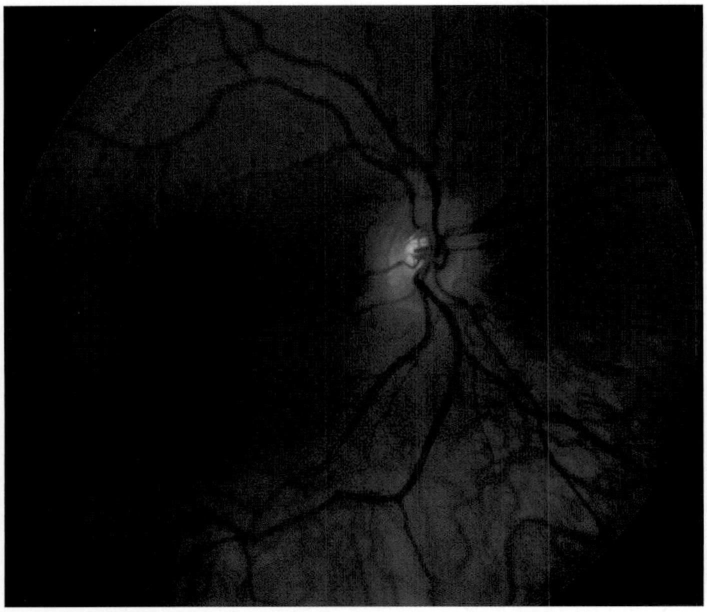

■ **Fig. 15.56** Small disc with normal calibre vessels.

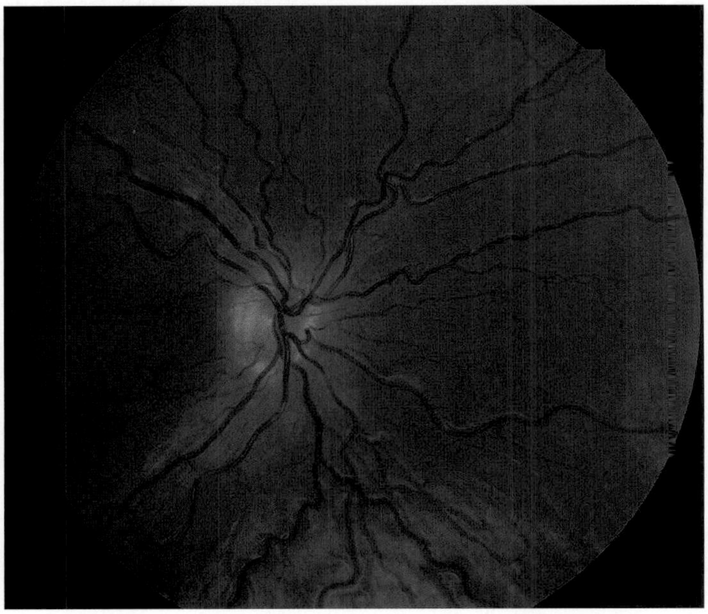

■ **Fig. 15.57** In some cases the blood vessels are tortuous.

Systemic association

De Morsier syndrome (septo-optic dysplasia)

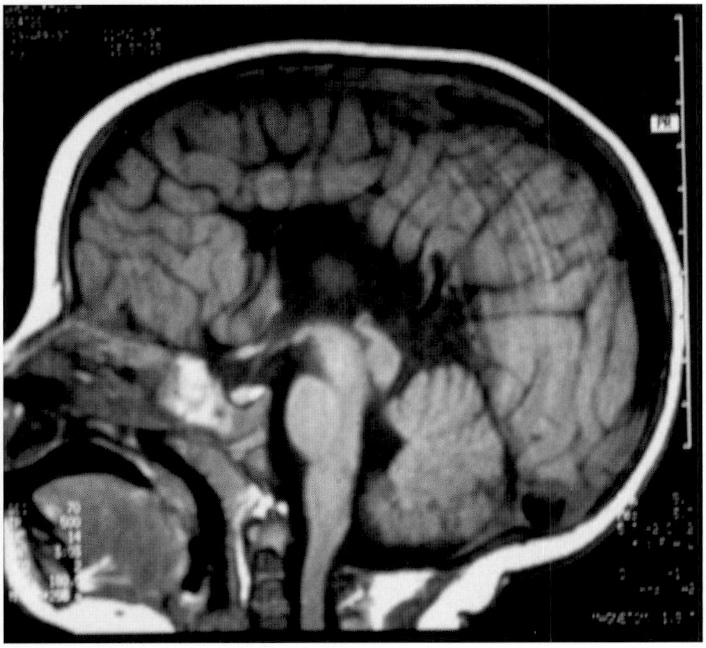

■ **Fig. 15.58** Sagittal MRI showing abscence of the corpus callosum. (Courtesy of K. Nischal.)

Megalopapilla

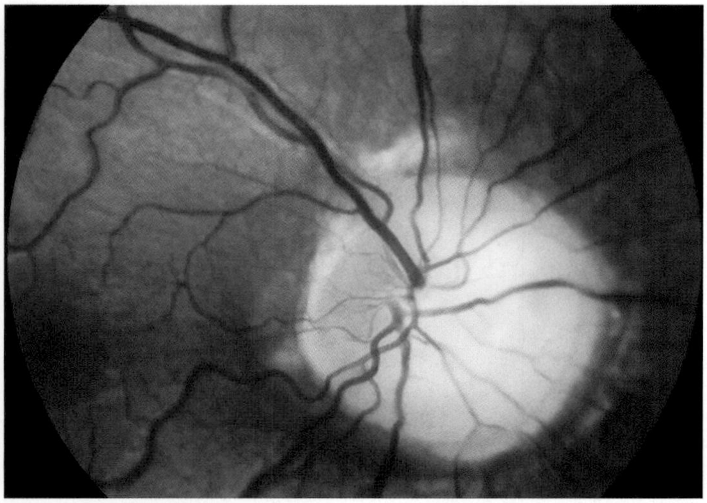

■ **Fig. 15.59** The horizontal and vertical disc diameters are 2.1 mm or more.

Peripapillary staphyloma

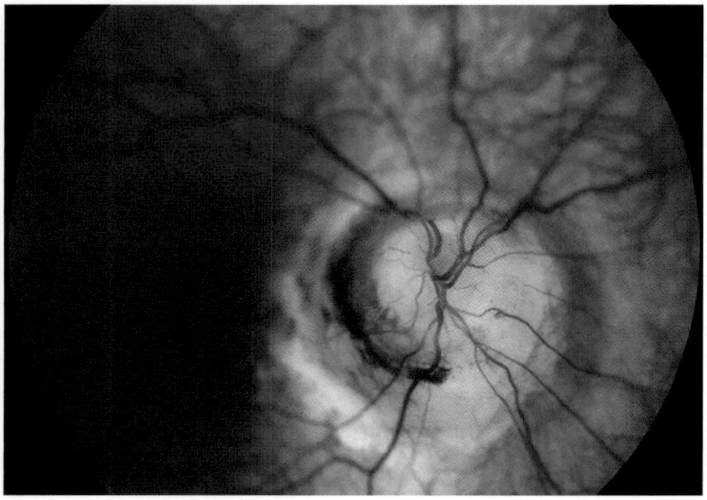

■ **Fig. 15.60** A relatively normal disc sits at the base of a deep excavation, which is surrounded by chorioretinal atrophy.

Dysplastic disc

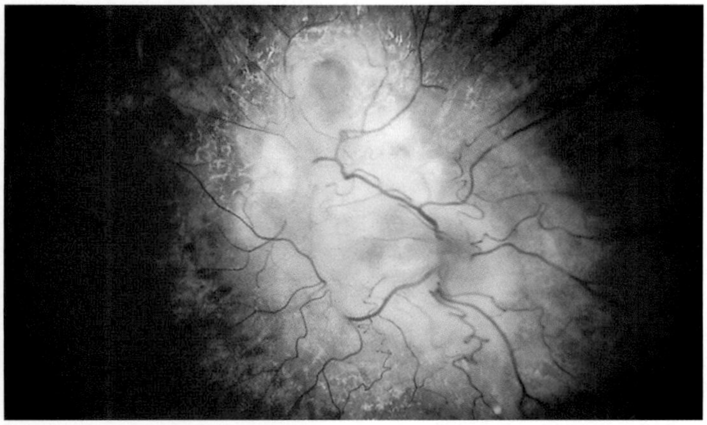

■ **Fig. 15.61** A markedly deformed disc that does not conform to any recognisable category described above. (Courtesy of C. Barry.)

VITREOUS

Persistent hyaloid artery

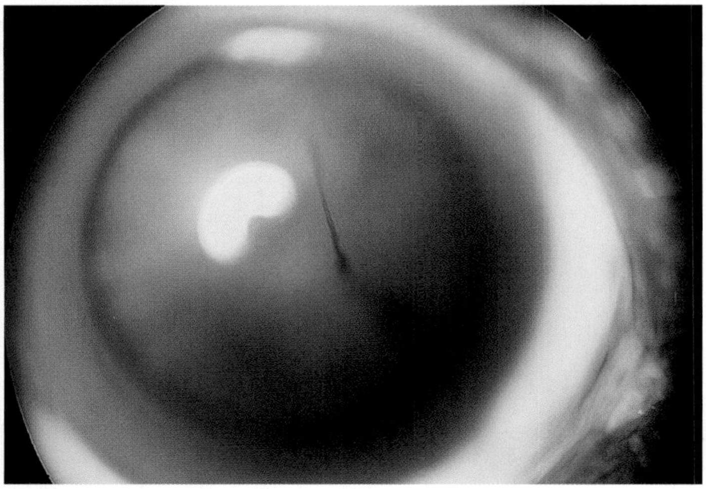

■ **Fig. 15.62** Glial remnants extending from the disc to the lens (Cloquet canal). The artery may contain blood at its point of attachment to the posterior lens capsule (Mittendorf spot).

Persistent hyperplastic primary vitreous (PHPV)

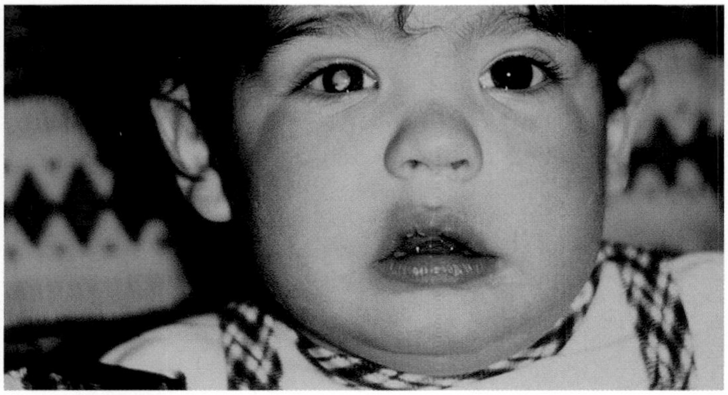

■ **Fig. 15.63** PHPV is an important cause of unilateral leukocoria in a microphthalmic eye.

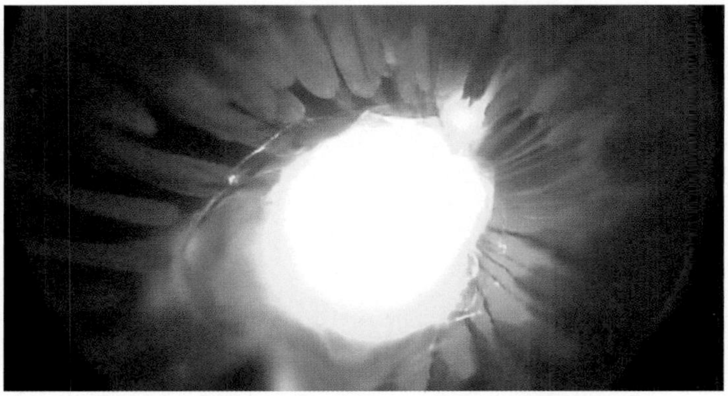

■ **Fig. 15.64** Retrolental mass into which elongated ciliary processes are inserted. (Courtesy of L. MacKeen.)

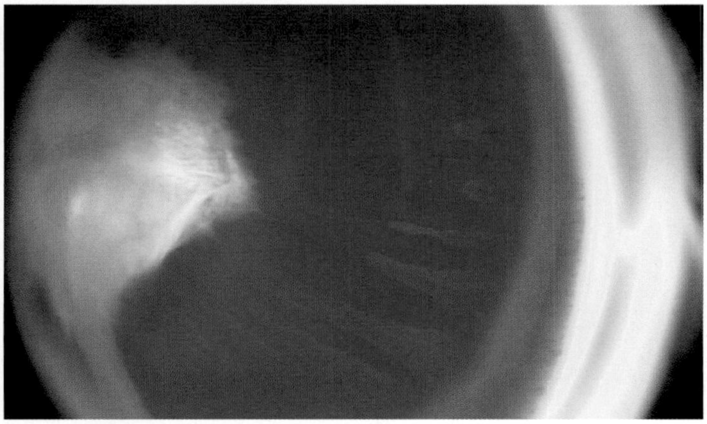

■ **Fig. 15.65** Contraction of the mass pulls the ciliary processes centrally so that they become visible through the pupil. (Courtesy of L. MacKeen.)

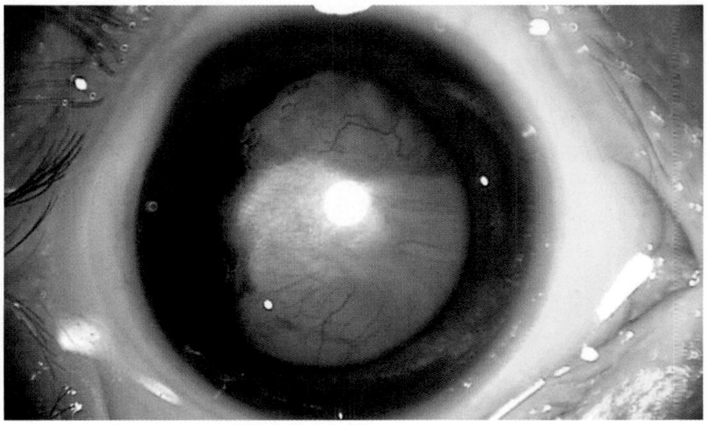

■ **Fig. 15.66** Vascularised retrolental mass and a shallow anterior chamber. (Courtesy of L. MacKeen.)

Posterior PHPV

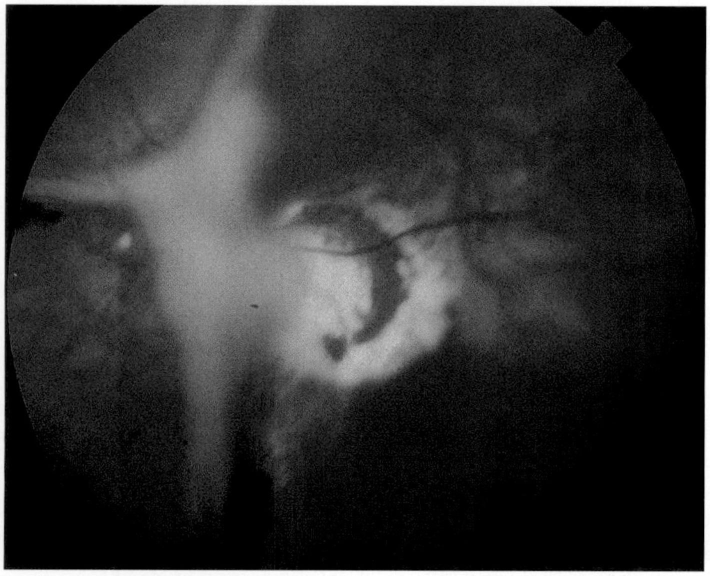

Fig. 15.67 A fold of condensed vitreous extends from the disc to the fundus periphery.

Congenital falciform fold

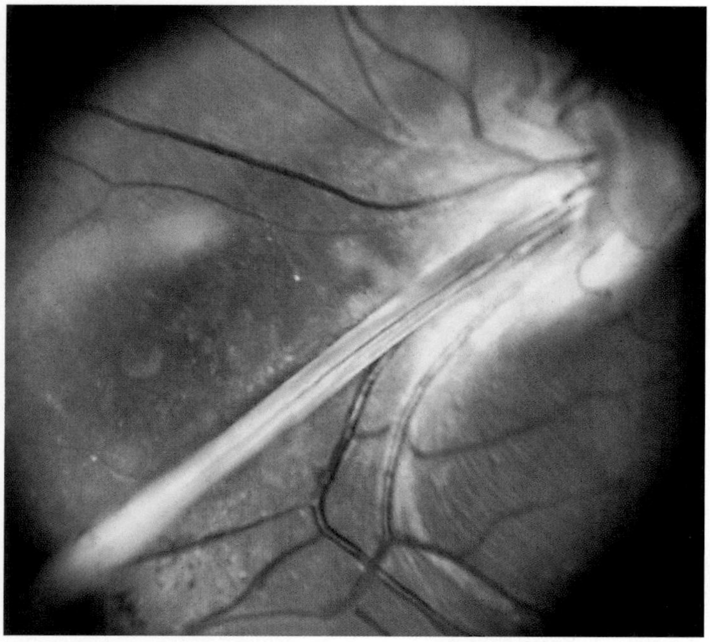

Fig. 15.68 Retinal fold extending from the optic disc to the peripheral retina or retrolental space, which may be a variant of posterior PHPV.

Incontinentia pigmenti (Bloch–Sulzberger syndrome)

Inheritance is X-LD; the condition is lethal in utero for boys.

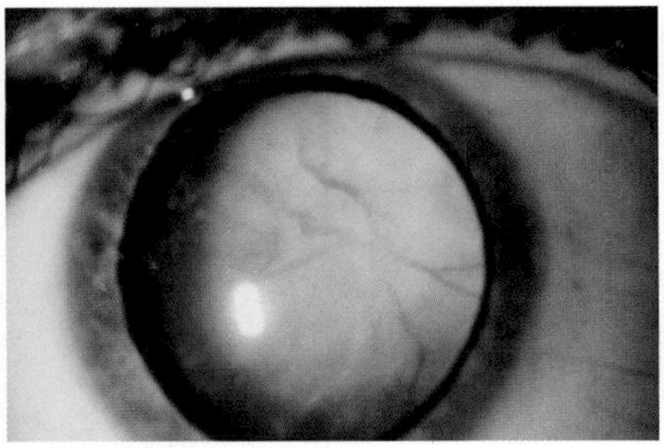

Fig. 15.69 Very severe unilateral or bilateral vascularised cicatricial retinal detachment which may give rise to leukocoria in the first year of life.

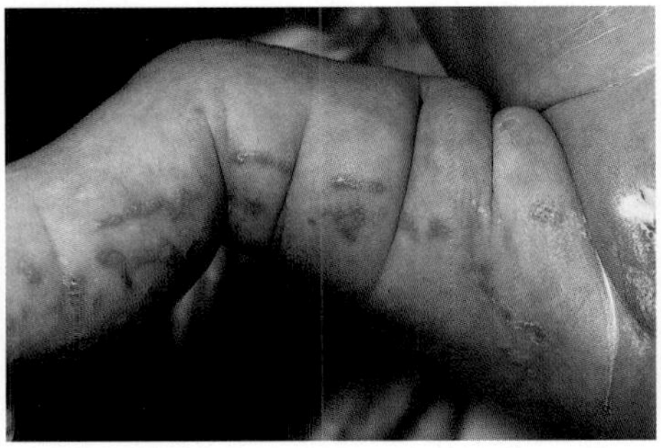

Fig. 15.70 Vesiculobullous rash on the trunk and extremities.

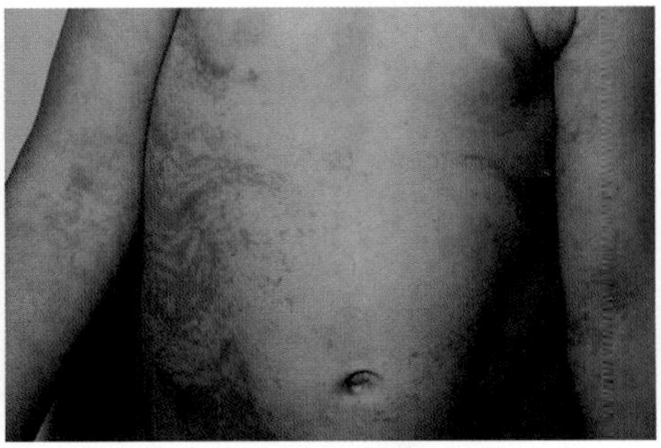

Fig. 15.71 Later linear pigmentation.

Congenital vitreous cyst

Congenital vitreous cysts may occur in eyes with remnants of the hyaloid system or in otherwise normal eyes.

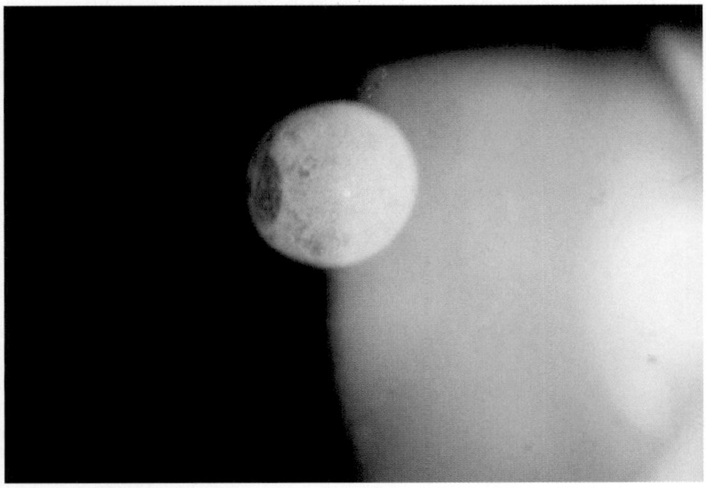

Fig. 15.72 Small cyst in the anterior v treous. (Courtesy of W. Lisch.)

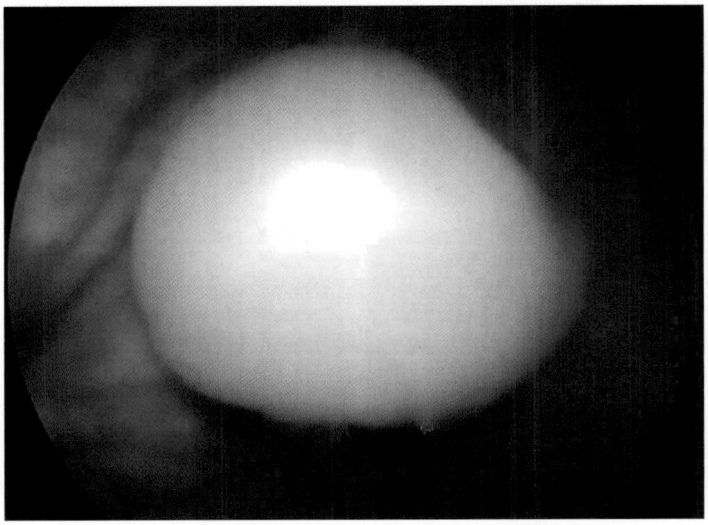

Fig. 15.73 White vitreous cyst in the posterior pole. (Courtesy of B. Chang.)

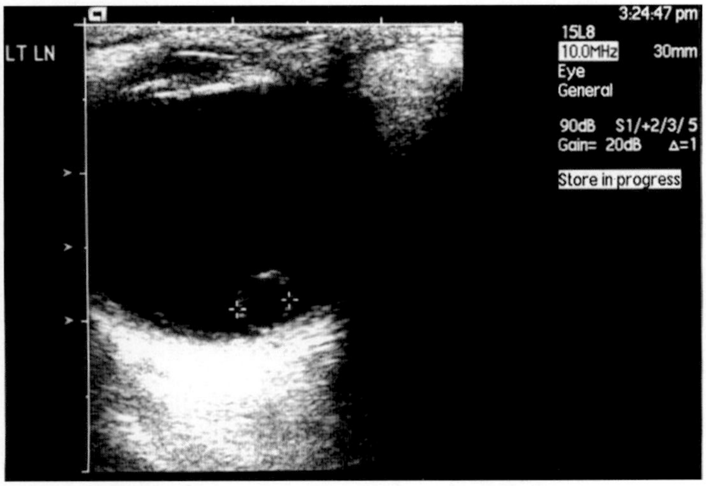

Fig. 15.74 US shows a cystic lesion at the posterior pole. (Courtesy of B. Chang.)

CHAPTER 16

NEURO-OPHTHALMOLOGY

OPTIC NERVE DISEASE

Optic atrophy

Primary

Primary optic atrophy occurs without antecedent swelling. Causes include retrobulbar neuritis, compressive lesions and hereditary optic neuropathy.

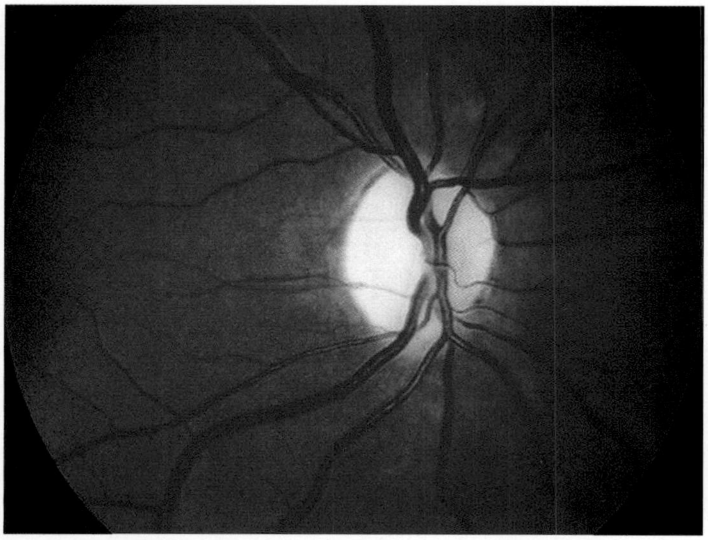

Fig. 16.1 Pale, flat disc with clearly delineated margins, reduction in number of small blood vessels on the disc surface (Kestenbaum sign), attenuation of peripapillary blood vessels, and thinning of the retinal nerve fibre layer.

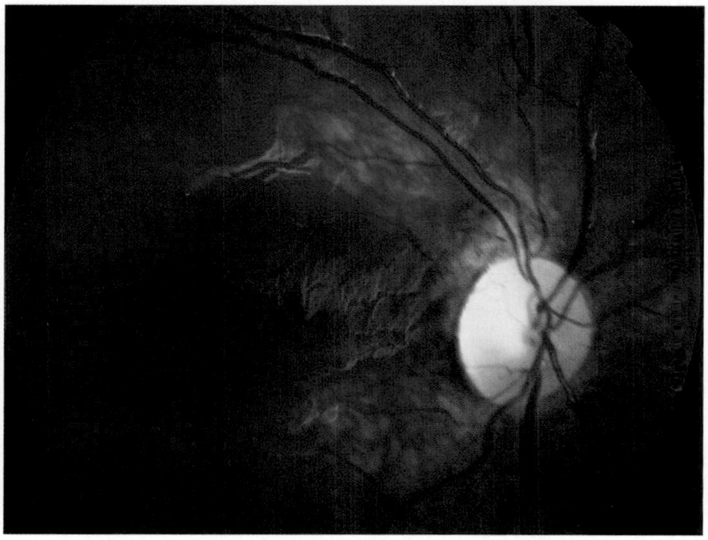

Fig. 16.2 Very severe primary optic atrophy.

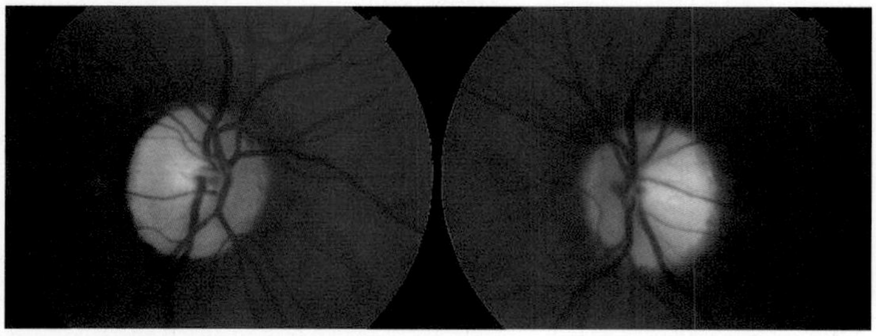

Fig. 16.3 Bilateral temporal pallor may indicate atrophy of fibres from the papillomacular bundle.

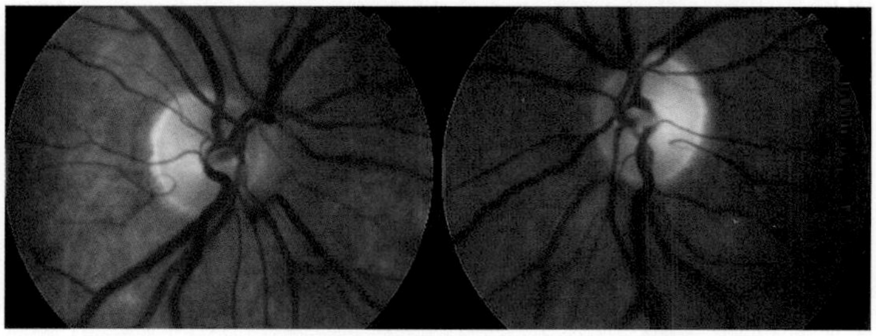

Fig. 16.4 Severe bilateral temporal pallor.

Secondary

Secondary optic atrophy is preceded by swelling of the optic nerve head. Causes include papilloedema, anterior ischaemic optic neuropathy and papillitis.

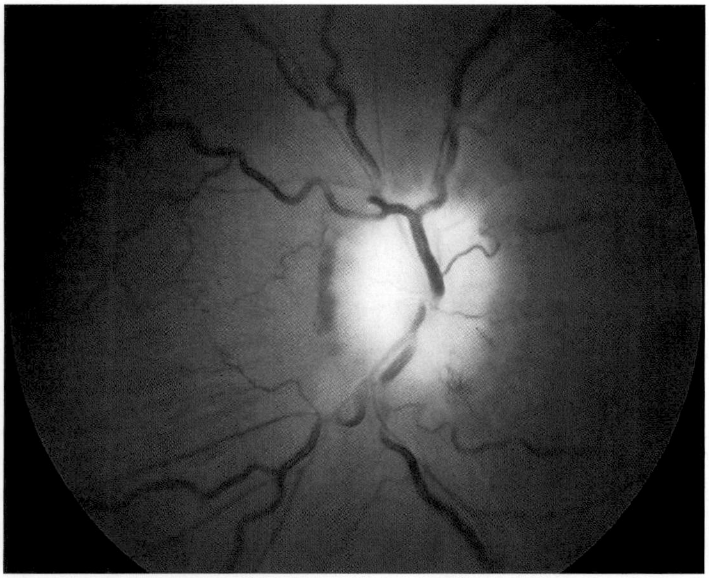

■ **Fig. 16.5** White or dirty grey, slightly raised disc with poorly delineated margins because of gliosis.

Optic neuritis

Retrobulbar neuritis

Retrobulbar neuritis is the most frequent type in young adults and is often associated with multiple sclerosis.

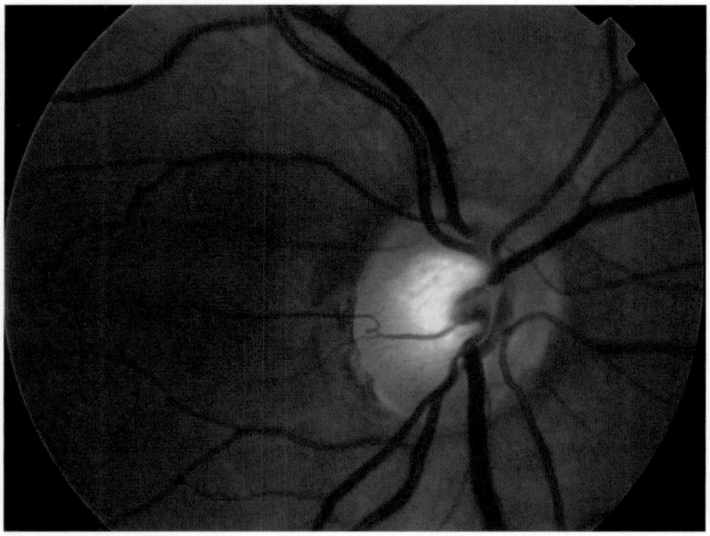

■ **Fig. 16.6** Normal optic disc associated with signs of optic nerve dysfunction.

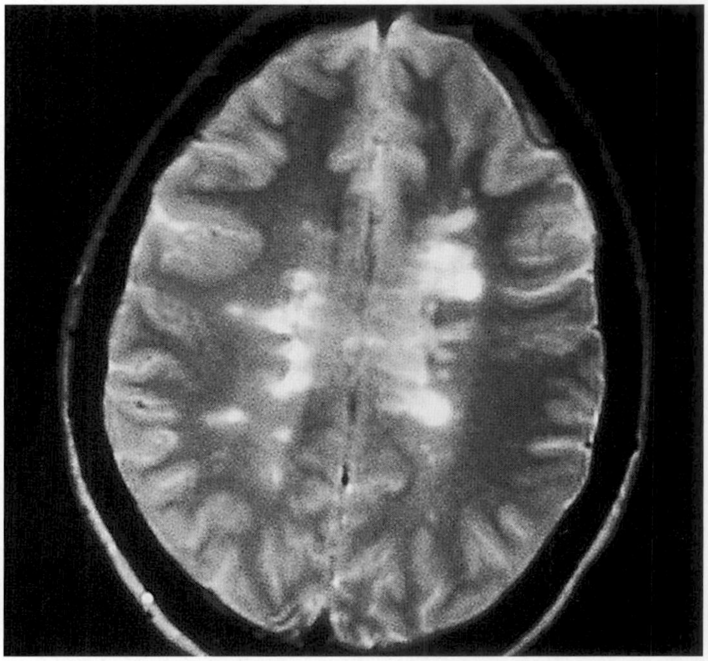

■ **Fig. 16.7** Axial T2-weighted MRI shows periventricular plaques of demyelination.

Papillitis

Papillitis is characterised by involvement of the optic nerve head, either primarily or secondary to contiguous retinal inflammation.

Primary papillitis

Primary papillitis is the most common type of optic neuritis in children and may be bilateral.

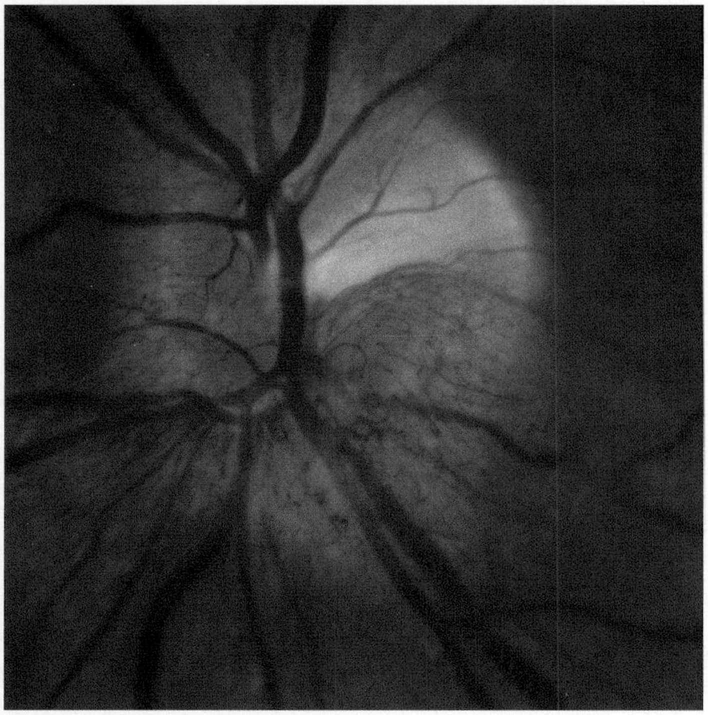

Fig. 16.8 Hyperaemia and oedema of the optic disc with cells in the posterior vitreous. (Courtesy of C. Barry.)

Secondary papillitis

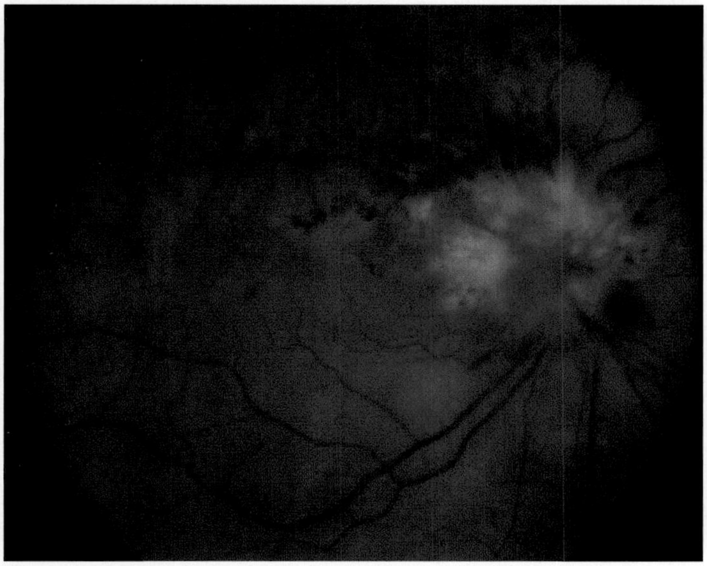

Fig. 16.9 Papillitis associated with cytomegalovirus retinitis. (Courtesy of S. Ford and R. Marsh.)

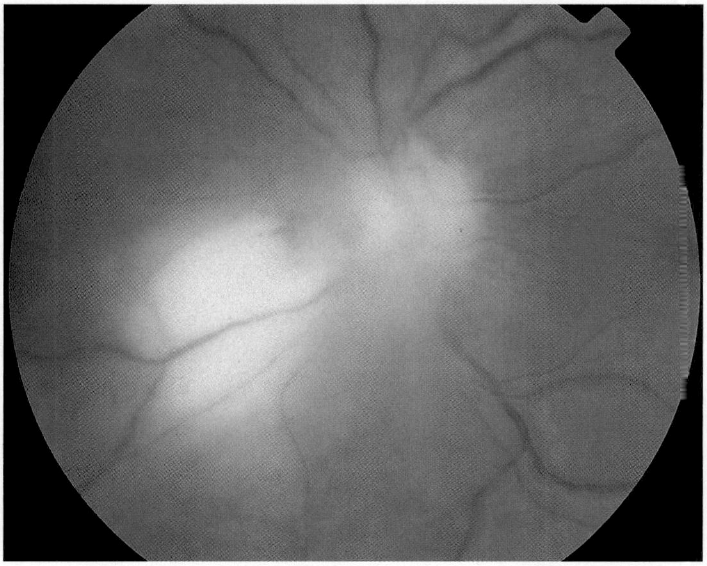

Fig. 16.10 Papillitis associated with juxtapapillary toxoplasma retinitis.

Neuroretinitis

Neuroretinitis is characterised by papillitis in association with inflammation of the retinal nerve fibre layer and a macular star figure. Causes include cat-scratch, Lyme disease and syphilis.

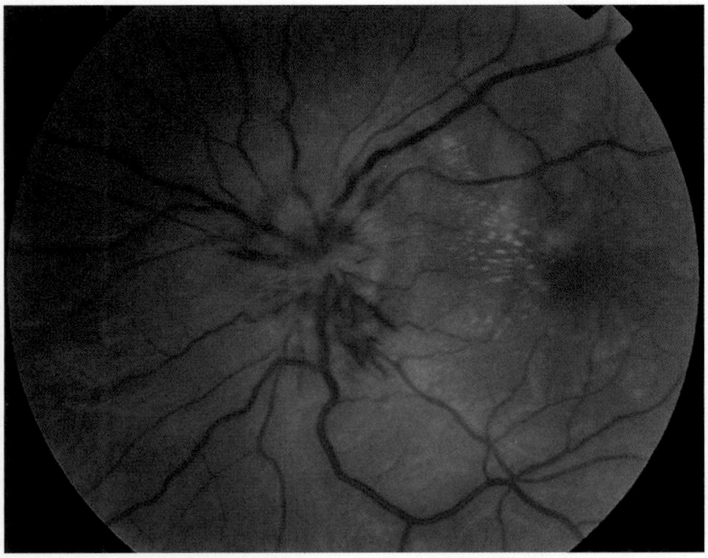

Fig. 16.11 Severe papillitis with flame-shaped haemorrhages and an early macular star. (Courtesy of R. Curtis.)

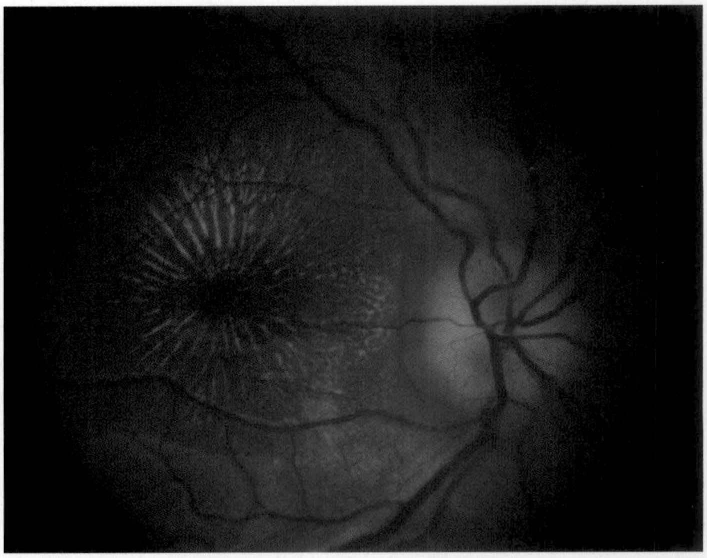

Fig. 16.12 Papillitis without haemorrhages associated with a complete macular star. (Courtesy of L. Merin.)

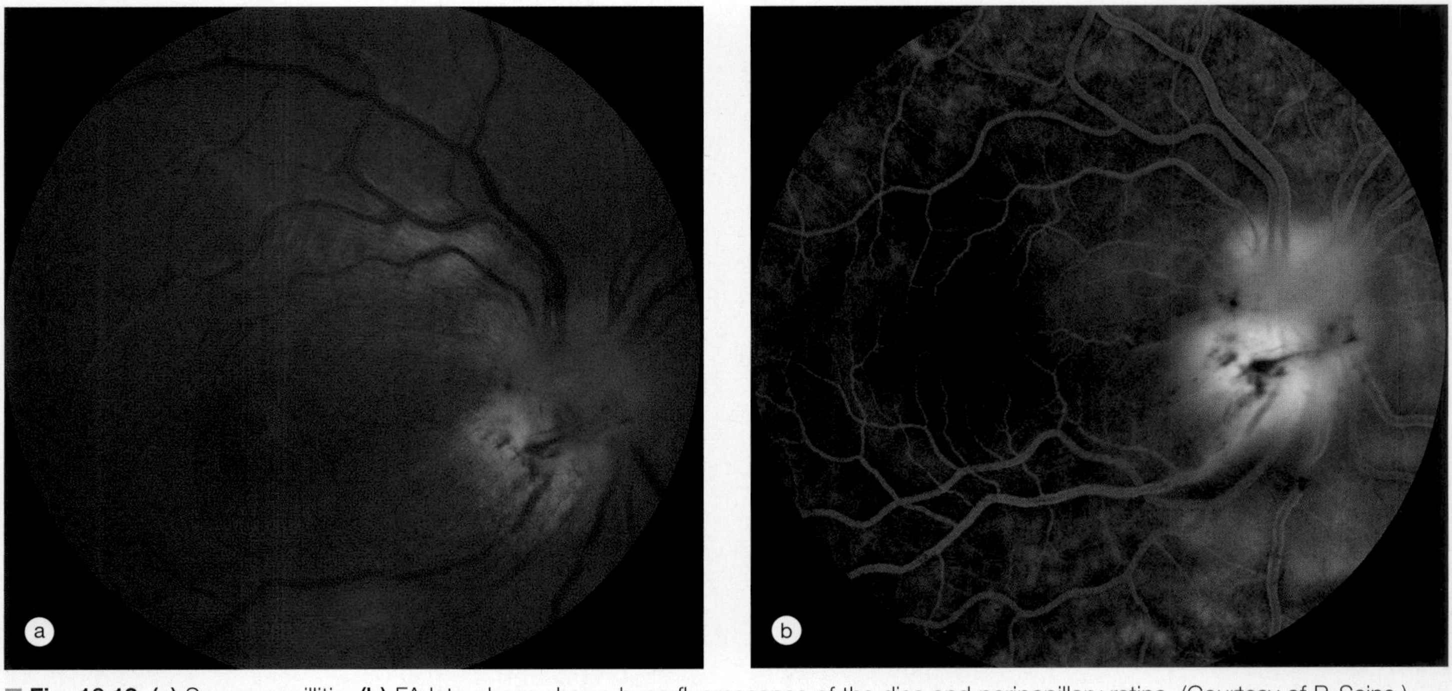

Fig. 16.13 **(a)** Severe papillitis. **(b)** FA late phase shows hyperfluorescence of the disc and peripapillary retina. (Courtesy of P. Saine.)

Ischaemic optic neuropathy

Non-arteritic anterior ischaemic optic neuropathy

This typically affects hypertensive adults.

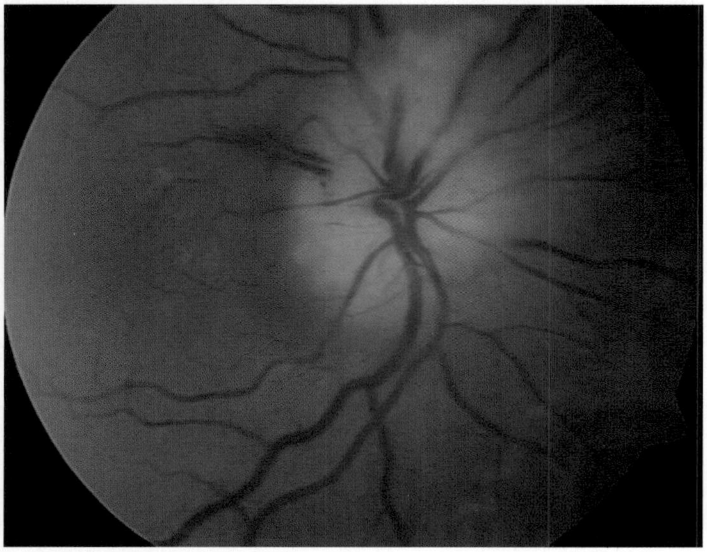

Fig. 16.14 Disc pallor associated with oedema and a few splinter-shaped haemorrhages. (Courtesy of P. Gili.)

Arteritic anterior ischaemic optic neuropathy

This typically affects patients with giant cell arteritis.

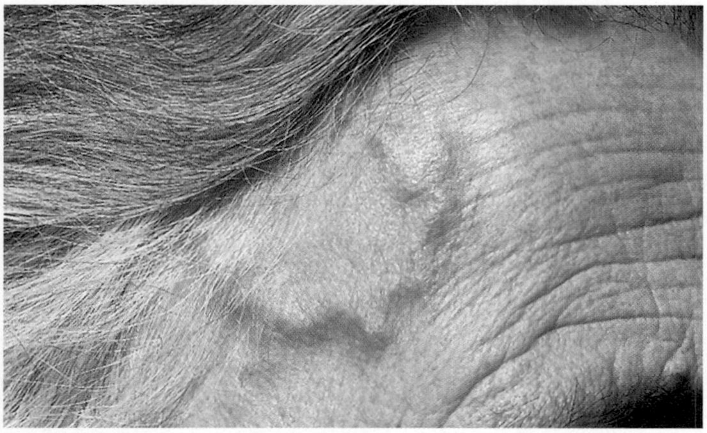

Fig. 16.15 Superficial temporal arteritis is characterised by thickened, tender, inflamed, nodular, non-pulsatile arteries that cannot be flattened against the skull.

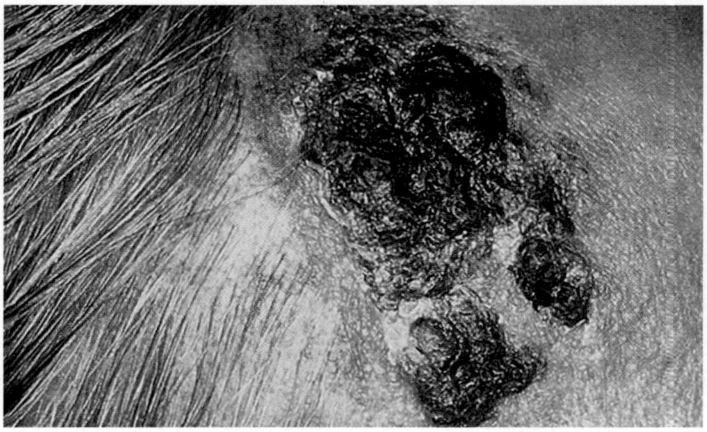

Fig. 16.16 In severe cases, scalp gangrene may ensue.

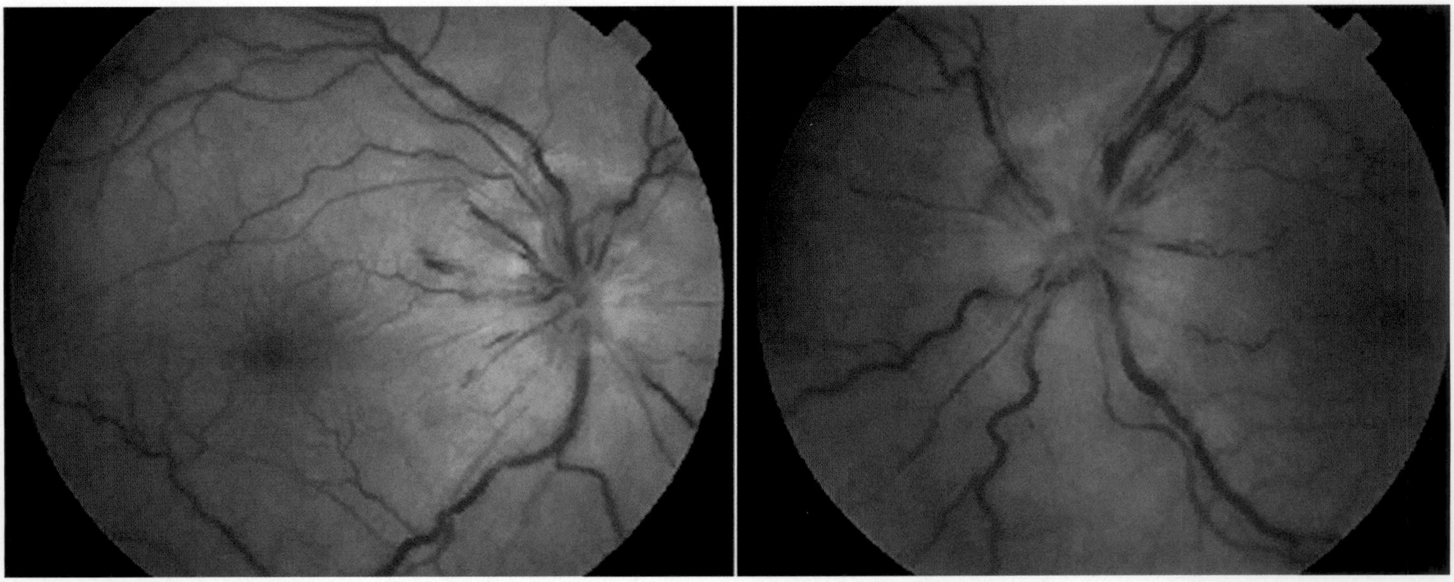

■ **Fig. 16.17** Bilateral involvement may result in blindness. (Courtesy of S. Ford and R. Marsh.)

Diabetic papillopathy

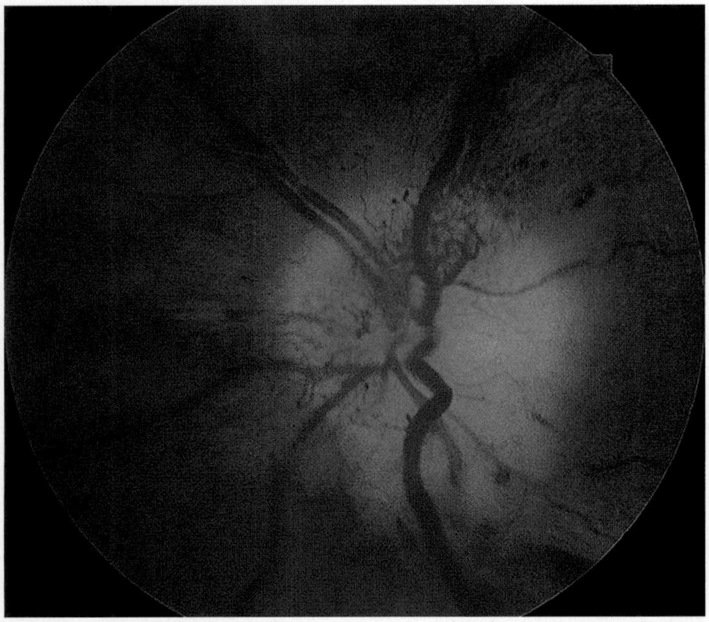

■ **Fig. 16.18** Mild disc swelling and hyperaemia with disc surface telangiectasia.

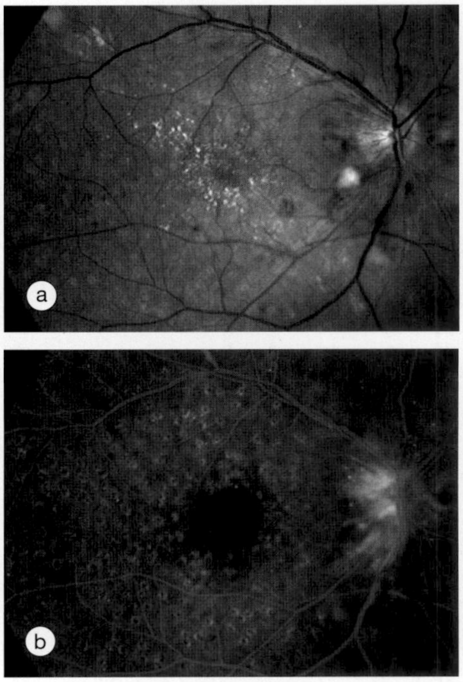

■ **Fig. 16.19** **(a)** Red-free image of diabetic papillopathy with laser scars following panretinal photocoagulation. **(b)** FA shows mild late hyperfluorescence. (Courtesy of Z. Bashshur.)

Leber hereditary optic neuropathy

This typically affects young adult males and results in severe bilateral visual loss.

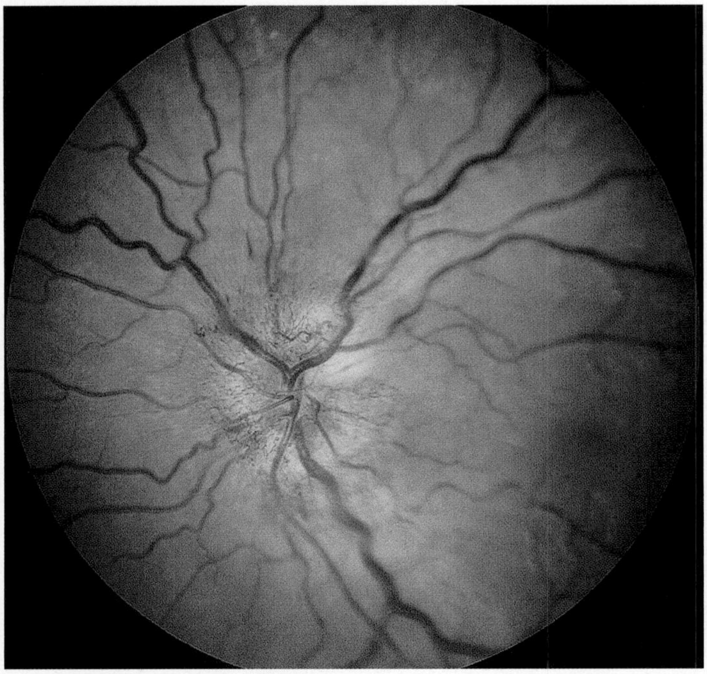

■ **Fig. 16.20** Dilated capillaries on the disc surface, which may extend on to adjacent retina (telangiectatic microangiopathy), vascular tortuosity and swelling of the peripapillary nerve fibre layer.

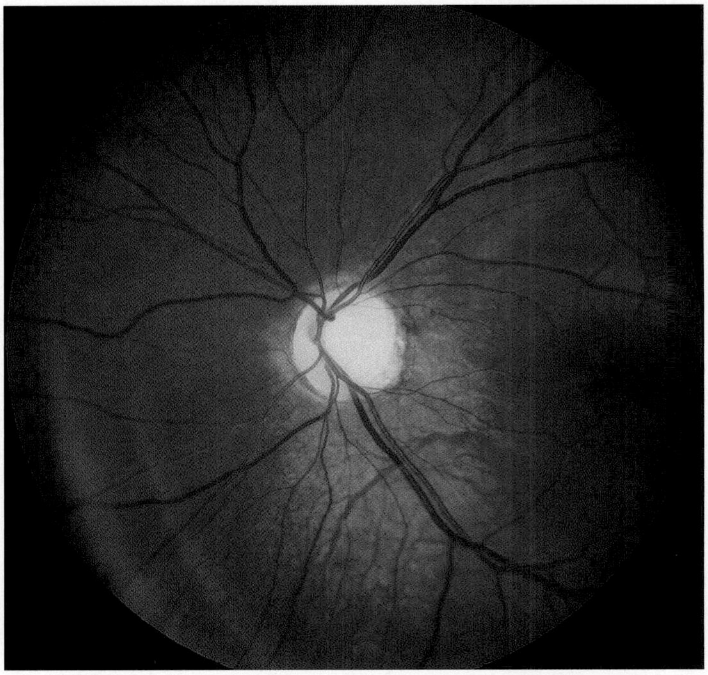

■ **Fig. 16.21** Subsequently, the telangiectatic vessels regress and severe optic atrophy ensues.

Papilloedema

Papilloedema is swelling of the optic nerve head, secondary to raised intracranial pressure. It is nearly always bilateral, although it may be asymmetrical.

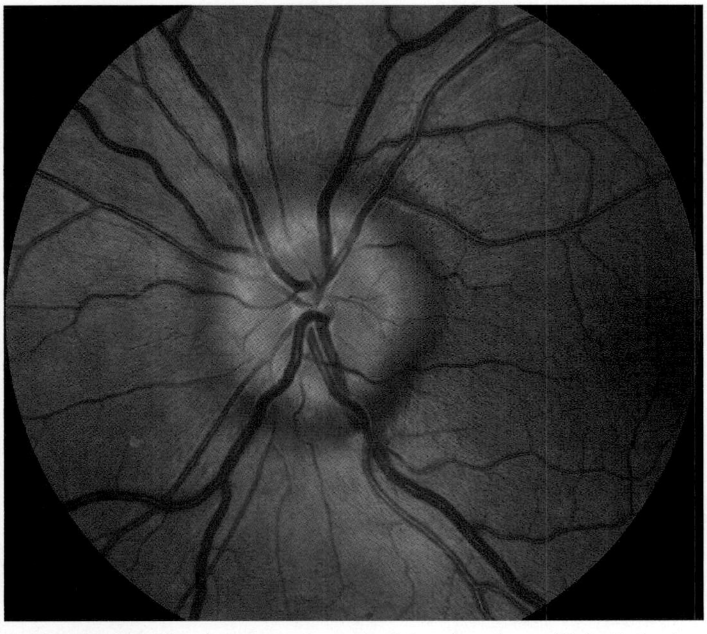

■ **Fig. 16.22** Disc hyperaemia and slight elevation with indistinct margins. (Courtesy of P. Saine.)

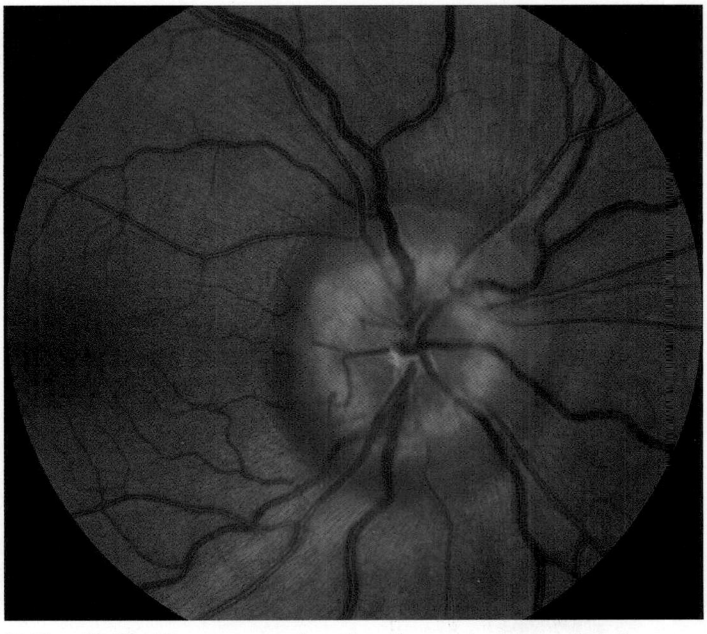

■ **Fig. 16.23** More severe disc elevation and venous dilatation. (Courtesy of P. Saine.)

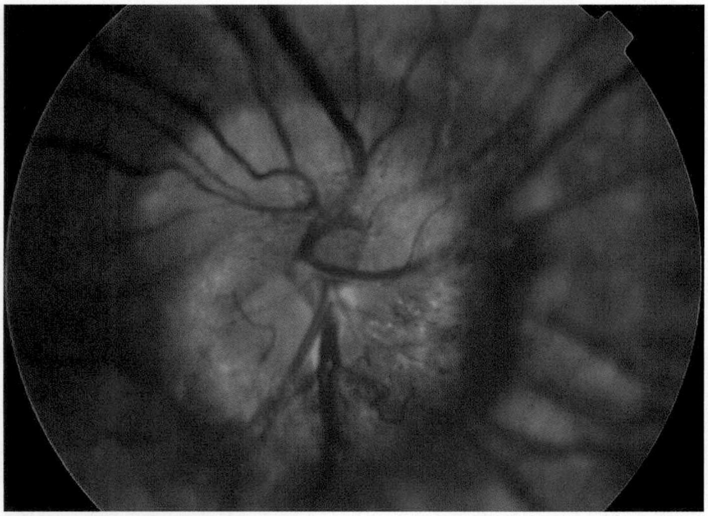

■ **Fig. 16.24** Severe disc hyperaemia.

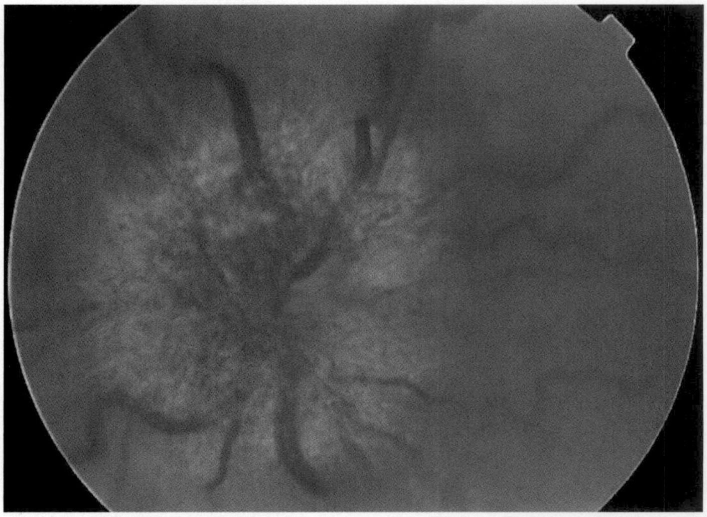

■ **Fig. 16.25** Severe hyperaemia and oedema with partial obscuration of disc vasculature.

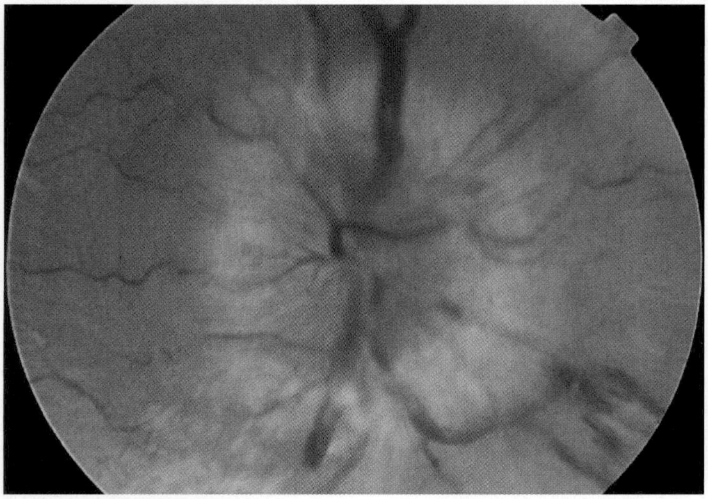

■ **Fig. 16.26** Severe oedema and peripapillary haemorrhages.

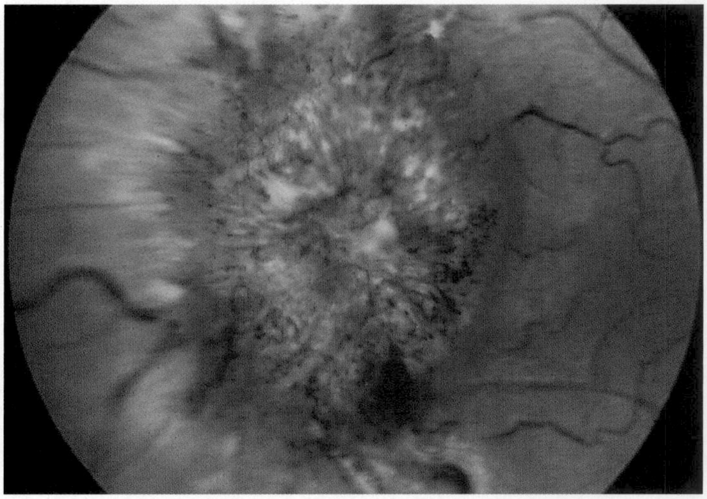

■ **Fig. 16.27** Very severe disc elevation.

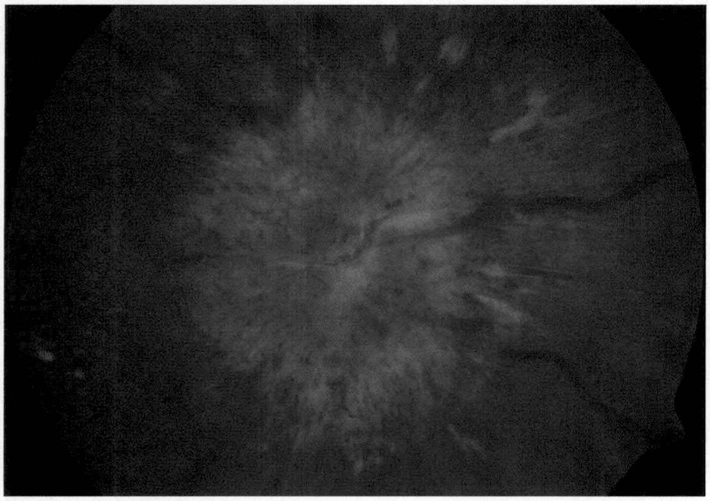

■ **Fig. 16.28** Total obscuration of the disc, peripapillary flame-shaped haemorrhages and cotton-wool spots, and small hard exudates at the macula. (Courtesy of P. Gili.)

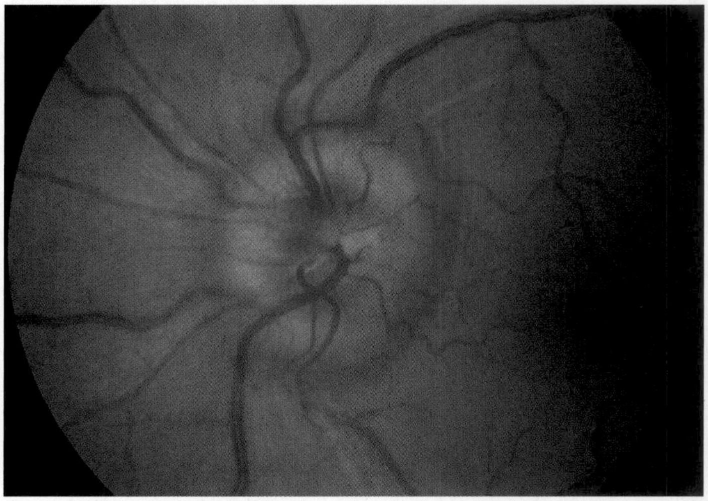

■ **Fig. 16.29** Champagne-cork-like disc elevation with resolution of vascular abnormalities.

PUPILLARY ABNORMALITIES

Oculosympathetic palsy (Horner syndrome)

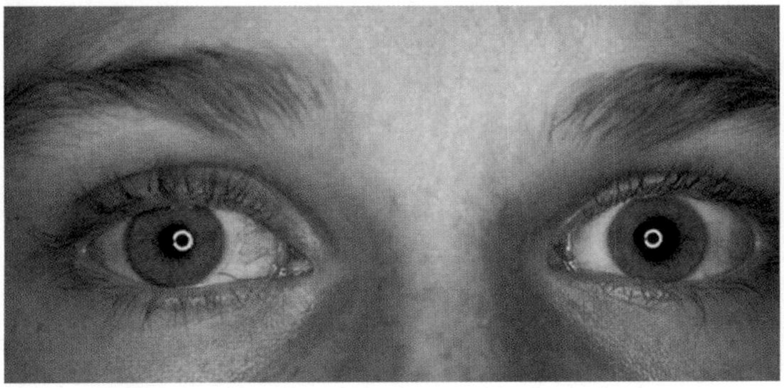

Fig. 16.30 Right Horner syndrome. Mild ptosis (usually 1–2 mm) as a result of weakness of Müller muscle; slight elevation of inferior eyelid as a result of weakness of inferior tarsal muscle; miosis resulting from unopposed action of the sphincter pupillae, with resultant anisocoria, which is accentuated in dim light, since the Horner pupil will not dilate like its fellow; normal reactions to light and near; reduced ipsilateral sweating, but only if the lesion is below the superior cervical ganglion, because the fibres supplying the skin of the face run along the external carotid artery.

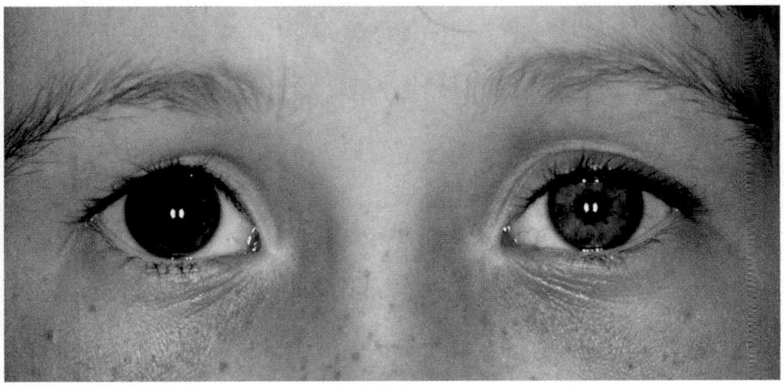

Fig. 16.31 Left Horner syndrome with left hypochromic heterochromia may be seen if the lesion is congenital or long-standing.

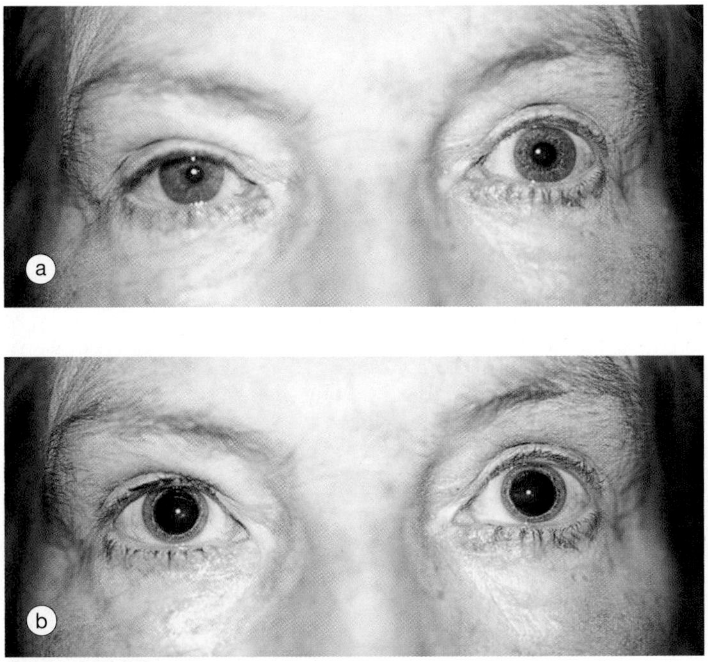

Fig. 16.32 Hydroxyamphetamine 1% may be used to differentiate a preganglionic from a postganglionic lesion. **(a)** Right preganglionic Horner syndrome. **(b)** Bilateral mydriasis following instillation of hydroxyamphetamine into both eyes. In a postganglionic lesion the Horner pupil will not dilate.

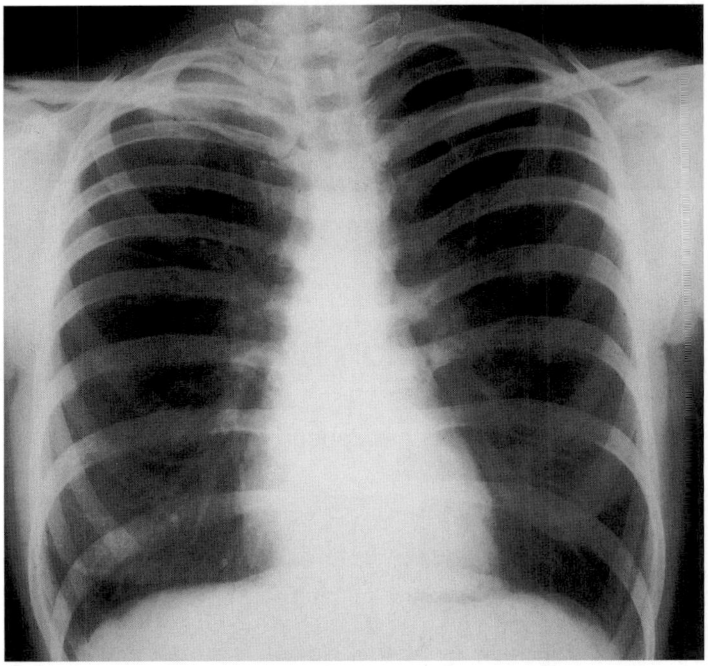

Fig. 16.33 Pancoast tumour (right apical shadow) is an important cause of preganglionic Horner.

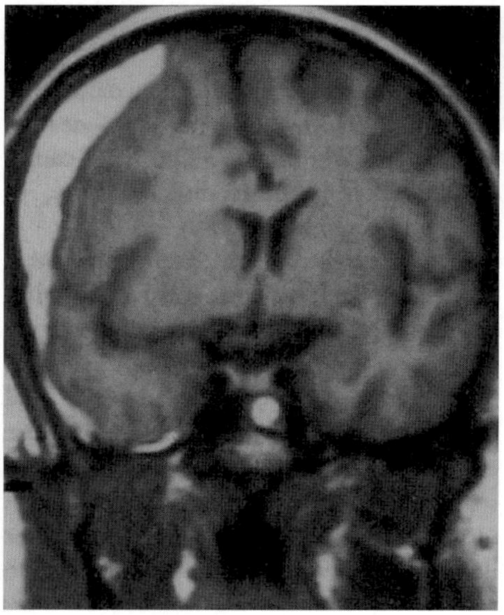

■ **Fig. 16.40** MRI showing a subdural haematoma, which will also cause a 'surgical' palsy. (Courtesy of C. D. Forbes and W. F. Jackson.)

Fourth nerve

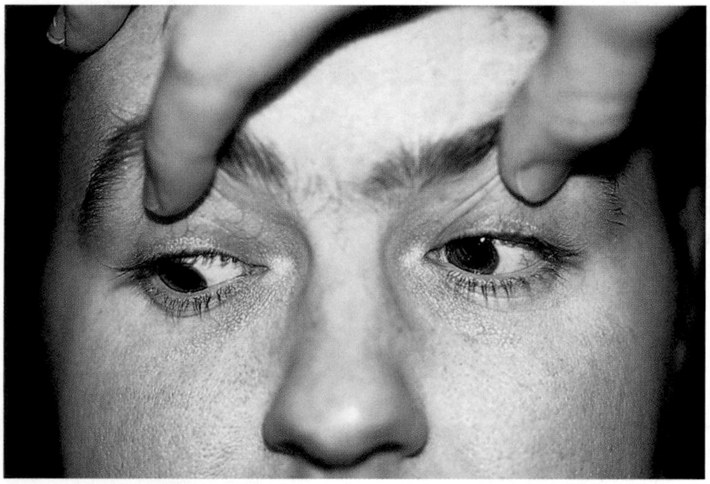

■ **Fig. 16.41** Left fourth nerve palsy. Limitation of left depression in adduction due to left superior oblique weakness.

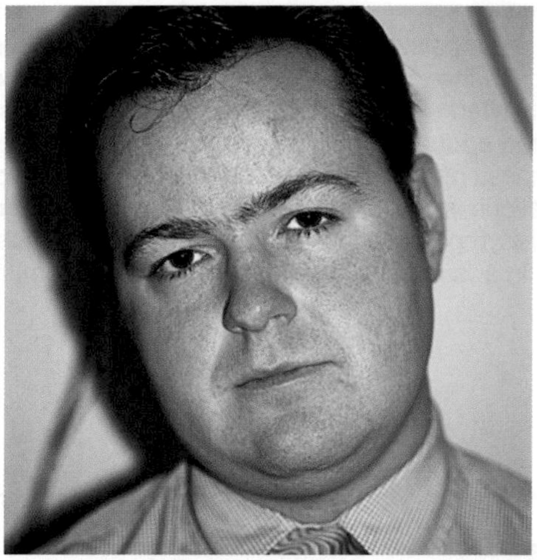

■ **Fig. 16.42** Compensatory head posture to avoid diplopia due to a left superior oblique palsy involves head tilt to the right to alleviate excyclotorsion as well as face turn to the right and depression of the chin to alleviate the inability to depress the eye in adduction.

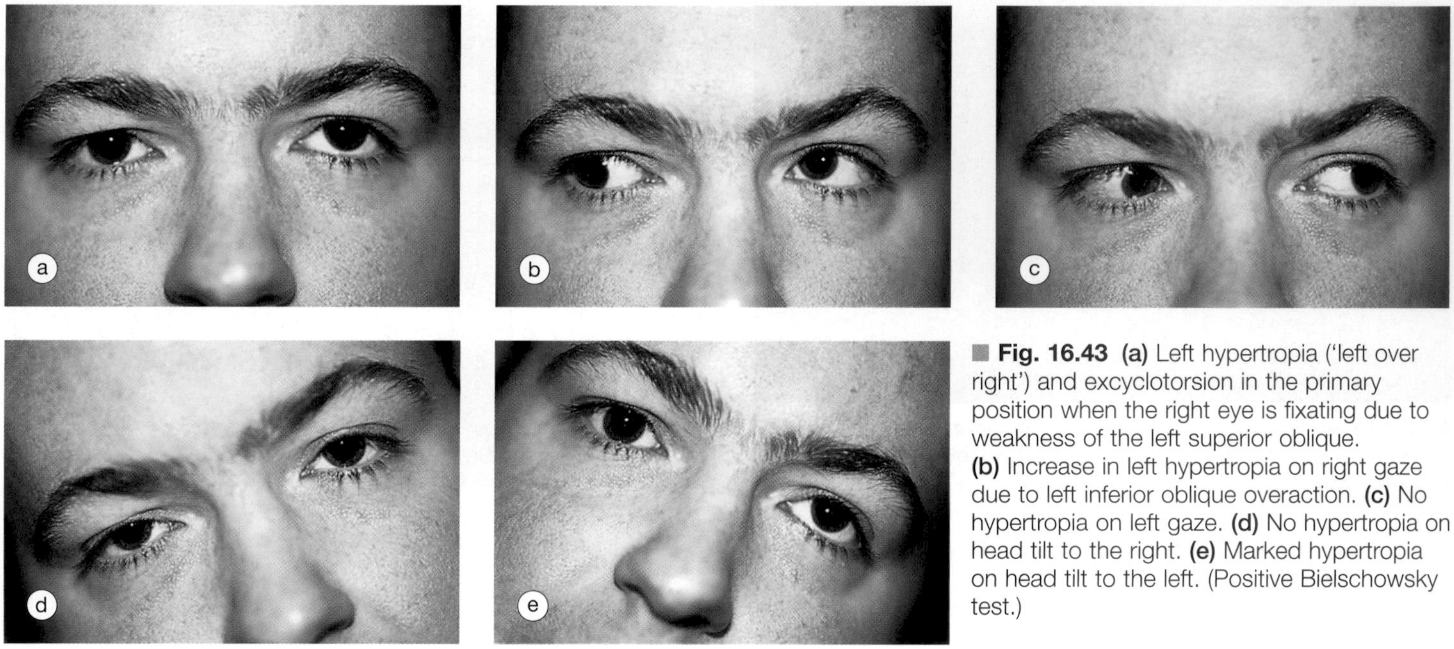

■ **Fig. 16.43** **(a)** Left hypertropia ('left over right') and excyclotorsion in the primary position when the right eye is fixating due to weakness of the left superior oblique. **(b)** Increase in left hypertropia on right gaze due to left inferior oblique overaction. **(c)** No hypertropia on left gaze. **(d)** No hypertropia on head tilt to the right. **(e)** Marked hypertropia on head tilt to the left. (Positive Bielschowsky test.)

Sixth nerve

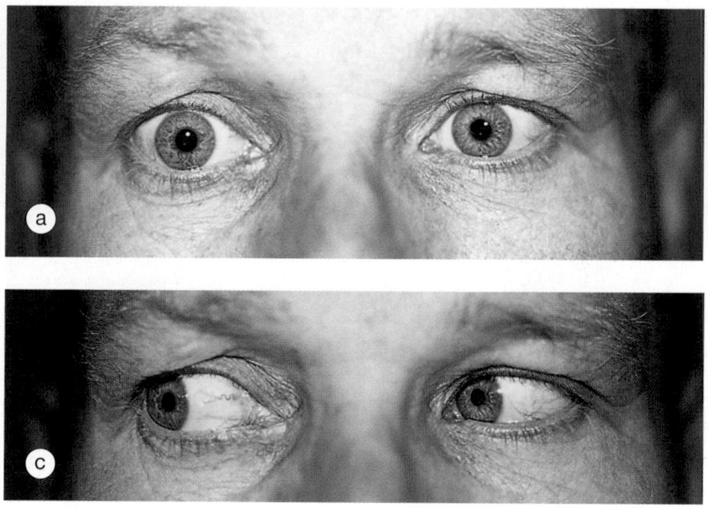

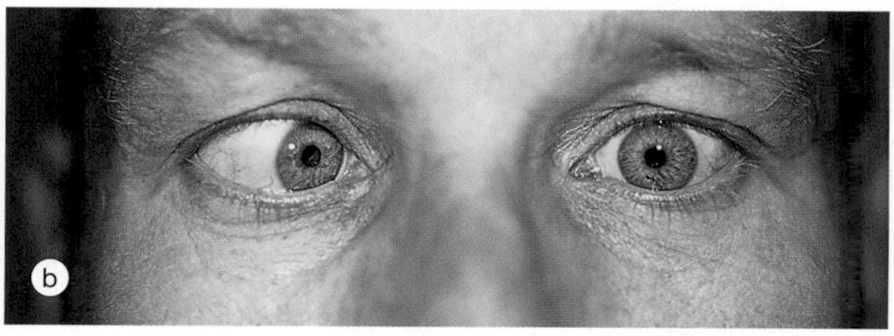

■ **Fig. 16.44** Left sixth nerve palsy. **(a)** Slight left esotropia in the primary position due to unopposed action of the left medial rectus. **(b)** Marked limitation of left abduction due to weakness of the left lateral rectus. **(c)** Normal left adduction. There will also be a compensatory face turn into the field of action of the paralysed muscle (i.e. to the right) to minimise diplopia, so that the eyes do not need to look towards the field of action of the paralysed muscle (i.e. to the right).

Causes

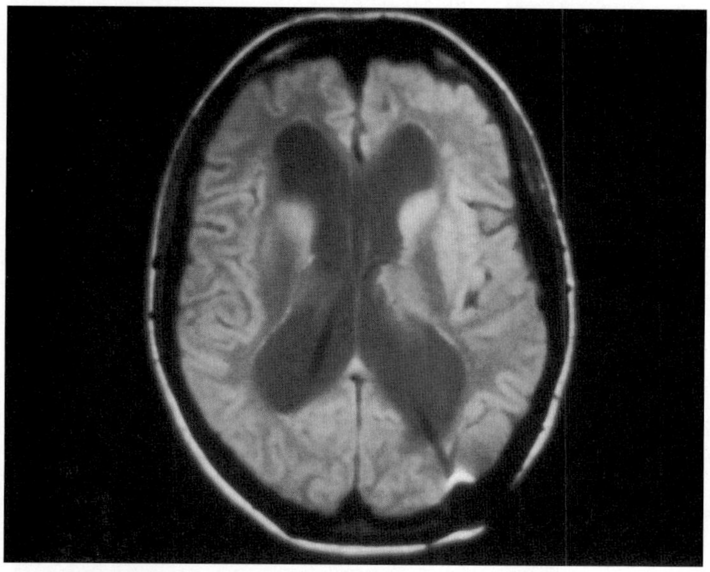

■ **Fig. 16.45** Raised intracranial pressure by an intracranial tumour or idiopathic intracranial hypertension may cause downward displacement of the brain stem and stretching of the sixth nerve over the petrous tip (a false localising sign). This axial MRI scan shows large ventricles due to raised intracranial pressure.

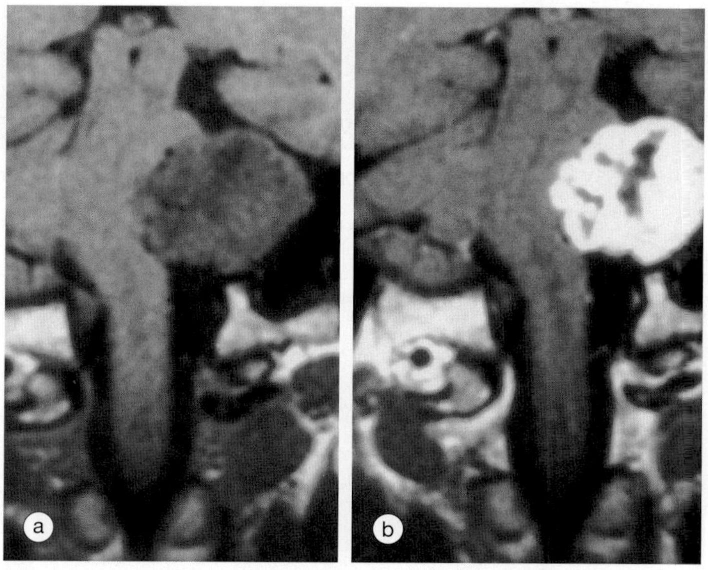

■ **Fig. 16.46** This sagittal MRI scan shows an acoustic neuroma. **(a)** Without enhancement. **(b)** Gadolinium enhance.

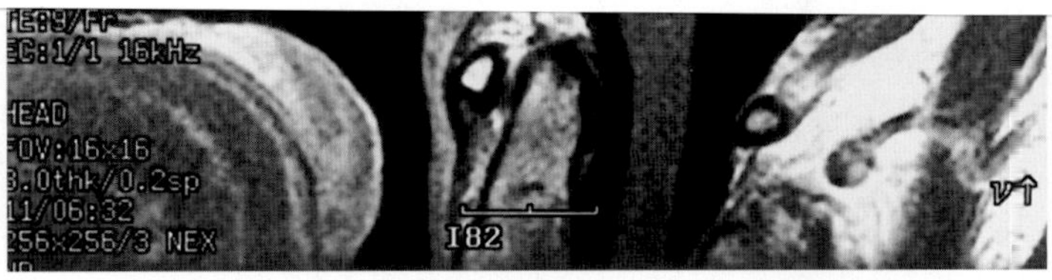

■ **Fig. 16.52** Sagittal T1-weighted gadolinium-enhanced MRI showing a pituitary adenoma (Courtesy of D. Thomas.)

Gaze palsy

Horizontal

Acidophil adenoma

Acidophil tumours secrete growth hormone, which causes gigantism in children and acromegaly in adults.

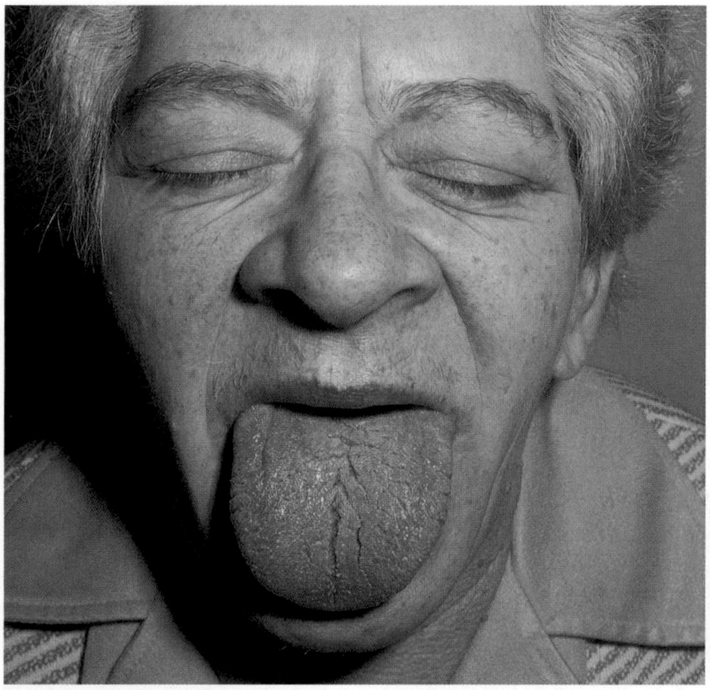

Fig. 16.53 Coarse facial features and macroglossia.

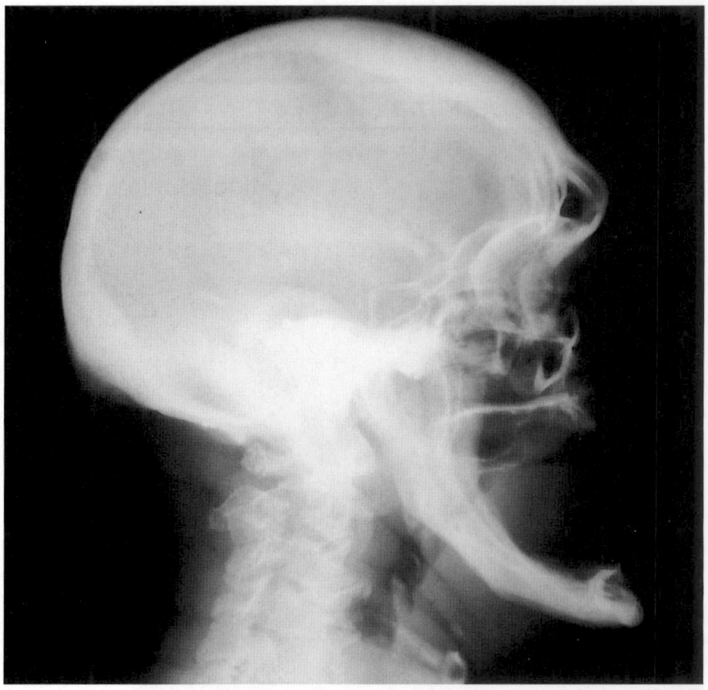

Fig. 16.54 Plain skull radiograph showing an enlarged mandible with widening of the mandibular angle, prognathism, enlarged frontal sinus, thickening of the skull vault and an enlarged pituitary fossa. (Courtesy of S. Ghiacy.)

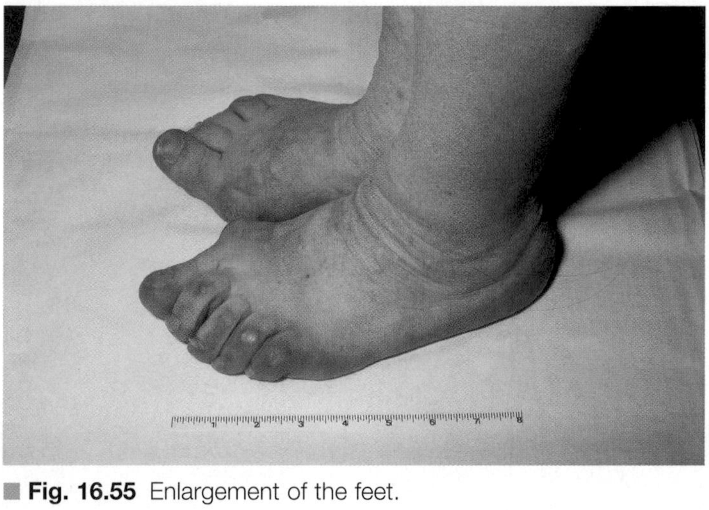

Fig. 16.55 Enlargement of the feet.

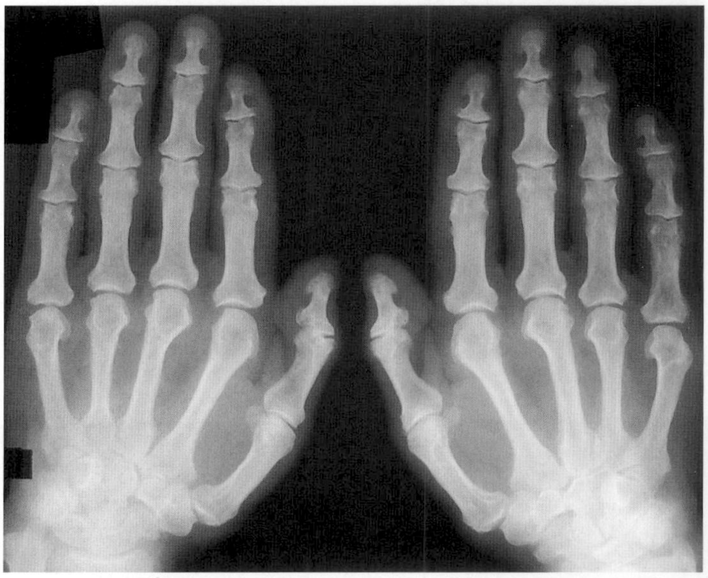

Fig. 16.56 Plain radiograph of the hands shows enlarged bones with prominent muscle attachments, lips and hooks of the terminal phalanges and early osteoarthritic changes of the wrists. (Courtesy of S. Ghiacy.)

Chromophobe adenoma

Chromophobe adenomas may secrete prolactin and are referred to as prolactinomas.

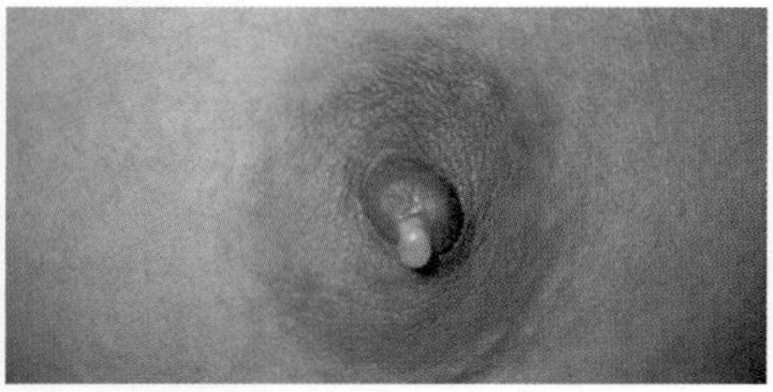

Fig. 16.57 Excessive levels of prolactin in women lead to the infertility–amenorrhoea–galactorrhoea syndrome. (Courtesy of P.-M. Bouloux.)

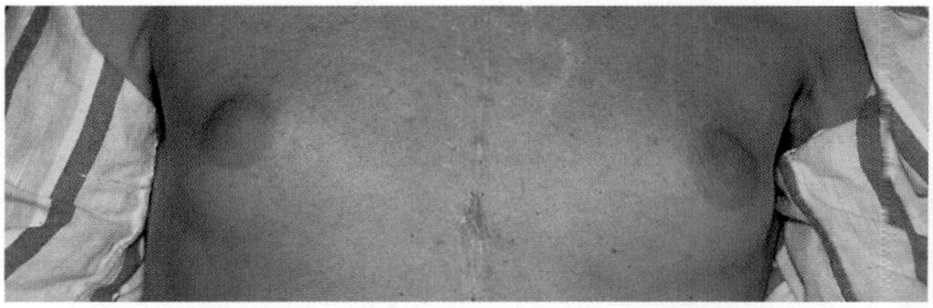

Fig. 16.58 Men may manifest gynaecomastia, impotence and sterility. (Courtesy of M. A. Mir.)

CHAPTER 17

STRABISMUS

ESOTROPIA

Pseudo-esotropia

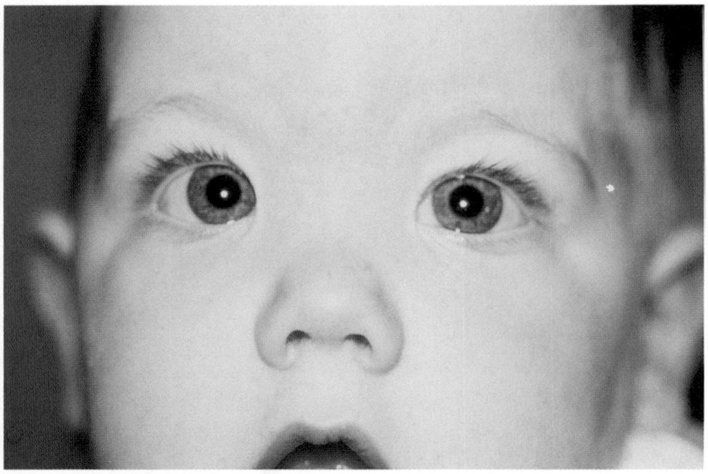

Fig. 17.1 False appearance of esotropia due to epicanthic folds and a flat nasal bridge; corneal reflexes are symmetrical.

Non-accommodative esotropia

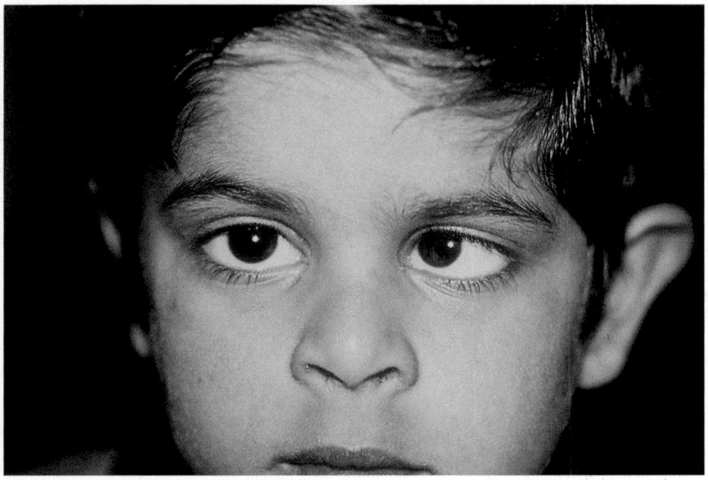

Fig. 17.2 Left esotropia without hypermetropia in which the distance and near deviations are the same.

Accommodative esotropia

Non-refractive

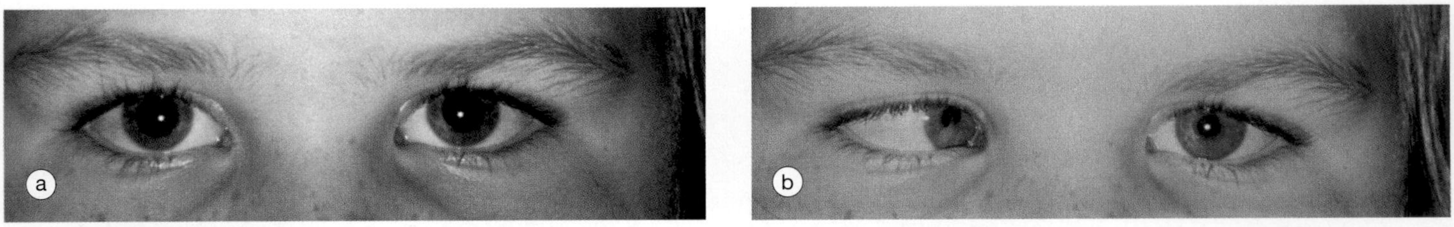

Fig. 17.3 This is caused by a high accommodative convergence/accommodation (AC/A) ratio without hypermetropia. **(a)** Straight for distance. **(b)** Right esotropia for near. (Courtesy of Wilmer Institute.)

Refractive

Fully accommodative

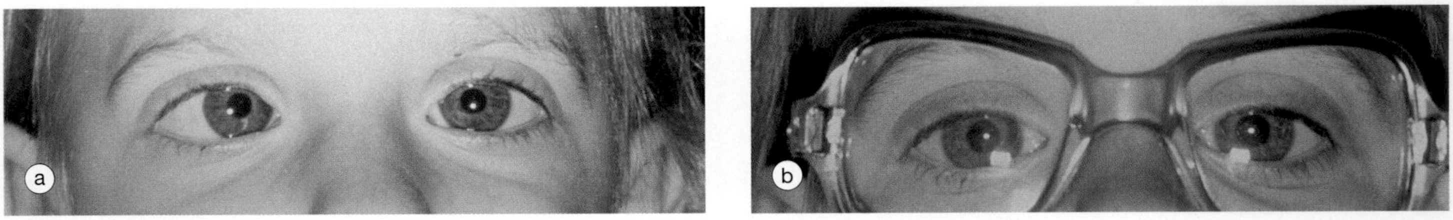

Fig. 17.4 This is caused by hypermetropia with a normal AC/A ratio. **(a)** Right esotropia for distance and near. **(b)** Straight for distance and near with spectacles. (Courtesy of Wilmer Institute.)

Partially accommodative

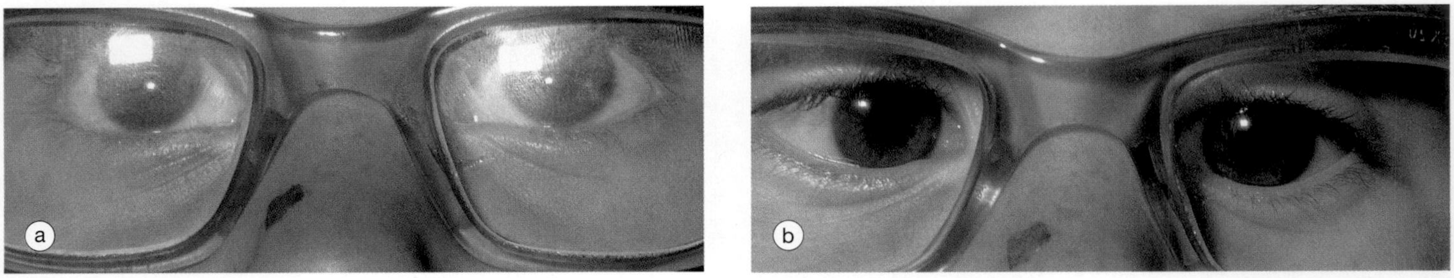

Fig. 17.5 **(a)** Straight for distance. **(b)** Right esotropia for near despite spectacles.

Mixed

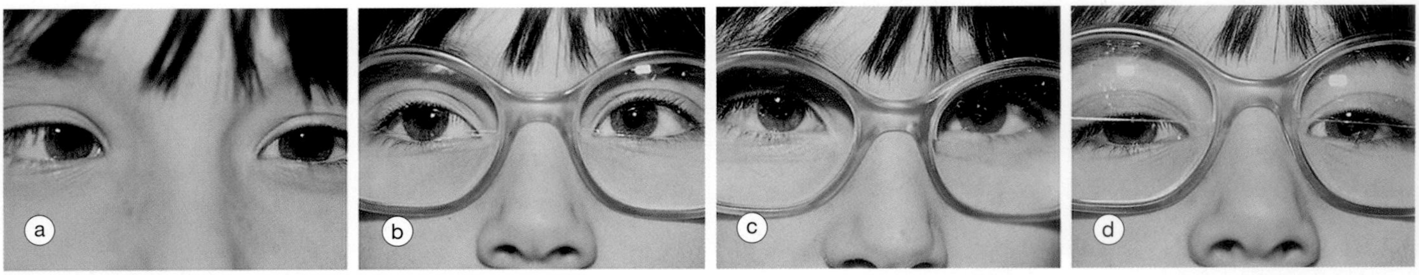

Fig. 17.6 This is caused by hypermetropia as well as a high AC/A ratio. **(a)** Right esotropia for distance that is worse for near. **(b)** Straight eyes for distance with spectacles. **(c)** Right esotropia for near despite spectacles. **(d)** Straight when looking through bifocals. (Courtesy of B. J. Zitelli and H. W. Davis.)

Essential infantile esotropia

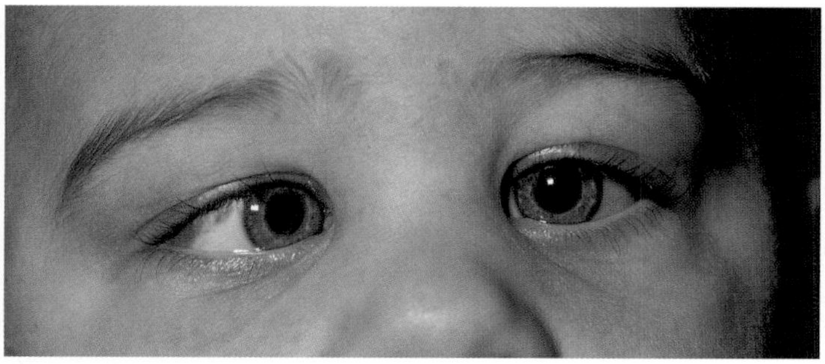

Fig. 17.7 Large angle.

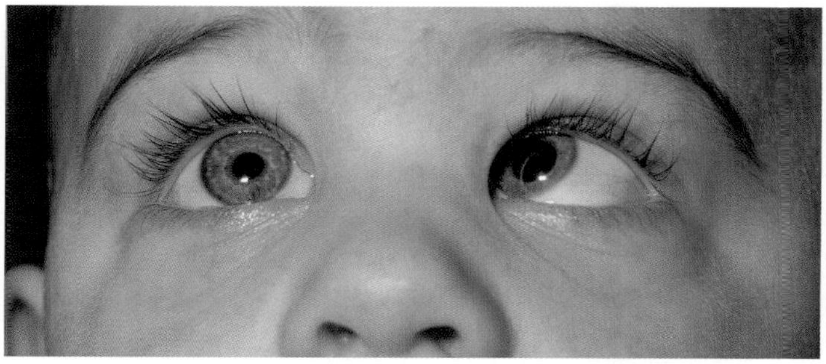

Fig. 17.8 Inferior oblique overaction is common.

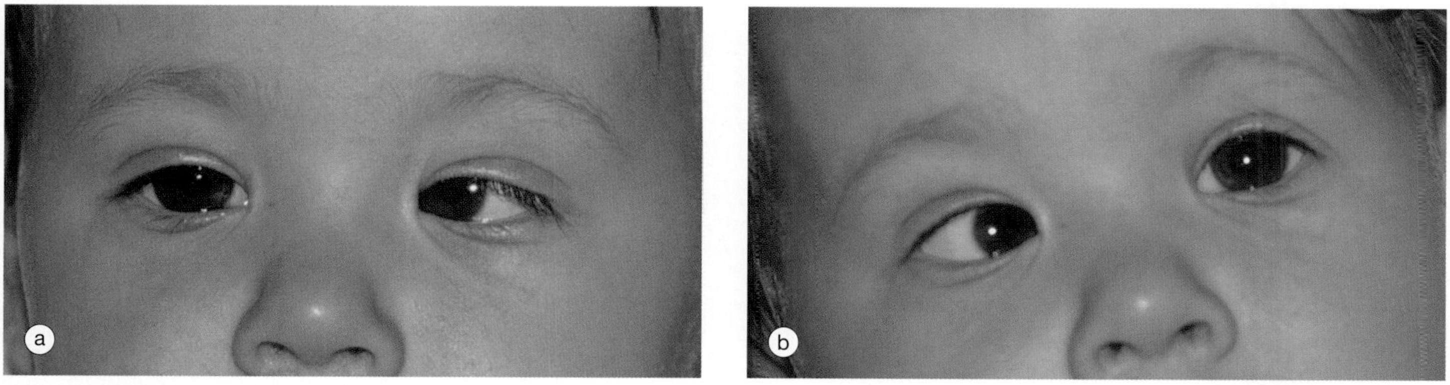

Fig. 17.9 Fixation is usually alternating in the primary position and cross-fixating in side gaze. **(a)** Left eye is used to fixate in right gaze. **(b)** Right eye is used to fixate in left gaze. (Courtesy of J. Yangüela.)

EXOTROPIA

Constant exotropia

Congenital

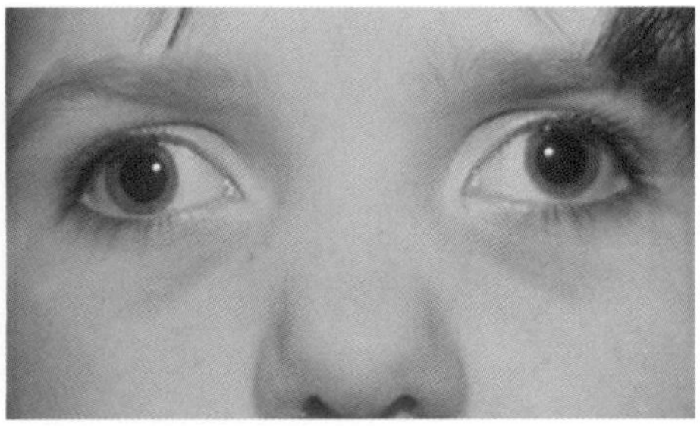

Fig. 17.10 The angle is large and refraction normal. (Courtesy of B. J. Zitelli and H. W. Davis.)

Sensory

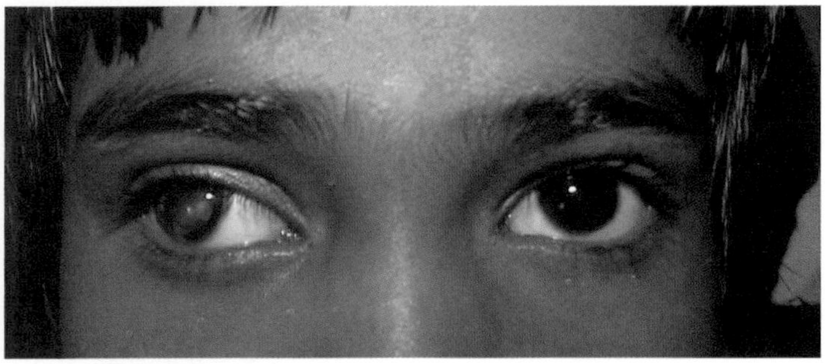

Fig. 17.11 Right sensory exotropia due to cataract. (Courtesy of M. Parulekar.)

Intermittent exotropia

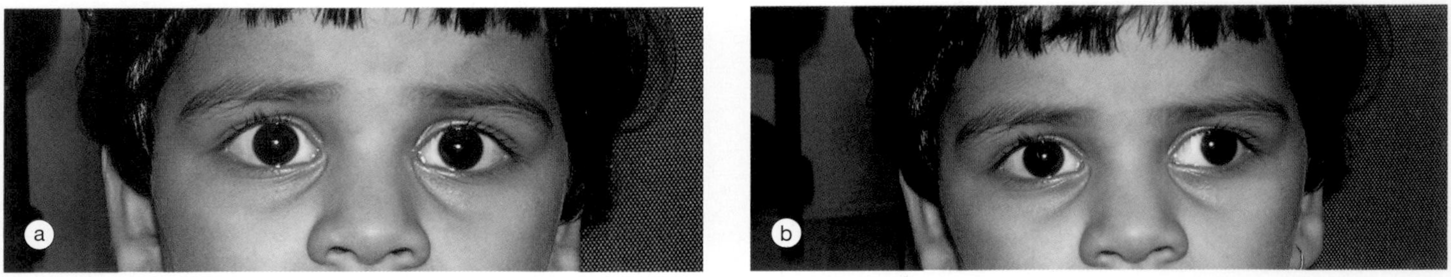

Fig. 17.12 Presentation is in childhood. **(a)** Straight eyes most of the time. **(b)** Exotropia under conditions of visual inattention, fatigue or ill-health. (Courtesy of M. Parulekar.)

Basic

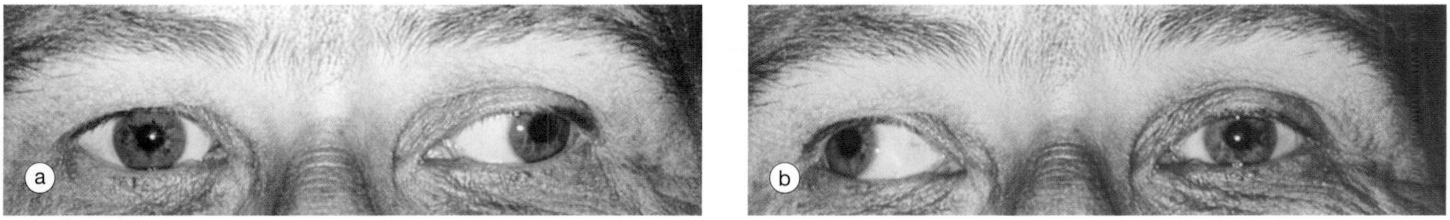

Fig. 17.13 Alternating fixation in which the angle is the same for distance **(a)** and near **(b)**. (Courtesy of Wilmer Institute.)

Convergent weakness

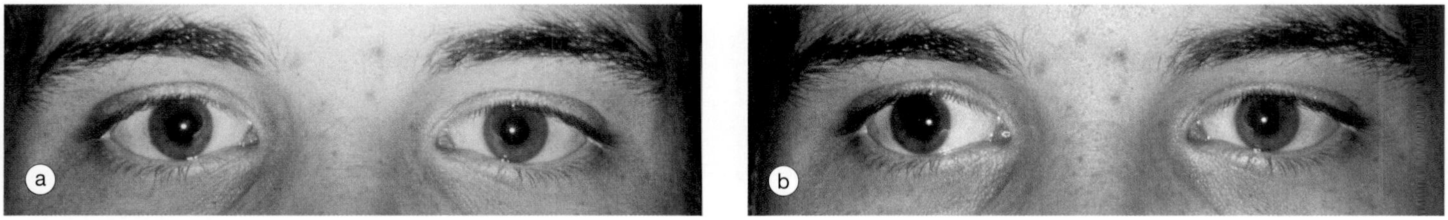

Fig. 17.14 The angle for distance **(a)** is less than for near **(b)**. (Courtesy of Wilmer Institute.)

Divergent excess

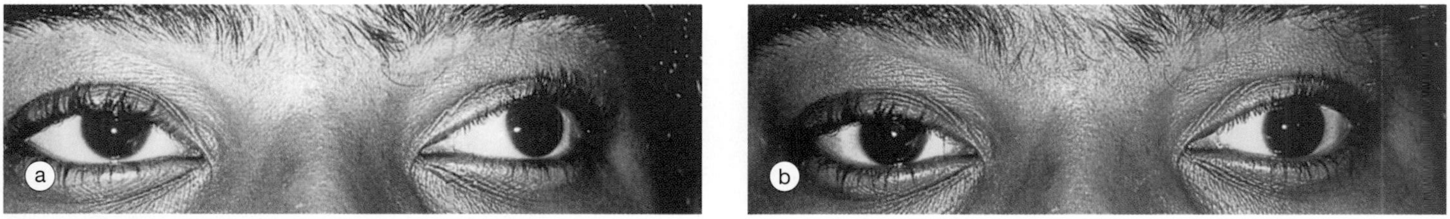

Fig. 17.15 The angle for distance **(a)** is greater than for near **(b)**. (Courtesy of Wilmer Institute.)

ALPHABET PATTERNS

'V' pattern

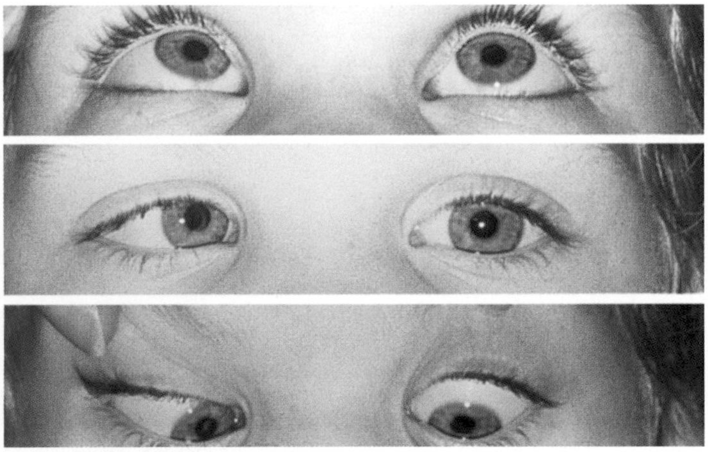

■ **Fig. 17.16** 'V' pattern esotropia; angle is greater in downgaze. (Courtesy of Wilmer Institute.)

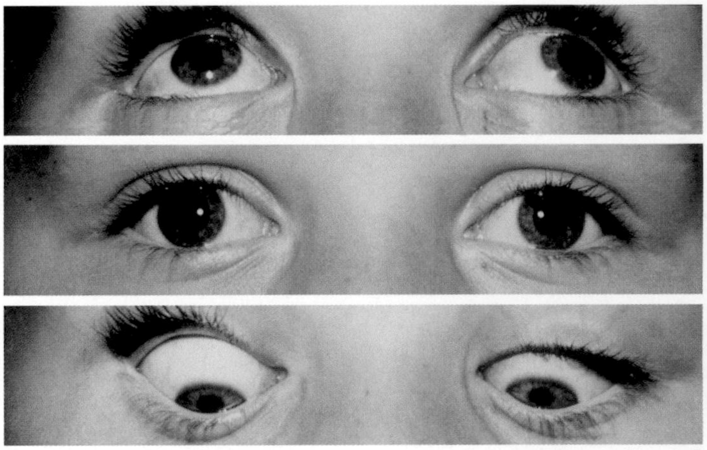

■ **Fig. 17.17** 'V' pattern exotropia; angle is greater in upgaze.

'A' pattern

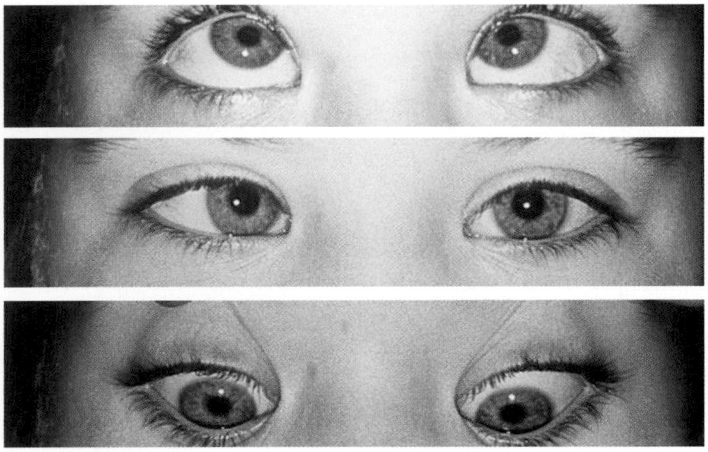

■ **Fig. 17.18** 'A' pattern esotropia; angle is greater in upgaze. (Courtesy of Wilmer Institute.)

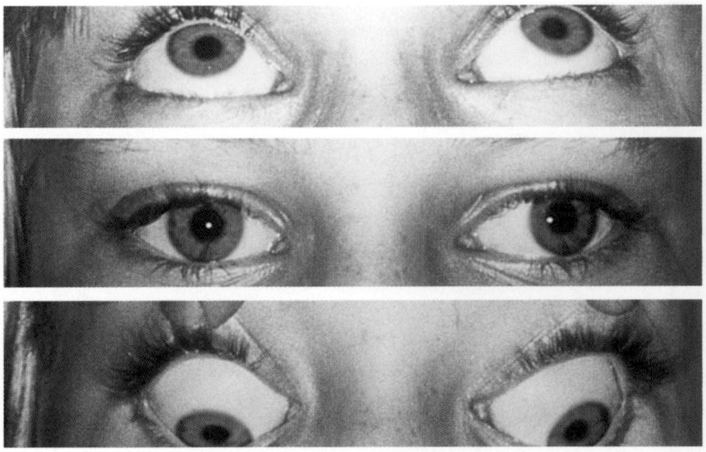

■ **Fig. 17.19** 'A' pattern exotropia; angle is greater in downgaze. (Courtesy of Wilmer Institute.)

SPECIAL SYNDROMES

Duane syndrome

The hallmark of Duane syndrome is retraction of the globe on attempted adduction, caused by co-contraction of the medial and lateral recti. The condition is often bilateral, although frequently involvement of one eye may be so subtle as to go unnoticed.

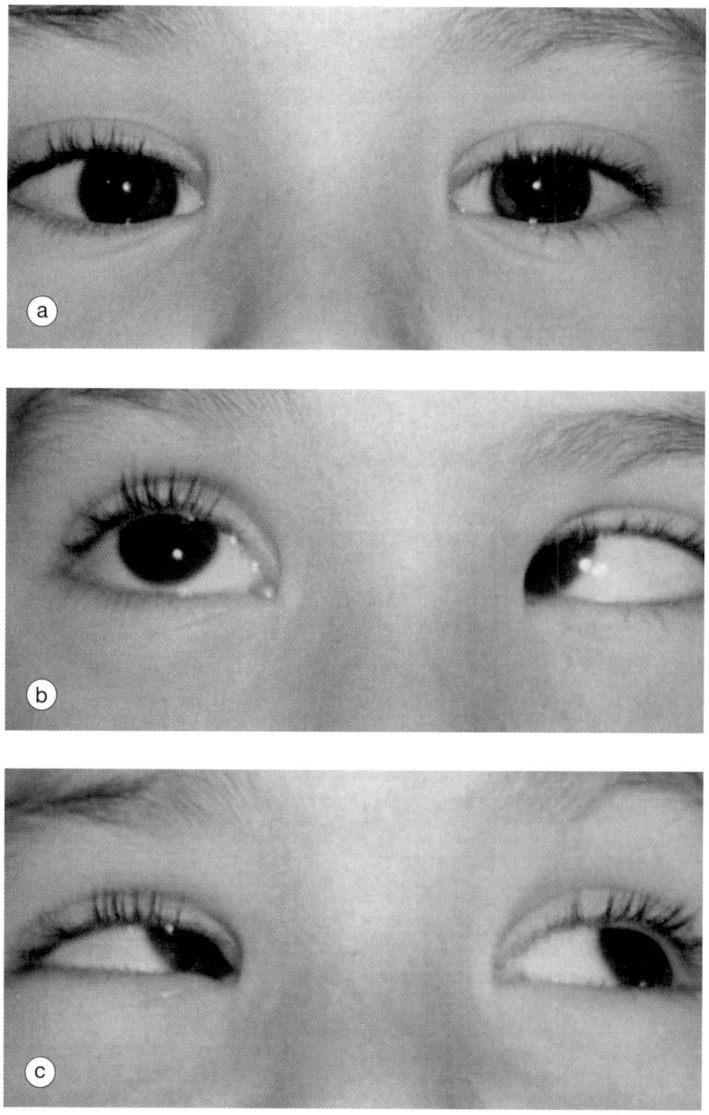

Fig. 17.20 Right Duane syndrome. **(a)** Slight right esotropia in the primary position. **(b)** Gross limitation of right abduction with slight widening of the right palpebral fissure. **(c)** Normal right adduction with narrowing of the right palpebral fissure.

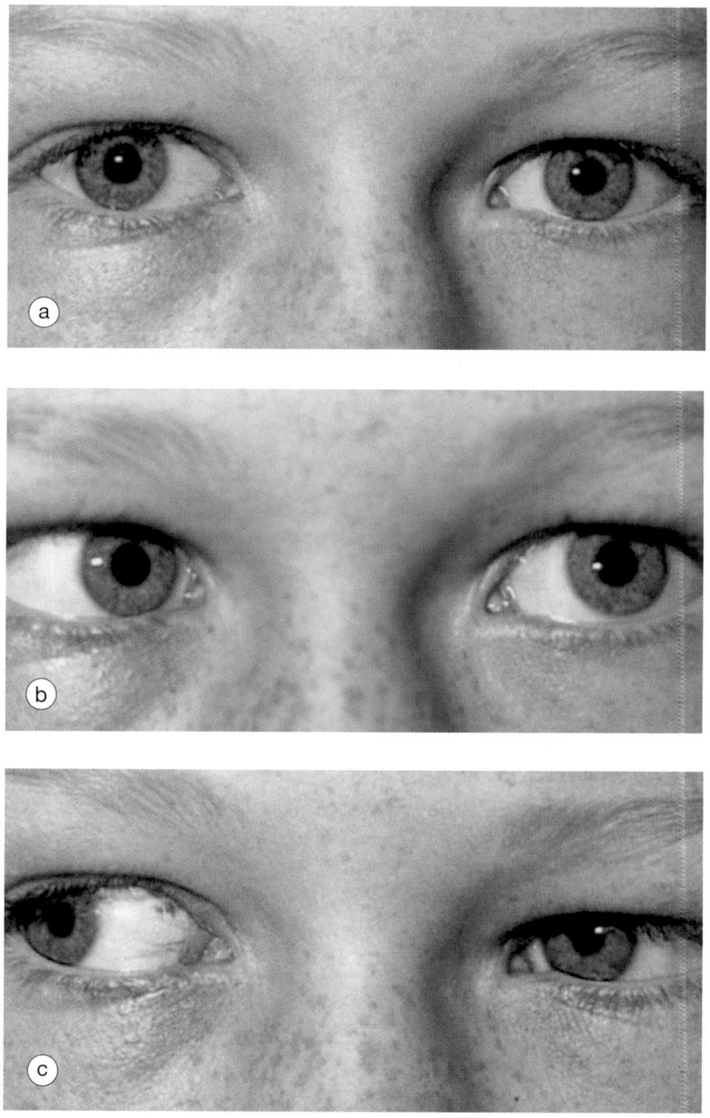

Fig. 17.21 Left Duane syndrome. **(a)** Straight in the primary position. **(b)** Severe limitation of left abduction. **(c)** Moderate limitation of left adduction with narrowing of the left palpebral fissure.

Monocular elevation defect

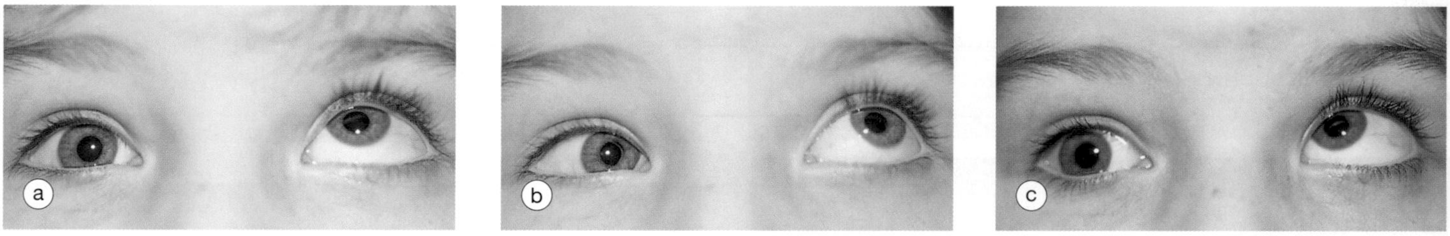

■ **Fig. 17.29** Defective elevation of the right eye in **(a)** upgaze; **(b)** gaze up and left; **(c)** gaze up and right.

Chronic progressive external ophthalmoplegia

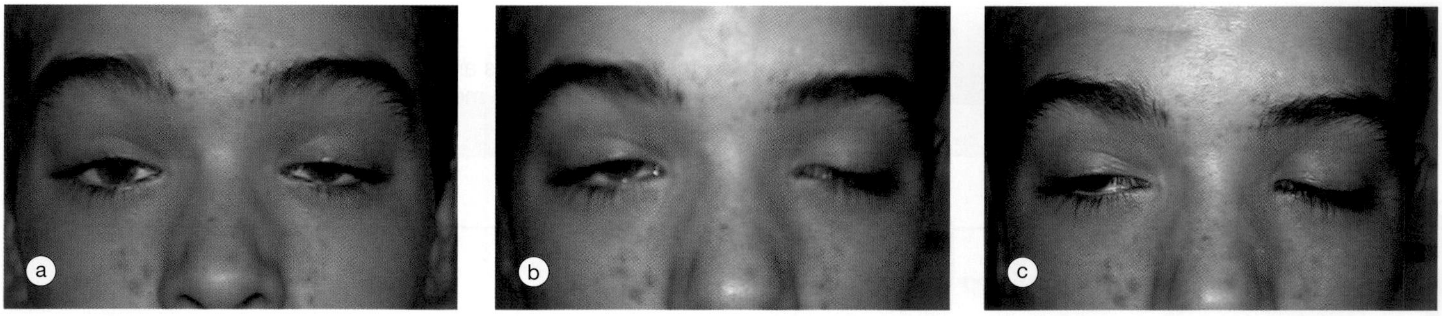

■ **Fig. 17.30** Ptosis and slowly progressive ocular immobility, which may occur in isolation or as part of oculopharyngeal dystrophy or Kearns–Sayre syndrome. **(a)** Primary position shows severe bilateral ptosis. **(b)** Gross limitation of left gaze. **(c)** Gross limitation of right gaze. (Courtesy of M. Parulekar.)

CHAPTER 18

TRAUMA

EYELID TRAUMA

Blunt trauma

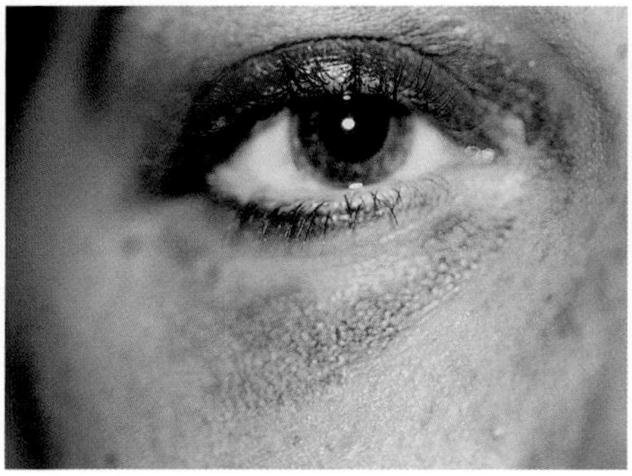

■ **Fig. 18.1** Mild periocular bruising.

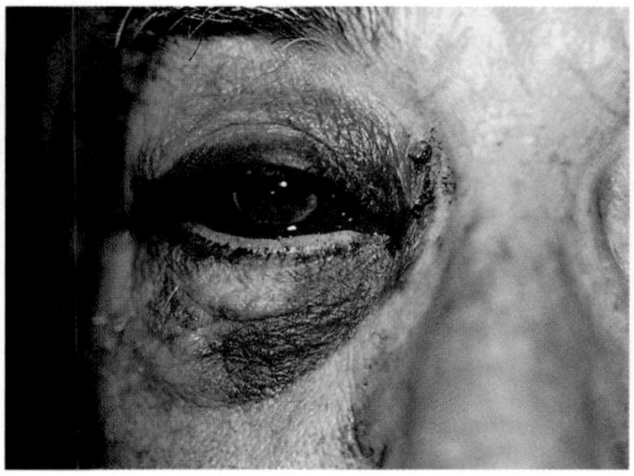

■ **Fig. 18.2** Periocular haematoma and subconjunctival haemorrhage.

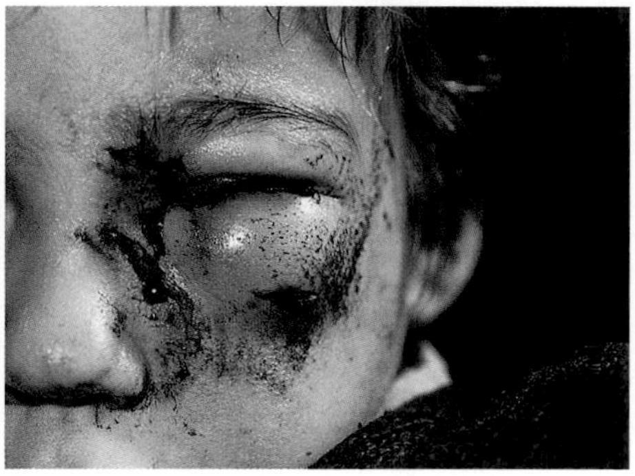

■ **Fig. 18.3** Very severe periocular haematoma and swelling, which may be associated with damage to the globe or orbit.

Laceration and avulsion

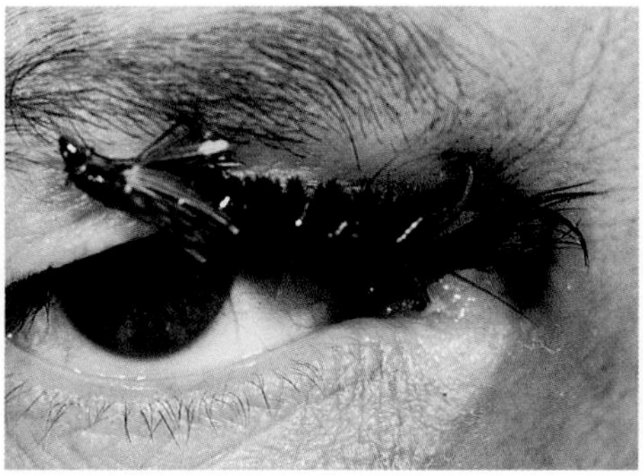

■ **Fig. 18.4** Fish hook injury.

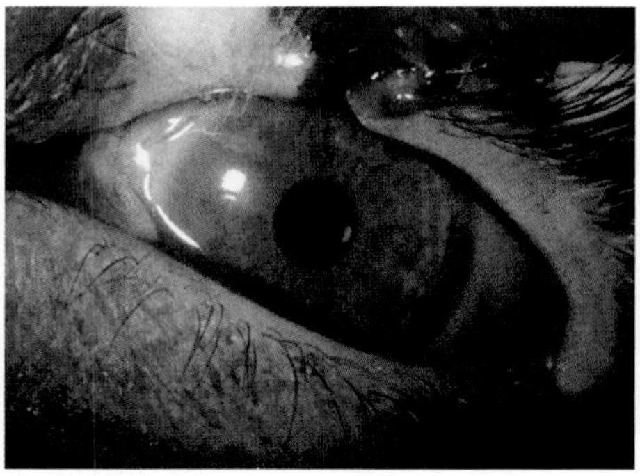

■ **Fig. 18.5** Laceration of the upper lid margin. (Courtesy of S Ford and R. Marsh.)

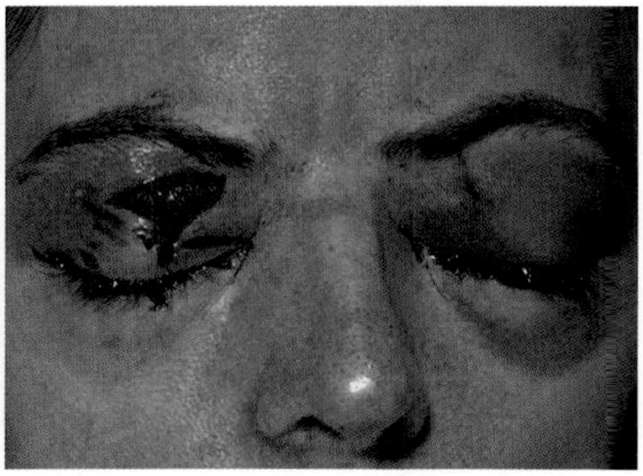

■ **Fig. 18.6** Two lacerations of the upper lid margin and tarsal plate. (Courtesy of S. Ford and R. Marsh.)

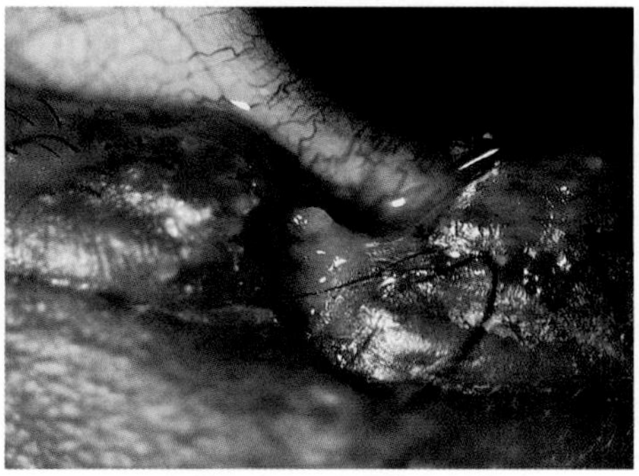

■ **Fig. 18.7** Laceration of the lower lid margin.

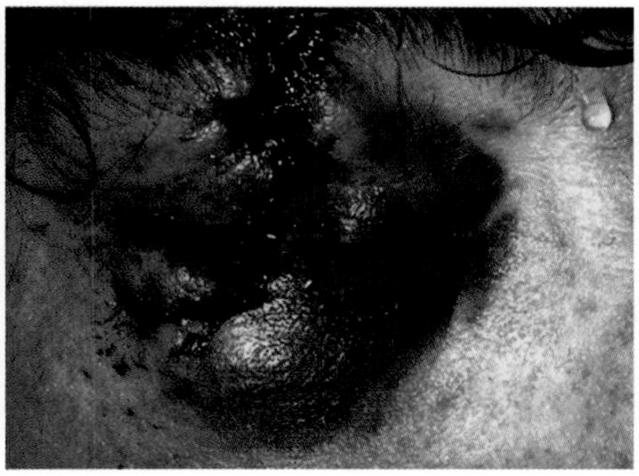

■ **Fig. 18.8** Laceration of upper and lower lids. (Courtesy of S. Ford and R. Marsh.)

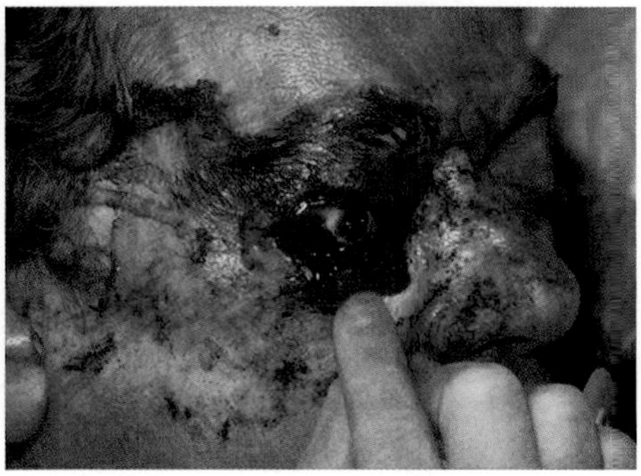

■ **Fig. 18.9** Avulsion of the lower lid. (Courtesy of S. Ford and R. Marsh.)

ORBITAL FRACTURES

Blowout orbital floor fracture

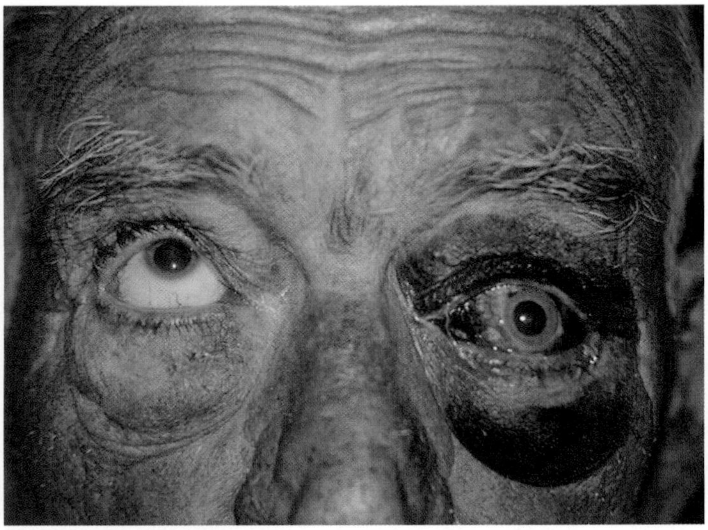

■ **Fig. 18.10** Restriction of upgaze due to entrapment within the fracture of the inferior rectus or inferior oblique muscle. (Courtesy of J. Yangüela.)

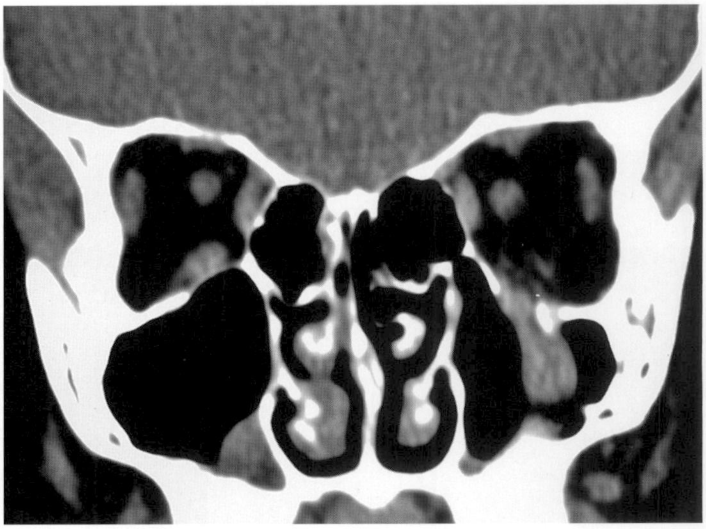

■ **Fig. 18.11** Coronal CT shows soft-tissue densities in the left maxillary antrum ('teardrop' sign), which may represent prolapsed orbital fat or extraocular muscles. (Courtesy of A. Pearson.)

Blowout fracture of the medial wall and floor

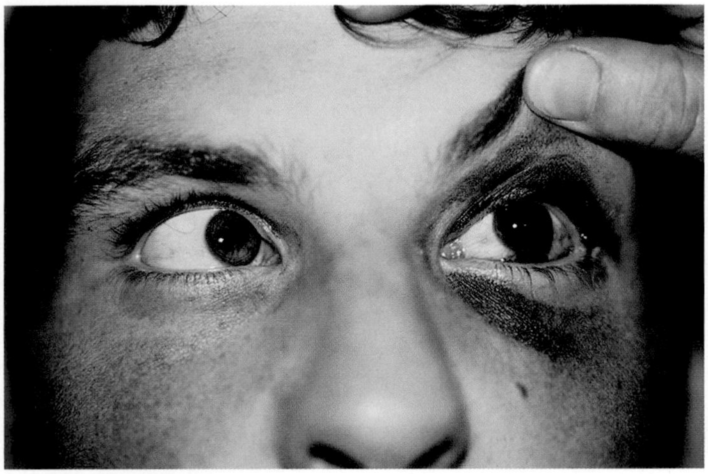

■ **Fig. 18.12** Restriction of abduction due to entrapment of the medial rectus. (Courtesy of A. Pearson.)

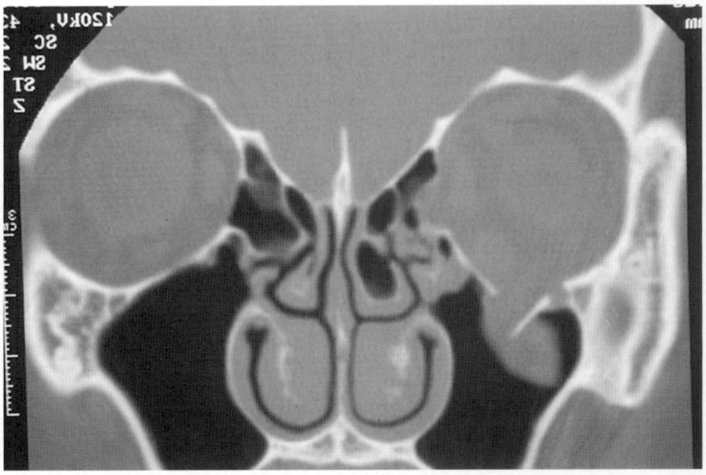

■ **Fig. 18.13** Coronal CT showing a fracture of the left medial wall and floor. (Courtesy of A. Pearson.)

Lateral wall fracture

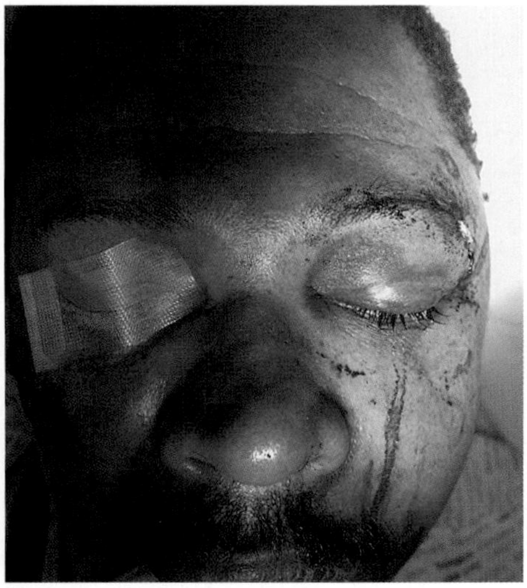

■ **Fig. 18.14** Lateral wall fractures are usually associated with severe facial damage. (Courtesy of A. Pearson.)

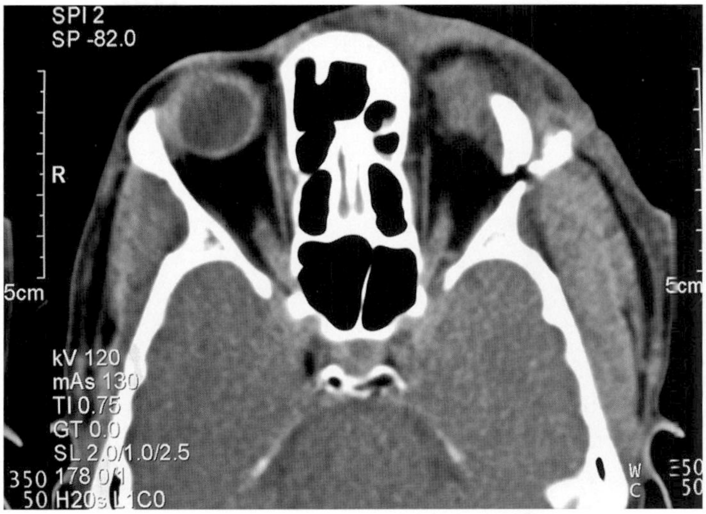

■ **Fig. 18.15** Axial CT showing a left lateral wall fracture. (Courtesy of A. Pearson.)

Roof fracture

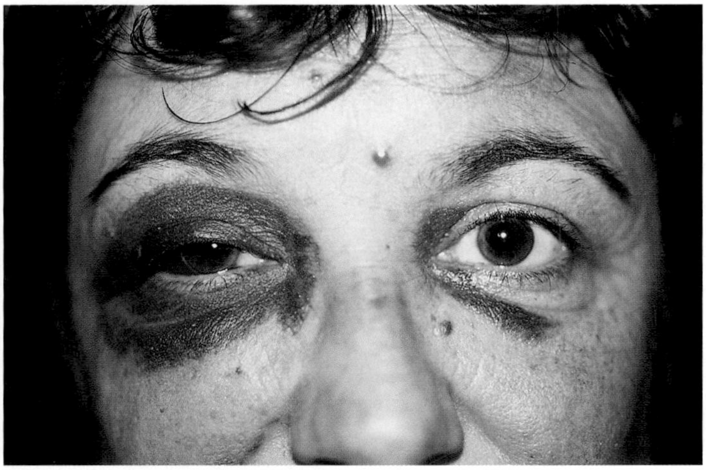

■ **Fig. 18.16** Periocular ecchymosis, which may spread to the uninvolved side.

BLUNT TRAUMA TO THE GLOBE

Anterior segment complications

Cornea

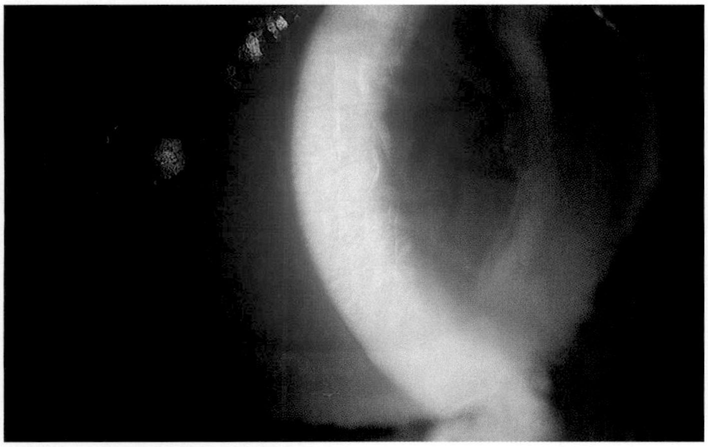

■ **Fig. 18.17** Corneal oedema associated with folds in Descemet membrane secondary to endothelial dysfunction.

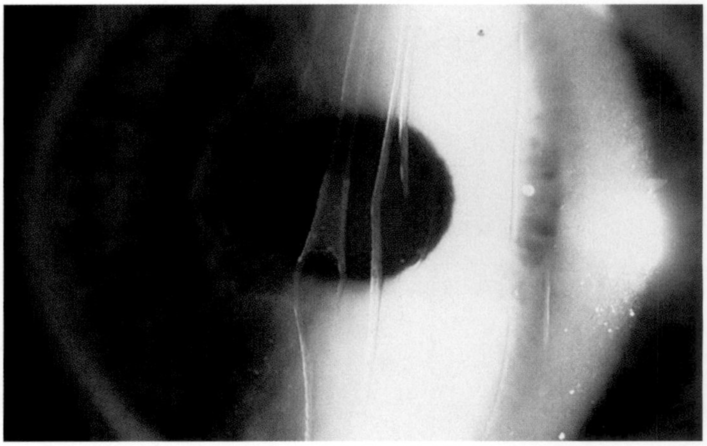

■ **Fig 18.18** Tears in Descemet membrane. (Courtesy of R. Curtis.)

Hyphaema

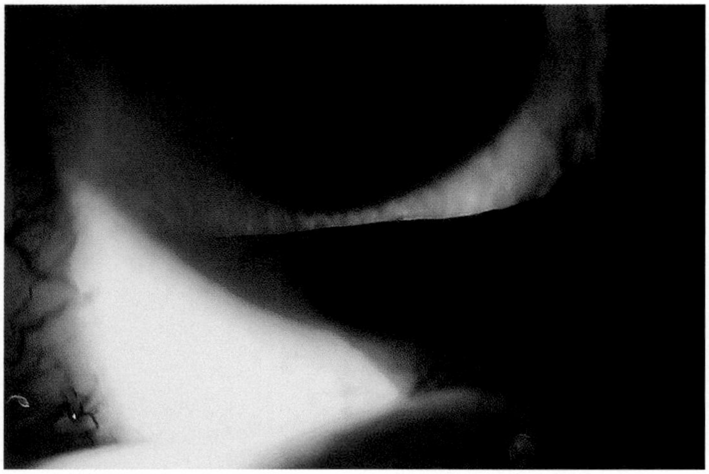

■ **Fig. 18.19** Hyphaema with a 'fluid level' resulting from sedimentation of red blood cells.

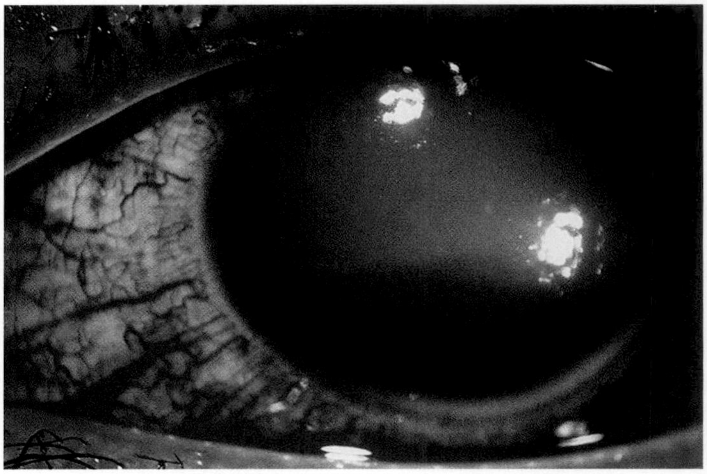

■ **Fig. 18.20** Total hyphaema.

Iris

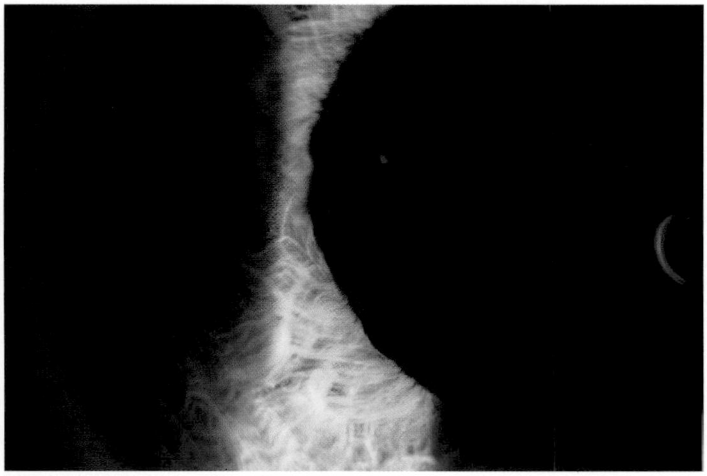

■ **Fig. 18.21** Mydriasis due to damage of the iris sphincter. It may be permanent and associated with sluggish pupillary reactions.

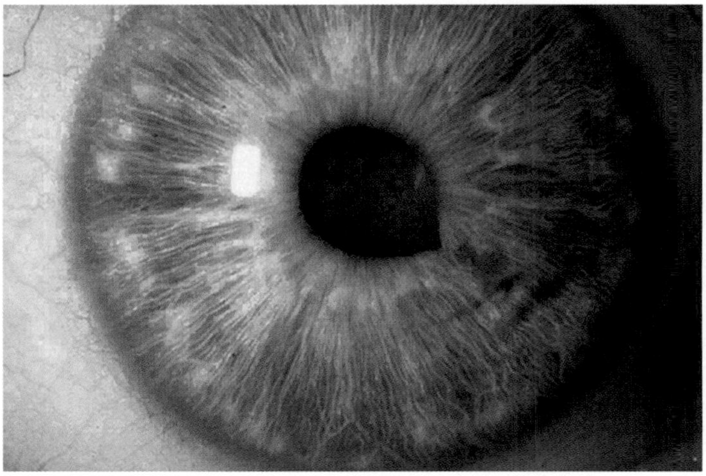

■ **Fig. 18.22** Radial tear in the pupillary margin. (Courtesy of S. Ford and R. Marsh.)

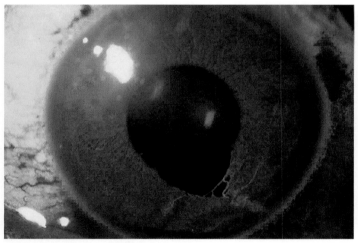

■ **Fig. 18.23** Large radial iris tear. (Courtesy of S. Ford and R. Marsh.)

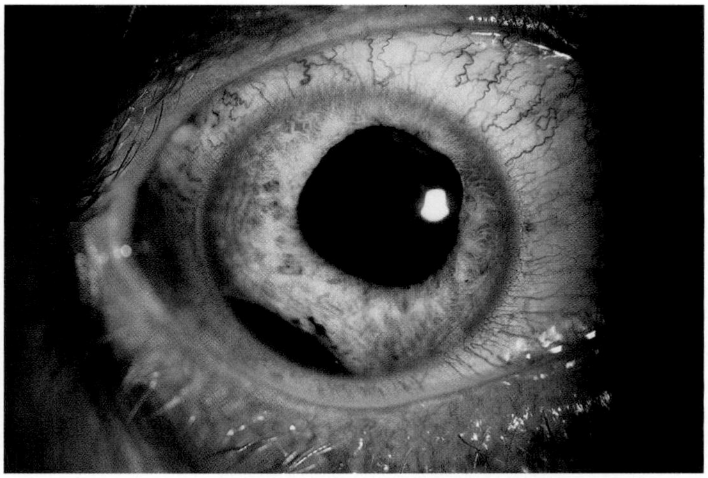

■ **Fig. 18.24** Iridodialysis is a dehiscence of the iris from the ciliary body at its root. The pupil is typically D-shaped and the dialysis is seen as a dark biconvex area near the limbus.

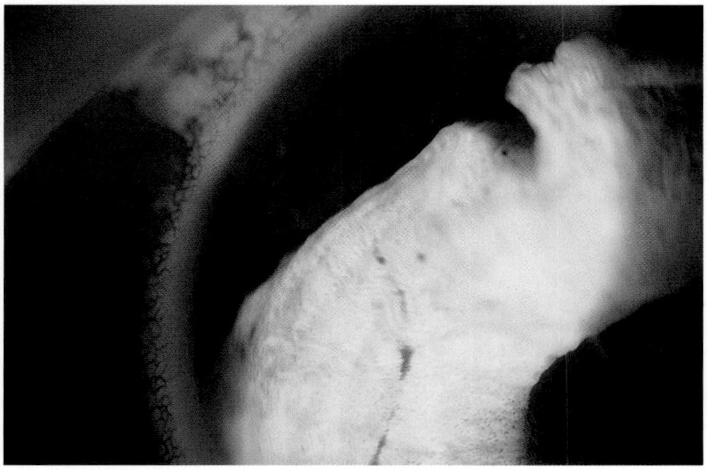

■ **Fig. 18.25** Large iridodialysis.

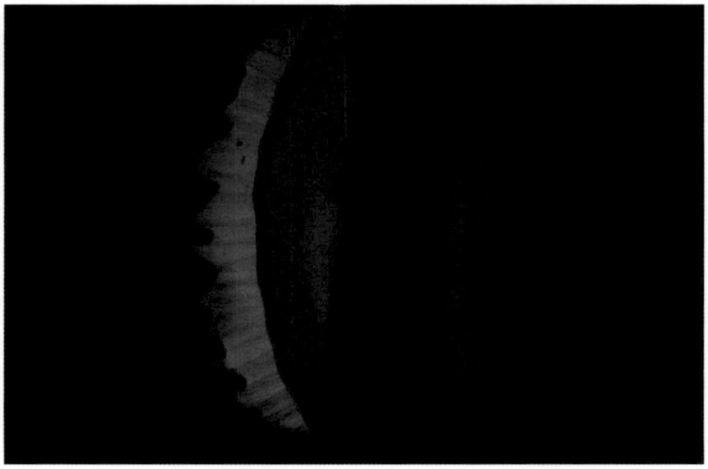

■ **Fig. 18.26** Very large iridodialysis seen on retroillumination. (Courtesy of P. Gili.)

Angle recession

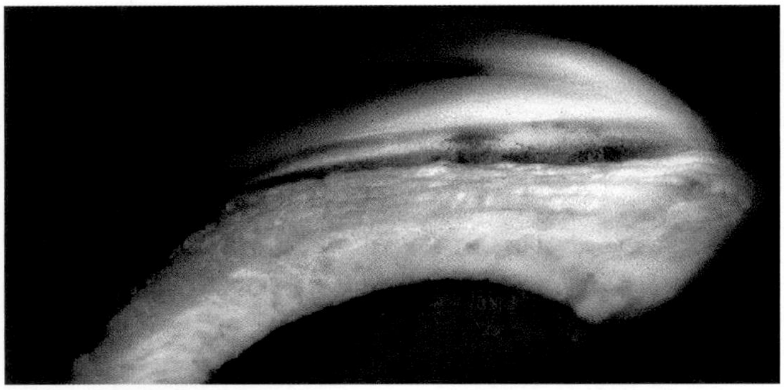

■ **Fig. 18.27** A tear extending into the face of the ciliary body with widening of the ciliary body band. (Courtesy of R. Curtis.)

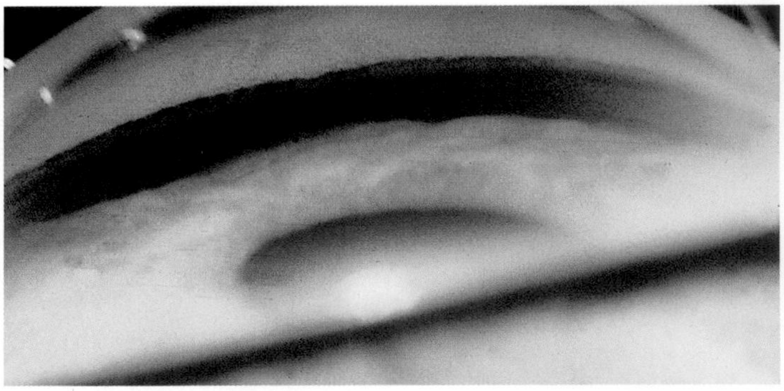

■ **Fig. 18.28** Very extensive angle recession.

Lens

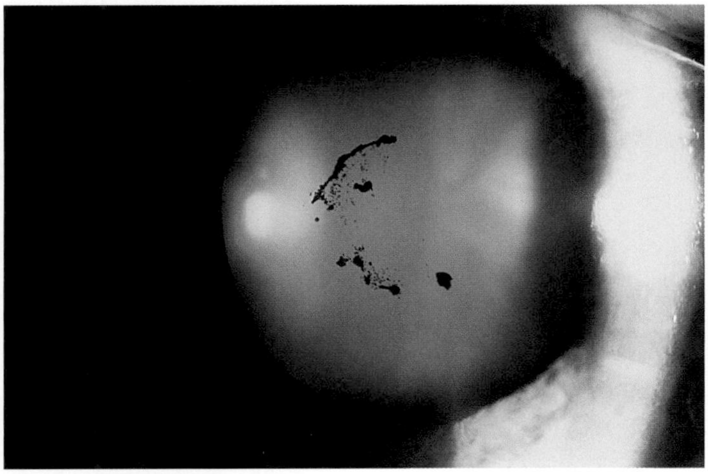

■ **Fig. 18.29** Ring-shaped 'imprinting' of iris pigment on the anterior lens capsule (Vossius ring).

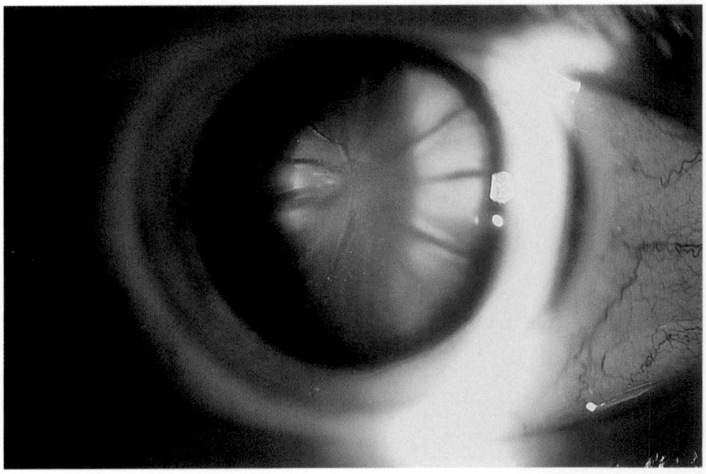

■ **Fig. 18.30** Opacification along the posterior sutures.

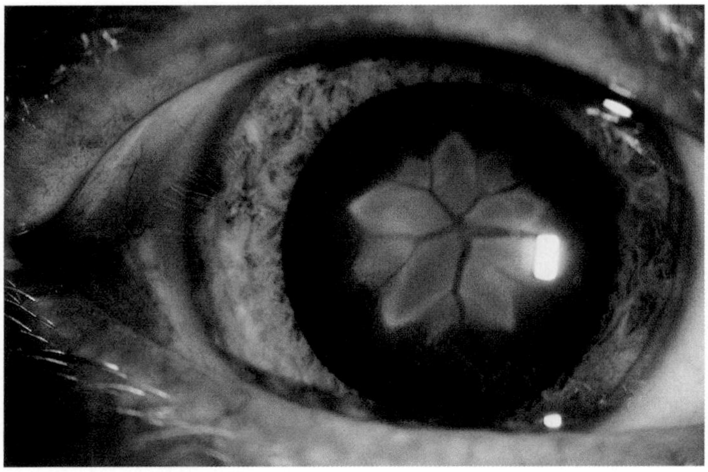

■ **Fig. 18.31** Flower-shaped cataract. (Courtesy of A. Shun-Shin.)

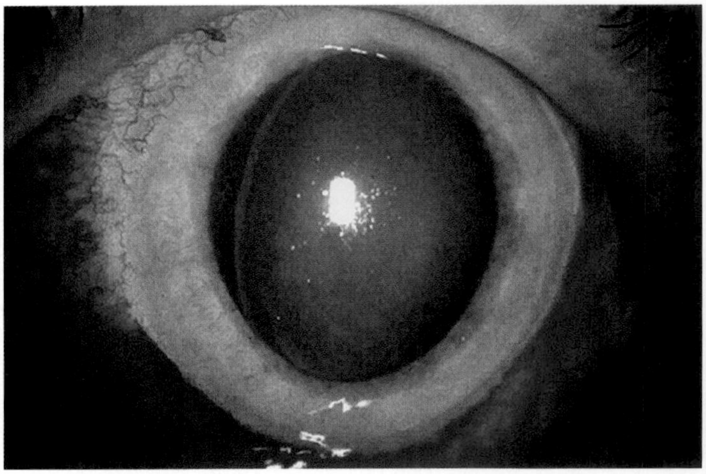

■ **Fig. 18.32** Lens subluxation and tilting. (Courtesy of S. Ford and R. Marsh.)

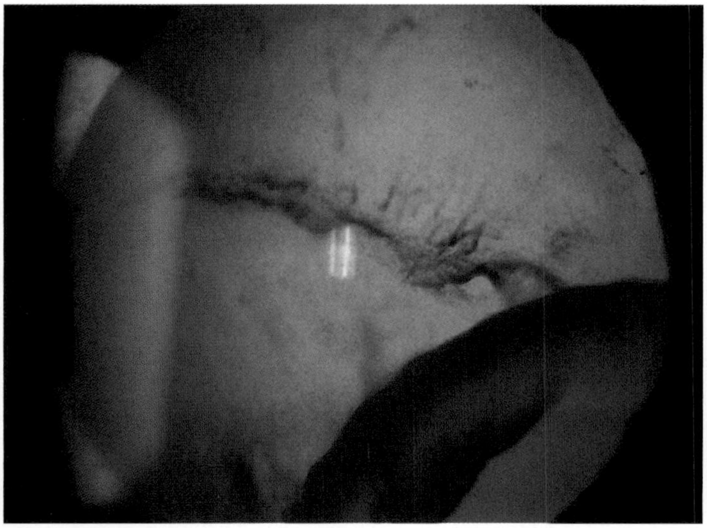

■ **Fig. 18.33** Inferior subluxation. (Courtesy of C. Barry.)

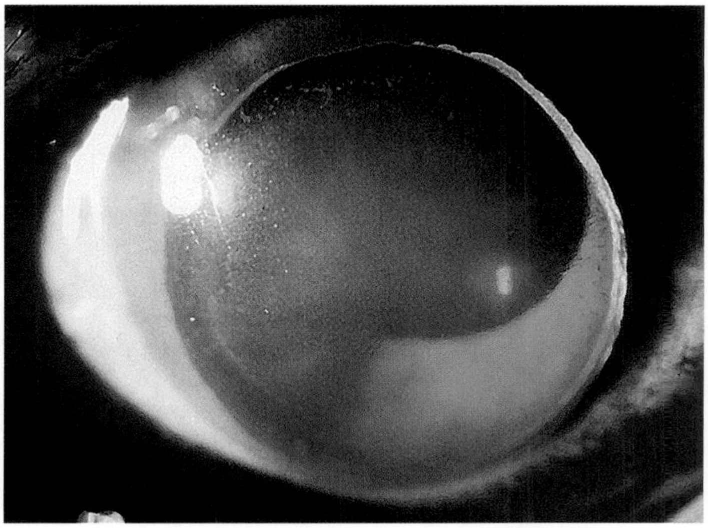

■ **Fig. 18.34** Dislocation into the anterior chamber is rare.

Globe rupture

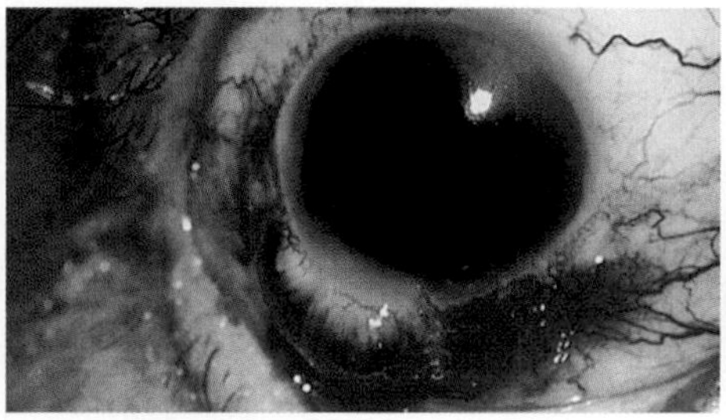

■ **Fig. 18.35** Total hyphaema and iris prolapse.

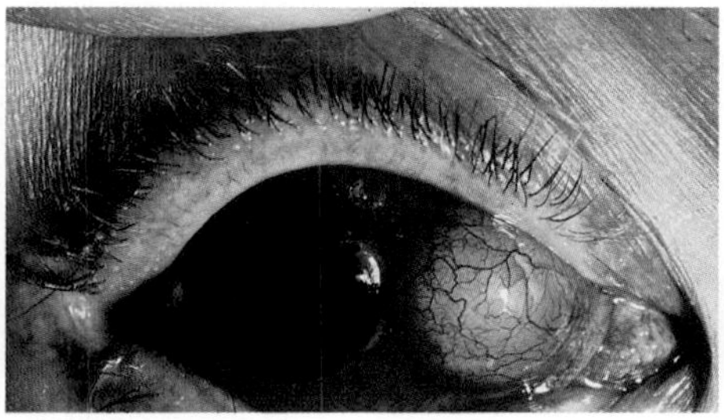

■ **Fig. 18.36** Total hyphaema and subconjunctival dislocation of the lens.

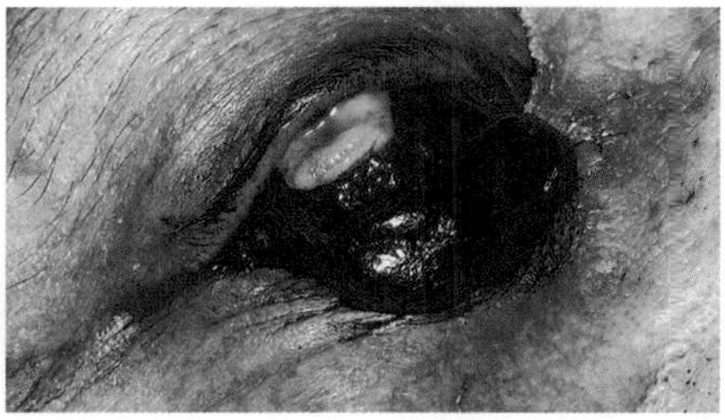

■ **Fig. 18.37** Very severe injury resulting in extrusion of all intraocular contents.

Posterior segment complications

Commotio retinae

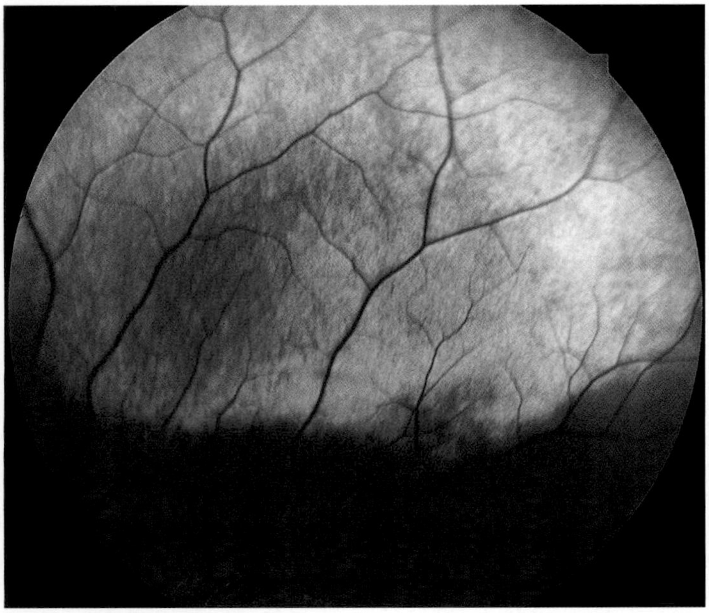

■ **Fig. 18.38** Opaque grey appearance to the involved retina resulting from cloudy swelling.

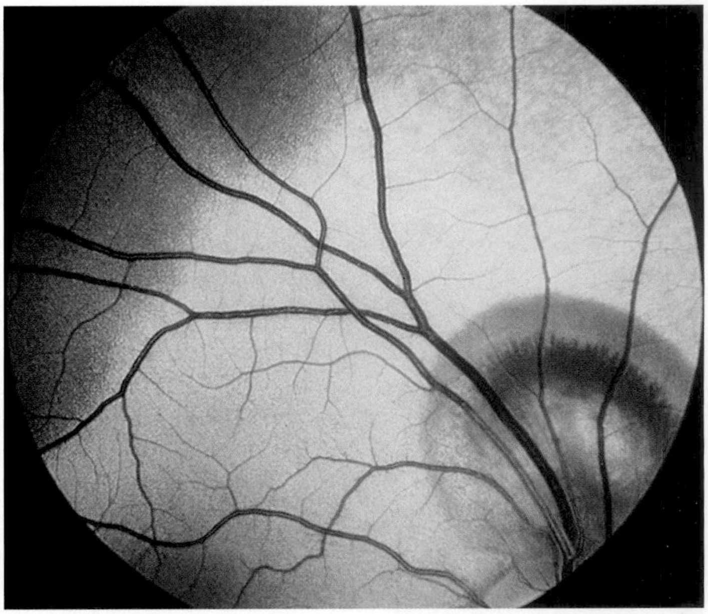

■ **Fig. 18.39** Commotio retinal and subretinal haemorrhage. (Courtesy of P. Morse.)

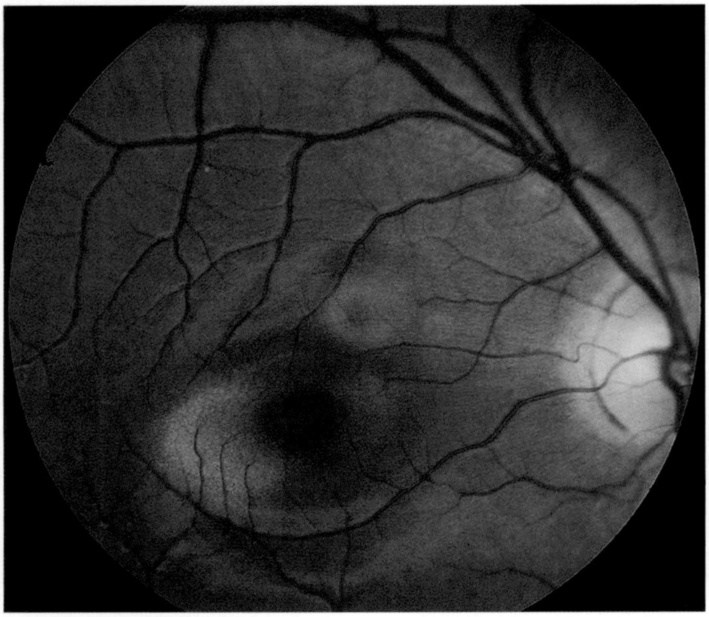

■ **Fig. 18.40** Mild commotio retinae at the macula.

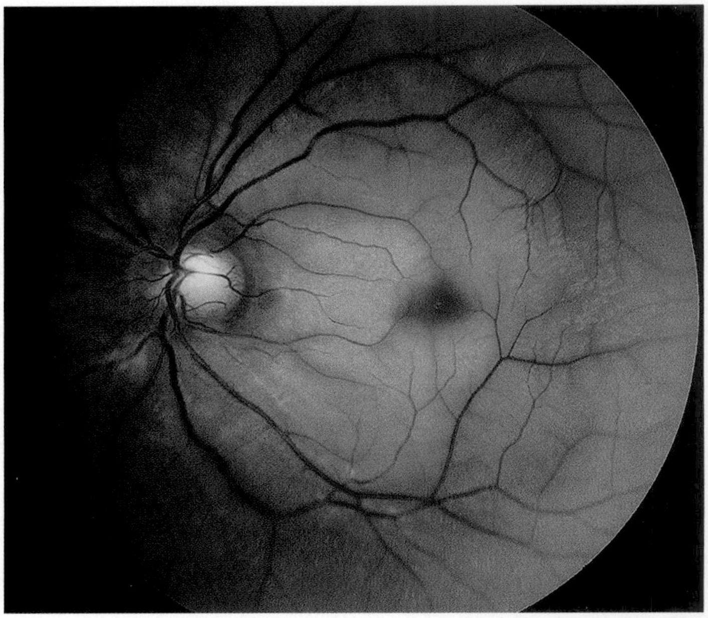

■ **Fig. 18.41** Severe commotio retinae involving the posterior pole with a 'cherry-red spot' at the fovea.

Macular hole

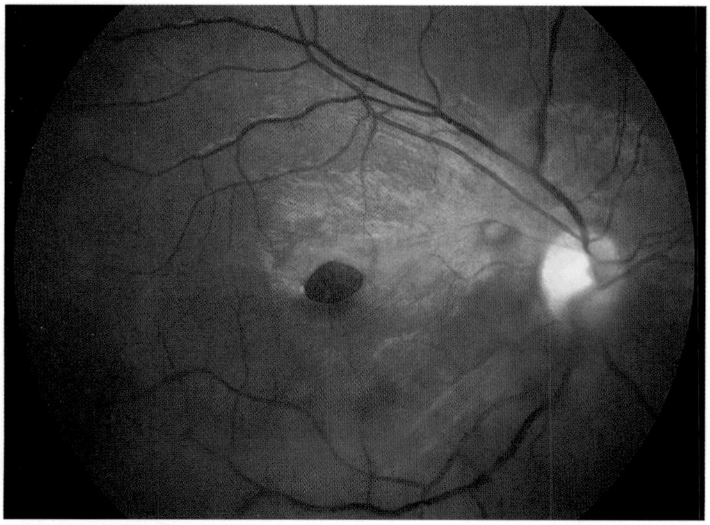

■ **Fig. 18.42** Macular hole and resolving commotio retinae. (Courtesy of C. Barry.)

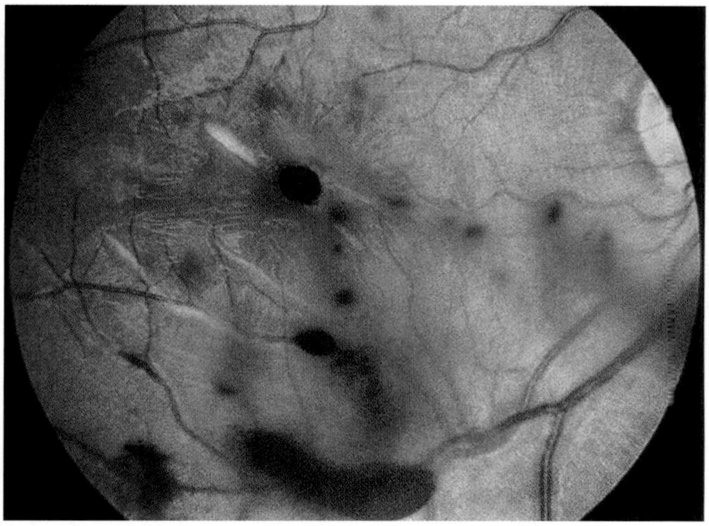

■ **Fig. 18.43** Macular hole and preretinal and vitreous haemorrhage.

Choroidal rupture

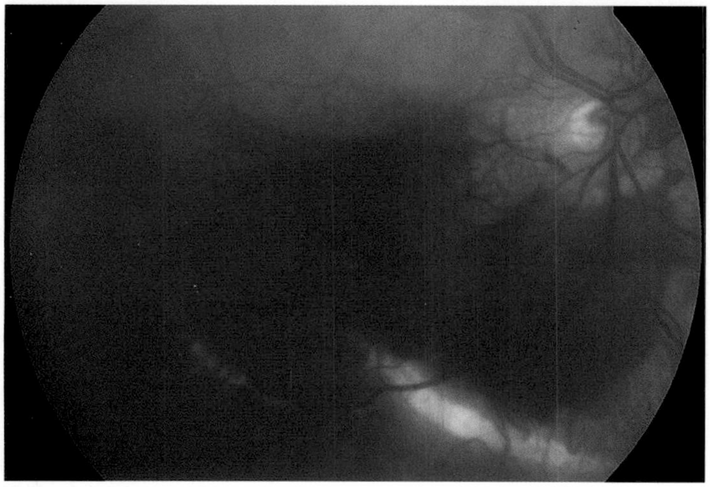

■ **Fig. 18.44** Two pale crescent-shaped lesion concentric with the optic disc associated with subretinal haemorrhage.

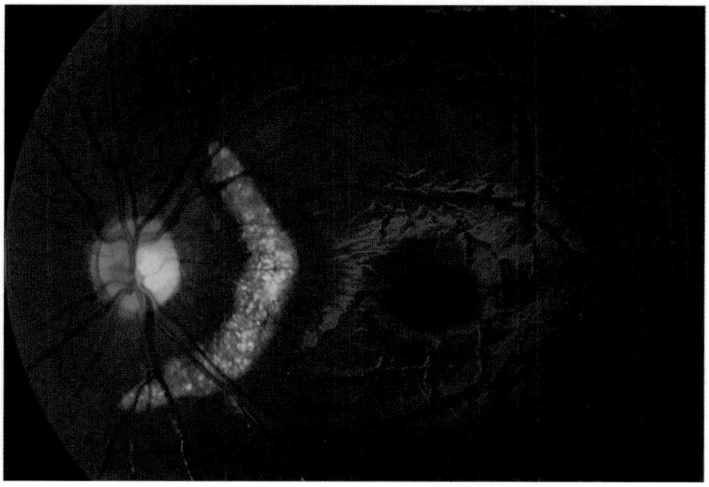

■ **Fig. 18.45** Old choroidal rupture characterised by a white, crescentic streak of exposed sclera.

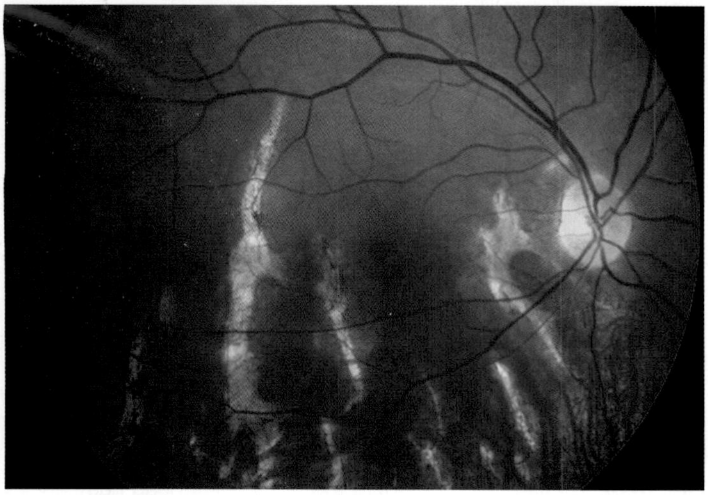

■ **Fig. 18.46** Multiple old choroidal tears. (Courtesy of C. Barry.)

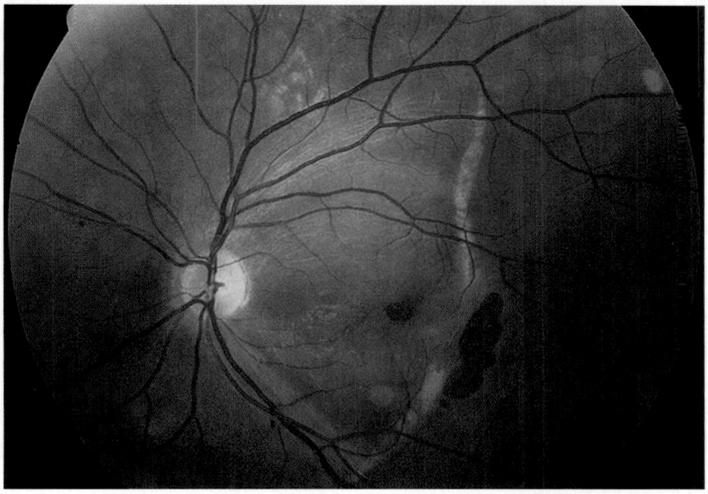

■ **Fig. 18.47** Old choroidal rupture associated with a macular hole and a larger hole at the edge of the tear. (Courtesy of B. Fleming.

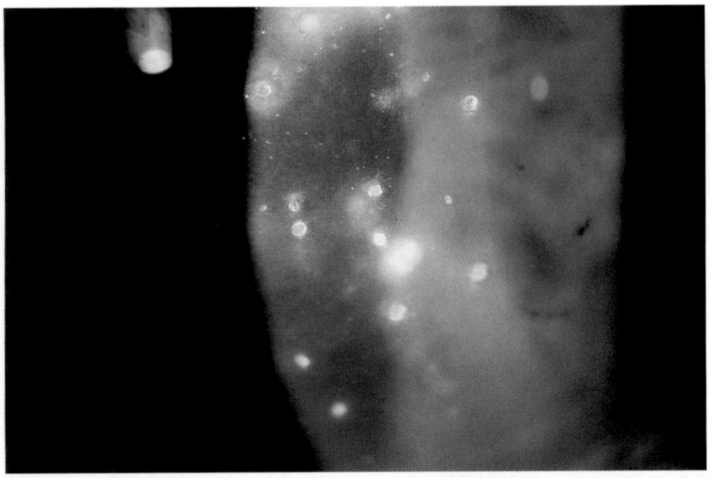

Fig. 18.59 Multiple corneal foreign bodies sustained during a grenade explosion.

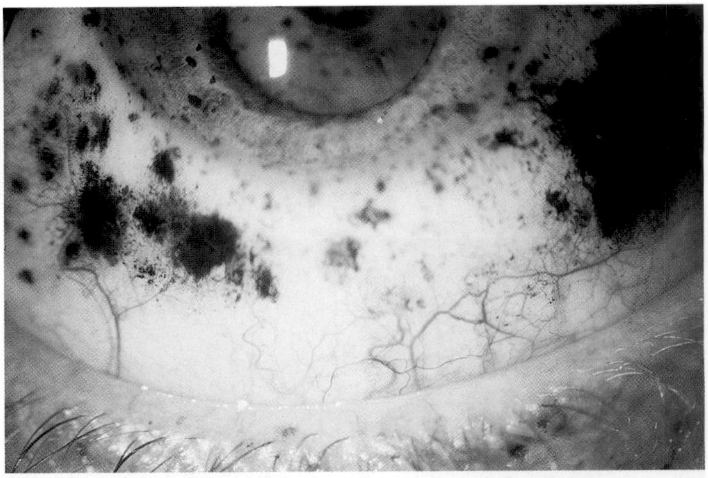

Fig. 18.60 Extensive conjunctival and corneal foreign bodies sustained during a tyre explosion.

Intraocular

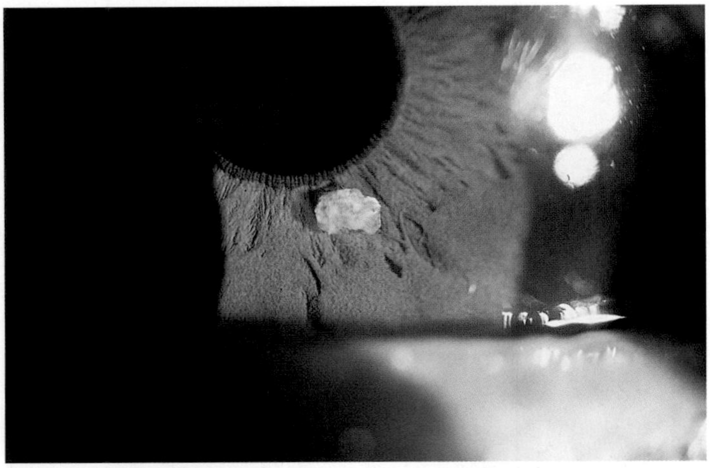

Fig. 18.61 Long-standing non-metallic foreign body in the anterior chamber.

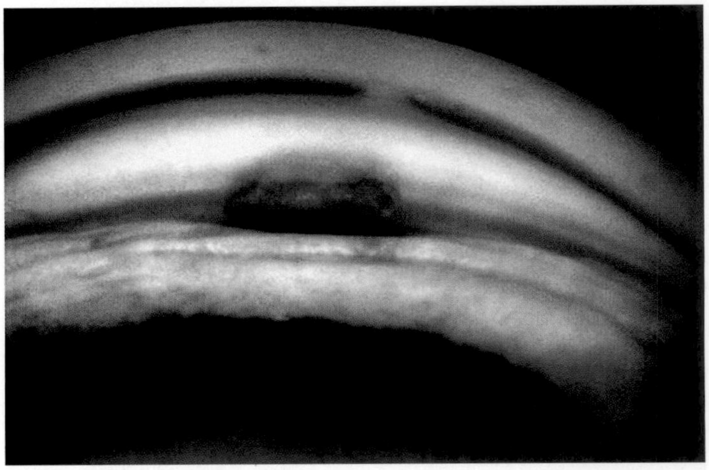

Fig. 18.62 Foreign body in the angle. (Courtesy of R. Curtis.)

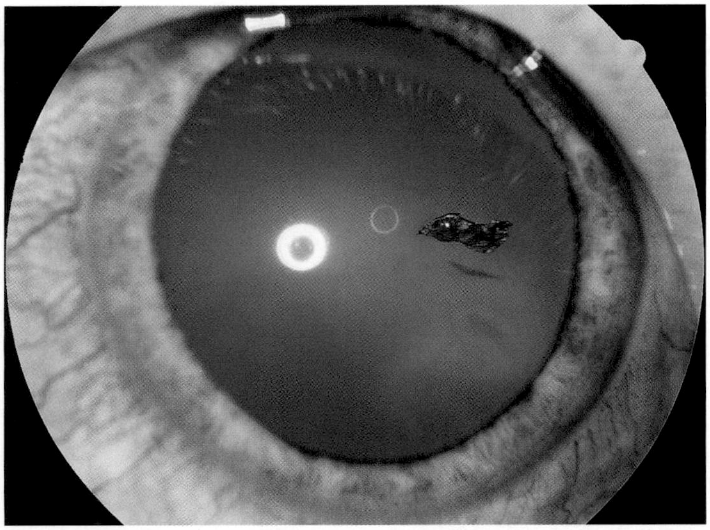

Fig. 18.63 Metallic intralenticular foreign body.

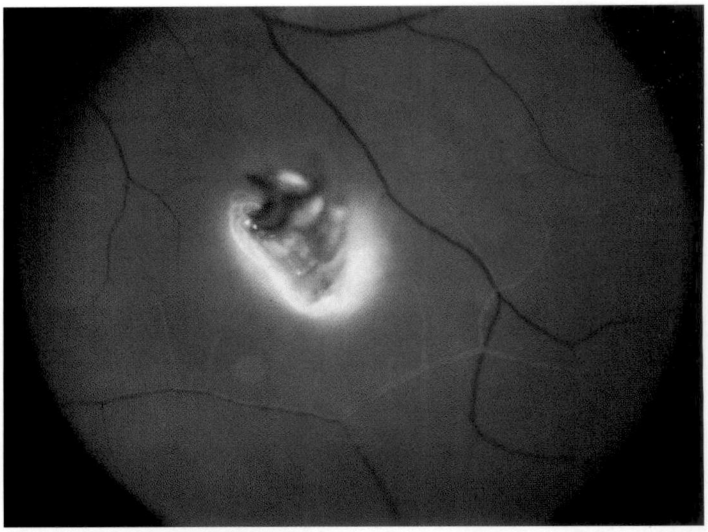

Fig. 18.64 Foreign body on the retina. (Courtesy of Wilmer Institute.)

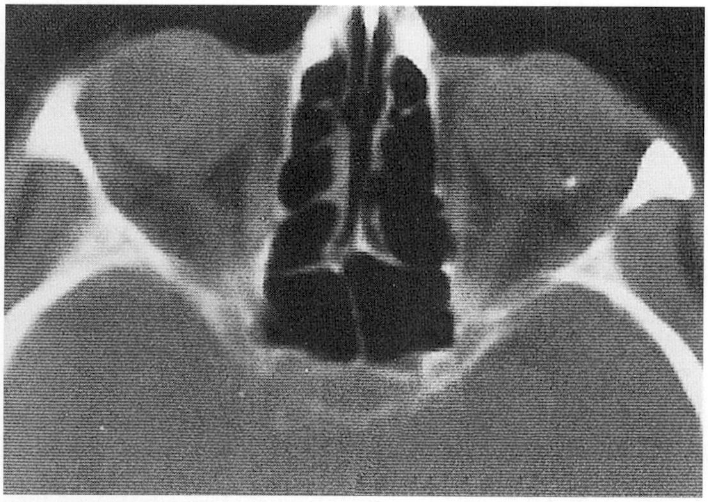

■ **Fig. 18.65** Axial CT scan showing a left intraocular foreign body. (Courtesy of Wilmer Institute.)

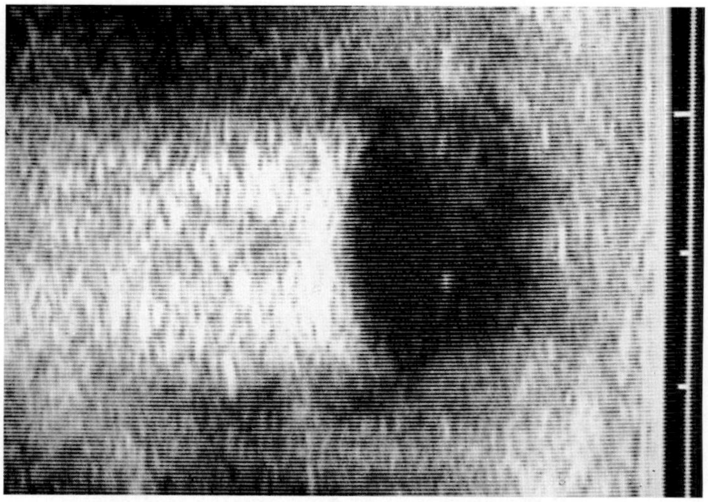

■ **Fig. 18.66** Ultrasound showing an intraocular foreign body.

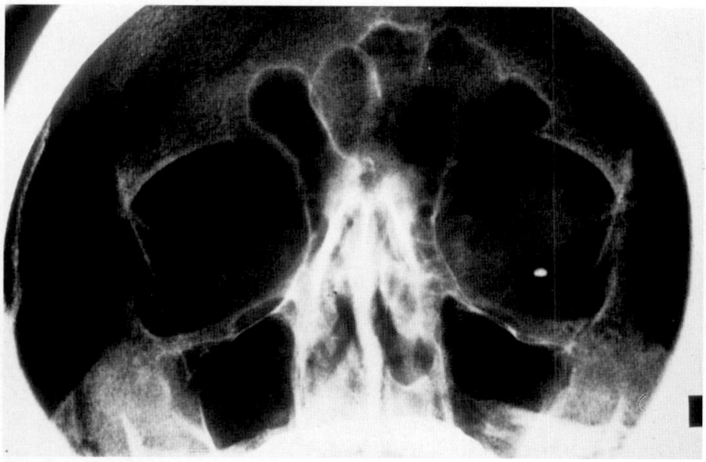

■ **Fig. 18.67** Plain radiograph showing a left intraocular foreign body.

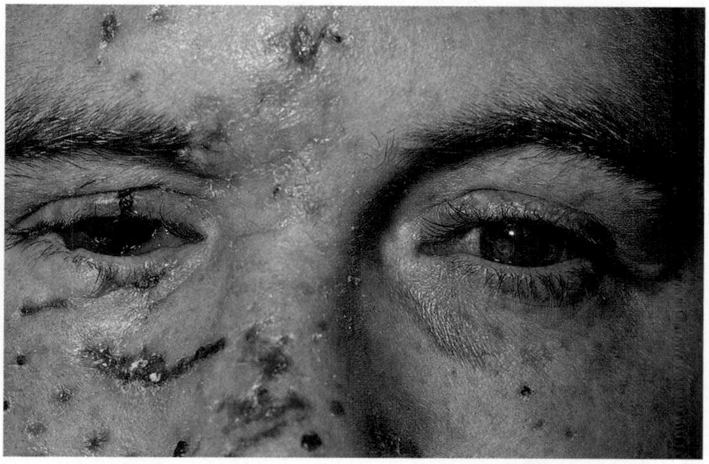

■ **Fig. 18.68** Multiple facial and intraocular foreign bodies due to a shotgun explosion.

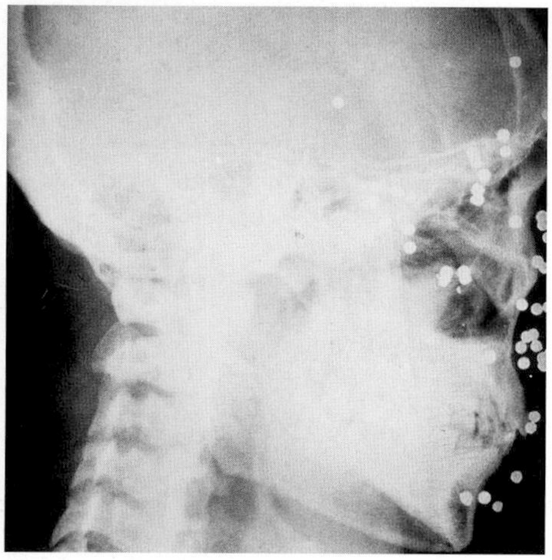

■ **Fig. 18.69** Plain radiograph showing multiple pellets.

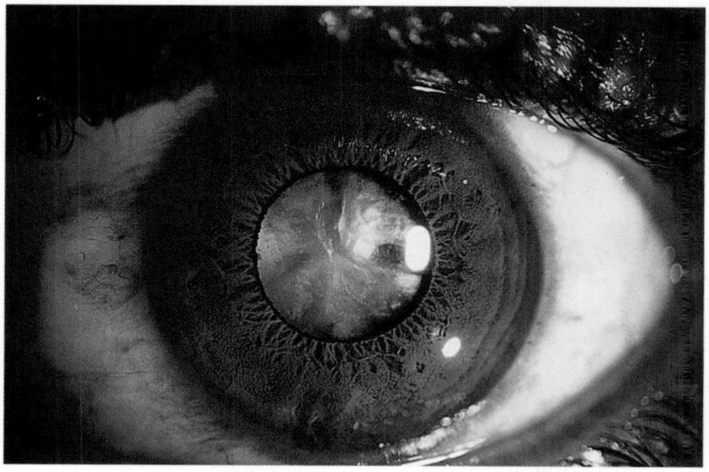

■ **Fig. 18.70** Cataract and reddish brown staining of the iris due to a retained ferrous foreign body (siderosis oculi). (Courtesy of J. Salmon.)

BURNS

Acute signs

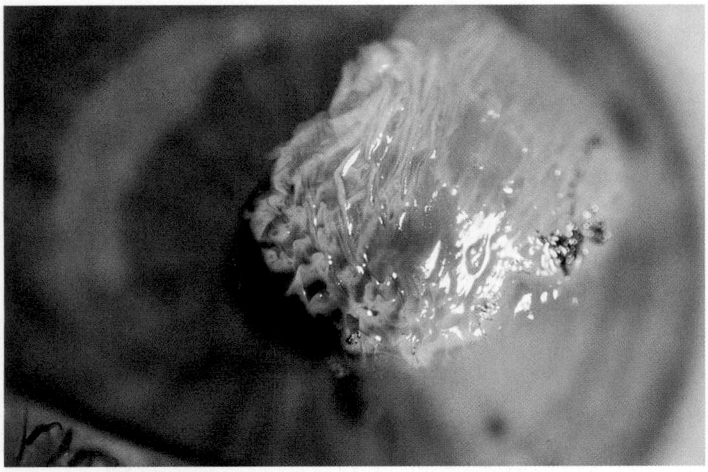

■ **Fig. 18.71** Thermal burn to the cornea.

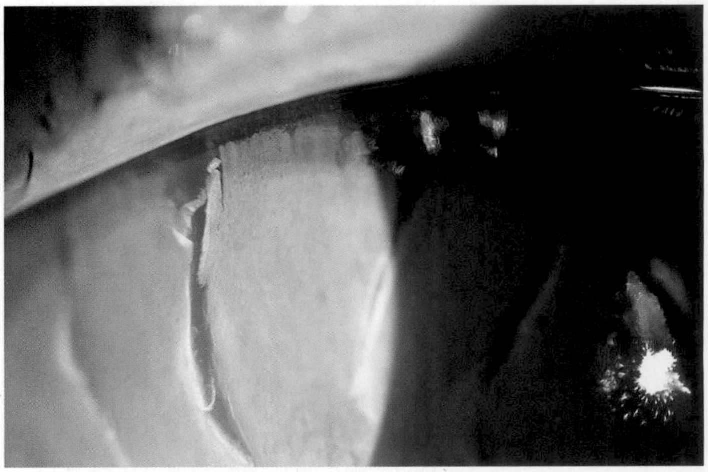

■ **Fig. 18.72** Severe thermal burn to the cornea.

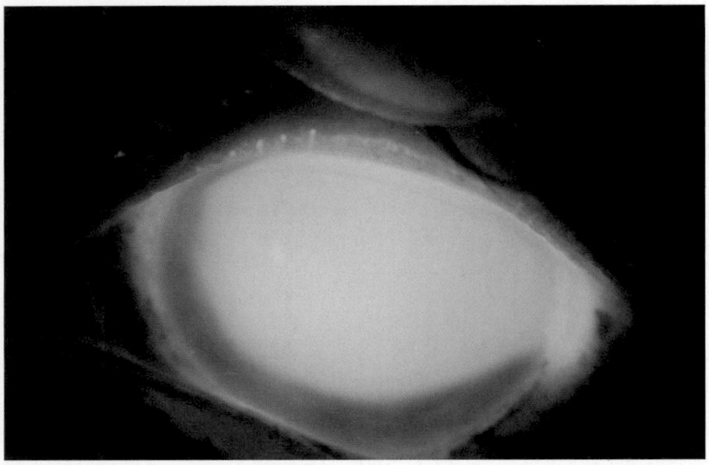

■ **Fig. 18.73** Chemical burn resulting in total epithelial loss. (Courtesy of S. Ford and R. Marsh.)

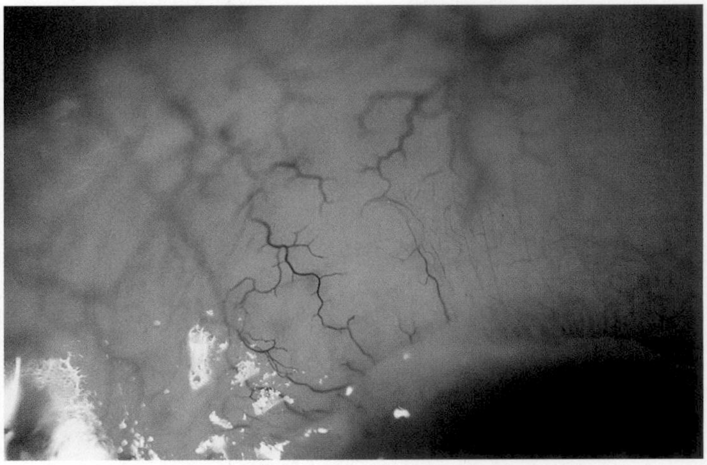

■ **Fig. 18.74** Chemical burn resulting in limbal ischaemia characterised by loss of patency of deep and superficial vessels at the limbus.

Grading of severity

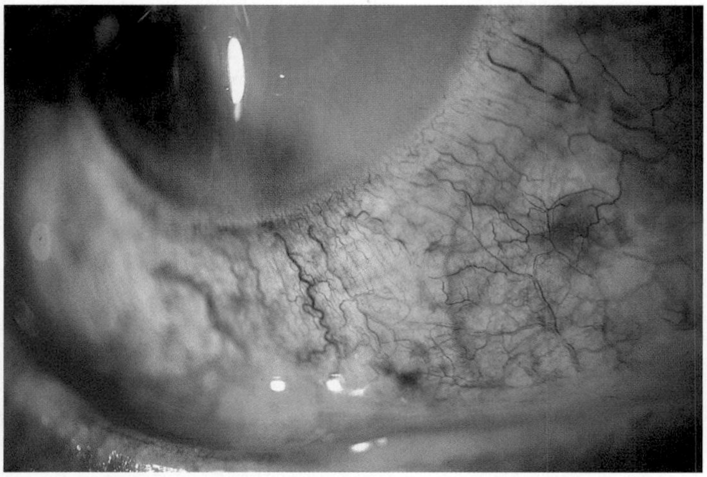

Fig. 18.75 Clear cornea and no limbal ischaemia (grade 1 – excellent prognosis).

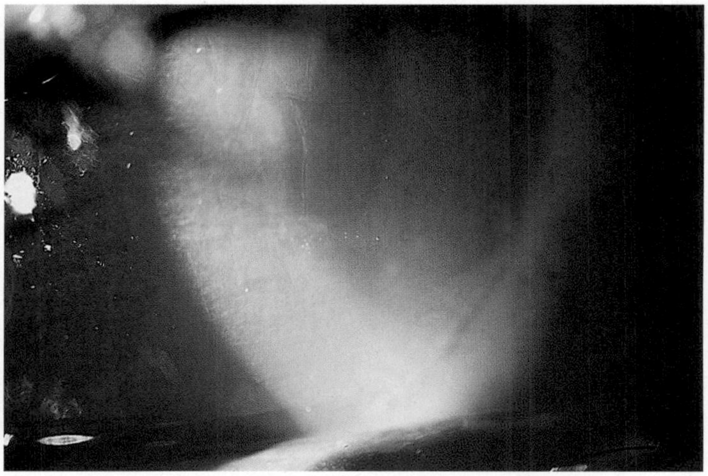

Fig. 18.76 Hazy cornea but with visible iris details and less than one-third of limbal ischaemia (grade 2 – good prognosis).

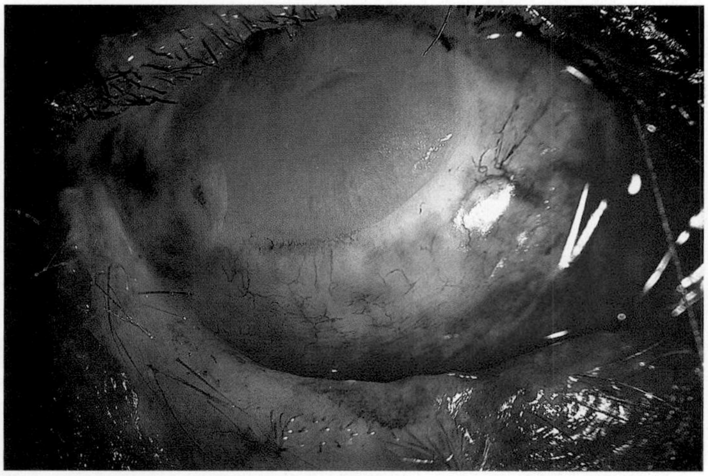

Fig. 18.77 Total loss of corneal epithelium, stromal haze obscuring iris details and one-third to a half of limbal ischaemia (grade 3 – guarded prognosis).

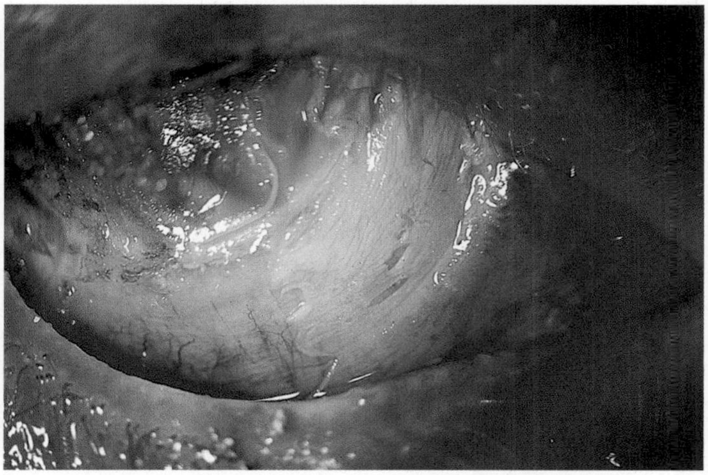

Fig. 18.78 Opaque cornea and more than half of limbal ischaemia (grade 4 – poor prognosis).

Late signs

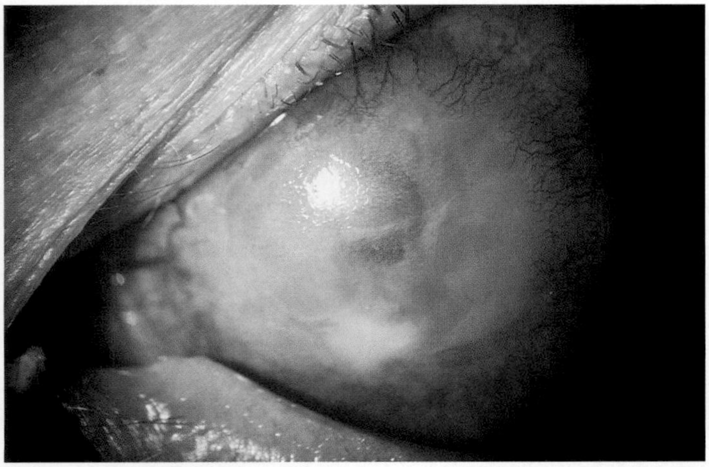

Fig. 18.79 Persistent epithelial loss, opacification and peripheral vascularisation. (Courtesy of S. Ford and R. Marsh.)

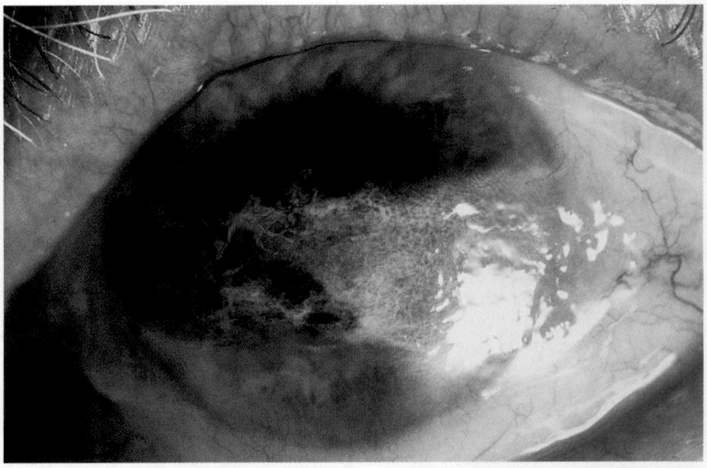

Fig. 18.80 Corneal opacification following exposure to mustard gas. (Courtesy of C. Barry.)

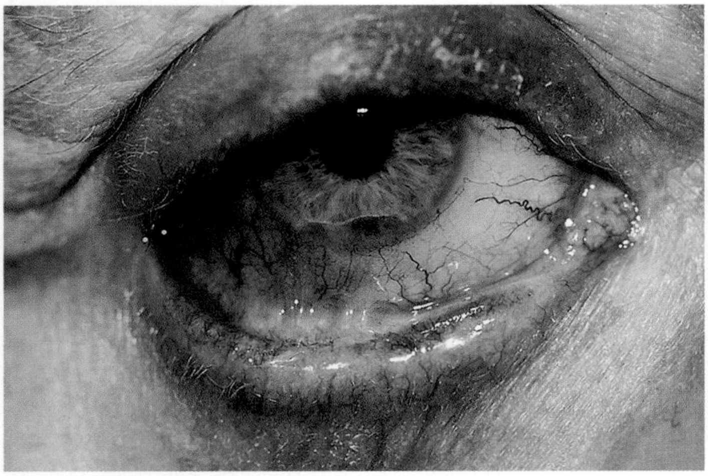

Fig. 18.81 Obliteration of the inferior fornix.

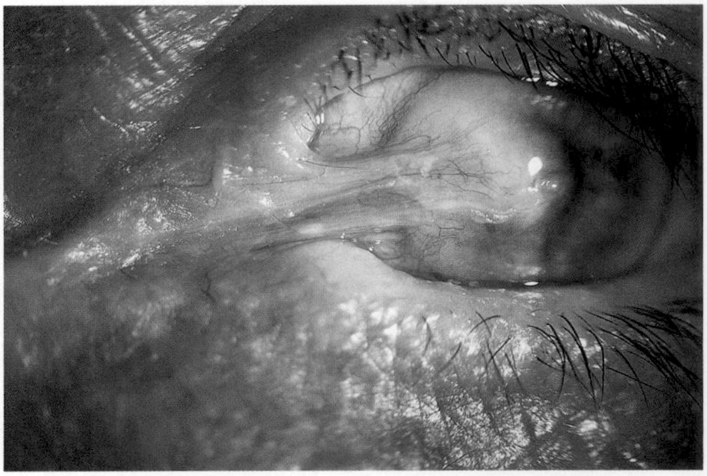

Fig. 18.82 Conjunctival adhesion to the cornea forming a pseudopterygium.

MISCELLANEOUS INJURIES

Non-accidental injury (shaken baby syndrome)

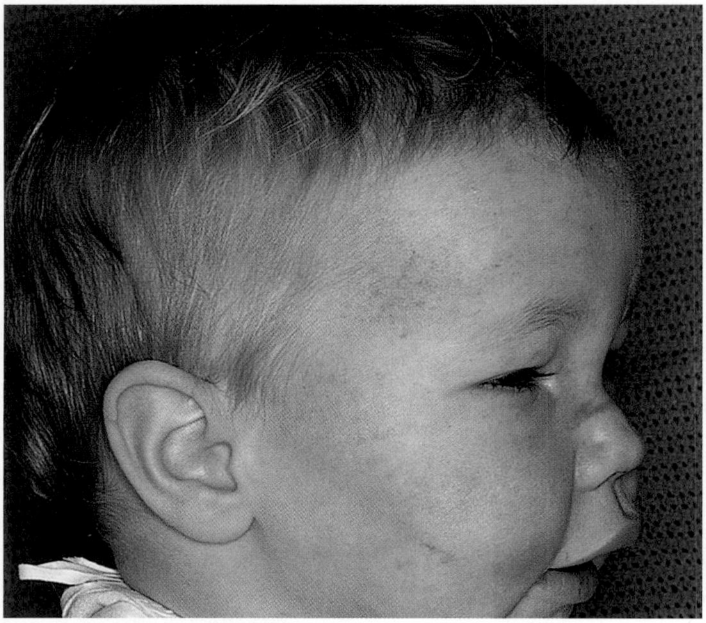

■ **Fig. 18.83** Facial and periocular bruising, which may be associated with neurological and skeletal damage.

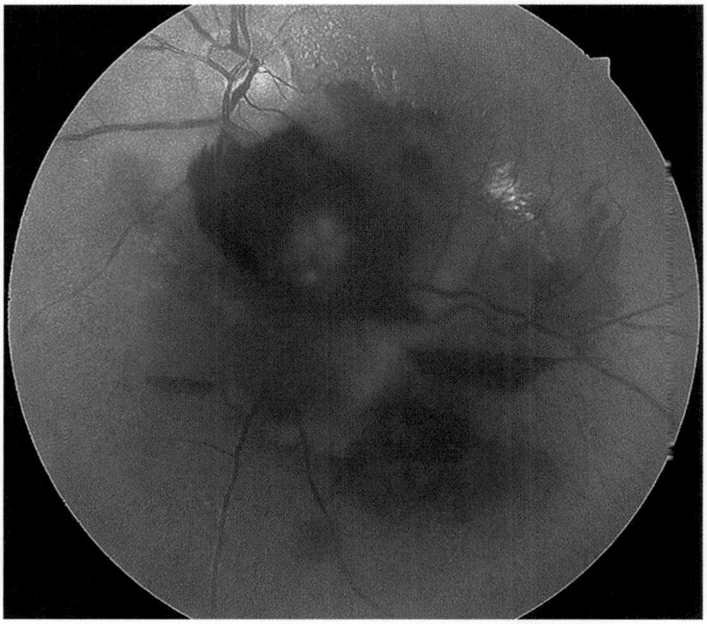

■ **Fig. 18.84** Fundus haemorrhages, which typically involve different layers of the retina and are most obvious in the posterior pole, although they often extend to the periphery.

Valsalva retinopathy

Valsalva retinopathy is caused by transmission of a sudden and severe increase in intrathoracic or intra-abdominal pressure to the eye resulting in intraocular bleeding.

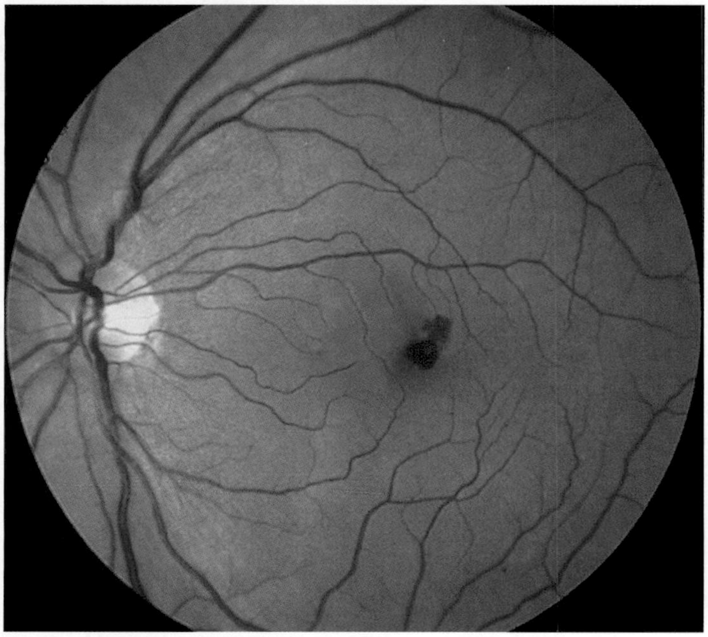

■ **Fig. 18.85** Two small macular haemorrhages.

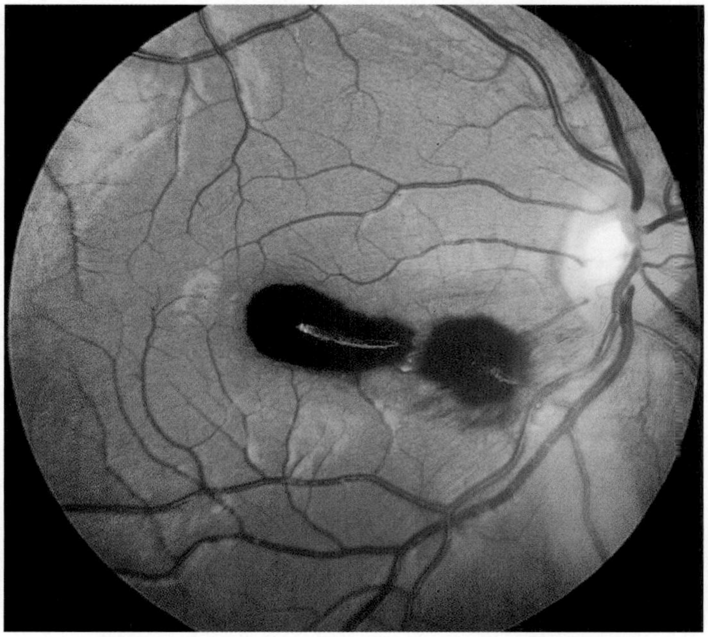

■ **Fig.18.86** Preretinal haemorrhage and a nerve fibre layer haemorrhage. (Courtesy of P. Morse.)

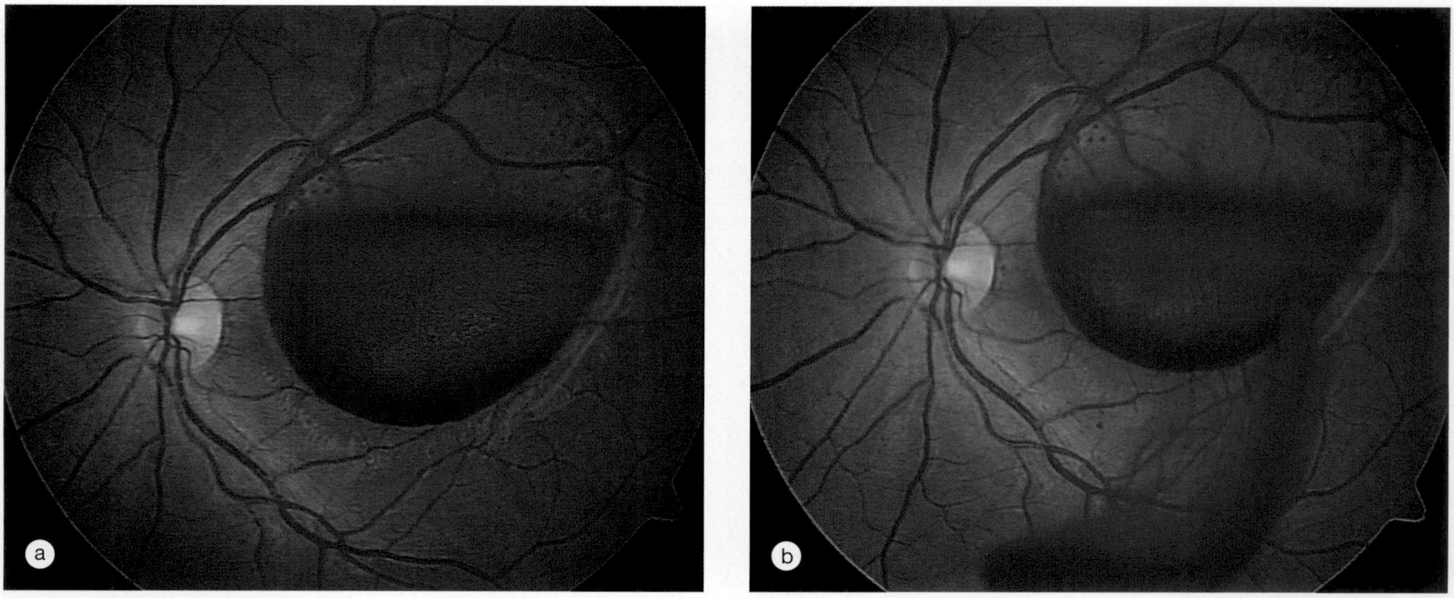

Fig. 18.87 **(a)** Large subhyaloid haemorrhage. **(b)** Immediately following treatment with a YAG laser in order to disperse the blood from in front of the macula. (Courtesy of P. Gili.)

Solar retinopathy

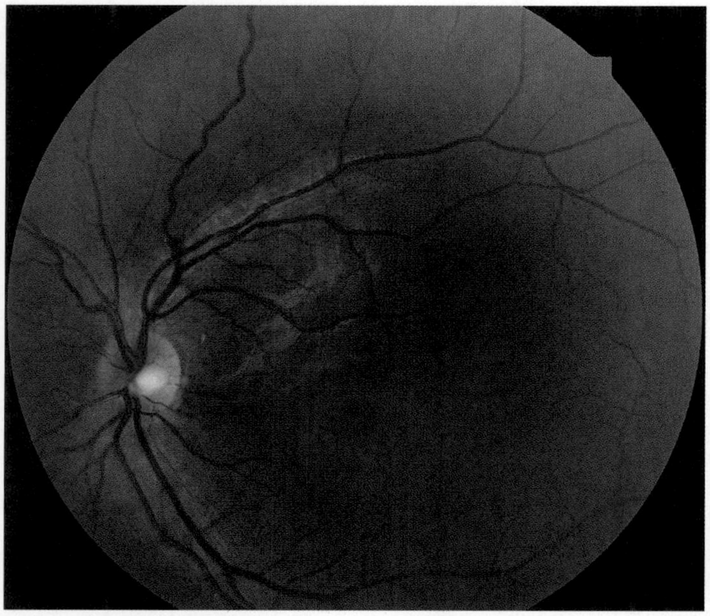

Fig. 18.88 Initially there are small, unilateral or bilateral, yellow foveolar spots with a grey margin.

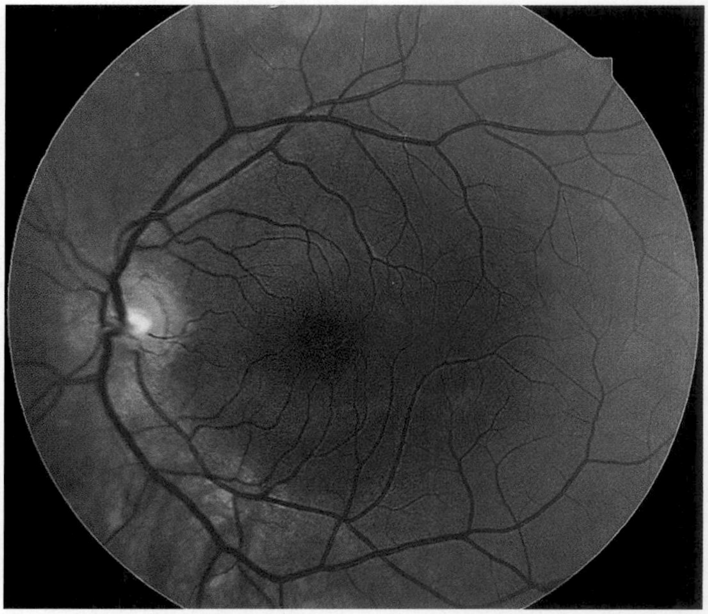

Fig. 18.89 This is followed about 2 weeks later by circumscribed RPE mottling or a lamellar hole.

INDEX